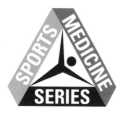

SPORTS MEDICINE SERIES

Keeping you one step ahead

McGraw-Hill Australia, market leader in this specialty, is proud to present the **Sports Medicine Series**.

Books published in this series have been specially commissioned and designed to reflect the learning needs of the diverse and growing sports medicine community. Reflecting a combination of sound research, international experience, current treatment and practical techniques, this is the series you can trust to deliver world class resources.

Look out for the following books in the **Sports Medicine Series**.

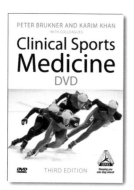

Clinical Sports Medicine Third edition DVD, by Brukner and Khan, is an innovative new tool to help students, patients and practitioners with the clinical aspects of sports-related injuries. The DVD has video sequences showing clinical examination of key anatomical parts.

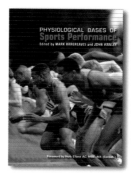

Clinical Sports Nutrition Third edition, by Burke and Deakin, is the definitive reference book for sports nutrition professionals, sports medicine clinicians, coaches, trainers and students of sports science. The book provides comprehensive coverage of the subject and successfully integrates the science and practice of sports nutrition.

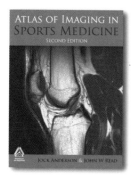

Atlas of Imaging in Sports Medicine Second edition, by Anderson and Read, is a comprehensive view of both the common and the unusual sports injury. With double the number of images of the first edition and new images from technologies such as MRI and ultrasound, this revision presents current developments in sports radiology and associated diagnostic tools.

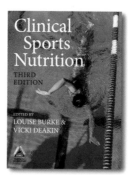

Physiological Bases of Sports Performance, by Hargreaves and Hawley who head a team of leading authorities in the fields of exercise science, nutrition and sports medicine to present research findings on the physiological bases of sports performance. This valuable reference book is essential reading for students, scientists and clinicians with an interest in understanding and optimizing sports performance.

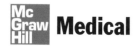

More titles are forthcoming and the publisher welcomes submissions for consideration of new and appropriate books for the **Sports Medicine Series**.

Clinical Sports
Medicine
REVISED
THIRD EDITION

45

l h a

PETER BRUKNER AND KARIM KHAN

WITH COLLEAGUES

Clinical Sports Medicine

REVISED
THIRD EDITION

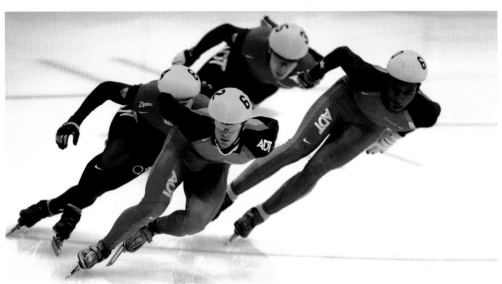

The McGraw·Hill Companies

Sydney New York San Francisco Auckland
Bangkok Bogotá Caracas Hong Kong
Kuala Lumpur Lisbon London Madrid
Mexico City Milan New Delhi San Juan
Seoul Singapore Taipei Toronto

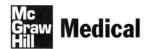

Medical

First published 1993
Second edition 2001
Revised second edition 2002
Third edition 2006
Revised third edition 2009
Reprinted 2010 (Twice)

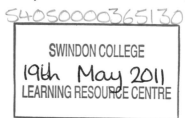

Text © 2006 Peter Brukner and Karim Khan
Illustrations and design © 2006 McGraw-Hill Australia Pty Ltd
Additional owners of copyright are named in on-page credits.

National Library of Australia Cataloguing-in-Publication data:

Brukner, Peter
Clinical sports medicine

3rd revised ed.
Includes index.
ISBN 978 0 070278 99 8.

1. Sports medicine. 2. Sports injuries. I. Khan, Karim. II. Title.

617.1027

Published in Australia by
McGraw-Hill Australia Pty Ltd
Level 2, 82 Waterloo Road, North Ryde NSW 2113
Publisher: Nicole Meehan
Production Editor: Sybil Kesteven
Editor: Carolyn Pike
Proofreader: Kerry Brown
Indexer: Max McMaster
Designer (cover and interior): Jan Schmoeger, Designpoint
Cover image: gettyimages
Illustrators: Vicky Earle (anatomical figures); Alan Laver, Shelly Communications
CD production: Midland Typesetters, Maryborough
Typeset in 10/11 pt Minion Pro by Midland Typesetters, Maryborough
Printed on 80 gsm matt art by 1010 Printing International Ltd, China

The McGraw·Hill Companies

Foreword to the first edition

Sport in Australia is ingrained in the national consciousness more widely, deeply and indelibly than almost anywhere else in the world. When a prominent sportsperson sustains a sporting injury either traumatically or from overuse, becomes excessively fatigued, or fails to live up to expectations, this assumes national importance. It is even more relevant nowadays with greater individual participation in sporting activities. The same type of problems occur for the recreational athlete, the middle-aged person wanting to become fit or the older person wishing to sustain a higher level of activity in their later years.

In *Clinical Sports Medicine* the authors define their topic as 'medicine of exercise' and the 'total medical care of the exercising individual'. They thus take sports medicine out of the realm of the elite athlete and place it fairly and squarely where it belongs—as a subspecialty to serve everyone in the community who wishes to be active.

The book is organized in a manner that is sensible and usable and differs in that way from many of the current sports medicine texts. The chapters are arranged according to the anatomical region of the symptom rather than diagnostic categories. This results in a very usable text for the sports physician, general/family practitioner, physiotherapist, masseur or athletic trainer whose practice contains many active individuals.

The authors also give coverage to nutritional and psychological techniques, as well as considering the special concerns of females, the young and the old. Individual chapters are devoted to important medical aspects of exercise, including emergencies, cardio-vascular, respiratory and gastrointestinal problems, epilepsy, diabetes and infection. The unique problems of exercising in the heat and cold are also included.

Practical aspects of sports medicine, which are not well covered in other texts, include the medical care of the sporting team and concerns that a physician might have when travelling with a team. Of particular relevance nowadays are drugs and exercise and, with the increasing number of Olympic-caliber athletes who need medication for legitimate conditions, the inclusion of this aspect together with an up-to-date list of medications permitted and restricted by the International Olympic Committee is very welcome.

In all, this is an eminently usable text which is timely in its production and will find an important place in the surgery or office of the sports medicine practitioner involved in the care of active individuals.

JOHN R SUTTON MD, FRACP
Professor of Medicine, Exercise Physiology
and Sports Medicine
Faculty of Health Sciences, University of Sydney
Past President, American College of Sports Medicine

This foreword was written by the late Professor
John Sutton before his untimely death in 1996;
it is retained in this textbook out of profound
respect for this champion of the integration
of science, physical activity promotion and
multidisciplinary patient care.

Foreword to the third edition

*C*linical Sports Medicine has become the gold standard of texts for clinicians and students interested in the field of sports medicine. In this third edition, Peter Brukner and Karim Khan have gathered together an impressive array of experienced researchers and clinicians, so this text builds on the previous editions by providing the latest evidence-based information without losing its practical clinical appeal. The multidisciplinary nature of the text allows the clinician to appreciate the intricacies of care for both the elite and recreational athlete from prescreening, to injury management, to returning to sport, involving the physical, psychological and nutritional aspects of the care.

The authors keep the reader abreast of the rapid advances in sports physiotherapy, particularly the scientific evidence validating various clinical approaches to treatment, as well as directing clinicians to the latest research in musculoskeletal pathology at both a macro and micro level. The addition of this cutting edge information has resulted in improved understanding and management of previously quite recalcitrant problems, such as tendinopathies. The very clear illustrations, full color plates, flow charts and summaries make *Clinical Sports Medicine* a very user-friendly text. With the addition of the clinical examination DVD, the third edition of *Clinical Sports Medicine* will become a 'must have' for every practicing sports clinician—doctor and physiotherapist. Clinicians will be able to instantly observe expert physical examinations, picking up useful tips to enhance their diagnosis and treatment.

In this third edition the authors have moved the sports medicine field forward, providing good science, great ideas and soundly based practise. The logical flow of the text covering all aspects of clinical management is a testament to the commitment of the authors to improve patient care by ensuring best practise. It is now up to the clinician to act on the information provided.

Jenny McConnell
McConnell & Clements Physiotherapy
Sydney
Australia

Brief contents

Contents

BRUKNER AND KHAN, CLINICAL SPORTS MEDICINE 3E REV, McGRAW-HILL PROFESSIONAL

BRUKNER AND KHAN, CLINICAL SPORTS MEDICINE 3E REV, McGRAW-HILL PROFESSIONAL

Preface

Clinical Sports Medicine is written for the clinician whose aim is to keep people active and injury free. We use the term 'medicine' broadly—to embrace all health professions which aim to harness that most powerful of all therapies—physical activity. With that in mind, this book has been written for physiotherapists, medical practitioners, osteopaths, massage therapists, podiatrists, sports/athletic trainers, fitness leaders, and nurses. We believe it is an ideal textbook for sports physiotherapy and medicine courses, both in the classroom and via distance education. We are gratified that it is a text in many Human Movement Studies/Kinesiology courses that focus on the crucial role of physical activity and injury prevention in health for all.

This rewritten, re-illustrated, and full-color edition of *Clinical Sports Medicine* remains practical and easy-to-read while capturing the many recent advances in the field. The book describes a completely symptom-oriented, integrated, multidisciplinary approach to treatment in the clinic or on the sidelines. It is designed so that the clinician can look at the chapter which describes the patient presentation (e.g. longstanding groin pain, acute ankle injury) and review the likely differential diagnoses, the clinical approach and the illustrated assessment. A major focus of this third edition is the clear presentation of treatment options which have been categorized as 'evidence-based' or 'expert-advocated', as well as annotated 'practise pearls' that are an essential part of high-quality clinical care.

For the reader's benefit, and thus for patient well-being, over 50 international colleagues, peers and pioneers in sports medicine helped to author this third edition of *Clinical Sports Medicine*; we are grateful to them for sharing their clinical wisdom with such alacrity. Our champion team includes world physiotherapy and medical authorities such as Håkan Alfredson, Elizabeth Arendt, Roald Bahr, Kim Bennell, Jill Cook, Kay Crossley, Sandra Hoffmann, Per Holmich, Mark Hutchinson, Pekka Kannus, Jon Karlsson, Ben Kibler, Nicola Maffulli, Jenny McConnell, Paul McCrory, George Murrell, Timothy Noakes, Joel Press and Kevin Singer. *Clinical Sports Medicine* authors now represent 12 countries and most continents.

The six parts of *Clinical Sports Medicine* provide comprehensive material for all aspects of the clinician's role. Part A details Fundamental Principles—the theoretical foundation for the remainder of the text. Part B addresses Regional Problems beginning with the head and ending at the toes. Each chapter provides a clinical perspective to aid with diagnosis, illustrates physical examination with color photographs, and details treatment of significant conditions in easy-to-read tables. The most common presentations are given the most attention. Exercise therapy is highlighted in text and illustration. Part C—Enhancing Sport Performance—summarizes a vast body of literature of great interest to all athletes. Part D discusses the sports medicine needs of Special Groups of Participants, such as the young, female, older and disabled person. Part E concerns the Management of Medical Conditions, such as diabetes and epilepsy—an area of particular importance for family practitioners and sports physicians. Part F provides what we hope is an essential guide to Practical Sports Medicine—working with teams, providing the coverage of events, drugs, ethics and the law.

Because of the rapid evolution of sports medicine, we have seen the need to add six new chapters in this third edition. These chapters are: Recovery

(Chapter 7), Diagnosis: Investigations including Imaging (Chapter 9), Core Stability (Chapter 11), Longstanding Groin Pain (Chapter 24), Maximizing Sporting Performance: To Use or Not to Use Supplements? (Chapter 38) and The Preparticipation Physical Evaluation (Chapter 56). We have also included substantial new sections within chapters that address new discoveries; for example, the prevention of lower limb injuries, particularly anterior cruciate ligament rupture (Chapter 27). We are particularly excited about the new material that reflects advances in the sports medicine care of patients with the following regional problems: concussion, management and rehabilitation of shoulder injuries, prevention of knee and ankle injuries, as well as the treatment of patello-femoral pain and tendinopathies. This book details programs for core stabilization and we emphasize the role of the kinetic chain in rehabilitation. All the medical management chapters have been revised and the chapters on emergency medicine, epilepsy, diabetes and heatstroke provide the latest evidence-based sports medicine information, which challenges many outdated beliefs. The chapters on practical sports medicine contain the essence of the experience of multiple authors who have cared for athletes on all continents and in a wide variety of settings, from the most remote to the Olympic Games.

All chapters contain substantial new text and most benefit from the 100-plus special color illustrations drawn by Vicky Earle. We note which treatments are supported by randomized controlled trials and which are based on expert opinion alone. All references have been updated; however, the classics are still highlighted where this is warranted. We include recommended readings for further study and, reflecting the increasing reliance on the Internet for information, we include web-based references and alert readers to recommended websites for information that is continually changing (e.g. drugs in sport). And you can view our website at <www.clinicalsportsmedicine.com>, which has links to key sports medicine websites and further educational opportunities.

In 1993 we wrote that no single profession has all the answers required to treat the ill or injured athlete. With the explosion since then in evidence for diagnosis and treatment of musculoskeletal conditions, this statement is even more relevant as we approach 2010, and is reflected in our seeking help from a champion team of coauthors and critical reviewers. As a result, we hope that whatever your training, *Clinical Sports Medicine* will help reinforce the knowledge and techniques you already use and will introduce you to other useful ideas to help with your clinical practise.

Guided Tour
of Your Book

The third edition of *Clinical Sports Medicine* is greatly enhanced from previous editions in three key areas. Look for the following features to maximize your learning and save you time.

Premium Content and Coverage

TREATMENT AND REHABILITATION is emphasized throughout the book. The book integrates coverage of differential diagnoses, the clinical approach and illustrated assessment.

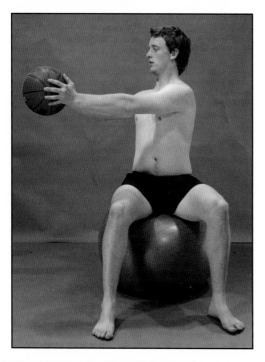

WORLD CLASS CONTRIBUTORS come from over 12 countries, and most continents, to share their knowledge and experience.

Team Doctor, World Track & Field Championships, Helsinki 2005

Garth Hunte MD, MSc, CCFP, CCFP(EM), FCFP, DipSportMed
Emergency Physician & Sports Medicine Physician. Department of Emergency Medicine, St Paul's Hospital, Vancouver. Clinical Assistant Professor, Department of Family Practice, University of British Columbia, Vancouver, Canada

Mark R. Hutchinson MD, FACSM
Professor of Orthopaedics and Sports Medicine and Head Team Physician, University of Illinois at Chicago, Chicago, Illinois; Head Team Physician, WNBA Chicago Sky, Chicago, Illinois; Volunteer event physician, LaSalle Bank Chicago Marathon, Chicago, Illinois, USA

Karen Inge APD, FASMF, FSDA
Sports Dietitian, Head of Nutrition, Victorian Institute of Sport, Melbourne, Australia

Pekka Kannus MD, PhD
Chief Physician, Accident and Trauma Research Center, UKK Institute, Tampere, Finland; Associate Professor (Docent) of Sports Medicine, University of Jyväskylä, Finland; Visiting Professor, Department of Orthopedics and Rehabilitation, University of Vermont College of Medicine, Burlington, Vermont, USA

Jon Karlsson MD, PhD
Orthopaedic Surgeon, Professor of Orthopaedics and Sports Traumatology, The Sahlgrenska Academy at Göteborg University, Göteborg, Sweden

W. Ben Kibler MD, FACSM
Medical Director, Lexington Clinic Sports Medicine Center, Kentucky, USA

Mary Kinch HDST(Phys Ed), BAppSc(Physio)
Physiotherapist, Olympic Park Sports Medicine Centre, Melbourne, Australia

Zoltan Kiss FRACP, FRANZCR, DDU
Radiologist, Mercy Private Hospital, Melbourne. Senior Fellow, Faculty of Medicine, Dentistry and Health Sciences, University of Melbourne, Australia

Michael S. Koehle MD, MSc, CCF DipSportMed(CASM)
Sport Physician, Clinical Assistant McGavin Sports Medicine Centre, Family Practice, University of Britt Vancouver, BC, Canada

Andrew Lambart B AppSc(Physic
Physiotherapist, Olympic Park Spc Centre, Melbourne; Team Physioth Hawthorn Football Club; Australia Physiotherapist, Athens 2004

Teresa Liu-Ambrose PhD, PT
Assistant Professor, University of E School of Rehabilitation Sciences, Physical Therapy; Head, Exercise a Function Unit, Centre for Hip Hea BC

Nicola Maffulli MD, MS, PhD, FR
Professor of Trauma and Orthopae Keele University School of Medici Trent, England

Merzesh Magra MBBS, MRCS
Orthopaedic Research Fellow, Dep Trauma and Orthopaedic Surgery, School of Medicine, Stoke on Tren

Jenny McConnell BAppSc(Physio
GradDipManipTher, MBiomedEn
Physiotherapist, McConnell & Cle Physiotherapy, Sydney, Australia.

Paul McCrory MBBS, PhD, FRAC
FACSM
Neurologist and Sports Physician; Professor, Centre for Health, Exerc Medicine, University of Melbourne

Chris Milne BHB, MBChB, Dip C
Med, FRNZCGP, FACSP
Sports Physician, Anglesea Sports Hamilton, New Zealand; Olympic

Bruce Mitchell MBBS, FACSP, MI
Sports Physician, Metro Spinal Cli CHESM, University of Melbourne Sports Medicine Australia

PRACTISE PEARLS provide tips and techniques for both the novice and experienced.

 Intervertebral joints, paraspinal muscles and local nerves may all contribute to the patient's low back pain and must be identified and corrected.

EVIDENCE-BASED PRACTISE is clearly presented with the scientific literature synthesized in a readable fashion.

Full Colour Presentation

COLOUR ILLUSTRATIONS AND PHOTO-GRAPHS highlight anatomy and physical examination to aid comprehension.

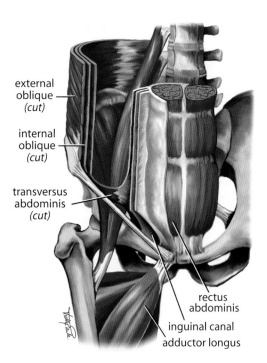

external oblique (cut)

internal oblique (cut)

transversus abdominis (cut)

rectus abdominis

inguinal canal

adductor longus

RADIOLOGICAL IMAGES include the latest MRI technologies and CT scanning techniques for accurate interpretation and diagnosis of sporting injuries.

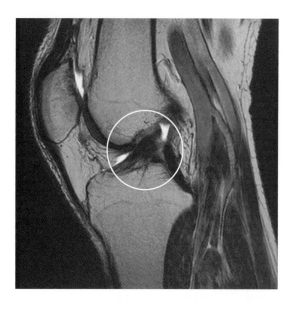

FLOW CHARTS AND TABLES present key information and steps in a visual format to aid understanding.

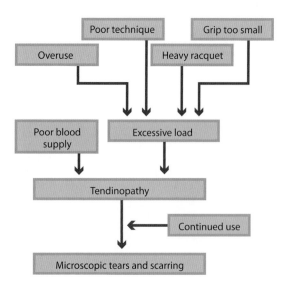

PATIENT INFORMATION SHEETS are included for the first time with the *bonus CD*. Presented in a consistent format, the Patient Information Sheets are a valuable summary of patient presentations and treatment options.

Innovative Learning Resources

RECOMMENDED READINGS, WEBSITES AND REFERENCES for each chapter provide additional resources for further study.

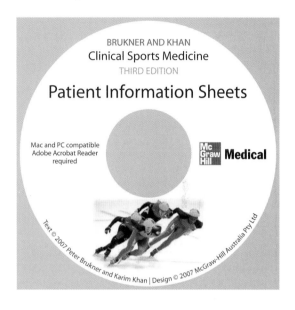

Recommended Reading

Bogduk N. *Clinical Anatomy of the Lumbar Spine and Sacrum.* 4th edn. Edinburgh: Churchill Livingstone, 2005.
Earl JE. Mechanical aetiology, recognition, and treatment of spondylolisthesis. *Phys Ther Sport* 2002; 3: 79–87.
George SZ, Delitto A. Management of the athlete with low back pain. *Clin Sports Med* 2002; 21: 105–20.
Hilde G, Bo K. Effect of exercise in the treatment of chronic low back pain: a systemic review, emphasising type and dose of exercise. *Phys Ther Rev* 1998; 3: 107–17.
Licciardone JC, Brimhall AK, King LN. Osteopathic manipulative treatment for low back pain: a systematic review and meta-analysis of randomized controlled trials. *BMC Musculoskelet Disord* 2005; 6: 43–54.
Lively MW, Bailes JE. Acute lumbar disk injuries in active patients. *Physician Sportsmed* 2005; 33: 000–00.
Maitland GD. *Vertebral Manipulation.* 5th edn. London: Butterworths, 1986.
McTimoney CAM, Micheli LJ. Current evaluation and management of spondylolysis and spondylolisthesis. *Curr Sports Med Rep* 2003; 2: 41–6.
Nadler SF, Malanga GA, DePrince M, et al. The relationship between lower extremity injury, low back pain, and hip muscle strength in male and female collegiate athletes. *Clin J Sport Med* 2000; 10(2): 89–97.
Richardson C, Jull G, Hodges P, et al. *Therapeutic Exercise for Spinal Segmental Stabilization in Low Back Pain.* 2nd edn. Edinburgh: Churchill Livingstone, 2004.
Standaert CJ. New strategies in the management of low back injuries in gymnasts. *Curr Sports Med Rep* 2002; 1: 293–300.
Standaert CJ, Herring SA, Pratt TW. Rehabilitation of the athlete with low back pain. *Curr Sports Med Rep* 2004; 3: 35–40.
Trainor TJ, Trainor MA. Etiology of low back pain in athletes. *Curr Sports Med Rep* 2004; 3: 41–6.
Urban J. Back to the future: what have we learned from 25 years of research into intervertebral disc biology? *J Back Musculoskel Rehabil* 1997; 9: 23–7.
Watkins RG. Lumbar disc injury in the athlete. *Clin Sports Med* 2002; 21: 147–65.

Recommended Website

An educational tool about low back pain can be found at:
<http://www.lowbackpain.tv>.

References

1. Hides JA, Stokes MJ, Saide M, et al. Evidence of lumbar multifidus muscle wasting ipsilateral to symptoms in patients with acute/subacute low back pain. *Spine* 1994; 19: 165–72.
2. Hodges PW, Richardson CA. Inefficient muscular stabilisation of the lumbar spine associated with low back pain: a motor control evaluation of transversus abdominis. *Spine* 1996; 21: 2640–50.
3. Hodges PW, Richardson CA. Delayed postural contraction of transversus abdominis in low back pain associated with movement of the lower limbs. *J Spinal Disord Tech* 1998; 11: 46–56.
4. Sihvonen T, Lindgren K, Airaksinen O, et al. Movement disturbances of the lumbar spine and abnormal back muscle electromyographic findings in recurrent low back pain. *Spine* 1997; 22: 289–95.
5. McGill S. *Low Back Disorders: Evidence-based Prevention and Rehabilitation.* Champaign, IL: Human Kinetics, 2002.
6. Donelson R, Aprill C, Medcalf R, et al. A prospective study of centralization of lumbar and referred pain. A predictor of symptomatic discs and annular competence. *Spine* 1997; 23: 2003–13.
7. Deyo RA, Diehl AK, et al. How many days of bed rest for acute low back pain? *N Engl J Med* 1986; 315: 1064–70.
8. Lord SM, Barnsley L, Bogduk N. The utility of comparative local anesthetic blocks versus placebo-controlled blocks for the diagnosis of cervical zygapophysial joint pain. *Clin J Pain* 1995; 11(3): 208–13.
9. Dreyfuss P, Halbrook B, Pauza K, et al. Efficacy and validity of radiofrequency neurotomy for chronic lumbar zygapophyseal joint pain. *Spine* 2000; 25: 1270–7.
10. Van Kleef M, Barendse GAM, Kessels A, et al. Randomised trial of radiofrequency lumbar facet joint denervation for chronic low back pain. *Spine* 1999; 24: 1937–42.
11. Yin W, Willard F, Carreiro J, et al. Sensory stimulation-guided sacroiliac joint radiofrequency neurotomy: technique based on neuroanatomy of the dorsal sacral plexus. *Spine* 2003; 28(20): 2419–25.
12. Pauza KJ, Howell S, Dreyfuss P, et al. A randomized, placebo-controlled trial of intradiscal electrothermal therapy for the treatment of discogenic low back pain. *Spine* 2004; 4(1): 27–35.
13. Carragee EJ. The surgical treatment of disc degeneration: is the race not to be swift? *Spine* 2005; 5: 587–8.
14. Deyo RA, Nachemson A, Mirza SK. Spinal-fusion surgery: the case for restraint. *N Engl J Med* 2004; 350: 643–4.
15. Brukner PD, Bennell KL, Matheson GO. *Stress Fractures.* Melbourne: Blackwell Scientific, 1999.

A **DVD** is available separately which presents the accurate techniques of tests and examinations, and rehabilitation.

A COMPANION WEBSITE provides specific tips for individual health professions, contains sample chapters and includes relevant conference proceedings. A comprehensive listing of online resources is available with current information for the sports medicine community. Go to www.clinicalsportsmedicine.com

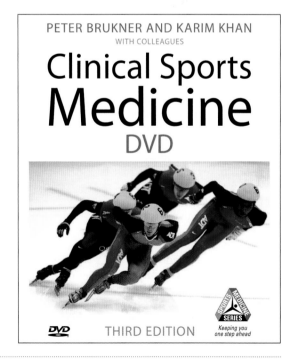

The authors

Peter Brukner
OAM, MBBS, DRCOG, FACSP, FASMF, FACSM
Sports Physician
Founding Partner, Olympic Park Sports Medicine
  Centre, Melbourne, Australia
Associate Professor, Centre for Health, Exercise
  and Sports Medicine, University of Melbourne
Honorary Fellow, Faculty of Law, University of
  Melbourne
Adjunct Professor, School of Human Movement
  Studies, University of Queensland
Visiting Associate Professor, Stanford University
  1997

Executive Member, Australian College of Sports
  Physicians 1985–2000
President, Australian College of Sports Physicians
  1991–92, 1999–2000.
Board of Trustees, American College of Sports
  Medicine, 2000–2002

Team Physician
  Australian Olympic Team, Atlanta 1996
  Australian Athletics Team, World Championships
    Tokyo 1991, Gothenburg 1995
  Australian Mens Hockey Team, 1995–96
  Australian Team World Cup Athletics, Havana
    1992
  Australian Team, World Student Games,
    Edmonton 1983, Kobe 1985, Zagreb 1987
  Australian Team, World Swimming
    Championships, Madrid 1986
  Melbourne Football Club (AFL) 1987–90
  Collingwood Football Club (AFL) 1996
  University Blues Football Club 1978–2006
  TEM Hockey Club 2001–2006

Medical Adviser
  Australian Paralympic Committee
  AFL Players Association

Senior Associate Editor
Clinical Journal of Sport Medicine
The Physician and Sportsmedicine
Current Sports Medicine Reports
Editor
Sport Health 1990–95

Co-author
Food for Sport 1987
Stress Fractures 1999
Drugs in Sport—What the GP needs to know 1996,
  2000
The Encyclopedia of Exercise, Sport and Health 2004
Essential Sports Medicine 2005

Medal of the Order of Australia
Inaugural Honour Award, *Australian College of
  Sports Physicians*, 1996
Citation Award, *American College of Sports
  Medicine*, 2000

Section Manager, Australian Athletics Team,
  Olympic Games, Sydney 2000
National Selector, Athletics Australia 2006
President, University Blues Football, 1974–76,
  78–79, 83–84
Juniors Vice-President TEM Hockey Club
  2000–2004
Mens Vice-President TEM Hockey Club 2004–2006

Media involvement includes ABC and SEN radio,
  The Age, Melbourne, and FoxFooty

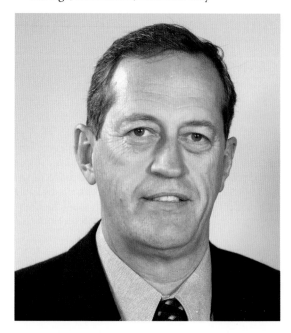

Karim Khan
BMedSci, MD, PhD, FACSP, FSMA (Australia) Dip
Sport Med (Canada) FACSM (US)
Sports Physician
Professor, University of British Columbia,
Vancouver Canada (Department of Family
Practice & School of Human Kinetics);
Associate Member, Departments of Physical
Therapy, Orthopaedics
Sports Physician
Allan McGavin Sports Medicine Centre,
Vancouver, Canada
Consultant: Osteoporosis Program. BC Women's &
Children's Hospital, Vancouver, Canada
Medical Advisor: Vancouver Coastal Health
Authority, Vancouver, Canada
Principal Investigator: Centre for Hip Health,
Vancouver, Canada
Committee Member, Osteoporosis Society of
Canada—Physical Activity and Fall Prevention
Subcommittee
Principal Fellow with title Associate Professor,
School of Physiotherapy, The University of
Melbourne, Melbourne, Australia
Honorary Visiting Fellow, School of Physiology &
Pharmacology, University of New South Wales,
Sydney, Australia
Adjunct Associate Professor, School of Human
Movement Studies, The University of
Queensland, Brisbane, Australia
Medical Education Committee, American College
of Sports Medicine 2002–2004
Research Evaluation Committee, American College
of Sports Medicine, 2005–

Sports Physician
Women's Field Hockey Canada 1999–2000
Olympic Games, Sydney, 2000, Basketball
Competition Venue
Australian Women's Basketball (The Opals)
1991–96
The Australian Ballet Company 1991–96
The Australian Ballet School 1991–96
Australian Team, World Student Games 1993
Australian Team, Junior World Cup Hockey
1993

Editorial Boards
*British Journal of Sports Medicine (North American
Editor)*
Journal of Science and Medicine in Sport 1997–2001
Clinical Journal of Sport Medicine 2003–2006
*Scandinavian Journal of Science and Medicine in
Sport*

Editor
Sport Health 1995–97

Co-author
Physical Activity and Bone Health 2001
The Encyclopaedia of Exercise, Sport and Health
2004

Prime Minister's Medal for Service to Australian
Sport
Sports Medicine Australia Fellows' Citation for
Service

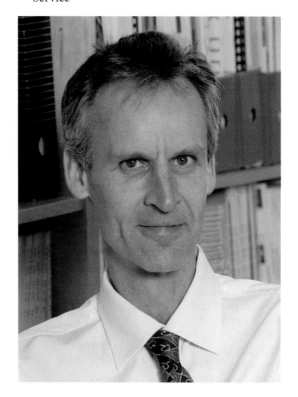

Chapter co-authors

Jason Agosta BAppScPodiatry
Podiatrist, Private practise, East Melbourne;
Podiatrist, Essendon Football Club and Melbourne
Storm Rugby League

Håkan Alfredson MD, PhD
Orthopaedic Surgeon. Professor Sports Medicine
Unit, Umeå University, Department of Surgical and
Perioperative Sciences, Umeå, Sweden

Julia Alleyne BHSc(PT), MD, CCFP, FACSM,
DipSportMed(CASM)
Assistant Clinical Professor; Chair Sport Medicine
Fellowship, Department of Family and Community
Medicine, University of Toronto. Assistant Clinical
Professor, Department of Rehabilitation, McMaster
University. Medical Director, Sport C.A.R.E.,
Women's College Hospital, Toronto. Past President,
Canadian Academy of Sport Medicine. Canadian
Olympic Committee, Medical Staff, Salt Lake City
2002, Turin 2006

Jock Anderson MBBS, FRANZCR, FACSP(Hon)
Consultant Radiologist. Associate Professor Sports
Medicine Program UNSW, Australia

Elizabeth Arendt MD, FACSM
Orthopaedic Surgeon, Professor, University of
Minnesota, USA. Medical Director of Men's and
Women's Intercollegiate Athletics at Univ. of
Minnesota. Vice Chair of the Dept of Orthopeadic
Surgery. Past team physician USA Soccer and
USA woman's hockey. Past member of President's
Council on Physical Fitness and Sports, AAOS
Task Force on Women's Issues, NCAA Medical
Safeguards Committee

Maureen C. Ashe PT, CHT, PhD
Physiotherapist, Certified Hand Therapist. Westside
Physiotherapy & Hand Clinic, Vancouver, Canada.
Michael Smith Foundation for Health Research
Postdoctoral Fellow, GF Strong Rehabilitation
Centre and Centre for Hip Health, Vancouver,
Canada

Roald Bahr MD, PhD
Professor of Sports Medicine, Norwegian
School of Sport Sciences; Chair, Oslo Sports
Trauma Research Center; Consultant physician,
Department of Sports Medicine, Olympic Training
Center, Norway

Simon Bell FRCS, FRACS, FAOrthA
Orthopaedic Surgeon, Olympic Park Sports
Medicine Centre; Senior Lecturer, Monash
University Department of Surgery; Head, Upper
Limb Unit, Monash Medical Centre, Clayton,
Australia

Kim Bennell BAppSc(Physio), PhD
Physiotherapist. Professor and Director, Centre
for Health, Exercise and Sports Medicine, School
of Physiotherapy, University of Melbourne,
Australia

Noel Blundell EdD, MSc, BEd, DipT(PhysEd)
Sports Psychologist. Director—High Five Sports
Psychology; Victorian Institute of Sport Australian
Institute of Sport; Tennis Australia; International
Tennis Federation; Australian Football League;
International Professional Golf and Tennis
circuits

Chris Bradshaw MBBS, FACSP
Sports Physician, Olympic Park Sports Medicine
Centre, Melbourne, Australia; Olympic Team
Physician, Sydney 2000; Team Physician, Geelong
Football Club

Nick Carter MB ChB, MRCP
Consultant in Rheumatology and Rehabilitation
Medicine, Defence Services Medical Rehabilitation
Centre, Headley Court, Surrey, UK

Jacqueline Close MBBS, MD, FRCP
Consultant Geriatrician and Conjoint Senior
Lecturer, Prince of Wales Hospital and Prince of
Wales Medical Research Institute, University of
New South Wales, Sydney, Australia

Emma Colson BAppSc(Physio),
GradDipManipPhysio
APA Sports Physiotherapist, Olympic Park Sports
Medicine Centre, Melbourne, Australia; Australian
Olympic Team Physiotherapist, Sydney 2000;
Australian representative, Mountain Bike Cross
Country, Commonwealth Games, Melbourne 2006

Jill Cook BAppSci(Physio),
GradDipManipTherapy, PhD
Physiotherapist. Associate Professor, La Trobe
University, Musculoskeletal Research Centre;
Associate Professor, Centre for Physical Health and
Nutrition, Deakin University, Australia. Australian
Olympic Team Physiotherapist, Olympic Games
Atlanta (1996), Sydney (2000)

Wendy L. Cook MD, MHSc, FRCPC
Geriatrician. Clinical Instructor, Division of
Geriatric Medicine, Faculty of Medicine, University
of British Columbia, Vancouver, BC, Canada

Randall Cooper BPhysio, MPhysio
Physiotherapist, Olympic Park Sports Medicine
Centre, Melbourne, Australia; Physiotherapist
Hawthorn Football Club; Physiotherapist,
Australian Winter Olympics team, Torino, 2006

Sallie Cowan BAppSc(Physio),
GradDipManipTher, PhD
Musculoskeletal Physiotherapist; NHMRC
Post Doctoral Research Fellow, Centre for
Health Exercise and Sports Medicine, School
of Physiotherapy, University of Melbourne,
Melbourne, Australia

Kay Crossley BAppSc(Physio), PhD
Physiotherapist, Olympic Park Sports Medicine
Centre, Melbourne, Australia; Australian Olympic
Team Physiotherapist, Sydney 2000; Senior
Research Fellow, Centre for Health, Exercise and
Sports Medicine, University of Melbourne

Bruce B. Forster MSc, MD, FRCP(C)
Associate Professor, Dept of Radiology, University
of British Columbia Hospital, Vancouver, Canada

Andrew Garnham MBBS, FACSP
Sports Physician. Senior Lecturer, Department
of Human Movement studies, Deakin University,
Burwood, Australia

Robert Granter BSocSci, DipAppSci
Soft Tissue Therapist, Victorian Institute of Sport,
Melbourne, Australia; Head of Massage Therapy
Services Australian Olympic Team 1996, 2000,
Head of Massage Therapy Services Melbourne 2006
Commonwealth Games

Peter T. Gropper MD, FRCSC
Clinical Professor, Department of Orthopaedics,
University of British Columbia, Vancouver, Canada

Peter Harcourt MBBS, DipRACOG, FACSP, FSMA
Sports Physician. Medical Director, Victorian
Institute of Sport. Australian Olympic Games
Medical Team 1992–2004 inclusive; Head—
Commonwealth Games Medical Team, 2006

Matt Hislop MBBS, MSc (Dublin), FACSP
Sports Physician, Brisbane Orthopaedic and Sports
Medicine Centre, Brisbane, Australia

Sandra J Hoffman MD, FACP, FACSM
Associate Professor Department of Family
Medicine, Idaho State University; Team Physician,
Idaho State University, Pocatello, Idaho, USA

Per Holmich MD
Orthopaedic Surgeon. Amager University Hospital,
Copenhagen, Denmark, Team Doctor for Emma
and Amelya's soccer and handball teams

Karen Holzer MBBS, FACSP, PhD
Sports Physician, Olympic Park Sports Medicine
Centre, Melbourne, Australia; NHMRC Senior
Research Fellow, Department of Respiratory
Medicine, Royal Melbourne Hospital; Australian

Team Doctor, World Track & Field Championships, Helsinki 2005

Garth Hunte MD, MSc, CCFP, CCFP(EM), FCFP, DipSportMed
Emergency Physician & Sports Medicine Physician. Department of Emergency Medicine, St Paul's Hospital, Vancouver. Clinical Assistant Professor, Department of Family Practice, University of British Columbia, Vancouver, Canada

Mark R. Hutchinson MD, FACSM
Professor of Orthopaedics and Sports Medicine and Head Team Physician, University of Illinois at Chicago, Chicago, Illinois; Head Team Physician, WNBA Chicago Sky, Chicago, Illinois; Volunteer event physician, LaSalle Bank Chicago Marathon, Chicago, Illinois, USA

Karen Inge APD, FASMF, FSDA
Sports Dietitian, Head of Nutrition, Victorian Institute of Sport, Melbourne, Australia

Pekka Kannus MD, PhD
Chief Physician, Accident and Trauma Research Center, UKK Institute, Tampere, Finland; Associate Professor (Docent) of Sports Medicine, University of Jyväskylä, Finland; Visiting Professor, Department of Orthopedics and Rehabilitation, University of Vermont College of Medicine, Burlington, Vermont, USA

Jon Karlsson MD, PhD
Orthopaedic Surgeon, Professor of Orthopaedics and Sports Traumatology, The Sahlgrenska Academy at Göteborg University, Göteborg, Sweden

W. Ben Kibler MD, FACSM
Medical Director, Lexington Clinic Sports Medicine Center, Kentucky, USA

Mary Kinch HDST(Phys Ed), BAppSc(Physio)
Physiotherapist, Olympic Park Sports Medicine Centre, Melbourne, Australia

Zoltan Kiss FRACP, FRANZCR, DDU
Radiologist, Mercy Private Hospital, Melbourne. Senior Fellow, Faculty of Medicine, Dentistry and Health Sciences, University of Melbourne, Australia

Michael S. Koehle MD, MSc, CCFP, DipSportMed(CASM)
Sport Physician, Clinical Assistant Professor, Allan McGavin Sports Medicine Centre, Department of Family Practice, University of British Columbia, Vancouver, BC, Canada

Andrew Lambart B AppSc(Physio)
Physiotherapist, Olympic Park Sports Medicine Centre, Melbourne; Team Physiotherapist, Hawthorn Football Club; Australian Olympic Team Physiotherapist, Athens 2004

Teresa Liu-Ambrose PhD, PT
Assistant Professor, University of British Columbia, School of Rehabilitation Sciences, Division of Physical Therapy; Head, Exercise and Cognitive Function Unit, Centre for Hip Health, Vancouver, BC, Canada

Nicola Maffulli MD, MS, PhD, FRCS(Orth)
Professor of Trauma and Orthopaedic Surgery, Keele University School of Medicine, Stoke on Trent, UK

Merzesh Magra MBBS, MRCS
Orthopaedic Research Fellow, Department of Trauma and Orthopaedic Surgery, Keele University School of Medicine, Stoke on Trent, UK

Jenny McConnell BAppSc(Physio), GradDipManipTher, MBiomedEng
Physiotherapist, McConnell & Clements Physiotherapy, Sydney, Australia.

Paul McCrory MBBS, PhD, FRACP, FACSP, FACSM
Neurologist and Sports Physician; Associate Professor, Centre for Health, Exercise and Sports Medicine, University of Melbourne

Chris Milne BHB, MBChB, Dip Obst, Dip Sports Med, FRNZCGP, FACSP
Sports Physician, Anglesea Sports Medicine, Hamilton. Olympic Team Physician, New Zealand

Bruce Mitchell MBBS, FACSP, MPainMed
Sports Physician, Metro Spinal Clinic; Fellow, CHESM, University of Melbourne; President, Sports Medicine Australia

Hayden Morris MBBS, Dip Anat, FRACS
Orthopaedic Surgeon, Olympic Park Sports
Medicine Centre, Melbourne, Australia

George Murrell MBBS, DPhil
Professor and Director, Department of
Orthopaedic Surgery, St George Hospital Campus,
University of New South Wales, Sydney, Australia

Timothy Noakes MBChB, MD, DSc, FACSM
Sports Physician & Exercise Physiologist,
Discovery Health Professor of Exercise and Sports
Science, University of Cape Town and Sports
Science Institute of South Africa, Cape Town,
South Africa

Stuart M. Phillips PhD
Associate Professor, Kinesiology—Exercise
Metabolism Research Group
McMaster University, Canada

Joel Press MD, FACSM
Medical Director, Spine & Sports Rehabilitation
Center, Rehabilitation Institute of Chicago, River
Forest, USA

Jaideep Rampure MD
MRI fellow, University of British Columbia,
Department of Radiology, Vancouver, Canada

Anthony Schache B.Physio(Hons), PhD
Physiotherapist, Olympic Park Sports Medicine
Centre & Richmond Football Club;
Research Fellow, Hugh Williamson Gait
Laboratory, Royal Children's Hospital, Melbourne,
& Centre for Health Exercise and Sports Medicine,
The University of Melbourne, Australia

Kevin P. Singer PhD, PT
Physiotherapist. Professor & Head of the Centre
for Musculoskeletal Studies, School of Surgery &
Pathology, The University of Western Australia,
Perth, Australia

Meena M. Sran PT, MPhty (Manips), PhD
Physiotherapist, BC Women's Health Centre,
Vancouver, BC, Canada
CIHR and MSFHR Postdoctoral Fellow, Simon
Fraser University, Burnaby, Canada

Lisa Sutherland BAppSci (Human Movement),
MND, GradCertSportsNutrition, Cert IV Fitness
Sports Dietitian & Fitness Consultant (Director—
Sports Dietitians Australia), Victorian Institute of
Sport/Deakin University, Melbourne, Australia

Jason E. Tang BSc
PhD candidate, Kinesiology—Exercise Metabolism
Research Group
McMaster University, Canada

Jack Taunton MSc, MD, DipSportMed(CASM),
FACSM
Sports Physician. Professor Department of
Family Practice and School of Human Kinetics
and Director, Allan McGavin Sports Medicine
Centre, University of British Columbia, Vancouver,
Canada. Chief Medical Officer, Olympic Winter
Games, Vancouver, 2010

Nick Webborn MBBS
Sports Physician & Medical Adviser to the British
Paralympic Association, The Sussex Centre for
Sport & Exercise Medicine, University of Brighton,
Eastbourne, UK

Other contributors

Riyad B. Abu-Laban MD, MHSc, FRCPC
Research Director, VGH Department of Emergency
Medicine. Scientist, VCHRI Centre for Clinical
Epidemiology & Evaluation; Assistant Professor,
University of British Columbia, Vancouver, Canada

Sally Child BAppSci(HmMvt), BPodiatry
Podiatrist, Olympic Park Sports Medicine Centre,
Melbourne, Australia; Richmond Football Club

Pierre Guy MD, MBA
Assistant Professor, Department of Orthopaedic
Surgery, University of British Columbia,
Vancouver, Canada

Gwendolen Jull MPhty, PhD, FACP
Professor, Division of Physiotherapy, School of
Health and Rehabilitation Sciences, University
of Queensland, Brisbane, Australia

Rebecca Morarty BAppSci(HmMvt), BPodiatry
Podiatrist, Olympic Park Sports Medicine Centre,
Melbourne, Australia; Collingwood Football Club

Moira O'Brien MB, BCh, FRCPI
Professor of Anatomy, Trinity College, Dublin, Ireland. President of the Irish Osteoporosis Society

Nadia Picco
Senior Graphic Designer, Digital Printing & Graphic Services, The Media Group, University of British Columbia, Vancouver, Canada

Nicki Quigley BAppSci(HmMvt), BPodiatry
Podiatrist, Olympic Park Sports Medicine Centre, Melbourne, Australia; Hawthorn Football Club

Aaron Sciascia MS, ATC
Program Coordinator, Lexington Clinic Sports Medicine Center, Lexington, KY, USA

Katerina Scott BA
Research Assistant, Bone Health Research Group, University of British Columbia, Vancouver, Canada

Justin Steer BPhysio
Physiotherapist, Olympic Park Sports Medicine Centre, Melbourne, Australia; Victorian Cricket team

Andy Stephens BAppSci(Physio)
Physiotherapist, Olympic Park Sports Medicine Centre, Melbourne, Australia

Paul Thompson MD, FACC, FACSM
Director, Preventive Cardiology, Hartford Hospital, Connecticut, USA

Larissa Trease BMedSci(Hons), MBBS(Hons)
Sports Medicine Registrar, Olympic Park Sports Medicine Centre, Melbourne, Australia

Susan White MBBS, FACSP
Sports Physician, Olympic Park Sports Medicine Centre, Melbourne, Australia; Member, Australian Sports Drug Medical Advisory Committee (ASDMAC)

The illustrator

Vicky Earle BSc(AAM), MET, Cert TBDL
Medical Illustrator, The Media Group, University of British Columbia, Vancouver, Canada

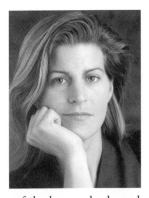

Vicky is a highly experienced medical illustrator who has been involved in the design and production of a wide variety of surgical procedural and medical illustrations which have been used in journals, books, conferences, lectures and legal presentations. Her keen interest in *Clinical Sports Medicine* stems not only from a great appreciation of the human body and its capabilities, but also from a decade of past racing experience as a canoeist, dragonboat racer and rower—and knowing first-hand the many injuries that accompany these activities.

Acknowledgments

This completely rewritten, full colour, third edition of *Clinical Sports Medicine* is unashamedly founded on the previous two editions. To date, this text has satisfied over 40 000 practitioners and provided core material for clinicians and students who care for active people in Australia, New Zealand, Africa, Asia, Great Britain and North America. A Portuguese translation is used in Brazil. The overwhelming support for this clinically-based textbook means we are particularly indebted to our partners in both the previous editions.

Specific thanks for the third edition go to chapter co-authors listed, with their affiliations, on the 'Chapter co-authors' on page xxxiv. We note that expert co-authors provide the crucial innovation and timeliness that users of *Clinical Sports Medicine* rely on. We emphasize this role on the cover and title page by reference to our esteemed 'with colleagues'. We would love to have listed each of your names on the cover—alas, the designer over-ruled us on that one! In addition to chapter co-authors, many other wonderful colleagues made this happen. It takes a community to create *Clinical Sports Medicine*—and we are grateful for every single member of that international community.

Because this edition was so much more than a text revision, we acknowledge especially those co-authors who contributed to the new colour photo shots and the DVD recording in Melbourne as well as to the final DVD production. For the production of the DVD we are indebted to our talented producer and editor Nick Ball, and Allyn Laing behind the camera; for the photos in Melbourne we thank Ryan Jaffe.

Vicky Earle is a gifted medical illustrator who already contributed to the second edition but who really embraced sports medicine once she received the colour licence from David Steele. We are sure he will never forget, or regret, that decision! Vicky committed to this book the same way that Steve Jobs is committed to Apple—we look forward to an ongoing partnership for various productions of *Clinical Sports Medicine*.

The University of British Columbia (Department of Family Practice—Faculty of Medicine as well as the Faculty of Education and The Media Group) provided essential support (KK) as did the Olympic Park Sports Medicine Centre and the University of Melbourne Centre for Health Exercise and Sports Medicine (PB).

Clinical Sports Medicine now benefits from the continuity, consistency, and integration of a dual-author book, while benefiting from the expertise that can only be achieved by multiple international contributors. We see this as the best of both worlds.

We give special thanks to our publishing team. Carolyn Pike—the medical editor extraordinaire for all three editions, Meiling Voon for emphasizing the need for a third edition, David Steele for having the faith that *Clinical Sports Medicine* warranted the full-colour treatment, Nicole Meehan for her support especially with the DVD, and Sybil Kesteven for constant encouragement and terrific production management; thank you for your patience and meticulous attention to making this book the best it could be, Sybil.

Most importantly, we most deeply thank our friends and families, especially Diana and Heather, thank you all for your tolerance, support (as before) and now endurance! We know there are not enough superlatives, so we will not try. We dedicate this third edition to our increasingly adult children—Bill Callista, Charles, Joe, Julia and Ryland. Thank you for tolerating our foibles (not just in book writing!).

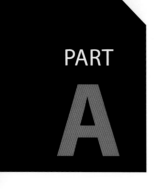

PART A

Fundamental Principles

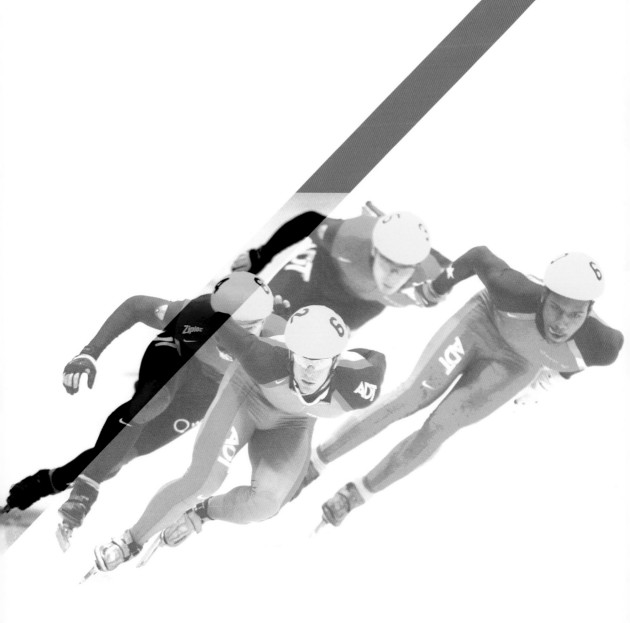

Sports Medicine: The Team Approach

Millions of people throughout the world perform physical exercise and play sport. These people have specific medical needs. To cater for these people a branch of medicine known as 'sports medicine' has evolved.[1, 2] Sports medicine includes: injury prevention, diagnosis, treatment and rehabilitation; performance enhancement through training, nutrition and psychology; management of medical problems; exercise prescription in health and in chronic disease states;[3] the specific needs of exercising in children, females, older people and those with permanent disabilities; the medical care of sporting teams and events; medical care in situations of altered physiology, such as at altitude or at depth; and ethical issues, such as the problem of drug abuse in sport.

Because of the breadth of content, sports medicine lends itself to being practiced by a multidisciplinary team of professionals with specialized skills who provide optimal care for the athlete and improve each other's knowledge and skills.[4] A sporting adage is that a 'champion team' would always beat a 'team of champions' and this also applies to sports medicine. Individuals who provide specialized skills and who utilize the skills offered by other members of the team provide the best athlete care. This team approach can be implemented in a multidisciplinary sports medicine clinic or by individual practitioners of different disciplines collaborating by cross-referral.

The sports medicine team

The most appropriate sports medicine team depends on the setting. In an isolated rural community, the sports medicine team may consist of a family physician or a physiotherapist/physical therapist alone. In a fairly populous city, the team may consist of:

- family physician
- physiotherapist/physical therapist
- sports physician
- massage therapist
- orthopedic surgeon
- radiologist
- podiatrist
- dietitian/nutritionist
- psychologist
- sports trainer/athletic trainer
- other professionals such as osteopaths, chiropractors, exercise physiologists, biomechanists, nurses, occupational therapists, orthotists, optometrists
- coach
- fitness adviser.

In the Olympic polyclinic, an institution that aims to serve all 10 000 athletes at the games, the sports medicine team includes 160 practitioners (Table 1.1).

Multiskilling

The practitioners in the team have each developed skills in a particular area of sports medicine. There may also be a considerable amount of overlap between the different practitioners. Practitioners should be encouraged to increase their knowledge and skills in areas other than the one in which they received their basic training. This 'multiskilling' is particularly important if the practitioner is geographically isolated or is travelling with sporting teams.

The concept of multiskilling is best illustrated by a number of examples. When an athlete presents with an overuse injury of the lower limb, it is the podiatrist or biomechanist who has the best knowledge

Table 1.1 Staff who provide medical coverage at an Olympic and Paralympic polyclinic

Administration/organization

Chief Medical Officer
Deputy Chief Medical Officer, and Chief, Athlete Services (sports physician)
Director of Clinical Services—Polyclinic (sports physician)
Director of Nursing
Director of Physiotherapy/Physical therapy
Director of Remedial Massage
Director of Podiatric Services
Director of Dental Services
Director of Emergency Services

Consulting

Medical practitioners: sports physicians; orthopedic surgeons; general practitioners; rehabilitation specialists;
  emergency medicine specialists; ear, nose and throat specialists; gynecologists; dermatologists; ophthalmologists;
  ophthalmic surgeons; radiologists; amputee clinic physician; spinal clinic physician
Physiotherapists/Physical therapists
Massage therapists
Podiatrists
Optometrists
Pharmacists
Dentists
Interpreters

of the relationship between abnormal biomechanics and the development of the injury, in clinical biomechanical assessment and in possible correction of any biomechanical cause. However, it is essential that other practitioners, such as a sports physician, orthopedic surgeon, physiotherapist/physical therapist and sports/athletic trainer, all have a basic understanding of lower limb biomechanics and are able to perform a clinical assessment. Similarly, in the athlete who presents complaining of excessive fatigue and poor performance, the dietitian is best able to assess the nutritional state of the athlete and determine if a nutritional deficiency is responsible for the patient's symptoms. However, other practitioners such as a sports physician, physiotherapist/physical therapist or trainer must also be aware of the possibility of nutritional deficiency as a cause of tiredness and be able to perform a brief nutritional assessment.

The sports medicine model

The traditional medical model (Fig. 1.1) has the physician as the primary contact practitioner with subsequent referral to other medical and paramedical practitioners.

The sports medicine model (Fig. 1.2) is different. The athlete's primary medical contact may be with a physician, however, it is just as likely to be a trainer, physiotherapist/physical therapist or massage

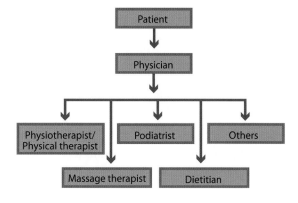

Figure 1.1 The traditional medical model

therapist. Athletes usually present to the practitioner with whom they have the best relationship or are most accustomed to seeing. Therefore, it is essential that all practitioners in the sports medicine team understand their own strengths and limitations and are aware of which other practitioners can offer the required skills for the best management of the patient.

If a patient is not responding to a particular treatment regimen, it is necessary to reassess the situation, reconsider the diagnosis and consider alternative methods of treatment. This may require referral to another member of the sports medicine team.

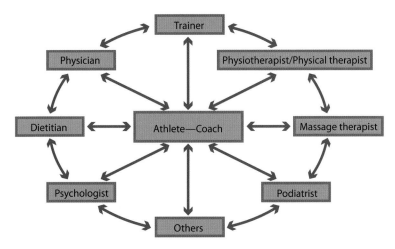

Figure 1.2 The sports medicine model. In professional sport the player's agent also features prominently in athlete–coach interaction

The challenges of management

The secret of success in sports medicine is to take a broad view of the patient and his or her problem. The narrow view may provide short-term amelioration of symptoms but will ultimately lead to failure. Examples of the narrow view may include a runner who presents with shin pain, is diagnosed as having a stress fracture of the tibia and is treated with rest until free of pain; a baseball pitcher who presents with shoulder pain, is diagnosed as having rotator cuff tendinitis and is treated with anti-inflammatory medication and rest from aggravating activities; or a triathlete who presents with excessive fatigue and poor performance and is treated with rest.

In all these examples, it is likely that in the short term each of these athletes will improve and return to activity. However, in each case there is a high likelihood of recurrence of the problem on resumption of activity. It is not adequate simply to diagnose the athlete's presenting problem and treat accordingly. The clinician must always ask 'Why has this injury/illness occurred?'. The cause may be obvious, for example, recent sudden doubling of training load, or it may be subtle and, in many cases, multifactorial.

The greatest challenge of sports medicine is to identify and correct the cause of the injury/illness. In the cases mentioned above, the runner with shin pain arising from a stress fracture will continue to have problems unless the cause is corrected. The cause may be one or more factors, such as abnormal biomechanics, inappropriate footwear, change of training surface or change in quantity or quality of training. The baseball pitcher may have shoulder tendinopathy because of poor throwing technique, excessive pitching or the presence of mild instability of the shoulder joint. The triathlete may have fatigue and impaired performance because of overtraining and/or inadequate recovery, poor nutrition, accompanying viral illness or a medical condition such as exercise-induced asthma. In each of these cases, it is essential to take a broad rather than narrow view of the problem.

In medicine, there are two main challenges—diagnosis and treatment. As mentioned, in sports medicine, it is necessary to diagnose both the problem and the cause. Treatment then needs to be focused on both these areas.

Diagnosis

Every attempt should be made to diagnose the precise anatomical and pathological cause of the presenting problem. With adequate knowledge of anatomy (especially surface anatomy) and an understanding of the pathological processes likely to occur in athletes, a precise diagnosis can usually be made. Thus, instead of using a purely descriptive term such as 'shin splints', the practitioner should attempt to diagnose which of the three underlying causes it could be—stress fracture, chronic compartment syndrome or periostitis—and use the specific term. Accurate diagnosis permits precise treatment.

There are, however, some clinical situations in which a precise anatomical and pathological diagnosis is not possible. For example, in many cases of low back pain, it is clinically impossible to differentiate between potential sites of pathology. In situations such as these, it is necessary to monitor symptoms and signs through careful clinical assessment and correct any abnormalities present (e.g. hypomobility of an intervertebral segment) using appropriate treatment techniques.

As mentioned, sports medicine often requires not only the diagnosis of the presenting problem but also the diagnosis of the cause of the problem. The US orthopedic surgeon, Ben Kibler, has coined the term 'victim' for the presenting problem and 'culprit' for the cause.[5] Diagnosis of the presenting problem requires a good knowledge of anatomy and possible pathology, while diagnosis of the cause often requires a good understanding of biomechanics, technique, training, nutrition and psychology. Just as there may be more than one pathological process contributing to the patient's symptoms, there may also be a combination of factors causing the problem.

As with any branch of medicine, diagnosis depends on careful clinical assessment, which consists of obtaining a history, physical examination and investigations. The most important of these is undoubtedly the history but, unfortunately, this is often neglected. It is essential that the sports clinician be a good listener and develop skills that enable him or her to elicit the appropriate information from the athlete. Once the history has been taken, an examination can be performed. It is essential to develop examination routines for each joint or region and to include in the examination an assessment of any potential causes.

Investigations should be regarded as an adjunct to, rather than a substitute for, adequate history and examination.[6] The investigation must be appropriate to the athlete's problem, provide additional information and should only be performed if it will affect the diagnosis and/or treatment.

Treatment

Ideally, treatment has two components—treatment of the presenting injury/illness and treatment to correct the cause. It is important to understand that no single form of treatment will correct all or even the majority of sports medicine problems. A combination of different forms of treatment will usually give the best results.

Therefore, it is important for the clinician to be aware of the variety of treatments and to appreciate when their use may be appropriate. It is also important to develop as many treatment skills as

possible or, alternatively, ensure access to others with particular skills. It is essential to evaluate the effectiveness of treatment constantly. If a particular treatment is not proving to be effective, it is important firstly to reconsider the diagnosis. If the diagnosis appears to be correct, other treatments should be considered (Chapter 36).

Meeting individual needs

Every patient is a unique individual with specific needs. Without an understanding of this, it is not possible to manage the athlete appropriately. The patient may be an Olympic athlete whose selection depends on a peak performance at forthcoming trials. The patient may be a non-competitive business executive whose jogging is an important means of coping with everyday life. The patient may be a club tennis player whose weekly competitive game is as important as a Wimbledon final is to a professional. Alternatively, the patient may be someone to whom sport is not at all important but whose low back pain causes discomfort at work.

The cost of treatment should also be considered. Does the athlete merely require a diagnosis and reassurance that he or she has no major injury? Or does the athlete want twice-daily treatment in order to be able to play in an important game. Obviously, the latter approach is more costly but may be what the patient wants. Treatment depends on the patient's situation, not purely on the diagnosis.

The coach, the athlete and the clinician

The relationship between the coach, the athlete and the clinician is shown in Figure 1.3. The clinician obviously needs to develop a good relationship with the athlete. A feeling of mutual trust and confidence would lead to the athlete feeling that he or she can confide in the clinician and the clinician feeling that the athlete will comply with advice.

As the coach is directly responsible for the athlete's training and performance, it is essential to involve

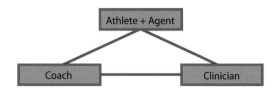

Figure 1.3 The coach, the athlete and the clinician

the coach in medical decision making. Unfortunately, some coaches have a distrust of clinicians, feeling, rightly or wrongly, that the main role of the practitioner is to prevent the athlete from training or competing. It is essential for the coach to understand that the practitioner is also aiming to maximize the performance and health of the athlete. When major injuries occur, professional athletes' agents will be involved in discussions.

Involving the coach in the decision-making process and explaining the rationale behind any recommendations will increase athlete compliance. The coach will also be a valuable aid in supervising the recommended treatment or rehabilitation program. Discussion with the coach may help to establish a possible cause for the injury as a result of faulty technique or equipment.

A good practitioner–coach relationship is a win–win situation. The coach will develop a better understanding of what the clinician has to offer and is more likely to seek help for minor problems which, if managed appropriately, may prevent subsequent major problems. The clinician will benefit from an increased understanding of the demands of the sport and may have an opportunity to institute various preventive measures.

'Love thy sport'

To be a successful sports clinician it is essential to know and love sport and to be an advocate for physical activity. The sports clinician needs to understand the importance of sport to the athlete and the demands of the sport. These demands may be physical, such as training and technique, or psychological. As well as understanding the general philosophy of sport and the athlete, it is important to have a thorough understanding of particular sports.

A good understanding of a sport and exercise confers two advantages. Firstly, if the clinician understands the physical demands and technical aspects of a particular sport, then this will improve his or her understanding of possible causes of injury and also facilitate development of sport-specific rehabilitation programs. Secondly, it will result in the athlete having increased confidence in the clinician.

The best way to understand the sport is to attend both training and competition or to actually participate in the sport. Thus, it is essential to be on site, not only to be available when injuries occur, but also to develop a thorough understanding of the sport.

References

1. Matheson GO, Pipe AL. Twenty-five years of sport medicine in Canada: thoughts on the road ahead. *Clin J Sport Med* 1996; 6: 148–51.
2. Blair SN, Franklin BA, Jakicic JM, Kibler WB. New vision for health promotion within sports medicine. *Am J Health Promot* 2003; 18(2): 182–5.
3. Chakravarthy MV, Booth FW. Eating, exercise, and 'thrifty' genotypes: connecting the dots toward an evolutionary understanding of modern chronic diseases. *J Appl Physiol* 2004; 96(1): 3–10.
4. Hahn A. Sports medicine, sports science: the multidisciplinary road to sports success. *J Sci Med Sport* 2004; 7: 275–7.
5. Kibler WB, Sciascia A. Kinetic chain contributions to elbow function and dysfunction in sports. *Clin Sports Med* 2004; 23(4): 545–52.
6. Khan KM, Tress BW, Hare WSC, et al. 'Treat the patient, not the X-ray': advances in diagnostic imaging do not replace the need for clinical interpretation. *Clin J Sport Med* 1998; 8: 1–4.

Sports Injuries

Regular physical activity is probably the most important overall determinant of a population's health. Unfortunately, physical activity may extract a cost in the form of an activity-related injury. Such an injury may be categorized as either being an acute injury or an overuse injury depending on the mechanism of injury and the onset of symptoms (Table 2.1).

Table 2.1 Classification of sporting injuries

Site	Acute injuries	Overuse injuries
Bone	Fracture Periosteal contusion	Stress fracture 'Bone strain', 'stress reaction' Osteitis, periostitis Apophysitis
Articular cartilage	Osteochondral/chondral fractures Minor osteochondral injury	Chondropathy (e.g. softening, fibrillation, fissuring, chondromalacia)
Joint	Dislocation Subluxation	Synovitis Osteoarthritis
Ligament	Sprain/tear (grades I–III)	Inflammation
Muscle	Strain/tear (grades I–III) Contusion Cramp Acute compartment syndrome	Chronic compartment syndrome Delayed onset muscle soreness Focal tissue thickening/fibrosis
Tendon	Tear (complete or partial)	Tendinopathy (includes paratenonitis, tenosynovitis, tendinosis, tendinitis)
Bursa	Traumatic bursitis	Bursitis
Nerve	Neuropraxia	Entrapment Minor nerve injury/irritation Adverse neural tension
Skin	Laceration Abrasion Puncture wound	Blister Callus

Acute injuries

Acute injuries may be due to extrinsic causes, such as a direct blow, either as a result of contact with another player or equipment, or intrinsic causes, such as a ligament sprain or muscle tear. As shown in Table 2.1, acute injuries may be classified according to the particular site injured (e.g. bone, cartilage, joint, ligament, muscle, tendon, bursa, nerve or skin) and the type of injury (e.g. fracture, dislocation, sprain or strain).

Bone

Fractures

Fractures may be due to direct trauma such as a blow, or indirect trauma such as a fall on the outstretched hand or a twisting injury. Fractures may be closed or open (compound), where the bony fragment punctures the skin.

Fractures are classified as transverse, oblique, spiral or comminuted (Fig. 2.1). Another type of fracture seen in athletes, particularly children, is the avulsion fracture, where a piece of bone attached to a tendon or ligament is torn away.

The clinical features of a fracture are pain, tenderness, localized bruising, swelling, and, in some cases, deformity and restriction of movement. Fractures are managed by anatomical and functional realignment. Non-displaced or minimally displaced fractures can be treated with bracing or casting. Displaced fractures require reduction and immobilization. A displaced, unstable fracture requires surgical stabilization.

There are a number of possible complications of fracture. These include:

- infection
- acute compartment syndrome
- associated injury (e.g. nerve, vessel)
- deep venous thrombosis/pulmonary embolism
- delayed union/non-union
- malunion.

Infection is most likely to occur in open (compound) fractures. Prophylactic antibiotic therapy is required in the treatment of any open fracture.

Occasionally a fracture may cause swelling of a muscle compartment that is surrounded by a non-distensible fascial sheath, usually in the flexor compartment of the forearm or the anterior compartment of the lower leg. This condition, acute muscle compartment syndrome (see below), causes pain out of proportion to the fracture, pain on passive stretch, pulselessness and paresthesia. This may require urgent

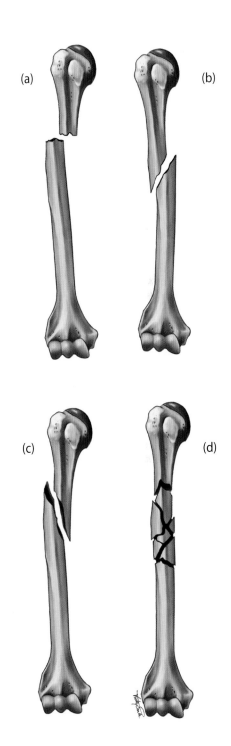

(a) (b) (c) (d)

Figure 2.1 Types of fracture

(a) transverse **(b)** oblique **(c)** spiral
(d) comminuted

fasciotomy, that is, release of the tight band of tissue surrounding the muscle compartment.

Occasionally, deep venous thrombosis and pulmonary embolism may occur after a fracture, especially a lower limb fracture. This should be prevented by early movement and active muscle contraction. Delayed union, or malunion, of a fracture causes persistent pain and disability that may require bone grafting, with or without internal fixation.

The problems of immobilization are discussed in Chapter 10. If immobilization is required for fracture healing, muscle wasting and joint stiffness will occur. Muscle wasting can be reduced by the use of electrical muscle stimulation and by isometric muscle contractions. Joint stiffness can be reduced by the use of limited motion braces instead of complete immobilization or by the use of surgical fixation, which allows early movement.

Growth plate fractures in children and adolescents present a particular problem. These fractures are reviewed in Chapter 40.

Soft tissue injury, such as ligament or muscle damage, is often associated with a fracture, and may cause more long-term problems than the fracture itself. Thus, it is important not to ignore the soft tissue components of any bony injury. Specific fractures that are common in athletes are discussed in Part B.

Periosteal injury

Acute periosteal injuries are uncommon. Like fractures, they can be extremely painful. Examples of periosteal injury include the condition known as a 'hip pointer', an injury to the periosteum of the iliac crest caused by a direct blow, and periosteal injury of the tibia resulting from a blow from a kick, stick or ball.

Articular cartilage

Articular cartilage lines the ends of long bones. It absorbs shock and compressive forces and permits almost frictionless movement of joints. These injuries are far more common than was previously realized.

With the advent of new imaging techniques such as magnetic resonance imaging (MRI) and the increasing availability of arthroscopy, it is now possible to distinguish three classes of articular cartilage injuries (Fig. 2.2):

1. disruption of the articular cartilage at its deeper layers with or without subchondral bone damage, while the articular surface itself remains intact (Fig. 2.2a)

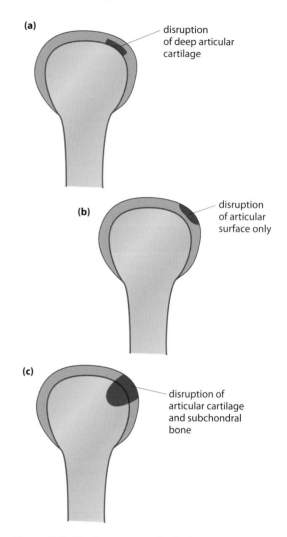

(a) disruption of deep articular cartilage

(b) disruption of articular surface only

(c) disruption of articular cartilage and subchondral bone

Figure 2.2 The three types of articular cartilage injury

2. disruption of the articular surface only (Fig. 2.2b)
3. disruption of both articular cartilage and subchondral bone (Fig. 2.2c).

Articular cartilage may be injured by acute shearing injuries such as dislocation and subluxation. Common sites of chondral and osteochondral injuries are the superior articular surface of the talus, the femoral condyles, the patella and the capitellum of the humerus. Osteochondral injuries may be associated with soft tissue conditions such as ligament sprains and complete ruptures (e.g. anterior cruciate ligament injury). As an initial X-ray examination is often normal, the clinician must maintain a high index of suspicion of osteochondral damage if an apparently 'simple joint sprain' remains painful and swollen for longer than expected. These injuries should be investigated with MRI. Arthroscopy may be required to assess the degree of damage and to remove loose fragments or to perform chondroplasty (smooth loose edges of damaged articular cartilage).

Acute damage to articular cartilage is present in association with complete ligament ruptures[1] and may predispose to premature osteoarthritis.[2] Therefore, every attempt should be made to restore the smooth surface of the articular cartilage. Immobilization has a detrimental effect on articular cartilage but continuous passive movement may help counter this effect.

Articular cartilage injuries generally do not heal fully. A variety of treatments have the potential to improve healing of articular surfaces, including perforation of subchondral bone, altered joint loading, periosteal and perichondral grafts, cell transplantation, growth factors, artificial matrices and mesenchymal stem cells. The latter treatments are still at an experimental stage and as yet no treatment can be said to restore a durable articular surface reliably.[3]

Joint

Dislocation/subluxation

Dislocation of a joint occurs when trauma produces complete dissociation of the articulating surfaces of the joint. Subluxation occurs when the articulating surfaces remain partially in contact with each other (Fig. 2.3).

The stability of a joint depends on its anatomy. The hip is relatively stable because it has a deep ball and socket configuration, whereas the shoulder is far

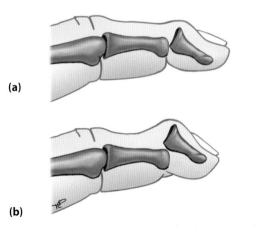

(a)

(b)

Figure 2.3 (a) Subluxation and **(b)** dislocation of a joint

less stable because it has a small area of bony contact. Less stable joints such as the shoulder and fingers are more likely to dislocate. More stable joints such as the hip, elbow, ankle and subtalar joints require much greater forces to dislocate and are, therefore, more likely to be associated with other injuries (e.g. fractures, nerve and vascular damage). All dislocations and subluxations result in injuries to the surrounding joint capsule and ligaments.

Complications of dislocations include associated nerve damage, for example, axillary nerve injury in shoulder dislocations, and vascular damage, for example, brachial artery damage in elbow dislocations. All dislocations should be X-rayed to exclude an associated fracture.

Dislocated joints, in most cases, may be reduced relatively easily. Occasionally, muscle relaxation is required and this is achieved either by the use of an injected relaxant such as diazepam or by general anesthetic. After reduction, the joint needs to be protected to allow the joint capsule and ligaments to heal. Where possible, early protected mobilization is encouraged. Subsequent muscle strengthening gives the joint increased stability. Management of the more common dislocations is discussed in Part B.

Ligament

The stability of a joint is increased by the presence of a joint capsule of connective tissue, thickened at points of stress to form ligaments. The ends of the ligament attach to bone.

Ligament injuries range from mild injuries involving the tearing of only a few fibers to complete tears of the ligament, which may lead to instability of the joint. Ligament injuries are divided into three grades (Fig. 2.4). A grade I sprain represents some stretched fibers but clinical testing reveals normal range of motion on stressing the ligament. A grade II sprain involves a considerable proportion of the fibers and, therefore, stretching of the joint and stressing the ligament show increased laxity but a definite end point. A grade III sprain is a complete tear of the ligament with excessive joint laxity and no firm end point. Although they are often painful conditions, grade III sprains can also be pain-free as sensory fibers are completely divided in the injury.

The management of acute ligament sprains is summarized in Figure 2.5. The initial management consists of first aid to minimize bleeding and swelling (Chapter 10). For grade I and II sprains, treatment aims to promote tissue healing, prevent joint stiffness, protect against further damage and strengthen

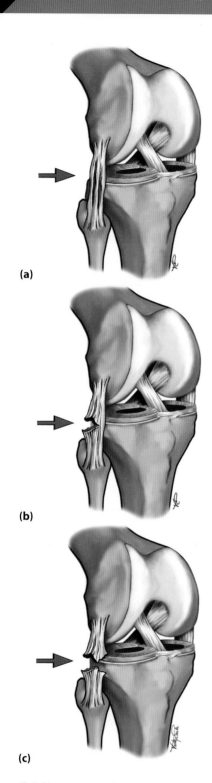

(a)

(b)

(c)

Figure 2.4 Ligament sprains

(a) Grade I **(b)** Grade II **(c)** Grade III

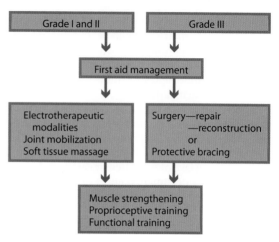

Figure 2.5 Management of acute ligament sprains

muscle to provide additional joint stability. The healing of collagen in a partial ligament tear takes several months.[4, 5] However, depending on the degree of damage, return to sport may be possible sooner than this, especially with protection against further injury.

The treatment of a grade III sprain may be either conservative or surgical. For example, the torn medial collateral ligament of the knee and the torn lateral ligament of the ankle may be treated conservatively with full or partial immobilization. Alternatively, the two ends of a torn ligament can be reattached surgically and the joint then fully or partially immobilized for approximately six weeks. In certain instances (e.g. anterior cruciate ligament rupture), torn ligament tissue is not amenable to primary repair and surgical reconstruction of the ligament, usually using tendon, may be performed instead.

Muscle

Strain/tear

Muscles are strained or torn when some or all of the fibers fail to cope with the demands placed upon them. Muscles that are commonly affected are the hamstrings, quadriceps and gastrocnemius; these muscles are all biarthrodial (cross two joints) and thus more vulnerable to injury. A muscle is most likely to tear during sudden acceleration or deceleration.

Muscle strains are classified in three grades (Fig. 2.6). A grade I strain involves a small number of muscle fibers and causes localized pain but no loss of strength. A grade II strain is a tear of a significant number of muscle fibers with associated pain and swelling. Pain is reproduced on muscle contraction.

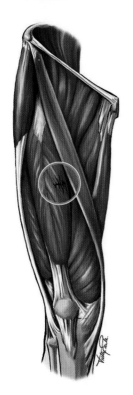 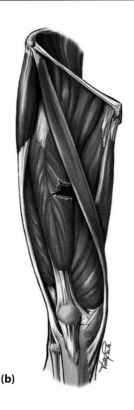 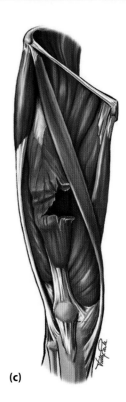

(a)   **(b)**   **(c)**

Figure 2.6 Muscle strains

(a) Grade I **(b)** Grade II **(c)** Grade III

Strength is reduced and movement is limited by pain. A grade III strain is a complete tear of the muscle. This is seen most frequently at the musculotendinous junction.

Management of muscle strains requires first aid to minimize bleeding, swelling and inflammation. Subsequent treatment promotes efficient scar formation through the use of strengthening exercises, electrotherapeutic modalities, soft tissue therapy and stretching.

A number of factors predispose to muscle strains:

- inadequate warm-up
- insufficient joint range of motion
- excessive muscle tightness
- fatigue/overuse/inadequate recovery
- muscle imbalance
- previous injury
- faulty technique/biomechanics
- spinal dysfunction.

Most muscle strains are preventable. Methods of injury prevention are discussed in Chapter 6.

Contusions

A muscle contusion usually results from a direct blow from an opposition player or firm contact with equipment in collision sports, such as football, basketball and hockey. The blow causes local muscle damage with bleeding. The most common site of muscle contusions is the front of the thigh in the quadriceps muscle. This injury is known as a 'cork thigh' or 'charley horse'.

Management of contusion includes minimization of bleeding and swelling, followed by encouragement of resorption of the blood clot with electrotherapeutic modalities, carefully controlled soft tissue therapy as well as stretching and strengthening. Although most of these injuries are relatively minor and do not limit participation in sport, occasionally a severe contusion may result in a large amount of bleeding, especially if the player continues in the game after sustaining the injury. Heat, alcohol and vigorous massage increase bleeding after a contusion and must be avoided.

Athletes playing sports with a high risk of contusions in a specific area, such as the thigh in some football codes, should consider the use of protective equipment such as padding. The athlete must weigh up the benefit of reducing injury risk versus the reduction in mobility that may result from wearing the equipment.

An occasional complication of a muscle hematoma is myositis ossificans. This occurs when the hematoma calcifies. Although this is most common following more severe muscle contusions, it may also occur in relatively minor cases. Myositis ossificans should be suspected in any muscle contusion that does not resolve in the normal time frame. An X-ray performed 10 to 14 days after the injury may show an area of calcification. Management of myositis ossificans is conservative and recovery is usually slow.

Cramps

Muscle cramps are painful, involuntary muscle contractions that occur suddenly and can be temporarily debilitating. The most common site of muscle cramps is the calf muscle but they may occur in any muscle. Disturbances at various levels of the central and peripheral nervous system and skeletal muscle are involved in the mechanism of cramp and may explain the diverse range of conditions in which cramp occurs.[4, 6] Other popular theories as to the cause of cramps include dehydration, low potassium or low sodium levels, inadequate carbohydrate intake or excessively tight muscles but these hypotheses appear to be falling out of favor as the weight of evidence supports the 'neural excitability' hypothesis.[7]

The treatment of cramps is aimed at reducing muscle spindle and motor neuron activity by reflex inhibition and afferent stimulation. There are no proven strategies for the prevention of exercise-induced muscle cramp but regular muscle stretching, correction of muscle balance and posture, adequate conditioning for the activity, mental preparation for competition and avoidance of provocative drugs may all be beneficial. Other strategies such as incorporating plyometrics or eccentric muscle strengthening into training programs, maintaining adequate carbohydrate reserves during competition or treating myofascial trigger points require further investigation.[8]

Prevention of cramps involves maintenance of normal muscle tissue through adequate recovery after training with stretching and massage. A high carbohydrate meal should be eaten 2 to 3 hours before exercise. Adequate fluid, carbohydrate and electrolyte intake is also helpful. True muscle cramps should be distinguished from cramp-like muscle pain that is commonly seen in referred pain from the spine to the extremities (Chapter 3).

Tendon

Complete or partial tendon ruptures may occur acutely (Fig. 2.7). Normal tendons consist of tight parallel bundles of collagen fibers. Injuries to tendons generally occur at the point of least blood supply, for example, with the Achilles tendon usually 2 cm (0.75 in.) above the insertion of the tendon, or at the musculotendinous junction.

A tendon rupture occurs without warning, usually in an older athlete without a history of injury in that particular tendon. The two most commonly ruptured tendons are the Achilles tendon and the supraspinatus tendon of the shoulder. The main objective of the treatment of tendon injuries is to restore full motion and function. Partial tears are characterized by the sudden onset of pain and by localized tenderness but they may be difficult to distinguish from tendinopathy (see below).

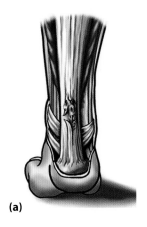

(a)

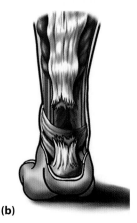

(b)

Figure 2.7 Tendon rupture

(a) Partial (b) Complete

When investigation is indicated, ultrasound and MRI can be useful. Both modalities can distinguish between a partial or complete tendon rupture and overuse tendinopathy. Generally, acute tendon rupture requires surgical treatment followed by progressive rehabilitation.

Bursa

Bursae are small fluid-filled sacs usually situated between a bone and a tendon. The role of a bursa is to reduce friction. There are numerous bursae around the hips, knees, feet, shoulders and elbows. Most injuries to bursae are associated with overuse but occasionally a direct fall onto a bursa may result in acute traumatic bursitis due to bleeding into the bursa. The management of acute hemorrhagic bursitis involves the application of ice and compression. Aspiration may be indicated if the condition does not resolve.

Nerve

Fortunately, major nerve injuries are unusual in athletes. However, a few nerves are relatively exposed and susceptible to injury from a direct blow. The nerves most often injured in this way are the ulnar nerve at the elbow and the common peroneal nerve at the neck of the fibula. The immediate symptoms are tingling, numbness and pain in the distribution of the nerve.

In minor nerve injuries the symptoms usually diminish quickly but in more severe injuries there will be persistent pain in the area of the distribution of the nerve. Occasionally, in severe injuries there will be paralysis or weakness of the muscles innervated by that nerve, in addition to sensory loss in the sensory distribution of the nerve. While this paralysis is present the area should be supported in a brace or cast. This injury, known as neuropraxia, usually resolves spontaneously but slowly.

There is increasing evidence that minor nerve injury is a common accompanying feature of many injuries. These nerve injuries are detected clinically by changes in neural tension and may make a significant contribution to the patient's symptoms. The concept of neural tension is discussed more fully in Chapter 3.

Skin

Injury to skin is common among athletes, especially those playing contact sports. Possible damage to underlying structures, such as tendons, muscles, blood vessels and nerves, should always be considered.

Open wounds may be abrasions, lacerations or puncture wounds. The principles of treatment of all open wounds are shown in Table 2.2.

Table 2.2 Principles of treatment of all open wounds

Principle	Details
1. Stop any associated bleeding	Apply a pressure bandage directly to the injured part and elevate it. If the wound is open and clean, bring the wound edges together using adhesive strips or sutures. A contaminated wound should not be closed.
2. Prevent infection	Remove all dirt and contamination by simple irrigation. Extensively wash and scrub with antiseptic solution as required as soon as possible. If the wound is severely contaminated, prophylactic antibiotic therapy should be commenced (e.g. flucloxacillin, 500 mg orally four times a day). If anaerobic organisms are suspected (e.g. wound inflicted by a bite), add an antibiotic such as metronidazole (400 mg orally three times a day).
3. Immobilization (where needed)	This applies when the wound is over a constantly moving part, for example, the anterior aspect of the knee. Certain lacerations, such as pretibial lacerations, require particular care and strict immobilization to encourage healing.
4. Check tetanus status	All contaminated wounds, especially penetrating wounds, have the potential to become infected with *Clostridium tetani*. Tetanus immunization consists of a course of three injections over 6 months given during childhood. Further tetanus toxoid boosters should be given at 5 to 10 year intervals. In the case of a possible contaminated wound, a booster should be given if none has been administered within the previous 5 years.

Overuse injuries

Overuse injuries present three distinct challenges to the clinician—diagnosis, treatment and an understanding of why the injury occurred. Diagnosis requires taking a comprehensive history of the onset, nature and site of the pain along with a thorough assessment of potential risk factors, for example, training and technique. Careful examination may reveal which anatomical structure is affected. It is often helpful to ask patients to perform the maneuver that produces their pain.

The treatment of overuse injuries may include relative rest, that is, avoidance of aggravating activities while maintaining fitness; the use of ice and various electrotherapeutic modalities; soft tissue techniques; and drugs, such as the non-steroidal anti-inflammatory drugs (NSAIDs) (Chapter 10).

A cause must be sought for every overuse injury. The cause may be quite evident, such as a sudden doubling of training quantity, poor footwear or an obvious biomechanical abnormality, or may be more subtle, such as running on a cambered surface, muscle imbalance or leg length discrepancy. The causes of overuse injuries are usually divided into extrinsic factors such as training, surfaces, shoes, equipment and environmental conditions, or intrinsic factors such as malalignment, leg length discrepancy, muscle imbalance, muscle weakness, lack of flexibility and body composition. Possible factors in the development of overuse injuries are shown in Table 2.3.

Bone

Stress fractures

Stress fractures, a common injury among sportspeople, were first reported in military recruits in the 19th century.[9] A stress fracture is a microfracture in bone that results from repetitive physical loading below the single cycle failure threshold. Overload stress can be applied to bone through two mechanisms:

1. the redistribution of impact forces resulting in increased stress at focal points in bone
2. the action of muscle pull across bone.

Histological changes resulting from bone stress occur along a continuum beginning with vascular congestion and thrombosis. This is followed by osteoclastic and osteoblastic activity leading to rarefaction, weakened trabeculae and microfracture and ending in complete fracture. This sequence of events can be interrupted at any point in the continuum if the process is recognized.

Table 2.3 Overuse injuries: predisposing factors

Extrinsic factors	Intrinsic factors
Training errors	Malalignment
Excessive volume	Pes planus
Excessive intensity	Pes cavus
Rapid increase	Rearfoot varus
Sudden change in type	Tibia vara
Excessive fatigue	Genu valgum
Inadequate recovery	Genu varum
Faulty technique	Patella alta
Surfaces	Femoral neck anteversion
Hard	Tibial torsion
Soft	Leg length discrepancy
Cambered	Muscle imbalance
Shoes	Muscle weakness
Inappropriate	Lack of flexibility
Worn out	Generalized muscle tightness
Equipment	Focal areas of muscle thickening
Inappropriate	
Environmental conditions	Restricted joint range of motion
Hot	
Cold	Sex, size, body composition
Humid	Other
Psychological factors	Genetic factors,
Inadequate nutrition	endocrine factors,
	metabolic conditions

Similarly, the process of bony remodeling and stress fracture in athletes is recognized as occurring along a clinical continuum with pain or radiographic changes presenting identifiable markers along the continuum. Since radioisotopic imaging and MRI can detect changes in bone at the phase of accelerated remodeling, these investigations can show stress-induced bony changes early in the continuum.

Stress fractures may occur in virtually any bone in the body. The most commonly affected bones are the tibia, metatarsals, fibula, tarsal navicular, femur and pelvis.[9-11] A list of sites of stress fractures and the likely associated sports or activities is shown in Figure 2.8. Table 2.4 lists the diagnostic features of a stress fracture.

It is important to note that a bone scan, although a routine investigation for stress fractures, is nonspecific, and other bony abnormalities such as tumors and osteomyelitis may cause similar pictures. It may also be difficult to localize the site of the area of increased uptake precisely, especially in an area such as the foot where numerous small bones are in close proximity.

Site of stress fracture	Associated sport/activity
Coracoid process of scapula	Trapshooting
Scapula	Running with hand weights
Humerus	Throwing; racquet sports
Olecranon	Throwing; pitching
Ulna	Racquet sports (esp. tennis); gymnastics; volleyball; swimming; softball; wheelchair sports
Ribs—1st	Throwing; pitching
Ribs—2nd–10th	Rowing; kayaking
Pars interarticularis	Gymnastics; ballet; cricket fast bowling volleyball; springboard diving
Pubic ramus *	Distance running; ballet
Femur—neck	Distance running; jumping; ballet
Femur—shaft	Distance running
Patella	Running; hurdling
Tibia—plateau	Running
Tibia—shaft	Running; ballet
Fibula	Running; aerobics; race-walking; ballet
Medial malleolus x	Running; basketball
Calcaneus	Long-distance military marching
Talus	Pole vaulting
Navicular	Sprinting; middle-distance running; hurdling; long jump; triple jump; football
Metatarsal—general	Running; ballet; marching
Metatarsal—2nd base	Ballet
Metatarsal—5th	Tennis; ballet
Sesamoid bone—foot	Running; ballet; basketball; skating

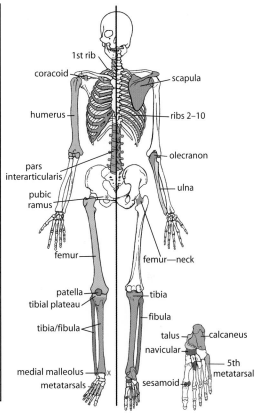

Figure 2.8 Stress fractures: site and common associated activity

Table 2.4 Diagnostic features of a stress fracture

Diagnostic features

- Localized pain and tenderness over the fracture site
- A history of a recent change in training or taking up a new activity
- X-ray appearance is often normal[12] or there may be a periosteal reaction (Fig. 2.9)
- Abnormal appearance on radioisotopic bone scan (scintigraphy) (Fig. 2.10),[13, 14] CT scan (Fig. 2.11) or MRI (Fig. 2.12)

MRI is being increasingly advocated as the investigation of choice for stress fractures. Even though MRI does not image fractures as clearly as do computed tomography (CT) scans, it is of comparable sensitivity to radioisotopic bone scans in assessing bony damage. The typical MRI appearance of a stress fracture shows periosteal and marrow edema plus or minus the actual fracture line (Fig. 2.12).

The treatment of stress fractures generally requires avoidance of the precipitating activity. The majority of stress fractures heal within six weeks of beginning relative rest. Healing is assessed clinically by the absence of local tenderness and functionally by the ability to perform the precipitating activity without pain. It is not useful to attempt to monitor healing with X-ray or radioisotopic bone scan.[9] CT scan appearances of healing stress fractures can be deceptive as in some cases the fracture is still visible well after clinical healing has occurred.[12]

The return to sport after clinical healing of a stress fracture should be a gradual process to enable the bone to adapt to an increased load (Chapter 12). An essential component of the management of an overuse injury is identification and modification of risk factors (Table 2.3).[14] There are, however, a number of sites of stress fractures in which delayed union or non-union of the fracture commonly occurs. These fractures need to be treated more aggressively. The sites of these fractures and the recommended treatments are shown in Table 2.5.

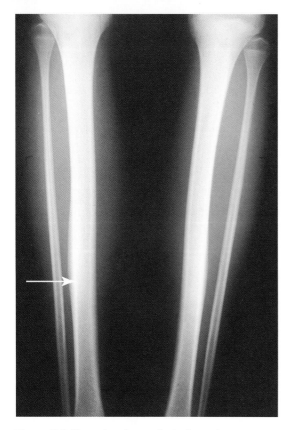

Figure 2.9 X-ray showing periosteal new bone formation indicative of a stress fracture

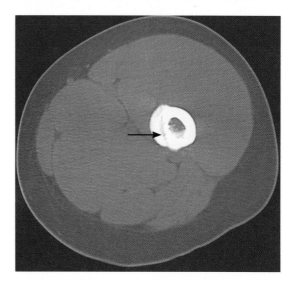

Figure 2.11 CT of a stress fracture showing a cortical defect (arrowed)

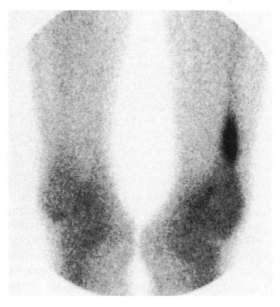

Figure 2.10 Stress fracture: radioisotopic bone scan appearance COURTESY OF Z. S. KISS

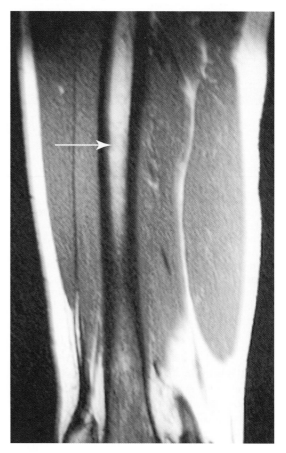

Figure 2.12 MRI of a stress fracture showing bony edema (white)

Table 2.5 Stress fractures that require specific treatment other than rest

Stress fracture	Treatment
Femoral neck	Undisplaced: initial bed rest for 1 week, then gradual weight-bearing Displaced: surgical fixation
Talus (lateral process)	Non-weight-bearing cast immobilization for 6 weeks, or surgical excision of fragment
Navicular	Non-weight-bearing cast immobilization for 6–8 weeks
Metatarsal—2nd base	Non-weight-bearing for 2 weeks; partial weight-bearing for 2 weeks
Sesamoid bone of the foot	Non-weight-bearing for 4 weeks
Metatarsal—5th base[a]	Cast immobilization or percutaneous screw fixation
Anterior tibial cortex	Non-weight-bearing on crutches for 6–8 weeks, or intramedullary screw fixation

(a) This is not a Jones' fracture, which is an acute fracture (see Chapter 35).

Bone strain

In some athletes bone scans show uptake of radio-isotope at non-painful sites. This is thought to represent bony remodeling at a very early subclinical level and has been termed 'bone strain'. Another situation encountered in clinical practice is the painful, tender focal area of bone that demonstrates a mildly increased uptake of radioisotope on bone scan, insufficient to be classified as a stress fracture. This has been termed 'stress reaction'. It would appear that there is a continuum of bone response to stress that ranges from mild (bone strain) to severe (stress fracture) (Fig. 2.13). The clinical features of bone strain, stress reaction and stress fractures are summarized in Table 2.6.

The presence of bone strain or a stress reaction are probably an indication that the patient is moving further along the continuum towards a stress fracture and should probably be an indication for reduction or modification of activity.

Osteitis and periostitis

Osteitis (impaction trauma or primary inflammation of bone) and periostitis (abnormal histological

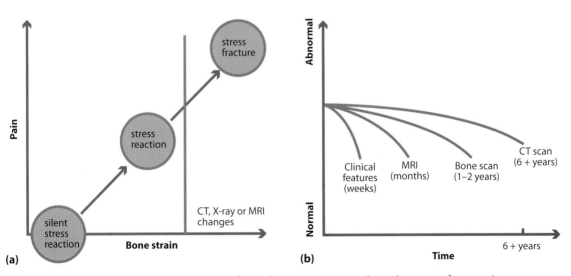

Figure 2.13 **(a)** The continuum of bone stress: from silent stress reaction through to stress fracture. At present, stress fracture is detected by changes on X-ray, CT scan or MRI. **(b)** MRI, bone scan and CT scan return to their normal appearance well after clinical union occurs

Table 2.6 Continuum of bony changes with overuse

Clinical features	Bone strain	Stress reaction	Stress fracture
Local pain	Nil	Nil	Nil
Local tenderness	Nil	Nil	Nil
X-ray appearance	Normal	Normal	Abnormal (periosteal reaction or cortical defect in cortical bone, sclerosis in trabecular bone)
Radioisotopic bone scan appearance	Increased uptake	Increased uptake	Increased uptake
CT scan appearance	Normal	Normal	Features of stress fracture (as for X-ray)
MRI appearance	May show increased high signal	Increased high signal	Increased high signal ± cortical defect

appearance of periosteal collagen) are also considered overuse injuries. The condition known as osteitis pubis occurs in the pubic bones of the pelvis and is characterized by deep-seated pain and tenderness of the symphysis pubis with generalized increased uptake on the radioisotopic bone scan. The exact pathogenesis of this injury remains in debate (Chapter 23).

Periostitis or tenoperiostitis (pain at the tendinous attachment to bone) occurs commonly, mainly at the medial border of the tibia, a condition often known as 'shin splints'. In this condition, tenderness along the medial border of the tibia corresponds with an area of increased uptake on bone scan.

The treatment of periostitis (or tenoperiostitis) consists of local symptomatic therapy as well as unloading the muscle contraction on the periosteum. In the shin, strain may be reduced by altering the biomechanics through controlling excessive pronation. Soft tissue therapy and stretching may also be effective.

Apophysitis

Bony inflammation and separation may occur at the attachment of the strong, large tendons to the growth areas. This condition is called 'apophysitis' and the most common examples are Osgood-Schlatter disease at the attachment of the patellar tendon to the tibial tuberosity and Sever's disease at the attachment of the Achilles tendon to the calcaneus. A full description of apophysitis is given in Chapter 40.

Articular cartilage

Overuse injury can affect the articular cartilage lining of joints, particularly in osteoarthritis. Changes range from microscopic inflammatory changes to softening, fibrillation, fissuring and ultimately to gross visible changes. In younger people, this pathology can arise at the patella (patellofemoral syndrome), but it is important to note that the pain of patellofemoral syndrome can occur in the presence of normal joint surfaces. This very common condition is discussed in Chapter 28.

Joint

Inflammatory changes in joints associated with overuse are classified as synovitis or capsulitis. Examples of these problems are the sinus tarsi syndrome of the subtalar joint and synovitis of the hip joint.

Ligament

Overuse injuries of ligaments are uncommon. The medial collateral ligament of the knee occasionally becomes inflamed, particularly in breaststroke swimmers.

Muscle

Focal tissue thickening/fibrosis

Repetitive microtrauma caused by overuse damages muscle fibers. This is thought by some to lead to development of adhesions between muscle fibers and the formation of cross-linkages in fascia (Fig. 2.14).

Clinically, these changes may be palpated as firm, focal areas of tissue thickening, taut, thickened bands arranged in the direction of the stress or as large areas of increased muscle tone and thickening.

These lesions may cause local pain or predispose other structures, such as tendons, to injury due to a reduction in the ability of the tissue to elongate under stretch or eccentric load. This will also compromise the ability of the affected muscle to contract and relax rapidly.

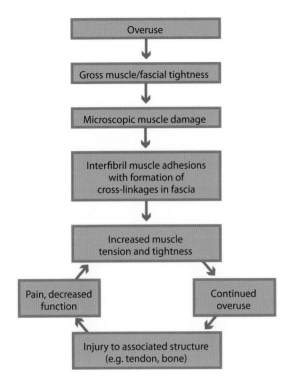

Figure 2.14 A theoretical model of the effect of overuse on muscle tissue

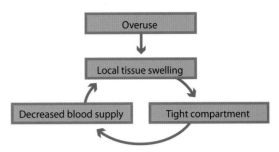

Figure 2.15 The development of increased muscle compartment pressure

These minor muscle injuries, which occur frequently in association with hard training, may respond to regular soft tissue therapy, strengthening and stretching (Chapter 10). Prevention of these injuries is discussed in Chapter 6.

Chronic compartment syndrome

Chronic compartment syndromes usually affect the lower leg but may also occur in the forearm. The muscles of the lower leg are divided into a number of compartments by fascial sheaths, which are relatively inelastic thickenings of collagenous tissue. Exercise raises the intracompartmental pressure and may cause local muscle swelling and accumulation of fluid in the interstitial spaces. The tight fascia prevents expansion. This impairs the blood supply and causes pain with exertion. A vicious cycle may occur (Fig. 2.15). Muscle hypertrophy may also be a precipitating factor in chronic compartment syndrome.

The main symptom of chronic compartment syndrome is pain that commences during activity and ceases with rest. This differs from other overuse injuries such as tendinopathies, where pain may be present with initial exercise, then diminish as the affected area warms up, only to return following cessation of activity. Compartment pressures may be measured both at rest and during pain-provoking exercise. Compartment pressure testing is described in Chapter 9.

Treatment of chronic compartment syndrome initially involves soft tissue therapy[15] and correction of biomechanical abnormalities where possible. If this fails, surgical treatment may be required—fasciotomy (release of the fascia) or fasciectomy (removal of the fascia).

Muscle soreness

Soreness accompanies muscle strains. A particular type of muscle soreness known as delayed onset muscle soreness (DOMS) develops 24–48 hours after unaccustomed physical activity. It appears to be more severe after eccentric exercise (involving muscle contraction while muscle is lengthening), such as downhill running.

The etiology of DOMS is unclear. Six theories have been proposed: lactic acid, muscle spasm, torn tissue, connective tissue, enzyme efflux and tissue fluid theories.[16] It is thought to occur less in those who train regularly, although even trained individuals may become sore after an unaccustomed exercise bout. Anti-inflammatory medication does not alleviate DOMS. Factors that appear to lessen DOMS include warm-down, post-event massage, active non-weight-bearing exercise, hydrotherapy and spa baths.

Tendon

Tendon injuries are among the most common overuse injuries.[17, 18] Tendons, which are made up of tight parallel collagen bundles, transmit forces from muscle to bone and are, therefore, subject to great tensile stresses. Tendons withstand strong tensile forces, resist shear forces less well and provide little resistance to compression force. The stress–strain curve for tendons is shown in Figure 2.16. As the strain increases, tissue

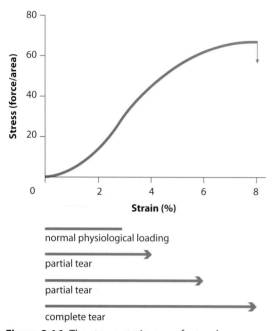

Figure 2.16 The stress–strain curve for tendons

deformation begins, some fibers begin to fail and ultimately macroscopic tendon failure occurs. There is, however, a large margin between the stresses that cause tendon failure and those that are experienced during normal physiological loading.

The vasculature of tendons is variable with the blood supply originating at both the musculotendinous and bone–tendon junctions. Vascular tendons are surrounded by a paratenon and avascular tendons are in sheaths. Tendon vascularity is compromised at sites of friction, torsion or compression.

Tendinosis

Collagen disarray and separation is the primary pathology in athletes who have undergone surgery for chronic tendinopathy of the rotator cuff, extensor carpi radialis brevis, patellar and Achilles tendons.[19] Histological examination of these tendons reveals separation of collagen bundles, increased hydrophilic ground substance, increased poor quality blood vessels (neovascularization) and absent inflammatory cells (Fig. 2.17). Other sites of tendinopathy that are likely to be due to tendinosis are the adductor longus, biceps, tibialis posterior and flexor hallucis longus tendons. It is uncertain whether tendinosis is preceded by acute inflammation. In animal models, acute inflammation lasts only five days after surgically induced tendon injury. Thus, even if inflammation precedes tendinosis, it is unlikely to be present for a

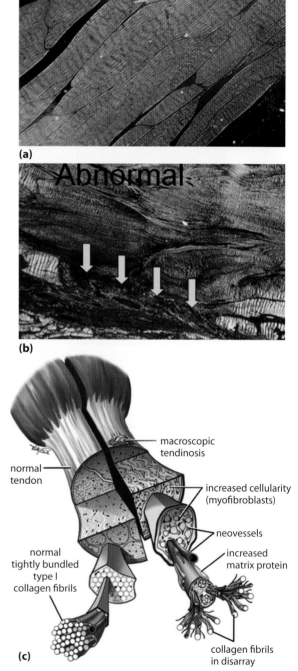

Figure 2.17 Tendon seen under polarized light microscopy. **(a)** Tightly bundled collagen of normal tendon compared with **(b)** collagen fibers in disarray. In three dimensions **(c)**, the tissue appears somewhat frayed; abnormal blood vessels are present in parts, and cells are abnormal in number (elevated in parts, absent in parts)

long period so clinicians should consider that they are treating the histopathological entity of tendinosis when they are confronted with a patient with overuse tendon pain (Table 2.7).

It would be ideal to grade tendinopathies but at present there is no reliable, widely accepted grading system that has been shown to provide useful guidance for treatment or prognosis. For patients with patellar tendinopathy or Achilles tendinopathy, we recommend the tendon-specific scoring systems called the VISA-P and VISA-A scores, respectively. These scoring system (range 0–100, see Chapters 28, 32) quantify the severity of symptoms and extent of loss of function.

Tendinosis often takes a long time to resolve, particularly if symptoms have been present for some months before presentation. The evidence-based treatments include exercise therapy (e.g. heel drops, partial squats, wrist exercises) and nitric oxide paste patches. There is emerging evidence for sclerosing therapy, a novel treatment (Chapter 10). Other commonly used treatments include relative rest, electrotherapeutic modalities and soft tissue therapy.[20, 21] Occasionally, tendinopathies do not respond to conservative management. Ultrasonography and MRI do not appear to predict which cases should be operated on,[22, 23] so the indication for surgery is clinical, based on failed conservative management. Tendon surgery may involve stripping of the paratenon, release of adhesions, removal of degenerative tissue, repair of a partial tear or excision of a torn flap. Overall, it appears that surgery relieves chronic tendon pain with 90% success or more, but only about 50–70%

Table 2.7 Clinical presentation of patients with overuse tendon pain (tendinosis)

- Pain some time after exercise or, more frequently, the following morning upon rising.
- Can be painful at rest and initially becomes less painful with use.
- Athletes can 'run through' the pain or the pain disappears when they warm up, only to return after exercise when they cool down.
- The athlete is able to continue to train fully in the early stages of the condition; this may interfere with the healing process.
- Examination, local tenderness and thickening.
- Frank swelling and crepitus may be present, although crepitus is more usually a sign of associated tenosynovitis or is due to the hydrophilic (water attracting) nature of the collagen disarray (it is not 'inflammatory fluid').

of patients who undergo tendon surgery return to sport at the previous level.

Tendinitis

Tendinitis refers to inflammation of the tendon itself and, despite the popularity of the diagnostic label, has rarely been proven to occur histologically. This may be because tissue is not obtained from tendons in humans who have only had tendon pain for a short time (days). Tendinitis may occur in association with paratendinitis. True inflammatory tendinitis may underpin the tendinopathies associated with the inflammatory arthritides.[24]

Paratenonitis

This term includes peritendinitis, tenosynovitis (single layer of areolar tissue covering the tendon) and tenovaginitis (double-layered tendon sheath). This is particularly likely to occur in situations where the tendon rubs over a bony prominence and directly irritates the paratenon. It is also seen in association with partial tears and tendinosis. Paratenonitis is also called tenosynovitis or tenovaginitis. A common example is de Quervain's tenosynovitis at the wrist. Clinically, it may be difficult to differentiate between tendinosis and paratenonitis. The principles of treatment are identical.

Partial tears

The term 'partial tear of a tendon' should be reserved for a macroscopically evident subcutaneous partial tear of a tendon, an uncommon acute, not overuse, injury, at least in the Achilles and patellar tendon.[25]

Bursa

The body contains many bursae situated usually between bony surfaces and overlying tendons. Their role is to facilitate movement of the tendon over the bony surface. Overuse injuries in bursae are quite common, particularly at the subacromial bursa, the greater trochanteric bursa, the bursa deep to the iliotibial band at the knee and the retrocalcaneal bursa separating the Achilles tendon from the calcaneus.

Bursitis is associated with local tenderness and swelling and pain on specific movements. Treatment involves the use of NSAIDs but this may be ineffective due to the poor blood supply of most bursae. Occasionally, a bursa needs to be drained of its fluid with or without subsequent corticosteroid infiltration.

Nerve

Nerve entrapment syndromes occur in athletes as a result of swelling in the surrounding soft tissues or anatomical abnormalities. These may affect the suprascapular nerve, the posterior interosseous, ulnar and median nerves in the forearm, the obturator nerve in the groin, the posterior tibial nerve at the tarsal tunnel on the medial aspect of the ankle and, most commonly, the interdigital nerves, especially between the third and fourth toes, a condition known as Morton's neuroma. This condition is not a true neuroma but rather a nerve compression. These nerve entrapments occasionally require surgical decompression.[26]

Chronic mild irritation of a nerve may result in damage manifested by an increase in neural tension. These may be the primary cause of the patient's symptoms or may contribute to symptoms. This concept is discussed more fully in Chapter 3.

Skin

Blisters may occur at any site of friction with an external source, such as shoes or sporting equipment. Foot blisters can be prevented by wearing-in new shoes, wearing socks, and smearing petroleum jelly over the sock at sites of friction. Strategies to prevent blisters also serve to prevent callus. Symptomatic callus can be pared down with a scalpel blade, taking care not to lacerate the normal skin.

At the first sign of a blister, the aggravating source should be removed and either adhesive tape applied over the blistered area or blister pads should be applied. Blister pads prevent blisters by acting as a barrier between skin and shoe. Treatment of blisters involves prevention of infection by the use of antiseptics and protection with sticking plaster. Fluid-filled blisters may be punctured and drained.

But it's not that simple …

While it is important to have a good understanding of the conditions outlined in this chapter, three important additional components are necessary for successful management of patients with musculoskeletal pain and sporting injuries.

Pain: where is it coming from?

The pain your patient feels at a particular site may not necessarily be emanating from that site. It is essential to understand the concept of referred pain, which is the topic of Chapter 3.

Masquerades

There are many medical conditions whose presentation may mimic a sporting injury. While many of these conditions are relatively rare, it is nevertheless important to keep them at the back of your mind. If the clinical pattern does not seem to fit the obvious diagnosis, then think of the conditions that may masquerade as sporting injuries. These are described in Chapter 4.

The kinetic chain

Every athletic activity involves movements of joints and limbs in coordinated ways to perform a task. These activities include running, jumping, throwing, stopping or kicking. The tasks may include throwing a ball, hitting a ball, kicking a ball, jumping over an object or propelling the body through air or water. Individual body segments and joints, collectively called links, must be moved in certain specific sequences to allow efficient accomplishment of the tasks.

The sequencing of the links is called the kinetic chain of an athletic activity.[27] Each kinetic chain has its own sequence but the basic organization includes proximal to distal sequencing, a proximal base of support or stability and successive activation of each segment of the link and each successive link. The net result is generation of force and energy in each link, summation of the developed force and energy through each of the links, and efficient transfer of the force and energy to the terminal link.

Injuries or adaptations in some areas of the kinetic chain can cause problems not only locally but distantly, as distal links must compensate for the lack of force and energy delivered through the more proximal links. This phenomenon, called catch-up, is both inefficient in the kinetic chain and dangerous to the distal link because it may cause more load or stress than the link can safely handle. These changes may result in anatomical or biomechanical situations that increase injury risk, perpetuate injury patterns or decrease performance. For example, a tennis player with stiffness of the lumbar spine may overload the rotator cuff muscles while serving in order to generate sufficient power and, thus, develop a tear of the rotator cuff muscles.

These deficits in the kinetic chain must be identified and corrected as part of the treatment and rehabilitation process. We will be constantly returning to the theme of the kinetic chain throughout the following chapters.

Recommended Reading

Bentley, S. Exercise-induced muscle cramp. Proposed mechanisms and management. *Sports Med* 1996; 21: 409–20.

Brukner P, Bennell K, Matheson G. *Stress Fractures.* Melbourne: Blackwell Scientific, Asia, 1999.

An easy-to-read, well-illustrated monograph that provides essential background for the clinician who commonly treats stress fractures.

Buckwalter, JA. Articular cartilage: injuries and potential for healing. *J Orthop Sports Phys Ther* 1998; 28: 192–202.

Coleman BD, Khan KM, Maffulli N, et al. Studies of surgical outcome after patellar tendinopathy: clinical significance of methodological deficiencies and guidelines for future studies. *Scand J Med Sci Sports* 2000; 10: 2–11.

A detailed outline of the limitations of surgical studies in tendinopathies that explains why the outcomes of tendon surgery cited in the literature may be overly optimistic.

Garrett WE Jr. Muscle strain injuries. *Am J Sports Med* 1996; 24: S2–S8.

Gulick DT, Kimura IF. Delayed onset muscle soreness: what is it and how do we treat it? *J Sport Rehab* 1996; 5: 234–43.

Józsa L, Kannus P. *Human Tendons.* Champaign, IL: Human Kinetics, 1997: 576.

This is the bible of books on tendons—a beautifully illustrated text that explains the anatomy, physiology and clinical aspects of tendinopathies. A must for the clinician interested in tendon conditions.

Kannus P. Tendon pathology: basic science and clinical applications. *Sports Exerc Injury* 1997; 3: 62–75.

Khan KM, Maffulli N. Tendinopathy: an Achilles' heel for athletes and clinicians. *Clin J Sport Med* 1998; 8: 151–4.

Khan K, McKay H, Kannus P, Bailey D, Wark J, Bennell K. *Physical Activity and Bone Health.* Champaign, IL: Human Kinetics, 2001.

Krivickas LS. Anatomical factors associated with overuse sports injuries. *Sports Med* 1997; 24: 132–46.

Mandelbaum BR, Browne JE, Fu F, et al. Articular cartilage lesions of the knee. *Am J Sports Med* 1998; 26: 853–61.

McCarthy P. Managing bursitis in the athlete: an overview. *Physician Sportsmed* 1989; 17(11): 115–25.

McCrory P, Bell S. Nerve entrapment syndromes as a cause of pain in the hip, groin and buttock. *Sports Med* 1999; 27: 261–74.

Neely FG. Intrinsic risk factors for exercise-related lower limb injuries. *Sports Med* 1998; 26: 253–63.

Neely FG. Biomechanical risk factors for exercise-related lower limb injuries. *Sports Med* 1998; 26: 395–413.

Newman AP. Articular cartilage repair. *Am J Sports Med* 1998; 26: 309–24.

Schwellnus MP, Derman EW, Noakes TW. Aetiology of skeletal muscle 'cramps' during exercise: a novel hypothesis. *J Sports Sci* 1997; 15: 277–85.

Walker JM. Pathomechanics and classification of cartilage lesions, facilitation of repair. *J Orthop Sports Phys Ther* 1998; 28(4): 216–27.

Wen DY, Puffer JC, Schmalzried TP. Injuries in runners: a prospective study of alignment. *Clin J Sport Med* 1998; 8: 187–94.

References

1. Engebretsen L, Arendt E, Fritts HM. Osteochondral lesions and cruciate ligament injuries. MRI in 18 knees. *Acta Orthop Scand* 1993; 64: 434–6.

2. Myklebust G, Bahr R. Return to play guidelines after anterior cruciate ligament surgery. *Br J Sports Med* 2005; 9(3): 127–31.

3. Buckwalter JA. Articular cartilage: injuries and potential for healing. *J Orthop Sports Phys Ther* 1998; 28: 192–202.

4. Frank CB. Ligament healing: current knowledge and clinical applications. *J Am Acad Orthop Surg* 1996; 4: 74–83.

5. Frank C, Shrive H, Hiraoka H, et al. Optimization of the biology of soft tissue repair. *J Sci Med Sport* 1999; 2: 190–210.

6. Schwellnus MP, Derman EW, Noakes TD. Aetiology of skeletal muscle cramps during exercise: a novel hypothesis. *J Sports Sci* 1997; 15: 277–85.

7. Schwellnus MP, Nicol J, Laubscher R, Noakes TD. Serum electrolyte concentrations and hydration status are not associated with exercise associated muscle cramping (EAMC) in distance runners. *Br J Sports Med* 2004; 38(4): 488–92.

8. Bentley S. Exercise-induced muscle cramp. Proposed mechanisms and management. *Sports Med* 1996; 21: 409–20.

9. Brukner P, Bennell K, Matheson G. *Stress Fractures.* Melbourne: Blackwell Scientific, Asia, 1999.

10. Brukner P, Bradshaw C, Khan KM, et al. Stress fractures: A review of 180 cases. *Clin J Sport Med* 1996; 6: 85–9.

11. Baquie P, Brukner P. Injuries presenting to an Australian sports medicine centre: a 12 month study. *Clin J Sport Med* 1997; 7: 28–31.

12. Khan KM, Fuller PJ, Brukner PD, et al. Outcome of conservative and surgical management of navicular stress fracture in athletes. Eighty-six cases proven with computerized tomography. *Am J Sports Med* 1992: 20(6): 657–66.

13. Matheson GO, Clement DB, McKenzie DC, et al. Scintigraphic uptake of 99mTc at non-painful sites in athletes with stress fractures. The concept of bone strain. *Sports Med* 1987; 4: 65–75.

14. Bennell KL, Malcolm SA, Thomas SA, et al. Risk factors for stress fractures in track and field athletes. A twelve-month prospective study. *Am J Sports Med* 1996; 24: 810–18.

15. Blackman PB, Simmons LR, Crossley KM. Treatment of chronic exertional anterior compartment syndrome with massage. A pilot study. *Clin J Sport Med* 1998; 8: 14–17.

16. Gulick DT, Kimura IF. Delayed onset muscle soreness: what is it and how do we treat it? *J Sport Rehab* 1996; 5: 234–43.

17. Kannus P. Tendons—a source of major concern in competitive and recreational athletes. *Scand J Med Sci Sports* 1997; 7: 53–4.

18. Józsa L, Kannus P. *Human Tendons*. Champaign, IL: Human Kinetics, 1997.

19. Khan KM, Cook JL, Bonar F, et al. Histopathology of common overuse tendon conditions: update and implications for clinical management. *Sports Med* 1999; 27: 393–408.

20. Alfredson H, Pietila T, Jonsson P, et al. Heavy-load eccentric calf muscle training for the treatment of chronic Achilles tendinosis. *Am J Sports Med* 1998; 26: 360–6.

21. Holmich P. Effectiveness of active physical training as treatment for long-standing adductor-related groin pain in athletes: randomised trial. *Lancet* 1999; 353: 439–53.

22. Cook JL, Khan KM, Harcourt PR, et al. Patellar tendon ultrasonography in asymptomatic active athletes reveals hypoechoic regions: a study of 320 tendons. *Clin J Sport Med* 1998; 8: 73–7.

23. Miniaci A, Dowdy PA, Willits KR, et al. Magnetic resonance imaging evaluation of the rotator cuff tendons in the asymptomatic shoulder. *Am J Sports Med* 1995; 23: 142–5.

24. Krishna Sayana M, Maffulli N. Insertional Achilles tendinopathy. *Foot Ankle Clin* 2005; 10: 309–20.

25. Maffulli N, Khan KM, Puddu G. Overuse tendon conditions. Time to change a confusing terminology. *Arthroscopy* 1998; 14: 840–3.

26. McCrory P, Bell S. Nerve entrapment syndromes as a cause of pain in the hip, groin and buttock. *Sports Med* 1999; 27: 261–74.

27. Kibler WB. Determining the extent of the functional deficit. In: Kibler WB, Herring SA, Press JM, eds. *Functional Rehabilitation of Sports and Musculoskeletal Injuries*. Gaithersburg, MD: Aspen Publishers, 1998: 16–19.

Pain: Where is it Coming From?

Just because a patient complains of pain at a certain site, it does not necessarily mean that site is the source of all, or even any, of the patient's pain. This is an essential concept for any clinician dealing with musculoskeletal pain.

Pain may be perceived via any of the pain-sensitive nerve endings that are present extensively throughout the body. These nerve endings, known as nociceptive nerve endings, are found within bone, cartilage, ligaments, muscle, tendon, fascia, bursa and neural structures. Stimulation of these nociceptive nerve endings will result in an individual perceiving pain. Nerve endings may be stimulated by chemicals such as potassium ions, histamine, 5-hydroxytryptophan, plasma kinins and prostaglandins released from damaged tissue. Nociceptors can also be stimulated by mechanical means.

In most cases of musculoskeletal injury, the nociceptive nerve endings of more than one structure are stimulated. The more severe the injury, the more likely that a greater number of structures will be damaged and contribute to the individual's pain. The longer the duration of the injury, the more likely that altered movement patterns and compensatory mechanisms will cause other structures to become damaged and painful. Therefore, the pain that the patient perceives and describes to the clinician is the sum total of all the stimulated pain-sensitive nerve endings.

The relative contribution of each structure to the overall perception of pain can be estimated from the clinical findings but can only be accurately assessed by the use of selective local anesthetic blocking techniques. Obviously this is not practical in a clinical setting. The other means of assessing the relative contribution to the perceived pain of the various structures is by treating each abnormality detected in these structures and assessing the effect on the total perceived pain.

Pain-producing structures

The three major groups of structures causing musculoskeletal pain are:

1. joints (including ligaments)
2. muscles (including tendons and fascia)
3. neural structures.

The pain perceived by the patient may arise from one of these groups or, more frequently, from two or three of the groups.

As an example, consider the patient who presents with low back pain. The initial incident may have involved a small tear of the outer part of the anulus fibrosus. Nociceptive nerve endings in the anulus may have been stimulated by the mechanical effect of the tear and by the chemicals released in the accompanying inflammatory process. In response to the localized pain and inflammation, there will be associated muscle spasm and possibly also direct chemical stimulation of nociceptive nerve endings in the muscles. As the pain and spasm persist, it is likely that small areas of fibrosis may develop within the muscle, further stimulating nociceptive nerve endings.

Because of the close proximity of the spinal cord and nerve roots to the primary site of injury, it is likely that neural structures such as the dura mater will also be stimulated, either by chemical or mechanical means, or both. As the pain and inflammation persist, local fibrosis, scarring and tethering may develop, resulting in further stimulation of the nociceptive nerve endings.

By the time the patient presents to the clinician there may be a contribution to the perceived pain from joint, muscle and neural structures. It is essential for the correct management of these conditions that each of these three elements is fully assessed and, if abnormalities are present, they are treated successfully. A major reason for unsuccessful treatment of musculoskeletal pain is a failure to recognize its multifactorial nature.

How does damage or abnormal function of joint, muscle and neural structures cause pain?

Joints

All joints within the body are richly innervated. These nerve endings may be stimulated chemically as a result of inflammation or mechanically as a result of stretch. Any abnormality of movement within a joint can result in stretching of the joint tissues and stimulation of nociceptive nerve endings. Examples of these abnormalities include hypomobility, hypermobility or abnormal quality of movement.

Abnormalities may occur either in physiological movements or accessory movements. Physiological movements are movements that patients can perform by themselves. However, in order to achieve a full range of physiological movement, it is necessary to have sufficient accessory movements.

Accessory movements are the involuntary, inter-articular movements, including glides, rotations and tilts, which occur in both spinal and peripheral joints during normal physiological movements. Loss of these normal accessory movements may cause pain, altered range or abnormal quality of movement. As all of these abnormal movements may produce pain, it is important to assess joints carefully and identify any abnormal movement during patient examination. Restoration of normal movement is an important part of the treatment of musculoskeletal injuries.

Muscle

Muscles, tendons and fascia are also richly supplied with nociceptive nerve endings. These structures may be damaged acutely (Chapter 2). They may also be damaged in association with other injuries. Muscle spasm occurs to protect underlying damaged tissue such as joints. If pain and inflammation from the joint injury persist, muscle spasm will also persist and the increase in muscle tension will lead to both chemical and mechanical stimulation of nociceptive nerve endings.

Chronic muscle tightness, abnormal movement or overuse may result in localized areas of muscle thickening that represent areas of inflammation and fibrosis. Lack of full pain-free motion will eventually cause stimulation of nociceptive nerve endings and pain. Successful treatment requires restoration of the full range of motion.

Palpation of these localized thickened areas within muscle tissue will usually reveal local tenderness. Occasionally, palpation of these areas will also produce pain referred in a characteristic pattern. These points are known as 'trigger points'.

Trigger points

Trigger points are present in all patients with chronic musculoskeletal pain. Travell and Simons have defined a trigger point as a discrete, focal, hyperirritable spot in a taut band of muscle.[1] The spots are painful on compression and can produce referred pain, referred tenderness, motor dysfunction, and autonomic phenomena. Trigger points are classified as being active or latent depending on their clinical characteristics.

An 'active' trigger point causes pain at rest. It is tender to palpation with a referred pain pattern that is similar to the patient's pain complaint. When stimulated, an active trigger point sets off a 'local twitch response' in the affected muscle. A local twitch response is defined as a transient visible or palpable contraction or dimpling of the muscle and skin. Evaluation of the electromyographic activity of the trigger point reveals unique, prolonged and rapid motor end-plate activity.[2]

A latent trigger point or 'tender point' is locally tender, does not refer pain and does not elicit a twitch response. Tender points may be associated with muscle tightness or weakness. Multiple tender points are present in fibromyalgia (see p. 32).

There are several proposed mechanisms to account for the development of trigger points and subsequent pain patterns, but scientific evidence is lacking. Both acute trauma and repetitive microtrauma may lead to the development of trigger points. Poor posture, sleep disturbance and anxiety may all predispose to their development.

Mense and Simons[3] proposed that a sensitization of nociceptors leads to local edema, venous congestion and ischemia. The ischemia interferes with normal energy (ATP) production, which leads to disturbance of the normal calcium pump activity, thus preventing actin and myosin filaments from releasing their contracted state. This is the hypothesized cause of the taut bands.

Patients with active trigger points present with persistent regional pain. It is usually related to activity although it can be constant. Occasionally it is worse at night and can interfere with sleep. It is frequently associated with muscle shortening and decreased range of motion. The most common areas affected, with the site of the trigger points in brackets, are the head and neck (upper trapezius, sternocleido-mastoid muscles), shoulder girdle (supraspinatus, infraspinatus), low back and pelvis (quadratus lumb-orum, gluteal muscles) and hamstring region (gluteal, piriformis).

Elimination of myofascial trigger points is an important component of the management of chronic musculoskeletal pain. Suggested methods of eliminat-ing trigger points include the cold and stretch tech-nique advocated by Travell and Simons,[1] application of various physical therapy modalities, soft tissue techniques such as myofascial release and ischemic pressure, and injections of local anesthetic or cortico-steroid. We have found ischemic pressure and dry needling to be the most effective (Chapter 10).

Neural structures

Injury to the structures of the nervous system may be the major source of the patient's perceived pain. More commonly, however, injury to neural structures accompanies joint or muscle injuries.[4, 5] Like the other structures, neural structures have nociceptive nerve endings that may be stimulated chemically by local inflammation from surrounding injured structures or mechanically, either by direct trauma or by acute or prolonged stretching. The most common example of mechanical nerve irritation is from nerve impinge-ment secondary to a prolapsed intervertebral disk or osteophyte. This impingement causes the classic radicular pain (see below).

Neural tension

Alteration to the mechanics of the nervous system, similarly to joints and muscles, may result in increased tension within the nervous system and, thus, pain. Butler[6] has shown that 'adverse tension' in the nervous system can impair its mobility and elasticity, and painful problems can arise as a result. He refers to the tissues that surround neural structures as the mechanical interface.

The assessment of neural mechanics and neural tension is an important component of the clinical examination. Neural provocation (or neural tension) tests assess the mobility of neural tissue in the extremi-ties and spinal canal. Positive adverse neural tension tests suggest poor mobility of neural tissue. Many factors cause hypomobility of neural tissue, includ-ing scar tissue, tight muscles, ectopic bone growth

and adhesions within nerves.[7] Ankle sprains[8] and hamstring strains,[9, 10] for example, have been shown to be associated with damage to neural tissues as well as muscle and ligamentous structures.

Tests to determine the presence of adverse neural tension are described in Chapter 8. They include the straight leg raise, slump test, neural Thomas test and the upper limb tension test. When the patient's pain is reproduced with increased tension and subsequently relieved when tension is decreased, abnormalities of neural structures are likely to be present.

Autonomic nervous system

While the central and peripheral nervous systems play an important role in pain production, the autonomic nervous system must not be overlooked. Autonomic fibers in the peripheral and central nervous system are also affected by abnormal neural mechanics and increased tension. The autonomic nervous system is particularly susceptible to abnormal mechanics where it is separate from the rest of the nervous system in the trunks, rami and ganglia. The sympa-thetic trunk, located just anterior to the mobile costo-vertebral joints, is particularly susceptible to damage. Involvement of the sympathetic trunk may explain the presence of unusual symptoms such as nausea, temperature changes and changes in the amount of sweating that may accompany pain. These can be affected by altering neural tension.

Referred pain

Pain is perceived by the patient as coming from a particular site. However, the patient's perception of the pain does not necessarily correspond to the source of the pain. Pain may indeed arise from a local struc-ture but, equally, it may be referred to that site from a structure some distance away. The best example of this concept occurs in amputees who perceive pain in their amputated limbs, known as 'phantom limb pain'. Another example occurs when pain is perceived in the neck or arm in patients with angina. An understanding of the concept of referred pain is vital for successful treatment of musculoskeletal pain.

Consider the following clinical presentations:

- A patient presents with a long history of intermittent, dull, occipital headache. The patient is thoroughly investigated for eye problems and the presence of intracranial pathology. All tests are normal.
- A patient presents with a history of an ache in the right shoulder that is difficult to localize and

is associated with pain on the medial aspect of the upper arm. There is some neck stiffness and tightness in the trapezius muscle.

- A 35-year-old executive complains of episodes of sharp, left-sided chest pain related to activity. The patient has already undergone extensive cardiological investigations that were all normal.
- A young athlete presents with a history of recurrent episodes of buttock and hamstring pain. There is no history of an acute tear and the patient describes the pain as deep-seated and dull with occasional sharp cramping in the hamstring. Examination of the hamstring shows some mild tenderness but full stretch and strength.

All of the above clinical presentations are common in sports medicine practise. All these patients are experiencing referred pain. Unless this is recognized, treatment will be unsuccessful.

It is important to remember that there is always a reason for pain. Because the pattern of pain does not fit a recognized diagnosis, it does not mean that the pain does not exist. It may mean that there is a lack of understanding by the clinician, rather than a problem being imagined by the patient. Obviously, many injuries are purely local problems, such as Achilles tendinopathy. Similarly, many problems are primarily referred, for example, dull hamstring ache. There is also a large group, probably the majority of patients with long-term pain, in which there is both a local and referred component. Unless both components are treated appropriately, the problem will not be resolved.

The concept of referred pain is not new. For many years clinicians have been familiar with a form of referred pain originating in the lumbar spine and shooting down the buttock and back of the leg. This was known as 'sciatica' and was attributed to nerve root compression, usually as a result of a herniated lumbar disk. For many years, any referred leg pain was thought to result from nerve root compression. However, nerve root compression is a relatively infrequent cause of leg pain referred from the lumbar spine.

Radicular pain

There are two types of referred pain. Radicular pain is the pain associated with nerve root compression and has the characteristic quality of sharp, shooting pain in a relatively narrow band. Radicular pain is caused by nerve root compression and must, therefore, be accompanied by other neurological abnormalities, for example, paresthesia corresponding to a dermatomal distribution or muscle weakness. Nerve root compression results in a fairly consistent pattern of pain distribution, known as a dermatome. These dermatomes are mapped out and used to determine the segmental level of the nerve root compression.

Somatic pain

The other type of referred pain is somatic pain. Somatic pain is pain perceived in one area that originates from another. Somatic referred pain may be from myofascial trigger points (see above) or from joints.

Pain perceived in the hamstring and buttock, for example, may arise from one of the pain-sensitive structures of the lumbar spine, such as the anulus fibrosus of the intervertebral disk or the apophyseal joint. Pain felt around the shoulder may originate from structures in the cervical spine.

The perception of pain at a point distant to the source of the pain is thought to be due to the brain misinterpreting the origin of a painful stimulus. For example, impulses from pain-sensitive structures in the lumbar spine may converge with impulses from the buttock or hamstring. The brain is, therefore, unable to distinguish between the two impulses. It is important to remember that it is possible to have pain at the site distant from the source without pain at the source itself. For example, lumbar spinal structures can be the source of pain in the hamstring region without causing low back pain.

Somatic pain is a static, dull ache that is hard to localize. It is not accompanied by neurological abnormalities. Thus, the possibility of referred somatic pain should be considered in any patient presenting with pain that is dull and poorly localized.

Local tenderness may occur even when the pain is referred from another source. However, the tenderness associated with referred pain will usually be considerably less than that found when pathology is local.

Pain referred from somatic structures, unlike radicular pain, does not have a consistent distribution. Fields of referred pain from particular segments overlap greatly, both in individuals and between individuals. Therefore, mapping of these areas of pain distribution (sclerotomes) should only be used as a guide.

Clinical assessment of referred pain

The possibility that some or all of the patient's pain may be referred from another source should be considered in all cases of musculoskeletal pain. Features of pain that suggest it is more likely to be referred include:

- a dull aching nature
- poorly localized
- deep-seated
- movement from point to point
- less local tenderness than expected
- longstanding pain
- a failure to respond to local treatment.

While it is not possible to map out distinct patterns of referred somatic pain, there are common sites of referred pain that tend to emanate from particular regions. These sites are shown in Table 3.1. The examination of any patient presenting with pain in one of these regions must include an examination of all possible sites of origin of the pain.

The aim of clinical assessment is to reproduce the referred pain by stressing the site of the source of the pain. This is achieved by local palpation if the

source is muscle, by passive or active joint movement (physiological or accessory) if the source is joint or by increasing neural tension if the source is neural. Inability to reproduce the referred pain does not necessarily exclude the diagnosis of referred pain.

Any significant abnormality of joints, muscle or neural structures at a site that is a possible source of the referred pain should be noted and considered a possible source of the patient's pain. The best means of confirming this is to treat the abnormality (e.g. restore full motion to the joint, eliminate active trigger points or restore normal neural tension) and then determine the effect on the pain. If the pain is modified or abolished, it is likely that the treated area was contributing significantly to the patient's pain.

Consider the example mentioned in the earlier part of this chapter of the patient presenting with low back pain with contributions from joint, muscle and neural structures. This patient later develops unilateral buttock and upper hamstring pain in addition to the low back pain. It is dull and aching in quality and poorly localized. On local examination, there is diffuse minimal local tenderness with good hamstring stretch and strength.

Assessment of possible sources of this patient's hamstring and buttock pain involves a neural tension test (the slump test) to assess the contribution of neural structures, palpation of the joints of the lumbar spine to assess the possible joint contribution and palpation of the paravertebral and gluteal muscles to assess the presence of active trigger points and taut bands. Any abnormalities found on assessment are then treated and the effect on the patient's symptoms and functional activity reviewed.

Table 3.1 Common sites of referred pain

Site of referred pain	Source of pain
Occipital headache	Upper cervical spine TrPs in upper trapezius, sternocleidomastoid
Shoulder	Lower cervical, upper thoracic spine TrPs in supraspinatus, infraspinatus
Lateral elbow	Lower cervical (C5–6), upper thoracic TrPs in forearm extensor muscles, supinator and triceps
Chest wall	Thoracic spine TrPs in pectoralis major, intercostal muscles
Sacroiliac region, loin, flank	Thoracolumbar junction (L4–5) TrPs in quadratus lumborum
Groin	Sacroiliac joint, thoracolumbar junction, upper lumbar spine TrPs in adductors, gluteal muscles
Buttock, hamstring	Lumbar spine, sacroiliac joint TrPs in gluteal muscles and piriformis
Lateral knee/thigh	Lumbar spine TrPs in tensor fascia lata, gluteus minimus

TrPs = trigger points.

Pain syndromes

The existence and definition of various pain syndromes has changed considerably in recent years. These syndromes include reflex sympathetic dystrophy, complex regional pain syndrome type 1, sympathetically maintained pain, sympathetically independent pain, causalgia, myofascial pain syndrome and fibromyalgia.

Complex regional pain syndrome type 1

For many years a syndrome of pain associated with unusual vasomotor (vascular-related) and sudomotor (sweat-related) features has been recognized and was until recently known as reflex sympathetic dystrophy (RSD). The International Association for the Study of Pain (IASP) has proposed the terminology 'complex regional pain syndrome' (CRPS) to replace the old terms RSD and causalgia.[11, 12]

CRPS type 1, formerly known as RSD, refers to a complex regional pain syndrome usually involving pain, swelling, stiffness and discoloration of an extremity that presents after trauma or disease. Typically in CRPS type 1, pain is out of proportion to the initial injury and is not attributable to a specific peripheral nerve injury. The pain associated with CRPS type 1 may be further divided into sympathetically maintained pain (SMP), in which pain is accompanied by signs of autonomic dysfunction and relieved by sympathetic blockade, and sympathetically independent pain (SIP), which is seen in treatment-resistant cases of CRPS type 1 suggesting some other neuropathic mechanism.

CRPS type 2, formerly known as causalgia, may present similarly to CRPS type 1 but it is differentiated by identification of a specific peripheral nerve injury. The ongoing pain usually exceeds the distribution of the injured nerve. It may also be associated with features of autonomic dysfunction.

CRPS type 1 occurs after trauma to either soft tissues, bone or nerves, or it may occur after surgery. It is unclear why a small proportion of those suffering these traumas go on to develop CRPS type 1. It may be that certain individuals have a genetic predisposition towards developing CRPS type 1.

A number of investigations, such as thermography, triple phase bone scan, quantitative sensory testing and sympathetic blockade, may help to confirm the diagnosis of CRPS type 1, but none has been shown to be reliable. These conditions are notoriously difficult to treat. The basis of treatment is an aggressive physiotherapy and exercise rehabilitation program. Patients must be encouraged to continue exercising in spite of their pain. Other treatments used with some success are drug treatments such as corticosteroids and tricyclic antidepressants, sympathetic blockade, continuous infusion of epidural opioids and local anesthetics, peripheral nerve stimulation, and spinal cord stimulation.[13]

Myofascial pain syndrome and fibromyalgia

Myofascial pain syndrome is a common local painful muscle disorder caused by myofascial trigger points (see above). Fibromyalgia is a generalized condition more common in females (4:1) and associated with the presence of multiple tender points. The features that differentiate the two conditions are shown in Table 3.2.

The American College of Rheumatology[14] introduced criteria for the diagnosis of fibromyalgia, which include a history of widespread pain that must be both above and below the waist and on both sides of the body, and the presence of at least 11 out of 18 designated tender points throughout the body. Fatigue, poor sleep and reduced muscle endurance are features of fibromyalgia. It is often associated with conditions such as irritable bowel syndrome, dysmenorrhea and a feeling of swollen joints.

Table 3.2 Differences between myofascial pain syndrome and fibromyalgia[15]

Feature	Myofascial pain syndrome	Fibromyalgia
Origin	Muscular	Systemic or central nervous system
Female:male ratio	1:1	4–9:1
Pain	Local or regional	Widespread, general
Tenderness	Focal	Widespread, most of body
Muscle palpation	Tense (taut bands)	Soft and doughy
Range of motion	Restricted stretch	Commonly hypermobile
Look for	Trigger points anywhere	Prescribed tender points
Response to trigger point treatment	Immediate	Delayed
Other	May also have fibromyalgia	Nearly all also have myofascial trigger points
	All myofascial trigger points are tender	Not all tender points are myofascial trigger points

Conclusion

Pain is often multifactorial in nature. The pain perceived by the patient may arise from a number of different structures, either locally or from some other point that may refer pain to the region perceived. Contributions to pain may be from joint, muscle and neural structures. Pain is usually associated with altered mechanics—commonly decreased but occasionally increased movement of these tissues. All abnormalities contributing to the patient's perceived pain require clinical assessment and treatment. Restoration of normal mechanics and full range of motion invariably leads to a significant reduction, if not complete resolution, of pain.

Recommended Reading

Alvarez DJ, Rockwell PG. Trigger points: diagnosis and management. *Am Fam Physician* 2002; 65(4): 653–60.

Bogduk N. *Clinical Anatomy of the Lumbar Spine and Sacrum.* 3rd edn. New York: Churchill Livingstone, 1997.

Brolinson PG, Sampson M. Pathophysiology of pain in sports. *Curr Sports Med Rep* 2003; 2: 310–14.

Butler D. *The Sensitive Nervous System.* Singapore: Noigroup Publications, 2000.

Chaitow L. *Modern Neuromuscular Techniques.* Singapore: Churchill Livingstone, 2003.

Gerwin RD. Myofascial pain and fibromyalgia: diagnosis and treatment. *J Back Musculoskel Rehabil* 1998; 11: 175–81.

Gerwin RD. Classification, epidemiology and natural history of myofascial pain syndrome. *Curr Pain Headache Rep* 2001; 5: 412–20.

Gunn C. *The Gunn Approach to the Treatment of Chronic Pain.* 2nd edn. New York: Churchill Livingstone, 1996.

Hall TM, Elvey RL. Nerve trunk pain: physical diagnosis and treatment. *Man Ther* 1999; 4(2): 63–73.

Hord E, Oaklander A. Complex regional pain syndrome: a review of evidence-supported treatment options. *Curr Pain Headache Rep* 2003; 7(3): 188–96.

Lew PC, Briggs CA. Relationship between the cervical component of the slump test and change in hamstring muscle tension. *Man Ther* 1997; 2: 98–105.

Starr M. Theory and practise of myofascial pain as both practicing clinician and patient. *J Back Musculoskel Rehabil* 1997; 8: 173–6.

Stephenson R. The complexity of pain: part 1. No pain without gain: the augmentation of nociception in the CNS. *Phys Ther Rev* 1999; 4: 105–16.

Travell JG, Simons DG. *Myofascial Pain and Dysfunction. The Trigger Point Manual.* Vol. 1. 2nd edn. Baltimore: Williams & Wilkins, 1998.

Travell JG, Simons DG. *Myofascial Pain and Dysfunction. The Trigger Point Manual.* Vol. 2. 2nd edn. Maryland: Williams & Wilkins, 1998.

Wheeler AH. Myofascial pain disorders: theory to therapy. *Drugs* 2004; 64(1): 45–62.

References

1. Travell JG, Simons DG. *Myofascial Pain and Dysfunction. The Trigger Point Manual.* Vol. 1. 2nd edn. Baltimore: Williams & Wilkins, 1998.

2. Gerwin RD. Myofascial pain and fibromyalgia: Diagnosis and treatment. *J Back Musculoskel Rehabil* 1998; 11: 175–81.

3. Mense S, Simons D. *Muscle Pain.* Philadelphia: Williams & Wilkins, 2001.

4. Greening J, Lynn B. Minor peripheral nerve injuries: an underestimated source of pain? *Man Ther* 1998; 3(4): 187–94.

5. Pahor S, Toppenberg R. An investigation of neural tissue involvement in ankle inversion sprains. *Man Ther* 1996; 1(4): 192–7.

6. Butler D. *Mobilisation of the Nervous System.* Singapore: Churchill Livingstone, 1991.

7. Gallant S. Assessing adverse neural tension in adults. *J Sport Rehabil* 1998; 9: 128–39.

8. Nitz A, Dobner JJ, Kersey D. Nerve injury and grade II and III ankle sprains. *Am J Sports Med* 1985; 13(3): 177–82.

9. Kornberg C, Lew P. The effect of stretching neural structures on grade one hamstring injuries. *J Orthop Sports Phys Ther* 1989; 10(12): 481–7.

10. Turl SE, George KP. Adverse neural tension: a factor in repetitive hamstring strain? *J Orthop Sports Phys Ther* 1998; 27(1): 16–21.

11. Merskey H, Bogduk N. *Classification of Chronic Pain: Description of Chronic Pain Syndromes and Definition of Pain Terms.* 2nd edn. Seattle: IASP Press, 1994.

12. Stanton-Hicks M, Janig W, Hassenbusch S, et al. Reflex sympathetic dystrophy: changing concepts and taxonomy. *Pain* 1995; 63: 127–33.

13. Hayek SM, Mekhail NA. Complex regional pain syndrome. *Physician Sportsmed* 2004; 32(5): 18–25.

14. Wolfe F, Smythe HA, Yunus MB, et al. The American College of Rheumatology 1990 criteria for the classification of fibromyalgia. *Arthritis Rheum* 1990; 33: 160–72.

15. Simons D. Understanding effective treatments of myofascial trigger points. *J Bodywork Movement Ther* 2002; 6: 81–8.

Beware: Conditions Masquerading as Sports Injuries

WITH NICK CARTER

Not every patient who presents to the sports medicine clinician has a sports-related condition. Sports medicine, like every branch of medicine, has its share of conditions that must not be missed but that may appear at first to be rather benign conditions. The aim of this chapter is to remind you that the patient with the minor 'calf strain' may, in fact, have a deep venous thrombosis, or that the young basketball player who has been labeled as having Osgood-Schlatter disease because of playing may actually have an osteosarcoma. The first part of the chapter outlines a clinical approach that should maximize your chances of recognizing a condition that is 'masquerading' as a sports-related condition. The second part of the chapter describes some of these conditions and illustrates how they can present in the sports medicine setting.

How to recognize a condition masquerading as a sports injury

The key to recognizing that everything is not as the first impression might suggest is to take a thorough history and perform a detailed physical examination. If the clinician has not recognized a masquerading condition from the history and examination, it is unlikely that he or she will order the appropriate investigations to make the diagnosis. For example, if a patient presents with tibial pain and it is, in fact, due to hypercalcemia secondary to lung cancer, a bone scan of the tibia looking for stress fracture will usually not help with the diagnosis, but a history of weight loss, occasional hemoptysis and associated abdominal pain may. In a basketball player with

shoulder pain, the history of associated arm tightness and the physical finding of prominent superficial veins are more important clues to axillary vein thrombosis than would be a gray-scale ultrasound scan looking for rotator cuff tendinopathy.

If there is something about the history and examination that does not fit the pattern of the common conditions, then consider alternative, less common conditions. To be able to make the diagnosis of a rare or non-musculoskeletal condition, you must ask yourself, 'Could this be a rare condition or unusual manifestation?' Then other options are entertained, and the appropriate diagnosis can be conceived. Thus, successful diagnosis of masquerading conditions requires recognition of a discrepancy between the patient's clinical features and the typical pattern that one is familiar with from clinical experience.

Conditions masquerading as sports injuries

Table 4.1 lists some of the conditions that may masquerade as sports medicine conditions. These are outlined below.

Bone and soft tissue tumors

Primary malignant tumors of bone and soft tissues are rare but when they occur it is most likely to be in the younger age group (second to third decade). Osteosarcomata can present at the distal or proximal end of long bones, more commonly in the lower limb, producing joint pain. Patients often recognize that pain is aggravated by activity and hence present to the sports medicine clinic. The pathological diagnosis of osteosarcoma is dependent on the detection of

Table 4.1 Conditions that may masquerade as sports medicine conditions

Bone and soft tissue tumors	Vascular disorders
Osteosarcoma Synovial sarcoma Synovial chondromatosis Pigmented villonodular synovitis Rhabdomyosarcoma Osteoid osteoma Ganglion cyst	Venous thrombosis (e.g. deep venous thrombosis, axillary vein thrombosis) Artery entrapment (e.g. popliteal artery entrapment) Peripheral vascular disease
Rheumatological conditions	**Genetic disorders**
Inflammatory monoarthritis Inflammatory polyarthritis Inflammatory low back pain (e.g. sacroiliitis) Enthesopathies (e.g. psoriatic, reactive arthritis)	Marfan's syndrome Hemochromatosis
	Granulomatous diseases
	Tuberculosis Sarcoidosis
Disorders of muscle	**Infection**
Dermatomyositis Polymyositis Muscular dystrophy	Osteomyelitis Septic arthritis Shingles
Endocrine disorders	**Regional pain syndromes**
Dysthyroidism Hypercalcemia Hypocalcemia Hyperparathyroidism Diabetes Cushing's syndrome Acromegaly	Complex regional pain syndrome type I Fibromyalgia/myofascial pain syndrome

tumor-producing bone and so an X-ray may reveal a moth-eaten appearance with new bone formation in the soft tissues and lifting of the periosteum (Codman's triangle, Fig. 4.1). In young patients, the differential diagnosis includes osteomyelitis. It is recommended that any child or adolescent with bone pain be X-rayed. Surgery is the preferred treatment.

Synovial sarcomata frequently involve the larger lower joints such as the knee and ankle. Patients present with pain, often at night or with activity, maybe with instability and swelling.

Trauma may result in hemorrhage into a rhabdomyosarcoma. In patients with hematomata that are slow to resolve or where the history of trauma does not fit with the clinical signs, the clinician should consider this alternative diagnosis.

Malignant tumors (e.g. of the breast, lung and prostate) may metastasize to bone. Patients may not recognize that a previously treated malignancy could be related to their limb pain. Breast carcinoma may also present as a frozen shoulder. An accurate history is, therefore, central to making an accurate diagnosis. Red flag signs for malignancy or infection include

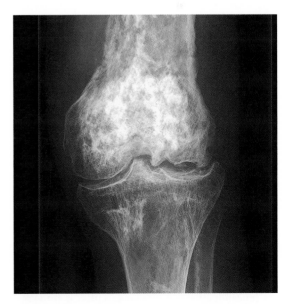

Figure 4.1 X-ray of an osteosarcoma in the distal femur of a 12-year-old boy presenting with knee pain with exercise

prominent night pain, often being woken at night with pain, fever, loss of appetite, weight loss and malaise. Patients exhibiting these symptoms should be examined and investigated thoroughly to determine the cause.

Synovial chondromatosis and pigmented villonodular synovitis are benign tumors of the synovium found mainly in the knee, which present with mechanical symptoms.

Osteoid osteoma (Fig. 4.2) is a benign bone tumor that often presents as exercise-related bone pain and tenderness and is, therefore, frequently misdiagnosed as a stress fracture. The bone scan appearance is also similar to that of a stress fracture, although the isotope uptake is more intense and widespread. This condition is characterized clinically by the presence of night pain and by the abolition of symptoms with the use of aspirin. The tumor has a characteristic appearance on CT scan (Fig. 4.2b) with a central nidus.

Ganglion cysts are lined by connective tissue, contain mucinous fluid and are found mainly around the wrist, hand, knee and foot (see also p. 323). They may be attached to a joint capsule or tendon sheath and may have a connection to the synovial cavity. They are usually asymptomatic but can occasionally cause pain and cosmetic deformity.[1]

Rheumatological conditions

These are dealt with in greater detail in the section on multiple joint problems (Chapter 50). Patients with inflammatory musculoskeletal disorders frequently present to the sports medicine clinic with a masquerading traumatic or mechanical condition. Low back pain of ankylosing spondylitis, psoriatic enthesopathy or early rheumatoid arthritis are common examples.

In patients presenting with an acutely swollen knee without a history of precipitant trauma or patellar tendinopathy without overuse, the clinician may be alerted to the possibility that these are inflammatory in origin. Prominent morning joint or back stiffness, night pain or extra-articular manifestations of rheumatological conditions (e.g. skin rashes, nail abnormalities, Fig. 4.3), bowel disturbance, eye involvement (conjunctivitis, iritis) or urethral discharge may all provide clues.

Inflammation of entheses (e.g. in lateral epicondylitis, patellar tendinopathy (Fig. 4.4), insertional Achilles tendinopathy and plantar fasciitis) is universal among those with HLA (human leukocyte antigens) B27-related, seronegative (for rheumatoid factor) arthropathies. Enthesopathy is usually associated

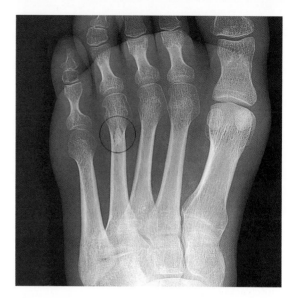

Figure 4.2 Osteoid osteoma

(a) X-ray of an osteoid osteoma

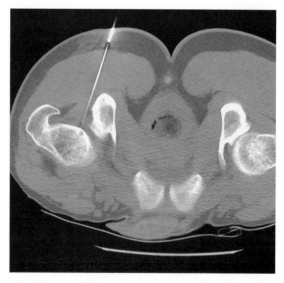

(b) CT scan of an osteoid osteoma about to undergo radioablation therapy

with other joint or extra-articular involvement, although a subgroup exists with enthesitis as the sole presentation.[2]

Disorders of muscle

Dermatomyositis and polymyositis are inflammatory connective tissue disorders characterized by proximal limb girdle weakness, often without

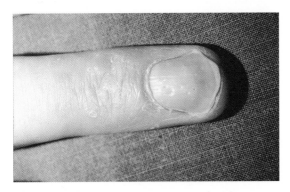

Figure 4.3 Typical pitted appearance of nails in a patient with psoriatic arthropathy

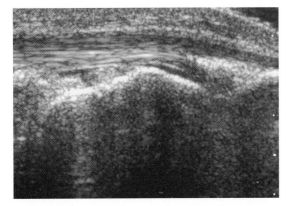

Figure 4.4 Calcific patellar tendinopathy in psoriatic arthropathy

pain. Dermatomyositis, unlike polymyositis, is also associated with a photosensitive skin rash in light-exposed areas (hands and face). In the older adult, dermatomyositis may be associated with malignancy in approximately 50% of cases. The primary malignancy may be easily detectable or occult. In the younger adult, weakness may be profound (e.g. unable to rise from the floor) but in the early stages may manifest only as under-performance in training or competition.

Dermatomyositis and polymyositis may also be associated with other connective tissue disorders such as systemic lupus erythematosus or systemic sclerosis, and muscle abnormality is characterized by elevated creatine kinase levels and electromyographic (EMG) and muscle biopsy changes.

Regional dystrophies such as limb girdle dystrophy and facio-scapulo-humeral dystrophy may also present with proximal limb girdle weakness in young adults. They are also associated with characteristic EMG changes.

Endocrine disorders

Several endocrine disorders, for example, hypothyroidism and hyperparathyroidism, may be associated with the deposition of calcium pyrophosphate in joints.[3] Patients may develop acute pseudogout or a polyarticular inflammatory arthritis resembling rheumatoid arthritis. X-rays of the wrists or knees may demonstrate chondrocalcinosis of the menisci or triangular fibrocartilage complex (Fig. 4.5).

Adhesive capsulitis or septic arthritis may be the presenting complaint in patients with diabetes mellitus and those with other endocrine disorders such as acromegaly may develop premature osteoarthritis or carpal tunnel syndrome. Patients with hypercalcemia secondary to malignancy (e.g. of the lung) or other conditions such as hyperparathyroidism can present with bone pain as well as constipation, confusion and renal calculi. A proximal myopathy may develop in patients with primary Cushing's syndrome or after corticosteroid use.

Vascular disorders

Patients with venous thrombosis or arterial abnormalities (Fig. 4.6) may present with limb pain and swelling aggravated by exercise. Calf, femoral or axillary veins are common sites for thrombosis. While a precipitant cause may be apparent (e.g. recent surgery or air travel), consider also the thrombophilias such as the antiphospholipid syndrome or deficiencies of protein C, protein S, antithrombin III or factor V Leiden.

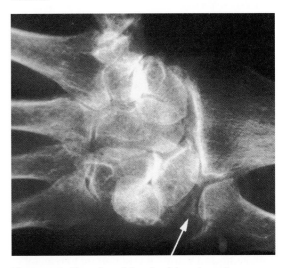

Figure 4.5 Chondrocalcinosis of the triangular fibrocartilage in calcium pyrophosphate dihydrate deposition disease

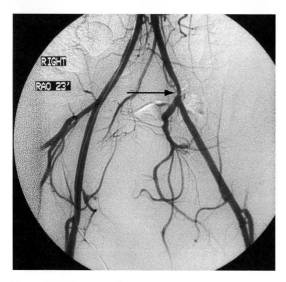

Figure 4.6 Common iliac artery stenosis

The claudicant pain of peripheral vascular disease is most likely to be first noticed with exercise and so patients may present to the sports medicine practitioner. Remember also that arteriopathy can occur in patients with diabetes. Various specific vascular entrapments are also found, such as popliteal artery entrapment, which presents as exercise-related calf pain, and thoracic outlet syndrome.

Genetic disorders

Marfan's syndrome is an autosomal dominant disorder of fibrillin characterized by musculoskeletal, cardiac and ocular abnormalities.[4] Musculoskeletal problems are common due to joint hypermobility, ligament laxity, scoliosis or spondylolysis. In patients with the Marfanoid habitus, referral for echocardiography and ophthalmological opinion should be considered as sudden cardiac death (Chapter 45) or lens dislocation may result.

Hemochromatosis is an autosomal recessive disorder of iron handling, which results in iron overload. Patients may present with a calcium pyrophosphate arthropathy with characteristic involvement of the second and third metacarpophalangeal joints and hook-shaped osteophytes seen on X-ray of these joints. While ferritin levels are raised in patients with hemochromatosis, it is important to remember that ferritin is also an acute-phase protein and so levels can be elevated in response to inflammatory arthropathy.

Granulomatous diseases

Tuberculosis is a granulomatous mycobacterial infection. Musculoskeletal involvement includes chronic septic arthritis and Pott's spine fracture.

Patients with acute sarcoidosis can present with fevers, lower limb (commonly) rash and ankle swelling. The rash of erythema nodosum (Fig. 4.7) may be mistaken for cellulitis and antibiotics have frequently been prescribed in error. The diagnosis is easily made by chest X-ray, which shows changes of bilateral hilar lymphadenopathy. The clinician should remember that the differential diagnosis of bilateral hilar lymphadenopathy includes tuberculosis and lymphoma. Chronic sarcoidosis is a systemic disorder involving the lungs, central nervous system, skin, eyes and musculoskeletal system. Patients can present with chronic arthropathy together with bone cysts or with bone pain due to hypercalcemia.

Infection

Bone and joint infections, while uncommon, may have disastrous consequences if the diagnosis is missed. Bone pain in children, worse at night or with activity, should alert the clinician to the possibility of osteomyelitis. Bone infection near a joint may result in a reactive joint effusion.

Septic arthritis is rare in the normal joint. In arthritic, recently arthrocentesed or diabetic joints, sepsis is much more common. Rapid joint destruction may follow if left untreated.

Even though *Staphylococcus aureus* is the causative organism in more than 50% of cases of acute septic joints, it is imperative that joint aspiration for Gram stain and culture and blood cultures are taken before commencement of antibiotic treatment. Once-only or repeated joint lavage may be considered in

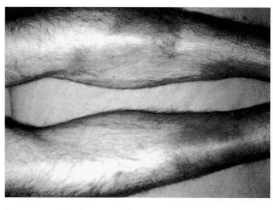

Figure 4.7 Erythema nodosum in acute sarcoidosis

patients receiving intravenous antibiotic treatment. The immunocompromised patient may present with a chronic septic arthritis. In this situation, tuberculosis or fungal infections should be considered.[5]

Regional pain syndromes

Complex regional pain syndrome type 1 (formerly known as reflex sympathetic dystrophy [RSD]), is a post-traumatic phenomenon characterized by localized pain out of proportion to the injury, vasomotor disturbances, edema and delayed recovery from injury. The vasomotor disturbances of an extremity manifest as vasodilatation (warmth, redness) or vasoconstriction (coolness, cyanosis, mottling). Early mobilization and avoidance of surgery are two important keys to successful management.[6]

Myofascial pain syndromes develop secondary to either acute or overuse trauma. They present as regional pain associated with the presence of one or more active trigger points (Chapter 3).

Fibromyalgia is a chronic pain syndrome characterized by widespread pain, chronic fatigue, decreased pain threshold, sleep disturbance, psychological stress and diffusely tender muscles. It is often associated with other symptoms, including irritable bowel syndrome, dyspareunia, headache, irritable bladder and subjective joint swelling and pain. Fibromyalgia is diagnosed on the examination finding of 11 of 18 specific tender point sites in a patient with widespread pain. Current treatment evidence is for a stepwise program emphasizing education, certain medications, exercise and cognitive therapy.[7] Chronic fatigue syndrome has many similarities to fibromyalgia[8] and may be the same disease process. It may present as excessive post-exercise muscle soreness but is always associated with excessive fatigue. Behavioral therapy and graded exercise therapy have shown promise as treatment.[8]

Recommended Reading

Abraham P, Bouye P, Quere I, Chevalier JM, Saumet JL. Past, present and future of arterial endofibrosis in athletes: a point of view. *Sports Med* 2004; 34(7): 419–25.

Biegle E, Lecocq J. Pseudotumoral osteochondromatosis of the hip in a soccer player. *Joint Bone Spine* 2000; 67(4): 331–3.

Echlin PS, Klein WB. Pancreatic injury in the athlete. *Curr Sports Med Rep* 2005; 4(2): 96–101.

Farrar KL, Gardiner L. Unresolving hip tendonitis leads to discovery of malignant tumor. *J Manipulative Physiol Ther* 2003; 26(3): 207.

Keisler BD, Armsey TD 2nd. Paget-Schroetter syndrome in an overhead athlete. *Curr Sports Med Rep* 2005; 4(4): 217–19.

Moses FM. Exercise-associated intestinal ischemia. *Curr Sports Med Rep* 2005; 4(2): 91–5.

Pogliacomi F, Vaienti E. Misdiagnosed juxta-articular osteoid osteoma of the calcaneus following an injury. *Acta Biomed Ateneo Parmense* 2003; 74(3): 144–50.

Wong CK, Restel BH. Unusual cause of knee pain mimicking meniscal pathology in a 14-year-old baseball player. *Clin J Sport Med* 2000; 10(2): 146–7.

References

1. Dallari D, Pellacani A, Marinelli A, Verni E, Giunti A. Deep peroneal nerve paresis in a runner caused by ganglion at capitulum peronei. Case report and review of the literature. *J Sports Med Phys Fitness* 2004; 44(4): 436–40.

2. Ozcakar L, Cetin A, Inanici F, et al. Ultrasonographical evaluation of the Achilles' tendon in psoriasis patients. *Int J Dermatol* 2005; 44(11): 930–2.

3. Canhao H, Fonseca JE, Leandro MJ, et al. Cross-sectional study of 50 patients with calcium pyrophosphate dihydrate crystal arthropathy. *Clin Rheumatol* 2001; 20(2): 119–22.

4. Maron BJ, Chaitman BR, Ackerman MJ, et al. Recommendations for physical activity and recreational sports participation for young patients with genetic cardiovascular diseases. *Circulation* 2004; 109(22): 2807–16.

5. Rollot K, Albert JD, Werner S, et al. *Campylobacter fetus* septic arthritis revealing a malignancy. *Joint Bone Spine* 2004; 71(1): 63–5.

6. Merritt WH. The challenge to manage reflex sympathetic dystrophy/complex regional pain syndrome. *Clin Plast Surg* 2005; 32(4): 575–604, vii–viii.

7. Goldenberg DL, Burckhardt C, Crofford L. Management of fibromyalgia syndrome. *JAMA* 2004; 292(19): 2388–95.

8. Whiting P, Bagnall AM, Sowden AJ, et al. Interventions for the treatment and management of chronic fatigue syndrome: a systematic review. *JAMA* 2001; 286(11): 1360–8.

Biomechanics of Common Sporting Injuries

WITH JASON AGOSTA

The term biomechanics can be used in a variety of ways. Most simply, biomechanics can be considered the evaluation of sporting technique (e.g. running biomechanics, swim stroke biomechanics) and this is how the term is often used in clinical circles. As this book is aimed at clinicians, we use the term in that way also. In the scientific world, the way we use the term biomechanics in this book would be referred to as 'subjective biomechanical analysis'. That is, we are describing movement such as walking, running or the tennis serve as it appears to direct observation.

The aim of this chapter is to provide clinically relevant and easily applicable descriptions of the common sporting techniques so that the clinician can better evaluate the sporting patient. It is becoming increasingly obvious that correct biomechanics plays a key role in both performance and injury prevention. For example, the javelin thrower with incorrect biomechanics will not only have a shorter throw than he or she could have but is also more prone to injury. In this chapter we explain how the thrower's injury may occur at the shoulder or elbow and, because of the interdependence of body parts in biomechanics, injury may also occur in the low back or lower limb.

Thus, an understanding of the biomechanics of different sporting activities is a vital foundation for the sports medicine practitioner—in the same way that an understanding of anatomy provides an important foundation for the surgeon. Once the practitioner understands normal sporting biomechanics, he or she is in a position to apply injury prevention strategies (Chapter 6).

Correct biomechanics

Correct biomechanics provides efficient movement and is likely to reduce injury risk. Abnormal biomechanics should always be considered as a potential cause of a non-traumatic sporting injury. Faulty biomechanics may result from static (anatomical) abnormalities or functional (secondary) abnormalities.

Static abnormalities such as leg length discrepancies or genu valgum cannot be altered. However, the secondary effects of these abnormalities can be minimized by compensatory devices such as a shoe build-up in the case of leg length discrepancy or an orthosis in the case of genu valgum.

Functional abnormalities may occur following injury or because of poor technique. For example, a ligament sprain may result in joint laxity, while a lengthy period of immobilization may lead to muscle imbalance.

Poor technique can cause abnormal biomechanics and contribute to subsequent injury.[1] Running with excessive anterior pelvic tilt and lumbar lordosis may result in hamstring strain, poor throwing technique may lead to the development of shoulder instability, and faulty backhand drive technique in tennis may cause extensor tendinopathy at the elbow. A list of technique faults and possible associated injuries is shown in Table 5.1.

Throughout this section, references will be made to the different planes of motion. These are shown in Figure 5.1.

The chapter first outlines normal and abnormal lower limb biomechanics before discussing biomechanics of various largely upper limb activities.

Table 5.1 Relationship of technique faults to injury

Sport	Technique	Injury
Tennis	Excessive wrist action with backhand Service contact made too far back (i.e. ball toss not in front)	Extensor tendinopathy of elbow Flexor tendinopathy of elbow
Swimming	Insufficient body roll Low elbow on recovery Insufficient external rotation of the shoulder	Rotator cuff tendinopathy
Diving	Shooting at the water too early (backward dives)	Lumbar spine injuries
Cycling	Incorrect handlebar and seat height Toe-in/toe-out on cleats	Thoracic/lumbar spine injuries Iliotibial band/patellofemoral syndrome
Weightlifting (Olympic)	Bar position too far in front of body in clean phase/jerk phase	Lumbar spine injuries Sacroiliac joint injury
Weightlifting (power lifting)	Grip too wide on bar in bench press Toes pointing forward on squatting	Pectoralis major tendinopathy Patellofemoral syndrome/medial meniscus injury
Javelin	Elbow 'dropped' Poor hip drive	Medial elbow pain Thoracic/lumbar spine dysfunction
Triple jump	'Blocking' on step phase	Sacroiliac/lumbar spine injuries, patellar tendinopathy, sinus tarsi syndrome
High jump	Incorrect foot plant	Patellar tendinopathy Sinus tarsi syndrome Fibular stress fracture
Pole vault	Too close on take-off Late plant	Lumbar spine injuries (e.g. spondylolysis) Ankle impingement Talar stress fracture Shoulder impingement
Running	Anterior pelvic tilt Poor lateral pelvic control	Hamstring injuries Iliotibial band friction syndrome
Cricket bowling	Mixed side-on/front-on action	Stress fracture pars interarticularis
Baseball pitching	Opening up too soon Dropped elbow 'hanging'	Anterior shoulder instability Medial collateral ligament sprains elbow Osteochondritis radiocapitellar joint Rotator cuff tendinopathy
Gymnastics	Excessive hyperextension on landing Tumble too short (not enough rotation)	Stress fracture pars interarticularis Anterior ankle impingement
Rowing	Change from bow side to stroke side	Stress fracture ribs
Ballet	Poor turnout 'Sickling' en pointe	Hip injuries Medial knee pain Stress fracture second metatarsal

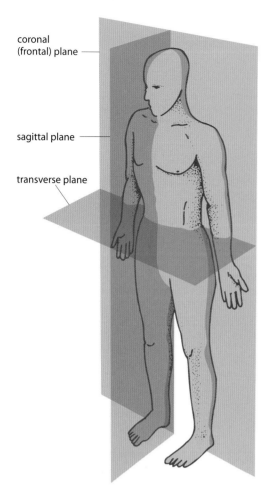

coronal
(frontal) plane

sagittal plane

transverse plane

Figure 5.1 Anatomical planes of the body

Lower limb biomechanics

An understanding of ideal lower limb biomechanics is essential to allow detection of excessive motion and asymmetrical mechanics.[2] The ideal stance position will be considered first, followed by the ideal position and range of motion of the joints of the lower extremity. The biomechanics of walking and running will also be considered. The clinician should always be aware that each individual has his or her own mechanical make-up due to structural characteristics and may never assume an ideal position.

Stance position

With the patient standing, the stance position may be examined. Ideal stance occurs when the joints of the lower limbs and feet are symmetrically aligned,

with the weight-bearing line passing through the anterior superior iliac spine, the patella and the second metatarsal (Fig. 5.2).

When the feet are in a symmetrical position, the subtalar (talocalcaneal) joint is neither pronated nor supinated and the midtarsal joint (talonavicular and calcaneocuboid joints) is maximally pronated. In the neutral foot, the forefoot is perpendicular to the bisection of the heel (Fig. 5.3), the ankle joint is neither plantarflexed nor dorsiflexed, the tibia is perpendicular to the supporting surface and the knee is fully extended. The hips are in neutral position (neither internally nor externally rotated, neither flexed nor extended). When the feet are in neutral position, both anterior superior iliac spines of the pelvis are level. A slight anterior tilt of the pelvis is normal.

Range of motion of joints in neutral position

The normal range of motion at the hip includes 120° flexion, 20° of extension in the sagittal plane, 40° abduction and 25° adduction in the frontal plane, and 45° internal rotation and 45° external rotation in the transverse plane. There should be no change in the degree of rotation of the hip with hip flexion or extension.

The ideal range of motion at the knee in the sagittal plane is approximately 135° flexion from a fully

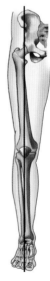

Figure 5.2 The alignment of the lower limb in neutral position. The weight-bearing line runs through the anterior superior iliac spine, patella and second metatarsal. The calcaneus is in line with the tibia and the forefoot is perpendicular to the calcaneus

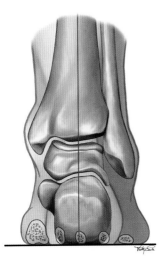

Figure 5.3 Normal relationship between the forefoot and rear foot when the foot is in neutral

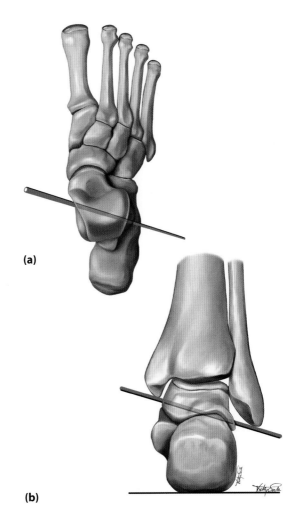

(a)

(b)

Figure 5.4 Axis of motion of ankle joint

(a) Superior view
(b) Posterior view

extended position. The knee is in a neutral position when fully extended. Normally, no hyperextension or frontal plane motion exists. The position of the knee in the frontal plane is often dictated by the angle between the neck and the shaft of the femur. No transverse plane movement occurs at the fully extended knee but up to 45° of transverse movement is available when the knee is flexed at 70°.

The normal range of motion of the ankle is approximately 45° of plantarflexion and 10–20° of dorsiflexion.[3] The ankle joint is in neutral position when the foot is perpendicular to the leg. There is normally very little transverse or frontal plane motion at the ankle joint, however, abduction of the foot occurs with dorsiflexion and adduction with plantarflexion. The minimum range of ankle dorsiflexion required for normal locomotion is 10–20°. The axis of motion of the ankle joint is shown in Figure 5.4.

Subtalar joint motion permits pronation and supination. Pronation consists of eversion, dorsiflexion and abduction of the foot. Supination consists of inversion, plantarflexion and adduction of the foot. The calcaneus will invert and evert with subtalar joint motion. The calcaneal inversion represents subtalar joint supination and pronation. The amount of inversion is usually twice that of eversion, approximately 20° inversion compared with 10° eversion (Fig. 5.5).

The midtarsal joint consists of two joints, the calcaneocuboid joint and the talonavicular joint. The midtarsal joint has two axes of motion, the oblique and the longitudinal axis. The oblique axis allows a large range of motion to occur, including dorsiflexion

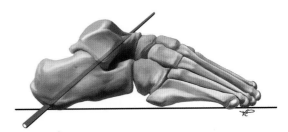

Figure 5.5 Axis of motion of subtalar joint

(a) Lateral view. Angle of inclination approximately 50° to transverse plane

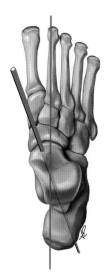

(b) Superior view. Angle between axis of motion of subtalar joint and longitudinal axis of the rear foot is approximately 15°

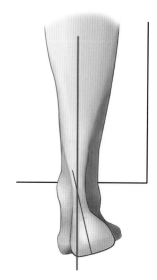

(d) Pronation at subtalar joint with 10° calcaneal inversion

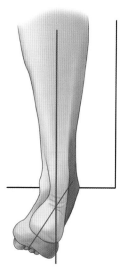

(c) Supination at subtalar joint with 20° calcaneal inversion

and abduction (with pronation), and plantarflexion and adduction (with supination). For every 1° of abduction there is 1° of dorsiflexion and for every 1° of adduction there is 1° of plantarflexion. The longitudinal axis has a small range of motion that consists of inversion and eversion of the forefoot (Fig. 5.6).

The range of motion of the midtarsal joint is dependent upon the subtalar joint. Pronation of the subtalar joint increases the range of motion of the midtarsal joint, whereas supination of the subtalar joint decreases midtarsal joint range of motion.

The first ray of the foot consists of the first metatarsal and the first (or medial) cuneiform bones. Dorsiflexion of the first ray is associated with an equal amount of inversion. Plantarflexion is accompanied by an equal amount of eversion. There should be equal amounts of both movements (dorsiflexion/inversion and plantarflexion/eversion) (Fig. 5.7).

The second ray consists of the second metatarsal and second (intermediate) cuneiform bones. The third ray consists of the third metatarsal and the third (lateral) cuneiform, while the fourth ray consists of the fourth metatarsal alone. Each of these rays exhibits plantarflexion and dorsiflexion only.

The fifth ray consists of the fifth metatarsal only. It exhibits equal amounts of plantarflexion and dorsiflexion with supination and pronation respectively. The neutral position is at the midpoint of the total range of motion of the fifth ray (Fig. 5.8).

The first metatarsophalangeal joint is the articulation between the head of the first metatarsal and the proximal phalanx. The most important motion at the first metatarsophalangeal joint is dorsiflexion. Dorsiflexion is necessary for toe-off and optimal function of the windlass mechanism during the gait cycle. The windlass mechanism is the direct relationship between the arch rising and the toe extending. With heel lift the toes are passively extended due to pressure against the ground. The normal range is approximately 65° (Fig. 5.9).

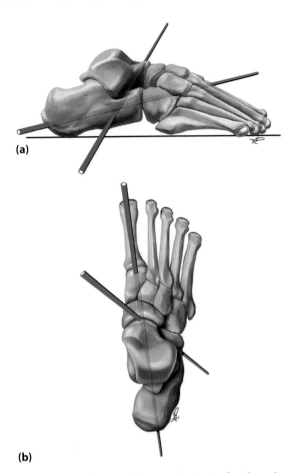

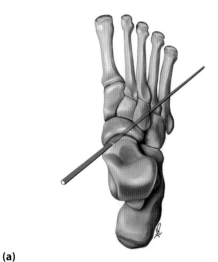

(a)

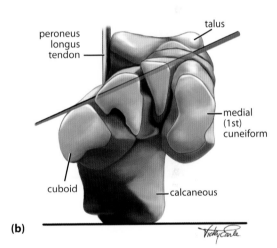

peroneus
longus
tendon

talus

medial
(1st)
cuneiform

cuboid

calcaneous

(b)

Figure 5.6 Oblique and longitudinal axis of midtarsal joint

(a) Lateral view
(b) Superior view

Figure 5.7 First ray axis of motion

(a) Superior view
(b) Anterior view

Biomechanics of walking

During normal walking, the gait cycle is divided into stance and swing phases.[4] One full gait cycle is the time from heel strike of one foot to the next heel strike of the same foot (Fig. 5.10).

The stance phase is divided into contact, midstance and propulsive phases. The stance phase begins and ends with the period where both feet are in contact with the ground. During this period the support of the body is being transferred from one foot to the other. This is known as the double support phase. The swing phase is divided into follow-through, forward swing and foot descent phases. The foot is in stance phase for 60% and in swing phase for 40% of the duration of each gait cycle.

Joint motion during walking

Movements of the pelvis occur during walking and are considered in three planes—sagittal, frontal and transverse. Posterior tilting of the pelvis occurs during the double support phase. Anterior tilting of the pelvis occurs during the single support phase of walking (Fig. 5.11). Sagittal plane motion increases with increased walking speed and the amount of motion appears to vary among individuals.

In the frontal plane, the pelvis tilts downward ('lateral tilting') on the non-weight-bearing limb side during the single support phase. Lateral tilting occurs

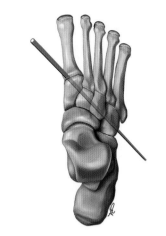

(a)

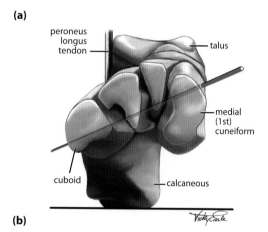

peroneus longus tendon

talus

medial (1st) cuneiform

cuboid

calcaneous

(b)

Figure 5.8 Fifth ray axis of motion

(a) Superior view
(b) Anterior view

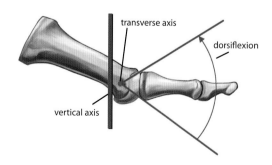

transverse axis

dorsiflexion

vertical axis

Figure 5.9 Motion of the hallux around the transverse axis of the first metatarsophalangeal joint

during the early stance phase as the body passes over the supporting limb.

Rotation of the pelvis also occurs in the transverse plane. This transverse rotation occurs at each hip joint and serves to reduce the fall in the center of gravity during the double support phase. Angular displacement during hip flexion and extension is also reduced.

The hip joint is flexed at heel contact and extends during midstance and toe-off. It is internally rotated during contact. During propulsion the hip extends and externally rotates in both the midstance and propulsive phases.

In the contact period, the knee flexes approximately 15° and the tibia internally rotates. The knee then extends from midstance until heel lift. The tibia externally rotates during midstance and propulsion. The knee flexes again throughout the propulsive period.

The ankle joint plantarflexes from heel contact to forefoot contact. The body and the lower limb then move forward, causing dorsiflexion at the ankle during the midstance period. Plantarflexion occurs again from heel lift to toe-off.

The subtalar joint is slightly supinated at heel strike and, therefore, the heel is inverted. During the contact phase the subtalar joint is pronated while the leg internally rotates. The heel is slightly everted. Pronation does not occur past the contact period in the normal foot.

From the beginning of midstance, the leg externally rotates and the subtalar joint supinates. The heel moves from a pronated position to a neutral position of the subtalar joint. During midstance, the subtalar joint continues to supinate and the heel becomes inverted. During the propulsion phase, the tibia continues to externally rotate and the subtalar joint supinates just before toe-off.

The forefoot is inverted around the long axis of the midtarsal joint at heel strike. As the forefoot is loaded, the heel is everting with subtalar pronation. When the subtalar joint is in neutral position, ground reaction locks the midtarsal joint around the long axis in pronation to lock the rear foot and forefoot in the necessary position for propulsion. During propulsion, external rotation causes supination of the forefoot at the midtarsal joint axis.

As the forefoot contacts the ground and the subtalar joint pronates, the first ray may dorsiflex and invert. If midtarsal joint inversion around the long axis is sufficient to compensate for the rear foot eversion, the first ray may not dorsiflex. Inadequate midtarsal inversion would allow ground reaction forces to dorsiflex and invert the first ray.

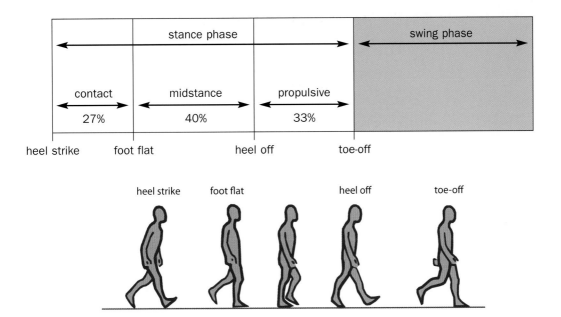

Figure 5.10 Phases of gait   ADAPTED FROM ROOT ET AL. 1977

(a) Normal gait cycle of walking

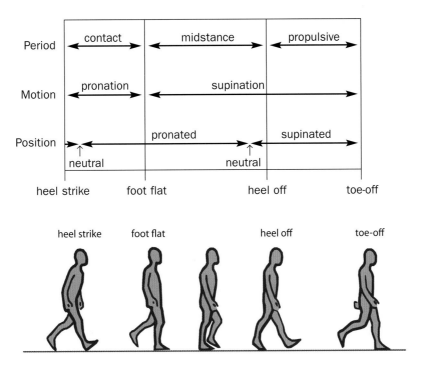

(b) Motion and position at subtalar joint during stance phase

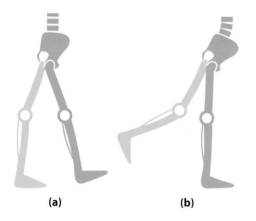

(a)   **(b)**

Figure 5.11 Tilting of the pelvis during walking

(a) Neutral position of the pelvis just before heel strike
(b) Anterior tilting of the pelvis occurs during single
support phase

Biomechanics of running

The phases of running are similar to walking
(Fig. 5.12). The stance phase is divided into contact,
midstance and propulsion. The swing phase is divided
into follow-through, forward swing and foot descent.
Whereas walking is the alternate placement of one foot
in front of the other separated by periods when both
feet are in contact with the ground, during running
there is a flight phase when neither foot is in contact
with the ground between stance phases.

In slower, longer running, the stance phase is
of longer duration than the flight phase. As running speed increases, stance phase and flight phase
times approach each other until the stance phase

becomes shorter than the swing phase in sprinting
(Fig. 5.13).

During running, there is an increased range of
pelvic, hip and knee rotation due to increases in joint
movements. This must be absorbed by increasing
muscle forces acting over these joints.[5] As running
speed increases, the foot maintains the same movements as in walking but with variations. In slower
running, the foot functions in a heel–toe manner. In
quicker running (striding), the foot may strike with
the heel and forefoot simultaneously prior to toe-off
or may strike with the forefoot initially and then the

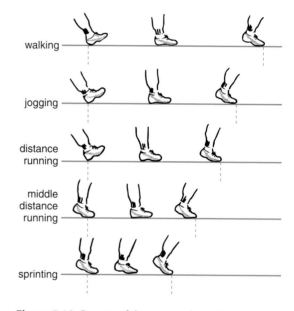

Figure 5.13 Pattern of the stance phase during
different speeds of walking and running

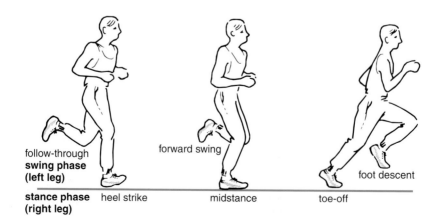

Figure 5.12 The swing and stance phases of running

heel lowering to the surface prior to toe-off. Sprinters maintain weight-bearing on the forefoot from contact to toe-off, although the heel may lower to the supporting surface at midstance.

Angle and base of gait in walking and running

The angle of gait is the angle between the longitudinal bisection of the foot and the line of progression (Fig. 5.14). The normal angle of gait is approximately 10° abducted from the line of progression in walking. Abducted gait describes an angle of gait greater than 10°. The angle of gait reflects the hip and tibial transverse plane positions. The base of gait is the distance between the medial aspect of the heels (Fig. 5.15). A normal base of gait is approximately 2.5–3.0 cm (~1 in.).

Changes from the normal angle and base of gait may be secondary to structural abnormalities or, more commonly, as compensation for another abnormality. For example, a wide base of gait may be necessary to increase stability. As speed increases while walking and running, the angle and base of gait decrease. While running, the angle of gait approaches zero and foot strike is on the line of progression. This limits deviation of the center of gravity as the lower limbs move beneath the body, thus allowing more efficient locomotion (Fig. 5.15b).

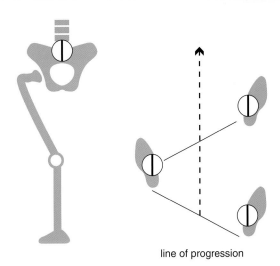

line of progression

Figure 5.15 Angle and base of gait

(a) Walking

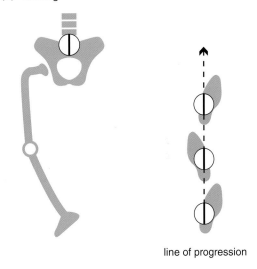

line of progression

(b) Running

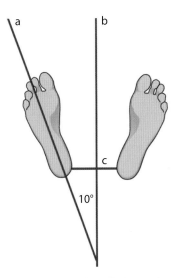

10°

Figure 5.14 The angle of gait is the angle between **(a)** the long axis at the foot and **(b)** the line of progression. **(c)** Base of gait is the distance between the medial aspect of the heels

Whenever possible, the practitioner should observe the patient running. Abnormal rotations of the lower limbs and feet may be seen from the front or rear. From a side-on position, anteroposterior posture as well as stride length may be observed.

Abnormal lower limb biomechanics

Overuse injuries have been linked with abnormal lower limb biomechanics. Recent studies suggest that many injuries can be the result of increased foot pronation.[6]

As the science of biomechanics advances and measurement of runners becomes more commonplace, researchers are confirming some of the clinically noted associations between biomechanics and injuries.[7,8] The area of biomechanics and injury prevention is a popular area of research that continues to provide interesting results, and hopefully in the future will provide more evidence-based practice.

A list of common lower limb injuries and the biomechanical abnormalities observed clinically is shown in Table 5.2.

There are three main biomechanical abnormalities affecting the lower limb: excessive pronation, excessive supination and abnormal pelvic movement.

Excessive pronation

Pronation of the foot occurs at the subtalar joint. Abnormal pronation occurs when the degree of pronation is excessive or when pronation occurs during the phase of gait when the foot should be supinating. An excessively pronated foot may cause excessive internal rotation of the entire lower limb during weight-bearing and this increases demands on numerous structures.

Excessive pronation causes increased ground reaction forces on the medial aspect of the foot. This contributes to the development of first metatarsophalangeal joint abnormalities, including exostoses and hallux valgus. Sesamoid pain is also commonly associated with excessive pronation. Due to the instability of the foot, callus and corn build-up is common. Interdigital (Morton's) neuroma may be caused by metatarsal hypermobility.

Excessive pronation also causes increased load on the medial longitudinal arch and increased strain on the plantar fascia and plantar musculature.

The gastrocnemius–soleus complex and tibialis posterior may eccentrically contract harder and longer in order to decelerate rotation of the leg and pronation of the foot. This may contribute to tendinopathy of the Achilles and tibialis posterior tendons. Overload of the long flexors of the leg may result in tibial periostitis presenting as medial shin pain.

Excessive pronation leads to an increased internal rotation of the tibia, a tendency to lateral subluxation of the patella, and muscle imbalance of the quadriceps, all of which contribute to patellofemoral joint dysfunction. Internal rotation of the tibia contributes to a change in alignment of the patellar tendon, which may predispose to patellar tendinopathy. Internal rotation of the tibia may also contribute to tightening of the iliotibial band.

Table 5.2 Lower limb injuries and associated biomechanical abnormalities often noted clinically

Injury	Common biomechanical abnormalities
Sesamoiditis	Pronated foot Abducted gait Limited first ray range of motion Forefoot valgus/plantarflexed first ray
Plantar fasciitis	Pronated foot/high arched foot Abducted gait Ankle equinus
Achilles tendinopathy	Pronated foot Ankle equinus
Peroneal tendinopathy	Pronated foot at toe-off Excessive supination
Medial shin pain	Pronated foot Ankle equinus Varus alignment Abducted gait
Patellar tendinopathy	Pronated foot Tight quadriceps, hamstrings, calves Anterior pelvic tilt Varus alignment
Patellofemoral pain	Pronated foot Anterior pelvic tilt Varus alignment Abducted gait
Iliotibial band friction syndrome	Lateral pelvic tilting Varus alignment
Hamstring strain	Anterior pelvic tilt Ankle equinus
Metatarsal stress fractures	Pronated foot Supinated foot
Navicular stress fractures	Pronated foot Varus alignment Ankle equinus
Fibular stress fractures	Supinated foot Pronated foot Varus alignment

Stress fractures are commonly associated with the unstable, pronated foot. Metatarsal fractures may occur due to uneven distribution of weight and excessive movement of the metatarsals with forefoot lowering. Stress fractures of the sesamoids may occur with greater loading of the first ray. Excessive pronation may lead to stress fractures of the tibia. Overuse of the tibialis posterior muscle and long flexor tendons may contribute to traction on the periosteum and bending of the tibia. As these muscles become increasingly fatigued due to excessive pronation, the tibia is subjected to greater impact.

With pronation of the foot through the propulsive phase of gait, the peroneal musculature attempts to stabilize the medial and lateral columns of the foot. Chronic overloading may result in stress fracture of the fibula.

Excessive supination

Excessive supination of the subtalar joint may occur to compensate for structural foot abnormalities. It also may occur as a result of weakness of the antagonist pronating musculature (e.g. peroneal) or as a result of spasm or tightness of the supinating musculature (e.g. tibialis posterior and the gastrocnemius–soleus complex). The supinated foot may be less mobile, which may result in poor shock absorption. It is possible that this may predispose to the development of stress fractures of the tibia, fibula, calcaneus and metatarsals (especially fourth and fifth metatarsals).

Lateral instability of the foot and ankle may be associated with excessive supination. A forefoot valgus foot type may be present. This results in an increased incidence of sprains of the ankle and the foot. Due to increased lateral stress on the lower limb, the iliotibial band becomes tighter and bursitis may occur at the femoral epicondyle.

Abnormal pelvic mechanics

In running, a certain amount of pelvic movement (rotation, anterior–posterior and lateral tilt) is required. However, there may be excessive movement in any of the three planes (sagittal, frontal and transverse) due to poor control of the stabilizing muscles. This poor control leads to less effective transmission of forces through the pelvis and less efficient movement. Frequently, abnormalities exist in more than one plane. Lack of stability in one plane may predispose to development of problems in another plane. The most common abnormalities are excessive anterior tilt, excessive lateral tilt and asymmetrical pelvic movement.

Excessive anterior tilt

An athlete with poor pelvic muscle control (abdominal, gluteus medius and minimus, hamstrings and external hip rotators) in combination with tightness of the hip flexors may be unable to dissociate active hip extension from pelvic movement, thus increasing

the anterior tilt or rotation while running. This may also increase the length and tension of the hamstrings and abdominal muscles.

The external rotator muscles of the hip become tight as they work excessively to provide pelvic stability to compensate for the reduced contribution by the gluteal muscles. Tight hip external rotators cause an abducted angle of gait.

Increased anterior pelvic tilt with hip extension leads to an increased lumbar lordosis and strain on the lumbar apophyseal joints and sacroiliac joints.

With anterior pelvic tilting, knee flexion is greater than normal at foot strike and midstance. This increases the eccentric load across the extensor mechanism of the knee, and may contribute to patellar tendinopathy. With greater knee flexion, the patella will be compressed against the femur with greater force, which may predispose to patellofemoral joint syndrome. The excessive anterior tilt may be bilateral or unilateral.

Excessive lateral tilt

Excessive lateral tilt occurs due to poor control of hip abductors and adductors of the weight-bearing limb allowing the contralateral hip to drop during its swing phase. This may lead to excessive strain and inflammation of lateral hip structures, adductors, tensor fascia lata, iliotibial band and other lateral knee structures as well as the lumbar spine.

Excessive anterior tilt of the pelvis results in increased gluteal muscle length and, therefore, reduced force of contraction. This also leads to increased lateral tilting of the pelvis.

Asymmetrical pelvic movement

Due to the large number of muscles that attach to the pelvis, asymmetry may be caused by:

- tight/shortened muscles
- incoordinate weakened muscles
- structural abnormalities (e.g. leg length discrepancy, scoliosis).

These may occur primarily as an adaptation to a previous injury. Asymmetry is commonly exacerbated by running and is often associated with osteitis pubis and lower limb overuse injuries.

Common structural abnormalities

Structural abnormalities of the foot, subtalar joint, ankle joint, lower leg bones and hip joint may contribute to abnormal biomechanics.

Forefoot varus

Forefoot varus is a structural abnormality in which the forefoot is inverted on the rear foot in the frontal plane at the midtarsal joint (Fig. 5.16a). The foot pronates excessively at the subtalar joint to compensate and allow the medial aspect of the foot to make ground contact (Fig. 5.16b).

Forefoot valgus

Forefoot valgus occurs when the forefoot is everted on the rear foot in the frontal plane (Fig. 5.17a). Supination occurs at the long axis of the midtarsal joint but is usually not sufficient to compensate for the abnormality and subtalar joint supination occurs (Fig. 5.17b).

Plantarflexed first ray

The first ray may be plantarflexed with regard to the other metatarsals. Supination around the long axis of the midtarsal joint and the subtalar joint occurs to compensate.

Rear foot varus

Rear foot varus occurs when the calcaneus is inverted in relation to the bisection of the tibia due to the position of the subtalar joint (Fig. 5.18a). To

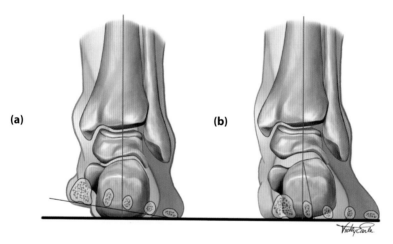

Figure 5.16 (a) Forefoot varus
(b) Compensated forefoot varus

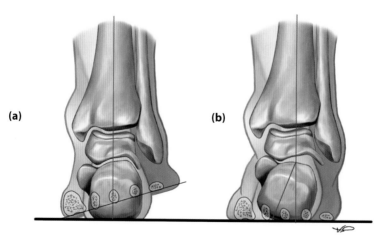

Figure 5.17 (a) Forefoot valgus
(b) Compensated forefoot valgus

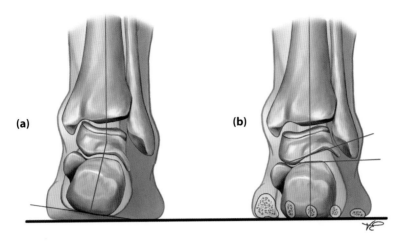

Figure 5.18 (a) Rear foot varus
(b) Compensated rear foot varus

compensate, the subtalar joint pronates excessively to allow the medial aspect of the foot to make ground contact (Fig. 5.18b).

Rear foot valgus

Rear foot valgus (Fig. 5.19a) is uncommon and may occur when the calcaneus is everted in relation to the bisection of the tibia due to the position of the subtalar joint. The midtarsal and subtalar joints supinate to compensate (Fig. 5.19b).

Ankle equinus

Ankle equinus (Fig. 5.20) occurs when there is less than 10–20° of dorsiflexion present. The 10–20° of ankle joint dorsiflexion is necessary for the tibia to rotate over the foot during the stance phase without early heel lift or pronation of the foot as compensation. Bony limitation of ankle joint motion may cause ankle equinus.

Ankle equinus may also be caused by tightness or shortening of the gastrocnemius or soleus muscles. With limited ankle joint dorsiflexion, the subtalar joint may pronate excessively in order to utilize the

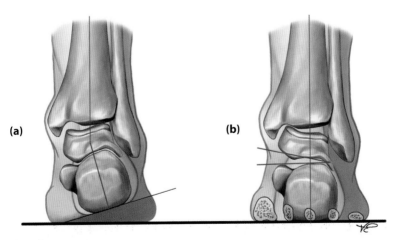

Figure 5.19 (a) Rear foot valgus
(b) Compensated rear foot valgus

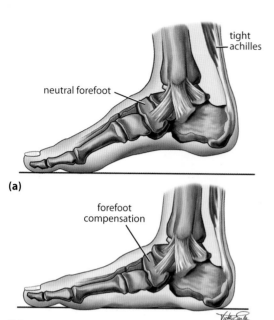

(a)

(b)

Figure 5.20 Ankle equinus

(a) Normal ankle dorsiflexion
(b) Abnormal ankle dorsiflexion

dorsiflexion component of pronation. The midtarsal joint may also collapse to utilize the sagittal plane motion associated with dorsiflexion around the oblique midtarsal joint axis.

A bouncy gait may be observed in athletes with limited ankle joint dorsiflexion as a result of the early heel lift caused by the equinus. Weight is then transferred prematurely to the forefoot, predisposing to injuries of the plantar fascia, metatarsals and toes. Compensatory mechanisms for limited ankle joint dorsiflexion may contribute to ligament sprains and muscle strains of the foot, Achilles tendon and calf muscle injuries, medial shin pain and stress fractures.

Tibial alignment

Tibia varum is a lateral deviation or bowing of the tibia causing inversion of the foot at heel strike. The foot pronates excessively to allow the medial aspect of the foot to contact the ground.

Increased tibial external torsion results in an abducted gait. This produces an excessive varus position at heel strike, greater lateral stress to the lower limb and possibly increased stress on lateral structures such as the iliotibial band. Excessive pronation of the foot follows. Internal tibial torsion results in an in-toed gait, lateral instability of the ankle, and supination

after contact. The foot may pronate to utilize the abduction component of pronation.

Genu varum

Genu varum (Fig. 5.21) or bowed legs causes increased varus heel strike and greater lateral stress. Varus strain at the knee may cause increased stress on the lateral knee structures and the development of patellofemoral pain. Excessive pronation occurs at the subtalar joint to allow the medial aspect of the foot to make ground contact.

Genu valgum

Genu valgum or 'knock knees' (Fig. 5.22) causes excessive pronation of the feet as the center of gravity during gait is medial to the subtalar joint.

Leg length differences

These may be structural or functional. Structural differences occur when different length osseous structures

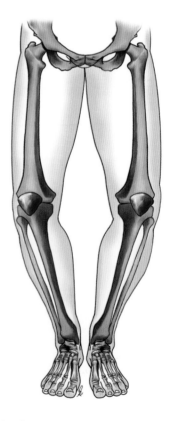

Figure 5.21 Genu varum

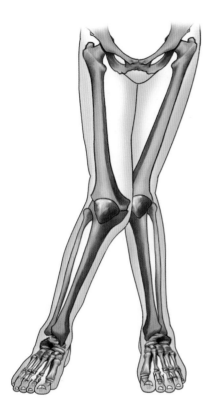

Figure 5.22 Genu valgum

are present. Functional differences occur with asymmetry of pelvic alignment, asymmetrical pronation or supination, or unilateral contractures. Structural and functional differences may both be present.

Manifestations of leg length differences include:

- head tilt and shoulder drop, often towards longer leg
- asymmetry of arm swing—abducted arm leads to increased deviation of center of gravity, often towards long side as center of gravity is deviated towards short side
- increased speed of arm swing due to increased elbow flexion—this indicates pelvis on opposite side is moving more quickly
- pelvis higher on long limb side
- circumduction of longer limb during swing phase
- increased stress on short side as weight falls to that side
- external rotation of hip to widen angle of gait to increase support on short side—increased angle of gait leads to increased base of support

- functional differences where one foot is pronating more, leading to a drop in the anterior pelvis and elevation of the posterior pelvis
- increased supination of one foot leading to increased elevation of the anterior and posterior superior iliac spines on this side.

Assessment of lower limb biomechanics

Biomechanical assessment is an important component of the examination of any athlete presenting with an overuse injury of the lower limbs. As with any examination procedure (Chapter 8) it is important to develop a routine. A routine for biomechanical lower limb assessment is shown in Figure 5.23. Clinically, measurements are not usually performed due to poor reliability and reproducibility, and rate of error.

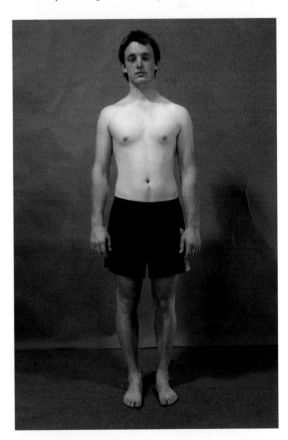

Figure 5.23 Biomechanical assessment

(a) Stance: front view. Assess the level of the anterior superior iliac spines, knee orientation, angle of stance, medial longitudinal arch and limb alignment

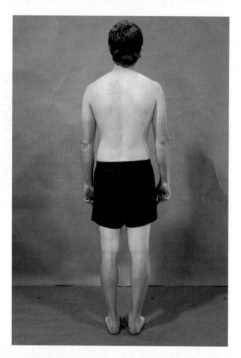

(b) Stance: rear view. Assess shoulder height, alignment of spine, level of posterior superior iliac spines, alignment of tibia in frontal plane, rear foot position and any medial ankle bulging

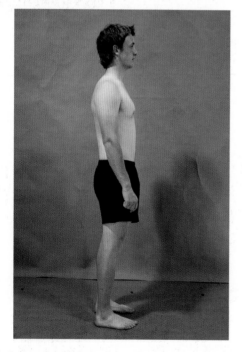

(c) Stance: lateral view. Assess lumbar lordosis, pelvic tilt and any hyperextension of the knee

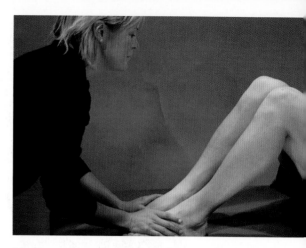

(d) Observation of lower limb alignment (supine) with knees flexed. Observe knee heights

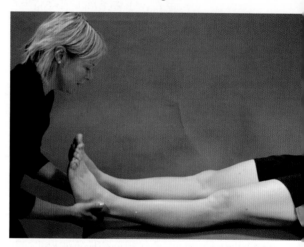

(e) Observation of lower limb alignment (supine)

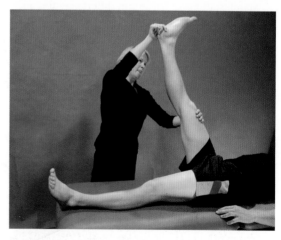

(f) Assessment of hamstring flexibility (supine)

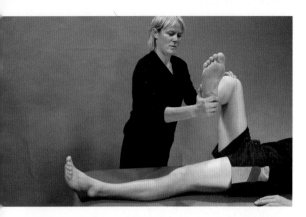

(g) Assessment of hip range of motion (supine). The leg is rotated outwards for internal hip rotation and inwards for external hip rotation

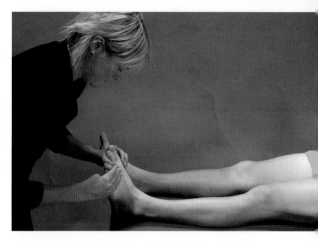

(j) First ray range of motion and position. With the subtalar joint in neutral and the midtarsal joint pronated, the first ray is dorsiflexed and plantarflexed through its range

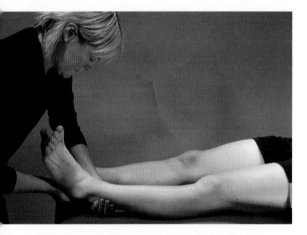

(h) Subtalar joint: range of motion. The quality of subtalar movement is assessed while inverting and everting

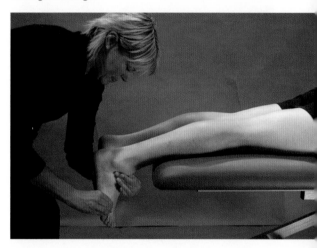

(k) Forefoot/rear foot positions. With the subtalar joint in neutral and the midtarsal joint pronated, the alignment of the rear foot to the leg is determined. The position of the forefoot on the rear foot is also determined

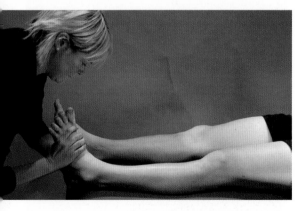

(i) Oblique and long axis (supine) of midtarsal joint. Subtalar joint is in neutral and foot is held just distal to talonavicular and calcaneocuboid joints

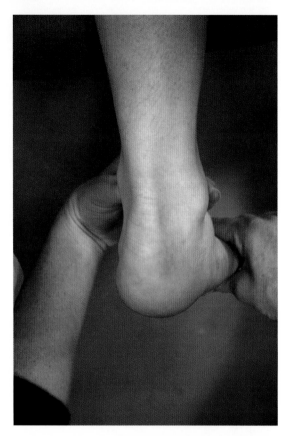

(l) Forefoot/rear foot positions looking from above

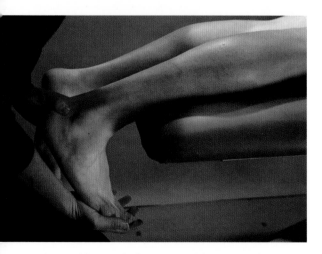

(m) Ankle: range of motion with knee extended (prone). With the subtalar joint in neutral, the angle between the lateral aspect of the leg and the fifth metatarsal is assessed

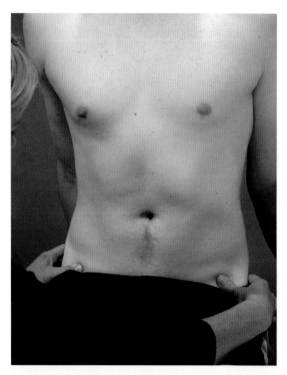

(n) Pelvic symmetry (standing)

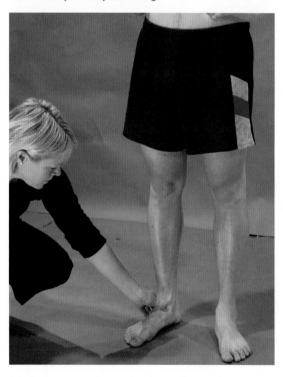

(o) Assessment of neutral calcaneal stance by palpation of talar heads

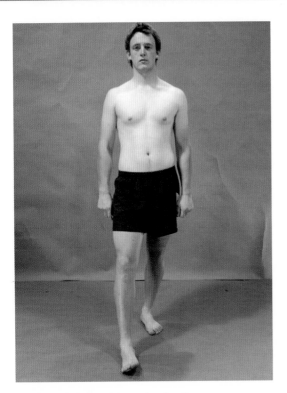

(p) Foot (right) position at heel strike

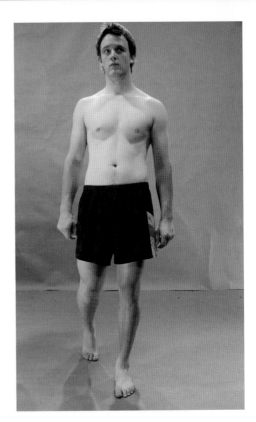

(r) Foot (right) position at toe-off

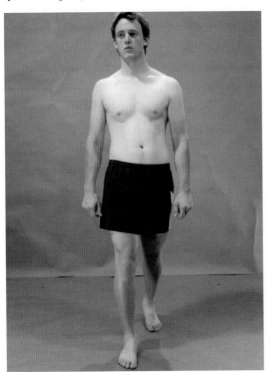

(q) Foot (right) position at midstance

Correction of biomechanics

Asymmetries detected in biomechanical assessment may require correction. These abnormalities include muscle tightness, weakness or incoordination, joint stiffness and increased neural tension (Chapter 3). Muscle tightness is corrected with appropriate stretching. Specific muscle weakness or incoordination require strengthening and retraining (Chapter 12). Joint stiffness may be treated with active or passive joint mobilization, while increased neural tension should be treated with appropriate neural stretching and correction of possible causes, for example, spinal hypomobility (Chapter 10).

Two important methods of correcting lower limb biomechanics are the use of orthoses and footwear and the correction of poor pelvic mechanics. A number of studies have investigated the effects of foot orthoses on the lower extremity, and many of these have documented the clinical efficacy of these devices.[9–15]

Orthoses

Orthoses are placed in the shoe to correct abnormal lower extremity mechanics and alignment. They control excessive subtalar and midtarsal movements that may occur to compensate for structural abnormalities. They do not change structural abnormalities and should not be considered the only means of treatment of excessive movement. It is important also to consider the influence of excessive muscle tightness and weakness, the influence of shoes and the influence of surfaces. Correct foot function is not achieved with orthoses alone and ideal control is achieved by using the appropriate orthosis with the appropriate footwear. It is important to note that, clinically, many athletes do not tolerate large degrees of control from orthoses and often a percentage of control is helpful. Adaption to one's own mechanics should never be underestimated. Orthoses may also assist in proprioceptive changes in controlling excessive motion. Orthoses should always be worn with complete comfort.

The factors influencing the type of orthoses used include foot type, severity of abnormal motion, sporting activity, footwear and weight of the patient. Orthoses range in material from flexible to semirigid devices, and may be casted or preformed.

Preformed orthoses

Preformed orthoses (Fig. 5.24) provide conservative control of the motion of the foot as they are most often flexible. The use of a preformed device is useful in determining whether control of motion can assist in injury management and can also indicate how tolerant an individual may be to changes in posture.

Preformed flexible orthoses are often relatively poor in durability but may give an indication of whether or not more rigid orthoses will be helpful in treating lower limb problems. Different materials used in preformed orthoses include EVA, polyurethane, cork, rubber and plasterzote.

Casted orthoses

Casted orthoses (Fig. 5.25) are manufactured from plaster impressions of the feet after biomechanical examination of the lower limbs and feet. Plaster impressions of the feet are taken and provide a means by which greater control of foot function may be restored. Casted orthoses may alter the mechanics of the foot significantly. The clinician should always be aware of an individual's tolerance to change in mechanics. Most often the materials used are polypropylene and carbon-fiber composites.

It is also useful to observe athletes participating in their sport to see the extent of abnormal movement that occurs during activity. Often, observations noted in stance and during walking may not reflect the extent of excessive motion during running.

Manufacture of casted orthoses

There are many different ways of manufacturing orthoses. It is important to prescribe a device that provides appropriate control of the structural abnormality.

After clinical examination and observation of the patient running and walking, plaster impressions of the feet (Fig. 5.26) are taken with the subtalar joint in the neutral position. Following the neutral casting, the orthosis is manufactured in the laboratory according to the prescription provided. The practitioner needs to determine how the device should control the foot, and how much pressure is required to control it. The

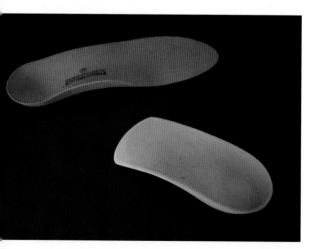

Figure 5.24 Preformed orthoses

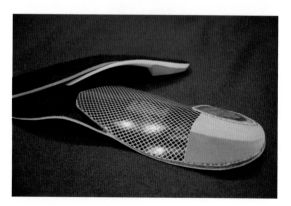

Figure 5.25 Casted orthoses

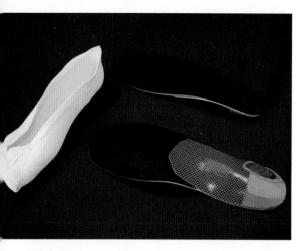

Figure 5.26 Plaster impression

prescription also includes recommendations regarding the materials to be used and the extent of accommodative postings, and takes into account shoe fit.

In the laboratory, the impression is filled with plaster to provide a solid model of the foot. From the solid model, additional plaster is used to provide the appropriate degrees of control. Once the plaster model has been modified, the material of choice is vacuum-pressed onto the plaster model. The molded firm plastic is then ground and covered to suit the individual.

Casted orthoses are durable and may influence lower limb function significantly. At times it may be necessary to reassess and evaluate the effectiveness of the orthosis by further gait analysis, including video analysis. Additional minor adjustments can be made to the orthosis.

Correction of abnormal pelvic biomechanics

Excessive pelvic movements, either bilateral or unilateral, are usually a result of poor control of the abdominals, gluteus minimus and medius, and external hip rotators in association with tightness of the postural muscles, for example, the hamstrings.

Correction is, therefore, directed at stretching the appropriate muscles, such as the psoas, rectus femoris, tensor fascia lata, hamstrings and hip adductors, to optimize hip and pelvic movement. This may require dissociating hip and pelvic movements. Soft tissue therapy is an important component of restoration of optimal tissue length.

Weak muscles require a strengthening program. This may initially be non-weight-bearing but should progress to weight-bearing functional positions as soon

as possible. As control improves, other components may be added gradually, such as hip movements. Large Swedish balls and the Pilates' method of exercise are just two of the many varieties of exercise programs currently used to achieve 'core' stability (Chapter 11).

The next stage involves the integration of this new control into functional activities, such as running. Small components of the overall movement should be incorporated initially. These movements may need to be performed slowly to allow them to be integrated successfully into the functional activity (Chapter 12).

Upper limb biomechanics
WITH W. BEN KIBLER

Correct biomechanics is as important in upper limb activities as it is in lower limb activities. For example, repeated throwing places tremendous stresses on the upper limb, especially the shoulder and elbow joints.[16] Throwing, however, is a 'whole body activity', involving the transfer of momentum from body to ball.

The biomechanics of throwing

Throwing is a whole body activity that commences with drive from the large leg muscles and rotation of the hips and progresses through segmental rotation of the trunk and shoulder girdle. It continues with a 'whip-like' transfer of momentum through elbow extension and through the small muscles of the forearm and hand, transferring propulsive force to the ball.

The skilled clinician should assess both the scapulohumeral and the truncal mechanics in a throwing athlete. The role of the scapula in throwing is discussed in more detail below, and the back, trunk and hips serve as a center of rotation and a transfer link from the legs to the shoulder.

Throwing can be divided into four phases:

1. preparation/wind-up } 80% time sequence
2. cocking
3. acceleration   2% time sequence
4. deceleration/follow-through 18% time sequence

Wind-up

Wind-up (Fig. 5.27) establishes the rhythm of the pitch or throw. During wind-up, the body rotates so that the hip and shoulders are at 90° to the target. The major forces arise in the lower half of the body and develop a forward-moving 'controlled fall'. In pitching, hip flexion of the lead leg raises the center

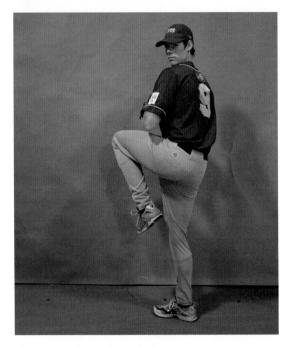

Figure 5.27 Throwing: wind-up

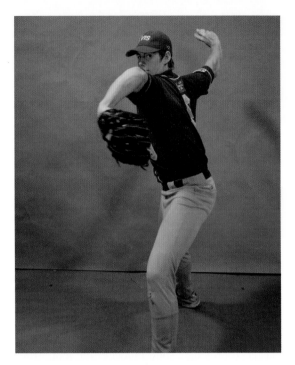

Figure 5.28 Throwing: cocking

of gravity. The wind-up phase lasts 500–1000 milliseconds. During this phase, muscles of the shoulder are relatively inactive.

Cocking

The cocking movement (Fig. 5.28) positions the body to enable all body segments to contribute to ball propulsion. In cocking, the shoulder moves into abduction through full horizontal extension and then into maximal external rotation. When the scapula is maximally retracted, the acromion starts to elevate. With maximal external rotation, the shoulder is 'loaded,' with the anterior capsule coiled tightly in the apprehension position storing elastic energy. The internal rotators are stretched.[17] At this stage, anterior joint forces are maximal and can exceed 350 newtons (N). Towards the end of cocking, the static anterior restraints (anterior inferior glenohumeral ligament and anterior inferior capsule) are under the greatest strain. Because of the repetitive nature of throwing, these structures can become attenuated and lead to subtle instability.[18] In the trunk, tensile forces increase in the abdomen, hip extensors and spine, with the lead hip internally rotating just prior to ground contact.

The cocking phase ends with the planting of the lead leg, with the body positioned for energy transfer through the legs, trunk and arms to the ball. This phase also lasts 500–1000 milliseconds. The wind-up and cocking phases together constitute 80% of the duration of the pitch (approximately 1500 milliseconds).

Shoulder cocking continues with the counterclockwise rotation of the pelvis and trunk (when viewed from above), which abruptly places the arm behind the body in an externally rotated position.

Lateral trunk flexion determines the degree of arm abduction. When viewed in the coronal plane, the relative abduction of the humerus to the long axis of the trunk is a fairly constant 90–100°, regardless of style. The overhand athlete leans contralaterally, while the side-arm or submarine thrower actually leans towards the throwing arm. Rotation of the trunk also aids in abduction. Although the muscles of the shoulder produce little abduction during the early cocking phase of a well-executed throw, the periscapular muscles are quite active. The force couple between the upper trapezius and serratus initiates acromial elevation and the lower trapezius maintains elevation at abduction angles greater than 65°.

Acceleration

The acceleration phase (Fig. 5.29) is extremely explosive. It consists of the rapid release of two forces—the stored elastic force of the tightly bound fibrous tissue of the capsule and forceful internal rotation from the internal rotators (subscapularis, pectoralis major,

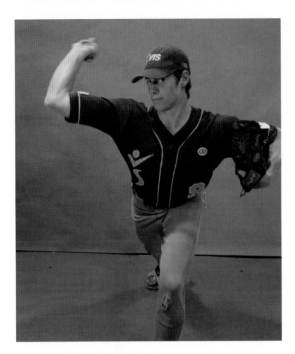

Figure 5.29 Throwing: acceleration

latissimus dorsi, teres major). This generates excessive forces at the glenohumeral articulation[19] and, thus, the cuff musculature remains highly active to keep the humeral head enlocated in the glenoid.

Large muscles outside the rotator cuff are responsible for the subsequent acceleration of the arm. This includes muscles of the anterior chest wall as well as the muscles and fascia that surround the spine. The critical role of the muscles controlling scapulothoracic motion—scapular positioning and stabilization against the thorax—is discussed below.

At the shoulder, acceleration is the shortest phase of the throwing motion, lasting only 50 milliseconds (2% of the overall time). In both the acceleration and the late cocking phases, muscle fatigue (which is accelerated if there is mild instability due to attenuated static restrains) can lead to loss of coordinated rotator cuff motion and, thus, decreased anterior shoulder wall support.

The acceleration phase concludes with ball release, which occurs at approximately ear level. The movements involved in acceleration place enormous valgus forces on the elbow, which tends to lag behind the inwardly rotating shoulder.

Deceleration/follow-through

Not all the momentum of the throw is transferred to the ball. In the deceleration/follow-through phase

(Fig. 5.30), very high forces pull forward on the glenohumeral joint following ball release, which places large stresses on the posterior shoulder structures. During this time both intrinsic and extrinsic shoulder muscles fire at significant percentages of their maximum, attempting to develop in excess of 500 N to slow the arm down. The force tending to pull the humerus out of the shoulder socket can exceed 500 N (roughly equivalent to 135 kg [300 lb]). The eccentric contraction of the rotator cuff external rotators decelerates the rapid internal rotation of the shoulder, as does eccentric contraction of the scapular stabilizers and posterior deltoid fibers. In the properly thrown pitch, the spine and its associated musculature have a significant role as a force attenuator.

Towards the end of the pitching motion, the torso, having decelerated so the arm could acquire kinetic energy in the arm acceleration phase, begins to rotate forward. The forward rotation of this larger link segment helps to reacquire some of this energy. This theoretically reduces the burden on the serratus anterior and other stabilizers, which are attempting to eccentrically maintain the position of the scapula and maintain the humeral head within the glenoid.

In addition to the high stresses on the posterior shoulder structures, this phase places large stresses

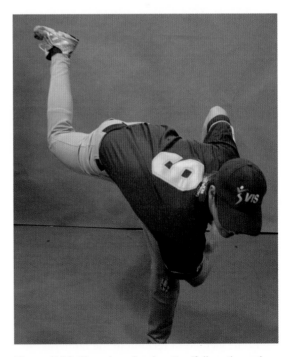

Figure 5.30 Throwing: deceleration/follow-through

on the elbow flexors that act to limit rapid elbow extension. This phase lasts approximately 350 milliseconds and constitutes approximately 18% of the total time.

The role of the trunk in throwing is clear. When trunk motion is inhibited or the potential ground reaction force reduced, throwing velocity is markedly lower. With a normal overhead throw rated at 100%, peak velocities dropped to 84% when a forward stride was not allowed and down to 63.5% and 53.1% when the lower body and lower body plus trunk were restricted, respectively.[20] Peak ball-release velocities attained by water polo players are approximately half the velocity that a thrown baseball might reach on land where a ground reaction force can be generated.

Normal biomechanics of the scapula in throwing

In recent years, the importance of the scapula in normal throwing biomechanics has been increasingly recognized. For optimal shoulder function, and to decrease injury risk, the scapula must move in a coordinated way (Fig. 5.31). This section outlines Ben Kibler's[21] description of the role of the scapula in throwing (Table 5.3). If the clinician understands the normal scapular biomechanics, he or she will be then able to detect abnormal scapular biomechanics in patients with upper limb injuries (for clinical implications of abnormal shoulder biomechanics, see p. 65).

The scapula provides a stable socket for the humerus

In normal shoulder function, the scapula forms a stable base for glenohumeral articulation. The glenoid is the socket of the ball-and-socket glenohumeral joint. Thus, the scapula must rotate as the humerus moves so that the center of rotation of the glenohumeral joint remains optimal throughout the throwing or serving motion. This coordinated movement keeps the angle between the glenoid and the humerus within the physiologically tolerable or 'safe zone', which extends about 30° of extension or flexion from neutral. In this range, there is maximal 'concavity/compression' of the glenohumeral joint, and the muscle constraints around the shoulder are also enhanced. The maximal concavity/compression results from the slightly negative intra-articular pressure of the normal joint, with optimal positioning of the glenoid in relation to the humerus, and coordinated muscle activity.

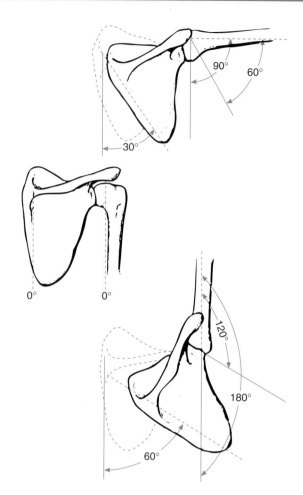

Figure 5.31 Normal scapulothoracic rhythm allows the scapula to rotate upwardly during abduction, bringing the glenoid fossa directly under the humeral head to lend stability to the glenohumeral joint

Table 5.3 Scapular function in normal shoulder mechanics

1. Provides a stable socket for the humerus.
2. Retracts and protracts along the thoracic wall.
3. Rotates to elevate the acromion.
4. Provides a base for muscle attachment.
5. Provides a key link in the kinetic chain.

The scapula must retract and protract along the thoracic wall

In the cocking phase of throwing (as well as in the tennis serve and swimming recovery), the scapula retracts (see above). Once acceleration begins, the scapula protracts smoothly laterally and then anteriorly around the thoracic wall to keep the scapula in a normal position relative to the humerus and also to dissipate some of the deceleration forces that occur in follow-through.

The scapula rotates to elevate the acromion

As almost all throwing and serving activities occur with a humerus-to-spine angle of between 85° and 100° of abduction, the scapula must tilt upwards to clear the acromion from the rotator cuff.

The scapula provides a base for muscle attachment

Stabilizing muscles attach to the medial, superior and inferior borders of the scapula to control its position and motion. The extrinsic muscles (deltoid, biceps and triceps) attach along the lateral aspect of the scapula and perform gross motor activities of the glenohumeral joint. The intrinsic muscles of the rotator cuff attach along the entire surface of the scapula and work most efficiently with the arm between 70° and 100° of abduction. In this position, they form a 'compressor cuff' enlocating the humeral head into the socket.

The scapula provides a key link in the kinetic chain

The scapula links the proximal-to-distal sequencing of velocity, energy and forces that optimize shoulder function. For most shoulder activities, this sequencing starts at the ground. Individual body segments, or links, move in a coordinated way to generate, summate and transfer force through various body segments to the terminal link. This sequencing is termed the 'kinetic chain.' Large proximal body segments provide the bulk of the force.

The scapula is pivotal in transferring the large forces and high energy from the legs, back and trunk to the arm and the hand. Forces generated in the proximal segments are transferred efficiently and regulated as they go through the funnel of the shoulder when the scapula provides a stable and controlled platform. The entire arm rotates as a unit around the stable base of the glenohumeral socket.

Thus, the scapula performs various interrelated functions to maintain the normal glenohumeral path and provide a stable base for muscular function. Abnormalities in scapular function that predispose to injury are discussed below.

Abnormal scapular biomechanics and physiology

The scapular roles can be altered by many anatomical factors to create abnormal biomechanics and physiology, both locally and in the kinetic chain (Table 5.4).

Clinical significance of scapular biomechanics in shoulder injuries

Abnormal shoulder biomechanics can compromise normal shoulder function. This observation has been given various descriptive titles, such as 'scapulothoracic dyskinesis', 'floating scapula' or 'lateral scapular slide'. It is important for the clinician to recognize that these are merely titles for the same phenomenon, that is, abnormal scapular function. We provide examples of how abnormal biomechanics can cause shoulder and elbow problems.

Lack of full retraction of the scapula on the thorax destabilizes the cocking point and prevents acceleration out of a fully cocked position. Lack of full scapular protraction increases the deceleration forces on the shoulder and alters the normal safe zone between the glenoid and the humerus as the arm moves through the acceleration phase. Too much protraction because of tightness in the glenohumeral capsule causes impingement as the scapula rotates down and forward. These cumulatively lead to abnormalities in concavity/compression due to the changes in the safe zone of the glenohumeral angle.

Loss of coordinated retraction/protraction in throwing opens up the front of the glenohumeral joint and, thus, provides an insufficient anterior bony buttress to anterior translation of the humeral head. This increases shear stress on the rest of the anterior stabilizing structure, the labrum and glenohumeral ligaments, which further decreases the stability of the glenoid for the rotating humerus.

Lack of acromial elevation leads to impingement in the cocking and follow-through phases. Impingement can also occur secondary to painful shoulder conditions that inhibit the function of the serratus and lower trapezius muscles. As these muscles normally act as a force couple to elevate the acromion, their inhibition commonly causes impingement. Thus, detecting and, if necessary, reversing serratus and trapezius inhibition is an important step in treating shoulder conditions.

If the scapula is unstable, the lack of an anchor affects the function of all scapula muscles. Muscles without a stable origin cannot develop appropriate or maximal torque and are predisposed to suffering muscular imbalance. If the scapula is truly unstable on the thoracic wall, as in spinal accessory nerve palsies or in extremely inhibited muscles, then the muscle origins and insertions are effectively reversed and the distal

Table 5.4 Alterations to scapular function

Scapular function alteration	Effect on scapular function
Anatomical factors	
Cervical spine lordosis	Excessive scapular protraction—leads to impingement with elevation
Thoracic spine kyphosis	Excessive scapular protraction—leads to impingement with elevation
Shoulder asymmetry (i.e. drooping of the shoulder or 'tennis shoulder')	Impingement/muscle function and fatigue
Injuries of scapula, clavicle	Alters orientation of scapula, length of clavicular strut; painful conditions that inhibit muscle function
Abnormalities in muscle function	
Overuse, direct trauma, glenohumeral causes (instability, labral lesions, arthrosis)	Muscle weakness or force couple imbalances. Serratus anterior and lower trapezius particularly susceptible. Can be a non-specific response to a variety of glenohumeral pathologies (this can be seen as analogous to the knee in that weakness of the vastus medialis obliquus can result in the patellofemoral syndrome)
Glenohumeral inflexibility, posterior (capsular or muscular)	Limits smooth glenohumeral joint motion and creates wind-up effect so that the glenoid and scapula get pulled in forward and inferiorly by the moving arm, leading to excessive protraction, which, in turn, holds the scapula and, importantly, the acromion inferiorly and, thus, makes it prone to impingement
Nerve injury (causes less than 5% of abnormal muscle function in shoulder problems)	Long thoracic nerve, serratus anterior, inhibited. Accessory nerve—trapezius function inhibited

end of the muscle becomes the origin. The scapula is then pulled laterally by the muscle, which contracts from the more stable distal humeral end rather than from the proximal scapular end. A further problem of the unstable scapula is that it does not provide a stable base for glenohumeral rotation during link sequencing. Therefore, the arm works on an unstable platform and loses mechanical efficiency.

One of the most important scapular biomechanical abnormalities is the loss of the link function in the kinetic chain. The kinetic chain permits efficient transfer of energy and force to the hand. The scapula and shoulder funnel forces from the large segments, the legs and trunk, to the smaller, rapidly moving small segments of the arm.

Scapular dysfunction impairs force transmission from the lower to the upper extremity. This reduces the force delivered to the hand or creates a situation of 'catch-up' in which the more distal links have to overwork to compensate for the loss of the proximally generated force. The distal links have neither the size, the muscle cross-sectional area, nor the time in which to develop these larger forces efficiently. For example, a 20% decrease in kinetic energy delivered from the hip and trunk to the arm necessitates an 80% increase in muscle mass or a 34% increase in rotational velocity at the shoulder to deliver the same amount of resultant force to the hand. Such an adaptation would predispose to overload problems.

This explains why injuries apparently unrelated to the upper limb, for example, decreased push-off due to Achilles tendinopathy, decreased quadriceps drive after a muscle strain or decreased segmental trunk rotation secondary to thoracic segmental hypomobility, can affect upper limb throwing mechanics and predispose to further, or more serious, upper limb injury.

Changes in throwing arm with repeated pitching

Repeated throwing causes adaptive changes to gradually develop in the shoulder and elbow. Changes occur in flexibility, soft tissue/muscle strength and bony contour.

At the shoulder, long-term throwing athletes have increased range of external rotation. This arises because of the repeated stress to the anterior capsule in the cocking phase and stretch or breakdown in the anterior static stabilizers of the shoulder joint (the inferior glenohumeral ligaments). This may compromise the dynamic balance that exists between shoulder function and stability. The combination of increased shoulder external rotation range of motion and breakdown of the static stabilizers may lead to anterior instability of the shoulder and secondary impingement.

The normal strength ratio of internal rotators to external rotators is approximately 3:2 but in throwers this imbalance is exaggerated and, over time, lack of external rotation strength may increase vulnerability to injury. These dynamic changes in the shoulder joint highlight the need for a structured exercise program to prevent or correct muscle imbalances.

Throwing also produces structural changes at the elbow. Due to the valgus stress applied in the throwing action there is a breakdown of the medial stabilizing structures (medial collateral ligament, joint capsule, flexor muscles). This leads to the development of an increased carrying angle at the elbow.

Less frequently, the eccentric overload on elbow structures causes anterior capsular strains, posterior impingement or forearm flexor strains and, subsequently, a fixed flexion deformity.

Common biomechanical abnormalities specific to pitching

One of the most common biomechanical problems is caused by the pitcher 'opening up too soon'. Normally the body rotates out of the cocking phase when the arm is fully cocked (externally rotated). If the body opens up too soon, the arm lags behind and is not fully externally rotated. This results in increased stress to the anterior shoulder structures and an increased eccentric load to the shoulder external rotators. It also results in increased valgus stress at the elbow.

The other common abnormality seen in pitchers is known as 'hanging', which is a characteristic sign of fatigue. Decreased shoulder abduction leads to dropping of the elbow and a reduction in velocity. There is an associated increase in the likelihood of injury, particularly to the rotator cuff as well as the shoulder joint and the elbow. It is normally related to excessive intensity, frequency or duration of activity.

The type of pitch is determined by the spin imparted onto the ball by the hands and fingers at ball release. The normal follow-through involves forearm pronation. In 'breaking' pitches, the forearm is relatively supinated at release and then pronates. 'Breaking' pitches are associated with an increased risk of injury. Some pitchers incorrectly forcefully supinate against the normal pronation of follow-through.

Biomechanics of swimming

Swimming relies on propulsion through the water using both the upper and lower limbs.[22] Approximately 90% of propulsion is generated by the upper limbs. The forward propulsive forces must overcome the drag force of the water. Therefore, when swimming front crawl (freestyle), the swimmer tries to maintain as horizontal a position as possible. If the head and shoulders are high in the water and the hips and legs are lower, or there is excessive side-to-side movement, there is an increased drag effect.

In freestyle, butterfly and backstroke there are two phases of the stroke—the pull-through and recovery. In simple terms, the pull-through involves adduction and internal rotation of the shoulder as the elbow flexes and then extends. The recovery phase involves abduction and external rotation of the shoulder, again followed by elbow flexion and then extension.

In all four competitive swimming strokes, swimmers do not simply pull the arm straight through the water. For example, pull-through is S-shaped in freestyle. Not all of the underwater phase of the stroke contributes to propulsion. In all strokes the beginning of propulsion, or catch point, begins approximately one-third of the way through the underwater phase. This represents the arm position where the elbow is above the hand. Understanding swimming biomechanics can aid stroke proficiency and minimizes risk of injury.

Swimming biomechanics and shoulder pain

Shoulder pain is extremely common among swimmers and is usually due to impingement and rotator cuff tendinopathy. Traditionally, anatomical factors were thought to cause impingement but it now appears that it is largely due to muscle weakness, dynamic muscle imbalance and biomechanical faults.

If the scapular stabilizing muscles are weak and the short scapulohumeral muscles tight, there will be insufficient scapular protraction and lateral rotation during the swimming stroke and, thus, a tendency for rotator cuff impingement. This problem is exacerbated if cervical and thoracic hypomobility is present. Dynamic imbalance between the internal and external shoulder rotators may also promote impingement in the pull-through phase of a stroke as the internal rotators are often excessively (>3:2 ratio) strong in swimmers.

Swimmers strive to have a long stroke as this improves propulsion but the resultant prolonged shoulder adduction and internal rotation may lead to hypovascularity of the supraspinatus muscle and increased risk of tendinopathy. This is exacerbated if hand paddles are used. Therefore, the stroke may need to be shortened to decrease injury risk. Other technique factors that predispose to impingement are an excessively straight arm during the recovery phase and insufficient body roll. Body roll also increases the efficiency of forward propulsion in freestyle and backstroke by allowing the shoulder to act in a more neutral position relative to the coronal plane, balancing the adductors and abductors.

To prevent shoulder injury in a swimmer, ensure that the athlete has adequate strength and control of the scapular stabilizing muscles and that the internal: external rotator strength ratio is normal (for the sport).[23] Ensure the athlete stretches the scapulo-humeral muscles, including the infraspinatus, teres minor and subscapularis muscles. Correct cervical and thoracic hypomobility.

When assessing swimming technique to prevent injury, the practitioner should look for good elbow height during the recovery phase of the stroke and adequate body roll. A bilateral breathing pattern increases body roll.

Common technical errors in specific swimming strokes that predispose to injury are shown in Table 5.5.

Biomechanics of tennis

Tennis places great stress on the shoulder and elbow. The shoulder receives maximal loads during the serve and overhead strokes and rotator cuff impingement may arise from a mechanism parallel to that in throwers and swimmers. The tennis service begins with 90° abduction and external rotation in the cocking phase. The shoulder then moves rapidly from external to internal rotation and from abduction into forward flexion. The deceleration or follow-through phase

is controlled by the external rotators. Impingement is exacerbated by increased internal rotation of the shoulder in forward flexion. Over 50% of the total kinetic energy and total force generated in the tennis serve is created by the lower legs, hips and trunk.

In many tennis serving motions, the feet and body are actually off the ground when this rotation reaches its maximum peak. The entire stable base of the arm, in this situation, rests on the scapula rather than on the feet or the ground. Therefore, stability of the scapula in relationship to the entire moving arm is the key point at this important time in the throwing sequence.

If we compare the biomechanics of serving to that of pitching, we find that the forces transmitted to the shoulder are lower in serving as the tennis racquet dissipates much of the impact force. This enables the tennis player to serve more than 100 times daily, whereas the pitcher can only pitch approximately every fourth day. Because of the racquet, tennis serving requires a smaller range of internal/external rotation than pitching. Nevertheless, shoulder instability may develop over time.

Tennis biomechanics and elbow pain

Elbow pain (Chapter 18) is extremely common among tennis players. This may be due to the dominant activity of the wrist extensors. Poor backhand technique is a major predisposing factor.[24] The role of racquets in the development of increased force through the elbow is discussed in Chapter 6. Commencing tennis late in life also appears to be a risk factor for elbow pain.

Tennis racquets

Tennis racquets can play an important role in injury and, although they could be categorized as a factor in tennis biomechanics, we discuss them in Chapter 6.

Table 5.5 Common technical errors in specific swimming strokes that predispose to injury

Swimming stroke	Common technical error that predisposes to shoulder injury
Butterfly	Entering the arms into the water too far outside the line of the shoulders or with the arms too close together
Backstroke	Pull-through with elbows extended, which results in a straight pull-through instead of an S-shaped pull-through Insufficient body roll
Freestyle	A line of pull-through that crosses far beyond the midline Striving for too much length in the stroke Insufficient body roll
Breaststroke	Excessive elbow extension

Biomechanics of other overhead sports

Any sport involving overhead activity may lead to the development of shoulder and elbow problems. Many of the principles of biomechanics discussed above apply to these sports. Water polo and volleyball provide the clinician with some specific challenges.

Water polo

Water polo players are particularly susceptible as the sport involves a combination of swimming and throwing. Shoulder impingement commonly occurs in association with anterior instability. Instability may be atraumatic or traumatic, for example, as a result of a block. Water polo players are susceptible to imbalance between internal and external rotators and they may have poor scapular control. Prevention of injury may be enhanced by prophylactic strengthening of the external rotators and scapular stabilizers.

Water polo players have a restricted throwing action due to the large ball size, the presence of the water and the lack of a base of support. This leads to poor throwing biomechanics—shoulder stabilizers must generate more forces and there is reduced elbow angular acceleration. They may attempt to overcome this by angling their bodies to become more horizontal in the water when shooting, thus enabling them to throw with the shoulder at 90° of abduction, reducing the likelihood of impingement.

Volleyball

The overhead spike in volleyball is associated with a high incidence of shoulder injury. The technique is similar to the throwing action. There is limitation in the amount of follow-through available with a spike due to the proximity of the net. Another potential hazard for the 'spiker' is that the spike may be blocked by an opponent. Internal and external rotator muscle balance must be maintained to prevent injury and the practitioner should also ensure that athletes have adequate scapular control.

An injury that is unique to volleyball, and results from specific biomechanics in association with an anatomical predisposition, is suprascapular nerve entrapment at the spinoglenoid notch.[25] Biomechanical and EMG studies showed that the muscle contraction pattern in players who use the 'float' serve and who have a suprascapular nerve that turns sharply after passing through the spinoglenoid notch are predisposed to traction-induced palsy of the suprascapular nerve.

Biomechanics of cycling
WITH EMMA COLSON

Cycling is unique due to the combination of extreme postural inertia of the upper and lower body together with excessive repetitious load on the lower limbs. A competitive road cyclist sits in the same position for 25–35 hours per week and cycles at a rate of 80–120 rpm, thus performing in excess of 150 000 lower limb repetitions per week. There are four main Olympic cycling disciplines: road, track, mountain bike and BMX. Within some of these disciplines, there are different events with different athlete types in competition (sprint, endurance and a mixture of both). There are also a huge variety of recreational cyclists.

As most kilometers are done on road bikes we present below the set-up basics of a road bike.

Set-up and positioning on the bike

Factors that the clinician must take into account when assessing bike set-up include seat height, seat fore/aft position and reach. When assessing set-up always ensure the cyclist has warmed up first.

Seat height

Incorrect seat height has several sequelae. If the seat is too high, power is diminished because lower limb muscles must work beyond their optimal length–tension range. Also, there is excess stress on the posterior structures (hamstrings, gastrocnemius and posterior knee joint capsule). Furthermore, compensatory excessive hip extension causes loss of the stable pelvic core.[26] In this situation, the rider often rocks the pelvis from side to side to maintain stability on the bicycle and this fatigues structures such as the adductors, gluteals, spine and even upper body musculature.

Conversely, a low seat increases knee flexion throughout the pedal cycle and increases patellofemoral and suprapatellar bursal loading.[27] It also places the hamstring, gluteal and gastrocnemius muscles in a suboptimal length–tension relationship.[26]

Measurement

- Foot at bottom stroke (Fig. 5.32a). With the elite cyclist, measurements are a guide but in the end this is the desired 'look'.
- In-seam measurement (Fig. 5.32b). A useful rough guide is the 'Le Mond' method first described by American cyclist Greg Le Mond. This measurement multiplied by a factor of 0.88 will roughly approximate the measurement of the center to top height (see Fig. 5.32c).

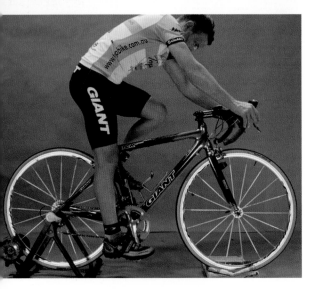

Figure 5.32 Measurement of seat height

(a) Elite rider extension of stroke

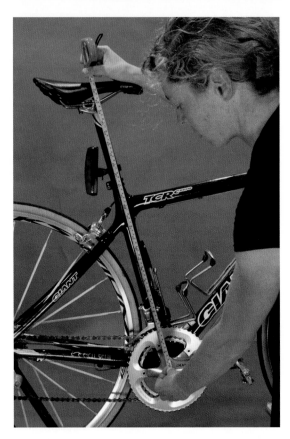

(c) Center to top measuring

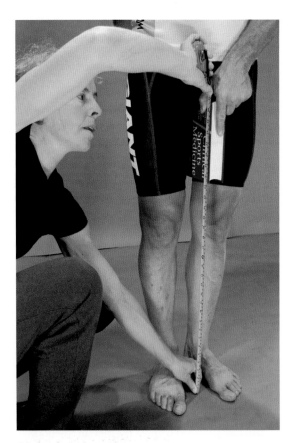

(b) In-seam measuring

- Center to top measurement (Fig. 5.32c). This height should be equal to the in-seam measurement multiplied by 0.88 (Le Mond method).

Variations to seat height measurement will be dependent upon:

- seat type and weight distribution
- cleat position—movement fore or aft will effectively alter leg length
- cleat stack height—will affect relative leg length
- personal preference—excessively plantarflexed riders might like a high seat
- seat fore/aft—a set-back seat may need to be lower
- crank length—smaller cranks will require a higher seat
- shoe thickness—thicker soles increase relative leg length
- rider experience—for the recreational cyclist or one new to the sport the first priority is the ability to safely dismount, so this type of cyclist

might ride with the seat at lower than optimum height.

Seat fore/aft position

Fore/aft position is important for knee loading.[27] A seat too far forward will result in increased patellofemoral compression forces. The seat fore/aft position also affects hip flexion and gluteal–hamstring muscle length. If the seat is too far back, the hamstring and gluteal muscles will be overlengthened, which appears to inhibit force production. If the seat is too far forward, the knees become more flexed, the hips more extended and the muscles of the lower limb are at a less than optimal length–tension relationship. In addition, the more upright position is less aerodynamic.

Seat inclination can also be varied from 0° of anterior tilt (i.e. a 'flat' seat) to about 15°, as inclination beyond this angle causes the rider to slip off the seat. Traditionally, it has been recommended that the seat be flat. A biomechanical study suggested that 10–15° of anterior inclination reduces low back pain.[28] Further study of this matter is required.

Measurement

- Plumb bolt method for saddle fore/aft measurement (Fig. 5.33). Here the bike is level and the plumb bolt is dropped from the posterior part of the tibial tuberosity to land either over the pedal axis or behind it. Landing in front of the axis will result in increased patellofemoral joint loading.

The amount of seat set-back is a personal one and will relate to the following:

- rider size—a larger cyclist will be more comfortable further back
- hip flexibility—a cyclist with poor hip range will need to be further forward
- bike handling—moving behind the bottom bracket may lighten the front end a little, which could feel unbalanced and less stable for a road bike but allow a mountain biker to lift the front and push the front wheel into corners more
- event type—time trial and triathlon cyclists are usually very far forward as they lean down and stretch out in front of the bike into an extreme aerodynamic position; this sort of riding is not comfortable for long distance, endurance training
- rider stability and flexibility—a cyclist needs flexibility and also stability to sustain a set-back seat position; this comes with years of cycling

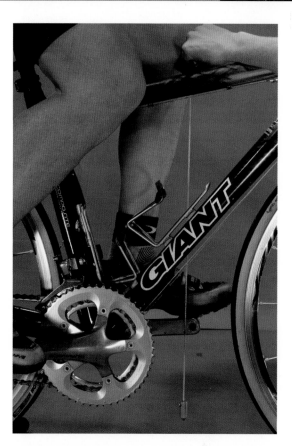

Figure 5.33 Measurement of seat fore/aft position: plumb bolt over axis

experience and can be assisted by specific exercises.

Reach

This measurement probably has the most variability with set-up. There is no measurement for reach as it will depend upon rider flexibility, experience, comfort, desired bike handling and desired aerodynamics. In Figure 5.34, it is clear that the same setting of reach can look right if the cyclist has the flexibility and control to maintain the position (Fig. 5.34a) or look wrong if the cyclist is stiff or unable to maintain the desired position (Fig. 5.34b).

Measurement

- Bar reach and drop—good positioning (Fig. 5.34a). With good positioning, the set-up allows the cyclist to attain an anteriorly tilted pelvis, a flat unkinked back, retracted scapulae, unlocked elbows and relaxed upper limbs.

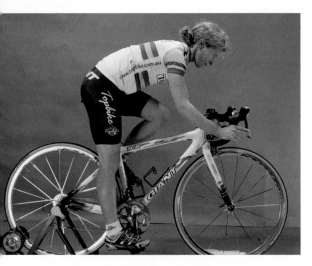

Figure 5.34 Measurement of reach

(a) Bar reach and drop—good positioning

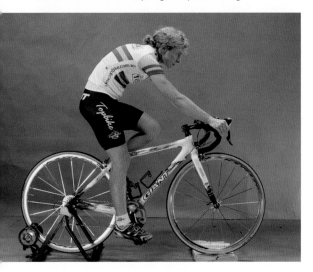

(b) Bar reach and drop—poor positioning

- Bar reach and drop—poor positioning
  (Fig. 5.34b). Poor positioning results when,
  for the same settings as those used in Figure
  5.34a, the cyclist has poor flexibility through the
  pelvis, hip and hamstrings. This pulls the cyclist
  backwards and makes the bike reach look too
  extreme.

Variations to reach will be dependent on the type
of cycling. Track riders and time trial athletes will be
very stretched out, whereas a mountain biker will
be more upright, reflecting less aerodynamic demand
and more about handling and maneuverability.

Cranks

Crank size is proportionate to trochanteric height (leg
length). In general the issue is really only for small
riders. Riders under about 165 cm (5 ft 5 in.) should
be on 170 length cranks or less. Very small riders of
160 cm (5 ft 3 in.) or less could be better on 167.5 or
even 165 cranks. If there is any issue of knee problems
in a smaller cyclist, this is one point to give early
consideration to. Conversely, very tall riders should
be on 175 cranks and those over 180 cm (6 ft) might
consider 177.5 cranks. Crank size seems unimportant
for people of average height.

Cleats/pedal interface

Cleats are the most finicky part of elite cycling. Effective force transference and hence less injury potential
is gained with a cleat with a low stack height. This
places the foot closer to the pedal.

Float has become a popular and controversial part
of cleat design. The desired outcome of float is motion
that allows the cyclist to move the foot unrestrained if
required. Getting out of the seat is one such example.
If the foot were fixed rigidly to the pedal, the knee
would be strained excessively. Float, however, should
not be confused with slop. Slop is undesired motion
of the foot while applying power to the pedals. Hence,
a good cleat design has a midpoint that the foot will
sit at most of the time with a small amount of force
required to move off that midpoint.

Cleat positioning

- Fore/aft. The cleat should allow the base of the
  first metatarsal to sit over the pedal axis. This
  facilitates maximum leverage though the foot
  (Fig. 5.35a).
- Medial and lateral. Most cleats allow adjustment
  towards the inside or outside of the shoe. Riders
  with narrow hips would place the cleats to
  the maximum outside position, thus allowing
  their legs to be close together–mimicking their
  standing alignment. Riders with wide hips or a
  wide natural stance would do the opposite.
- Rotation. In general the feet should be pointing
  straight ahead. However, if the cyclist has a
  natural toe-out position, then the cleat needs
  to be rotated in to accommodate that. Many
  cyclists ride quite comfortably hitting the crank
  with their heel slightly on each pedal stroke.

The main aim of cleat setting is to align the hip,
knee and ankle (Fig. 5.35b). However, should the
natural stance of the cyclist be poorly aligned, then
the cleats will be set to allow for this.

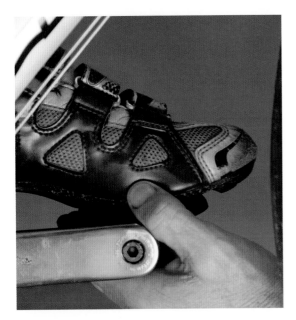

Pedal and cleat systems mostly go together. The size of the pedal platform might be relevant for very tall cyclists who find smaller cleat systems too unstable. Similarly, very small riders might find a large pedal platform reduces their foot leverage.

Cyclists with narrow hips may also have problems with the increased Q angle of some pedal systems that are set along way out from the crank. This situation is aggravated by a wide bottom bracket (on many mountain bikes) and also cranks that angle outwards at the pedal end.

Seats

Comfort on the seat is imperative to endurance cycling. Seats should be set horizontal as mentioned above. A slight downward tilt can be useful with aerobar use or for someone with limited hip motion. Seats should be narrow enough to allow the legs to pedal freely without impingement (Fig. 5.36).

Figure 5.35   (a) Cleat position. Note the therapist's thumb is over the base of the first metatarsal, which lines up with the center point of the pedal spindle

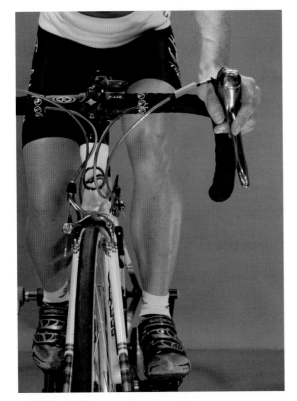

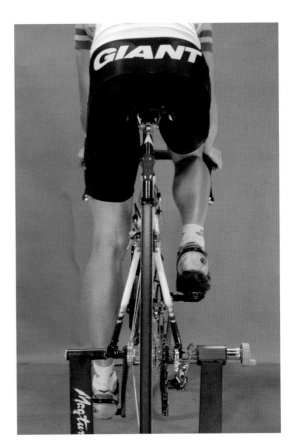

(b) Limb alignment. Note the alignment of the hip, knee and ankle

Figure 5.36 Seat width. Note how the narrow seat allows the cyclist's legs to drop down unimpeded

Shoes

Many road shoes have a poor foot bed and may require the addition of an orthosis, especially for riders with pronation. Also assess the different shoe shapes. Recreational cyclists riding 'street wear' bike shoes sacrifice rigidity and will overload the knees if they do any substantial distance in them.

Handlebars

Handlebars come in different shapes and sizes. The addition of aerobars to a road bike without any adjustment to seat position will probably create over-stretching and neck problems.

Bike set-up in other forms of cycling

Other forms of riding follow this basic bicycle set-up but alter some aspects because of the specifics of the sport. In mountain biking, the aerodynamic positioning is less important than control (depending upon the technical difficulty of the course). Thus, the rider is more upright and maneuverability of the bicycle becomes paramount. Hence, the frames tend to be small in comparison to the rider and reach is often shortened to make the front end easier to position and lift over objects. For the same reason trick/trial bikes look ridiculously small for the rider. For downhill mountain biking, power generation is not as important as stability and control, so the seat is positioned to maintain a center of gravity as low as possible. Downhill cyclists usually have another bike with a 'correct' seat set-up for fitness training as distance training with their competition bike set-up would predispose to knee problems.

For time trial, track sprinting and triathlons, the relative height of the seat to handlebars is sometimes increased to improve aerodynamics. These athletes need good flexibility and excellent stability. Aerobars are added in triathlons to enhance aerodynamics. Triathletes tend to ride with the seat positioned higher and further forward than recommended and hence 'toe' more (i.e. paddle using the toe rather than dipping the heel to plantar grade). This most likely increases the contribution of their quadriceps at the expense of underutilization of the hamstring, gastrocnemius and gluteal muscles.[26] Anecdotally, triathletes report that their hamstrings feel better for the running section after using this position in the ride.

Aerodynamics and wind resistance

Wind resistance is the primary retarding force in road cycling.[29] The single most important factor in reducing the effect of wind resistance is the front-on surface area that the cyclist exposes to the wind. This becomes particularly important for the cyclist involved in time trial events. The rider must be able to position the pelvis in an anterior tilt to flatten out the lumbar spine and so reduce his or her front-on surface area. It appears that there is a metabolic cost for the cyclist to attain such a position but this is far outweighed by the aerodynamic power savings.[30]

Road bikes are designed with this ideal in mind, and hence an inability to attain an aerodynamic posture can result in injuries. Physical assessment and rehabilitation of the road cyclist should be directed towards the cyclist attaining an efficient aerodynamic posture without placing strain on his or her body to do so. This requires flexibility, strength and motor control. Should the cyclist be unable to control a posture to fit the bike, then the setting of the bicycle needs to be modified to ensure injury-free cycling.

Pedaling technique

Motion of the pedal stroke needs to appear (and sound) smooth and continuous. Trying to create an upstroke can be injurious to the cyclist. Cleats aid proprioception to stop the foot falling off the pedal and during high-intensity pedaling.[31]

An upstroke utilizes the psoas and hamstrings at their less than optimal length–tension range and so will destabilize the pelvis, providing an ineffective base for generation of leg muscle power. The last 'up' phase of the pedal cycle is very short. It corresponds to the power phase of the opposite pedal in steady state riding. The momentum of the ascending leg and drive of the opposite leg creates a negative torque situation that drives the ascending leg through to the top stroke.

Assessment

The practitioner needs to understand the cycling discipline of the injured athlete. Athlete experience, phase of training program and current goals must be established. As always, the history of the injury is important, with special attention to recent crashes, equipment modifications, training spikes or training variations. The important components of the physical assessment are:

- body type and size—big sprinters will have very different issues to small hill climbers; very small females are often riding equipment designed for much larger people

- physical alignment (or malalignment) and how that might relate to the injury
- flexibility and stability—to attain the on-bike posture (Fig. 5.37) the cyclist needs to be flexible through:
  — arm overhead
  — thoracic spine
  — pelvis anterior tilt
  — hamstrings in tilt position
  — gluteals/hips (tightness here will affect knee tracking)
  — iliotibial band
  — knee range
  — ankle dorsiflexion range.

The cyclist also needs the appropriate muscle strength to hold the on-bike position (Fig. 5.37) and dissociation of the hip motion from the pelvis and trunk to deliver power.

Strength imbalances in cycling can result in over-loading of one leg or other regions of the body. Assessment should be made of right versus left leg, the lower nerve roots, the vastus medialis obliquus, gluteus maximus, gluteus medius, erector spinae, pelvic floor, transversus abdominis, pelvic floor, the upper body stabilizers (the retractor group) and also single leg balance and control.

Rehabilitation

The key to the management of cycling injuries is to identify and treat the cause. It is important for the cyclist to continue riding, in a modified form, if at all possible.

Rehabilitation exercises should, as much as possible, mimic the on-bike demands. Hence, working the body while maintaining an on-bike anterior tilt position is useful. Examples of important rehabilitation exercises for the cyclist are shown in Figure 5.38.

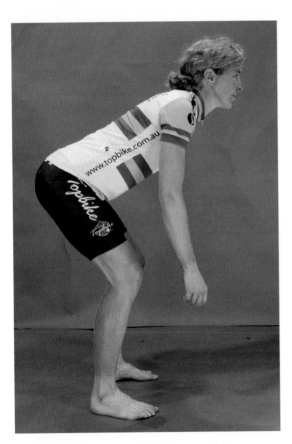

Figure 5.37 Cyclist in 'on-bike' posture. Maintenance of this posture requires both flexibility and stability. The ability to deliver power in the posture requires dissociation of the hips from a stable pelvis and trunk

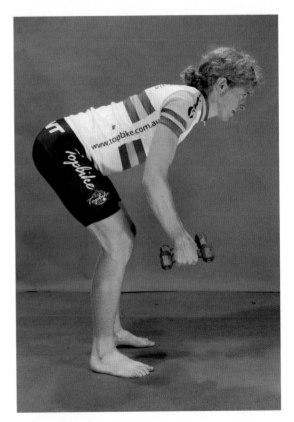

Figure 5.38 (a) Scapular strengthening exercises. Cyclists with neck problems should strengthen the scapular retractors while maintaining an anterior pelvic tilt

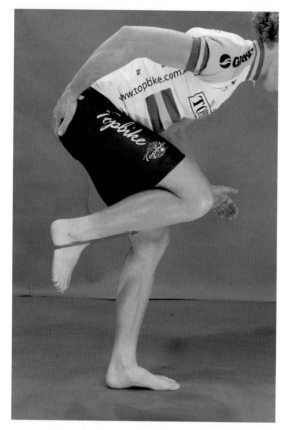

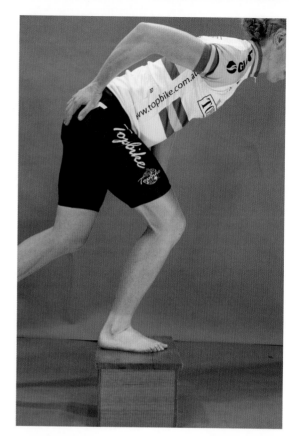

(b) Gluteal strengthening exercise. A weak gluteal muscle can be worked in this on-bike position. Thus, the rehabilitation aims of stability (holding the pelvis in single leg stance), strengthening of the gluteals and rehearsing dissociation of the limb from the pelvis are incorporated

(c) High box step-ups. Strength imbalances in the right quadriceps are addressed in this high stepping activity. The cyclist maintains an anterior tilt to mimic the on-bike position

Conclusion

An appreciation of the postural/biomechanical and physical demands of the sport of cycling will enhance the practitioner's ability to diagnose and manage cycling injuries.

Recommended Reading

Kaufman KR, Brodine SK, Shaffer RA, Johnson CW, Cullison TR. The effect of foot structure and range of motion on musculoskeletal overuse injuries. *Am J Sports Med* 1999; 27(5): 585–93.

Lang LMG, Volpe RG, Wernick J. Static biomechanical evaluation of the foot and lower limb: the podiatrist's perspective. *Man Ther* 1997; 2(2): 58–66.

Mellion MB, Burke ER. Bicycling injuries. *Clin Sports Med* 1994; 13: 1–258.

This entire issue of Clinics in Sports Medicine *is devoted to cycling and, although not a recent publication, covers subjects from bike fit and cycling physiology to injuries. Contains 14 separate chapters by various experts.*

Neely FG. Biomechanical risk factors for exercise-related lower limb injuries. *Sports Med* 1998; 26: 395–413.

A thorough review of which biomechanical factors are, and are not, risk factors for injury.

Werner SL, Plancer KD. Biomechanics of wrist injuries in sports. *Clin Sports Med* 1998; 17: 407–20.

A good overview of anatomy, biomechanics and mechanisms of injuries in various sports; 52 references.

Yates B, White S. The incidence and risk factors in the development of medial tibial stress syndrome among naval recruits. *Am J Sports Med* 2004; 32(3): 772–80.

References

1. Maloney MD, Mohr KJ, el Attrache NS. Elbow injuries in the throwing athlete. Difficult diagnoses and surgical complications. *Clin Sports Med* 1999; 18: 795–809.

2. Ounpun S. The biomechanics of walking and running. *Clin Sports Med* 1994; 13: 843–63.

3. Khan K, Roberts P, Nattrass C, et al. Measurement of lower limb range of motion in elite fulltime classical ballet dancers. *Clin J Sport Med* 1997; 7: 174–9.

4. Chan CW, Rudins A. Foot biomechanics during walking and running. *Mayo Clin Proc* 1994; 69: 448–61.

5. Winter DA, Bishop PJ. Lower extremity injury. Biomechanical factors associated with chronic injury to the lower extremity. *Sports Med* 1992; 14: 149–56.

6. Williams DS 3rd, McClay IS, Hamill J. Arch structure and injury patterns in runners. *Clin Biomech* 2001; 16: 341–7.

7. Clement DB, Taunton JE, Smart GW. Achilles tendinitis and peritendinitis. Etiology and treatment. *Am J Sports Med* 1984; 12: 179–84.

8. McCrory JL, Martin DF, Lowery RP, et al. Etiologic factors associated with Achilles tendinitis in runners. *Med Sci Sports Exerc* 1999; 31: 1374–81.

9. Williams DS, Davis I, Baitch SP. Effect of inverted orthoses on lower-extremity mechanics in runners. *Med Sci Sports Exerc* 2003; 35(12): 2060–8.

10. Astrom M, Arvidson R. Alignment and joint motion in the normal foot. *J Orthop Sports Phys Ther* 1995; 22: 216–22.

11. Crossley K, Bennell K, Green S, McConnell J. A systematic review of physical interventions for patellofemoral pain syndrome. *Clin J Sport Med* 2001; 11: 103–10.

12. Gross M, Napoli R. Treatment of lower extremity injuries with orthotic shoe inserts. *Sports Med* 1993;15: 66–70.

13. Landorf K, Keenan A. Efficacy of foot orthoses: what does the literature tell us? *J Am Podiatr Med Assoc* 2000; 90: 149–58.

14. Lynch D, Goforth W, Martin J, Odom R, Preece C, Kotter M. Conservative treatment of plantar fasciitis: a prospective study. *J Am Podiatr Med Assoc* 1998; 88: 375–80.

15. Novick A, Kelley D. Frontal plane movement changes about the rearfoot with orthotic intervention. *Phys Ther* 1992; 72: S78

16. Arroyo JS, Hershon SJ, Bigliani LU. Special considerations in the athlete throwing shoulder. *Orthop Clin North Am* 1997; 28: 69–78.

17. Harrington L. Glenohumeral joint: internal and external rotation range of motion in javelin throwers. *Br J Sports Med* 1998; 32: 226–8.

18. Kvitne RS, Jobe FW, Jobe CM. Shoulder instability in the overhand or throwing athlete. *Clin Sports Med* 1995; 14: 917–35.

19. Cavallo RJ, Speer KP. Shoulder instability and impingement in throwing athletes. *Med Sci Sports Exerc* 1998; 30: S18–S25.

20. Toyoshima S, Hoshikawa T, Miyashita M, Aguri T. Contribution of the body parts to throwing performance. *Biomechanics IV.* Baltimore: University Park Press, 1974: 169–74.

21. Kibler BW. The role of the scapula in athletic shoulder function. *Am J Sports Med* 1998; 26: 325–37.

22. Troup JP. The physiology and biomechanics of competitive swimming. *Clin Sports Med* 1999; 18: 267–85.

23. Bak K, Magnusson SP. Shoulder strength and range of motion in symptomatic and pain-free elite swimmers. *Am J Sports Med* 1997; 25: 454–9.

24. Knudson D, Blackwell J. Upper extremity kinematics of the one-handed backhand drive in tennis players with and without tennis elbow. *Int J Sports Med* 1997; 18: 79–82.

25. Ferretti A, De Carli A, Fontana M. Injury of the suprascapular nerve at the spinoglenoid notch. The natural history of infraspinatus atrophy in volleyball players. *Am J Sports Med* 1998; 26: 759–63.

26. Brown D, Kautz S, Dairaghi C. Muscle activity patterns altered during pedaling at different body orientations. *J Biomech* 1996; 29: 1349–56.

27. McLean B, Blanch P. Bicycle seat height: a biomechanical consideration when assessing and treating knee pain in cyclists. *Sport Health* 1993; 11: 12–15.

28. Salai M, Brosh T, Blankstein A, et al. Effect of changing the saddle angle on the incidence of low back pain in recreational bicyclists. *Br J Sports Med* 1999; 33: 398–400.

29. Faria I. Energy expenditure, aerodynamics and medical problems in cycling—an update. *Sports Med* 1992; 14: 43–63.

30. Gnehm P, Reichenbach S, Altpeter E, et al. Influence of different racing positions on metabolic cost in elite cyclists. *Med Sci Sports Exerc* 1997; 29: 813–23.

31. Capmal S, Vandewalle H. Torque–velocity relationships during ergometer sprints with and without toe clips. *Eur J Appl Physiol* 1997; 76: 375–9.

Principles of Injury Prevention

WITH ROALD BAHR

An important role for the sports medicine practitioner is to minimize activity-related injury, that is, to improve the benefit:risk ratio associated with physical activity and sport. There have been many advances in the field of sports injury prevention in the past decade.

Sports injury prevention can be characterized as being 'primary', 'secondary' or 'tertiary'. In this book, we use the term 'prevention' synonymously with what is technically known as 'primary prevention'.[1] Examples of primary prevention include health promotion and injury prevention (e.g. ankle braces being worn by an entire team, even those without previous ankle sprain). Secondary prevention can be defined as early diagnosis and intervention to limit the development of disability or reduce the risk of reinjury. We to refer to this as 'treatment' in this book (e.g. early RICE treatment of an ankle sprain, see Chapter 10). Finally, tertiary prevention is the focus on rehabilitation to reduce and/or correct an existing disability attributed to an underlying disease. We refer to this as 'rehabilitation' (Chapter 12); in the case of a patient who has had an ankle sprain, this would refer to wobble board exercises and graduated return to sport after the initial treatment for the sprain. The proactive clinician will initiate injury prevention strategies, give prevention advice during consultations where treatment is being sought and devise in-season strategy planning sessions with coaches and during screening of athletes (Chapter 57).

This chapter begins with a widely used model of how sports injuries occur. This is a very useful guide to ways to prevent sport injuries in a systematic manner. From there, we direct the reader to review the importance of correct biomechanics of sports for injury prevention, as outlined in Chapter 5. Then, we discuss other important factors that may assist in the prevention of injury:

- warm-up
- stretching
- taping and bracing
- protective equipment
- suitable equipment
- appropriate surfaces
- appropriate training
- adequate recovery
- psychology
- nutrition.

Systematic injury prevention

Research on sports injury prevention typically follows a sequence described by van Mechelen et al. (Fig. 6.1).[2] This conceptual model can be applied successfully by sports clinicians as well. Firstly, the magnitude of the problem must be identified and described in terms of the incidence and severity of sports injuries. If you are responsible for a team, this would involve recording all injuries within the squad, as well as training and match exposure. Secondly, the risk factors and injury mechanisms that play a part in causing sports injuries must be identified. For the clinician, this could involve systematic steps to examine the athletes and their training and competition program (see below). The third step is to introduce measures that are likely to reduce the future risk and/or severity of sports injuries. Such measures should be based on information about the etiological factors and the injury mechanisms as identified in the second step. Finally, the effect of the measures must be evaluated by repeating the first step. From

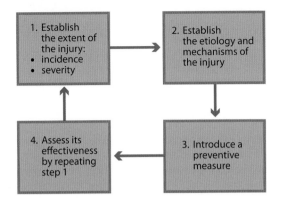

Figure 6.1 The sequence for prevention of sports injuries[2]

model not only takes into account the multifactorial nature of sports injuries, but also the time sequence of events leading to injuries.

Firstly, it considers the internal risk factors—factors that may predispose to or protect the athlete from injury. This includes athlete characteristics, factors such as age, maturation, gender, body composition and fitness level. One factor that consistently has been documented to be a significant predictor is previous injury—almost regardless of the injury type studied. Internal factors such as these interact to predispose to or protect from injury. Internal risk factors can be modifiable and non-modifiable, and both are important from a prevention point of view. Modifiable risk factors may be targeted by specific training methods. Non-modifiable factors (such as gender) can be used to target intervention measures to those athletes who are at an increased risk.

The second group of risk factors is the external factors the athletes are exposed to, for example, floor friction in indoor team sports, snow conditions in alpine skiing, a slippery surface (running track), very cold weather, or inappropriate footwear. Exposure to such external risk factors may interact with the internal factors to make the athlete more or less susceptible to injury. When intrinsic and extrinsic risk factors act simultaneously, the athlete is at far greater

a research standpoint, it is preferable to evaluate the effect of preventive measures by means of a randomized controlled trial. For the medical practitioner responsible for a team, continuous surveillance of the injury pattern within the team will reveal whether changes occur in the injury risk.

Sports clinicians who want to prevent injuries in a systematic way could base their approach on a model of potential causative factors for injury, which was first described by Meeuwisse,[3] and later expanded by Bahr and Holme[4] and Bahr and Krosshaug[5] (Fig. 6.2). The

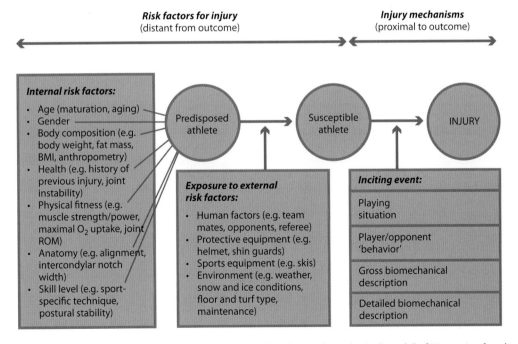

Figure 6.2 A comprehensive injury causation model based on the epidemiological model of Meeuwisse[3] and modified by Bahr and Krosshaug[5]   BMI = body mass index; ROM = range of motion

risk of injury than when risk factors are present in isolation.

The final link in the chain of events is the inciting event, which is usually referred to as the injury mechanism—what we see when watching an injury situation. Again, it may be helpful to use a comprehensive model to describe the inciting event, which accounts for the events leading to the injury situation (playing situation, player and opponent behavior), as well as includes a description of whole body and joint biomechanics at the time of injury (Chapter 5).[5] Each injury type and each sport does have its typical patterns, and for team medical staff it is important to consult the literature to reveal the typical injuries and their mechanisms for the sport in question. However, one limitation of the model is that it is not obvious how the team's training routine and competitive schedule can be taken into consideration as potential causes, and the model has therefore traditionally been mainly used to describe the causes of acute injuries. For overuse injuries, the inciting event can sometimes be distant from the outcome. For example, for a stress fracture in a long distance runner, the inciting event

is not usually the single training session when pain became evident but the training and competition program he or she has followed over the previous weeks or months.

For clinicians, this model can be used to identify potential causes of injury. The key questions to ask are: Who is at increased risk? Why? How do injuries typically occur? When caring for a defined group of athletes, such as a soccer team or an alpine skiing team, this can be done using a systematic risk management approach. Individual risk factors (and protective factors) can be mapped during the pre-season physical examination (e.g. history of previous injury, malalignment) or tested as part of the team's fitness testing program (e.g. strength, flexibility, neuromuscular control). Then it is possible to do a risk analysis to document the parts of the season when athletes are at the greatest risk of sustaining injuries as a result of the training or competitive programs (Fig. 6.3). Examples of situations in which risk increases are when athletes switch from one training surface to another (e.g. from grass to gravel) or to new types of training (e.g. at the start of a strength training period). This type of

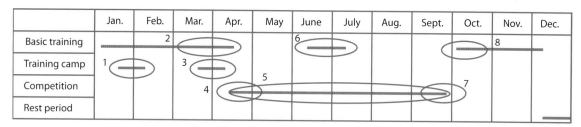

	Jan.	Feb.	Mar.	Apr.	May	June	July	Aug.	Sept.	Oct.	Nov.	Dec.
Basic training		2				6					8	
Training camp	1		3									
Competition				4	5					7		
Rest period												

Figure 6.3 Risk profile. Examples of periods of the season when a college basketball team may be at particular risk of injury. The comments below concern the risk periods that are circled:

1. Change of time zone, off-court training surface, climate, and altitude during training camp in Colorado. Emphasis on defensive stance training and quick lateral movements could lead to acute groin injuries (Chapter 23). Athletes should not increase the amount or intensity of training too much.
2. Transition to greater amount of on-court training and intensity, combined with several practise games. Floor surface quite hard. Risk of lower leg overuse injuries such as Achilles tendinopathy, shin splints.
3. New training camp to fine-tune players before beginning the competitive season; practise games on unusually slippery courts. Competition to avoid being cut from the squad leads to increased intensity during training and competition.
4. The beginning of the competitive season. A higher tempo and a packed competitive schedule to which the athlete is unaccustomed. Risk of overuse injury (e.g. patellar tendinopathy, tibial stress fracture) compounded by heavy academic program, leading to additional fatigue.
5. High risk of acute ankle and knee injuries during the competitive season and a tough competition schedule at full intensity.
6. Interposed period of hard basic training, strength exercises to which the athlete is not accustomed, and plyometric training increases risk of tendinopathy and muscle strain.
7. The end of the competitive season. Worn out and tired players? This is an important time to treat low-level 'grumbling' injuries aggressively. Waiting for the injury to heal simply with 'rest' is not recommended.
8. Transition to basic training period with running on trails.

analysis is an important basis for planning preventive measures, particularly for the purpose of avoiding overuse injuries. The analysis is based on the idea that the risk of injuries is greater during transitional periods and that each stage has certain characteristics that may increase risk. The risk profile usually varies from sport to sport. Healthcare personnel responsible for teams or training groups should do this type of analysis in collaboration with the coaches and athletes and create a plan for relevant preventive measures based on the risk analysis. In this chapter we examine strategies that are often used to ameliorate intrinsic and extrinsic sports injury risk factors or prepare the athlete for potential inciting events.

Warm-up

Warm-up prepares the body for exercise. The type of exercise to be performed determines the type of warm-up. The most effective warm-up consists of both general and specific exercises. General exercises may include jogging, general stretching and resistance exercises. Specific exercises include stretches and movements that are appropriate for the particular activity about to be undertaken.

The possible benefits of warm-up prior to physical activity include:[6-8]

- increased blood flow to muscles
- increased oxyhemoglobin breakdown, with increased oxygen delivery to muscles
- increased circulation leading to decreased vascular resistance
- increased release of oxygen from myoglobin
- enhanced cellular metabolism
- reduced muscle viscosity leading to smoother muscle contraction and increased mechanical efficiency
- increased speed of nerve impulses
- increased sensitivity of nerve receptors
- decreased activity of alpha fibers and sensitivity of muscles to stretch
- decreased number of injuries due to increased range of motion
- decreased stiffness of connective tissue leading to decreased likelihood of tears
- increased cardiovascular response to sudden strenuous exercise
- increased relaxation and concentration.

There are no data on which to prescribe intensity and duration of a warm-up. Thus, it may make sense to allow athletes to determine their own warm-up

regimen. In team sports there can be a group regimen with a built-in period of 'free warm-up'. One guideline for the intensity of the warm-up is to produce some mild sweating without fatigue. The effect of a warm-up lasts approximately 30 minutes, so it is important not to warm up too early.[6]

Several clinical studies, including a recent high-quality randomized trial,[9] have shown that structured warm-up programs designed to prevent injuries can reduce injury risk by 50% or more. However, it is not known whether it is the physiological effects of the warm-up program as described above which confer the effect on injury risk, or whether the reduced risk results from training effects on strength, neuromuscular control, technique or other factors.

Stretching

The ability to move a joint smoothly throughout a full range of movement is considered an important component of good health. There is a hereditary component to general flexibility, and specific joints or muscles may become stiff as a result of injury, over-activity or inactivity. Although increased flexibility attained through stretching was widely believed to decrease musculotendinous injuries, and minimize and alleviate muscle soreness, and perhaps even improve performance, research by Peter Magnusson and others has thrown enormous doubt on these widely held dogmas.[10-17] Such relationships are difficult to prove,[3, 6] and studies on military personnel have not shown any effect from general, systematic stretching programs on the overall injury risk.[18, 19] It is not known whether a specific stretching program to prevent a particular injury type, such as stretching the hamstrings to prevent hamstring strains, is effective. Because of the need to randomize elite athletes to a trial of 'not stretching' and 'stretching' specific muscles, and then waiting to see whether there are more injuries of that muscle in the non-stretching group, it may be difficult to obtain definitive data on the 'stretching prevents injury' hypothesis. It, does, however, seem unlikely that stretching, per se, improves performance in sports,[20-25] except in sports where range of motion is a key performance factor, such as gymnastics and diving.

Witvrouw et al.[26] have raised an interesting hypothesis that stretching may be more important for preventing injury in sports that have a high intensity of stretch–shortening cycles (e.g. football, basketball) than in sports with relatively low demands on the muscle–tendon stretch–shortening cycle (e.g. jogging, cycling, swimming).

There are two types of flexibility—static and dynamic. Static flexibility describes the degree to which joints may be passively moved to the end points of range of motion. Dynamic flexibility is the degree to which a joint can be moved as a result of muscle contraction. Low static or dynamic flexibility may be an intrinsic risk factor for some injury types.

Athletes commonly perform three different types of stretching exercises—static, ballistic and proprioceptive neuromuscular facilitation (PNF).

Static stretching

In static stretching, the stretch position is assumed slowly and gently and held for 30–60 seconds.[7] The athlete should not experience any discomfort in the stretched muscle. As the position is held, tension from the stretch becomes strong enough to initiate the inverse myotatic stretch reflex with subsequent muscle relaxation. The muscle can then be stretched a little further, again without discomfort. This increased stretch should also be held for approximately 30 seconds, then relaxed. If, during either stage of the stretch, there is a feeling of tension or pain, overstretching is occurring and this may cause injury. The athlete should ease off to a more comfortable position. Of the different types of stretches, static stretch produces the least amount of tension and is probably the safest method of increasing flexibility.

Ballistic stretching

In a ballistic stretch, the muscle is stretched to near its limit, then stretched further with a bouncing movement. The disadvantage of this stretch is that the quick bouncing causes a strong reflex muscle contraction. Stretching a muscle against this increased tension heightens the chances of injury. Therefore, this technique is not commonly used.

Ballistic stretching may be used, however, by athletes in the latter stages of a stretching program. It should be preceded by an adequate warm-up and slow static stretching. It is used particularly in gymnastics, ballet and dance where maximal range of motion is advantageous.

Proprioceptive neuromuscular facilitation stretching

PNF stretching is performed by alternating contraction and relaxation of both agonist and antagonist muscles. PNF stretching is based on the observations

that muscle relaxation is increased both after agonist contraction and antagonist muscle contraction.

There are a number of different PNF stretching techniques (Fig. 6.4). PNF stretching may produce greater flexibility gains than other stretching techniques. Its major disadvantage is that there is a tendency to overstretch. PNF stretches should ideally be performed with a partner who is aware of the potential dangers of the technique.

Principles of stretching

The basic principles of stretching are:

- warm-up prior to stretching
- stretch before and after exercise
- stretch gently and slowly
- stretch to the point of tension but never pain.

A general stretching program involving stretches of the major muscle groups is shown in Figure 6.5. Specific stretches used in the prevention or rehabilitation of specific injuries are shown in the relevant chapters in Part B.

Taping and bracing

Taping (or strapping) and bracing are used to restrict undesired, potentially harmful motion and allow desired motion. There are two main indications for the use of tape and braces:

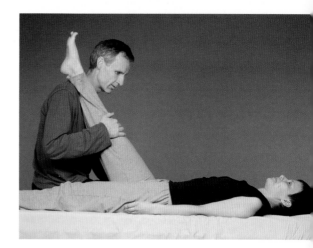

Figure 6.4 PNF hamstring stretch. The partner passively stretches the hamstring to the onset of discomfort. The athlete then performs isometric hamstring contraction against the partner's shoulder. The partner then passively stretches the hamstring further to the point of discomfort

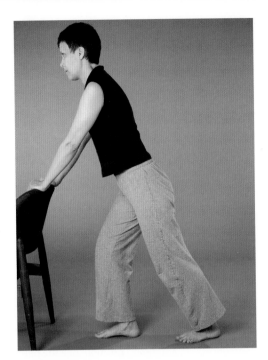

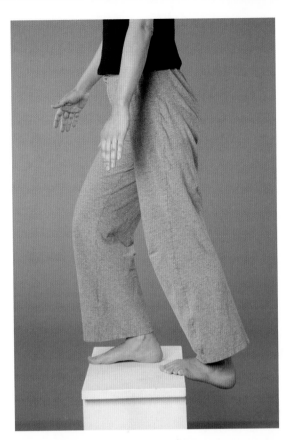

Figure 6.5 General stretching program

(a) Gastrocnemius. Pushing against a wall or fence with leg straight out behind, feeling a gentle calf stretch

(c) Calf (general). With the toes supported on a step or gutter, allow the heel to drop beneath the level of the toe. Allow gravity to impart a gentle stretch

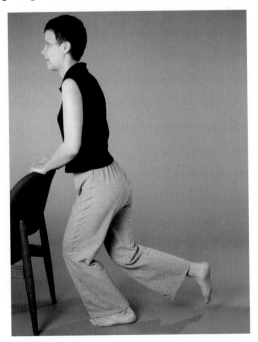

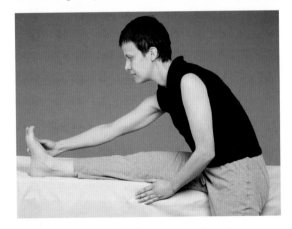

(d) Hamstring. With the leg supported on a beam or bench and keeping the leg straight, gently bend forward at the hips until a stretch is felt at the hamstring. Do not bend the back in order to get the chest closer to the knee; rather bend at the hips with the back kept straight

(b) Soleus. Supported by a wall or fence with knee flexed, bring leg to be stretched underneath body and lunge forward, again feeling a gentle steady calf stretch

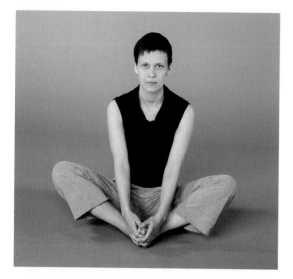

(e) Groin. Sitting on the floor with the knees flexed, soles of feet together and the back kept straight, gently push the outside of the knees towards the ground until a stretch is felt in the groin

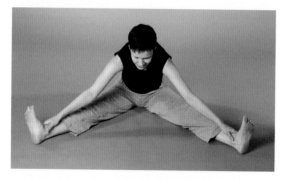

(f) Groin. Sitting on the floor with the legs straight and the hips abducted, bend forward at the hips until a stretch is felt in the groin. By bending towards either leg, this stretch can be used to stretch the hamstrings

1. prevention—taping is used as a preventive measure in high-risk activities, for example, basketball players' ankles
2. rehabilitation—taping is used as a protective mechanism during the healing and rehabilitation phases.[27, 28]

Although taping and bracing are used in the injury management of conditions in numerous joints, they have not been proven to be effective for primary injury prevention in the shoulder, elbow, knee and spinal joints. However, there is good evidence to suggest that bracing may prevent reinjuries in athletes with a history of a previous ankle sprain.

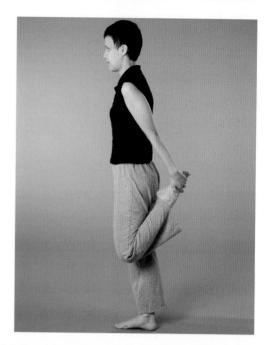

(g) Quadriceps. In a standing position, pull the heel to the buttock until a stretch is felt at the front of the thigh. The stretch can be increased if necessary by pressing the hips forward. Attempt to keep the knees together and do not rotate at the pelvis

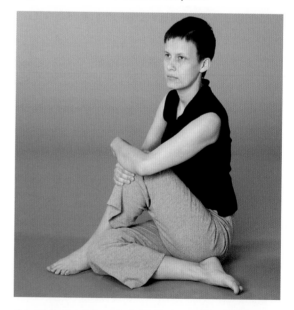

(h) Gluteals/piriformis (left). Sitting on the floor, bend the left leg up in front. Place the left heel over the thigh of the right leg and pull the left knee towards the chest, until a stretch is felt in the left gluteal region. Attempt to keep both buttocks square on the ground

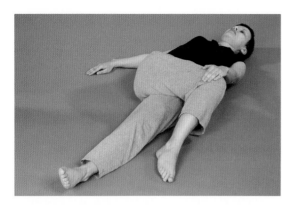

(i) Low back. Lying on the ground or the bed, bend up one knee and rotate towards the opposite side until the knee touches the floor. Keep the shoulders flat on the ground. A gentle stretch should be felt in the lower back

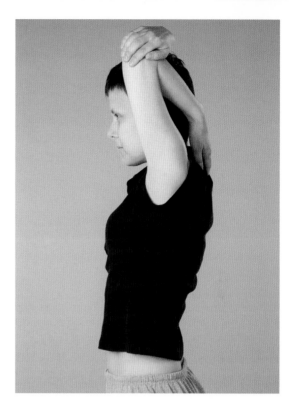

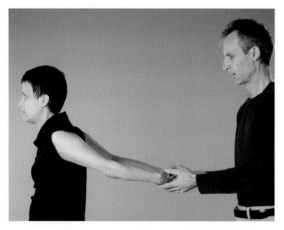

(j) Pectoral girdle. Standing or in a seated position, clasp both hands behind the back and straighten the elbows. A partner then lifts the hands gently. Keep the back straight. A stretch should be felt in the front of the shoulder and in the chest

(k) Triceps. Lifting the arm into maximum flexion and abduction, bend the elbow to its fully flexed position. Then, placing the opposite hand on the elbow, pull across and back until a stretch is felt in the triceps and shoulders

Taping

There are many different tapes and bandages available for use by athletes. However, when the purpose is to restrict undesired motion, only adhesive, non-stretch (rigid) tape is appropriate (Fig. 6.6). Elastic tape is inappropriate for restricting motion. Good tape should be adhesive, strong, non-irritant and easily torn by the therapist.

Tape is ideally applied over joints where skin sliding can be limited to one direction. The joints most suitable for taping are the ankle, wrist, finger, acromioclavicular joint and the first metatarsophalangeal joint.

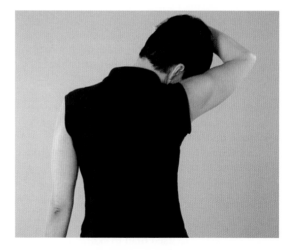

(l) Levator scapulae. To stretch the levator scapulae, place the chin on the chest and then rotate the head away from the side to be stretched. Then apply a stretch with the hand on the side of the head. A stretch should be felt in the neck and shoulder

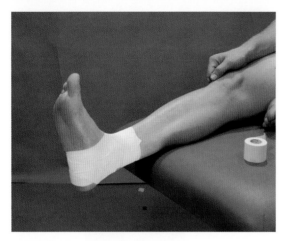

Figure 6.6 Taping application—an example of ankle taping

As well as providing mechanical support, tape may enhance proprioception. Guidelines for tape application are given below.

Preparation

- The athlete and the therapist should be in a comfortable position for tape application.
- Tailor the taping to the needs of the individual and the sport being played. It is important to provide support but not restrict essential movement.
- Injured ligaments should be held in a shortened position during taping. Ligaments that have not previously been injured should be held in neutral position.
- Shave body hair, preferably at least 8 hours prior to tape application to avoid skin irritation.
- Clean skin, remove grease and sweat.
- Apply an adhesive skin spray prior to taping, especially if sweating is likely to reduce the adhesiveness of the tape.
- Use an underwrap if a skin allergy exists.
- Care should be taken with the use of non-stretch tape around swollen joints.
- Use tape of appropriate width.

Application

- Use anchors proximally and distally, as tape adheres better to itself than to skin.
- Unroll the tape before laying it upon the skin to ensure correct tension.
- Apply even pressure.
- Overlap the previous tape by one-half to ensure strength and even application.

- Smooth out all folds and creases to prevent blisters and lacerations.
- If discomfort is present after tape application, adjust the tape.

Removal

- Remove tape carefully with the use of tape cutters or tape scissors.

Complications

Complications of tape application include reduced circulation from tight taping, skin irritation due to mechanical or allergic phenomena, and decreased effectiveness of tape with time. Tape provides substantial material support but, as with any material, does have a threshold where it fails.[29] It may be necessary to reapply tape at a suitable break during the athletic activity, for example, at half-time. Tape application requires practise to perfect technique.

Bracing

Bracing has several advantages over taping. An athlete can put a brace on by himself or herself and although the initial cost of a brace may be high, a good quality, strong brace will last a considerable time and may prove to be cheaper than repeated taping.

Bracing also has a number of disadvantages. These include possible slipping of the brace during use, the weight of the brace, problems with exact sizing and the risk of the brace wearing out at an inopportune moment. Sometimes it may be necessary for braces to be custom-made.

A number of different types of braces are available. Heat-retaining sleeves are commonly used in the treatment of many chronic inflammatory conditions. These sleeves are commonly made out of neoprene. The neoprene support offers increased warmth and comfort over the affected area and may improve proprioception but provides little or no mechanical support. The sleeves are available for most joints and muscles. Increased mechanical support can be gained by the use of harder material or the addition of straps or laces. Certain braces are used only to restrict movement, such as a hinged knee brace (Fig. 6.7).[30–32]

Braces can be custom-made by molding thermoplastic material over the affected part. Such splints are commonly used in the hand and wrist, particularly over the first carpometacarpal joint after a Bennett's fracture or at the first metacarpophalangeal joint after a hyperextension sprain or ulnar collateral ligament sprain (Fig. 6.8).

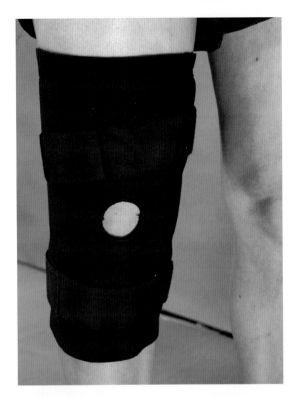

Figure 6.7 Hinged knee brace

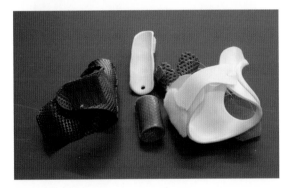

Figure 6.8 Molded braces

Protective equipment

Protective equipment has been designed to shield various parts of the body against injury without interfering with sporting activity. Protective equipment can also be used on return to activity after injury in situations where direct contact may aggravate the injury.

Helmets are mandatory in certain sports such as motor racing, motor cycling, cycling, ice hockey, horse riding and American football (Fig. 6.9). In other sports the use of helmets is not universally accepted, such

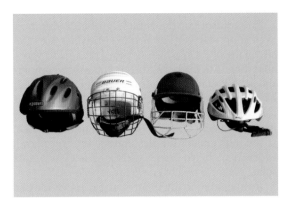

Figure 6.9 Helmets

as in rugby football and skateboarding. The role of helmets, and face shields[33] in protection against head injuries is discussed in Chapter 13.

Other protective equipment commonly worn includes: mouthguards in most collision sports; shoulder pads in American and rugby football; chest, forearm and groin protectors in ice hockey; knee pads when playing on artificial surfaces or while rollerblading; wrist guards in rollerblading and snowboarding; and shin pads in soccer and hockey. It is important that protective equipment fits correctly. Protective equipment may provide a psychological benefit by increasing a player's confidence.

Suitable equipment

Running shoes, football boots, ski boots and tennis racquets are important elements that contribute to, or prevent, sports injuries.

Running shoes

The sports clinician must be able to assess foot type and advise athletes on the type of shoe most suited to their needs. The optimum shoe for a runner is one that matches the runner's specific mechanical features. Several features of shoes may affect foot function. The first part of the shoe to be considered is the heel counter, the upper rear part of the shoe. The heel counter should be made of rigid, firm plastic to assist in rear foot stability.[34]

Forefoot flexibility (Fig. 6.10a) must be adequate to allow easy motion of the foot flexing at toe-off. With a rigid sole, the calf muscles may need to perform extra work in order to plantarflex the foot during propulsion. A shoe with a lack of flexibility in the forefoot may help the individual with metatarsalgia (Chapter 35).

The midsole of the shoe is probably the most important feature (Fig. 6.10b). Midsoles are usually made of EVA, which is light and a good shock absorber. The midsole houses the more complex shock-absorbing materials such as gel pads and air bladders. The most important feature of the midsole is its density (durometer). It should be appropriately firm or soft depending on the mechanics and weight of the individual. Midsoles that are too soft permit excessive mobility, whereas firmer ones allow a more stable platform and often extended wear.

Runners requiring control of excessive motion should use a midsole of dual density that is harder on the medial aspect of the foot (Fig. 6.10c). Runners requiring extra shock absorption should choose a shoe with a soft midsole that still provides lateral stability. Maximum impact forces vary little in magnitude between soft and hard midsoles but the maximal forces occur at a later stage in the soft shoes.

Midsoles that are flared promote rapid and excessive pronation of the foot and should be avoided. This negative aspect of lateral flaring outweighs the advantage of decreased impact forces.

Last construction refers to the method used to join the upper of the shoe to the midsole. Shoes are generally slip lasted where the upper is sewn together and glued directly to the sole. This promotes shoe flexibility but may reduce stability. Stroebel lasting is a technique whereby canvas or foam is perimeter-stitched to the base of the upper and then glued to the midsole. This lasting technique became popular when manufacturers replaced the fiber boards with rigid plates lodged directly in the midsole to increase torsional rigidity. Last construction, once the primary feature in footwear design, is now seen as a prime factor influencing the fit of a shoe (Fig. 6.10d) but it has

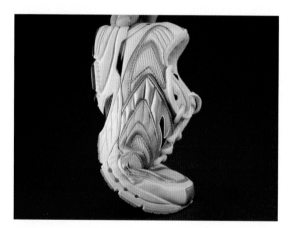

Figure 6.10 Characteristics of a running shoe

(a) Forefoot flexibility

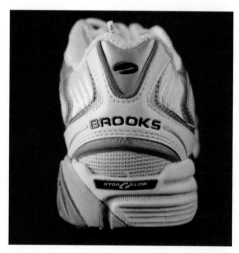

(c) Midsole: dual density. Medial side of the midsole is harder than the lateral side. This promotes stability

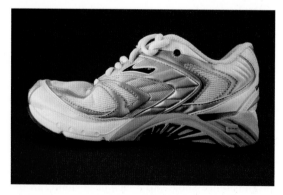

(b) Midsole: this is the part between the upper and the outsole

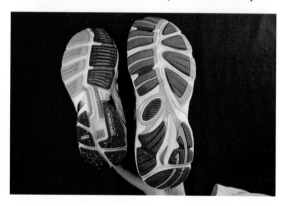

(d) Last shape. Shoe on the left is straight while shoe on the right is curved

little influence on mechanics and foot function. There is no evidence to support the commonly held view that the shape of a shoe influences foot function.

There is a range of last shapes available in today's shoe market. It is important that the athlete is fitted by a professional and is comfortable with the 'feel' of the running shoes before they are purchased. Note that footwear brands differ in their construction.

A summary of the recommended features of the running shoe for different foot types is shown in Table 6.1.

 There is no optimal running shoe, per se. However, certain shoes are optimal for an individual.

Running spikes

Poorly designed running spikes may contribute to foot and lower limb injuries but there is a dearth of published literature in this field. The majority of running spikes are designed so that the spike plate is plantar grade in relation to the heel. When running on a flat surface the heel lift is negligible and, thus, the heel is lower than the forefoot, which we call 'negative heel' (Fig. 6.11). This phenomenon is the opposite of a heel 'raise', as used in the treatment of Achilles' problems.

When running in spikes, the athlete strikes the ground on the forefoot and midfoot with the heel off the ground. The heel does not usually make contact with the ground while running at or near top speed. However, at lesser speeds, as the body weight moves over the foot, the foot lowers to the ground with little stability due to the negative heel.

The calf muscles may be subject to greater eccentric load due to the negative heel lift as the tibia is required to dorsiflex over the foot through a greater range. In addition, the small heel provides little stability for the eccentric lowering of the heel by the calf muscles. These factors may predispose to the development of Achilles tendinopathy and shin pain in runners, as well

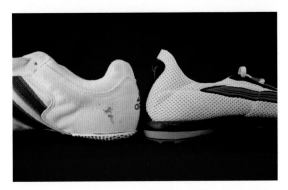

Figure 6.11 Running spikes with negative heel (left) compared with modified heel lifted with EVA material (right)

as increasing the amount of compensatory pronation and midtarsal joint dorsiflexion. Running spikes may be modified to provide more stability by increasing the heel lift and balancing the shoe (Fig. 6.11).

Football boots

Football boots (Fig. 6.12) require all the features of a good running shoe in addition to features that will allow kicking and rapid changes of direction, particularly on soft surfaces.

The construction of many types of football boots provides inadequate support for the lower limb. Common structural features found in football boots and the problems associated with each particular feature are summarized in Table 6.2.

The ideal football boot should be of adequate foot depth in the upper, have a rigid heel counter, have sufficient forefoot flexibility, have a wide sole, be slightly curved in shape and the 'stops' or cleats should be placed to allow adequate forefoot flexibility.

Ski boots

Generally, ski boots have become stiffer. However, a stiff ski boot does not allow adequate compensatory

Table 6.1 Shoe features appropriate for different foot types

Shoe features	Excessive pronator	Normal	Excessive supinator
Heel counter	Rigid	Rigid	Rigid
Forefoot flexibility	Yes	Yes	Yes
Midsole density	Hard dual density	Intermediate	Soft
Last construction	Combination	Slip or combination	Slip
Shape of last	Straight or slightly curved	Slightly curved	Curved or slightly curved

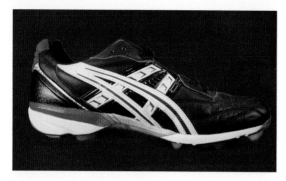

Figure 6.12 Football boots

(a) Midsole cushioned boot

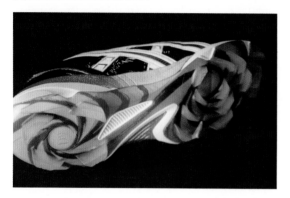

(b) Thermoplastic outsole with cleats designed to enhance rotation

movement at the midtarsal and subtalar joint and places additional stress on the bones and joints of the lower limb. More advanced skiers require stiff boots. Ski boots should be individually fitted and boots are available that allow individual molding to the shape of the skier's foot.

During skiing, control is maintained by pronating the foot to edge the downhill ski into the slope. Skiers who have certain biomechanical abnormalities (e.g. forefoot varus, rear foot varus) already have their foot fully pronated in a flat position in the boot. This forces the skier to internally rotate the lower limb and adopt a valgus knee position to maintain edge control. This may lead to inefficient skiing, fatigue and medial knee pain.

Excessive foot pronation may be corrected with an orthosis placed in the ski boot to restore the foot to a neutral position. As the degree of correction possible with orthoses is limited by boot fit, additional control is sometimes required by the use of canting or wedging of the underside of the boot. These changes to the boot may affect the release mechanism of the binding.

Most equipment-related skiing injuries occur when the ski acts as a lever to turn or twist the lower leg, and many can be prevented with appropriate binding release. Beginners are particularly at risk as they have relatively tighter bindings and boots and bindings of lower quality than the intermediate level skier.[35, 36]

Tennis racquets

In tennis, the impact between ball and racquet produces a significant amount of force, and how much force reaches the tennis player's arm depends on how hard the player swings, the speed of the incoming ball, where on the racquet face the ball is struck, the qualities of the racquet, the string tension and the stroke mechanics.

Table 6.2 Problems associated with certain structural features of football boots

Structural features	Associated problems
Soft heel counter	Decreased rear foot support
Narrow heel counter	Heel irritation
Reinforced rigid heel counter	Heel friction and irritation (especially on bony prominences)
Outsole in two pieces	Decreased midfoot stability
Narrow sole (width)	Decreased stability Skin lesions—blisters
Curved shape	Decreased stability/poor fit
Rigid sole	Decreased forefoot flexibility
Shallow upper	Decreased stability/poor fit
'Stop'/cleat placement	Often at point of forefoot flexibility Sometimes causes pain under first metatarsophalangeal joint

Each racquet has an area where the initial shock is at a minimum—the center of percussion or 'sweet spot'. When the ball is hit in the sweet spot, the shot feels good. If the ball is not hit in the sweet spot, there is increased shock transmitted to the hand, wrist and elbow.

The major factor in the etiology of tennis-related elbow pain is incorrect stroking technique, especially the backhand drive. However, the characteristics of the racquet may also contribute. The older style wooden racquets were heavy and flexible, both of which reduced shock on impact. The modern wide-body racquets are lighter and stiffer in order to generate increased power but these racquets do not absorb the shock of impact as well as wooden racquets.

There are a number of ways of altering the tennis racquet to reduce the shock at impact and lessen the force transmitted to the player's arm:

- lower string tension
- increase flexibility of the racquet
- increase the size of the racquet head
- increase the weight (add lead tape to head and handle)
- increase the grip size (Fig. 6.13)
- grip higher on the handle of the racquet.

The tennis player should choose the largest comfortable grip size (Fig. 6.13). A larger grip size prevents the player gripping the racquet too tightly. Players should also be encouraged to loosen their grip on the racquet. It is only necessary to squeeze firmly on the grip during the acceleration phase of the stroke.

Appropriate surfaces

The surface on which sportspeople play is under the spotlight as it may be a major contributor to injury risk through excessive shoe–surface traction. This possibility was proposed as a mechanism for anterior cruciate ligament (ACL) rupture in European handball as early as 1990,[37] and has later been examined in a large, epidemiological study where the ACL injury rate was compared between two different floor types—wooden floors (parquet, generally having lower friction) and artificial floors (generally having higher friction).[38] These results indicated that the risk of ACL injury among female team handball players is higher on high-friction artificial floors than on wooden floors. However, other factors also have a significant role in shoe–surface friction, principally shoe type and floor maintenance.

In Australian football, Orchard and colleagues[39] noted the greater rate of ACL injuries in the northern

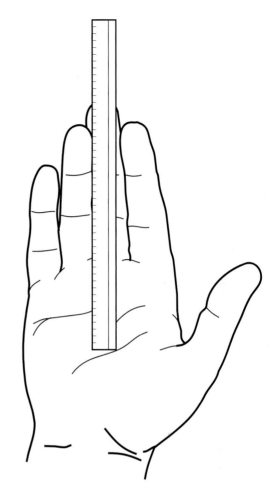

Figure 6.13 Grip size. Optimal racquet grip circumference should equal the distance from the proximal palmar crease to the tip of the ring finger

(warmer) climes. Although it was tempting to attribute this to hotter weather, thus leading to drier, harder ground,[40] that hypothesis was not supported by data from American football teams where games were played on natural grass. Further analysis of both the Australian and the US data suggested that the type of grass itself and, thus, the tightness of the thatch, may influence ACL risk; the more northern Australian venues had types of grass that permitted excessive shoe–surface traction (Fig. 6.14).

According to turf authority McNitt,[41] perennial rye grass is associated with lower shoe–surface traction than Kentucky blue grass or bermuda grass because it creates less thatch. These studies suggest that rye grass generally offers a safer surface with respect to ACL injuries for football than some other grasses.

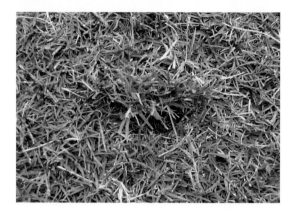

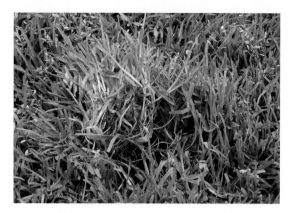

Figure 6.14 Four different types of grasses that provide the surface for Australian Rules football and have been associated with different rates of ACL injury.

(a) Bermuda ('couch') grass surface, showing a thick thatch layer between grass leaves and soil

(d) Annual blue grass surface, showing a moderate thatch layer

WITH PERMISSION FROM ORCHARD ET AL. 2005[39]

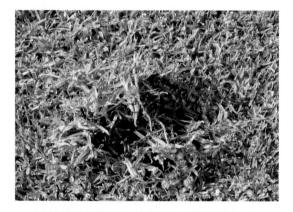

(b) Kikuyu grass, also showing a thick thatch layer

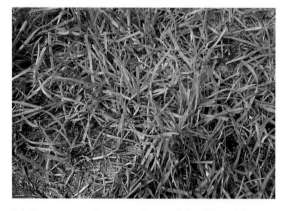

(c) Rye grass surface, showing a minimal thatch layer. This is probably a safer surface than the others as the blades or cleats of the football boot are less likely to be 'gripped' by the surface

To prevent all possible injuries, it is important to consider playing surface hardness because of its association with overuse injuries such as stress fractures, shin pain and tendinopathy. A hard surface such as concrete generates greater force through the musculoskeletal system than a forgiving surface such as grass. Sporting activities can generate extremely high loads that may, or may not, be modulated by the surface. Maximal impact forces during walking have been shown to approach twice body weight, during running three to four times and during jumping five to 12 times.[42]

Appropriate training

It is essential for sports clinicians to understand the different elements of training and their possible relationship to injury. This familiarity facilitates clinicians obtaining a full training history from an injured athlete or learning about the longer term training strategy from a coach. This makes it possible to determine where training error occurred and to take active steps to prevent this recurring.

Principles of training

'Training' is the pursuit of activity that will ultimately lead to an increase in performance in a given sport. A number of general principles of training apply to all sports:

- periodization
- specificity
- overload
- individuality.

Periodization

Periodization is an important component of all training programs, both in the long term and short term. Training can be divided into three distinct phases: conditioning (preparation), pre-competition (transitional) and competition.

The conditioning phase emphasizes developing aerobic and anaerobic fitness, strength and power. Often during this period, the athlete is 'training tired' and if required to compete would probably perform poorly. During the pre-competition phase of training, the emphasis switches from pure conditioning to technique work. During the competition phase, the emphasis is on competitive performance while maintaining basic conditioning (Table 6.3).

In many sports, for example, basketball, football and hockey, a four to six month competition season is usual. In some instances, an athlete is required to undertake two periods of competition in the one year. A suggested program for athletes in these types of sports is shown in Figure 6.15. In other instances, the competition period may last as long as eight to 10 months and conditioning work must extend into the competitive season. However, the same principles of training apply. The athlete should aim for a peak performance at a predetermined time in a competitive season, such as a specific championship or final.

To ensure complete recovery from the physical and mental stress of competition, adequate time should be allowed between the end of one season and the start of the next. This period may last four to six weeks.

In the intermediate time frame, it is important to introduce easy weeks into the training program; these give the athlete time to recover (Chapter 7) and diminish the risk of injury. During these easy weeks, the volume and intensity of training may be decreased and the opportunity may be taken to test the athlete's

Table 6.3 Different types of training are performed during the three phases of the yearly cycle

Training phase	Aerobic training	Anaerobic training	Plyometrics training	Weight training	Technique training	Competition
Preparation/ conditioning	+++	++	++	+++	+	−
Transitional/ pre-competition	++	+++	++	++	+++	−
Competition	+	+	−	+	++	+++

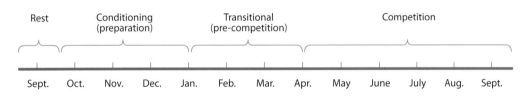

Figure 6.15 Periodization of training

(a) Team sports (e.g. basketball) with five to six month season

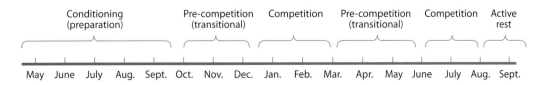

(b) Eighteen month program for an athlete who wishes to peak twice in that period

progress in the form of a time trial, mini competition or practise match. The optimal spacing of these easy weeks is probably every third or fourth week.

In the short term, the training program must allow for adequate recovery between training sessions. For example, an athlete whose training program involves weight training, aerobic and anaerobic training as well as technique work might plan to combine aerobic work with a weight session and technique work with an anaerobic session. A suggested weekly program for such an athlete is shown in Table 6.4.

Overload

Overload is a variable that athletes and coaches manipulate to allow the athlete to perform work at a greater intensity or to perform a greater volume of work at a given intensity, or to decrease recovery time between efforts of a given volume and intensity.

Overload principles include the following:

- Apply stress to the body over and above that which is normally encountered.
- If increased stress is not excessive and adequate adaptation time is allowed, the work capacity of the athlete will be increased ('supercompensation').
- Allow adequate recovery time to produce a training effect.

- Increase training load by changing the volume (quantity or duration) or the intensity (quality) of training.
- Only increase volume or intensity at any particular time (increases in volume should precede increases in intensity).
- Progress new training activities slowly so as not to cause injury to muscle groups and joints unaccustomed to that activity.
- Titrate overload to maximally improve performance without incurring injury (this is an art!).
- Monitor the athlete closely for signs of decreased performance or overtraining (Chapter 52).

Specificity

Specificity refers to the principle of directing training to performance in the athlete's given sport. It is important, therefore, to identify the most important components of fitness for each particular sport and tailor the athlete's training towards improving these particular components. There is no advantage for a power athlete in doing large amounts of endurance training, nor for an endurance athlete to spend considerable time on strength training. Some sports, for example, football, require both strength and endurance training.

Table 6.4 Suggested three-weekly cycle for a track and field athlete[a]

Week	1	2	3
Monday	Jog Weights	Jog Weights (pyramid)	Jog Test bench press Light weights
Tuesday	Interval	6 × 120 m Technique Plyometrics	2 × 150 m (timed) Technique
Wednesday	Jog Weights	Jog Weights (pyramid)	Jog Test power clean Light weights
Thursday	Interval (e.g. 4 × 300 m) Plyometrics	400 m + 300 m + 200 m + 100 m Technique	1 × 300 m (timed) Technique
Friday	Jog Weights	Jog Weights	Jog Gymnastics Swim
Saturday	Interval (e.g. 6 × 100 m)	4 × 200 m	6 × 20 m
Sunday	Rest	Rest	Rest

(a) For example, a pole vaulter, whose training requires aerobic and anaerobic training, weight training, plyometrics and technique work. The third week of the cycle is a 'recovery week'.

Individuality

As individual differences between athletes are great, training must be tailored to the individual's needs. Individuals differ in their tolerance of particular training loads, response to specific training stimuli, speed of recovery, psychological make-up, nutritional intake and lifestyle habits. Individual responses to training are influenced by previous training history, age, current state of fitness and genetic make-up.

Training methods

Types of training include endurance or aerobic training, anaerobic training, strength and power training, flexibility training, speed and agility training, specific skill training and cross-training.

Aerobic training

Aerobic training is performed to increase aerobic capacity or fitness. The aerobic capacity of an individual is the ability to utilize the body's glycogen stores via the aerobic metabolic pathway. An individual's aerobic capacity is measured by the maximum oxygen consumption, better known as the Vo_{2max}—the maximum amount of oxygen an individual is able to utilize in one minute per kilogram of body weight. This can be measured in the laboratory by exercising the individual to exhaustion and directly measuring the amount of oxygen consumed and carbon dioxide produced. From this procedure, the maximum amount of oxygen consumed can be determined accurately. A simpler, but less exact, method known as 'the predicted Vo_{2max}' is estimated by measuring the heart rate at a specific workload. This predicted Vo_{2max} is commonly performed in health and fitness centers. Alternatively, the rating of perceived exertion (RPE) can also be measured at a series of submaximal workloads so that the maximal workload predicted to occur at a maximal RPE of 20 units can be estimated. Although the athlete is unable to monitor oxygen consumption directly during training he or she can monitor heart rate or RPE or both, which correlates well with oxygen consumption during submaximal activity. Thus, heart rate or RPE can be used to monitor the intensity of aerobic training (see box).

In muscle, aerobic activity increases mitochondrial number and activity, glycogen storage, ability to use free fatty acids and vascularity. Cardiovascular effects include decreased heart rate and blood pressure with increased cardiac stroke volume and improved endothelial function.[43]

Guide to aerobic training

Aerobic training effects occur while maintaining a heart rate of between 70% and 85% of the maximum heart rate.

Maximum heart rate is estimated by subtracting the age of the athlete from 220 (e.g. a 30-year-old athlete has a maximum heart rate of approximately 190 (220 − 30). The ideal range of heart rate for a 30-year-old to gain an aerobic effect would, therefore, be between 135 and 160 beats per minute.

Anaerobic training

Anaerobic exercise utilizes the anaerobic (oxygen independent, i.e. without the need for oxygen) metabolism of glucose to produce energy. This pathway utilizes ATP as its energy substrate and, as a result, produces less energy per molecule of glucose utilized than does aerobic exercise.

Anaerobic training improves the capacity to maintain a high rate of power production for short durations of exercise at very high intensities. This requires that muscle recruitment and muscle contractile function be better maintained after training so that the onset of fatigue is developed. This may result, in part, from the increased efficiency of the body's anaerobic metabolism while also improving its tolerance of lactic acidosis. The level of discomfort experienced in training correlates well with measured serum lactate concentrations. Physiologists and coaches regularly measure blood lactate concentrations during training to assess progress. This usually occurs in submaximal exercise where the blood lactate concentration is plotted against speed of movement (e.g. in swimming, rowing, running, cycling). However, many other variables probably contribute to the superior performance seen after 'anaerobic' training.

The concept of maximum oxygen consumption (Vo_{2max}) and lactic acidosis limiting athletic performance is currently undergoing critical evaluation.[44-46] The 'classic' model of Hill, which still enjoys support among a substantial number of exercise physiologists, suggests that:

1. progressive muscle hypoxia limits maximal exercise performance; as a result, the main determinant of exercise performance is the heart's ability to supply sufficient blood (and oxygen) to the exercising muscles
2. anaerobiosis (lack of muscle oxygen) secondary to the inability to further increase the cardiac output (producing a 'plateau' in cardiac output)

explains the onset of lactate production by skeletal muscle at the 'anaerobic threshold'
3. mitochondrial adaptation in the exercising muscles alone explains changes in performance with endurance training.

This model has been challenged with the contemporary, but certainly not universally accepted, model of Timothy Noakes, the South African physician and exercise physiologist. Noakes' data refute the classic model and he concludes that skeletal muscle recruitment and contractile function are regulated by a hierarchy of controls (conceptually 'the governor') specifically to prevent damage to any number of different organs.[46–52] He argues that, according to the Hill model in which a plateau in cardiac output precedes the development of skeletal muscle anaerobiosis and lactic acidosis, the first organ to be threatened by the plateau in cardiac output would be the heart, not skeletal muscle. The plateau in cardiac output would prevent any further increase in blood flow to the heart, leading to myocardial ischemia, the onset of chest pain (angina pectoris) and heart failure. He also provides evidence that this was, in fact, the belief of the early exercise physiologists, including Hill in England and Dill at the Harvard Fatigue Laboratory in the United States, and was a central component of their teachings. Hill conceived the presence of a 'governor' in either the heart or the brain that would reduce heart function as soon as myocardial ischemia developed. Noakes and colleagues have extended this interpretation to suggest that the governor exists in the central nervous system, hence the central governor, and that it responds to the input of multiple sensory inputs from all the organs in the body. In response to those inputs the central governor regulates the number of motor units that can be recruited in the exercising limbs, reducing or limiting the number that can be recruited when their continued recruitment, necessary to maintain the work output or exercise intensity, threatens whole-body homeostasis. Hence, Noakes suggests that during maximal exercise the progressive myocardial ischemia that precedes skeletal muscle anaerobiosis must be prevented so that 'neither the heart nor the skeletal muscle develop irreversible rigor and necrosis with fatal consequences'. The reader is directed to the publications that summarize this argument to date.[46–48, 50–52]

Irrespective of the theoretical background that underpins the physiology, the most efficient method of increasing anaerobic fitness is to undertake a form of intermittent exercise or interval training. Interval training involves a number of bouts of exercise that are separated by periods of rest or recovery. The principle of such training is to achieve a level of lactic acidosis with one individual effort and then allow the body to recover from its effects before embarking on another bout of exercise. There is scope for enormous variation in the intensity and duration of the exercise bouts and the duration of the recovery period.

Interval training must be activity-specific. It is also important to note that interval training is only one component of an athlete's training, often undertaken in conjunction with an aerobic program. Because of its increased intensity, the potential for injury or accelerated chronic fatigue while undertaking interval training is relatively greater than for aerobic training.

Strength and power training

Muscular strength is the amount of force that may be exerted by an individual in a single maximum muscular contraction. Power is the maximum amount of work an individual can perform in a given unit of time. Both of these qualities are inherent to many athletic pursuits; therefore, the development of muscular strength and power is an important component of training.

Muscular strength may be increased by utilizing one of three different resistance training techniques. These are summarized in the box.

Isotonic strength training

Isotonic strength training is a commonly utilized strength technique.

- It may be concentric (in which the muscle shortens as it contracts to move a weight) or

---

Three different resistance training techniques

1. Isotonic ('same rate of contraction') exercise: resistance to movement is constant and the speed of movement is varied.
2. Isokinetic ('same speed of movement') exercise: a muscle group contracts to move through a range of motion at a constant speed with variable resistance. To achieve this, the resistance must be increased as the movement progresses (i.e. with an isokinetic machine).
3. Isometric ('same length', i.e. muscle does not change length) exercise: maximal muscular contraction against immovable resistance.

eccentric (in which the muscle contracts as it lengthens) or utilize a combined movement.

- Resistance can be provided by free weights, rubber bands, pulleys, weight machines or the individual's own body weight.
- Examples include the bench press, the dumbbell curl, the power squat and the calf raise.

The advantages of isotonic weight training over isometric and isokinetic techniques include:

- tend to be more functional, natural movements
- athlete can observe the work being done as the weight is lifted
- may be performed over a full range of movement or, alternatively, over a specific limited range of movements
- athlete/coach can measure the amount of weight lifted and the number of repetitions performed.

The potential dangers of isotonic weight training include:

- athletes require adequate supervision in the gymnasium
- athlete should never attempt to lift a maximal weight without a 'spotter'—an assistant who is able to help the athlete if problems arise
- isotonic machines such as the Universal or Nautilus machines may provide a safe alternative to free weights but these machines limit the range of motion and are unable to provide truly constant resistance through the lift.

Isotonic exercises in which the body weight of the individual is used as resistance are also safer than free weights and are often more convenient to perform. Exercises such as sit-ups, push-ups and chin-ups can be done almost anywhere and require no supervision. However, it is difficult to increase the resistance of the exercise and the only way to increase the effort is to increase the number of repetitions performed.

Isokinetic and isometric strength training

Because of the need for specialized equipment, the use of isokinetic training by athletes is usually limited to rehabilitation from injury (Chapter 12). Isometric training is usually discouraged because it develops strength in a very small range of motion but it is used in rehabilitation after injury where range of motion may be restricted.

Olympic-type weightlifting

Olympic-type weightlifting is often used as part of a strength training program. Olympic lifting involves the lifting of a weight from the floor to a position above the ground. The Olympic-type lifts are the power clean, snatch, and clean and jerk. These lifts exercise a greater number of muscle groups than conventional weightlifting, exercising them both concentrically and eccentrically. The potential for injury is high and athletes must learn correct lifting techniques before attempting large weights. It is advisable to wear a weight belt to prevent back injuries. Because of the explosive nature of the lift, Olympic-type lifting is an excellent means for improving power as well as strength.

Plyometric training

Another technique of increasing power is plyometric training. Plyometric exercises (plyometrics) use the natural elastic recoil elements of human muscle and the neurological stretch reflex to produce a stronger, faster muscle response. Plyometrics is a form of resistance training that combines a rapid eccentric muscle contraction followed by a rapid concentric contraction to produce a fast forceful movement. It must be performed in conjunction with a resistance training program as athletes need to have minimum basic strength levels before commencing plyometrics.

There are a number of plyometric exercises available. These include hopping and bounding drills, jumps over hurdles and depth jumps (see Fig. 11.18). All of these activities emphasize spending as little time as possible in contact with the ground.

Because of the explosive nature of the exercise, plyometrics has a great potential for injury and, therefore, an athlete's plyometrics program should be carefully supervised. Delayed onset muscle soreness (Chapter 2) may occur following this form of exercise.

Plyometric training should only be performed one to two times per week and when the athlete is fresh. The surface must be firm, but forgiving, such as sprung basketball floors. Injury risk is minimized if the athlete warms up and warms down correctly and the volume of work is built up gradually. When technique begins to deteriorate, the exercise should be stopped.

Flexibility training

Flexibility training using one or more of the stretching techniques mentioned earlier in this chapter is an important component of training. In developing an increased range of motion across a joint, it is also important to develop muscle strength and power through this newly acquired range of motion to avoid muscle injuries.

Speed training

Running speed, a largely inherited ability, is an important component of many sports. Athletes can, however, develop speed by improving muscular power and strength, thus increasing stride length and cadence, as well as by improving technique, which increases the efficiency of ground coverage. Therefore, running speed can be increased by undertaking resistance and power training as well as by performing running drills. These drills may include 'high knees', 'heel to buttock' and 'overspeed' work, for example, downhill running.

Agility training

Agility and rapid reflexes are also inherited characteristics. However, like speed, they can be improved somewhat by training and, thus, are included in training programs of all sports. There is an increasing emphasis on agility training for exercise prescription among seniors to prevent falls.[53] Examples of specific agility exercises include the classic military stepping exercises and figure of eight running. These exercises should be sport-specific whenever possible.

Specific skill training

Sports have specific skills that require training in order to achieve a high level of efficiency. A proportion of training time must be devoted to developing these specific skills, preferably with the aid of a coach. Often, skill training requires the repetition of explosive movements and, therefore, has a high risk of injury. To prevent injury, a proportion of skill training should be done at an intensity level below normal competition conditions.

Cross-training

To prevent injury it may be beneficial to reduce the amount of weight-bearing exercise. Cross-training enables the athlete to maintain aerobic fitness while reducing stress on weight-bearing joints, muscles and tendons.

In athletes with a chronic condition such as articular cartilage damage to a weight-bearing joint, cross-training may be used to reduce the impact load while maintaining adequate training volume. Similarly, in a patient returning to sport from an overuse injury, such as a stress fracture, cross-training can reduce the risk of recurrence.

Runners may wish to introduce one to two sessions per week of activities such as cycling, swimming or water running. These alternative work-outs can mirror the athlete's usual training session (e.g. interval training, aerobic or anaerobic training).

Adequate recovery

Adequate recovery is essential if the athlete is to benefit fully from training and prevent injuries from occurring. This is discussed in Chapter 7.

Psychology and injury prevention

Excessive psychological arousal (Chapter 39) can not only impair sporting performance but is also likely to increase the risk of injury. Overarousal is associated with impairment of natural technique, which players describe as a 'loss of rhythm'. Loss of concentration can also predispose to injury by giving the athlete less time to react to cues. This is clearly a risk in contact and collision sports but can also cause injury in non-contact sports. For example, an overaroused tennis player who does not react optimally to an opponent's serve will then be forced to return from a biomechanically poor position, which increases stress on certain muscle groups.

Underarousal can also predispose to injury. For example, if a player has been relegated to a lower level of competition, he or she may not warm up as diligently as normal. Furthermore, visual cues may not cause as rapid a response as when truly focused. This may lead to injury in a body contact sport or technical errors that can lead to falls in a sport such as gymnastics.

Nutrition and injury prevention

Inadequate nutrition may increase the risk of injury due to its effect on recovery (Chapter 7). Inadequate glycogen repletion causes a reliance on fat and protein stores and this may result in increased protein breakdown, which, in turn, may lead to soft tissue injury.

There are several mechanisms by which inadequate dietary protein intake may lead to muscle injury. Intense training causes skeletal muscle breakdown, which can be exacerbated by inadequate dietary protein. Inadequate hydration may compromise blood flow to working muscle, which may increase susceptibility to injury. Hydration is thought to influence the amount and composition of joint fluid, which helps to nourish articular cartilage.

Calcium is the major mineral component of bone but inadequate dietary intake does not appear to be directly associated with bony injury, such as stress fracture.[54] Because of the role of micronutrients in bone and/or muscle metabolism, deficiencies in nutrients such as potassium, iron, zinc, magnesium, chromium, copper and various vitamins may increase susceptibility to injury. However, at present no data demonstrate this to be the case.

Maintaining low weight and low body fat is important in many sports and confers an advantage in sports such as running and gymnastics. In sports such as rowing and wrestling, weight limits are set. Athletes may have rapid, large fluctuations in weight immediately prior to competition, which is associated with significant losses of lean body tissue and water. Another group of athletes constantly strives to lower weight. Certain female athletes with chronic low-energy diets are at risk of menstrual disturbance and reduced bone formation (Chapter 41). These women have an increased risk of stress fracture. Similarly, people suffering from eating disorders such as anorexia nervosa and bulimia have low bone density and increased risk of bony injury.

Recommended Reading

Ahern DK, Lohr BA. Psychosocial factors in sports injury rehabilitation. *Clin Sports Med* 1997; 16: 755–68.
An overview of a variety of psychological techniques that have a role in prevention and rehabilitation.

Arnason A, Engebretsen L, Bahr R. No effect of a video-based awareness program on the rate of soccer injuries. *Am J Sports Med* 2005; 33(1): 77–84.

Bahr R, Maehlum S. *Clinical Guide to Sports Injuries: An Illustrated Guide to the Management of Injuries in Physical Activity.* Champaign, IL: Human Kinetics Publishers, 2004.
The authoritative text on a number of fronts, and injury prevention is at the heart of this beautifully illustrated book.

Barbic D, Pater J, Brison RJ. Comparison of mouth guard designs and concussion prevention in contact sports: a multicenter randomized controlled trial. *Clin J Sport Med* 2005; 15(5): 294–8.

Emery CA, Cassidy JD, Klassen TP, Rosychuk RJ, Rowe BH. Effectiveness of a home-based balance-training program in reducing sports-related injuries among healthy adolescents: a cluster randomized controlled trial. *Can Med Assoc J* 2005; 172(6): 749–54.

Murphy DF, Connolly DA, Beynnon BD. Risk factors for lower extremity injury: a review of the literature. *Br J Sports Med* 2003; 37(1): 13–29.

Noakes TD. *Lore of Running.* 4th edn. Champaign, IL: Human Kinetics Publishers, 2003.
A classic book on a number of fronts but particularly relevant to anyone interested in the history, and the physiology, behind training regimens for running.

Olsen OE, Myklebust G, Engebretsen L, Holme I, Bahr R. Exercises to prevent lower limb injuries in youth sports: cluster randomized controlled trial. *BMJ* 2005; 330(7489): 449.

Shrier I. Does stretching help prevent injuries. In: MacAuley D, Best T, eds. *Evidence-Based Sports Medicine.* London: BMJ Books, 2002: 97–116.

Sulheim S, Holme I, Ekeland A, Bahr R. Helmet use and risk of head injuries in alpine skiers and snowboarders. *JAMA* 2006; 295(8): 919–24.

Thacker SB, Stroup DF, Branche CM, Gilchrist J, Goodman RA, Porter Kelling E. Prevention of knee injuries in sports. A systematic review of the literature. *J Sports Med Phys Fitness* 2003; 43(2): 165–79.

Verhagen E, van der Beek A, Twisk J, Bouter L, Bahr R, van Mechelen W. The effect of a proprioceptive balance board training program for the prevention of ankle sprains: a prospective controlled trial. *Am J Sports Med* 2004; 32(6): 1385–93.

Yeung EW, Yeung SS. Interventions for preventing lower limb soft-tissue injuries in runners. *Cochrane Database Syst Rev* 2001; 3: CD001256.

The five-part British Journal of Sports Medicine series outlining the 'central governor' model of skeletal muscle recruitment and regulation is listed below:

St Clair Gibson A, Noakes TD. Evidence for complex system integration and dynamic neural regulation of skeletal muscle recruitment during exercise in humans. *Br J Sports Med* 2004; 38(6): 797–806.

Lambert EV, St Clair Gibson A, Noakes TD. Complex systems model of fatigue: integrative homoeostatic control of peripheral physiological systems during exercise in humans. *Br J Sports Med* 2005; 39(1): 52–62.

Noakes TD, St Clair Gibson A, Lambert EV. From catastrophe to complexity: a novel model of integrative central neural regulation of effort and fatigue during exercise in humans. *Br J Sports Med* 2004; 38(4): 511–14.

Noakes TD, St Clair Gibson A. Logical limitations to the 'catastrophe' models of fatigue during exercise in humans. *Br J Sports Med* 2004; 38(5): 648–9.

Noakes TD, St Clair Gibson A, Lambert EV. From catastrophe to complexity: a novel model of integrative central neural regulation of effort and fatigue during exercise in humans: summary and conclusions. *Br J Sports Med* 2005; 39(2): 120–4.

References

1. Vaz D, Santos L, Carneiro AV. Risk factors: definitions and practical implications. *Rev Port Cardiol* 2005; 24(1): 121–31.

2. van Mechelen W, Hlobil H, Kemper HC. Incidence, severity, aetiology and prevention of sports injuries. A review of concepts. *Sports Med* 1992; 14(2): 82–99.

3. Meeuwisse WH. Predictability of sports injuries. What is the epidemiological evidence? *Sports Med* 1991; 12(1): 8–15.

4. Bahr R, Holme I. Risk factors for sports injuries—a methodological approach. *Br J Sports Med* 2003; 37(5): 384–92.

5. Bahr R, Krosshaug T. Understanding injury mechanisms: a key component of preventing injuries in sport. *Br J Sports Med* 2005; 39(6): 324–9.

6. Green JP, Grenier SG, McGill SM. Low-back stiffness is altered with warm-up and bench rest: implications for athletes. *Med Sci Sports Exerc* 2002; 34(7): 1076–81.

7. Rosenbaum D, Hennig EM. The influence of stretching and warm-up exercises on Achilles tendon reflex activity. *J Sports Sci* 1995; 13(6): 481–90.

8. Stewart IB, Sleivert GG. The effect of warm-up intensity on range of motion and anaerobic performance. *J Orthop Sports Phys Ther* 1998; 27(2): 154–61.

9. Olsen OE, Myklebust G, Engebretsen L, Holme I, Bahr R. Exercises to prevent lower limb injuries in youth sports: cluster randomised controlled trial. *BMJ* 2005; 330(7489): 449.

10. Magnusson SP. Passive properties of human skeletal muscle during stretch maneuvers. A review. *Scand J Med Sci Sports* 1998; 8(2): 65–77.

11. Magnusson SP, Aagaard P, Larsson B, Kjaer M. Passive energy absorption by human muscle-tendon unit is unaffected by increase in intramuscular temperature. *J Appl Physiol* 2000; 88(4): 1215–20.

12. Magnusson SP, Aagaard P, Nielson JJ. Passive energy return after repeated stretches of the hamstring muscle-tendon unit. *Med Sci Sports Exerc* 2000; 32(6): 1160–4.

13. Magnusson SP, Aagard P, Simonsen E, Bojsen-Moller F. A biomechanical evaluation of cyclic and static stretch in human skeletal muscle. *Int J Sports Med* 1998; 19(5): 310–16.

14. Magnusson SP, Simonsen EB, Aagaard P, Dyhre-Poulsen P, McHugh MP, Kjaer M. Mechanical and physical responses to stretching with and without preisometric contraction in human skeletal muscle. *Arch Phys Med Rehabil* 1996; 77(4): 373–8.

15. Magnusson SP, Simonsen EB, Aagaard P, Gleim GW, McHugh MP, Kjaer M. Viscoelastic response to repeated static stretching in the human hamstring muscle. *Scand J Med Sci Sports* 1995; 5(6): 342–7.

16. Magnusson SP, Simonsen EB, Aagaard P, Sorensen H, Kjaer M. A mechanism for altered flexibility in human skeletal muscle. *J Physiol* 1996; 497(part 1): 291–8.

17. Magnusson SP, Simonsen EB, Dyhre-Poulsen P, Aagaard P, Mohr T, Kjaer M. Viscoelastic stress relaxation during static stretch in human skeletal muscle in the absence of EMG activity. *Scand J Med Sci Sports* 1996; 6(6): 323–8.

18. Herbert RD, Gabriel M. Effects of stretching before and after exercising on muscle soreness and risk of injury: systematic review. *BMJ* 2002; 325(7362): 468.

19. Pope RP, Herbert RD, Kirwan JD, Graham BJ. A randomized trial of preexercise stretching for prevention of lower-limb injury. *Med Sci Sports Exerc* 2000; 32(2): 271–7.

20. Shrier I. Stretching before exercise does not reduce the risk of local muscle injury: a critical review of the clinical and basic science literature. *Clin J Sport Med* 1999; 9(4): 221–7.

21. Shrier I. Stretching before exercise: an evidence based approach. *Br J Sports Med* 2000; 34(5): 324–5.

22. Shrier I. Flexibility versus stretching. *Br J Sports Med* 2001; 35(5): 364.

23. Shrier I. Meta-analysis on preexercise stretching. *Med Sci Sports Exerc* 2004; 36(10): 1832; author reply 1833.

24. Shrier I. Does stretching improve performance? A systematic and critical review of the literature. *Clin J Sport Med* 2004; 14(5): 267–73.

25. Shrier I. Stretching perspectives. *Curr Sports Med Rep* 2005; 4(5): 237–8.

26. Witvrouw E, Mahieu N, Danneels L, McNair P. Stretching and injury prevention: an obscure relationship. *Sports Med* 2004; 34(7): 443–9.

27. Bahr R, Lian O, Bahr IA. A twofold reduction in the incidence of acute ankle sprains in volleyball after the introduction of an injury prevention program: a prospective cohort study. *Scand J Med Sci Sports* 1997; 7(3): 172–7.

28. Verhagen E, van der Beek A, Twisk J, Bouter L, Bahr R, van Mechelen W. The effect of a proprioceptive balance board training program for the prevention of ankle sprains: a prospective controlled trial. *Am J Sports Med* 2004; 32(6): 1385–93.

29. Bragg RW, Macmahon JM, Overom EK, et al. Failure and fatigue characteristics of adhesive athletic tape. *Med Sci Sports Exerc* 2002; 34(3): 403–10.

30. Beynnon BD, Ryder SH, Konradsen L, Johnson RJ, Johnson K, Renstrom PA. The effect of anterior cruciate ligament trauma and bracing on knee proprioception. *Am J Sports Med* 1999; 27(2): 150–5.

31. Fleming BC, Renstrom PA, Beynnon BD, Engstrom B, Peura G. The influence of functional knee bracing on the anterior cruciate ligament strain biomechanics in weightbearing and nonweightbearing knees. *Am J Sports Med* 2000; 28(6): 815–24.

32. Swirtun LR, Jansson A, Renstrom P. The effects of a functional knee brace during early treatment of patients with a nonoperated acute anterior cruciate ligament tear: a prospective randomized study. *Clin J Sport Med* 2005; 15(5): 299–304.

33. Benson BW, Mohtadi NG, Rose MS, Meeuwisse WH. Head and neck injuries among ice hockey players wearing full face shields vs half face shields. *JAMA* 1999; 282(24): 2328–32.

34. Wilk BR, Fisher KL, Gutierrez W. Defective running shoes as a contributing factor in plantar fasciitis in a triathlete. *J Orthop Sports Phys Ther* 2000; 30(1): 21–8; discussion 29–31.

35. Finch CF, Kelsall HL. The effectiveness of ski bindings and their professional adjustment for preventing alpine skiing injuries. *Sports Med* 1998; 25(6): 407–16.

36. Natri A, Beynnon BD, Ettlinger CF, Johnson RJ, Shealy JE. Alpine ski bindings and injuries. Current findings. *Sports Med* 1999; 28(1): 35–48.

37. Strand T, Tvedte R, Engebretsen L, Tegnander A. [Anterior cruciate ligament injuries in handball playing. Mechanisms and incidence of injuries.] *Tidsskr Nor Laegeforen* 1990; 110(17): 2222–5.

38. Olsen OE, Myklebust G, Bahr R. Effect of floor type on injury risk in team handball. *Scand J Med Sci Sports* 2003; 13(5): 299–304.

39. Orchard JW, Chivers I, Aldous D, Bennell K, Seward H. Rye grass is associated with fewer non-contact anterior cruciate ligament injuries than bermuda grass. *Br J Sports Med* 2005; 39(10): 704–9.

40. Orchard J. Is there a relationship between ground and climatic conditions and injuries in football? *Sports Med* 2002; 32(7): 419–32.

41. McNitt A, Waddington D, Middour R. *Traction Measurement on Natural Turf*. West Conshohocken, PA: American Society for Testing and Materials, 1997.

42. Whiting WC, Zernicke RF. *Biomechanics of Musculoskeletal Injury*. Champaign, IL: Human Kinetics Publishers, 2006.

43. Maeda S, Tanabe T, Miyauchi T, et al. Aerobic exercise training reduces plasma endothelin-1 concentration in older women. *J Appl Physiol* 2003; 95(1): 336–41.

44. Noakes TD. 1996 J. B. Wolffe Memorial Lecture. 'Challenging beliefs: ex Africa semper aliquid novi'. *Med Sci Sports Exerc* 1997; 29: 571–90.

45. Noakes TD. Maximal oxygen uptake: 'classical' versus 'contemporary' views: a rebuttal. *Med Sci Sports Exerc* 1998; 30: 1381–98.

46. Noakes TD, St Clair Gibson A, Lambert EV. From catastrophe to complexity: a novel model of integrative central neural regulation of effort and fatigue during exercise in humans. *Br J Sports Med* 2004; 38(4): 511–14.

47. Noakes TD, Peltonen JE, Rusko HK. Evidence that a central governor regulates exercise performance during acute hypoxia and hyperoxia. *J Exp Biol* 2001; 204(part 18): 3225–34.

48. Noakes TD, St Clair Gibson A. Logical limitations to the 'catastrophe' models of fatigue during exercise in humans. *Br J Sports Med* 2004; 38(5): 648–9.

49. Noakes TD. Physiological factors limiting exercise performance in CFS. *Med Sci Sports Exerc* 2004; 36(6): 1087.

50. Noakes TD, St Clair Gibson A, Lambert EV. From catastrophe to complexity: a novel model of integrative central neural regulation of effort and fatigue during exercise in humans: summary and conclusions. *Br J Sports Med* 2005; 39(2): 120-4.

51. Lambert EV, St Clair Gibson A, Noakes TD. Complex systems model of fatigue: integrative homoeostatic control of peripheral physiological systems during exercise in humans. *Br J Sports Med* 2005; 39(1): 52–62.

52. St Clair Gibson A, Noakes TD. Evidence for complex system integration and dynamic neural regulation of skeletal muscle recruitment during exercise in humans. *Br J Sports Med* 2004; 38(6): 797–806.

53. Liu-Ambrose T, Khan KM, Eng JJ, Janssen PA, Lord SR, McKay HA. Resistance and agility training reduce fall risk in women aged 75 to 85 with low bone mass: a 6-month randomized, controlled trial. *J Am Geriatr Soc* 2004; 52(5): 657–65.

54. Nattiv A. Stress fractures and bone health in track and field athletes. *J Sci Med Sport* 2000; 3(3): 268–79.

Recovery

In recent years there has been an increased emphasis on recovery following bouts of heavy training or competition, and the possible means by which recovery can be enhanced. There are a number of situations where enhancing recovery can be helpful for the athlete.

The athlete may have to perform again in a few hours time, such as running a heat of an event in the morning and then the final later in the day. Occasionally in tournaments, individuals or teams have to compete twice in one day. A tennis player may have to play a singles match and then a doubles match a few hours later, or a team sport athlete may have a number of games in a day as part of a weekend round robin tournament. Even though playing another high-intensity competition the same day is the exception rather than the rule, it is not uncommon to have to play on consecutive days or at least two or three times a week. Full recovery is obviously very important.

Even for those playing weekly, it is important to be fully recovered as quickly as possible to enable the athlete to train effectively during the week. In all these situations, recovery from exhaustive activity is important and coaches and conditioning staff have, in recent times, implemented post-game programs to enhance recovery.

Overall the aim is to maximize performance and minimize potential for injury at the next event. There are a number of specific objectives in the recovery process:

- restoration of function
- neuromuscular recovery
- tissue repair
- resolution of muscle soreness
- psychological recovery.

Unfortunately there is limited research into the various recovery methods. Current research has a number of limitations:

- poor study design:
  — often not randomized
  — lack appropriate control populations
- small numbers:
  — increased likelihood of chance findings
  — difficulty finding statistical benefit
  — confusing statistical and clinical benefit
- optimum regimen unknown for most techniques
- sports have different requirements
- underlying mechanisms unclear/speculative
- indirect outcome measures.

A number of methods are commonly used to hasten the recovery process. These include warm-down (active recovery), the use of ice baths, contrast baths, whirlpools or spas, and soft tissue massage, as well as nutritional and psychological techniques.

Ensuring adequate recovery

Warm-down or active recovery

Most serious athletes perform a warm-down or active recovery following the conclusion of intense exercise. The length of warm-down generally varies with the level of the participant's activity but ranges from 5 to 15 minutes. This is usually followed by stretching of the muscles used in training or competition.

Active recovery has been shown to remove lactate from the circulation more quickly than does passive recovery.[1] The clearance of lactate appears to be related to the intensity of the exercise performed in the warm-down up to about 50% of maximal oxygen uptake

($V_{O_{2max}}$), which is a higher intensity than routinely practiced by most sportspeople. The warm-down appears particularly important if the next bout of activity is within 2–4 hours.

The benefits of warm-down on muscle soreness and performance after 24–48 hours are not clear from current research. Dawson et al. compared immediate recovery procedures to next-day recovery training (25 minutes of pool exercise) and found no difference in recovery of muscle soreness, flexibility and power at 48 hours after an Australian football match.[2]

Deep-water running

Deep-water running involves 'running' in the deep end of a swimming pool using a buoyancy vest. This technique can be used to maintain fitness during recovery from lower limb injury (Chapter 12), and as a form of cross-training to reduce impact with the aim of reducing overuse injuries (Chapter 6). Its use has also been advocated as part of the recovery program either immediately after the bout of strenuous exercise or the following day. Reilly et al. showed that a regimen of deep-water running for three consecutive days after intense exercise reduced muscle soreness and appeared to speed up the restoration of muscle strength.[3]

Ice immersion, contrast baths, whirlpools and spas

The use of ice immersion, contrast baths, whirlpools and spas has become common among athletes attempting to enhance the recovery process. Despite this, there is little evidence for their efficacy. Most of the research has looked at the effect of these various treatments in delayed onset muscle soreness (DOMS)—one of but by no means the only feature of muscle damage following intense exercise.

Cryotherapy has long been used to treat musculoskeletal injury (Chapter 10) due to its effect on reducing the hemodynamic response to injury. Decreasing tissue temperature results in constriction of local blood vessels, thus reducing the accumulation of edema. Through predominantly vascular effects, cold application is thought to diminish the edema response to musculoskeletal trauma and decrease metabolism in injured tissues, thus lowering the oxygen requirement and limiting the inflammatory response in the tissues. It is thought that cold application has various other effects on injured tissues, such as reduction of muscle spasm and slowing of nerve conduction velocity, thus altering perceived pain.[4]

There is much variation in the preferred method of ice or cold application. Research has thus far failed to show convincing evidence for a positive effect from ice massage,[5, 6] crushed ice,[7] ice water immersion[8–12] or contrast water immersion.[2, 13]

There are currently two common methods used. The simplest and easiest method involves use of an ice bath (2–10°C). Although no specific protocol exists, in current practice the regimen commonly used involves the athlete standing waist deep in the ice bath for 1 minute followed by a minute out of the bath. This is repeated two or three times. The second common technique is the contrast bath, alternating warm and cold baths for a minute each, repeated three or four times. Despite the lack of scientific evidence, these techniques are widely used and may have a significant placebo effect. Anecdotally, players invariably report that they believe these techniques help their recovery.

The use of whirlpools and spas appears to improve the recovery process. These baths may have both a physiological effect on muscle and other soft tissue as well as a psychological effect by decreasing arousal.

Soft tissue massage

Regular soft tissue massage contributes to soft tissue recovery from intense athletic activity. Intense training causes prolonged elevation of muscle tone in both the resting and the contractile states. This is often felt as muscle 'tightness' by athletes and occurs particularly during periods of adaptation to increased volume and intensity of training.

It is thought that hard training and 'abnormal tone' have numerous effects. These may impair the delivery of nutrients and oxygen to the cells and slow the removal of metabolites. They may contribute to biomechanical abnormalities, particularly if muscle tightness is asymmetrical. Increased tone also limits the extensibility and shock absorbency of soft tissue and thus predisposes the tissue to strain. Fatigue associated with hard training also impairs proprioceptive mechanisms and may directly trigger nociceptors.

Intense training also causes irritation of previously inadequately treated soft tissue lesions. Repetitive microtrauma of these lesions may cause bulky connective tissue to develop, which further compromises muscle function and flexibility. Fascial tissue may become less pliable due to cross-linkages developing. Active trigger points that result from heavy training may reduce muscle strength. These problems can impair training and competition and can progress to injury if they are not resolved.

Although not entirely clear, soft tissue massage is thought to work by reducing excessive post-exercise muscle tone, increasing muscle range of motion, increasing the circulation and nutrition to damaged tissue and deactivating symptomatic trigger points. As well as improving soft tissue function, regular soft tissue massage provides the opportunity for the massage therapist to identify any soft tissue abnormalities, which, if untreated, could progress to injury.

Once again there is little scientific evidence as to the efficacy of soft tissue massage in enhancing recovery, although it would appear to have a positive psychological effect.[14, 15] One study has shown that a combination of active recovery and soft tissue massage was more effective than single interventions of passive recovery, active recovery or soft tissue massage in maintaining performance time in two simulated 5 km maximal cycling tests separated by 20 minutes.[1]

Lifestyle factors

Adequate rest and sleep are thought to be important in the recovery process although there has been little research into this area. It has been shown that sleep loss following a match can interfere with performance at training the next day; however, any loss of sleep is likely to be compensated for the next night.[16]

It is traditional in certain sports to overindulge in alcohol following a competition. This can have a significant negative effect on recovery. Studies in cyclists showed that muscle glycogen storage was impaired when alcohol was consumed immediately after exercise and displaced carbohydrate intake from the recovery diet.[17] It is likely, however, that the most important effects of alcohol intake on glycogen resynthesis are indirect—by interfering with the athlete's ability, or interest, to achieve the recommended amounts of carbohydrate required for optimal glycogen restoration.[18] Athletes are therefore encouraged to follow the guidelines for sensible use of alcohol in sport.[19]

The role of nutrition in aiding recovery

Nutrition aids recovery from intense exercise by replenishing glycogen stores and by providing necessary protein and water.

Glycogen replacement

Glycogen is the major energy source for muscular activity (Chapter 37). Training depletes muscle and liver glycogen stores. Repetitive bouts of activity can cause profound glycogen depletion and impair sporting performance.

The aim of a high-carbohydrate diet is to restore glycogen levels to normal within 24 hours of strenuous exercise. The type, amount and timing of carbohydrate ingestion influences glycogen replenishment. The guidelines for carbohydrate needs in training and recovery have recently been revised and are shown in Table 7.1.

Protein replacement

Intense exercise results in breakdown of muscle tissue. Intake of protein in recovery meals is recommended to enhance net protein balance, tissue repair and adaptations involving synthesis of new proteins.

The co-ingestion of protein with carbohydrate will increase the efficiency of muscle glycogen storage when the amount of carbohydrate ingested is below the threshold for maximum glycogen synthesis or when feeding intervals are more than 1 hour apart. The effectiveness of protein to enhance muscle glycogen storage appears limited to the first hour after supplementation. It has been shown that glycogen storage during the first 40 minutes of recovery after exercise was twice as fast after a carbohydrate–protein feeding than after an isoenergetic carbohydrate feeding, and four times faster than after a carbohydrate feeding of the same carbohydrate concentration. This trend also continued following the second feeding 2 hours into recovery.[20] These results have important implications for sports with very short recovery periods during competition, such as soccer and ice hockey.[18]

The consumption of excessively large amounts of protein and fat in an athlete's diet is discouraged because they may displace carbohydrate foods within the athlete's energy requirements and affect gastric comfort, thereby indirectly interfering with glycogen storage by preventing adequate carbohydrate intake.[18]

Rehydration

Large amounts of fluid may be lost during exertion, particularly with increasing intensity and in hot or humid conditions. It can be difficult for athletes to maintain fluid balance in certain environmental conditions. Athletes should weigh themselves before and after exercise and replace the weight lost with water.

Restoration of fluid balance after exercise is an important part of the recovery process and becomes even more important in hot, humid conditions. If a second bout of exercise has to be performed after a relatively short interval, the rate of rehydration is of crucial importance. Rehydration after exercise requires not only replacement of volume losses, but

Table 7.1 Revised guidelines for the intake of carbohydrate in the everyday or training diets of athletes[18]

- Athletes should aim to achieve carbohydrate intakes to meet the fuel requirements of their training program and to optimize restoration of muscle glycogen stores between work-outs. General recommendations can be provided but should be fine-tuned with individual consideration of total energy needs, specific training needs and feedback from training performance.
  - Immediate recovery after exercise (0–4 hours): 1.0–1.2 g/kg/h consumed at frequent intervals
  - Daily recovery for moderate duration/low intensity training: 5–7 g/kg/day
  - Daily recovery for moderate-to-heavy endurance training: 7–12 g/kg/day
  - Daily recovery for extreme exercise program (4–6 hours per day): 10–12+ g/kg/day
- It is valuable to choose nutrient-rich carbohydrate foods and to add other foods to recovery meals and snacks to provide a good source of protein and other nutrients. These nutrients may assist in other recovery processes and, in the case of protein, may promote additional glycogen recovery when carbohydrate intake is suboptimal or when frequent snacking is not possible.
- When the period between exercise sessions is <8 hours, the athlete should begin carbohydrate intake as soon as practical after the first work-out to maximize the effective recovery time between sessions. There may be some advantages in meeting carbohydrate intake targets as a series of snacks during the early recovery phase.
- During longer recovery periods (>24 hours), the athlete should organize the pattern and timing of carbohydrate-rich meals and snacks according to what is practical and comfortable for the individual situation. There is no difference in glycogen synthesis when liquid or solid forms of carbohydrate are consumed.
- Carbohydrate-rich foods with a moderate-to-high glycemic index (GI) provide a readily available source of carbohydrate for muscle glycogen synthesis and should be the major carbohydrate choices in recovery meals.
- Adequate energy intake is important for optimal glycogen recovery; the restrained eating practises of some athletes, particularly females, make it difficult to meet carbohydrate intake targets and to optimize glycogen storage from this intake.
- Guidelines for carbohydrate (or other macronutrients) should not be provided in terms of percentage contributions to total dietary energy intake. Such recommendations are neither user-friendly nor strongly related to the muscle's absolute needs for fuel.
- Athletes should not consume excessive amounts of alcohol during the recovery period since it is likely to interfere with their ability or interest to follow guidelines for post-exercise eating. Athletes should follow sensible drinking practises at all times, but especially in the period after exercise.

also replacement of the electrolytes, mainly sodium lost in the sweat.

Daily sweat and sodium losses vary widely among individuals and depend on many factors, including the environment, diet, physical fitness and heat acclimatization status. However, when sweat losses are large, the total sodium loss will generally be high.

The replacement of sweat losses with plain water will lead to hemodilution. The fall in plasma osmolality and sodium concentration that occurs reduces the drive to drink and stimulates urine output, and has potentially more serious consequences such as hyponatremia. Hyponatremia is a major problem in ultra-endurance events. A moderate excess of salt intake would appear to be beneficial as far as hydration status is concerned without any detrimental effects on health. Any excess sodium ingested will be excreted in the urine. Drinks intended for rehydration should therefore have a higher electrolyte content than drinks formulated for consumption during exercise.[21]

The addition of an energy source is not necessary for rehydration, although intake of a small amount of carbohydrate may improve the rate of intestinal uptake of sodium and water, and will improve palatability. Where sweat losses are high, rehydration with carbohydrate solutions has implications for energy balance (e.g. 10 L of soft drink will provide approximately 1000 g of carbohydrate, which is equivalent to about 17 000 kJ or 4000 calories). The volume of beverage consumed should be greater than the volume of sweat lost to allow for ongoing obligatory urine losses, and palatability of the beverage is a major issue when large volumes of fluid have to be consumed.[21]

Intravenous rehydration appears equally effective in rehydration and has the added advantage of speed in situations where time is limited and rehydration is required. There is no evidence that intravenous rehydration is more effective than oral rehydration in recovery after 24 hours or more.[22]

The role of psychology in aiding recovery

As the nervous system controls cardiovascular function, respiration and metabolism during and after exercise, psychological factors play an important role in recovery (Chapter 39).

The function of the autonomic nervous system

After exercise, the nervous system, which functions by releasing neurotransmitters, may be substantially fatigued. The efferent cells of the peripheral nervous system are categorized into those that control skeletal muscle (somatic nerves) and those that control glands, cardiac muscle and smooth muscle found in the walls of body organs such as the gastrointestinal tract, the blood vessels and airways (autonomic nerves).

Autonomic nerves themselves are divided into sympathetic and parasympathetic nerves according to both anatomical and physiological differences. Some organs receive input from both sympathetic and parasympathetic nerves.

Effect of exercise on the autonomic nervous system

The sympathetic nervous system controls the 'fight or flight' reaction, which is characterized by an adrenalin rush, tachycardia, increased cardiac output and bronchodilation. At the same time, blood is shunted away from the gastrointestinal organs to enhance muscle blood flow. Liver glycogen stores are used up to provide blood glucose.

After exercise, this automatic effect should be reversed to allow muscles to relax and to replenish body stores of glycogen. If there is insufficient recovery of the nervous system, the athlete may remain sympathetically aroused. This manifests as increased resting heart rate, muscle tiredness and insomnia. Sympathetic overarousal may delay absorption of nutrients from the gastrointestinal tract as well as elevating the metabolic rate. Over time, the sympathetic nervous system can become exhausted and the patient develops bradycardia, an inability to utilize glycogen and a diminution in work capacity. This psychological state parallels depression.

Techniques that aid psychological recovery

Athletes who have a good understanding of their arousal level are generally calm and stable. They, thus, tend to place less stress on their autonomic nervous system. Specific techniques can lower arousal level. These include the use of soft tissue massage, spas, warm baths and showers, flotation tanks, music, visualization and relaxation tapes, all of which are discussed in Chapter 39. As recovery is vital for optimal performance, coaches should be encouraged to incorporate recovery time into athletes' schedules.

Recommended Reading

Burke LM, Kiens B, Ivy JL. Carbohydrates and fat for training and recovery. *J Sports Sci* 2004; 22(1): 15–30.

Hemmings BJ. Physiological, psychological and performance effects of massage therapy in sport: a review of the literature. *Phys Ther Sport* 2001; 2: 165-170.

Reilly T, Ekblom B. The use of recovery methods post-exercise. *J Sports Sci* 2005; 23(6): 619–27.

Shirreffs SM, Armstrong LE, Cheuvront SN. Fluid and electrolyte needs for preparation and recovery from training and competition. *J Sports Sci* 2004; 22(1): 57–63.

References

1. Monedero J, Donne B. Effect of recovery interventions on lactate removal and subsequent performance. *Int J Sports Med* 2000; 21(8): 593–7.

2. Dawson B, Cow S, Modra S, et al. Effects of immediate post-game recovery procedures on muscle soreness, power and flexibility levels over the next 48 hours. *J Sci Med Sport* 2005; 8(2): 210–21.

3. Reilly T, Cable NT, Dowzer CN. The efficacy of deep water running. In: McCabe PT, ed. *Contemporary Ergonomics*. London: Taylor & Francis, 2002: 162–6.

4. Macauley D. Do textbooks agree on their advice on ice? *Clin J Sport Med* 2001; 11: 67–72.

5. Yackzan L, Francis KT. The effects of ice massage on delayed onset muscle soreness. *Am J Sports Med* 1984; 12: 159–65.

6. Howatson G. Ice massage: effects on exercise-induced muscle damage. *J Sports Med Phys Fitness* 2003; 43(4): 500–5.

7. Denegar CR. Effect of transcutaneous electrical nerve stimulation, cold, and a combination treatment on pain, decreased range of motion, and strength loss associated with delayed onset muscle soreness. *J Athl Train* 1992; 27(3): 200–6.

8. Paddon-Jones DJ. Effect of cryotherapy on muscle soreness and strength following eccentric exercise. *Int J Sports Med* 1997; 18(8): 588–93.

9. Eston RG. Effects of cold water immersion on the symptoms of exercise-induced muscle damage. *J Sports Sci* 1999; 17(3): 231–8.

10. Byrnes WC, White JS, Hsieh SS, et al. Delayed onset muscle soreness following repeated bouts of downhill running. *J Appl Physiol* 1985; 59(3): 710–15.

11. Papalia S. Is post exercise cold water immersion cryotherapy to reduce post exercise muscle damage worth the discomfort? *J Sci Med Sport* 2003; 6(4): 265.

12. Sellwood K, Brukner PD, Hinman R, et al. Ice water immersion and delayed onset muscle soreness: a randomised controlled trial. *J Sci Med Sport* 2005; 8(4): 223.

13. Kuligowski LA, Giannantonio FP, Blanc RO. Effect of whirlpool therapy on the signs and symptoms of delayed-onset muscle soreness. *J Athl Train* 1998; 33(3): 222–8.

14. Hemmings B, Smith M, Graydon J, et al. Effects of massage on physiological restoration, perceived recovery, and repeated sports performance. *Br J Sports Med* 2000; 34(2): 109–14.

15. Robertson A, Watt JM, Galloway SD. Effects of leg massage on recovery from high intensity cycling exercise. *Br J Sports Med* 2004; 38(2): 173–6.

16. Reilly T, Piercy M. The effects of partial sleep deprivation on weight-lifting performance. *Ergonomics* 1994; 37: 107–15.

17. Burke LM, Collier GR, Davis PG, et al. Muscle glycogen storage after prolonged exercise: effect of the frequency of carbohydrate feedings. *Am J Clin Nutr* 1996; 64: 115–19.

18. Burke LM, Kiens B, Ivy JL. Carbohydrates and fat for training and recovery. *J Sports Sci* 2004; 22(1): 15–30.

19. Burke LM, Maughan RJ. Alcohol in sport. In: Maughan RJ, ed. *Nutrition in Sport*. Oxford: Blackwell Science, 2000: 405–14.

20. Ivy JL, Goforth HW Jr, Damon BM, et al. Early postexercise muscle glycogen recovery is enhanced with a carbohydrate-protein supplement. *J Appl Physiol* 2002; 93(4): 1337–44.

21. Shirreffs SM, Armstrong LE, Cheuvront SN. Fluid and electrolyte needs for preparation and recovery from training and competition. *J Sports Sci* 2004; 22(1): 57–63.

22. Neal A, Brukner P, Nicol A, et al. Comparison of the effectiveness of oral and intravenous rehydration in recovery following exercise. *J Sci Med Sport* 2005; 8(4): 223.

Principles of Diagnosis: Clinical Assessment

The importance of making an accurate, pathological diagnosis cannot be overemphasized. This chapter addresses what physicians call the history and physical examination and what physiotherapists/physical therapists consider as the subjective and objective assessment. Chapter 9 addresses investigations.

Far too often sporting injuries are given descriptive labels such as 'swimmer's shoulder' or 'tennis elbow'. These terms do not represent diagnoses. Accurate pathological diagnosis is essential because it enables:

1. the clinician to explain the problem and the natural history of the condition to the athlete, who will want to know precisely for how long he or she will be affected. A patient may present with an acute knee injury but the diagnosis of anterior cruciate ligament tear has markedly different implications to the diagnosis of minor meniscal injury.
2. optimum treatment. Numerous conditions have similar presentations but markedly different treatments. For example, consider the differences in treatment between: lateral ligament sprain of the ankle and osteochondral fracture of the talus; patellofemoral joint syndrome and meniscal tear; hamstring tear and hamstring pain referred from the lumbar spine.
3. optimum rehabilitation prescription. For example, rehabilitation after shin pain due to stress fracture will be more gradual than that after identical shin pain due to chronic compartment syndrome.

 When a patient presents with an overuse injury, an accurate pathological diagnosis must be supplemented by assessment of the etiologic factors underlying the condition, otherwise the injury is likely to be slow to recover and highly likely to recur.

Etiologic factors include training error, malalignment, faulty technique and inappropriate equipment. An important etiologic factor can sometimes be identified by examining the entire 'kinetic chain'.

Occasionally, it may be impossible to make a precise pathological diagnosis. For example, in a patient with low back pain, the exact source of the pain is often difficult to isolate. In such cases it is still possible to exclude certain causes of low back pain (e.g. spondylolysis) and identify abnormalities such as areas of focal tenderness, altered soft tissue consistency or abnormalities of range of motion. Treatment then aims to correct these abnormalities. How treatment affects symptoms and signs can help determine how each particular abnormality contributes to the overall picture.

Making a diagnosis

Diagnosis relies on taking a careful history, performing a thorough physical examination and using appropriate investigations. There is a tendency for clinicians to rely too heavily on sophisticated investigations and to neglect their clinical skills.[1]

Keys to accurate diagnosis in patients presenting with apparent musculoskeletal pain include:

- whether the symptoms are of musculoskeletal origin (Chapter 4)
- possible local causes of the patient's symptoms
- sites that could be referring pain to the site of the symptoms (Chapter 3)

- the relevant kinetic chain (e.g. the back and lower limb in a shoulder injury of a tennis player)
- biomechanics (Chapter 5)
- other possible causative factors (e.g. metabolic).

History

History remains the keystone of accurate diagnosis; it will provide the diagnosis in the majority of cases. Please consider the following principles when taking a history.

Allow enough time

The patient must feel that the clinician has time available to allow the story to unfold, otherwise important symptoms will not surface.[2] In addition to the details of the injury, there must be time to take the history of the training program or diet as appropriate. Look into possible causes of injury. As a minimum, 30 minutes is required to assess a patient with a new injury but in complex chronic cases up to 1 hour may be necessary.

Be a good listener

The clinician must let the story unravel. Appropriate body language and focus on the patient (not the medical record) will aid this.[3] The sports clinician is in the fortunate position that many patients have good body awareness and are generally able to describe symptoms very well. When seeing inactive patients for exercise prescription, take the time to listen to their goals and fears (Chapter 55).

Know the sport

It is helpful to understand the technical demands of a sport when seeing an athlete as this engenders patient confidence. More importantly, knowledge of the biomechanics and techniques of a particular sport can assist greatly in both making the primary diagnosis and uncovering the predisposing factors.

Discover the exact circumstances of the injury

The first task in history taking is to determine the exact circumstances of the injury. Most patients will be able to describe in considerable detail the mechanism of injury. In acute injuries this is the single most important clue to diagnosis. For example, an inversion injury to the ankle strongly suggests a lateral ligament injury, a valgus strain to the knee may cause a medial collateral ligament injury, and a pivoting injury accompanied by a 'pop' in the knee and followed by rapid swelling suggests an anterior cruciate ligament injury.

Obtain an accurate description of symptoms

An accurate description of the patient's symptoms is essential. Common musculoskeletal symptoms include pain, swelling, instability and loss of function.

Pain

Consider the characteristics of the patient's pain.

1. Location. Note the exact location of pain. A detailed knowledge of surface anatomy will enable you to determine the structures likely to be involved. If the pain is poorly localized or varies from site to site, consider the possibility of referred pain.
2. Onset. Speed of onset helps determine whether the pain is due to an acute or overuse injury. Was the onset of pain associated with a snap, crack, tear or other sensation?
3. Severity. Severity may be classified as mild, moderate or severe. Assess the severity of the pain immediately after the injury and subsequently. Was the patient able to continue activity?
4. Irritability. This refers to the level of activity required to provoke pain and how long it subsequently takes to settle. The degree of irritability is especially important because it affects how vigorously the examination should be performed and how aggressive the treatment should be.
5. Nature. This refers to the quality of the pain. It is important to allow patients to describe pain in their own words.
6. Behavior. Is the pain constant or intermittent? What is the time course of the pain? Is it worse on waking or does it worsen during the day? Does it wake the patient at night?
7. Radiation. Does the pain radiate at all? If so, where?
8. Aggravating factors. Which activity or posture aggravates the pain?
9. Relieving factors. Is the pain relieved by rest or the adoption of certain postures? Do certain activities relieve the pain? Is the pain affected by climatic changes, for example, cold weather?
10. Associated features. These include swelling, instability, sensory symptoms, such as pins and needles, tingling or numbness, and motor symptoms, such as muscle weakness.

11. Previous treatment. What was the initial treatment of the injury? Was ice applied? Was firm compression applied? Was the injured part immobilized? If so, for how long? What treatment has been performed and what effect did that treatment have on the pain?

Swelling

Immediate swelling following an injury may indicate a severe injury such as a fracture or major ligament tear accompanied by hemarthrosis. Record the degree of swelling—mild, moderate or severe—and subsequent changes in the amount of swelling.

Instability

Any history of giving way or feeling of instability is significant. Try to elicit the exact activity that causes this feeling. For example, in throwing, does the feeling of instability occur in the cocking phase or the follow-through?

Function

It is important to know whether the athlete was able to continue activity without any problems immediately after the injury, was able to continue with some restriction or was unable to continue. Note subsequent changes in function with time.

History of a previous similar injury

If the athlete has had a previous similar injury, record full details of all treatment given, response to each type of treatment and whether any maintenance treatment or exercises have been performed following initial rehabilitation. Previous injury is a major risk factor for recurrence.[4]

Other injuries

Past injuries may have contributed to the current injury, for example, an inadequately rehabilitated muscle tear that has led to muscle imbalance and a subsequent overuse injury. Because of the importance of spinal abnormalities as a potential component of the athlete's pain (Chapter 3), the patient should always be questioned about spinal symptoms, especially pain and stiffness in the lower back or neck. Past or present injuries in body parts that may at first seem unrelated to the present injury may also be important. For example, a hamstring injury in a throwing athlete can impair the kinetic chain leading to the shoulder, alter throwing biomechanics and, thus, contribute to a rotator cuff injury.

General health

Is the patient otherwise healthy? The presence of symptoms such as weight loss and general malaise may suggest a serious abnormality, for example, a tumor. It must be remembered that musculoskeletal symptoms are not always activity-related (Chapter 4).

Work and leisure activities

Work and leisure activities can play a role in both the etiology and subsequent management of an injury. For example, a patient whose job involves continual bending or who enjoys gardening may aggravate his or her low back pain. It is important to know about these activities and to ascertain whether they can be curtailed.

Consider why the problem has occurred

Predisposing factors should be considered not only in overuse injuries but also in medical conditions and in acute injuries. In an athlete suffering from exercise-induced asthma, symptoms may occur only during important competition if there is an underlying psychological component. Alternatively, the asthma may occur only at a particular time of the year or at a particular venue if allergy is present.

An athlete with an acute hamstring tear may have a history of low back problems or, alternatively, a history of a previous inadequately rehabilitated tear. Recurrence can only be prevented by eliminating the underlying cause.

Training history

In any overuse injury, a comprehensive training history is required. This is best done as a weekly diary as most athletes train on a weekly cycle (Chapter 6). It should contain both the quantity and quality of training and describe any recent changes. Note the total amount of training (distance or hours depending on the sport) and training surfaces. Continual activity on hard surfaces or a recent change in surface may predispose to injury. In running sports, pay particular attention to footwear (Chapter 6). For both training and competition shoes, note the shoe type, age and the wear pattern. Record recovery activities such as massage, spa/sauna and hours of sleep.

Equipment

Inappropriate equipment may predispose to injury (Chapter 6). For example, a bicycle seat that is set too low may contribute to patellofemoral pain.

Technique

Patients should discuss technique problems that either they, or their coach, have noted. Faulty technique may contribute to injury. For example, a 'wristy' backhand drive may contribute to extensor tendinopathy at the elbow.

Overtraining

Symptoms such as excessive fatigue, recurrent illness, reduced motivation, persistent soreness and stiffness may point to overtraining as an etiologic factor (Chapter 6).

Psychological factors

Injury can be caused or exacerbated by a number of psychological factors that may relate to sport (i.e. pressure of impending competition) or may concern personal or business life. The clinician needs to consider this possibility and approach it sensitively.

Nutritional factors

Inadequate nutrition can predispose to the overtraining syndrome and may play a role in the development of musculoskeletal injuries. In an athlete presenting with excessive tiredness (Chapter 52), a full dietary history is essential.

Determine the importance of the sport to the athlete

The level of commitment to the sport, which will not necessarily correlate with the athlete's expertise, has a bearing on management decisions. Be aware of the athlete's short- and long-term future sporting commitments to schedule appropriate treatment and rehabilitation programs.

At the conclusion of taking the history, it is important to consider the differential diagnosis and the possible etiologic factors. Then proceed to a thorough focused examination.

Examination

A number of general principles should be followed in an examination[5] and these are outlined below.

Develop a routine

Use a specific routine for examining each joint, region or system as this forms a habit and allows you to concentrate on the findings and their significance rather than thinking of what to do next. In Part B, we outline a routine for examining each body part.

Where relevant, examine the other side

With some aspects of the examination, for example, ligamentous laxity or muscle tightness, it is important to compare sides using the uninjured side as a control.

Consider possible causes of the injury

Try to ascertain the cause of the injury. It is not sufficient to examine the painful area only (e.g. the Achilles tendon). Examine joints, muscles and neural structures proximal and distal to the injured area, seeking predisposing factors (e.g. limited dorsiflexion of the ankle, tight gastrocnemius–soleus complex, lumbar facet joint dysfunction).

Attempt to reproduce the patient's symptoms

It is helpful to reproduce the patient's symptoms if possible. This can be achieved both by active and/or passive movements and by palpation either locally or, in the case of referred pain, at the site of referral. It may require you to send the patient for a run or some other test of function prior to examination (see below).

Assess local tissues

Assess the joints, muscles and neural structures at the site of pain for tenderness, tissue feel and range of motion.

Assess for referred pain

Assess the joints, muscles and neural structures that may refer to the site of pain (Chapter 3).

Assess neural tension

Neural tension (Chapter 3) should be assessed using one or more of the neural tension tests (see below).

Examine the spine

Many injuries have a spinal component to the pain or dysfunction. The presence of abnormal neural tension suggests a possible spinal component. In lower limb injuries, examine the lumbar spine and the thoracolumbar junction. In upper limb injuries, examine the cervical and upper thoracic spines. In particular, it is important to seek hypomobility of isolated spinal segments as this may contribute to distant symptoms.

Biomechanical examination

As biomechanical abnormalities are one of the major causes of overuse injuries, it is essential to include this examination in the assessment of overuse injuries (Chapter 5). The biomechanical examination of the lower limb is illustrated in Chapter 5.

Functional testing

If a particular maneuver reproduces the patient's pain, then have the patient perform that maneuver in an attempt to understand why the pain has occurred. This can sometimes be done in the office, for example, a deep squat, or it may be necessary to watch the athlete perform the activity at a training venue, for example, a long jumper taking off or a gymnast performing a backward walkover. Video analysis may be helpful.

The examination routine

Inspection

It is important to observe the individual walking into the office or walking off the field of play as well as inspecting the injured area. Note any evidence of deformity, asymmetry, bruising, swelling, skin changes and muscle wasting. There may, however, be a degree of asymmetry due to one side being dominant, such as the racquet arm in a tennis player.

Range of motion testing (active)

Ask the athlete to perform active range of motion exercises without assistance. Look carefully for restriction of range of motion, the onset of pain at a particular point in the range and the presence of abnormal patterns of movement. In many conditions, such as shoulder impingement or patellofemoral pain, the pattern of movement is critical to making a correct diagnosis.

If a patient's pain is not elicited on normal plane movement testing, examine 'combined movements' (i.e. movements in two or more planes). By combining movements and evaluating symptom response, additional information is gained to help predict the site of the lesion. Other movements, such as repeated, quick or sustained movements, may be required to elicit the patient's pain.

Range of motion testing (passive)

Passive range of motion testing is used to elicit joint and muscle stiffness. Injury may be the cause of joint stiffness. Alternatively, stiffness may already have been present and predisposed to injury by placing excessive stress on other structures (e.g. a stiff ankle joint can predispose to Achilles tendinopathy). Range of motion testing should include all directions of movement appropriate to a particular joint and should be compared both with normal range and the unaffected side. Overpressure may be used at the end of range to elicit the patient's symptoms.

Palpation

Palpation is a vital component of examination and precise knowledge of anatomy, especially surface anatomy, optimizes its value. At times it is essential to determine the exact site of maximal tenderness, for example, in differentiating between bony tenderness and ligament attachment tenderness after a sprained ankle. When palpating soft tissues, properties of the soft tissue that need to be assessed include:

- resistance
- muscle spasm
- tenderness.

Palpate carefully and try to visualize the structures being palpated. Commence with the skin, feeling for any changes in temperature or amount of sweating, infection or increased sympathetic activity. When palpating muscle, assess tone, focal areas of thickening or trigger points, muscle length and imbalance.

It is important not only to palpate the precise area of pain, for example, the supraspinatus tendon attachment, but also the regions proximal and distal to the painful area, such as the muscle belly of the trapezius muscle. Determine whether tenderness is focal or diffuse. This may help differentiate between, for example, a stress fracture (focal tenderness) and periostitis (diffuse tenderness).

To palpate joints correctly, it is important to understand the two different types of movement present at a joint. Physiological movements are movements that patients can perform themselves. However, in order to achieve a full range of physiological movement, accessory movements are required.

Accessory movements are the involuntary, inter-articular movements, including glides, rotations and tilts, that occur in both spinal and peripheral joints during normal physiological movements. Loss of these normal accessory movements may cause pain, altered range or abnormal quality of physiological joint movement. Palpation of the spinal and peripheral joints is based on these principles. An example of palpation of accessory movements involves postero-anterior pressure over the spinous process of the vertebra, producing a glide between that vertebra and the ones above and below.

Ligament testing

Ligaments are examined for laxity and pain. Specific tests have been devised for all the major ligaments of the body. These involve moving the joint to stress a particular ligament. This may cause pain or reveal laxity in the joint. Laxity is graded into +1 (mild), +2 (moderate) and +3 (severe). Pain on stressing the ligament is also significant and may indicate, in the absence of laxity, a mild injury or grade I ligament sprain. A number of different tests may assess a single ligament: for example, the anterior drawer, Lachman's and pivot shift tests all test anterior cruciate ligament laxity.

Strength testing

Muscles or groups of muscles should be tested for strength and compared with the unaffected side. Muscle weakness may occur as a result of an injury, for example, secondary to a chronic joint effusion, or may be a predisposing factor towards injury.

Neural tension testing

Advances in the understanding of neural tension have led to improved awareness of why pain occurs in chronic overuse injuries and pain syndromes. Changes in neural tension are an important component of these disorders (Chapter 3).

Just as restrictions of the normal mechanics of joints and muscles may contribute to symptoms, restriction of the normal mechanics of the nervous system may also produce pain. Certain movements require considerable variations in nerve length. Neural tension testing examines restriction of these normal mechanics and their effect on the patient's symptoms. Treatment aims to restore normal nerve mechanics.

Neural tension tests produce systematic increases in neural tension by successive addition of movements that increase neural tension. The tests may provoke the presenting symptoms or, alternatively, other symptoms such as pins and needles or numbness. The amount of resistance encountered during the test is also significant, especially when compared with the uninjured side. The assessment of symptom production and resistance may be affected by each step in the neural tension test (see Figs 8.1–8.4). This may give an indication of the location of the abnormality.

The main neural tension tests are:

- straight leg raise (SLR) (Fig. 8.1)
- slump test (Fig. 8.2)

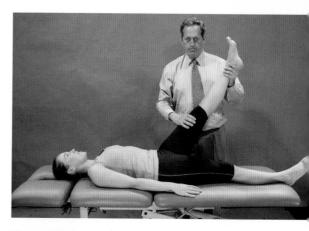

Figure 8.1 Straight leg raise

(a) Patient lies supine. The examiner places one hand under the Achilles tendon and the other above the knee. The leg is lifted perpendicular to the bed with the hand above the knee preventing any knee flexion

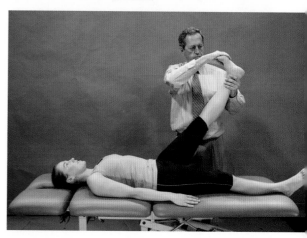

(b) Dorsiflexion of the ankle is added. Eversion and toe extension may sensitize this test further. Other variations can be added (Table 8.1)

- neural Thomas test (Fig. 8.3)
- upper limb tension test (ULTT) (Fig. 8.4).

A summary of the tests, the methods, indications for their use, normal responses and variations of each test is shown in Table 8.1.

A tension test can be considered positive if:

- it reproduces the patient's symptoms
- the test response can be altered by movements of different body parts that alter the neural tension
- differences in the test occur from side to side and from what is considered normal.

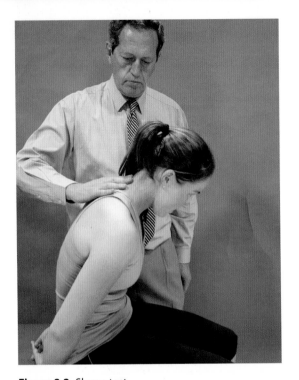

Figure 8.2 Slump test

(a) Patient slumps forward and overpressure is applied. The sacrum should remain vertical

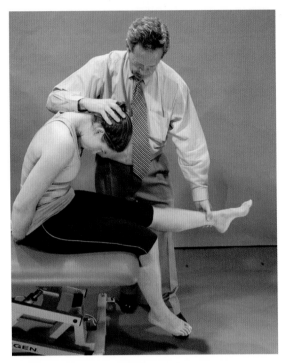

(c) Patient actively extends one knee

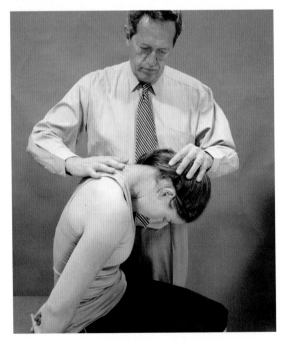

(b) Patient is asked to put chin on chest and overpressure is applied

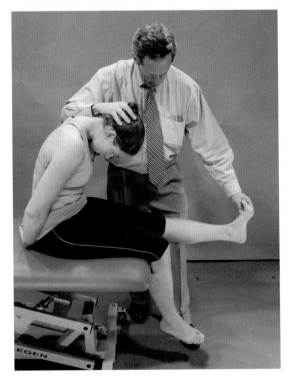

(d) Patient actively dorsiflexes the ankle and overpressure may be applied

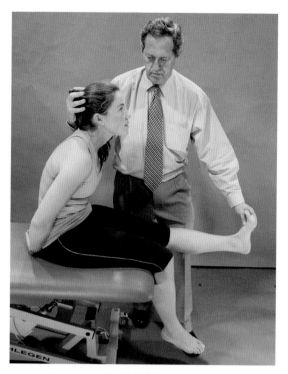

(e) Neck flexion is slowly released. Steps (d), (e) and (f) are repeated with the other knee. Other variations can be added (Table 8.1)

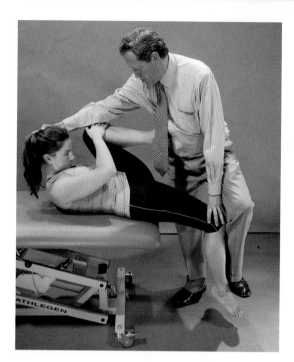

(b) Patient's neck is passively flexed by the examiner, then the examiner passively extends the patient's (right) knee with his or her leg

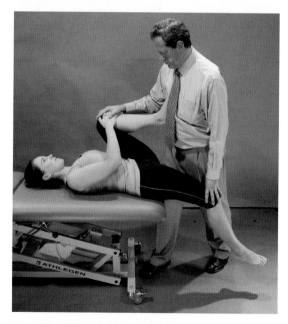

Figure 8.3 Neural Thomas test

(a) Patient lies supine over the end of the couch in the Thomas position

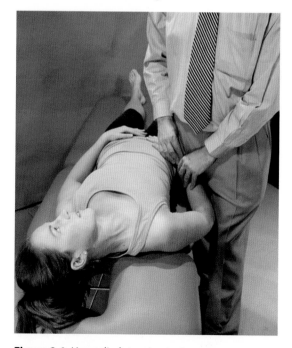

Figure 8.4 Upper limb tension test

(a) Patient lies supine close to the edge of the couch. Neck is laterally flexed away from the side to be tested

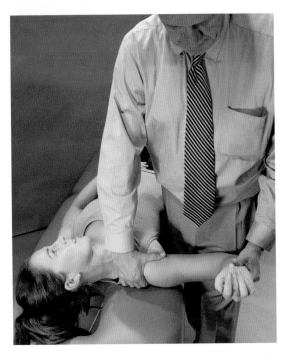

(b) The shoulder is depressed by the examiner's hand (left) and the arm abducted to approximately 110° and externally rotated

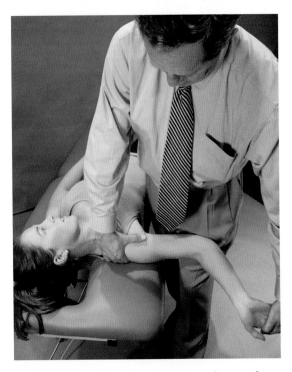

(d) The elbow is extended to the point of onset of symptoms

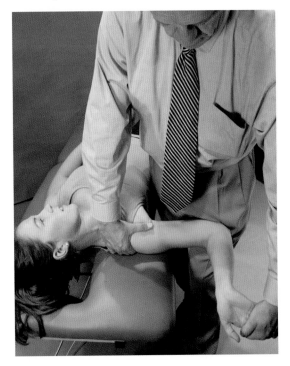

(c) The forearm is supinated and the wrist and fingers extended

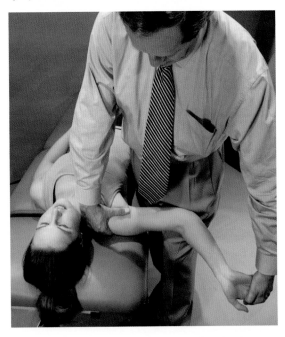

(e) The neck position returns to neutral and is then laterally flexed towards the side of the test. Any change in symptoms is noted. Other variations can be added (Table 8.1)

Table 8.1 Neural tension tests

Test	Method	Indications	Normal response	Variations
Straight leg raise (Fig. 8.1)	Patient lies supine Leg extended Clinician lifts leg	Leg pain Back pain Headache	Tightness and/or pain in posterior knee, thigh and calf	Ankle dorsiflexion Ankle plantarflexion/inversion Hip adduction Hip medial rotation Passive neck flexion
Slump test (Fig. 8.2)	Patient sitting Slumps Neck flexion Knee extension Ankle dorsiflexion Release neck flexion	Back pain Buttock pain Leg pain	Upper thoracic pain Posterior knee pain Hamstring pain	Leg abduction (obturator nerve) Hip adduction Hip medial rotation Ankle and foot alterations
Neural Thomas test (Fig. 8.3)	Patient lies supine Hip extension Neck flexion Knee flexion	Groin pain Anterior thigh pain	Quadriceps pain and/or tightness	Hip abduction/adduction Hip medial/lateral rotation
Upper limb tension test (Fig. 8.4)	Patient supine towards side of couch Cervical contralateral flexion Shoulder girdle depression Shoulder abducted to 110° and externally rotated Forearm supination Wrist/fingers extended Elbow extended	Arm pain Neck/upper thoracic pain Headache	Ache in cubital fossa Tingling in thumb and fingers	Forearm pronation Wrist deviation Shoulder flexion/extension Add straight leg raise

Neural tension tests are non-specific but form an extremely useful part of the examination. Abnormalities of neural tension should lead the clinician to examine possible sites producing the abnormal tension, especially the spine. Neural tension tests can also be used as a treatment procedure. This is discussed in Chapter 10.

Spinal examination

Clinical experience suggests that spinal abnormality (e.g. hypomobility) can present in various ways. The presentation may be as pain or injury and this may occur either locally (at the spine) or distantly. Examples for both upper limb and lower limb spinal abnormalities are given in Table 8.2. The pathophysiology underlying these concepts has been discussed in Chapter 3.

In patients presenting with upper limb pain, the cervical and upper thoracic spines must be examined. Examine the lumbar spine (including the thoracolumbar junction) in any patient presenting with lower limb pain. An abnormal neural tension test strongly indicates a spinal component to the pain. However, a negative neural tension test does not exclude the possibility of a spinal component.

Begin examining the relevant area of the spine by assessing range of movement with the patient standing. The patient should then lie prone on a firm examination table so the examiner can palpate the vertebrae centrally over the spinous processes and laterally over the apophyseal joints to detect any hypomobility and/or tenderness. Hypomobility or tenderness at a level appropriate to that of the patient's symptoms indicate the site is a possible source of referred pain (Chapter 3).

After detecting spinal abnormality on examination, perform a trial treatment (Chapter 10) and then reassess the patient's symptoms and signs. If there is a change in the pain and/or range of movement, then this strongly suggests that the spine is contributing to the symptoms.

Occasionally, palpation of a particular site in the spine will actually reproduce the patient's symptoms distant from the spine. It is important to understand that, even if the symptoms are not produced by palpation of the spine, this does not rule out the possibility of a spinal component.

Biomechanical examination

The role of abnormal biomechanics in the production of injuries, especially overuse injuries, is discussed in Chapter 5. Because abnormal biomechanics can contribute to any overuse injury, all clinicians need to perform a biomechanical examination.

As with other components of the examination, it is important to develop a routine for the assessment of biomechanical abnormalities. A routine for the assessment of lower limb biomechanics is illustrated in Chapter 5.

Technique

Faulty technique is another common cause of injury. A list of technique faults associated with particular injuries is shown in Table 5.1. While the clinician cannot be aware of all techniques in various sports, he or she should be able to identify the common technique faults in popular activities, for example, pelvic instability while running or faulty backhand drive in tennis. Clinicians should seek biomechanical advice and assistance with assessment from the athlete's coach or a colleague with expertise in the particular area. Video analysis with slow motion or freeze frame may be helpful.

Table 8.2 Examples of how spinal abnormality can manifest locally or distantly, with either pain or injury in the upper limb and lower limb

Presentation	Local manifestation	Distant manifestation
Upper limb		
Pain	Hypomobility of C5–6 joint presenting as neck pain	Hypomobility of C5–6 joint presents as elbow pain
Injury		Hypomobility of C5–6 joint predisposing to lateral elbow tendinopathy in a tennis player
Lower limb		
Pain	Hypomobility of L5–S1 joint presenting as lumbosacral pain	Hypomobility of L5–S1 joint presents as buttock and hamstring pain
Injury		Hypomobility of L5–S1 joint predisposing to a hamstring tear in a sprinter

Equipment

Inappropriate equipment predisposes to injury (Chapter 6). Inspect the athlete's equipment, such as running shoes, football boots, tennis racquet, bicycle or helmet.

At the conclusion of the examination, consider the differential diagnosis and possible predisposing factors. If the practitioner is certain of the diagnosis and of the predisposing factors, then counseling and treatment can begin. However, in many cases, further information may be required and the practitioner must decide what, if any, investigations may be needed.

Recommended Reading

Murtagh J. *General Practice*. 3rd edn. Sydney: McGraw-Hill, 2003. *An excellent symptom-based approach to diagnosis in family medicine. A must for all physicians.*
Stanitski CL. Correlation of arthroscopic and clinical examinations with magnetic resonance imaging findings of injured knees in children and adolescents. *Am J Sports Med* 1998; 26(1): 2–6.

References

1. Khan K, Tress B, Hare W, et al. 'Treat the patient, not the X-ray': advances in diagnostic imaging do not replace the need for clinical interpretation. *Clin J Sport Med* 1998; 8: 1–4.
2. Vernec A, Shrier I. A teaching unit in primary care sports medicine for family medicine residents. *Acad Med* 2001; 76: 293–6.
3. Ruusuvuori J. Looking means listening: coordinating displays of engagement in doctor–patient interaction. *Soc Sci Med* 2001; 52: 1093–108.
4. Orchard JW. Intrinsic and extrinsic risk factors for muscle strains in Australian football. *Am J Sports Med* 2001; 29: 300–3.
5. Plastaras CT, Rittenberg JD, Rittenberg KE, et al. Comprehensive functional evaluation of the injured runner. *Phys Med Rehabil Clin North Am* 2005; 16: 623–49.

Principles of Diagnosis: Investigations including Imaging

WITH BRUCE FORSTER, JAIDEEP RAMPURE, ZOLTAN KISS AND JOCK ANDERSON

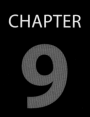

Investigations

Appropriate investigations can confirm or exclude a diagnosis suggested by the history and physical examination but should never be a substitute for careful history taking and a comprehensive examination (Chapter 8). We begin with seven principles that may help clinicians maximize the utility of investigations. We then detail the utility of current radiological investigations, before outlining a broad range of laboratory and special investigations that can add detail to the sports medicine diagnosis.

Understand the meaning of test results

The sports clinician should be able to interpret investigation results and not rely blindly on the investigation report. For example, a clinician who is aware that stress fractures are rarely demonstrated on plain X-rays is better able to help an athlete with bony tenderness and a normal plain X-ray than one who assumes a normal X-ray excludes the possibility of a fracture. A clinician who knows that about a quarter of asymptomatic elite jumping athletes have ultrasound abnormalities in their patellar tendons can reassure the patient that the imaging finding is not an indication for surgery. This is an example of a false positive investigation. Many such examples exist.

Know how soon changes can be detected by investigations

To detect certain abnormalities, the timing of an investigation may need to be appropriate. A female gymnast must have hormone levels tested in the second half of her menstrual cycle to detect low progesterone levels in luteal deficiency. Likewise, there is nothing to be gained by repeating a radioisotopic bone scan or a CT scan to assess fracture healing two months after diagnosing a lumbar pars interarticularis defect in a tennis player.

Only order investigations that will influence management

It is inappropriate to perform extensive (and expensive) investigations to confirm an already obvious diagnosis. If a stress fracture is seen on a plain X-ray, there is rarely anything to be gained from a radioisotopic bone scan, CT scan or MRI. On the other hand, if plain X-ray reveals a fractured dome of the talus, further tests may be indicated to stage the fracture as this affects treatment.

Provide relevant clinical findings on the requisition

The written requisition should contain a brief summary of the patient's condition and your differential diagnosis to aid correct imaging interpretation.[1] If particular X-ray views are required, they should be requested. If you cannot remember the names of certain views, write that down on the request forms—generally the radiographer will know and, if not, the radiologist will! It is often helpful to call the radiologist in advance to discuss the best way to image a patient. Remember that weight-bearing views are important to assess suspected osteoarthritis at the hip, knee and ankle. 'Functional' views (with the patient placing the joint in the position of pain) are useful for anterior and posterior impingement of the ankle (Chapter 34).

Do not accept a poor quality test

Inappropriate views or investigations performed on inferior equipment can lead to more diagnostic confusion than no investigation at all.

Develop a close working relationship with the investigators

Clinicians and investigators can learn from each other and assist the patient maximally by discussing clinical problems when this is appropriate.[1] Regular clinico-radiological rounds or case presentations should be encouraged. The advent of digital imaging has made discussion of images easier; the clinician and radiologist can be separated by miles and each can be viewing the images on his or her own monitor.

Explain the investigations to the patient

Give the patient an understanding of the rationale behind each investigation. An athlete who complains of persistent ankle pain and swelling several months after an ankle sprain may need an X-ray, a radioisotopic bone scan and possibly a CT scan or MRI. If the patient is merely told that an X-ray is necessary to exclude bony damage, he or she might become confused when told that the X-ray is normal but that further investigations are required to exclude bony or osteochondral damage. Also, be sure to alert patients who are going for a minimally invasive procedure (e.g. MR arthrogram), that there will be an 'injection'. Otherwise our radiologist and radiography colleagues are put in the awkward position of having to explain this to the patient de novo.

The patient should understand exactly what is involved in each procedure as well as why the procedure is being performed. It is helpful to give the patient a leaflet explaining the investigation, how long it will take and when he or she should be reviewed with the results of the investigation.

Radiological investigation

Plain X-ray

Despite the availability of sophisticated imaging techniques, plain film radiography often provides diagnostic information about bony abnormalities, such as fractures, dislocations, dysplasia and calcification (Fig. 9.1).[2] Correctly positioning the patient is vital for a useful X-ray. A minimum of two perpendicular views is required to evaluate any bone adequately. Complex joints such as the ankle, wrist or the elbow may require additional or specialized

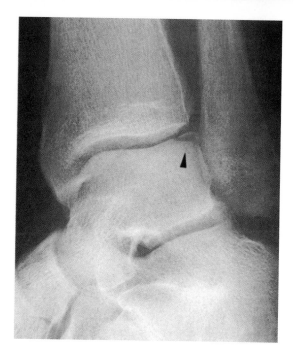

Figure 9.1 X-ray of an osteochondral fracture of the talar dome (COURTESY OF I.F. ANDERSON)

views. Weight-bearing or 'stress' views may give further information.

Radioisotopic bone scan

Radioisotopic bone scan (scintigraphy) (Fig. 9.2) is a highly sensitive but non-specific nuclear medicine investigation used to detect areas of increased blood flow (inflammation, infection) and bone turnover (fractures and other bone lesions, including tumors).

Nuclear medicine provides physiological rather than anatomical information. In contrast to routine radiography and CT, which measure X-ray transmission through a patient, nuclear medicine detects gamma ray emission from a patient following intravenous administration of a radiopharmaceutical. The radiopharmaceutical contains a radioactive atom that decays, resulting in gamma ray photon emission. These emitted photons are detected by a gamma camera imaging system.[3]

A triple-phase bone scan is performed after the injection of a technetium-labeled bone-seeking agent. Scans are obtained immediately (isotope angiogram), after 2 minutes (blood pool phase) and after 2 hours (bone phase). This sequence of scans allows

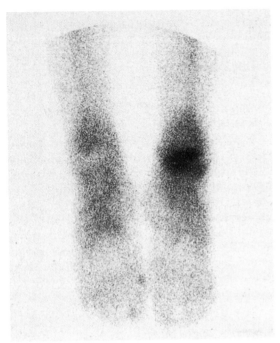

Figure 9.2 Radioisotopic bone scan of an osteochondral fracture of the talar dome

COURTESY OF I. F. ANDERSON

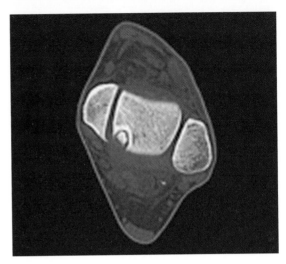

Figure 9.3 CT scan of an osteochondral fracture of the talar dome

differentiation between soft tissue and bone injury. Radioisotopic bone scans are particularly useful for the detection of stress fractures and osteochondral lesions[4, 5] but give little information regarding soft tissue and mean significant radiation exposure. The blood pool phase can show hyperemia. Bone scans are particularly useful when seeking hook of hamate fractures as these subtle fractures can be overlooked when using CT scans or MRI.

Single photon emission computed tomography (SPECT) techniques are also used in sports medicine. In SPECT, gamma cameras are mounted on a rotating gantry, and a full 360° acquisition can be obtained.[3] The main advantage of SPECT over planar imaging is enhanced tissue contrast, resulting in improved sensitivity and specificity of lesion detection and localization.[6] The main use of SPECT in sports medicine is in the detection of stress fractures of the pars interarticularis of the lumbar spine. In some centers, SPECT bone scan for pars injuries is more sensitive than MRI.

Computed tomographic scanning

CT scanning (Fig. 9.3) allows cross-sectional imaging of soft tissue, calcific deposits and bone. Conventional CT scanning consists of a rotating X-ray tube emitting a collimated radiation beam and multiple detectors to measure transmission through a stationary patient. A computer then processes the data to provide a two-dimensional or simulated three-dimensional image. Technical advances have led to the development of helical or spiral CT scanning.

CT scanning is particularly useful in evaluation of the spine, fractures in small bones and fractures in anatomically complex regions, such as the ankle, foot or pelvis. Newer multi-detector scanners have 4, 16 or 64 rows of detectors, and are capable of providing high-resolution reconstructions of the imaging data in any plane.

CT arthrography is performed after an injection of radio-opaque contrast medium into the joint cavity—most commonly the shoulder or ankle. This procedure is becoming superseded by MR arthrograms (MRA) with gadolinium in centers where MRI is readily available (see below). The disadvantage of CT scanning is the significant radiation dose, especially in children.

Magnetic resonance imaging

MRI (Fig. 9.4) is based on the number of free water protons present within a tissue sample. When a patient is placed in a strong magnetic field, the free water protons align with the external magnetic field. In MRI a series of radiofrequency (RF) pulses are applied to the tissue sample, which causes the protons to change their alignment relative to the external magnetic field. The energy released during this realignment of protons is used to create the image.

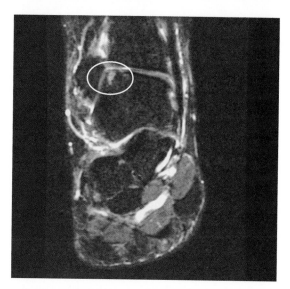

Figure 9.4 MRI of an osteochondral fracture (circled) of the talar dome. The plain X-rays and CT were normal

A pulse sequence is a specific series of RF pulses or gradient changes that result in excitation and realignment of water protons in a predictable fashion, allowing for the creation of an image. Spin echo (SE), gradient echo (GRE) and inversion recovery (IR) sequences are the basic types of sequences used in musculoskeletal imaging.[3] T1-weighted, T2-weighted, proton density and short T1 inversion recovery (STIR) sequences are often taken (Table 9.1). Fat-suppressed and fat-saturated sequences can also be taken.

MRI is not dependent on ionizing radiation and is not invasive. Compared with CT scanning, it is less capable of defining bone details and detecting small areas of calcification, but it is nevertheless very useful at revealing occult bony abnormalities,[7-9] and its superior contrast resolution allows the detection of subtle soft tissue changes. This latter property, together with its multiplanar scanning capability, is most valuable in detecting spinal disk/root abnormalities, avascular necrosis and bone marrow tumors, and in evaluating soft tissue masses. MRI is commonly used to assess internal derangement of joints.[10, 11]

 There are a few strict contraindications to MRI (e.g. certain brain aneurysm clips, neurostimulators and cardiac pacemakers) but, contrary to popular medical opinion, patients with metallic orthopedic hardware and metallic surgical clips outside the brain, in place for more than six weeks, can be safely scanned.

Sports clinicians must be aware that MRI can be overly sensitive to abnormal tissue signals and, thus, provide false positive results. In asymptomatic athletes in numerous studies, MR images are consistent with significant injury but none exists.[12, 13] This emphasizes the need for the appropriate selection of patients for investigation and careful clinical–imaging correlation.[1] As with any medical investigation, errors can occur; ideally, images should be read by an experienced musculoskeletal MRI radiologist.

Ultrasound scan

High-resolution ultrasound scanning (Fig. 9.5) with 10–12 megahertz (MHz) probes is a painless method of imaging tendons, muscles and other soft tissues without exposing the patient to any radiation. Other

Table 9.1 Different MRI images

Image	Signal intensity	Clinical use
T1-weighted image	Fat: bright Muscle: intermediate Water, tendons and fibrocartilage: dark	Good for anatomical detail, bone marrow Lacks sensitivity in detecting soft tissue injury Good for meniscal pathology
T2-weighted image	Water: bright Fat: intermediate Muscle, fibrocartilage: dark	Good for most soft tissue injury, especially tendons
Proton density (PD)	Fat: bright Calcium, tendons, fibrocartilage: dark Water: intermediate	Good for menisci and ligaments
Short T1 inversion recovery (STIR)/ Fat saturated T2 sequence	Water: very bright Fat, muscle, fibrocartilage: dark	Good for bone marrow and soft tissue pathology

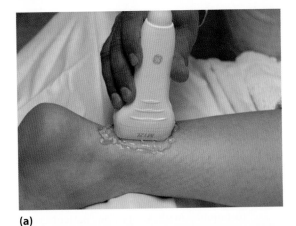

(a)

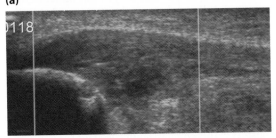

(b)

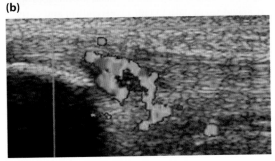

(c)

Figure 9.5 (a) Method of imaging tendons.
(b) Gray-scale ultrasound scan and **(c)** color
Doppler ultrasound scan of the patellar tendon

advantages include its dynamic nature, short examination time and ability to guide therapeutic injection under real time. Disadvantages include the less graphic images, the fact that it is more operator-dependent with respect to image quality than any other modality, and the fact that it cannot penetrate tissues to show deeper structures, such as shoulder/hip labra or anterior cruciate ligaments/menisci. The most commonly examined areas are large tendons, for example, the Achilles, patellar and rotator cuff tendons, and the muscles of the thigh and calf. Ultrasound can also demonstrate muscle tear, hematoma formation

or early calcification, and may be useful in localizing foreign bodies.

Ultrasound scanning is able to distinguish complete tendon rupture from other tendon abnormalities (e.g. tendinopathy). As with MRI, ultrasound imaging of elite athletes reveals morphological 'abnormalities' that are not symptomatic and do not appear to predict imminent tendon pain.[14]

Real-time ultrasound examination during active movement (dynamic ultrasound) is particularly helpful in the evaluation of shoulder impingement. In recent years, color Doppler ultrasound has gained popularity in sports medicine for the assessment of tendons as innovative research suggested that the abnormal flow detected using the color Doppler feature provided a better guide as to whether tendons were painful or not.[15] Although this had been the case in cross-sectional studies,[16] longitudinal studies have failed to show that color Doppler ultrasound findings of vascularity predict changes in symptoms.[16-18] Also, exercise affects the level of vascularity.[19] Thus, as this text goes to print, the jury is still out as to the additional clinical utility of this modality. New data that come to hand, including standardized exercise protocols and warm-up techniques for assessing this interesting phenomenon, will be summarized in updates to this chapter at <http://www.clinicalsportsmedicine.com>. Also, in several studies ablation of this abnormal flow using the sclerosing agent polidocanol was shown to reduce tendon pain.[20, 21]

Neurological investigations

Electromyography

Electromyography (EMG) measures muscle activity by recording action potentials from the contracting fibers, either by using surface electrodes or by inserting needle electrodes into the muscle. After an electrical stimulus is applied to muscle, the type of response provides information regarding the nature of the dysfunction.

Nerve conduction studies

Motor and sensory nerve conduction studies aim to recognize and localize peripheral nerve abnormalities. After a stimulus (either electrical or mechanical) is applied to a distant part of the nerve, electrical action potentials are measured. Characteristic changes in the amplitude or velocity of action potential conduction reflect abnormalities of nerve function, for example, demyelination or axonal damage.

Neuropsychological testing

Neuropsychological testing is used to assess the severity of and recovery from minor head injury. The specific techniques used are discussed in Chapter 13.

Muscle assessment

Compartment pressure testing

Intracompartmental pressures are measured at rest and during exercise using a Stryker catheter. The patient then exercises the muscles of the specific compartment either to exhaustion or until symptoms are reproduced. Post-exercise resting pressure is monitored for 5 minutes. The diagnosis of compartment pressure syndrome is confirmed when the compartment pressures reach a diagnostic threshold during and after exercise (Chapter 30).

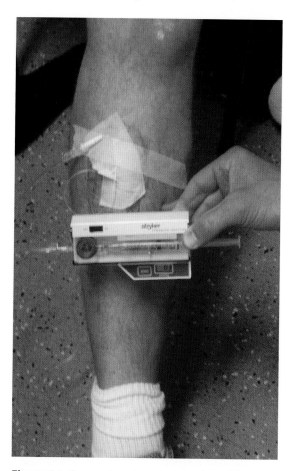

Figure 9.6 Compartment pressure testing of the anterior compartment of the lower limb

Cardiovascular investigations

Electrocardiography

Electrocardiography (ECG/EKG) measures the electrical activity and function of the heart via surface electrodes. A number of recognizable electrical deflections (P wave, QRS complex, T wave) are observed. Characteristic ECG abnormalities may reflect underlying cardiac disease.

Ambulatory ECG monitoring is the long-term ECG monitoring of patients during normal daily activity. The patient wears a portable monitor that records the ECG changes. This technique may be useful in the diagnosis of arrhythmia or intermittent ischemia, the evaluation of drug therapy and in detecting pacemaker malfunction.

Stress electrocardiography

Stress or exercise ECG is performed by monitoring the patient electrocardiographically while exercising. It is used to investigate ischemic heart disease. This procedure is discussed further in Chapter 45.

Echocardiography

Echocardiography is the clinical application of ultrasound to the diagnosis of heart disease. Ultrasound waves reflected from the different parts of the heart can map out the normal anatomical structure of the heart in two dimensions. Doppler echo techniques enable accurate measurements of intracardiac blood velocity and, therefore, enable the clinician to determine the gradients across valves or shunts.

Respiratory investigations

Pulmonary function tests

There are a number of simple tests of ventilatory capacity, such as forced expiratory volume in one second (FEV_1) and vital capacity (VC), which require relatively simple apparatus. Coupled with arterial blood gas measurements, these tests provide information on the mechanical characteristics of the ventilatory pump and the adequacy of pulmonary gas exchange. Carbon monoxide transfer indicates the gas exchange mechanisms and may detect subtle changes in function. More sophisticated techniques enable measurement of lung compliance, peripheral airway disease, airway reactivity, mucociliary clearance, respiratory muscle function and work of breathing.

Bronchial provocation challenge tests used in the diagnosis of exercise-induced bronchospasm (EIB) are discussed fully in Chapter 46.

The diagnosis

As a result of careful clinical assessment (Chapter 8) and the judicious use of investigations, the diagnosis should be evident. The next step is to discuss the diagnosis, the possible causes of the problem and an outline of the treatment program with the patient. Muscle charts and models of particular joints can assist the athlete understand the condition. Internet links can often provide the athlete with a lot of information; this will be appreciated.

Once the diagnosis is made and a clear explanation given to the patient, it is time to consider what treatment is appropriate for the condition. Chapter 10 provides an overview of current treatment alternatives.

Recommended Reading

Anderson J, Read JW, Steinweg J. *Atlas of Imaging in Sports Medicine*. Sydney: McGraw-Hill, 1998.

Calkins C, Sartoris DJ. Imaging acute knee injuries: direct diagnostic approaches. *Physician Sports Med* 1992; 20(6): 91–8.

Cross TM, Smart RC, Thomson JEM. Exposure to diagnostic ionizing radiation in sports medicine: assessing and monitoring the risk. *Clin J Sport Med* 2003; 13: 164–70.

Interesting article highlighting concerns about multiple procedures exposing athletes to high levels of ionizing radiation.

Halpern B, Herring SA, Altchek D, et al. *Imaging in Musculoskeletal and Sports Medicine*. Malden, MA: Blackwell Scientific, 1997.

Ishibashi Y, Okamura Y, Otsuka H, et al. Comparison of scintigraphy and magnetic resonance imaging for stress injuries of bone. *Clin J Sport Med* 2002; 12: 79–84.

Sanders TG, Fults-Ganey C. Imaging of sports-related injuries. In: DeLee JC, Drez D Jr, eds. *Orthopaedic Sports Medicine*. 2nd edn. Philadelphia: Saunders Elsevier Science, 2003.

Spritzer CE. Impact of magnetic resonance imaging in sports medicine. In: Garrett WE, Speer KP, Kirkendall DT, eds. *Principles and Practice of Orthopaedic Sports Medicine*. Philadelphia: Lippincott, Williams & Wilkins, 2000.

Stanitski CL. Correlation of arthroscopic and clinical examinations with magnetic resonance imaging findings of injured knees in children and adolescents. *Am J Sports Med* 1998; 26(1): 2–6.

Stoller DW, Tirman PFJ, Bredella MA. *Diagnostic Imaging Orthopaedics*. Salt Lake City, UT: Amirsys, 2004.

Outstanding textbook with excellent images and adjacent beautiful diagrams.

References

1. Kilhenny C. Improving communications between team physician and radiologist. *Am J Sports Med* 1972; 1: 20.

2. Taljanovic MS, Hunter TB, Fitzpatrick KA, et al. Musculoskeletal magnetic resonance imaging: importance of radiography. *Skeletal Radiol* 2003; 32: 403–11.

3. Spritzer CE. Impact of magnetic resonance imaging in sports medicine. In: Garrett WE, Speer KP, Kirkendall DT, eds. *Principles and Practice of Orthopaedic Sports Medicine*. Philadelphia: Lippincott, Williams & Wilkins, 2000.

4. Shikare S, Samsi AB, Tilve GH. Bone imaging in sports medicine. *J Postgrad Med* 1997; 43: 71–2.

5. Ishibashi Y, Okamura, Y, Otsuka, H, et al. Comparison of scintigraphy and magnetic resonance imaging for stress injuries of bone. *Clin J Sport Med* 2002; 12: 79–84.

6. Groshar D, Gorenberg M, Ben Haim S, et al. Lower extremity scintigraphy: the foot and ankle. *Semin Nucl Med* 1998; 28: 62–77.

7. Bencardino J, Rosenberg ZS, Delfaut E. MR imaging in sports injuries of the foot and ankle. *Magn Reson Imaging Clin N Am* 1999; 7: 131–49, ix.

8. Ascenti G, Visalli C, Genitori A, et al. Multiple hypervascular pancreatic metastases from renal cell carcinoma: dynamic MR and spiral CT in three cases. *Clin Imaging* 2004; 28: 349–52.

9. Gaeta M, Minutoli F, Scribano E, et al. CT and MR imaging findings in athletes with early tibial stress injuries: comparison with bone scintigraphy findings and emphasis on cortical abnormalities. *Radiology* 2005; 235: 553–61.

10. De Smet AA, Norris MA, Yandow DR, et al. MR diagnosis of meniscal tears of the knee: importance of high signal in the meniscus that extends to the surface. *Am J Roentgenol* 1993; 161: 101–7.

11. De Smet AA, Tuite MJ, Norris MA, et al. MR diagnosis of meniscal tears: analysis of causes of errors. *Am J Roentgenol* 1994; 163: 1419–23.

12. Miniaci A, Mascia AT, Salonen DC, et al. Magnetic resonance imaging of the shoulder in asymptomatic professional baseball pitchers. *Am J Sports Med* 2002; 30: 66–73.

13. Ludman CN, Hough DO, Cooper TG, et al. Silent meniscal abnormalities in athletes: magnetic resonance imaging of asymptomatic competitive gymnasts. *Br J Sports Med* 1999; 33: 414–6.

14. Cook JL, Khan KM, Harcourt PR, et al. Patellar tendon ultrasonography in asymptomatic active athletes reveals hypoechoic regions: a study of 320 tendons. Victorian Institute of Sport Tendon Study Group. *Clin J Sport Med* 1998; 8: 73–7.

15. Weinberg EP, Adams MJ, Hollenberg GM. Color Doppler sonography of patellar tendinosis. *Am J Roentgenol* 1998; 171: 743–4.

16. Zanetti M, Metzdorf A, Kundert HP, et al. Achilles tendons: clinical relevance of neovascularization diagnosed with power Doppler US. *Radiology* 2003; 227: 556–60.

17. Khan KM, Forster BB, Robinson J, et al. Are ultrasound and magnetic resonance imaging of value in assessment of Achilles tendon disorders? A two year prospective study. *Br J Sports Med* 2003; 37: 149–53.

18. Reiter M, Ulreich N, Dirisamer A, et al. Colour and power Doppler sonography in symptomatic Achilles tendon disease. *Int J Sports Med* 2004; 25: 301–5.

19. Cook JL, Kiss ZS, Ptasznik R, et al. Is vascularity more evident after exercise? Implications for tendon imaging. *Am J Roentgenol* 2005; 185: 1138–40.

20. Alfredson H, Ohberg L. Neovascularisation in chronic painful patellar tendinosis—promising results after sclerosing neovessels outside the tendon challenge the need for surgery. *Knee Surg Sports Traumatol Arthrosc* 2005; 13: 74–80.

21. Alfredson H, Ohberg L. Sclerosing injections to areas of neovascularisation reduce pain in chronic Achilles tendinopathy: a double-blind randomised controlled trial. *Knee Surg Sports Traumatol Arthrosc* 2005; 13: 338–44.

Treatments Used for Musculoskeletal Conditions: More Choices and More Evidence

WITH ROBERT GRANTER

Treatment begins when the patient first presents with symptoms. But the boundary between the end of treatment and the start of rehabilitation is blurry. In many conditions that are managed conservatively (e.g. hamstring muscle strain, tendinopathy) the exercises that are started for 'treatment' also contribute to the rehabilitation process. If one were required to make a distinction, it might be that the treatment exercises are focused on the pathological structure, whereas the rehabilitative exercises have a wider scope and ensure that other structures are not suffering from the injury-related immobility.

For the reader's convenience, we discuss therapies that apply to both 'treatment' and 'rehabilitation' in just one of the relevant chapters. For example, manual therapy is covered in this chapter even though it can be an important part of ongoing rehabilitation. On the other hand, exercise prescription (resistance exercises, proprioceptive training, flexibility training and activities that combine these elements), an essential 'treatment' of musculoskeletal conditions, is covered in Chapter 12.

Evidence for treatment effectiveness is continually changing

The purpose of this chapter is to provide the essential background information regarding various treatments that are referred to in Part B. Here we define and describe specific treatments, we report the level of evidence for their effectiveness and we aim to provide a clinical perspective on their use in musculoskeletal

medicine. For therapies that have uniform doses of treatment (e.g. glyceryl trinitrate [GTN] patches for various tendinopathies) the doses are specified in this chapter. Where treatment instructions vary by body part (e.g. electrotherapy modes and doses), specifics are held over to the chapter dealing with treatment of that region.

Overall, the past decade has seen an augmentation of evidence for many treatments in sports medicine (see box).

Some people believe that no treatment is really effective for any condition. This view is captured in the aphorism 'Time heals and the physician sends the bills' (note that other members of the clinical team are not guilty of this!). Another term for this philosophical position is 'therapeutic nihilism'. Such a position has little merit in the 21st century with the increasing evidence for successful treatments for musculoskeletal conditions and the overwhelming evidence for physical activity as a very major determinant of all-system health.

Our final introductory point regarding treatment, and evidence or absence of it, is to remind the reader that there has been no randomized controlled trial evidence suggesting that, when jumping from an airplane, using a parachute provides superior outcomes to jumping without one. All evidence of harm to those who jumped without a parachute has been in retrospective case series (level 4 evidence; Fig. 10.1). As clinicians, we should take note of the evidence that has been gathered but celebrate that our craft remains as much art as science.

Part of the art of musculoskeletal medicine is ensuring that patients can benefit from the appropriate

Examples of treatments with a long history of 'clinical use' which were investigated in randomized controlled trials (RCTs)

RCTs found that the established treatment was effective

Manual therapy in neck pain[1, 2]
Manual therapy in back pain[3, 4]
Resistance training for adductor tendinopathy[5]
McConnell program for patellofemoral pain[6]
McConnell program for knee osteoarthritis[7]
Strength and balance exercises after ankle sprain[8]
Early mobilization after injury[9]
Strength and balance training for fall prevention in seniors[10]

RCT(s) found that the established treatment was ineffective (at 1 April 2006)

Corticosteroid injection for early lateral elbow tendinopathy[11]
When the knee is mobilized with exercise after knee replacement, adding continuous passive motion or slider
board therapy did not provide additional benefit[12]
NSAIDs in Achilles tendinopathy[13]
Low-intensity infra-red laser for plantar fasciitis[14]

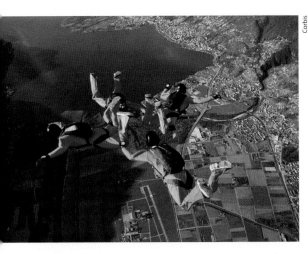

Corbis

Figure 10.1 Skydiving. There is only level 4 evidence (case reports) to suggest that wearing a parachute is associated with outcomes superior to those when not wearing one when jumping from an airplane

elements of a large menu of available treatments. This chapter discusses this menu according to the following subheadings:

- minimizing extent of injury (RICE)
- immobilization and early mobilization
- therapeutic drugs, including glyceryl trinitrate (GTN), sclerosing therapy, glucosamine
- heat and cold
- electrotherapeutic modalities

- extracorporeal shock wave therapy
- manual therapy
  — joints
    – mobilization
    – manipulation
    – traction
  — muscles
    – soft tissue therapy
    – muscle energy techniques
  — neural—stretching
- acupuncture
- dry needling
- hyperbaric oxygen
- surgery.

The clinician should evaluate the effectiveness of each type of treatment by comparing symptoms and signs before and after treatment (i.e. both immediately after treatment and again at the next visit). This enables the clinician to choose the most appropriate mode of treatment for the specific injury and the specific individual.

Minimizing extent of injury (RICE)

The most important time in the treatment of acute soft tissue injuries is in the 24 hours immediately following injury. When soft tissue is injured, blood vessels are usually damaged too. Thus, blood accumulates around damaged tissue and compresses adjoining tissues, which causes secondary hypoxic injury and further tissue damage. Consequently, every effort should be made to reduce bleeding at the site of injury. The most appropriate method of doing this is summarized by the letters RICE.

R Rest
I Ice
C Compression
E Elevation

Rest

Whenever possible following injury, the athlete should cease activity to decrease bleeding and swelling. For example, with a thigh contusion, bleeding will be increased by contraction of the quadriceps muscle during running. Where necessary, complete rest can be achieved with the use of crutches for a lower limb injury or a sling for upper limb injuries.

Ice

Immediately after injury, ice is principally used to reduce tissue metabolism.[15] Ice is also used in the later stages of injury treatment as a therapeutic modality (this is discussed further under heat and cold on page 137).

Ice can be applied in a number of forms:

- crushed ice can be wrapped in a moist cloth or towel and placed around the injured area, held in place with a crepe bandage
- reusable frozen gel packs
- instant ice packs that do not need pre-cooling
- ice immersion in a bucket (useful for treatment of injuries of the extremities)
- cold water and cooling sprays, which are often used in the immediate treatment of injuries but are unlikely to affect deeper tissues.

Although there is no high-quality evidence for how long, and how often, to apply ice after an acute injury,[15, 16] a systematic review suggested that intermittent 10-minute ice treatments are most effective at cooling injured animal tissue and healthy human tissue.[17] Many practitioners apply ice for 15 minutes every 1–2 hours initially and then gradually reduce the frequency of application over the next 24 hours. Ice should not be applied where local tissue circulation is impaired (e.g. in Raynaud's phenomenon, peripheral vascular disease) or to patients who suffer from a cold allergy. Other adverse effects of prolonged ice application are skin burns and nerve damage.[18]

Compression

Compression of the injured area with a firm bandage reduces bleeding and, therefore, minimizes swelling. Compression should be applied both during and after ice application. The width of the bandage applied varies according to the injured area.

The bandage should be applied firmly but not so tightly as to cause pain. Bandaging should start just distal to the site of bleeding with each layer of the bandage overlapping the underlying layer by one-half. It should extend to at least a hand's breadth proximal to the injury margin.

Elevation

Elevation of the injured part decreases hydrostatic pressure and, thus, reduces the accumulation of interstitial fluid. Elevation can be achieved by using a sling for upper limb injuries and by resting lower limbs on a chair, pillows or bucket. It is important to ensure that the lower limb is above the level of the pelvis.

Other minimizing factors

In the initial phase of injury (first 24 hours), heat and heat rubs, alcohol, moderate/intense activity and vigorous soft tissue therapy should all be avoided. Whether or not electrotherapeutic modalities (e.g. magnetic field therapy, interferential stimulation, TENS) provide effective pain relief and reduction of swelling in the initial period is a subject of debate. These modalities are described later in this chapter.

Immobilization and early mobilization

Immobilization has beneficial effects in the early phase of muscle regeneration and is crucial for fracture healing. However, lengthy immobilization has detrimental effects; it causes joint stiffness, degenerative changes in articular cartilage, muscle atrophy, weakness and stiffness.

Complete immobilization is primarily required for acute fractures. Certain stress fractures, for example, tarsal navicular fractures, also require immobilization. Occasionally in severe soft tissue injuries, it may be helpful to immobilize the injured area for up to 48 hours to limit pain and swelling.

Immobilization can be obtained through the use of rigid braces, air splints, taping, thermoplastic materials or, most commonly, with the use of a plaster cast. Plaster casts have the disadvantages of being relatively heavy, prone to damage and not water-resistant. For undisplaced fractures and immobilization of soft tissue injuries, fiberglass casts are preferred. Fiberglass casting material is light, strong and waterproof. A waterproof underwrap is available that enables the athlete to bathe without the need to protect the cast. This allows those with lower limb casts to exercise in water to maintain fitness.

Protected mobilization

Mobilization, on the other hand, has numerous tissue benefits.[19] One way to achieve early, but safe, mobilization is by 'protected mobilization'. This term refers to the use of protective taping or bracing to prevent movement in a direction that would cause excessive stress on an injured structure. For example, a hinged knee brace prevents valgus strain in a second degree medial collateral ligament injury. Non-injured structures are allowed to move (i.e. the knee joint continues to function), and this feature distinguishes protected mobilization from complete immobilization. This allows enough movement to prevent stiffness, maintain muscle strength and improve the nourishment of the articular cartilage, while still protecting the damaged ligament.

Early mobilization in patients with acute limb injuries (e.g. ankle sprains, stable factures and after surgical tendon repair), decreases pain and swelling, and improves functional outcomes compared to cast immobilization.[9]

Continuous passive motion

Continuous passive motion (CPM) may be used after surgery using a specific CPM machine. It is particularly beneficial when pain limits active range of motion exercises or when there is a need to control the range of movement to allow wound healing. CPM may also encourage nourishment of articular cartilage and minimize joint stiffness. CPM may have a role in the early stages of treatment of second or third degree muscle tears, for example, in the hamstring or quadriceps, to encourage alignment of healing fibers.

Mobilization and exercise therapy

Whether 'early mobilization' or exercise therapy is 'treatment' or rehabilitation remains a gray area; it is covered in Chapter 12. However, we emphasize that exercise therapy itself may provide a tissue regenerative stimulus. For example, with respect to muscle, early mobilization promotes rapid and intensive capillary ingrowth into the injured area, regeneration of muscle fibers and more parallel orientation of

myofibers compared with immobilization.[20] In tendon, it appears that certain 'strengthening' protocols (e.g. heavy resistance training heel drops; Fig. 10.2) may stimulate collagen synthesis among tendon cells which, in turn, strengthen tendon.[21, 22]

Therapeutic drugs

Drugs commonly used in the treatment of sporting injuries include analgesics, NSAIDs, corticosteroids; novel therapies include hyaluronic acid injections, glyceryl trinitrate (GTN) patches and sclerosing agents such a polidocanol.

Analgesics

Analgesics are used in the acute phase immediately after injury to reduce pain. Subsequent use depends on the degree and duration of pain. Pain reduction during rehabilitation may facilitate movement. Aspirin (ASA), paracetamol (acetaminophen) and codeine are the most commonly used analgesics, either singly or in combination.

At low dosages (250–300 mg), aspirin (ASA) has an analgesic and antipyretic effect. At higher dosages aspirin also has an anti-inflammatory effect but these dosages are associated with a significant incidence of side-effects, particularly of the gastrointestinal system.

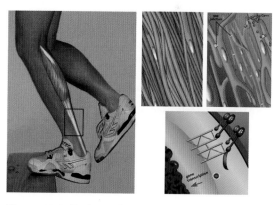

Figure 10.2 Evidence that exercise therapy (heel drops) acts as a stimulus for tendon tissue repair (treatment). Exercise (macroscopic view, heel drop, left panel) causes sliding of collagen fibers (microscopic view, top center panel), that leads to intercellular communication via gap junctions (top right panel) and communication with the cell nucleus to upregulate protein synthesis (lower right panel). This is the process of mechanotransduction. Thus, exercise therapy is not just part of 'rehabilitation' but can act as a therapy itself through the process of mechanotransduction

We advise against the use of aspirin in acute injuries because it inhibits platelet aggregation and, thus, may increase bleeding associated with the injury.

Paracetamol (acetaminophen) has an analgesic and antipyretic effect but has no influence on the inflammatory process and no effect on blood clotting. It is safe to use in the acute phase of injuries; the standard dose is up to 3–4 g per day.

Codeine is a more potent analgesic. It is a narcotic analgesic and was formerly listed as a banned substance by the International Olympic Committee (Chapter 61). This ban was lifted in the mid 1990s.

Topical analgesics

Topical analgesics are used extensively by athletes and are known as 'sports rubs', 'heat rubs' and 'liniments'. Most commercially available topical analgesics contain a combination of substances such as menthol, methyl salicylate, camphor and eucalyptus oil.

The majority act as skin counterirritants. Most products contain two or more active ingredients that produce redness, dilate blood vessels and stimulate pain and temperature receptors. The type and intensity of the effect depends on the particular counterirritant, its concentration, dosage and method of application. The exact mechanism of action of counterirritants is unknown.

Counterirritants should not be used to replace a proper warm-up as they do not penetrate to deeper muscles but they may be of use as an adjunct to warm-up. Counterirritants may irritate the skin and occasionally cause blistering or contact dermatitis.

Non-steroidal anti-inflammatory drugs

NSAIDs are widely used in the treatment of sporting injuries. The first NSAIDs used were aspirin and the salicylates, while more recently other NSAIDs have been introduced. All these drugs have analgesic, anti-inflammatory and antipyretic properties. They are also widely used in the treatment of arthritis.

Inflammation occurs at the site of acute injury. A local soft tissue injury such as a ligament tear causes the release of arachidonic acid from cell walls. Arachidonic acid is converted by a number of enzymes, in particular cyclo-oxygenase (COX), to prostaglandins, thromboxane and prostacyclins. These substances mediate the inflammatory response. NSAIDs block the conversion of arachidonic acid to prostaglandin by inhibiting the action of cyclo-oxygenase. NSAIDs may also have other effects on the inflammatory response.[23]

In spite of the widespread clinical use of NSAIDs, there are no convincing research data proving their effectiveness in the treatment of acute soft tissue injuries. Most studies lacked a placebo group and compared the effectiveness of one NSAID with another.[23] They do not appear to be any more effective than simple analgesics in the management of acute muscle injuries.[24] The lack of scientific support for the use of NSAIDs in acute injury may reflect biological reality or may be due to the methodological difficulties in performing randomized placebo-controlled trials in the diverse range of acute sporting injuries.

More studies are needed to investigate the effectiveness of NSAIDs, particularly in the management of overuse injuries. In the meantime, the precise criteria for the use of NSAIDs in the management of sporting injuries remain a matter for debate. There are a large number of NSAIDs currently available (Table 10.1) and there are considerable differences in their dosage schedules (Table 10.1).[25]

In general, the NSAIDs have minimal adverse effects; the most common are gastrointestinal symptoms, especially epigastric pain, nausea, indigestion and heartburn. There appears to be considerable individual variation of side-effect profiles among the different NSAIDs.

Table 10.1 Commonly used NSAIDs

Drug	Some trade names	Usual dose (mg)	Daily doses
Acetylsalicylic acid (ASA)	Aspirin	650	3–4
Celecoxib	Celebrex	100–200	1–2
Diclofenac	Voltaren	25–50	2–3
Ibuprofen	Brufen, Motrin, Advil	400	3–4
Meloxicam	Mobic	7.5–15	1
Naproxen	Naprosyn, Anaprox	250–1000	1–4

The risk of dyspeptic side-effects can be lowered by using the minimum effective dose, taking the drug with or immediately after food or milk, or by the use of antacids. Alcohol, cigarettes and coffee may aggravate the dyspepsia. To our knowledge, frank peptic ulceration with the short-term use of NSAIDs has not been reported among sportspeople. Occult bleeding may contribute to iron depletion in athletes. The clinician should be wary of prescribing long-term use of these drugs in iron-depleted sportspeople.

Other occasional side-effects include asthma, allergic rhinitis, rashes, tinnitus, deafness, headache and confusion. The NSAIDs have a number of important drug interactions with anticoagulants, antihypertensives, diuretics and peripheral vasodilators. Older patients with a history of hypertension, congestive heart failure or coronary artery disease are at particular risk of adverse cardiovascular events with NSAIDs. Patients with impaired renal function are at risk of fluid retention, hyperkalemia (increased serum potassium level) and hypertension.

A group of anti-inflammatory medications, the selective COX-2 inhibitors, have been available since the late 1990s. These drugs appeared to be effective in the management of osteoarthritis with a reduction of the side-effects associated with the non-selective NSAIDs. There were concerns regarding their effectiveness in the management of acute musculoskeletal injuries as they had been shown, in animal models of acute injury, to be detrimental to tissue-level repair.[26]

Two of these medications, rofecoxib and valdecoxib, were withdrawn from the market in 2004 because of an increased risk of cardiovascular complications[27] associated with long-term use.[28, 29] Note that COX-2 blockade promotes thrombosis. The future role of COX-2 inhibitors is unclear at this time.[30]

A recent study suggested that two commonly used non-selective NSAIDs (diclofenac and ibuprofen) may also be associated with a higher risk of myocardial infarction.[31]

Topical anti-inflammatory agents

A number of topical anti-inflammatory products are available. These include benzydamine, adrenocortical extract, indomethacin and diclofenac gel. Traditionally these topical drugs have been administered through creams, gels and sprays which often required three to four applications per day. More recently, anti-inflammatory drugs have been applied through a patch which releases the drug over 24 hours. Early trials have shown a ketoprofen patch[32] and a diclofenac patch[33] to be effective in the treatment of ankle sprain and acute impact injuries, respectively.

Corticosteroids

The use of corticosteroids, which are potent anti-inflammatory drugs, is controversial due to the incidence of side-effects and concern regarding the effect of corticosteroids on tissue healing. Corticosteroids may be administered either by local injection, orally or by iontophoresis. We found no randomized controlled trials of iontophoresis for sports medicine conditions. A goal of the use of local corticosteroid injection is to reduce pain and inflammation sufficiently to allow a strengthening program to commence. Corticosteroid injections should be considered a 'bridge' treatment that provides immediate symptomatic relief while the underlying cause of the problem is addressed with definitive, disease-modifying therapy.

Local injection for various pathologies

Local injection of corticosteroid agents maximizes the concentration at the site of the injury and minimizes the risk of side-effects associated with systemic administration. Clinicians often use local injection of corticosteroids in conditions that include bursitis, paratenonitis, tenosynovitis, joint synovitis, osteoarthritis, chronic muscle strain and trigger points.

Local corticosteroid injection may be particularly effective in the treatment of bursitis. Conditions such as subacromial, olecranon, pre-patellar and retrocalcaneal bursitis may be resistant to standard physiotherapy/physical therapy combined with NSAIDs. Side-effects of corticosteroid injections include the potential systemic effects of absorbed cortisone, and local effects of injection. Corticosteroids inhibit collagen synthesis and tissue repair. As deleterious effects of corticosteroids appear to be dose-related, repeated injections are discouraged.

Intra-articular injections, particularly into weight-bearing joints, must be approached with considerable caution because of possible long-term damage to articular cartilage. They should be performed only when the condition has proven refractory to treatments such as physiotherapy and NSAIDs. Rheumatologists have long used corticosteroids intra-articularly in acute monoarticular exacerbations of osteoarthritis. An acute attack of gouty arthritis may also respond well to aspiration and corticosteroid injection as part of the overall management.

Apophyseal joint injections have been used in the management of patients with back pain and who have only a short-term response to manual therapy, but the efficacy of such treatment at the lumbar spine is no better than placebo.[25] Controversy surrounds the use of injectable corticosteroid into the epidural space.

The role of corticosteroids in the treatment of tendon conditions has been the subject of considerable debate but very few well-designed studies have been performed.[34] The main concern is a possible increase in the incidence of tendon rupture following injection, but as the tendons being injected are already compromised it is not clear whether the injection has led to the tendon rupture or the damaged tendon was already predisposed to rupture.

Corticosteroid injection *into* tendon tissue was generally contraindicated; recently, Danish investigators actively injected the area of tendinosis with corticosteroid and reported symptomatic relief and no complications.[35] This approach requires further research before entering the mainstream of therapy.

As tendinopathy is not associated with inflammatory cells (Chapter 2), corticosteroid therapy is generally falling out of favor for this condition, although there is evidence for one injection as part of the treatment of supraspinatus tendinopathy (Chapter 17). In a rabbit study, corticosteroids made the tendon more vulnerable to failure.[36] Nevertheless, some practitioners advocate the injection of tendon sheaths with corticosteroid, whereas others advocate the 'bathing' of the tendon with corticosteroid by injection around, but not into, the tendon. The long-term effects of these practices are unknown.

Some clinicians recommend the injection of trigger points with corticosteroid. Soft tissue therapy, dry needling or local anesthetic injection appear to be equally as effective.

The main side-effect of corticosteroid injection, apart from the possible damage to articular cartilage and tendon, is infection. This is a rare occurrence and should be prevented by the use of strict aseptic technique, particularly when performing intra-articular injections. The presence of an overlying skin infection is a contraindication to injection.

Corticosteroid injections commonly cause a short-term exacerbation of symptoms, a phenomenon known as 'post-injection flare'. This may commence soon after injection and usually subsides within 24 hours. This phenomenon is thought to be due to a crystalline synovitis and is considered by some to be a positive sign of a favorable outcome to the treatment. Patients should always be warned that this may occur.

Corticosteroid injections have a reputation of being a particularly painful procedure but this can be minimized by adding local anesthetic (0.5–1.0 mL 1% lignocaine [lidocaine]) to the injection. The abolition of pain after the local anesthetic injection may be diagnostically significant.

Traditionally, patients have been advised to rest and minimize activity for three to seven days following corticosteroid injection, but the advantages of this protocol have recently been questioned.[37]

There are a number of different forms of injectable corticosteroid available. They include hydrocortisone, betamethasone, methylprednisolone and triamcinalone. The main differences are in the speed of onset and half-life of action. There is no convincing evidence that their efficacy differs.

In summary, the use of local corticosteroid injections should be restricted to conditions that have not responded to other forms of treatment, such as bursitis. The number of injections to any one site should be restricted and successive injections should not be performed within three to four weeks.

Oral corticosteroids

Despite their effectiveness as an anti-inflammatory agent, clinicians have traditionally been reluctant to use oral corticosteroids for the treatment of musculoskeletal inflammation probably because of potential side-effects.[38] The most common conditions for which they are used are acute cervical or lumbar radiculopathy/diskogenic pain, osteitis pubis, adhesive capsulitis (frozen shoulder) and chronic tendinopathies.

Possible complications include avascular necrosis of the femoral head.[39] However, the use of short courses (five to seven days) of oral prednisolone (25–50 mg) appears to be associated with minimal detrimental effects.

Note that the use of oral corticosteroids is still banned by the International Olympic Committee in competition.

Iontophoresis

Iontophoresis is a process by which drugs can be transmitted through the intact skin via electrical potential. Drugs such as corticosteroids, salicylates, local anesthetics and NSAIDs can thus be administered locally without the traumatic effects of injection, with no pain for the patient and no risk of infection. This process has been shown to deliver the drugs through skin and subcutaneous tissue. In this way, the drug can reach tissue that may have markedly reduced vascularity, for example, a bursa or tendon. As with all pharmacological agents, it should only be considered as part of the overall management of the patient.

The results of well-controlled studies suggest that iontophoresis with diclofenac or salicylates improves symptoms in lateral epicondylitis. Iontophoresis with corticosteroid appears to give rapid-onset analgesia in both lateral epicondylitis and plantar fasciitis. Short-term iontophoresis (two weeks) improves pain and facilitates rehabilitation.[40]

Ketorolac tromethamine

Ketorolac tromethamine is a potent analgesic and anti-inflammatory medication that can be administered orally, intravenously and intramuscularly. It acts by blocking the synthesis of prostaglandins in the cyclo-oxygenase pathway.[41]

A survey of US National Football League teams revealed that 28 out of the 30 teams that responded to the survey used ketorolac with 93% game-day usage.[42]

Side-effects include headache, vasodilatation, asthma, bleeding and kidney dysfunction. Of particular concern in the sporting context is the bleeding tendency.

Nitric oxide donor

Glyceryl trinitrate (GTN), or nitroglycerin, is a nitric oxide donor used for over 100 years as a vasodilator and for symptomatic treatment of angina. But why does it rate a mention in a 21st century sports medicine book? The mechanism of action of organic nitrates is through the production of nitric oxide, a highly reactive free radical that is an important mediator in many physiological and pathophysiological processes. One action of nitric oxide is to stimulate collagen synthesis by wound fibroblasts, so it is proposed that nitric oxide may modulate tendon healing by stimulating fibroblasts to repair collagen. Thus, organic nitrates such as GTN may be viewed as prodrugs of endogenous nitric oxide, an endothelial cell-derived relaxing factor. Transdermal GTN patches are a simple way of applying and dosing nitric oxide.

Evidence for the effectiveness of nitric oxide in sports medicine conditions is accumulating. Topical GTN improved immediate short-term pain scores in patients with acute supraspinatus tendinopathy.[43] In recent years, Paoloni et al. provided level 2 evidence that use of nitric oxide donor (GTN patches applied locally 1.25 mg/day) was an effective treatment for Achilles, supraspinatus and lateral elbow tendinopathy.[44-46] About 20% more patients prescribed the GTN patches were asymptomatic at six months than

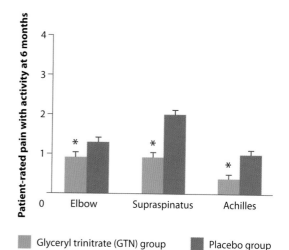

Figure 10.3 At six months GTN patches provided outcomes superior to those from the placebo patch for three different tendinopathies (elbow, shoulder and Achilles)

control group participants who received 'best-practise' care (i.e. rehabilitation alone) (Fig. 10.3).

Sclerosing therapy

A new treatment for tendinopathy is sclerotherapy of abnormal vessels (Fig. 10.4) that are associated with painful tendons (tendinosis, Chapter 2); this sports medicine use of a traditional treatment for varicose veins was pioneered by the Swedes, Hakan Alfredson and Lars Ohberg. They hypothesized that abnormal vessels, and possibly nerves accompanying the vessels, were involved in the pain mechanisms in chronic painful Achilles tendinosis. To eliminate these painful structures, they studied the effect of sclerosing the abnormal vessels. Sclerosis is widely used for treating varicose veins and telangiectasia.[47]

Sclerosing abnormal vessels (termed 'neovessels'), firstly in Achilles tendons[48] but then also in patellar tendons,[49] significantly decreased pain and allowed the patients to return to pain-free tendon loading activity. Reduction in the number of abnormal neovessels by color Doppler ultrasound correlated well with reduced pain from tendons. Polidocanol irritates the vascular intima to cause vessel thrombosis. Polidocanol may also sclerose nerves adjacent to the neovessels, either directly (by destruction) or indirectly (by ischemia). The Swedish protagonists of the therapy would be the first to agree that there is a need for further investigation of the mechanism by which polidocanol injection reduces tendon pain.

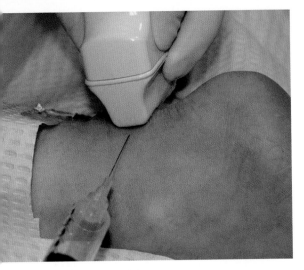

Figure 10.4 Sclerosing therapy under ultrasound control

Prolotherapy

Prolotherapy, an injection-based treatment of chronic musculoskeletal pain, has grown in popularity and has received significant recent attention.[50] This treatment involves a small volume of an irritant solution being injected at multiple sites on painful ligament and tendon insertions, and in adjacent joint spaces. The three commonly used prolotherapy solutions are purported to act in different ways: dextrose 10% by osmotic rupture of cells, phenol-glycerine-glucose (P2G) by local cellular irritation, and sodium morrhuate by chemotactic attraction of inflammatory mediators. The volume depends on the region of injection but 9 mL was used in one randomized control trial of intra-articular prolotherapy at the knee.

Best and colleagues reviewed data from 34 case reports and case series and two non-randomized controlled trials;[50] these suggested that prolotherapy was efficacious for many musculoskeletal conditions. However, results from six randomized controlled trials are conflicting. Two trials on osteoarthritis reported decreased pain, increased range of motion, and increased patellofemoral cartilage thickness after prolotherapy, and two on low back pain reported significant improvements in pain and disability compared with control subjects, whereas two others did not. They concluded that further investigation with high-quality randomized controlled trials was required before it would be possible to determine whether or not, and in which clinical settings, prolotherapy was effective.

Glucosamine and chondroitin sulfate

Glucosamine sulfate and chondroitin are compounds extracted from animal products that have been used in various forms for osteoarthritic symptoms in Europe for more than a decade. They are absorbed from the gastrointestinal tract and appear to be capable of increasing proteoglycan synthesis in articular cartilage. Whether or not they are effective, and in whom, remains controversial.

The 2005 Cochrane systematic review included 20 studies with 2570 patients.[51] Their authors conclude that the company that formulated the glucosamine was an important factor! Preparations made by companies other than one Canadian company failed to show benefit in pain and in the widely accepted measure of function (WOMAC score). Studies showed that Rotta-prepared glucosamine was superior to placebo in the treatment of pain and functional impairment that is seen in osteoarthritis. Clinical experience is that it may take two months for the benefits to be felt.

As for chondroitin, which is commonly packaged with glucosamine as a remedy for joint pain, a recent analysis of the combined results of seven randomized controlled trials indicated that the supplement may reduce osteoarthritis symptoms and improve function by an average of some 50%, although the studies had flaws that may exaggerate the benefits.

No study so far has found any serious side-effects from either glucosamine or chondroitin. The most common side-effects are increased intestinal gas and softened stools.

Hyaluronic acid therapy

Hyaluronic acid is a polysaccharide member of the family of glycosaminoglycans. It is a naturally occurring substance found in many extracellular tissues, including synovial fluid, the aqueous humor of the eye, skin and cartilage. It is produced in normal joints but breaks down in patients with osteoarthritis and this appears to increase the susceptibility of articular cartilage to injury.

In recent years, hyaluronic acid, obtained either from humans or genetically engineered, has been given as an intra-articular injection for patients with osteoarthritis of the knee. Some studies suggest a long-term benefit of three to five once-weekly injections with regard to clinically relevant outcome measures.[52-56] Side-effects are uncommon but include gastrointestinal discomfort, knee swelling and/or effusion (incidence rate less than 1% per year). It appears that hyaluronic acid may be a safe therapy for patients with osteoarthritis of the knee and it remains to be further studied at the hip.

Antidepressants

Antidepressants, especially the tricyclics and the selective serotonin reuptake inhibitors (SSRI), are widely used in the treatment of chronic pain. Originally, the therapeutic effect of these drugs was thought to be related to their antidepressant properties, but their analgesic efficacy at doses below those needed for a reduction of depression and their relatively rapid effect suggest another mechanism of action. They can also improve sleep, which can be a boon to patients with chronic pain.

Treatment should commence with a low (amitryptyline, 10 mg) bedtime dosage, which is titrated slowly upwards depending on patient response. Side-effects vary but include excess daytime sedation, dry mouth, constipation, weight gain and, in older patients, urinary retention. Antidepressants can be administered in conjunction with other analgesics and anti-inflammatory medications.

There is limited evidence for the use of tricyclic antidepressants in chronic musculoskeletal pain[57] but more convincing evidence in fibromyalgia.[58, 59]

Local anesthetic injections

Local anesthetic pain-killing injections are part of professional contact sports such as football. The aim of such injections is to lower the rate of players missing matches through injury. The most common injuries that are treated in this way are acromioclavicular joint sprains, finger and rib injuries, and iliac crest hematoma. Clinicians expert in these injections recommend against intra-articular injections to the knee, ankle, wrist, joints of the foot, and to the pubic symphysis and major tendons of the lower limb. In one physician's six-year case series, local anesthetic was used for 268 injuries (about 10% of players each week).[60] These injections were associated with four major complications (chronic tendinopathies, bursal infection, worsening ligament tears and osteolysis of the distal clavicle).

Players requesting injections should be made well aware of the possible complications. The joints affected by long-term injury sequelae of professional football, such as increased rates of osteoarthritis of the knee (in particular), hip, ankle and lumbar spine, are not the joints associated with injuries for which local anesthetic is commonly used.

To enable the benefit and risk profile of local anesthetic injections to be better understood, it has been argued that professional football competitions make local anesthetics legal only with compulsory notification.

Heat and cold

Cryotherapy

This section focuses on the use of cryotherapy for the treatment of acute or chronic injury; its role in the RICE regimen was discussed earlier (p. 129). It has been argued that the main role of cryotherapy in the treatment phase is to provide analgesia by decreasing motor and sensory nerve conduction velocity, thus decreasing the rate of firing of muscle spindle afferents and stretch reflex responses, decreasing acetylcholine levels and, therefore, decreasing pain and muscle spasm. The indications, contraindications and complications of cryotherapy are shown in Table 10.2. The different methods of using cryotherapy are summarized in Table 10.3.

Ice massage is used in the treatment of specific superficial conditions such as tendinopathy or tenoperiostitis. Ice massage may be performed with ice blocks or, more commonly, by water frozen in a polystyrene cup and rubbed directly onto the affected area. The massage is usually performed in a circular motion for 5–10 minutes.

Superficial heat

Appropriate warm-up (Chapter 6) and superficial heat may contribute to improved treatment of soft tissue injuries. Stimulated warm muscles absorb more energy than do unstimulated muscles.[20] The indications, contraindications and side-effects of superficial heat therapy are shown in Table 10.2. Heat should not be applied in the first 24 hours following an acute injury.

Heat can be applied in a number of different ways including warm showers and baths, warm whirlpools and heat packs. These are summarized in Table 10.4. Heat packs are canvas bags filled with hydrophilic silicone gel stored in hot water and wrapped in towels. They are then applied for 15 minutes.

Contrast baths

Contrast baths aim to decrease swelling by alternating heat and cold to create an alternating mechanical force. These baths are used after the acute phase of injury to reduce swelling. The injured part is immersed in a hot bath for 4 minutes, followed by a cold bath with ice and water for 1–2 minutes. This should be repeated

Table 10.2 Features of electrotherapeutic and thermal modalities

Modality	Effects	Clinical indications	Contraindications	Danger
Cryotherapy (ice)	Decreases pain Decreases swelling/bleeding (vasoconstriction) Decreases cellular metabolism	Muscle spasm Trigger point pain Acute swelling/edema Inflammation Heat illness Contusion (e.g. cork thigh) Acute injuries Pre- and post-massage	Cold hypersensitivity Raynaud's phenomenon Circulatory insufficiency	Ice burns Anesthesia (masks pain) Increased edema after prolonged use Superficial nerve damage
Superficial heat	Pain relief Increases local blood flow	Pain Muscle spasm Cervical pain Chronic pain and swelling	Sensory changes Circulatory problems Heat injury Hyper- or hyposensitivity to heat	Increased bleeding and swelling (if used in first 48 hours after acute injury) Burns
Ultrasound	*Thermal* Increases local blood flow Increases cellular metabolism Increases extensibility of connective tissue Decreases pain	Muscle spasm Contusion Localized inflammation and pain (e.g. ligament sprains, muscle strains)	Acute phase of injury Deep venous thrombosis, acute infection, post-laminectomy, pacemaker Should not be used over open epiphyses, broken skin, major nerves, cranium, fractures, eyes, gonads, malignancies or post-radiotherapy areas Myositis ossificans (early stages)	Burns
	Non-thermal Micro massage Increases cell permeability Decreases pain	Acute injuries		
TENS	*High frequency* Pain relief (immediate and short term) Muscle stimulation	Decreases acute pain and muscle spasm	Over carotid sinus Cardiac pacemaker Sensory deficit	Removal of protective influence of pain
	Low frequency Latent pain relief	Muscle re-education Trigger points Acupuncture points Muscle spasm Chronic pain		

continues

Table 10.2 Features of electrotherapeutic and thermal modalities *(continued)*

Modality	Effects	Clinical indications	Contraindications	Danger
Interferential stimulation	Pain relief Decreases edema and swelling Muscle stimulation Increases cellular activity	Acute soft tissue injuries Swelling/edema Muscle spasm Pain, especially deep (e.g. acute knee, ankle, shoulder injuries)	Use over carotid sinus Cardiac pacemaker Sensory deficit Arterial disease Deep venous thrombosis Pregnancy Local infection Malignant tumor	Electrical burns may occur (due to increased skin resistance)
High voltage galvanic stimulation	Pain relief Decreases swelling/edema Decreases inflammation Muscle stimulation	Pain Muscle spasm Swelling/edema Muscle inhibition Inflammation (e.g. tendinitis) Post-operative muscle disuse atrophy	Sensory deficit Increased skin resistance Broken skin As for TENS	
Laser	Pain relief Decreases muscle spasm Increases cell regeneration Decreases inflammation	Localized, superficial pain and inflammation Trigger points Superficial ligaments and tendon injuries Superficial wound healing	Pregnancy Patients receiving photosensitive medication Malignancies Infants	Retinal damage with prolonged exposure
Magnetic field therapy	Decreases swelling and edema Decreases inflammation	Acute soft tissue injury Edema (e.g. acute joint sprain, contusion)	Pregnancy Tuberculosis	Gastrointestinal symptoms with treatment of chronic pain

Table 10.3 Superficial cold modalities used for treating sports-related injuries

Modality	Description	Special concerns	Temperature	Duration	Exercise during application	Expense
Reusable cold packs	Durable plastic packs containing silica gel that are available in many sizes and shapes	Apply a towel between the bag and skin to avoid nerve damage or frostbite	≤15°C (59°F)	20–30 min	No	Inexpensive
Endothermal cold packs	Packets are squeezed or crushed to activate: convenient for emergency use	Single use only	20°C (68°F)	15–20 min	No	Expensive
Crushed ice bags	Crushed ice molds easily to body parts	Apply a towel between the bag and skin to avoid nerve damage or frostbite	0°C (32°F)	5–15 min	No	Inexpensive
Vapulocoolant sprays	Easily portable therapy for regional myofascial pain syndrome, acute injuries, pain relief, and in rehabilitation with spray and stretch techniques	Intermittently spray the area for <6 s to avoid frostbite	Varies depending on duration of treatment	Multiple brief sprays	Spray <6 s and stretch to increase range of motion	Expensive
Ice water immersion	Whenever uniform cold application to an extremity is desired	Carries the most risk of hypersensitivity reactions; restrict amount of extremity immersion	0°C (32°F)	5–10 min	Allows motion of the extremity during treatment	Inexpensive
Ice massage	Used to produce analgesia: freeze water in a foam cup, then peel back cup to expose the ice; massage area as often as needed	Apply for short intervals to avoid frostbite; avoid excess pressure	0°C (32°F)	5–10 min	Can allow supervised, gentle, stretching during analgesia	Inexpensive
Refrigerant inflatable bladders	When cold and compression are needed	Avoid excess compression	10–25°C (50–77°F)	Depends on temperature	No	Expensive
Thermal cooling blankets	To provide constant temperature, such as after surgery	Scrutinize temperature settings	10–25°C (50–77°F)	Depends on temperature	No	Expensive
Contrast baths	Transition treatment between cold and heat for a subacute injury, sympathetic mediated pain, stiff joints	Do not use in acute setting due to potential to increase blood flow	Hot bath 40.5°C 105°F) Cold bath 15.5°C (60°F)	4 min hot, 1 min cold	Allows motion of the extremity during treatment	Inexpensive

Table 10.4 Superficial heat modalities used for treating sports-related injuries

Modality	Description	Special concerns	Temperature	Duration	Exercise during application	Expense
Heat packs	Vigorous heating for superficial injuries; mild effects reduce muscle spasm in deeper tissues	Layers of towel must be placed between hot pack and skin to avoid burns; size precludes use for superficial joints	149°F (65°C)	5 min, then check for mottled erythema	No	Requires physiotherapy
Fluidotherapy	Vigorous heating, ideal for hand or foot; allows high temperature without discomfort	Avoid contact with open wounds	35–45°C (95–113°F)	10–30 min	Yes	Requires physiotherapy
Hydrotherapy	Whirlpool tanks combine thermal, pressure and buoyancy effects of water	As with all heat modalities, use caution with peripheral vascular disease and sensory loss; avoid full body immersion	35.5–40.5°C (95.9–104.9°F)	10–20 min	Gravity-free exercise	Requires physiotherapy
Radiant heat	Heat from infra-red lamp; no discomfort of weight, good for treating large areas	Only penetrates a few millimeters	Depends on intensity, distance from source	Up to 20 min	Yes	Requires physiotherapy

three to seven times. A cold bath should be used to finish to encourage vasoconstriction.

Electrotherapeutic modalities

A large number of different electrotherapeutic modalities are available for the treatment of sporting injuries. Their use varies widely between therapists and is based on clinical experience rather than scientific evidence. Although electrotherapeutic modalities are claimed to decrease inflammation and promote healing, there is only limited evidence as yet to support many of these claims. In any case, such modalities should not be relied on as the sole form of treatment. A summary of the different electrotherapeutic modalities, their clinical indications, contraindications and side-effects is shown in Table 10.2.

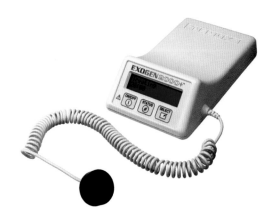

Figure 10.5 Exogen 2000 low-intensity pulsed ultrasound machine

Ultrasound

The effects, clinical indications, contraindications and side-effects of ultrasound therapy are shown in Table 10.2. There is little evidence to support ultrasound treatment on overuse soft tissue injuries,[61] including lateral elbow tendinopathy, shoulder pain,[62] low back pain, patellofemoral pain[63] and osteoarthritis of the knee. Most clinical trials investigating its efficacy have small sample sizes and are poorly designed and reported. Therefore, it is difficult to make valid, irrefutable conclusions regarding its efficacy.

Phonophoresis is the use of ultrasound therapy in combination with a pharmacological coupling medium, usually either an analgesic or anti-inflammatory medication. The clinical effect of this method of treatment is unknown.

Low-intensity (<0.1 W/cm^2) pulsed ultrasound (LIPUS) (Fig. 10.5) has been used successfully in the treatment of acute fractures as well as those that show delayed or non-union.[64, 65] LIPUS is performed using a stationary treatment head over the fracture site. The low intensity of the treatment means there is no risk of tissue damage. LIPUS is introduced daily for 20 minutes in contrast to traditional ultrasound practice, which is usually for no more than 5 minutes, no more than three times a week. It is possible that the reason conventional ultrasound machines do not have the same effect is that the treatments have been too short and infrequent.[66]

The use of LIPUS in sports medicine is growing. A significant reduction in healing time and thus time to return to sport has been shown in acute fractures and its use in the management of stress fractures, especially those with a tendency to delayed or non-

union (e.g. navicular, anterior cortex of tibia), is becoming widespread. Initial case reports suggest a reduction in time to return to sport.[65] There have also been suggestions that LIPUS may have similar effects with ligament, tendon, muscle and articular cartilage injuries.

TENS

Transcutaneous electrical nerve stimulation (TENS) is a modality used commonly to treat sporting injuries. It provides pain relief and has the advantage of being portable. A direct current is applied across the skin to cause electrical stimulation.

There are two commonly used types of TENS—high frequency (conventional) or low frequency (acupuncture-like).

High-frequency currents generated by a portable stimulating unit are administered via conducting pads (electrodes) placed on the intact surface of the skin. Research into the effectiveness of TENS treatment in patients with both acute (mainly post-operative) pain and chronic pain has produced conflicting results.[67] Some patients obtain good pain relief, some respond initially but then become tolerant, and others fail to respond at all.

Acupuncture-like TENS (AL-TENS) describes high-intensity, low-frequency currents passed across the surface of the skin to elicit strong but comfortable phasic muscle contractions at sites myotomally related to the origin of the pain.[68] AL-TENS appears to be mediated through the release of endorphins within the central nervous system. This form of TENS is often used to stimulate trigger points or acupuncture points. The indications and contraindications for TENS are shown in Table 10.2.

Interferential stimulation

Interferential stimulation is a form of TENS in which two alternating medium-frequency currents are simultaneously applied to the skin. The two sinusoidal currents become superimposed on each other where they intersect and cause wave interference, which in turn results in a modulated frequency equal to the difference in frequency of the two original waves (beat frequency).

Interferential therapy stimulates muscle in a similar manner to normal voluntary muscle contraction. It has an effect on pain similar to conventional TENS and varying effects on circulation depending on the frequency used. Vasodilatation occurs at frequencies of 90–100 Hz, whereas at low frequencies of 0–10 Hz, muscle stimulation occurs to assist removal of fluid in venous and lymph channels. The clinical indications and contraindications for interferential stimulation are shown in Table 10.2.

High voltage galvanic stimulation

High voltage galvanic stimulation (HVGS) is also a form of TENS and has two distinct specifications. It transmits voltage greater than 100 V and it has a twin-peaked monophasic current with a high peak but low average current.

The treatment is not actually galvanic but is called galvanic due to its monophasic current. The low average current density results in minimal charge build-up on the electrodes, thus minimizing the possibility of chemical burns. There are two methods of HVGS application. Pads or a probe are used over muscles requiring stimulation or local painful sites.

The clinical indications and contraindications for HVGS are shown in Table 10.2.

Low voltage stimulation

Low voltage stimulators were the earliest forms of electrical stimulation used for pain relief. They stimulate innervated or denervated muscles and can also be used as a medium for iontophoresis.

There are three types of currents—faradic (now rarely used), sinusoidal and galvanic (direct). Wave forms can deliver high average currents to produce chemical and thermal responses. However, this modality is more likely to cause thermal and chemical burns.

Neuromuscular stimulators

Neuromuscular electrical stimulators (NMES) are primarily used to maintain strength and flexibility, minimize atrophy during the healing process and for re-education of weak or poorly controlled muscles. They are similar to conventional TENS units and the units are interchangeable. The difference lies in the fact that the NMES have an interruption (on–off) mode in the current to allow the muscle to contract for a set period of time and then relax. This prevents fatigue and maximizes strengthening. NMES is used to improve muscle control in situations where active control is reduced, for example, vastus medialis obliquus and scapular retraction muscles.

Point stimulators

Point stimulators or hyperstimulation analgesia is a form of electroacutherapy, similar to acupuncture except that the points are stimulated with electrical current instead of needles. Small electrodes deliver current to a well-defined focal region which is perceived by the patient as a stinging sensation. It is thought that pain may be modulated when noxious stimuli cause descending tract inhibition.

Laser

Laser is an acronym for Light Amplification by Stimulated Emission of Radiation. Laser is pure light or amplified luminous energy produced by a series of reactions causing emission of photons. The type of atom stimulated determines the wavelength of the laser.

There are two categories of lasers. High-powered lasers with an output of up to 100 milliwatts (mW) are used extensively in industry, military services, engineering and some branches of medicine. Low- and mid-powered lasers (also known as cold or soft lasers) have a maximum output of less than 50 mW. There is no measurable heat associated with their use. One feature of laser light is that it has a single, well-defined wavelength.

Two types of cold lasers are used in the treatment of soft tissue injuries. The gallium arsenide (GaAs) laser has a wavelength of 904 nm and is not visible. The helium neon (HeNe) laser has a wavelength of 632.8 nm and is visible. Laser light waves travel unidirectionally and symmetrically with minimal diversion.

The clinical indications and contraindications of laser are shown in Table 10.2.

Various dosages are used depending on factors such as the depth of the lesion, the age of the patient, the amount of adipose tissue overlying the injury, the response to biostimulation and the temperature of the diode. Generally there is little evidence from clinical trials that laser therapy is helpful in the treatment of musculoskeletal pain, however, there is evidence to suggest that low-level laser therapy is effective in the treatment of subacute tendinopathy if a location-specific dose and valid treatment procedure are used.[69]

Diathermy

Microwave and short-wave diathermies use high-frequency electromagnetic waves to create heat in superficial muscles. A review of clinical trials using short-wave diathermy showed a lack of conclusive evidence but overall showed a trend in favor of the use of short-wave diathermy in the management of chronic pain conditions and wound healing.[70]

Magnetic therapy

Magnetic therapy is a widely used treatment, particularly in those with chronic pain. There are two ways in which magnetic therapy is delivered: pulsed electromagnetic fields (PEMF), using an alternating current through a coil applicator, or static magnetic fields (SMF).

Various studies claim a positive effect of PEMF in conditions such as low back pain, osteoarthritis, ankle sprains and whiplash injuries, however, the studies are generally of poor quality.[71] The evidence for the use of SMF is inconclusive,[72] although a recent critical review suggested that the majority of studies demonstrated a positive effect of static magnets in achieving analgesia across a broad range of different types of pain.[73] The clinical indications and contraindications of magnetic field therapy are shown in Table 10.2.

Extracorporeal shock wave therapy

Extracorporeal shock wave therapy has been used in the treatment of non-unions of fractures[74] and tendinopathy.[75] The jury is still out as to the effectiveness of shock wave therapy in tendinopathy; there are several papers showing its effectiveness and others that do not agree.[76–78] There is a vigorous debate regarding its efficacy in the treatment of chronic extensor tendinopathy at the elbow ('tennis elbow')[79] but the treatment has gained US Food and Drug Administration (FDA) approval for plantar fasciitis. Details of its effectiveness at specific sites are discussed in the relevant chapters in Part B.

Manual therapy

Manual therapy is a broad group of treatments in which the clinician applies forces directly to the musculoskeletal system. The aim of all manual therapy is to restore pain-free full range of motion.

The discipline of manual therapy relies on careful clinical assessment and particular attention to identifying abnormalities of tissue texture, tenderness, pain and restricted movement. Manual therapy is used to correct these abnormalities. Each abnormality detected in the clinical assessment must be considered as a possible contributor to the patient's symptoms and signs.

An essential component of all manual therapy is to assess pain and restriction of movement before and after each specific type of treatment so that treatment efficacy can be evaluated immediately. Before performing any manual therapy, the practitioner should explain the procedure to the patient. If the patient is aware of what is about to occur, he or she will be more likely to relax and gain maximum benefit from the treatment.

Manual therapy can be applied to joints, muscles (including tendons and fascia) and neural structures. The different types of manual therapy used in the treatment of abnormalities of each of these systems is shown below.

1. Joints: mobilization
   manipulation
   traction
2. Muscles: soft tissue therapy
   muscle energy techniques
3. Neural structures: neural stretching

Joint mobilization

Mobilization is a passive movement technique applied to a spinal or peripheral joint in which an oscillatory movement is performed within the control of the patient, who can prevent the movement if desired (Fig. 10.6).

Mobilization aims to restore full range of motion to a joint that is noted to be stiff and/or painful on clinical examination. Reduced range of motion (stiffness) may result from restriction of either physiological movements of the joint or accessory movements of the joint.

Physiological joint movements are those that can be performed actively by the patient. For example, physiological movements at the shoulder are flexion/extension, abduction/adduction and internal/external rotation.

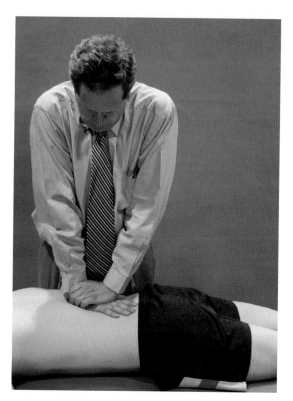

Figure 10.6 Mobilization

Accessory movements cannot be performed voluntarily by the patient but are a necessary component of normal joint function. Although their range of movement is small, a full range of accessory movements is essential for normal active and passive joint movements. The clinician can detect loss of an accessory movement by observing or palpating restriction in normal joint range of motion. Accessory movements in the shoulder include posteroanterior and anteroposterior movement, longitudinal movements (both superiorly and inferiorly) and lateral movement.

Mobilization is commonly performed at the vertebral joints. The exact physiological mechanism by which mobilization exerts a beneficial effect on these joints is uncertain but may include:

- an effect on the hydrostatics of the intervertebral disk and intervertebral bodies
- activation of type I and II mechanoreceptors in the capsule of the apophyseal joint
- alteration of the activity of the neuromuscular spindle in the intrinsic muscles
- assistance in the pumping effect on the venous plexus of the vertebral segment.

Common mobilizing techniques

A large number of mobilizing techniques are available to the clinician. These include those recommended by Maitland, Kaltenborn, Cyriax, McKenzie and others.[80–83] The aim of all these techniques is to restore normal pain-free range of motion. Maitland techniques involve mobilization in either physiological or accessory ranges of motion using rhythmic, oscillating movements.[80] Numerous randomized controlled trials have been performed with the majority of high-quality trials demonstrating mobilization to be an effective treatment for spinal pain.[84] Mobilization appears to be particularly effective when combined with other treatments such as soft tissue and muscle stabilizing techniques,[1] and with exercise therapy.[2]

Grades of mobilization

When using mobilizing techniques, treatment will usually begin with a gentle grade of movement, particularly if there is local pain and tenderness. The intensity of the treatment will gradually increase until normal movement is restored. For a stiff, pain-free joint, more vigorous mobilization may be performed from the commencement of treatment.

Maitland describes different types of mobilization at different ranges of movement and different amplitudes (Table 10.5). Treatment grade depends on whether pain or stiffness is the main problem. In painful joints, grades I and II are most commonly used (Fig. 10.7). In pain-free stiff joints, grades III and IV are used. Often when treating painful joints, initial grade I and grade II treatment will improve the patient's pain-free range and eventually allow grade III and IV movements to be performed.

Indications and contraindications for mobilization

Any joint in which there is pain or stiffness on physiological and/or accessory movements can be treated

Table 10.5 Grades of mobilization

Grade	Degree of mobilization
I	Small amplitude movement performed at the beginning of range
II	Large amplitude movement performed within the free range but not moving into any resistance or stiffness
III	Large amplitude movement performed up to the limit of range
IV	Small amplitude movement performed at the limit of range

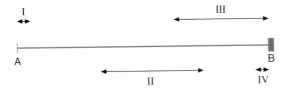

Figure 10.7 Grades of mobilization (A: beginning of range of movement; B: end of range of movement)

with mobilization. Contraindications to mobilization are:

- local malignancy
- local bony infection, for example, osteomyelitis, tuberculosis
- fractures
- spinal cord compression
- cauda equina compression.

Joint manipulation

Manipulation is a sudden movement or thrust of small amplitude performed at high speed at the end of joint range such that the patient is unable to prevent the movement. Manipulation is performed primarily at the intervertebral joints but may also be performed at peripheral joints.

Manipulation can be a very effective method of treatment.[3, 4, 85] It is, however, associated with considerable risks if performed inappropriately or with faulty technique. Manipulation should only be performed by fully qualified practitioners who have had formal training in manipulative skills.

Manipulation techniques

A number of different spinal manipulation techniques have been described. These include cervical rotation, cervical transverse thrust, thoracic posteroanterior rotation, thoracic rotation and lumbar rotation.

Indications and contraindications for manipulation

There are two main indications for manipulation. The first is a stiff pain-free joint that has been mobilized to the full extent of range possible. The second is an acute, locked joint such as a cervical apophyseal joint. The contraindications for manipulation are:

- all the contraindications for mobilization
- vertebral artery insufficiency (test prior to cervical manipulation; Chapter 16)
- rheumatoid arthritis of the atlanto-occipital and C1–2 joints

- spondylolisthesis (if symptoms arise from the slip)
- acute nerve root compression
- children whose epiphyseal plates have not closed
- joint instability
- pregnancy (last trimester)
- recent 'whiplash' injury
- hemophilia.

Joint traction

Traction, which involves intermittent or sustained pressure in a direction to distract joint surfaces, is used with variable success to treat patients with spinal pain. Spinal traction may result in distraction of the vertebral bodies or facet joints, widening of the intervertebral foramen and stretching of the spinal musculature.

This may be performed manually or by a traction apparatus, which may be either the use of weights or an electrical machine. Manual traction may have increased effectiveness with the use of a belt.

Types of traction

Continuous traction is applied with small weights for long periods of time (hours). This form of traction does not appear to be effective, possibly because insufficient force is applied to separate the vertebrae.

A heavier weight is used for shorter duration (minutes) in sustained traction. This can be performed with hanging weights or a mechanical device. Intermittent mechanical traction is provided by a device that alternately applies and releases tension.

Manual traction can be applied by the therapist usually for a short period of time (seconds). Gravity traction is provided by inversion machines. The patient is usually strapped into the machine at the ankles.

Indications for traction

Traction has traditionally been recommended in the treatment of nerve root compression due to either herniated disc material or narrowing of the intervertebral foramen, although the evidence for its use is not convincing. Its role in the treatment of hypomobile intervertebral segment(s) and muscle spasm is unclear.

Contraindications for traction

Traction is contraindicated in the presence of local tumor or infection. Symptoms associated with segmental spinal instability may be aggravated by traction.

Soft tissue therapy

Soft tissue therapy, also known as massage therapy, is a very popular clinical treatment for abnormalities such as:

- increased muscle tone/tension
- myofascial trigger points, active or latent
  —refer pain in a regular pattern
  —inhibit local muscle contraction
- palpably abnormal thickening of connective tissue.

In this section we touch on the biological rationale for soft tissue therapy in musculoskeletal medicine, provide an overview of several key soft tissue techniques, which are used as specific treatments in Part B, and alert the reader to some self-treatment options.

Any assessment of soft tissue must identify regions of abnormal tension and focal abnormalities such as trigger points by range of motion testing and precise, systematic palpation.

Soft tissue abnormalities may be a cause of pain and, importantly, adversely affect neuromuscular control. Areas of increased muscle tone, connective tissue thickening, and pain-producing or inhibitory trigger points[86] may reduce muscle power and endurance and lead to abnormalities of muscle activation. As such, soft tissue therapy may play an important role in correcting the inhibition of healthy activation patterns.[87]

As described in Chapter 3, it is important to look for both proximal and distal contributions to the patient's pain. Pain may refer directly to the site, for example, from spinal structures or myofascial trigger points. Similarly, pain may develop indirectly from altered muscle activation patterns caused by the inhibitory effect of inflammation, active trigger points and pain behavior.

Position of treatment

For successful soft tissue therapy, the 'target tissue' should be placed in an ideal position, either under tension or laxity. The advantages of treating soft tissue in a position of stretch include:

- focal sites of abnormality, taut bands, or areas of increased tension will often become more easily palpable
- myofascial trigger points may become more clearly evident and refer more dramatically in positions of stretch
- positions of increased neural tension will often facilitate palpation of the soft tissue abnormalities that contribute to improved neural mechanics

- enhanced effectiveness of rupturing abnormal cross-linkages between collagen fibers.

Digital ischemic pressure

Digital ischemic pressure describes the application of direct pressure perpendicular to the skin towards the center of a muscle with sufficient pressure to evoke a temporary ischemic reaction (Fig. 10.8). The aims of this technique are to stimulate the tension-monitoring receptors within muscle to reduce muscle tone, to provide an analgesic response in soft tissue by eliciting a release of pain-mediating substances and to deactivate symptomatic trigger points.

Digital ischemic pressure may be performed either using the therapist's thumb (Fig. 10.8a), elbow (Fig. 10.8b) or a hand-held device such as a T-shaped bar.

Sustained myofascial tension

Sustained myofascial tension is performed by applying a tensile force with the thumb, braced digits or forearm in the direction of greatest fascial restriction or in the direction of elongation necessary for normal

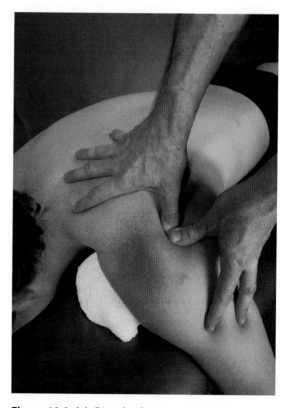

Figure 10.8 (a) Digital ischemic pressure to the infraspinatus trigger point using the therapist's thumb

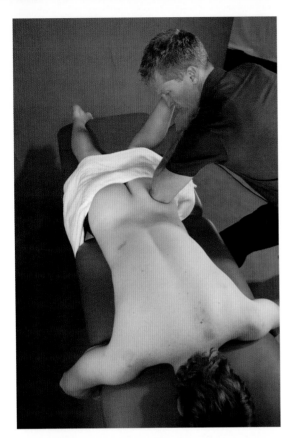

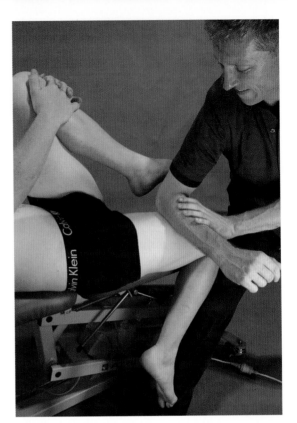

Figure 10.9 Sustained myofascial tension

(b) Digital ischemic pressure to the gluteus medius trigger point using the therapist's elbow

function. The aim of this technique is to restore the optimal length of tissue in the exact location where abnormal structural thickening is present.

By inducing a prolonged tensile force, the aim is to rupture abnormal cross-linkages between collagen fibers that limit the ability of connective tissue to elongate. The cross-linkages form as a result of the inflammatory response to acute or overuse injury.

Tension is developed in the tissue by blocking or anchoring one thumb proximal or distal to the lesion and moving the other thumb or braced digit through the region of dysfunction to impart a shear force. Greater shear force can be imparted by using passive or active joint movement in conjunction with local tissue contact (Fig. 10.9).

Depth of treatment

Granter and King developed a grading system for depth of soft tissue therapy (Table 10.6).

The scale of treatment depth is based on the patient's level of pain (I–IV) and the therapist's sense

Table 10.6 Granter-King scale for grading the depth of soft tissue therapy

Pain grade (P)	Patient's perception of pain
I	No pain perceived
II	Commencement of pain
III	Moderate level of pain
IV	Severe level of pain (seldom used)
Resistance grade (R)	**Therapist's perception of tissue resistance**
A	No sense of tissue resistance
B	Onset of tissue resistance
C	Moderate tissue resistance

of resistance to palpation (A–C). Post-acute lesions are first treated without pain to gauge the response to treatment without a sense of tissue resistance, that is, P—IA depth. Progression of treatment would be to IB and then IIB about one week after the injury.

A chronic lesion requires deep pressure such as IIC progressing to IIIC. This grading system permits clinicians to record depth of treatment consistently.

Combination treatment

Following these techniques aimed at restoring muscle length, sustained stretching can be performed to maximize the goal of restoring muscle length.

Soft tissue treatment must be used in combination with other forms of treatment, especially muscle retraining and strengthening to improve muscle activation patterns in chronically inhibited muscles.

Lubricants

Many soft tissue techniques require a lubricant applied to the skin to aid both patient comfort and the therapist's ability to palpate the tissue for abnormalities. There should be sufficient lubricant to prevent excessive resistance, particularly when palpating areas with large amounts of hair. Irritation of hair follicles may result in contact dermatitis.

With techniques such as sustained myofascial tension, skin contact should be maximal; therefore, no lubricant (or a dense cream) is required. Because repetitive movements are not used in this technique, there is little risk of irritation to hair follicles.

Vacuum cupping

The aim of vacuum cupping is to stretch soft tissue. Oil is applied to the skin to contain the negative pressure created in the cup by a vacuum pump. In the vacuum the soft tissue is 'drawn' upwards, thereby stretching the soft tissue in a regulated sustained stretch. The cup contains a one-way valve that allows the pump to be removed.

Vacuum cupping has been used in, for example, anterior compartment syndrome of the lower limb, thickening of the medial aponeurosis of the soleus or muscle tightness in the iliotibial band.

Cupping can cause significant capillary rupture and damage to the periosteum if used with excessive vacuum or with incorrect placement. The skin color should be monitored closely and the cup removed if the skin becomes more deeply rose-colored than normal reactive hyperemia.

Initial application should be for 15 seconds at a degree of suction such that the patient does not perceive a stretch in the tissue. The procedure can be repeated. Subsequent application can progress to a duration of 90 seconds at a degree of vacuum suction where comfortable tissue stretch is perceived by the patient.

Self treatment

The patient can work on his or her own soft tissue using various techniques designed to reduce muscle tone/tension and deactivate symptomatic myofascial trigger points (Fig. 10.10). Self treatment can be undertaken daily and should not cause a pain response that is excessive, which would adversely affect training, or result in an increase in symptoms. Typically, self treatment would involve the application of a sustained force (digital ischemic pressure) to the identified lesion, with pressure sustained until tone/tension reduces and pain or referred symptoms resolve.

Muscle energy techniques

Muscle energy techniques are osteopathic techniques for the assessment and correction of asymmetry or dysfunction (or both) of the musculoskeletal system. They are based on the principle that optimal static and dynamic body posture should be symmetrical.

Dysfunction and asymmetry may develop either as a result of a major traumatic event, such as a major muscle tear or severe fall, or by gradual decompensation. This results in changes in tissue adaptability and resting length. These changes may occur in response to pain, functional loss or stiffness. Muscle

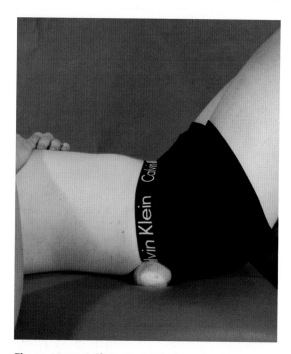

Figure 10.10 Self treatment. Treating the gluteus medius with a tennis ball

energy techniques involve detection of asymmetry or dysfunction (or both) and then correction of the abnormality without identification of specific tissues or spinal levels responsible for the abnormality. Thus, the unit is treated as a whole and corrected for adaptive changes in both normal as well as abnormal tissue.

For example, a moderately severe hamstring muscle tear may result in an adaptive posterior rotation of the ilium on the sacrum. Local treatment of the hamstring muscle tear may assist in healing of the tear but will not correct the adaptive change in the pelvis. Thus, further problems may arise.

Muscle energy techniques are used most commonly around the pelvis, spine, shoulder and lower limb. Most clinical experience has been with lower limb problems associated with abnormalities in the pelvis.

Muscle energy techniques utilize the concept of reciprocal innervation in which contraction of agonist muscles reflexly inhibits the antagonist muscle. They also make use of the principle that contraction of facilitated muscle in a lengthened position to activate the Golgi tendon organ will result in reflex muscle inhibition. As a result of these two principles, accurately localized, low intensity, isometric contractions of the agonist or antagonist muscle may lead to relaxation of that muscle and, therefore, correction of the asymmetry and dysfunction.

Despite its widespread use in clinical practice, there has been only one small clinical trial investigating its efficacy. This trial demonstrated that treatment with muscle energy techniques coupled with supervised neuromuscular re-education and resistance training resulted in significantly reduced disability in patients with low back pain compared to a control group with supervised neuromuscular re-education and resistance training alone.[88]

Neural stretching

Abnormalities of neural tension and restriction of normal movement of the structures of the nervous system may make a significant contribution to the patient's symptoms and signs in certain injuries (Chapter 3). Unless these abnormalities are corrected in addition to other soft tissue abnormalities associated with the injury, full recovery, as indicated by full pain-free range of motion, may not occur.

Abnormalities of neural tension may be secondary to an associated soft tissue lesion or, alternatively, due to primary damage to neural tissues. Treatment needs to be directed at the soft tissue lesion and the neural tissue itself.

Neural stretching (mobilization) is an effective method of restoring normal neural tension and mechanics of the nervous system. These stretches are adaptations of the neural tension tests (Chapter 8). The two most commonly used neural stretches are adaptations of the upper limb tension test (Fig. 10.11) and the slump test (Fig. 10.12). These stretches can often

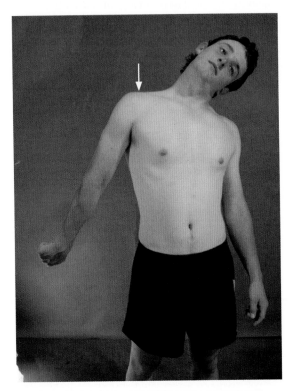

Figure 10.11 Upper limb tension test stretch. Athlete adopts the position illustrated. The degree of stretch can be increased by shoulder depression

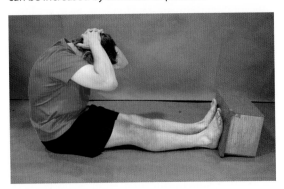

Figure 10.12 Slump stretch. Athlete adopts the position illustrated. The degree of stretch can be increased by forward flexion of the trunk

be helpful in the treatment of conditions in which neural tension is abnormal. Variations of these tests may be used for both diagnosis and treatment.

Particular care must be taken in acute or irritable conditions, as neural stretches may aggravate the patient's symptoms. Stretches should always begin gently and gradually increase under the close supervision of an experienced clinician. As with other methods of treatment, neural stretches alone are rarely sufficient to correct all abnormalities present. They are particularly effective in longstanding, chronic conditions where increased neural tension is common.

Acupuncture

Acupuncture is a medical tradition dating back to the most ancient times in China. In an ancient Chinese classic, the Yellow Emperor is quoted as saying to his physicians:

> I who am chief of a great people and who should receive taxes from them find myself afflicted by not being able to collect them because my people are sick. I desire, therefore, that the employment of remedies cease and that only the needles be used. I order that this method be transmitted to all future generations and that the laws concerning it be clearly defined so that it will be easy to practice it, hard to forget it and that it will not be abandoned in the future.

Historical anatomical drawings exist of points along lines called meridians or *zing*. During the Sung Dynasty (960–1279 AD), Emperor Wei-yi ordered a bronze statue to be cast on which all acupuncture points were located. This statue remains famous today and is still used by students of acupuncture.

At approximately the same time, treatises were written that established the relationship between the 12 meridians or *zing* and the body organs, which are divided into five *zsang* (heart, liver, spleen, lungs and kidneys) and the six *fu* (stomach, gall bladder, large intestine, small intestine, bladder and the function known as triple warmer). To these 11 organs or functions, a twelfth meridian was added—that of the pericardium.

The word 'acupuncture' is derived from the Latin word *acus* (the needle) and means 'puncturing of bodily tissue for the relief of pain'. Acupuncture is performed by inserting needles of various lengths and diameters into acupuncture points located all over the body. The needles are inserted to various depths, rotated and either immediately withdrawn or left in place. The needles may also be stimulated electrically (electroacupuncture) or by moxibustion (application

of heat to acupuncture points by burning moxa, the dried leaves of *Artemisia vulgaris*).

The exact mechanism of action of acupuncture is uncertain. Its effects may be explained by the gate control of pain in which stimulation of one part of the body may block pain from other parts of the body. The autonomic nervous system may also play an important role in mediating the acupuncture effect. In addition, acupuncture causes the body to release endorphins from the pituitary gland and other organs that may block signals in the pain pathways.

Dry needling

A number of techniques have been advocated for the elimination of active trigger points. Dry needling is, in our experience, an effective way to eliminate trigger points in taut muscle bands found in chronic musculoskeletal pain syndromes.[89] Needles are inserted perpendicularly through the skin down on to the tender, palpable taut band (Fig. 10.13). Usually, there is increased resistance to the needle in the area of the trigger point compared to the surrounding 'normal' muscle. If resistance and pain is not encountered at

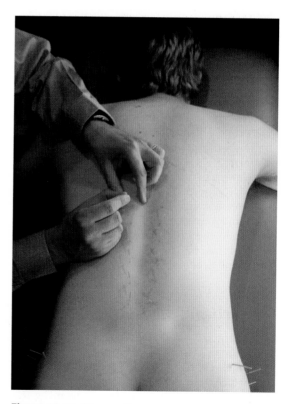

Figure 10.13 Dry needling

the first attempt, it may be necessary to draw back slightly and move the needle around to find the trigger point.

Originally we used 21-gauge hypodermic needles but in recent years we have used thin acupuncture needles. These needles have the advantage of less local muscle fiber trauma with less bleeding.

We have also changed our technique from the traditional method of inserting the needle into the taut band and leaving it in place for a few minutes. Instead, we introduce the needle into the taut band within the muscle and then repeatedly move the needle in and out of the muscle (but not back through the skin), constantly trying to find points within the band that reproduce the patent's pain and also produce a 'twitch' response.

When the needle makes contact with the trigger point, the patient feels an acute pain of varying intensity at the site of injection, in the area of pain referral, or both. Frequently, a twitch response will occur in the muscle when contact is made. Initially, the needle may be grasped by the muscle, followed by gradual relaxation and lengthening of the muscle.

Dry needling of a number of trigger points can be done at each treatment session. Usually after the first treatment session, pain relief lasts three to four days. Then following each subsequent session the duration of the pain relief is longer. Up to three or four treatment sessions may be required initially to eliminate the trigger point. A single trigger point should not be needled more than twice in a week.

Following dry needling there will be some residual local pain and tenderness. If the needling has elicited a particularly painful response, then it is helpful to apply a heat pack to the area for 10 minutes after treatment.

Following dry needling treatment it is important to passively stretch the affected muscles to maximize the increased range of motion.

Various research studies have compared dry needling to injection of local anesthetic and various other substances. The results of dry needling have been found to be just as effective.[90, 91]

Hyperbaric oxygen

Hyperbaric oxygen therapy refers to the medical procedure in which patients inspire 100% oxygen while their entire bodies are subjected to pressure greater than ambient barometric pressure at sea level, that is, greater than 1 atmosphere or 760 mmHg. This treatment is widely accepted as a primary treatment for decompression sickness, air embolism and carbon monoxide poisoning. It also appears to improve recovery after severe burns and crush injuries.

Hyperbaric oxygen may work by reducing the inflammatory response and enhancing collagen deposition or, alternatively, by inhibiting the release of oxygen free radicals.

Anecdotal evidence suggests that hyperbaric oxygen may assist in the healing of soft tissue injuries, however, well-designed studies[92] have failed to show any beneficial effect in the treatment of ankle sprains[93] and delayed-onset muscle soreness.[94] More positive evidence from well-designed studies in which treatment is initiated in the first 24 hours after injury are required before this treatment can be recommended.

Surgery

Despite the many advances in the non-operative management of sports injuries, surgery has a major role to play in the management of both acute injuries and overuse injuries. Surgery is used to remove, repair, reconstruct or realign damaged tissue. Sports surgery can be classified as arthroscopic surgery or open surgery.

Arthroscopic surgery

Arthroscopy involves the introduction of a fiber-optic telescope into a joint space to provide diagnostic information and afford the opportunity to undertake minimally invasive surgery.

Arthroscopy is a well-established procedure for the knee, shoulder, elbow, ankle and hip, and, more recently, the wrist. Arthroscopy of the shoulder, elbow, knee and ankle is performed with a standard 3.2 mm (1.3 in.) fiber-optic telescope inserted into a sheath. The procedure is performed using fluid to distend the joint, provide irrigation and remove debris.

Arthroscopy utilizes a light source to illuminate the joint and a video camera to capture the image, which is then displayed on one or more screens. The arthroscope is introduced through a standard portal, while another portal or portals are used to introduce operating instruments. The location of portals is important to minimize the risk of damage to vessels and nerves. A number of instruments are available for use in arthroscopic procedures.

Arthroscopy can be carried out under local, regional or, often, general anesthesia as a day procedure. The main areas of interest to be viewed through the arthroscope are the articular surfaces, the synovium and intra-articular structures such as the meniscus and cruciate ligaments of the knee, the glenoid labrum, rotator cuff tendons of the shoulder and the acetabular labrum of the hip. In most joints, the majority of the articular surfaces can be viewed. Assessment of stability can be aided by combining a direct view of the joint with maneuvers that place the joint under stress.

Common procedures performed through the arthroscope include removal of loose bodies within the joint, separation of and removal of the torn part of a meniscus, repair of a torn structure such as a peripheral tear of the meniscus, a labral detachment in the shoulder or dividing a tight structure such as the glenohumeral joint capsule in the shoulder or scar tissue in the knee. There is level 2 evidence that debridement of arthritic lesions is of no value in the knee. This may also be the case with other joints. More complex reconstructive joint procedures (anterior cruciate ligament reconstruction, rotator cuff repair) can be performed with the aid of an arthroscope.

Arthroscopy has a low complication rate. There is a small incidence of infection and delayed portal healing. Occasionally, arthroscopy can produce a persistent joint reaction manifesting as prolonged joint effusion, persistent pain and muscle wasting. Whether this is due to the arthroscopy itself or to the underlying joint pathology is sometimes difficult to determine. Complex regional pain syndrome type 1 may occasionally develop after arthroscopy.

Open surgery

The open surgical treatment of sports-related problems includes surgery related to acute trauma and surgery for the treatment of overuse injuries. Surgery after an acute injury aims to recreate the pre-injury anatomy by the repair of damaged tissues. This may require internal bone fixation for an unstable fracture or repair of torn ligaments or tendons. If repair of the damaged tissue is not possible, a reconstructive procedure may be performed, for example, anterior cruciate ligament reconstruction.

Following an acute injury, the athlete may develop chronic problems, such as instability, that may require surgical repair or reconstruction. Chronic ligamentous or capsular inadequacy may develop following an injury or as a gradual process. Surgery may be required to tighten the stretched tissue, either by moving the attachment of the tissue or by a shortening procedure, such as plication, reefing or shifting.

Overuse injuries that have failed to respond to conservative measures are sometimes managed by surgical tissue release, division or excision. Excision

may be performed if impingement is present or if degenerative change has led to tissue necrosis. In nerve compression, decompression or transposition of the nerve may be required. Stress fractures that fail to heal (non-union) are treated by fixation or bone graft.

With all surgical procedures, arthroscopic or open, the surgery must be considered as only a part of the treatment. Adequate post-surgical rehabilitation is equally as important as the procedure itself. Rehabilitation following injury and surgery is discussed in Chapter 12.

Recommended Reading

Boyling JD, Jull GA. *Grieve's Modern Manual Therapy. The Vertebral Column.* 3rd edn. Edinburgh: Churchill Livingstone, 2004.

Cameron MH. *Physical Agents in Rehabilitation.* Philadelphia, PA: WB Saunders, 1999.

Excellent, well-referenced overview.

Hunter G. Specific soft tissue mobilization in the management of soft tissue dysfunction. *Man Ther* 1998; 3(1): 2–11.

Jarvinen TA, Jarvinen TL, Kaariainen M, Kalimo H, Jarvinen M. Muscle injuries: biology and treatment. *Am J Sports Med* 2005; 33(5): 745–64.

Kaltenborn FM. *Manual Therapy of the Extremity Joints.* Oslo: Bokhandel, 1975.

Kannus P, Parkkari J, Jarvinen T, Jarvinen T, Jarvinen M. Basic science and clinical studies coincide: active treatment approach is needed after a sports injury. *Scand J Med Sci Sports* 2003; 13: 150–4.

Maitland GD. *Vertebral Manipulation.* 5th edn. London: Butterworths, 1986.

Classic text.

McKenzie R. *The Lumbar Spine: Mechanical Diagnosis and Therapy.* Waikane: Spinal Publications, 1981.

Classic text.

Refshauge K, Gass E. *Musculoskeletal Physiotherapy. Clinical Science and Evidence-Based Practice.* 2nd edn. Oxford: Butterworth-Heinemann, 2004.

Simons DG, Travell JG, Simons LS. *Myofascial Pain and Dysfunction. The Trigger Point Manual.* 2nd edn. Baltimore, MA: Williams & Wilkins, 1999.

Weerapong P, Hume PA, Kolt GS. The mechanisms of massage and effects on performance, muscle recovery and injury prevention. *Sports Med* 2005; 35(3): 235–56.

Recommended Websites

The *British Medical Journal*'s 'Clinical Evidence' site—musculoskeletal subsection. This contains abbreviated evidence based on the Cochrane Collaboration and other systematic reviews so that the clinician can readily access information for the specific conditions listed: <http://www.clinicalevidence.com/ceweb/conditions/msd/msd.jsp>

References

1. Hoving JL, Koes BW, de Vet HC, et al. Manual therapy, physical therapy, or continued care by a general practitioner for patients with neck pain. A randomized, controlled trial. *Ann Intern Med* 2002; 136(10): 713–22.
2. Jull G, Trott P, Potter H, et al. A randomized controlled trial of exercise and manipulative therapy for cervicogenic headache. *Spine* 2002; 27(17): 1835–43.
3. Aure OF, Nilsen JH, Vasseljen O. Manual therapy and exercise therapy in patients with chronic low back pain: a randomized, controlled trial with 1-year follow-up. *Spine* 2003; 28(6): 525–31.
4. Mior S. Manipulation and mobilization in the treatment of chronic pain. *Clin J Pain* 2001; 17: S70–76.
5. Holmich P, Uhrskou P, Ulnits L, et al. Effectiveness of active physical training as treatment for long-standing adductor-related groin pain in athletes: randomised trial. *Lancet* 1999; 353(9151): 439–43.
6. Crossley K, Bennell K, Green S, Cowan S, McConnell J. Physical therapy for patellofemoral pain: a randomized, double-blinded, placebo-controlled trial. *Am J Sports Med* 2002; 30(6): 857–65.
7. Hinman RS, Crossley KM, McConnell J, Bennell KL. Efficacy of knee tape in the management of osteoarthritis of the knee: blinded randomised controlled trial. *BMJ* 2003; 327(7407): 135.
8. Verhagen E, van der Beek A, Twisk J, Bouter L, Bahr R, van Mechelen W. The effect of a proprioceptive balance board training program for the prevention of ankle sprains: a prospective controlled trial. *Am J Sports Med* 2004; 32(6): 1385–93.
9. Nash CE, Mickan SM, Del Mar CB, Glasziou PP. Resting injured limbs delays recovery: a systematic review. *J Fam Pract* 2004; 53(9): 706–12.
10. Robertson MC, Campbell AJ, Gardner MM, Devlin N. Preventing injuries in older people by preventing falls: a meta-analysis of individual-level data. *J Am Geriatr Soc* 2002; 50(5): 905–11.
11. Newcomer KL, Laskowski ER, Idank DM, McLean TJ, Egan KS. Corticosteroid injection in early treatment of lateral epicondylitis. *Clin J Sport Med* 2001; 11(4): 214–22.
12. Beaupre LA, Davies DM, Jones CA, Cinats JG. Exercise combined with continuous passive motion or slider board therapy compared with exercise only: a randomized controlled trial of patients following total knee arthroplasty. *Phys Ther* 2001; 81(4): 1029–37.
13. Astrom M, Westlin N. No effect of piroxicam on Achilles tendinopathy. A randomized study of 70 patients. *Acta Orthop Scand* 1992; 63: 631–4.
14. Basford JR, Malanga GA, Krause DA, Harmsen WS. A randomized controlled evaluation of low-intensity laser therapy: plantar fasciitis. *Arch Phys Med Rehabil* 1998; 79(3): 249–54.
15. Bleakley C, McDonough S, MacAuley D. The use of ice in the treatment of acute soft-tissue injury: a systematic review of randomized controlled trials. *Am J Sports Med* 2004; 32(1): 251–61.
16. Hubbard T, Aronson S, Denegar C. Does cryotherapy hasten return to participation? A systemative review. *J Athl Train* 2004; 39: 88–94.
17. MacAuley DC. Ice therapy: how good is the evidence? *Int J Sports Med* 2001; 22(5): 379–84.
18. Moeller JL, Monroe J, McKeag DB. Cryotherapy-induced common peroneal nerve palsy. *Clin J Sport Med* 1997; 7(3): 212–6.
19. Kannus P, Parkkari J, Jarvinen T, Jarvinen T, Jarvinen M. Basic science and clinical studies coincide: active treatment approach is needed after a sports injury. *Scand J Med Sci Sports* 2003; 13: 150–4.
20. Jarvinen TA, Jarvinen TL, Kaariainen M, Kalimo H, Jarvinen M. Muscle injuries: biology and treatment. *Am J Sports Med* 2005; 33(5): 745–64.
21. Kongsgaard M, Aagaard P, Kjaer M, Magnusson SP. Structural Achilles tendon properties in athletes subjected to different exercise modes and in Achilles tendon rupture patients. *J Appl Physiol* 2005; 99(5): 1965–71.
22. Miller BF, Olesen JL, Hansen M, et al. Coordinated collagen and muscle protein synthesis in human patella tendon and quadriceps muscle after exercise. *J Physiol* 2005; 567(Pt 3): 1021–33.
23. Radi Z, Khan N. Effects of cyclooxygenase inhibition on bone, tendon, and ligament healing. *Inflamm Res* 2003; 54: 358–66.
24. Rahusen FT, Weinhold PS, Almekinders LC. Nonsteroidal anti-inflammatory drugs and acetaminophen in the treatment of an acute muscle injury. *Am J Sports Med* 2004; 32(8): 1856–9.
25. Bogduk N. A narrative review of intra-articular corticosteroid injections for low back pain. *Pain Med* 2005; 6(4): 287–96.
26. Warden SJ. Cyclo-oxygenase-2 inhibitors: beneficial or detrimental for athletes with acute musculoskeletal injuries? *Sports Med* 2005; 35(4): 271–83.

27. Brophy JM, Solomon SD, Wittes J, et al. Cardiovascular risk associated with celecoxib. *N Engl J Med* 2005; 352(25): 2648–50.

28. Horton R. Vioxx, the implosion of Merck, and aftershocks at the FDA. *Lancet* 2004; 364(9450): 1995–6.

29. Juni P, Nartey L, Reichenbach S, Sterchi R, Dieppe PA, Egger M. Risk of cardiovascular events and rofecoxib: cumulative meta-analysis. *Lancet* 2004; 364(9450): 2021–9.

30. Kaplan RJ. Current status of nonsteroidal anti-inflammatory drugs in physiatry: balancing risks and benefits in pain management. *Am J Phys Med Rehabil* 2005; 84(11): 885–94.

31. Hippisley-Cox J, Coupland C. Risk of myocardial infarction in patients taking cyclo-oxygenase-2 inhibitors or conventional non-steroidal anti-inflammatory drugs: population based nested case-control analysis. *BMJ* 2005; 330(7504): 1366.

32. Mazieres B, Rouanet S, Velicy J, Scarsi C, Reiner V. Topical ketoprofen patch (100 mg) for the treatment of ankle sprain: a randomized, double-blind, placebo-controlled study. *Am J Sports Med* 2005; 33(4): 515–23.

33. Predel HG, Koll R, Pabst H, et al. Diclofenac patch for topical treatment of acute impact injuries: a randomised, double blind, placebo controlled, multicentre study. *Br J Sports Med* 2004; 38(3): 318–23.

34. Shrier I, Matheson GO, Kohl HW. Achilles tendonitis: are corticosteroid injections useful or harmful. *Clin J Sport Med* 1996; 6: 245–50.

35. Koenig MJ, Torp-Pedersen S, Qvistgaard E, Terslev L, Bliddal H. Preliminary results of colour Doppler-guided intratendinous glucocorticoid injection for Achilles tendonitis in five patients. *Scand J Med Sci Sports* 2004; 14(2): 100–6.

36. Hugate R, Pennypacker J, Saunders M, Juliano P. The effects of intratendinous and retrocalcaneal intrabursal injections of corticosteroid on the biomechanical properties of rabbit Achilles tendons. *J Bone Joint Surg Am* 2004; 86A(4): 794–801.

37. Charalambous C, Paschalides C, Sadiq S, Tryfonides M, Hirst P, Paul AS. Weight bearing following intra-articular steroid injection of the knee: survey of current practice and review of the available evidence. *Rheumatol Int* 2002; 22(5): 185–7.

38. Brukner P, Nicol A. Use of oral corticosteroids in sports medicine. *Curr Sports Med Rep* 2004; 3(4): 181–3.

39. Gebhard KL, Maibach HI. Relationship between systemic corticosteroids and osteonecrosis. *Am J Clin Dermatol* 2001; 2(6): 377–88.

40. Bolin DJ. Transdermal approaches to pain in sports injury management. *Curr Sports Med Rep* 2003; 2(6): 303–9.

41. Dietzel D, Hedlund E. Injections and return to play. *Curr Pain Headache Rep* 2005; 9(1): 11–16.

42. Tokish JM, Powell ET, Schlegel TF, Hawkins RJ. Ketorolac use in the National Football League: prevalence, efficacy, and adverse effects. *Physician Sportsmed* 2002; 30(9): 19–24.

43. Berrazueta JR, Losada A, Poveda J, et al. Successful treatment of shoulder pain syndrome due to supraspinatus tendinitis with transdermal nitroglycerin. A double blind study. *Pain* 1996; 66(1): 63–7.

44. Paoloni JA, Appleyard RC, Nelson J, Murrell GA. Topical glyceryl trinitrate treatment of chronic noninsertional Achilles tendinopathy. A randomized, double-blind, placebo-controlled trial. *J Bone Joint Surg Am* 2004; 86A(5): 916–22.

45. Paoloni JA, Appleyard RC, Nelson J, Murrell GA. Topical nitric oxide application in the treatment of chronic extensor tendinosis at the elbow: a randomized, double-blinded, placebo-controlled clinical trial. *Am J Sports Med* 2003; 31(6): 915–20.

46. Paoloni JA, Appleyard RC, Nelson J, Murrell GA. Topical glyceryl trinitrate application in the treatment of chronic supraspinatus tendinopathy: a randomized, double-blinded, placebo-controlled clinical trial. *Am J Sports Med* 2005; 33(6): 806–13.

47. Winter H, Drager E, Sterry W. Sclerotherapy for treatment of hemangiomas. *Dermatol Surg* 2000; 26: 105–8.

48. Ohberg L, Alfredson H. Ultrasound guided sclerosis of neovessels in painful chronic Achilles tendinosis: pilot study of a new treatment. *Br J Sports Med* 2002; 36(3): 173–5, discussion 176–7.

49. Alfredson H, Ohberg L. Sclerosing injections to areas of neo-vascularisation reduce pain in chronic Achilles tendinopathy: a double-blind randomised controlled trial. *Knee Surg Sports Traumatol Arthrosc* 2005; 13(4): 338–44.

50. Rabago D, Best TM, Beamsley M, Patterson J. A systematic review of prolotherapy for chronic musculoskeletal pain. *Clin J Sport Med* 2005; 15(5): E376.

51. Towheed TE, Maxwell L, Anastassiades TP, et al. Glucosamine therapy for treating osteoarthritis. *Cochrane Database Syst Rev* 2005; 2: CD002946.

52. Lo GH, LaValley M, McAlindon T, Felson DT. Intra-articular hyaluronic acid in treatment of knee osteoarthritis: a meta-analysis. *JAMA* 2003; 290(23): 3115–21.

53. Aggarwal A, Sempowski IP. Hyaluronic acid injections for knee osteoarthritis. Systematic review of the literature. *Can Fam Physician* 2004; 50: 249–56.

54. Arrich J, Piribauer F, Mad P, Schmid D, Klaushofer K, Mullner M. Intra-articular hyaluronic acid for the treatment of osteoarthritis of the knee: systematic review and meta-analysis. *CMAJ* 2005; 172(8): 1039–43.

55. Bellamy N, Campbell J, Robinson V, Gee T, Bourne R, Wells G. Viscosupplementation for the treatment of

osteoarthritis of the knee. *Cochrane Database Syst Rev* 2005; 2: CD005321.

56. Conrozier T, Vignon E. Is there evidence to support the inclusion of viscosupplementation in the treatment paradigm for patients with hip osteoarthritis? *Clin Exp Rheumatol* 2005; 23(5): 711–16.

57. Moulin DE. Systemic drug treatment for chronic musculoskeletal pain. *Clin J Pain* 2001; 17(4 suppl.): S86–S93.

58. O'Malley PG, Balden E, Tomkins G, Santoro J, Kroenke K, Jackson JL. Treatment of fibromyalgia with antidepressants: a meta-analysis. *J Gen Intern Med* 2000; 15(9): 659–66.

59. Tofferi JK, Jackson JL, O'Malley PG. Treatment of fibromyalgia with cyclobenzaprine: a meta-analysis. *Arthritis Rheum* 2004; 51(1): 9–13.

60. Orchard JW. Benefits and risks of using local anaesthetic for pain relief to allow early return to play in professional football. *Br J Sports Med* 2002; 36(3): 209–13.

61. Gam AN, Johannsen F. Ultrasound therapy in musculoskeletal disorders: a meta-analysis. *Pain* 1995; 63(1): 85–91.

62. Green S, Buchbinder R, Glazier R, Forbes A. Systematic review of randomised controlled trials of interventions for the painful shoulder: selection criteria, outcome assessment, and efficacy. *BMJ* 1998; 316: 354–60.

63. Brosseau L, Casimiro L, Robinson V, et al. Therapeutic ultrasound for treating patellofemoral pain syndrome. *Cochrane Database Syst Rev* 2001; 4: CD003375.

64. Warden SJ, McMeeken JM. Ultrasound usage and dosage in sports physiotherapy. *Ultrasound Med Biol* 2002; 28(8): 1075–80.

65. Warden SJ. A new direction for ultrasound therapy in sports medicine. *Sports Med* 2003; 33(2): 95–107.

66. Gebauer D, Mayr E, Orthner E, Ryaby JP. Low-intensity pulsed ultrasound: effects on nonunions. *Ultrasound Med Biol* 2005; 31(10): 1391–402.

67. Khadilkar A, Milne S, Brosseau L, et al. Transcutaneous electrical nerve stimulation (TENS) for chronic low-back pain. *Cochrane Database Syst Rev* 2005; 3: CD003008.

68. Bjordal JM, Johnson MI, Ljunggreen AE. Transcutaneous electrical nerve stimulation (TENS) can reduce postoperative analgesic consumption. A meta-analysis with assessment of optimal treatment parameters for postoperative pain. *Eur J Pain* 2003; 7(2): 181–8.

69. Bjordal JM, Couppe C, Chow RT, Tuner J, Ljunggren EA. A systematic review of low level laser therapy with location-specific doses for pain from chronic joint disorders. *Aust J Physiother* 2003; 49(2): 107–16.

70. Shields N, Gormley J, O'Hare N. Short-wave diathermy: current clinical and safety practices. *Physiother Res Int* 2002; 7(4): 191–202.

71. Vallbona C, Richards T. Evolution of magnetic therapy from alternative to traditional medicine. *Phys Med Rehabil Clin N Am* 1999; 10(3): 729–54.

72. Hinman M. The therapeutic use of magnets: a review of recent research. *Phys Ther Rev* 2002; 7: 33–43.

73. Eccles NK. A critical review of randomized controlled trials of static magnets for pain relief. *J Altern Complement Med* 2005; 11(3): 495–509.

74. Haupt G, Haupt A, Ekkernkamp A, Gerety B, Chvapil M. Influence of shock waves on fracture healing. *Urology* 1992; 39(6): 529–32.

75. Haupt G. Use of extracorporeal shock waves in the treatment of pseudarthrosis, tendinopathy and other orthopedic diseases. *J Urol* 1997; 158(1): 4–11.

76. Buchbinder R, Green S, White M, Barnsley L, Smidt N, Assendelft WJ. Shock wave therapy for lateral elbow pain. *Cochrane Database Syst Rev* 2002; 1: CD003524.

77. Gerdesmeyer L, Wagenpfeil S, Haake M, et al. Extracorporeal shock wave therapy for the treatment of chronic calcifying tendonitis of the rotator cuff: a randomized controlled trial. *JAMA* 2003; 290(19): 2573–80.

78. Rompe JD. Shock wave therapy for calcific tendinitis of the shoulder: a prospective clinical study with two-year follow-up. *Am J Sports Med* 2003; 31(6): 1049–50, author reply 1050.

79. Bisset L, Paungmali A, Vicenzino B, Beller E. A systematic review and meta-analysis of clinical trials on physical interventions for lateral epicondylalgia. *Br J Sports Med* 2005; 39(7): 411–22.

80. Maitland GD. *Vertebral Manipulation*. 5th edn. London: Butterworths, 1986.

81. Kaltenborn F. *Manual Therapy of the Extremity Joints*. Oslo: Bokhandel, 1975.

82. Cyriax J. *Textbook of Orthopaedic Medicine*. 6th edn. London: Bailliere Tindall, 1975.

83. McKenzie R. *The Lumbar Spine: Mechanical Diagnosis and Therapy*. Waikane: Spinal Publications, 1981.

84. Sran MM. To treat or not to treat: new evidence for the effectiveness of manual therapy. *Br J Sports Med* 2004; 38(5): 521–5.

85. Cleland JA, Childs JD, McRae M, Palmer JA, Stowell T. Immediate effects of thoracic manipulation in patients with neck pain: a randomized clinical trial. *Man Ther* 2005; 10(2): 127–35.

86. Gerwin RD, Shannon S, Hong CZ, Hubbard D, Gevirtz R. Interrater reliability in myofascial trigger point examination. *Pain* 1997; 69(1–2): 65–73.

87. Lucas KR, Polus BI, Rich PA. Latent myofascial trigger points: their effects on muscle activation and movement efficiency. *J Bodywork Movement Ther* 2004; 8: 160–6.

88. Wilson E, Payton O, Donegan-Shoaf L, Dec K. Muscle energy technique in patients with acute low back pain: a pilot clinical trial. *J Orthop Sports Phys Ther* 2003; 33(9): 502–12.

89. Huguenin LK. Myofascial trigger points: the current evidence. *Phys Ther Sport* 2004; 5: 2–12.

90. Garvey TA, Marks MR, Wiesel SW. A prospective, randomized, double-blind evaluation of trigger-point injection therapy for low-back pain. *Spine* 1989; 14(9): 962–4.

91. Hong CZ. Lidocaine injection versus dry needling to myofascial trigger point. The importance of the local twitch response. *Am J Phys Med Rehabil* 1994; 73(4): 256–63.

92. Bennett M, Best T, Babul S, Taunton J, Lepawsky M, Bennett M. Hyperbaric oxygen therapy for delayed onset muscle soreness and closed soft tissue injury. *Cochrane Database Syst Rev* 2005; 4: CD004713.

93. Borromeo CN, Ryan JL, Marchetto PA, Peterson R, Bove AA. Hyperbaric oxygen therapy for acute ankle sprains. *Am J Sports Med* 1997; 25(5): 619–25.

94. Staples JR, Clement DB, Taunton JE, McKenzie DC. Effects of hyperbaric oxygen on a human model of injury. *Am J Sports Med* 1999; 27(5): 600–5.

Core Stability

In recent years an understanding of the concept of core stability has changed the way in which we rehabilitate our patients. We have chosen to use the term 'core stability' in this book but there are many other interchangeable terms (Table 11.1).

All these terms are a description of the muscular control required around the lumbopelvic–hip region to maintain functional stability. Particular attention has been paid to the core because it serves as a muscular corset that works as a unit to stabilize the body and spine with and without limb movement. In short, the core serves as the center of the functional kinetic chain. The core has been referred to as the 'powerhouse', the foundation or engine of all limb movement. All movements are generated from the core and translated to the extremities.

We use the term 'stability' rather than 'strength' because strength is just one component of the dynamic stability required. Dynamic stabilization refers to the ability to utilize strength and endurance in a functional manner through all planes of motion and action despite changes in the centre of gravity.[1] A comprehensive strengthening or facilitation of these core muscles has been advocated as a preventive, rehabilitative and performance-enhancing program for various lumbar spine and musculoskeletal injuries.

The 'core' has been described as a box with the abdominals in the front, paraspinals and gluteals in the back, diaphragm as the roof, pelvic floor and hip girdle musculature as the bottom, and hip abductors and rotators laterally.[2] All these muscles have direct or indirect attachments to the extensive thoracolumbar fascia and spinal column, which connect the upper and lower limbs.

Stability of the lumbar spine involves both passive stiffness, through the osseous and ligamentous structures, and active stiffness, through muscles. A bare spine, without muscles attached, is unable to bear much of a compressive load.[3, 4] Spinal instability occurs when either of these components is disturbed. *Gross instability* is true displacement of vertebrae, such as with traumatic disruption of two out of three vertebrae. On the other hand, *functional instability* is defined as a relative increased range of the neutral zone (the range in which internal resistance from active muscular control is minimal).[5] Active stiffness or stability can be achieved through muscular co-contraction, akin to tightening the guys of a tent to unload the center pole (Fig. 11.1).[6]

A major advance in our understanding of how muscles contribute to lumbar stabilization came from recognizing the difference between local and global muscles. Global (dynamic, phasic) muscles are the large, torque-producing muscles, such as the rectus abdominis, external oblique and the thoracic part of lumbar iliocostalis, which link the pelvis to the thoracic cage and provide general trunk stabilization as well as movement.

Local (postural, tonic) muscles are those that attach directly to the lumbar vertebrae and are responsible for

Table 11.1 Terms used to describe core stability

Lumbar/lumbopelvic stabilization
Dynamic stabilization
Motor control
Neuromuscular training
Neutral spine control
Muscular fusion
Trunk stabilization
Core strengthening

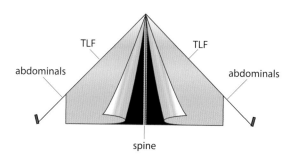

Figure 11.1 Active stability is achieved through muscular co-contraction via the thoracolumbar fascia (TLF). This is similar to the stability imparted by the guys of a tent ADAPTED FROM PORTERFIELD[6]

providing segmental stability and directly controlling the lumbar segments during movement. These muscles include lumbar multifidus, psoas major, quadratus lumborum, the lumbar parts of iliocostalis and longissimus, transversus abdominis, the diaphragm and the posterior fibers of internal oblique (Fig. 11.2).

Whereas previously the major emphasis in rehabilitation has been to strengthen the global muscles (e.g. the use of sit-ups as a treatment for low back pain), we now understand that both groups of muscles must be working efficiently. We have also come to realize that strength is not the only, nor indeed the most important, quality of the muscle. Muscle activation and endurance are probably more important than strength and any rehabilitation program should reflect this.

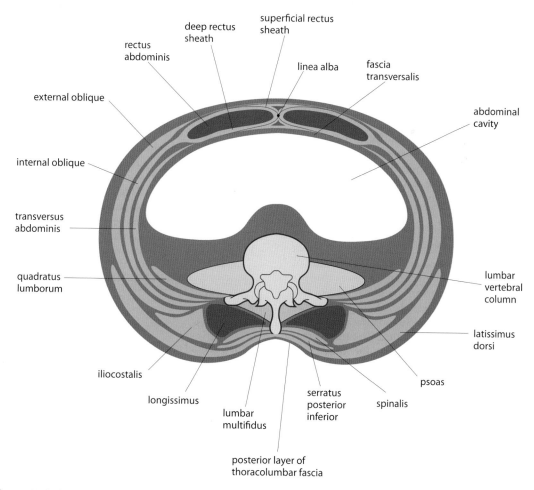

Figure 11.2 Cross-sectional anatomy of the lumbar spine

Anatomy

Stability and movement are critically dependent on the coordination of all the muscles surrounding the lumbar spine. Even though recent research has advocated the importance of a few muscles in particular (transversus abdominis and multifidi), all core muscles are needed for optimal stabilization and performance.[7] To achieve muscular co-contraction precise neural input and output (which has also been referred to as proprioceptive neuromuscular facilitation by neurorehabilitationists) is needed.[8]

Osseous and ligamentous structures

Passive stiffness is imparted to the lumbar spine by the osseoligamentous structures. Tissue injury to any of these structures may cause functional instability. The posterior elements of the spine include the pedicle, lamina and pars interarticularis. These structures are, in fact, flexible. However, too much load causes failure, typically at the pars. The intervertebral disk is composed of the anulus fibrosus, nucleus pulposus and the end plates. Compressive and shearing loads can cause injury initially to the end plates and ultimately to the anulus such that posterior disk herniations result. Excessive external loads on the disk may be caused by weak muscular control, thus causing a vicious cycle where the disk no longer provides optimal passive stiffness or stability. The spinal ligaments provide little stability in the neutral zone. Their more important role may be to provide afferent proprioception of the lumbar spine segments.[9]

The thoracolumbar fascia

The thoracolumbar fascia (TLF) acts as 'nature's back belt'. It works as a retinacular strap of the muscles of the lumbar spine. The thoracolumbar fascia consists of three layers: the anterior, middle and posterior layers. Of these three layers the posterior layer has the most important role in supporting the lumbar spine and abdominal musculature. The transversus abdominis has large attachments to the middle and posterior layers of the TLF.[2] The posterior layer consists of two laminae: a superficial lamina with fibers passing downward and medially, and a deep lamina with fibers passing downward and laterally. The aponeurosis of the latissimus dorsi muscle forms the superficial layer. In essence, the TLF provides a link between the lower limb and the upper limb.[10] With contraction of the muscular contents, the TLF acts as an activated proprioceptor, like a back belt providing feedback in lifting activities.

Paraspinals

There are two major groups of the lumbar extensors: the erector spinae and the so-called local muscles (rotators, intertransversi, multifidi). The erector spinae in the lumbar region are composed of two major muscles: the longissimus and iliocostalis. These are actually primarily thoracic muscles which act on the lumbar region via a long tendon that attaches to the pelvis. This long moment arm is ideal for lumbar extension and for creating posterior shear with lumbar flexion.[4]

Deep and medial to the erector spinae muscles lie the local muscles. The rotators and intertransversi muscles do not have a great moment arm. It is likely that they represent length transducers or position sensors of a spinal segment by way of their rich composition of muscle spindles. The multifidi pass along two or three spinal levels. They are theorized to work as segmental stabilizers. Due to their short moment arms, the multifidi are not involved much in gross movement. Multifidi have been found to be atrophied in individuals with low back pain.[11]

Quadratus lumborum

The quadratus lumborum is a large, thin, quadrangular-shaped muscle that has direct insertions to the lumbar spine. There are three major components or muscular fascicles to the quadratus lumborum: the inferior oblique, superior oblique and longitudinal fascicles. Both the longitudinal and superior oblique fibers have no direct action on the lumbar spine. They are designed as secondary respiratory muscles to stabilize the twelfth rib during respiration. The inferior oblique fibers of the quadratus lumborum are generally thought to be a weak lateral flexor of the lumbar vertebrae. McGill believes the quadratus lumborum is a major stabilizer of the spine, typically working isometrically.[12]

Abdominals

The abdominal muscles serve as a vital component of the core. The transversus abdominis has received particular attention. Its fibers run horizontally around the abdomen, allowing hoop-like stresses with contraction. Isolated activation of the transversus abdominis is achieved through 'hollowing in' of the abdomen. As well, the transversus abdominis has been shown to activate prior to limb movement, theoretically to stabilize the lumbar spine. Patients with low back pain have delayed activation of the transversus abdominis.[1]

The internal oblique has similar fiber orientation to the transversus abdominis, yet receives much less attention in regards to its creation of hoop stresses. Together, the internal oblique, external oblique and transversus abdominis increase the intra-abdominal pressure, thus imparting functional stability to the lumbar spine.[4]

Finally, the rectus abdominis is a paired, strap-like muscle of the anterior abdominal wall. Contraction of this muscle predominantly causes flexion of the lumbar spine. Most fitness programs incorrectly emphasize rectus abdominis and internal oblique development, thus creating an imbalance with the relatively weaker external oblique.[13]

Hip girdle musculature

The hip musculature plays a significant role within the kinetic chain, particularly for all ambulatory activities, stabilization of the trunk/pelvis, and in transferring force from the lower extremities to the pelvis and spine.[14] Poor endurance and delayed firing of the hip extensor (gluteus maximus) and abductor (gluteus medius) muscles have previously been noted in individuals with lower extremity instability or low back pain.[15, 16] Nadler et al. demonstrated a significant asymmetry in hip extensor strength in female athletes with reported low back pain.[17] In a prospective study, Nadler et al. demonstrated a significant association between hip strength imbalance of the hip extensors measured during the pre-participation physical examination and the occurrence of low back pain in female athletes over the ensuing year.[18] Overall, the hip appears to play a significant role in transferring forces from the lower extremities to the pelvis and spine, acting as one link within the kinetic chain.

The psoas major is a long, thick muscle whose primary action is flexion of the hip. However, based upon its attachment sites into the lumbar spine it has the potential to aid in spinal biomechanics. Anatomical dissections have shown that the psoas muscle has three proximal attachment sites: the medial half of the transverse processes from T12 to L5, the intervertebral disk, and the vertebral body adjacent to the disk.[19] However, it is not likely that the psoas provides much stability to the lumbar spine except in increased lumbar flexion.[4] Increased stability requirements or a tight psoas will concomitantly cause increased compressive injurious loads to the lumbar disks.

Diaphragm and pelvic floor

The diaphragm serves as the roof of the core. Stability is imparted to the lumbar spine by contraction of the diaphragm and increasing intra-abdominal pressure. Recent studies have indicated that individuals with sacroiliac pain have impaired recruitment of the diaphragm and pelvic floor.[20] Likewise, ventilatory challenges on the body may cause further diaphragm dysfunction and lead to more compressive loads on the lumbar spine.[21] Thus, diaphragmatic breathing techniques may be an important part of a core strengthening program. Furthermore, the pelvic floor musculature is coactivated with transversus abdominis contraction.[22]

Assessment of core stability

While there is no single measure of core stability, a few simple tests will provide an indication of the endurance of certain key muscle groups. The four tests advocated are the prone and lateral bridges, and the torso flexor and extensor endurance tests. The bridge tests are functional in that they assess strength, muscle endurance and how well the athlete is able to control the trunk by the synchronous activation of many muscles.[23]

The prone bridge (Fig. 11.3) is performed by supporting the body's weight between the forearms and toes and primarily assesses the anterior and posterior core muscles. Failure occurs when the athlete loses neutral pelvis and falls into a lordotic position with anterior rotation of the pelvis.

The lateral bridge (Fig. 11.4) assesses the lateral core muscles. Failure occurs when the patient loses the straight posture and the hip falls towards the table.

Testing of the torso flexors (Fig. 11.5) can be done by timing how long the patient can hold a position of seated torso flexion at 60°. Failure occurs when the athlete's torso falls below 60°.

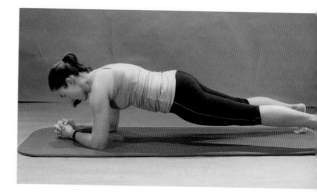

Figure 11.3 Prone bridge. Patients support themselves on the forearms, with the pelvis in the neutral position and the body straight

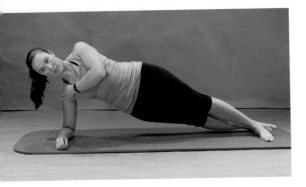

Figure 11.4 Lateral bridge. Legs are extended and the top foot placed in front of the lower foot for support. Patients support themselves on one elbow and on their feet while lifting their hips off the floor to create a straight line over their body length. The uninvolved arm is held across the chest with the hand placed on the opposite shoulder

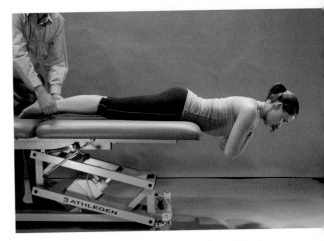

Figure 11.6 Extensor endurance test. The athlete is prone over the edge of the couch with the pelvis, hips and knees secured. The upper limbs are held across the chest with the hands resting on the opposite shoulders

Table 11.2 Mean endurance times in seconds and flexion/extension ratio in young healthy subjects (mean age 21 years)[4]

	Men	Women
Extension	161	185
Flexion	136	134
Right side bridge	95	75
Left side bridge	99	78
Flexion/extension ratio	0.84	0.72

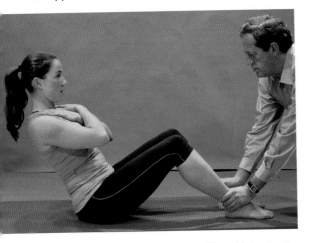

Figure 11.5 Flexor endurance test. The athlete sits at 60° with both hips and knees at 90°, arms folded across the chest with the hands placed on the opposite shoulder, and toes secured under toe straps or by the examiner

The endurance of the torso extensors can be tested with the athlete prone, as shown in Figure 11.6. Failure occurs when the upper body falls from horizontal into a flexed position.

McGill[4] has published normative data for the lateral, flexor and extensor tests for young healthy individuals and this is shown in Table 11.2. McGill has further shown that the relationship of endurance among the anterior, lateral and posterior musculature is upset once back troubles begin and persists long after symptoms have resolved. Typically, the extensor endurance is diminished relative to flexor endurance (e.g. flexion/extension ratio >1.0) and lateral musculature.[4]

The single-legged squat exercise (Fig. 11.7) is also used as an indicator of lumbopelvic–hip stability. The single-legged squat is functional, requires control of the body over a single weight-bearing lower limb and is frequently used clinically to assess hip and trunk muscular coordination and/or control.

Ultrasound imaging is also used as an assessment technique (see p. 164).

Exercise of the core musculature

Exercise of the core musculature is more than trunk strengthening.[7] In fact, motor relearning of inhibited

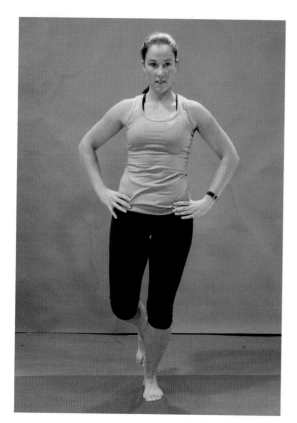

Figure 11.7 Single-legged squat exercise

muscles may be more important than strengthening in patients with low back pain. In athletic endeavors, muscle endurance appears to be more important than pure muscle strength.[24]

The overload principle advocated in sports medicine is a nemesis in the back. In other words, the progressive resistance strengthening of some core muscles, particularly the lumbar extensors, may be unsafe to the back. In fact, many traditional back strengthening exercises may also be unsafe. For example, Roman chair exercises or back extensor strengthening machines require at least torso mass as resistance, which is a load often injurious to the lumbar spine.[3]

Traditional sit-ups are also unsafe because they cause increased compression loads on the lumbar spine.[25] Pelvic tilts are utilized less often than in the past because they may increase spinal loading. In addition, all these traditional exercises are non-functional.[4] In individuals suspected to have instability, stretching exercises should be used with caution, particularly ones encouraging end-range lumbar flexion. The risk of lumbar injury is greatly increased when the spine

is fully flexed and with excessive repetitive torsion.[26] Exercise must progress from training isolated muscles to training as an integrated unit to facilitate functional activity.

The neutral spine has been advocated by some as a safe place to begin exercise.[27] The neutral spine position is a pain-free position that should not be confused with assuming a flat back posture. It is said to be the position of power and balance. However, because functional activities move through the neutral position, exercises should be progressed to non-neutral positions.

Decreasing spinal and pelvic viscosity

Spinal exercises should not be done in the first hour after awakening due to the increased hydrostatic pressures in the disk during that time.[28] The 'cat/camel' (Fig. 11.8) and the pelvic translation exercises are ways to achieve spinal segment and pelvic accessory motion prior to starting more aggressive exercises. As well, improving hip range of motion can help dissipate

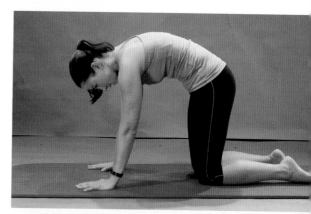

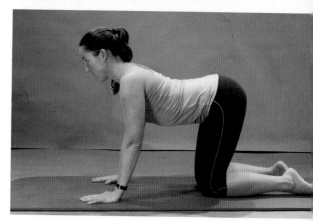

Figure 11.8 Cat/camel exercise

forces from the lumbar spine. A short aerobic program may also be implemented to serve as a warm-up. Fast walking appears to cause less torque on the lower back than slow walking.[29]

Grooving motor patterns

The initial core strengthening protocol should allow for individuals to become aware of motor patterns. Some individuals who are not adept at volitionally activating motor pathways require facilitation in learning to recruit muscles in isolation or with motor patterns. As well, some individuals with back injury will fail to activate core muscles due to fear–avoidance behavior.[30] More time will need to be spent with these individuals at this stage. Prone and supine exercises to train the transversus abdominis and multifidi are described below.

Biofeedback units are used to help facilitate the activation of the multifidi and transversus abdominis.[2] Verbal cues may also be useful to facilitate muscle activation. For example, abdominal 'hollowing' is performed by transversus abdominis activation; abdominal 'bracing' is performed by co-contraction of many muscles including the transversus abdominis, external obliques and internal obliques. However, most of these isolation exercises of the transversus abdominis are in non-functional positions. When the trained muscle is 'awakened', exercise training should quickly shift to functional positions and activities.

Ultrasound imaging in rehabilitation

The use of real-time ultrasound imaging has become increasingly popular as a means of assessing muscle size and activity during the rehabilitation process. Most emphasis has been on the assessment of muscle size and muscle activation in the transversus abdominis and multifidus muscles. These measures have been shown to be valid.[31]

Ultrasound imaging may improve treatment from two perspectives: as a measure of muscle dysfunction and outcome, and as a tool for provision of feedback. There is some evidence that the use of ultrasound to both guide treatment and assess outcome has been successful in monitoring multifidus[32] and transversus abdominis function[33] with positive clinical outcomes in patients with chronic low back pain.

Accurate feedback is critical for skill learning and feedback with ultrasound imaging may increase the quality of training, particularly for that group of patients who find it difficult to activate these muscles. Several studies using ultrasound imaging in the training of muscle control in patients with low back pain have reported positive outcomes.[32] However, whether the outcome with inclusion of ultrasound was improved above that which could be achieved without ultrasound feedback has not been established.

Stabilization exercises

Stabilization exercises can be progressed from a beginning level to more advanced levels. There are many different programs published, however, the general principles are common to all. Initially the motor skill (e.g. activation of transversus abdominis and multifidus) must be learned, but ultimately the activation must become automatic without conscious effort when performing the patient's sporting activity.

Rehabilitation of these muscles takes place in three distinct stages:

1. formal motor skill training
2. functional progression
3. sport-specific training.

Most clinicians agree that motor education, especially teaching patients to activate their deep stabilizing muscles (transversus abdominis and multifidus), is the first stage of the program. Richardson et al.[2] advocate the co-contraction of transversus abdominis and multifidus and also stress the importance of co-contraction of the pelvic floor musculature and transversus abdominis. The most significant motor skill that is linked to the stability of these two muscles is the action of abdominal 'drawing in' (Fig. 11.9).

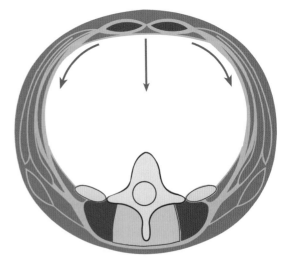

Figure 11.9 Diagrammatic representation of the muscle contraction of 'drawing in' of the abdominal wall with an isometric contraction of the lumbar multifidus

The aim is for the patient to use the correct muscles in response to the command 'draw in your abdominal wall without moving your spine or pelvis and hold for 10 seconds while breathing normally'. The four-point kneeling position (Fig. 11.10) is the best position to teach the patient the action. Ask the patient to take a relaxed breath in and out and then draw the abdomen up towards the spine without taking a breath. The contraction must be performed in a slow and controlled manner. At the same time the patient contracts the pelvic floor and slightly anteriorly rotates the pelvis to activate the multifidi. Assessment of optimal recruitment of these muscles can be done through palpation or with the use of biofeedback or ultrasound imaging. Once the contraction has been achieved, the patient should commence breathing in a slow and controlled manner, holding the contraction for 10 seconds.

Once the action is understood by the patient, the formal test is conducted with the patient lying prone and using a pressure biofeedback unit. The patient lies prone with arms by the side and the pressure biofeedback unit is placed under the abdomen with the navel in the center and the distal edge of the pad in line with the right and left anterior superior iliac spines. The pressure pad is inflated to 70 mmHg and allowed to stabilize. The patient is again instructed to breathe in and out and then, without breathing in, to slowly draw in the abdomen so that it lifts up off the pad, keeping the spinal position steady. Once the contraction has been achieved, the patient should commence normal relaxed breathing. The contraction is held for 10 seconds and the procedure repeated up to 10 times.

A successful performance of the test reduces the pressure by 6–10 mmHg. This pressure change indicates that the patient is able to contract the transversus abdominis into its shortened range independently of the other abdominal muscles. Once the abdominal drawing in technique is successfully learned in the prone position, the patient is encouraged to continue the exercise while in the sitting and standing positions.

Others have a different approach to the 'drawing in' exercise. McGill advocates bracing of the spine,[4] which activates all the abdominal musculature and extensors at once. This is usually performed with the patient in a standing position by simultaneously contracting the abdominal musculature and the extensors. Bracing activates all three layers of the abdominal musculature, not just the transversus abdominis.

Once the patient has learned to stabilize the lumbo-pelvic region with the above isometric exercises to create a functional muscle corset, he or she can progress towards dynamic stabilization. McGill advocates early incorporation of his 'big three' exercises into the program.[4] These are outlined below:

1. Curl-ups for the rectus abdominis (Fig. 11.11). The rectus abdominis is most active during the initial elevation of the head, neck and shoulders. The lumbar spine should stay in neutral. The exercise can be advanced by asking the patient to raise the elbows a couple of centimeters.
2. Side bridge exercises for the obliques, quadratus lumborum and transversus abdominis (Fig. 11.12). Abdominal bracing is also required. The exercise can be advanced initially by placing the free arm along the side of the torso, and subsequently by straightening the legs.

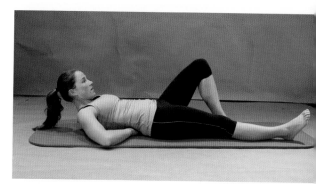

Figure 11.11 Curl-ups. Patient lies supine with the hands supporting the lumbar region. Do not flatten the back to the floor. One leg is bent with the knee flexed to 90°. Do not flex the cervical spine. Leave the elbows on the floor while elevating the head and shoulders a short distance off the floor

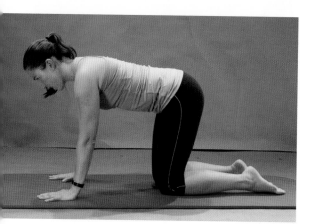

Figure 11.10 The four-point kneeling position

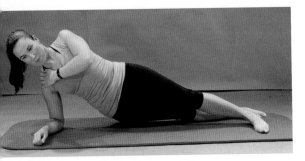

(a)

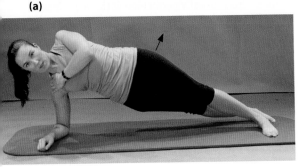

(b)

Figure 11.12 Side bridges. **(a)** In the beginning, position the patient on the side supported by the elbow and hip. The free hand is placed on the opposite shoulder pulling it down. **(b)** The torso is straightened until the body is supported on the elbow and feet

3. Bird dog exercise (Fig. 11.13). Leg and arm extensions in a hands–knees position eventually leading to the 'bird dog' exercise for the back extensors.

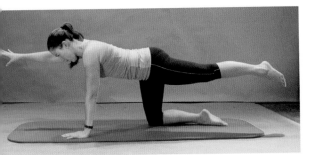

Figure 11.13 Bird dog exercise. The bird dog position is with hands under the shoulders and knees directly under the hips. Initially, simply lift one hand or knee a couple of centimeters off the floor. The patient can progress to raising the opposite hand and knee simultaneously, then raising one arm or leg at a time and then raising the opposite arm and leg simultaneously, as shown.

Other frequently used exercises include the 'clam' (Fig. 11.14) and the bridge (Fig. 11.15). It is important to avoid incorrect techniques (Fig. 11.15c).

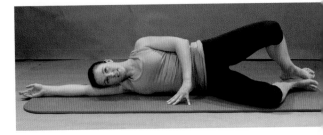

Figure 11.14 Clam

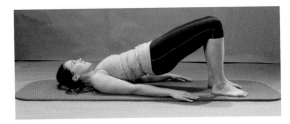

Figure 11.15 Bridging

(a) Supine bridging

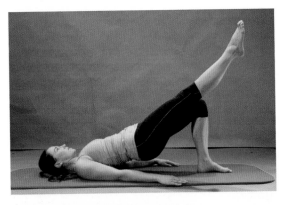

(b) Supine bridging with leg extension

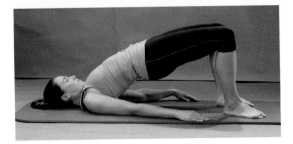

(c) Incorrect bridging technique

Many clinicians base their progressive exercises on Saal and Saal's seminal dynamic lumbar stabilization efficacy study (Table 11.3).[33]

Sahrmann also describes a series of progressive lower abdominal muscle exercises (Table 11.4).[13]

Functional progression

The initial basic strengthening exercises described above are initiated on the ground. The exercises must

Table 11.3 Stabilization and abdominal program described by Saal and Saal[27]

Finding neutral position
Sitting stabilization
Prone gluteal squeezes
Supine pelvic bracing
Pelvic bridging progression
Quadruped
Kneeling stabilization
Wall slide quadriceps strengthening
Position transition with postural control
Curl-ups
Dead bugs
Diagonal curl-ups
Straight leg lowering

Table 11.4 Sahrmann's lower abdominal exercise progression[13]

Position	Exercise
Base position	Supine with knee bent and feet on floor; spine stabilized with 'navel to spine' cue
Level 0.3	Base position with one foot lifted
Level 0.4	Base position with one knee held to chest and other foot lifted
Level 0.5	Base position with one knee held *lightly* to chest and other foot lifted
Level 1A	Knee to chest (>90° of hip flexion) held actively and other foot lifted
Level 1B	Knee to chest (at 90° of hip flexion) held actively and other foot lifted
Level 2	Knee to chest (at 90° of hip flexion) held actively and other foot lifted and slid on ground
Level 3	Knee to chest (at 90° of hip flexion) held actively and other foot lifted and slid *not* on ground
Level 4	Bilateral heel slides
Level 5	Bilateral leg lifts to 90°

progress to positions of function, from a stable ground environment to a progressively less stable environment, and movements must increase in complexity.[23] In other words, the athlete must progress from muscle activation and strengthening to a program of dynamic stabilization.

Several important principles must be applied to exercise progression. These include dynamic exercises, multiplanar exercises, balance, proprioception, power exercises (plyometrics), sport specificity and motor programming.

When the athlete has first mastered proper activation and control of the lumbopelvic region, he or she should progress from a stable surface to a labile surface. Eventually, external input can be added to challenge the athlete even more (Fig. 11.16).

Secondly, exercises must be performed in all planes. While sagittal (sit-ups, lunges) and frontal plane (side walking, side bridges) exercises are popular, the transverse/rotational plane is frequently neglected.

Thirdly, proprioceptive training should be incorporated (Fig. 11.17). Balance board or dura disk training improves proprioception in all the joints, tendons and muscles, not just those at the ankle.

Plyometrics should also be incorporated (Fig. 11.18) as jumping exercises require a strong and stable core. Advancement to a physioball (Fig. 11.19) can be done at this stage (Table 11.5).

Core strengthening for sports

Core training programs for sports are widely used by strengthening and conditioning coaches at the collegiate and professional levels. An example of Vern Gambetta's program is provided in Table 11.6.[34]

Different fitness programs incorporate various aspects of core strengthening and may be a useful way to maintain compliance in many individuals (Table 11.7).

Efficacy of core strengthening exercise

Core strengthening programs have not been well researched for clinical outcomes. Studies are hampered by the lack of consensus on what constitutes a core strengthening program. For example, some studies describe remedial neuromuscular retraining, some describe sport-specific training and others describe functional education. No randomized controlled trial has been conducted on the efficacy of core strengthening. Most studies are prospective, uncontrolled case series.

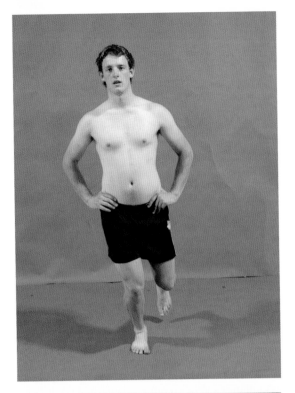

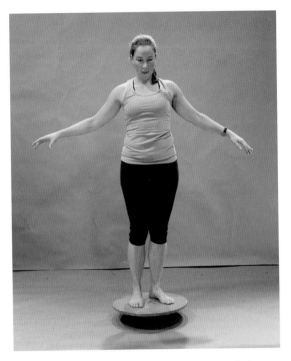

Figure 11.17 Proprioceptive training using a balance board

(a) Balance board with both legs

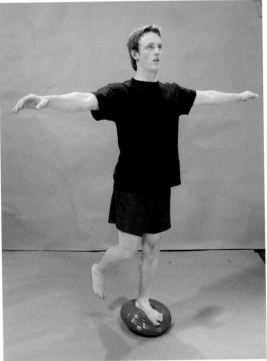

Figure 11.16 Progression from single-leg squat on the floor to a single-leg squat on a dura disk

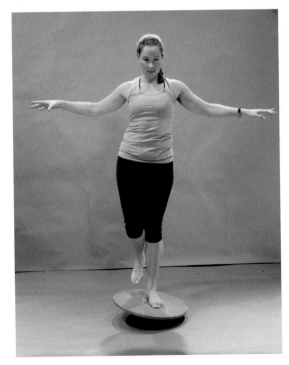

(b) Balance board on single leg

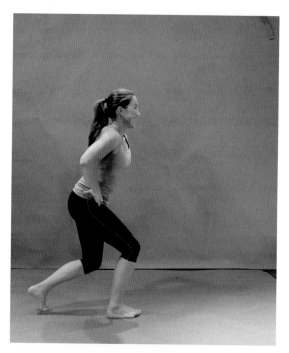

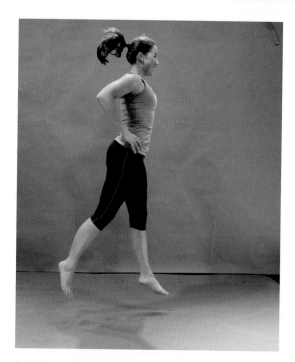

Figure 11.18 Plyometric exercises. These exercises should be multiplanar and upgraded to include labile surfaces

(a) Preparing for take-off

(c) Maintaining good core control

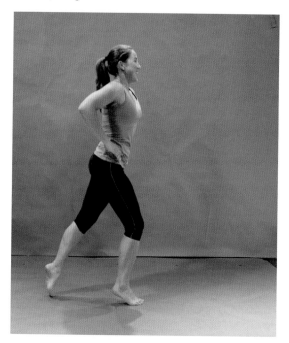

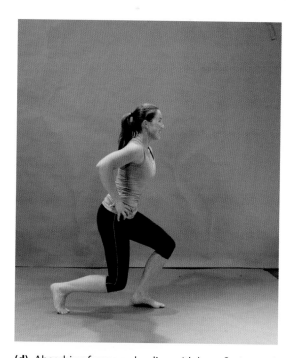

(b) Explosive movement

(d) Absorbing forces on landing with knee flexion and activation of deep abdominal muscles

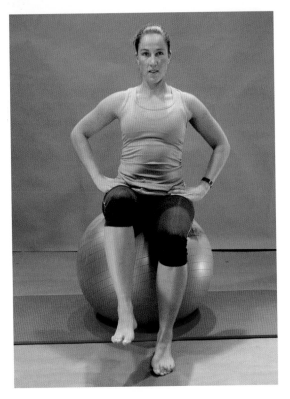

Figure 11.19 Use of physioball

(a) Leg lift seated on ball

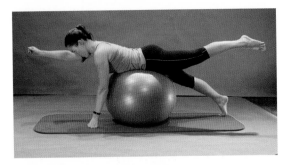

(b) Bird dog or superman on ball

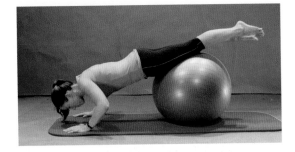

(c) Push-ups

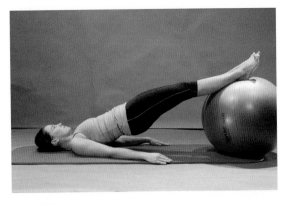

(d) Bridging on ball

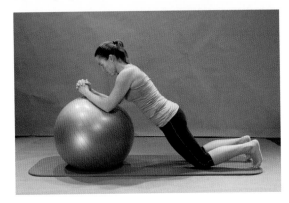

(e) Plant on the ball, moving hips forward

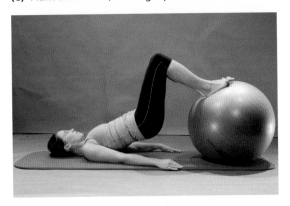

(f) Hamstring pull in

Table 11.5 Physioball exercises for the core

Abdominal crunch
Balancing exercise while seated
'Superman' prone exercise
Modified push-up
Pelvic bridging

Table 11.6 Advanced core program used by Vern Gambetta[34]

Body weight and gravitational loading—push-ups, pull-ups, rope climbs
Body blade exercises
Medicine ball exercises—throwing and catching
Dumbbell exercises in diagonal patterns
Stretch cord exercises
Balance training with labile surfaces
Squats
Lunges

Table 11.7 Fitness programs utilizing core strengthening principles

Pilates
Yoga (some forms)
Tai-Chi
Feldenkrais
Somatics
Matrix dumbbell program[35]

Prevention of injury and performance improvement

In 2001, Nadler et al. attempted to evaluate the occurrence of low back pain before and after incorporation of a core strengthening program.[18] The core strengthening program included sit-ups, pelvic tilts, squats, lunges, leg presses, dead lifts, hang cleans and Roman chair exercises. Although the incidence of low back pain decreased by 47% in male athletes, this was not statistically significant. In female athletes the overall incidence of low back pain slightly increased despite core conditioning. This negative result may have been due to the use of some unsafe exercises (e.g. Roman chair extensor training).[4, 36] In addition, the exercises chosen for this study included only frontal and sagittal plane movements, which may have affected the results. Future studies incorporating exercises in the transverse plane may help to solve the issue surrounding core strengthening exercise and low back pain.

A study comparing 'core stability measures' between male and female athletes and their incidence of lower extremity injury found that reduced isometric hip abductor and external rotation strength were predictors of injury. From this the authors claimed that 'core stability has an important role in injury prevention'.[37] While the findings of this study may be important, core stability was not measured.[38]

Another study found a rehabilitation program consisting of progressive agility and trunk stabilization exercises more effective than a program emphasizing isolated hamstring stretching and strengthening in promoting return to sports and preventing injury recurrence in athletes suffering an acute hamstring strain.[39]

Treatment of low back pain

The first study conducted of a core stability program was an uncontrolled prospective trial of 'dynamic lumbar stabilization' for patients with lumbar disk herniations creating radiculopathy.[33] The impact of therapeutic exercise alone was difficult to ascertain in this study due to other non-operative interventions being offered, such as medication, epidural steroid injections and back school. The exercise training program was well outlined and consisted of a flexibility program, joint mobilization of the hip and the thoracolumbar spinal segments, a stabilization and abdominal program (see Table 11.3), gym program, and aerobic activity. Successful outcomes were apparently achieved in 50 of 52 (96%) individuals. The described dynamic lumbar stabilization program resembles the current concept of a core stability program without the higher level sport-specific core training. Several other authors have since described similar programs.[40, 41]

Effectiveness in sports injuries

To date, the only studies to have shown a positive benefit of core stability training in the management of sporting injuries are Sherry and Best's study[39] on the treatment of hamstring strains and a study by Holmich et al.[42] on the rehabilitation of athletes with chronic groin pain which incorporated some stability training into its program. However, a number of other sporting pathologies theoretically would benefit from this mode of training. Theses include stress fractures of the pars interarticularis of the lumbar spine, a common injury among cricket fast bowlers and other sports that involve repetitive hyperextension and rotation. The positive results from O'Sullivan et al.'s study[41] in non-sporting patients with spondylolysis would suggest that core stability training may be effective in this condition. Lumbar instability seen commonly in gymnasts is another condition for which theoretically a core stability program may be helpful. Many physiotherapists now incorporate an element of core stability training in the rehabilitation of a wide variety of lower limb injuries.

Conclusion

The concept of core stability has a theoretical basis in the treatment and prevention of various musculoskeletal conditions. However, other than studies in the treatment of low back pain, research is severely lacking. With the advancement in knowledge of motor learning theories and anatomy, core stability programs appear on the cusp of innovative new research.

Recommended Reading

Akuthota V, Nadlet S. Core strengthening. *Arch Phys Med Rehabil* 2004; 85: S86–S92.

Bliss LS, Teeple P. Core stability: the centerpiece of any training program. *Curr Sports Med Rep* 2005; 4: 179–83.

Bogduk N. *Clinical Anatomy of the Lumbar Spine and Sacrum.* 3rd edn. New York: Churchill Livingstone, 1997.

McGill S. *Low Back Disorders: Evidence-Based Prevention and Rehabilitation.* Champaign, IL: Human Kinetics, 2002.

Richardson C, Jull G, Hodges P, et al. *Therapeutic Exercise for Spinal Segmental Stabilization in Low Back Pain.* 2nd edn. Edinburgh: Churchill Livingstone, 2004.

Sahrmann S. *Diagnosis and Treatment of Movement Impairment Syndromes.* St Louis: Mosby, 2002.

Sherry M, Best T, Heiderscheit B. The core: where are we and where are we going? *Clin J Sport Med* 2005; 15: 1–2.

References

1. Hodges PW, Richardson CA. Inefficient muscular stabilization of the lumbar spine associated with low back pain. A motor control evaluation of transversus abdominis. *Spine* 1996; 21(22): 2640–50.

2. Richardson C, Jull G, Hodges P, et al. *Therapeutic Exercise for Spinal Segmental Stabilization in Low Back Pain.* Edinburgh: Churchill Livingstone, 1999.

3. Lucas D, Bresler B. *Stability of the Ligamentous Spine.* San Francisco: Biomechanics Laboratory, University of California—San Francisco, 1961.

4. McGill S. *Low Back Disorders: Evidence-Based Prevention and Rehabilitation.* Champaign, IL: Human Kinetics, 2002.

5. Panjabi MM. Clinical spinal instability and low back pain. *J Electromyogr Kinesiol* 2003; 13(4): 371–9.

6. Porterfield J, DeRosa C. *Mechanical Low Back Pain: Perspectives in Functional Anatomy.* 2nd edn. Philadelphia: WB Saunders, 1998.

7. Akuthota V, Nadlet S. Core strengthening. *Arch Phys Med Rehabil* 2004; 85: S86–S92.

8. Ebenbichler GR, Oddsson LI, Kollmitzer J, et al. Sensory-motor control of the lower back: implications for rehabilitation. *Med Sci Sports Exerc* 2001; 33(11): 1889–98.

9. Solomonow M, Zhou BH, Harris M, et al. The ligamentomuscular stabilizing system of the spine. *Spine* 1998; 23(23): 2552–62.

10. Vleeming A, Pool-Goudzwaard AL, Stoeckart R, et al. The posterior layer of the thoracolumbar fascia. Its function in load transfer from spine to legs. *Spine* 1995; 20(7): 753–8.

11. Hides JA, Richardson CA, Jull GA. Multifidus muscle recovery is not automatic after resolution of acute, first-episode low back pain. *Spine* 1996; 21(23): 2763–9.

12. McGill SM. Low back stability: from formal description to issues for performance and rehabilitation. *Exerc Sport Sci Rev* 2001; 29(1): 26–31.

13. Sahrmann S. *Diagnosis and Treatment of Movement Impairment Syndromes.* St Louis: Mosby, 2002.

14. Lyons K, Perry J, Gronley JK, et al. Timing and relative intensity of hip extensor and abductor muscle action during level and stair ambulation. An EMG study. *Phys Ther* 1983; 63(10): 1597–605.

15. Beckman SM, Buchanan TS. Ankle inversion injury and hypermobility: effect on hip and ankle muscle electromyography onset latency. *Arch Phys Med Rehabil* 1995; 76(12): 1138–43.

16. Devita P, Hunter PB, Skelly WA. Effects of a functional knee brace on the biomechanics of running. *Med Sci Sports Exerc* 1992; 24(7): 797–806.

17. Nadler SF, Malanga GA, DePrince M, et al. The relationship between lower extremity injury, low back pain, and hip muscle strength in male and female collegiate athletes. *Clin J Sport Med* 2000; 10(2): 89–97.

18. Nadler SF, Malanga GA, Feinberg JH, et al. Relationship between hip muscle imbalance and occurrence of low back pain in collegiate athletes: a prospective study. *Am J Phys Med Rehabil* 2001; 80(8): 572–7.

19. Bogduk N. *Clinical Anatomy of the Lumbar Spine and Sacrum.* 3rd edn. New York: Churchill Livingstone, 1997.

20. O'Sullivan PB, Beales DJ, Beetham JA, et al. Altered motor control strategies in subjects with sacroiliac joint pain during the active straight-leg-raise test. *Spine* 2002; 27(1): E1–E8.

21. McGill SM, Sharratt MT, Seguin JP. Loads on spinal tissues during simultaneous lifting and ventilatory challenge. *Ergonomics* 1995; 38(9): 1772–92.

22. Sapsford RR, Hodges PW, Richardson CA, et al. Co-activation of the abdominal and pelvic floor muscles during voluntary exercises. *Neurol Urodyn* 2001; 20(1): 31–42.

23. Bliss LS, Teeple P. Core stability: the centerpiece of any training program. *Curr Sports Med Rep* 2005; 4: 179–83.

24. Taimela S, Kankaanpaa M, Luoto S. The effect of lumbar fatigue on the ability to sense a change in lumbar position. A controlled study. *Spine* 1999; 24(13): 1322–7.

25. Juker D, McGill S, Kropf P, et al. Quantitative intramuscular myoelectric activity of lumbar portions of psoas and the abdominal wall during a wide variety of tasks. *Med Sci Sports Exerc* 1998; 30(2): 301–10.

26. Farfan HF, Cossette JW, Robertson GH, et al. The effects of torsion on the lumbar intervertebral joints: the role of torsion in the production of disc degeneration. *J Bone Joint Surg Am* 1970; 52(3): 468–97.

27. Saal JA. Dynamic muscular stabilization in the nonoperative treatment of lumbar pain syndromes. *Orthop Rev* 1990; 19(8): 691–700.

28. Adams MA, Dolan P, Hutton WC. Diurnal variations in the stresses on the lumbar spine. *Spine* 1987; 12(2): 130–7.

29. Callaghan JP, Patla AE, McGill SM. Low back three-dimensional joint forces, kinematics, and kinetics during walking. *Clin Biomech* 1999; 14(3): 203–16.

30. Klenerman L, Slade PD, Stanley IM, et al. The prediction of chronicity in patients with an acute attack of low back pain in a general practice setting. *Spine* 1995; 20(4): 478–84.

31. Hodges PW. Ultrasound imaging in rehabilitation. Just a fad? *J Orthop Sports Phys Ther* 2005; 35: 333–7.

32. Hides JA, Stokes MJ, Saide M, et al. Evidence of lumbar multifidus muscle wasting ipsilateral to symptoms in patients with acute/subacute low back pain. *Spine* 1994; 19: 165–72.

33. Saal JA, Saal JS. Nonoperative treatment of herniated lumbar intervertebral disc with radiculopathy. An outcome study. *Spine* 1989; 14(4): 431–7.

34. Gambetta V. The core of the matter. *Coaching Management* 2002; 10.5.

35. Gray G. *Chain Reaction Festival*. Michigan: Adrian Wynn Marketing, 1999.

36. Kollmitzer J, Ebenbichler GR, Sabo A, Kerschan K, Bochdansky T. Effects of back extensor strength training versus balance training on postural control. *Med Sci Sports Exerc* 2000; 32(10): 1770–6.

37. Leetun DT, Ireland ML, Willson JD, et al. Core stability measures as risk factors for lower extremity injury in athletes. *Med Sci Sports Exerc* 2004; 36: 926–34.

38. Sherry M, Best T, Heiderscheit B. The core: where are we and where are we going? *Clin J Sport Med* 2005; 15: 1–2.

39. Sherry MA, Best TM. A comparison of 2 rehabilitation programs in the treatment of hamstring strains. *J Orthop Sports Phys Ther* 2004; 34: 116–25.

40. Manniche C, Lundberg E, Christensen I, et al. Intensive dynamic back exercises for chronic low back pain: a clinical trial. *Pain* 1991; 47(1): 53–63.

41. O'Sullivan PB, Twomey LT, Allison GT. Evaluation of specific stabilizing exercise in the treatment of chronic low back pain with radiologic diagnosis of spondylolysis or spondylolisthesis. *Spine* 1997; 22(24): 2959–67.

42. Holmich P, Uhrskov P, Ulnits L, et al. Effectiveness of active physical training for long standing adductor-related groin pain in athletes: randomised trial. *Lancet* 1999; 353: 439–43.

Principles of Rehabilitation

WITH MARY KINCH AND ANDREW LAMBART

A dictionary definition of rehabilitation is the 'restoration to a former capacity or standing, or to rank, rights and privileges lost or forfeited'. This is the essence of sports medicine rehabilitation. While the treatment described in Chapter 10 may lead to an athlete becoming pain-free and able to return to activities of daily living, rehabilitation is required to return the athlete to the previous level of function.

All musculoskeletal injuries require active rehabilitation. Rehabilitation is also necessary following surgery. The primary aim of injury rehabilitation is to enable the athlete to return to sport with full function in the shortest possible time. If rehabilitation is inadequate the athlete is:

- prone to reinjury of the affected area
- incapable of performing at pre-injury standard
- predisposed to injuring another part of the body.

The rehabilitation program

Although sports medicine is readily classified as a science, devising a successful rehabilitation program should be considered an art. Skilful rehabilitation cannot be replaced by a recipe approach as each athlete is an individual who brings very different personality and lifestyle factors to the therapy room. Furthermore, each athlete has different post-injury sporting goals, levels of skill and degrees of competitiveness, all of which influence the rehabilitation program. Several general principles should underpin every rehabilitation program.

Every athlete is an individual

To prescribe rehabilitation requires high-level people skills as the psychological make-up of each athlete is different. As some athletes are highly motivated and become overzealous, they may need to be held back throughout rehabilitation. Other athletes are hesitant and lack confidence and require considerable psychological support and encouragement.

Each athlete has a different lifestyle. Some have considerable career or job commitments whereas others are full-time professionals. Some athletes have good support from their family and peers, whereas others are loners. The therapist must establish a caring, trusting relationship with the patient and be aware of the psychological effects of the patient's injury throughout the rehabilitation period. It may also be appropriate for the therapist to communicate regularly with the athlete's coach or parent and keep them informed of progress.

Because of the individual differences between athletes, and also to improve compliance, the therapist must customize each rehabilitation program. The program should be monitored and may need to be modified throughout the rehabilitation period, based on subjective and objective assessment findings.

Once the diagnosis has been made (Chapters 8, 9) and initial therapy instituted (Chapter 10), the therapist performs a comprehensive baseline assessment from which to measure progress. An appropriate, individualized rehabilitation plan is then formulated.

Keys to a successful rehabilitation program

Explanation

The rehabilitation plan should be explained to the patient with realistic, approximate time frames. It should be emphasized that the time frames are only approximate and not 'promises'. It is important to set short-term goals, for example, the removal of a brace or the commencement of jogging, and long-term goals, such as a return to sport.

It is also important to explain the rationale behind the program. This is only possible if the therapist has first formulated a hypothesis as to why the injury occurred. For example, if lack of flexibility contributed to injury, the therapist should include an ongoing program to gradually improve the athlete's flexibility beyond the pre-injury level. If dynamic joint instability was a precipitating factor, or a result of injury, rehabilitation should emphasize muscle control and strengthening. If incorrect biomechanics and poor muscle control were important factors in the etiology of the injury, these components should be addressed.

Provide precise prescription

During the rehabilitation program, the therapist must emphasize correct exercise technique and carefully apply principles for the progression and limitation of exercises and activities. The therapist must also constantly monitor and, if necessary, modify the program as required. This requires one-to-one attention, and cannot be 'supervised' while attending to several other patients.

Make the most of the available facilities

If facilities such as a gymnasium, pool or biofeedback devices are available, the program may take advantage of these facilities. If sophisticated equipment is not available, however, simple equipment, such as an exercise bike, rubber tubes, steps, free weights, and the use of appropriate functional exercises incorporating body position and body weight, can all be incorporated in the program.

Begin as soon as possible

The rehabilitation program should start as early as possible following injury or surgery.[1] Pain, inflammation, swelling or joint effusion must be controlled in the early stages as they inhibit optimal function. Rest from aggravating activities, ice, electrotherapeutic modalities and anti-inflammatory medications will help reduce these factors (Chapter 10).

In the past, it has been customary to begin rehabilitation with range of motion exercises (e.g. stretching) and introduce strength training later. A variation to this approach has recently been presented in acute hamstring strains,[2] indicating that a rehabilitation program consisting of progressive agility and trunk stabilization exercises is more effective than a program that consists of hamstring stretching and strengthening in regards to promoting return to sport and preventing recurrence of injury. This approach may well be the way of the future, but more research is required into this area.

The important components of rehabilitation are:

- muscle conditioning
- flexibility
- neuromuscular control (balance, proprioception)
- functional exercises
- sport skills
- correction of abnormal biomechanics
- maintenance of cardiovascular fitness
- psychology.

These components are incorporated into the overall rehabilitation program (Fig. 12.1).

Soft tissue response to injury

Understanding the pathophysiology, phases and time frames of soft tissue healing following injury improves the therapist's ability to construct a successful rehabilitation program. These phases (Fig. 12.2) are outlined below.

1. Acute inflammatory phase (0–72 hours): Damaged tissue is filled immediately with erythrocytes and inflammatory cells. Phagocytosis of necrotic cells occurs within 24 hours. Fibroblasts slowly lay down collagen scar.
2. Proliferation/repair phase (2 days – 6 weeks): Fibroblasts are the predominant cells, initially resulting in large amounts of scar collagen with

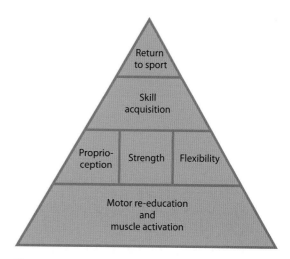

Figure 12.1 Integration of individual components into a progressive rehabilitation program

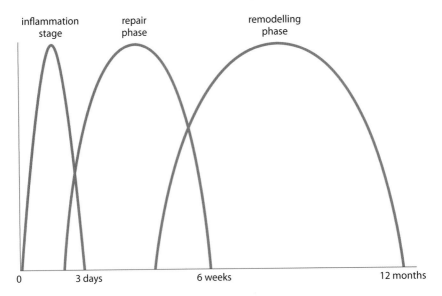

Figure 12.2 Stages of soft tissue response to injury

excessive cross-links. As stress is applied to the healing tissue, the amount of cross-links is reduced and the tensile strength on the tissue is increased.

3. Remodeling/maturation phase (4 weeks – 12 months): Total collagen content within the tissue is slowly reduced, and the scar tends towards assuming the structure of the pre-injured tissue. The initial severity of the injury will largely influence the time taken for complete remodeling to occur.

Muscle conditioning

The effect of injury upon muscle

After injury, there is rapid muscle atrophy due to a cellular response to pain, inflammation and immobility. Muscle strength decreases after relatively short periods of immobilization. Muscles also show increased fatigability and, therefore, less endurance after immobilization.

Persistent pain alone will cause muscle weakness due to decreased neural input. However, there does not appear to be a direct relationship between the intensity of pain and the amount of muscle inhibition. A joint effusion, however small, may also lead to reflex inhibition of surrounding muscles.

Muscle atrophy patterns appear to depend on the relative length of the immobilized muscle and, therefore, the type and amount of impulses from the stretch receptors. Muscle immobilized in a lengthened position maintains muscle weight and fiber cross-sectional area better than muscles immobilized in a shortened position.

In chronic injuries, measurement of limb circumference underestimates the true extent of muscle wasting because the width of the subcutaneous fat increases when muscle is lost. On the other hand, the clinician should not automatically assume that reduced muscle mass means reduced muscle strength. A muscle may regain full strength at the end of the rehabilitation process, yet still appear smaller than the other side. The clinician should look for subtle evidence of muscle dysfunction such as differences in muscle tone, endurance, fine control and timing of action.

There are several methods of assessing deficits in muscle strength. These include manual muscle testing (e.g. comparing muscle strength against resistance provided by the therapist), functional testing (e.g. standing jump, quarter squat, hops) and isokinetic testing (e.g. on computerized devices such as KinCom).

Apart from the obvious wasting following acute injury or surgery, specific patterns of muscle wasting are also noted in association with overuse injuries, for example, wasting of the vastus medialis obliquus and gluteus medius in patients with patellofemoral joint pain.

In patients with chronic lumbar spine, hip and lower leg problems, weakness and wasting in the phasic muscles (quadriceps, gluteals, peroneals and tibialis anterior) is often found in conjunction with tight postural muscles (gastrocnemius, hamstrings and psoas muscles) and weak stabilizing muscles (transversus abdominis, lumbar multifidus). Similarly, in cases of chronic shoulder impingement or instability, weakness, wasting and alterations of muscle timing occur in the scapular stabilizers (rhomboids, serratus anterior, lower and mid trapezius, latissimus dorsi) in conjunction with poor rotator cuff function.

It is important for the clinician to recognize these common patterns of weakness either in association with, or as a possible predisposing factor to, injury. Adequate rehabilitation requires careful assessment, strengthening of the weak muscle groups, stretching of the tight structures and gradual motor re-education to facilitate correct timing of muscle activity.

Principles of muscle conditioning

The two basic principles of muscle conditioning are:

1. specific adaptation to imposed demand (SAID)
2. overload.

Specific adaptation to imposed demand

The aim of the training program is to adapt the individual to the demands of performance. The strengthening program should be injury-specific and sport-specific.

The type of muscle contraction and the speed and intensity of the exercise will cause specific training effects. If a patient exercises at submaximal levels for a lengthy period of time, the recruitment of motor units will be limited to slow oxidative fibers, in contrast to high-intensity, brief bouts of training that recruit mainly fast twitch motor units. Specificity of function means that in the more advanced stages of rehabilitation, the athlete must simulate the task required in the sport to ensure optimal neural patterning and correct timing of all the muscle groups involved in the action.

Overload

A muscle must be overloaded in order to gain increases in strength, power or endurance. Muscle is constantly being broken down and resynthesized. Depending on the nature of the imposed stress, muscle will become stronger, more powerful or develop improved endurance.

A muscle can be overloaded by:

- increasing the speed of movement
- increasing resistance

- increasing the number of repetitions
- increasing the frequency or duration of work-outs
- decreasing the recovery time between work-outs
- altering the form of exercise
- altering the range through which a muscle is being worked.

The most common error in muscle conditioning is doing 'too much too soon'. A high repetition, low resistance regimen should be used initially and then progressed to a low repetition, higher resistance program performed less frequently. As function and strength improve, the athlete may progress to faster, functional and eccentric exercises in the advanced stage.

Components of muscle conditioning

There are four components of muscle conditioning:

1. muscle activation and motor re-education
2. muscle strength
3. muscle power
4. muscle endurance.

Each of these components is necessary to varying degrees in both activities of daily living and sport. Each component may be affected by injury and, therefore, must be assessed and, if necessary, rehabilitated.

Muscle activation and motor re-education

Muscle activation and motor re-education are crucial, but often overlooked, aspects of muscle conditioning. Injury causes pain and swelling, both of which have an inhibitory effect on muscle's ability to contract. Furthermore, certain injuries are often associated with abnormal motor patterns in groups of muscles, so therapy aimed at individual muscles will not be effective. Stability is as important as muscle strength, because muscle acting on a joint with reduced stability will be less effective.

Muscle conditioning must commence with teaching the patient how to activate an inhibited muscle. For example, following an anterior cruciate ligament reconstruction, the quadriceps muscles are inhibited, and the patient is taken through a series of progressive exercises that result in a solid isometric contraction being achieved. This is essential before other forms of muscle conditioning can be commenced.

It is important to understand the difference between local and global muscles.[3] Global muscles are the large, torque-producing muscles, whereas local muscles are responsible for local stability. In recent years there has been an increased understanding of the important role the local muscles play in providing joint stability.

Motor re-education is particularly important in the rehabilitation of injuries of the shoulder region (Chapter 17), groin and pelvis (Chapters 23, 24) and low back (Chapter 21). For example, if chronic shoulder impingement leads to a decrease in the effectiveness in the scapular stabilizers (local muscles), the result is incorrect timing. The scapula protracts and elevates excessively, so that the long muscles (global muscles) attached to the scapula have reduced leverage. This leads to a reduction in the size of the subacromial space and an increase in impingement on the rotator cuff tendon. The vicious cycle is complete.

The pelvis provides another example of the problem of abnormal movement patterns. Lack of pelvic control (in any of the planes of the pelvis) while running places increased stress on lower limb muscles and tendons. This may lead to overuse injuries, for example, hamstring injuries associated with excessive anterior pelvic tilt. More recently, Hodges[4] has demonstrated an association between low back pain and abnormal functioning of the transversus abdominis and lumbar multifidus muscles (local muscles) (Chapter 21).

Rehabilitation of these incorrect motor patterning syndromes relies on careful assessment of the pattern of movement, the individual strength and function of the involved muscles and the flexibility of the muscles and joints. As this abnormal movement pattern has developed over a lengthy period, it is necessary for the patient to learn a new movement pattern. This takes time and patience. The movement should be broken down into its components and the patient must initially learn to execute each component individually. Eventually, the complete correct movement will be learned.

Lack of flexibility in muscles and muscle groups may prevent correct execution of a particular movement. This tightness should gradually be corrected. In addition, weak, poorly functioning muscles require specific, localized strengthening initially in isolation. Various methods are used to assist the patient to isolate the particular muscle or muscle groups. These include palpation of the muscle by the patient or therapist, verbal feedback from the therapist, the use of a mirror, muscle stimulation and biofeedback. Applying strapping tape to the skin when the patient is in a desired position may help to increase postural awareness (Fig. 12.3). This may facilitate correct muscle contraction and inhibit overuse of muscle groups. Initially, the movement should not be resisted as resistance may cause the patient to compensate or return to the previous movement pattern.

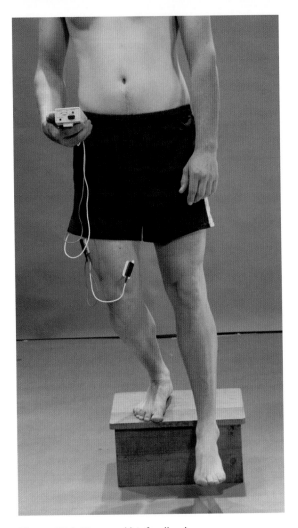

Figure 12.3 Tape and biofeedback

The starting position of the exercise should facilitate the exercise. For example, pelvic tilt exercises should be commenced lying supine. As timing, strength and endurance improve, the patient progresses to kneeling and standing and eventually incorporates the correct pelvic position into functional exercises (e.g. step-downs, pulley work, jogging).

During shoulder re-education, scapular stabilization is begun in isolation without glenohumeral movements (Chapter 17). Exercises in some degree of elevation are introduced when adequate movement patterns are established. Gradual loading, such as with free weights, is introduced with strict adherence to the correct movement pattern. Eventually, the athlete should return to sport using the new movement. When recommencing sport drills, the athlete should commence with simple activities or drills and gradually progress to more complex activities.

The supervision of a stability program requires skill and patience from the therapist. It is important that the patient understands the concept of stability and what you are trying to achieve. Many athletes, in particular, are used to strengthening their global muscles and have difficulty with the concepts of stability training. Many people also have poor body awareness and have difficulty isolating the necessary muscles. Pressure biofeedback can be extremely useful in this education process.

Other techniques used to facilitate this learning are listed below.[5]

- Visualization of the correct muscle action. The therapist should demonstrate and describe the muscle action to the patient. Anatomical illustrations of the muscles involved are an effective teaching aid.
- Use of instructions that cue the correct action. Phrases such as 'pull your navel up towards your spine' can be used to cue the patient to the muscle action (transversus abdominis) required.
- Focus on precision. The patient has to concentrate and focus on the precise muscle action to be achieved. It should be stressed that activation of these muscles is a gentle action. Other muscles should remain relaxed during this localized exercise.
- Facilitation techniques. Show the patient how to feel the muscle contracting.

Pilates' method

Joseph Pilates (1880–1967) had a lifelong interest in body conditioning and the exercises he developed are being used in many rehabilitation programs to improve muscle control. His philosophy and techniques were adapted by many ballet dancers and performers at his New York clinic, which he established in 1923. Initially, his exercise programs for these dancers were extremely complex but in recent years his principles have been adapted and the exercise programs simplified and broken down into stages. The basis of Pilates' work is his eight principles:

1. relaxation
2. concentration
3. alignment
4. breathing
5. centering
6. coordination
7. flowing movements
8. stamina

Initially, many of Pilates' exercises were performed on special machines (Fig. 12.4a) but, more recently, mat-work exercises (Fig. 12.4b) are being used to equal effect.

Muscle strength training

Muscle strength is the muscle's ability to exert force. Muscle hypertrophy and increase in strength are dependent on five biochemical and physiological factors that are all stimulated by conditioning:

1. increased glycogen and protein storage in muscle
2. increased vascularization
3. biochemical changes affecting the enzymes of energy metabolism
4. increased number of myofibrils
5. recruitment of neighboring motor units.

As strength can be gained rapidly and before hypertrophy occurs, it appears that initial strength improvement in response to exercise is related to increased neuromuscular facilitation.

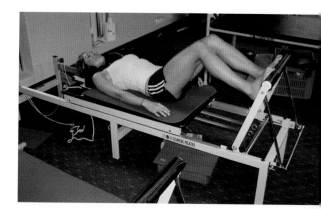

Figure 12.4 Pilates exercises

(a) Specially designed machines

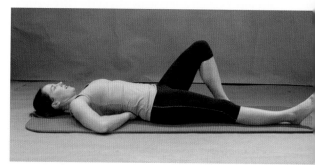

(b) Mat exercises

The following factors will help maximize strength gains during rehabilitation:

- adequate warm-up to increase body temperature and metabolic efficiency
- good quality, controlled performance of the exercise
- pain-free performance of exercise
- use of a slow, pain-free pattern initially with little or no resistance to develop a good base for neural patterning to occur
- comprehensive stretching program to restore/maintain full range of motion
- muscle strengthening throughout the entire range of motion available.

Types of exercise

The three main types of exercise used in muscle conditioning are:

1. isometric
2. isotonic
3. isokinetic.

Exercises can also be open chain or closed chain.

Isometric exercise

An isometric exercise occurs when a muscle contracts without associated movement of the joint on which the muscle acts. Isometric exercises are often the first form of strengthening exercise used after injury, especially if the region is excessively painful or if the area is immobilized. They are commenced as soon as the athlete can perform them without pain.

Isometric exercises may also be used later in the rehabilitation process when a muscle is too weak to perform range of motion exercise, in conditions where other forms of exercise are not possible, such as patellar dislocation and shoulder dislocation, or when isometric contraction is required in activities, for example, stabilizing. Isometric exercises prevent atrophy by increasing static strength, lessen swelling through a pumping action to remove accumulated fluid and may also limit neural dissociation of proprioceptors.

Ideally, isometric exercises are held for 5 seconds with a rest of 10 seconds. They should be performed frequently during the day in sets of 10 repetitions. The number of sets will vary at different stages of the rehabilitation program. The quality of exercise is more important than the quantity.

Isometric exercises should be carried out at multiple angles if possible, as strength gain is fairly specific to the angle of exercise, with an approximate 15°

overflow effect on either side. The patient should progress from submaximal to maximal isometric exercise slowly within the limitations of pain. When significant isometric effect is tolerated at multiple joint angles, dynamic exercises may begin.

An example of an isometric exercise for the quadriceps muscle is shown in Figure 12.5. If a patient has difficulty accomplishing this type of exercise, it may be performed against the resistance of an immovable object.

Isotonic exercise

Isotonic exercises are performed when the joint moves through a range of motion against a constant resistance or weight. Isotonic exercises may be performed with free weights, such as dumbbells or sandbags, or with weight devices (Fig. 12.6).

The use of free weights has a number of advantages. Exercises with free weights result in strengthening of both the primary and synergistic stabilizing muscles as well as providing stress on ligaments and tendons. With free weights it is possible to simulate athletic activities as the body position can be varied. The strength gains from free weights translate well to the playing field.

Isotonic exercises may be:

- concentric—a shortening isotonic contraction in which the origin and insertion of the muscles approximate. Individual muscle fibers shorten during concentric contraction.
- eccentric—a lengthening isotonic contraction where the origin and insertion of the muscles separate. The individual muscle fibers lengthen during eccentric contraction.

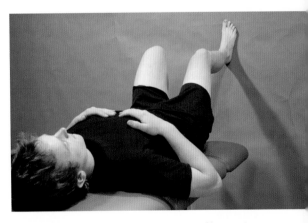

Figure 12.5 Isometric co-contraction of hamstrings, gluteals and quadriceps muscles with patient pushing foot into wall

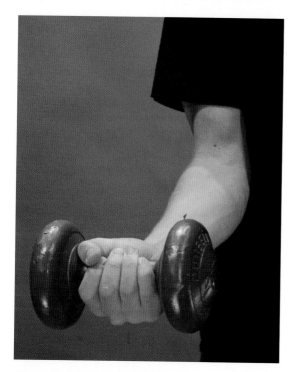

Figure 12.6 Isotonic exercises

(a) Dumbbell

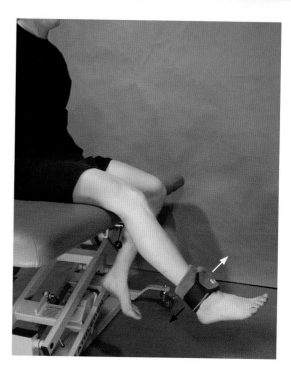

Figure 12.7 Concentric (white arrow) and eccentric (black arrow) exercises—quadriceps

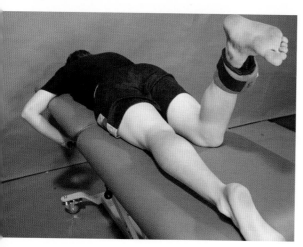

(b) Sandbag

A comparison of concentric and eccentric exercises for the quadriceps is shown in Figure 12.7.

The intramuscular force produced per motor unit during an eccentric contraction is larger than that during a concentric contraction.[6] Eccentric contractions may generate high tension within the series elastic component. The series elastic component consists of connective tissue and the actin–myosin cross-bridges in muscles. It has been implicated in the recurrent injury of muscles used in speed/power activities such as sprinting or jumping. The use of eccentric exercise programs helps prevent recurrence of musculotendinous injuries. Eccentric training has also been advocated in the rehabilitation of tendon injuries.[7, 8]

Eccentric muscle contraction immediately preceding concentric contraction significantly increases the forces generated concentrically. This eccentric–concentric coupling in muscle action is used in many sporting activities, such as the eccentric quadriceps contraction performed before performing a standing jump. Incorporating this coupling of movement into a training program forms the basis of plyometric training discussed previously in Chapter 6.

Eccentric work has the potential to cause delayed onset muscle soreness or muscle damage if used inappropriately. Consequently, eccentric programs should commence at very low levels and progress gradually to higher intensity and volume.

A variation of isotonic exercise is exercise against variable resistance. These exercises are performed using variable resistance devices, such as Nautilus and Eagle Universal. Although the specific amount of weight is constant, the resistance varies through-out the range of motion in an attempt to match the length–tension ratio of the muscle. This results in the muscle working at, or near, maximal resistance throughout the range of motion.

Isokinetic exercises

Isokinetic exercises are performed on devices at a fixed speed with a variable resistance that is totally accommodative to the individual throughout the range of motion. The velocity is, therefore, constant at a preselected dynamic rate, while the resistance varies to match the force applied at every point in the range of motion. This enables the patient to perform more work than is possible with either constant or variable resistance isotonic exercise.

A number of isokinetic devices are available and include the Ariel, Biodex, Cybex, KinCom, Lido and Merac machines. These devices can be used for testing and rehabilitation, although they are slowly becoming less common in mainstream rehabilitation.

Open chain and closed chain exercises

An open (kinetic) chain exercise is performed when the limb is not fixed and allowed to move freely through space. A closed (kinetic) chain exercise is performed when the limb is fixed or maintains contact with a ground reactive force. The advantages and disadvantages of these two types of exercise are shown in Table 12.1. For example, Figure 12.8a shows an open chain knee extension with the foot moving freely, whereas Figure 12.8b shows a closed chain exercise with the foot immobile. Rather than the near isolation of the large muscle groups seen during open chain exercises, performance of closed chain knee flexion and extension results in coactivation of both hamstrings and quadriceps muscle groups.[9, 10] Both agonists and antagonists are simultaneously strengthened through co-contraction, which mimics

the real-life situation in lower limb sports such as running.

Closed chain exercises can also be performed for the upper limb. Closed chain upper limb exercises are particularly useful during the early recovery period from shoulder surgery (Chapter 17) as there is less shear force imparted across the glenoid labrum, whereas multiple muscles around the scapula and glenohumeral joint can be simultaneously activated.[11] An example of a rehabilitation technique that demon-strates open (right arm) and closed (left arm) chain exercises is shown in Figure 12.8c.

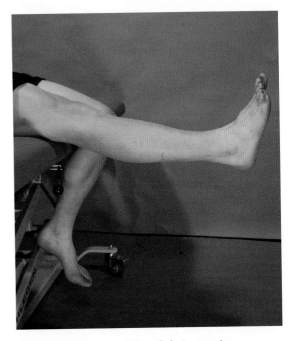

Figure 12.8 Open and closed chain exercises

(a) Open chain knee extension with the foot moving freely

Table 12.1 Advantages and disadvantages of open and closed chain exercises

	Advantages	Disadvantages
Open chain exercises	Decreased joint compression Can exercise in non-weight-bearing positions Able to exercise through increased ROM Able to isolate individual muscles	Increased joint translation Decreased functionality
Closed chain exercises	Decreased joint forces in secondary joints (e.g. less patellofemoral force with squat) Decreased joint translation Increased functionality	Increased joint compression Not able to exercise through increased ROM Not able to isolate individual muscles

ROM = range of motion.

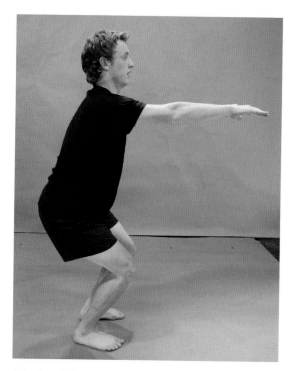

(b) Closed chain knee extension with the feet immobile

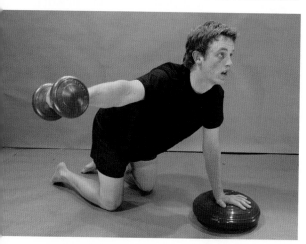

(c) Open chain (right arm) and closed chain (left arm) exercises on unstable surface

Muscle power training

Muscle power is the muscle's rate of doing work. It is equivalent to explosive strength. When injury has decreased muscle power or when the athlete's sport includes explosive activities, power activities should be emphasized in the later stages of the rehabilitation program. These may include:

- fast speed isotonic or isokinetic exercises (concentric or eccentric)
- increased speed of functional exercises, for example, faster reverse calf raise, drop squat, hop and so on
- plyometric activities, for example, hopping, bounding and depth jumps.

These should be as appropriate to the athlete's sport as possible (e.g. bounding for a sprinter, jump and land for a basketballer).

Muscle endurance training

Muscle endurance is the muscle's ability to sustain contraction or perform repeated contractions. Endurance conditioning should be included in conjunction with the strengthening program.

To gain muscle endurance it is necessary to stress the aerobic pathways to improve the oxidative enzyme capacity of the slow twitch muscle fibers and increase the density of mitochondria in the muscle fibers. This requires low load, high repetition exercise. The amount of resistance can be increased gradually. This will stimulate cellular adaptation and facilitate strength gains.

Means of improving muscle endurance include riding a stationary bike, swimming, and specific low load, high repetition isotonic or isokinetic exercise or circuit training. The muscular endurance response to training only occurs in the specific muscles used in the exercise; there is no cross-over effect.

Flexibility

Regaining full flexibility of joints and soft tissues is an essential component of the rehabilitation process. Following injury, musculotendinous flexibility is decreased as a result of spasm of surrounding muscles. Similarly, when inflammation, pain or stiffness limit joint range of motion, normal extensibility of the musculotendinous unit cannot be maintained. This may result in dysfunction of adjacent joints and soft tissues, for example, of the lumbar spine following knee surgery or foot stiffness after immobilization.

Adequate soft tissue extensibility after injury or surgery is essential for pain-free tissue excursion during movements. Adequate joint mobility allows normal kinesiological relationships between limb segments during activity. Following injury, both the joint and surrounding soft tissues must be gradually mobilized and stretched. Joint mobilization is used to regain full joint range of motion. Stretching is used primarily to regain musculotendinous flexibility.

Joint range of motion

Joint range of motion is frequently decreased in association with painful injury and/or inflammation. Pain inhibits normal muscle function around the joint and swelling causes increased intra-articular pressure. Both these processes limit joint motion.

Prolonged limitation of motion secondary to full immobilization in a cast or relative immobilization due to pain causes adaptive tightening of the joint capsule and pericapsular tissues (ligaments, muscles and tendons). Articular cartilage is also adversely affected if joint motion is reduced.

There is considerable variation among patients in the amount of joint stiffness that occurs following injury or immobilization. Intrinsic soft tissue stiffness or laxity appears to depend on the nature of the patient's collagen. Those patients with a known tendency to develop stiffness require intensive preventive measures, for example, early mobilization.

Wherever possible, early restoration of range of motion is an important component of the rehabilitation process. A number of techniques of joint mobilization may be used at different stages of the rehabilitation process.

Continuous passive motion

CPM devices are used in the post-operative or post-acute injury phase to maintain joint range of motion. The range of motion is usually increased progressively but should always be pain-free. CPM appears to reduce the amount of stiffness as well as protect and nourish the articular cartilage. CPM may be commenced immediately after surgery or injury and continued for up to one week.

Passive mobilization

Passive mobilization of accessory or physiological movement (Chapter 10) may be helpful in regaining or maintaining range of motion when active movements cannot be performed due to pain or when active movements are insufficient to mobilize the joint fully. Initially, in the presence of pain, these movements should be gentle but may be quite vigorous during the later stages of rehabilitation or in cases where range of motion is severely restricted.

Passive exercises

In passive exercises, the joint is moved through the available range of motion with the assistance of gravity, the patient's other limb(s), or an outside force, such as a therapist. Passive exercises may be used to regain range of motion when active exercises are too painful to perform or when end of range is restricted (Fig. 12.9).

Active exercises

Active exercises are used to regain range of motion and maintain normal function. They should be commenced as soon as possible within the limits of pain. The therapist should emphasize a progressive increase of range of motion without increasing symptoms. In the early stages, ice and appropriate electrotherapeutic modalities following exercise may help control inflammation, pain and swelling, thereby minimizing the risk of exercise aggravating symptoms (Fig. 12.10).

Active-assisted exercises

Active-assisted exercise occurs when the joint is actively moved through the available range of motion with assistance from an outside force, such as a therapist (Fig. 12.11) or a pulley system.

Musculotendinous flexibility

Tight or shortened muscles are commonly associated with sporting injury. This shortening may be present at the site of the injury (e.g. hamstring) or proximally (e.g. paraspinal and gluteal muscles in hamstring injury). Traditionally, stretching has been the primary method of restoring normal flexibility. However, if the

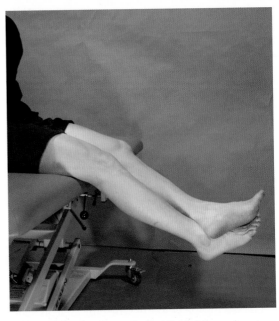

Figure 12.9 Passive exercises—the left leg rests on the right, which takes the left leg through a range of motion

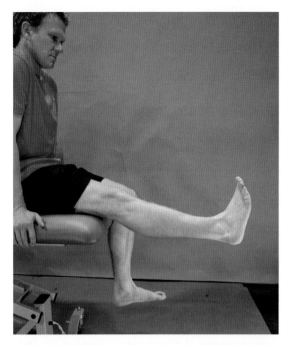

Figure 12.10 Active exercise—knee extension/flexion

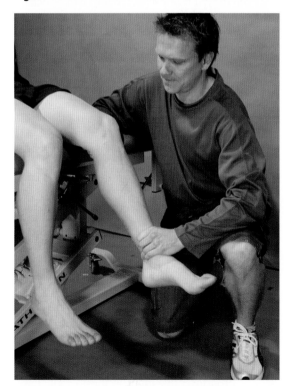

Figure 12.11 Active-assisted exercise—the leg is passively moved through a range of motion with some active contraction of the hamstring

muscle tightness is secondary to neural restriction or trigger points, these must be corrected first if stretching is to be fully effective. The spinal and trigger point contribution to muscle tightness must be assessed (Chapter 8) and treated with pressure techniques or dry needling (Chapter 10), in conjunction with an appropriate stretching program.

Lack of flexibility may be associated with specific injuries. Some examples are shown in Table 12.2.

Stretching has a number of possible beneficial effects:[12]

- increases flexibility
- increases muscle relaxation
- decreases muscle soreness
- improves circulation
- helps prevent excessive adhesion
- promotes a flexible, strong scar
- reduces muscle resistance.

The three different types of stretching—static, ballistic and proprioceptive neuromuscular facilitation—are described in Chapter 6. All these stretches may be used in the rehabilitation process.

Recommendations for effective stretching

A stretching program should be designed for the individual, taking into consideration the nature and stage of the injury, the athlete's sport and the athlete's abilities and deficits.

- Stretching should be preceded by an adequate warm-up involving activities such as jogging, cycling or swimming until there is mild sweating.
- Heat may be applied to the area prior to stretching. Increased tissue temperature facilitates stretching. The choice of superficial or deep heating methods depends on the structures contributing to the restriction of range of motion.

Table 12.2 Tight muscle(s) and possible associated injuries

Tight muscles	Possible associated injury
Sternocleidomastoid	Cervical apophyseal joint injuries
Psoas	Lumbar apophyseal joint, hamstring injuries
Quadriceps vastus group	Patellar tendinitis
Vastus lateralis, iliotibial band, tensor fascia lata	Patellofemoral syndrome
Soleus	Achilles tendinopathy

- Cryotherapy may overcome pain and spasm more effectively than heat. However, care must be taken not to overstretch injured parts while the pain threshold is eliminated by the application of ice. Gentle stretching may be performed while ice is applied early in the post-injury phase.
- Athletes should be carefully instructed regarding the correct stretching position for the particular muscle. Incorrectly performed stretching is common. The stretch should be held with a slow sustained stretch for a minimum of 15 seconds. The patient should feel stretch in the appropriate area. As athletes progress through a stretching program, they may sustain stretches for 1 minute or longer.
- As stretching is more effective when the muscle is relaxed, elimination of antigravity reflexes by appropriate starting positions may be helpful, for example, lumbar stretching may be more effective in a sitting or lying position than standing.
- To make gains in flexibility, the stretching program should be based on the overload principle, similar to that used to develop strength and endurance. Overload requires increases in intensity, duration, frequency and type of stretch. As the athlete's flexibility improves, these factors should be gradually and systematically increased.
- Stretching should always be pain-free.

Although ballistic stretching involving rapid application of force in a repeated bouncing or jerky manner is not universally recommended as a means of injury prevention (Chapter 6), it may have a role in injury rehabilitation.

Most athletic activities incorporate fast and forceful stretching, therefore, ballistic stretching does promote specific adaptation to these imposed demands (SAID principle). The dangers of ballistic stretching include overstretching, which may result in soreness or injury, and initiation of the stretch reflex. There is probably no permanent soft tissue lengthening as there is insufficient time for neurological adaptation to occur with ballistic stretching.

Ballistic stretching may be performed provided the following criteria are met:

- the athlete is thoroughly warmed up
- it is preceded by slow static stretching
- it is only introduced in the advanced stages of a stretching program
- it is taught carefully and performed with accuracy and care

- it is performed slowly and in a controlled manner, gradually increasing speed.

The dangers of stretching

Regardless of which type of stretching is used, overstretching and subsequent injury can occur. This depends on the intensity, duration and velocity of the stretch as well as the number of movements performed in a given period. These factors should be closely monitored and progressed gradually as the rehabilitation program proceeds. Stretching should not be performed into pain. Specific stretching may be contraindicated in hypermobility syndromes or in the presence of instability, for example, anterior instability of the shoulder in baseball pitchers.

Neuromuscular control (proprioception and balance)

Neuromuscular retraining following injury is another important component of the rehabilitation process. Proprioception describes nerve impulses originating from the joints, muscles, tendons and associated deep tissues, which are then processed in the central nervous system to provide information about joint position, motion, vibration and pressure.

In acute and overuse soft tissue injuries, nerve endings and nerve pathways are damaged and, thus, impair segmental transmission of nerve impulses in a reflex action. This may result in impaired balance and decreased coordination, diminished joint position sense, tendency for the joints to give way and altered reflexes when performing specific or general movements.

Impaired proprioception and balance is a common sequel to lower limb injuries. When early and comprehensive neuromuscular training is undertaken, objective improvement in proprioception and balance can be demonstrated and there is a reduced rate of recurrence of injuries.

Proprioceptive and balance exercises should begin as early as possible in the rehabilitation program. They act to restore the athlete's kinesthetic awareness. Neuromuscular retraining is not stressful to the healing tissues and enhances general coordination as well as facilitating the effectiveness of the strength and endurance exercises.

As soon as patients are weight-bearing, they are gaining proprioceptive input. A most simple lower limb neuromuscular exercise is to stand on one leg. The degree of difficulty of these exercises may be slowly increased by introducing movements of other body parts, performing toe-raising exercises and balancing with closed eyes.

The addition of a moving surface, such as ski simulators (Fitters), a rocker or balance board (Fig. 12.12a), a dura disk (Fig. 12.12b) or a Swiss ball (Fig. 12.12c), makes neuromuscular exercises more challenging.

Balancing on the rocker board or disk should commence with two legs, then one leg only, with gradual progression in difficulty.

Once these simple tasks are mastered, more complex tasks such as hopping, exercising on a minitrampoline (Fig. 12.12d) and walking on soft, uneven or sloped surfaces may be introduced. In the later stages of rehabilitation, agility and sport-specific drills encourage improvement in proprioception and balance. Detailed progression of lower limb neuromuscular exercises is shown in the box.

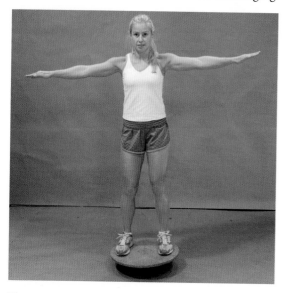

Figure 12.12 Proprioceptive aids

(a) Rocker board

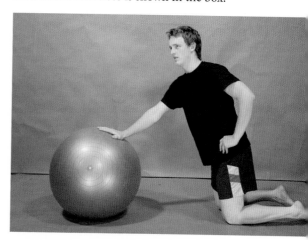

(c) Swiss ball

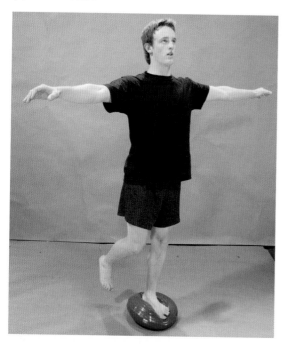

(b) Dura disk

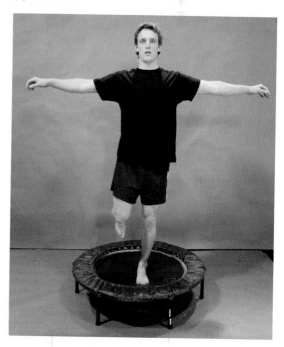

(d) Minitrampoline

Progression of neuromuscular exercises

Partial weight-bearing

- Walking with support (crutches) ensuring correct heel–toe movement
- Seated with feet on rocker board, forward/backwards rocking for 2 minutes pain-free, first with both legs, then with one leg

Full weight-bearing

- Multiaxial rocker or dura disk (both legs)
  - 2–3 minutes each way circling
  - Attempt to balance for 15 seconds, rest 10 seconds
  - Progressively increase complexity—arms out in front of body
    - arms crossed
    - eyes closed
    - knee bends
    - other leg swinging
    - bounce/catch ball
- Balance on minitrampoline
  - Same progression as above
  - Hop and land
  - Hop and land with one-quarter turn and return
  - Progress to half turn, three-quarter turn and full turn
  - Rhythmical hopping, alternatively placing toe forwards and sideways
  - Rhythmical hopping across a line, forward/backwards, sideways
- Jumping
  - Various patterns
- Hopping without rebounder
  - Alternatively two hops on one leg, two hops on other leg
- Skipping
  - On spot, both legs, forwards/backwards/sideways
  - Single leg, two hops on one leg, two hops on other leg
- Advanced tasks
  - Walk/run across a steep hill each way
  - Run sideways up and down hill, each way
  - Walk along balance beam, then bounce and throw ball while walking
  - Sideways step-ups, gradually increasing height of step
- Running drills
  - Straight
  - Backwards
  - Sideways
  - Circle (5 m diameter)
  - Cutting 90°
  - Zigzag through cones set at 45°

Neuromuscular exercises are also important in the rehabilitation of upper limb injuries. Initially, exercises are performed with light weights in the available pain-free range. These exercises give proprioceptive input through the hand, wrist, elbow and shoulder girdle. Exercises may progress to weight-bearing exercises in different positions, for example, push-ups either seated, kneeling, prone or standing against a wall or on a Swiss ball.

Functional exercises

Once a reasonable level of strength, power, endurance, flexibility and neuromuscular control has been achieved, the athlete should be gradually reintroduced to the functional activities that form the basis of his or her sport. These activities prepare the athlete physically and mentally for the demands of the sport. Depending on the nature of the activity, functional exercises will enhance all the other components of the rehabilitation.

Basic functional activities (e.g. walking, jogging, striding) commence early in the rehabilitation program and are gradually progressed. They may be performed alone or in the company of team mates.

Agility drills relevant to the sport are gradually introduced. These are initially performed in isolation and then with appropriate equipment, for example, a basketball or hockey stick. As the athlete's functional level improves, drills may be performed with a team mate or in team training. These functional exercises will be supplemented by continued progressive strength, power, endurance, flexibility and neuromuscular exercises that slowly become more sport-specific. Functional exercises are not a substitute for the more advanced stages of these other programs. An example of progression of functional exercises for an athlete recovering from a serious lower limb injury is shown opposite.

- Walking
- Jogging
  — Jog 200 m, walk 200 m
  — Increase jog to 400 m, walk nil
  — Increase jog to 1500 m
  — Increase jog to 3 km
- Running
  — Increase pace during 3 km run intermittently for 100 m at a time (surge)
- Sprint
  — Accelerate for 20 m, half pace for 40 m, decelerate for 30 m
  — Repeat up to 10 times
  — Gradually increase pace to 60, 70, 80, 90 and 100%
- Figure of eight
  — Run large (25 m) figure of eight, 5 times
  — Gradually increase speed
  — Progress to smaller (15 m, 10 m, 5 m) figures
- Agility drills
  — 45° zigzag slowly increasing speed
  — 90° cutting
  — Run around square (forwards, sideways, backwards)
  — Side to side (e.g. across tennis court)

Sport skills

When athletes sustain serious injuries requiring lengthy rehabilitation, they often harbor the fear that they will not regain their pre-injury skill level, even if the physical deficits are corrected. An important part of the initial discussions with the athlete should consist of reassurance that talent is not lost overnight and that the rehabilitation process will permit sport-specific skill training as soon as possible.

Once adequate strength, flexibility and proprioception have been regained, these components must be combined to perform the relevant sport skills. With graduated training, the athlete relearns the various motor patterns necessary for his or her sport.

For tissues that have not been subjected to performance level stress for some time, the program must be progressed gradually through tasks of increasing difficulty. The athlete begins with the most basic level in the program and works until the necessary level is reached. The athlete can only progress if there is no increase in the signs and symptoms of the injury following activity. If there is any exacerbation of symptoms, the level of activity must be reduced. The athlete should incorporate skills into the program as soon as he or she is able. Examples include a tennis player recovering from a knee injury hitting shots while seated in a wheelchair, a basketballer shooting foul shots while recovering from lower limb stress fracture, a footballer jogging and stretching with the rest of the team while recovering from a hamstring injury. By performing these activities, the athlete feels more motivated and skill levels are maintained as much as possible. Normal function will return more quickly to the athlete who is allowed to continue with activities that permit near-normal function without compromising the healing process.

During this sport skills phase of the rehabilitation program, careful attention must be paid to correct form and technique. Constant repetition is required as part of the relearning process. Examples of sport skills programs for a basketball player and a tennis player returning after serious lower limb injury are shown in the boxes below. The athlete should be closely observed to ensure that substitution patterns and compensatory movements do not occur.

Return to sport skills program after lower limb injury: basketball player

Individual drill

Defensive stance
- Stationary
- Side to side
- Pivoting

Dribbling
- Forwards/backwards
- Side to side
- Zigzag
- Cross-overs

Shooting
- Foul shots (no jump)
- Dribble and shoot (no jump)
- Dribble, jump shot, rebound alone

Lay ups
- Alone

Rebounding
- Post moves
- High post
- Low post

Team drills
- Set play
- One on one
- Half court play
- Full court scrimmage
- Match practise
- Match (off bench)
- Match (start)

Ground strokes
- Forehand, backhand, gradually increase time from 5 to 20 minutes

Serving
- Service action without ball, 10 repetitions
- Half pace serves, 10 repetitions
- Gradually increase 50% to 100% serves, 10 repetitions
- Gradually increase repetitions to 40 with break after each set of 20

Overhead shots
- Slow at first, 15 repetitions
- Gradually increase speed

Match practise
- Initially 15 minutes
- Gradually progress to one set, two sets, full match

Correction of biomechanical abnormalities

Biomechanical abnormalities are an important predisposing factor to injury, especially overuse injuries (Chapter 5). Normal lower limb biomechanics and the mechanics of walking and running are discussed on pages 45–49. The biomechanics involved in throwing activities are discussed on pages 61–7.

Biomechanical examination must form part of the assessment of every overuse injury. If an abnormality is detected, the clinician must determine whether the abnormality is contributing to the injury, either directly or indirectly. This requires a good understanding of both biomechanics and the pathology of the injury.

If abnormal biomechanics is contributing to an injury, its correction is a vital part of treatment and rehabilitation. An athlete should not be allowed to return to the same activity that produced the overuse injury without the cause of the injury having been removed.

Abnormal biomechanics may be due to a structural abnormality, such as genu valgum, or secondary to muscle weakness, muscle imbalance or incoordinate muscle action. A number of treatment methods are available for the correction of these abnormalities. They include muscle stretching, strengthening and motor re-education, taping, padding, shoe modifications and orthoses (casted or non-casted).

Cardiovascular fitness

The maintenance of cardiovascular fitness is another essential component of the rehabilitation process. No matter what type of injury the athlete has sustained, it should always be possible to design an exercise program to enable cardiovascular fitness to be maintained.

In injuries to the lower limb that require a period of restricted weight-bearing activity, cardiovascular fitness may be maintained by performing activities such as cycling, swimming or water exercises. These activities can be used in a training program that follows the same principles as the athlete's normal training. Depending on the athlete's particular sport, this may include a combination of endurance, interval, anaerobic and power work.

It is important to maintain these alternative training methods for cardiovascular fitness even after the patient has resumed some weight-bearing training of his or her own. The clinician must explain to the patient that while he or she is gradually returning to weight-bearing activity, the cardiovascular endurance aspect of training should be performed as non-weight-bearing.

Following complete recovery and return to sport, it may be advantageous, particularly in patients who have had an overuse injury, to incorporate some of these non-weight-bearing forms of training as a substitute for some weight-bearing training.

Deep-water running

Deep-water running, or aqua running, consists of simulated running in the deep end of a pool, aided by a flotation device (vest or belt) that maintains the head above water (Chapter 7). The form of running in the water is patterned as closely as possible after the pattern used on land, but therapists should be aware that for most athletes deep-water running will provide a new stress to the body, hence the risk of new injury caused by deep-water running will be increased. Athletes should therefore undergo a conditioning phase of deep-water running to lessen the risk of injury. The participant may be held in one location by a tether cord or by the force of a wall jet, or may actually run through the water. As there is no contact with the bottom of the pool, impact is eliminated.

A greater physiological response in terms of maximum oxygen uptake and heart rate can be obtained by adhering strictly to proper technique. The water line should be at the shoulder level, the mouth should be comfortably out of the water without having to tilt the head back. The head should be straight, not down. The body should assume a position slightly forward of the vertical, with the spine maintained in a neutral position.[13] Arm and leg motion should be identical to that used on land.

Studies have shown that in spite of slightly lower heart rates (80–95%) and maximum oxygen uptake (83–89%) for a given level of perceived exertion, deep-water running elicits a sufficient cardiovascular response to result in a training effect. Several possible explanations exist for the differences in metabolic response to deep-water running and land-based running. Differences in muscle use and activation patterns contribute to these differences in exercise response. Furthermore, as weight-bearing is eliminated but replaced with resistance, larger muscle groups of the lower extremities perform relatively less work and the upper extremities perform comparatively more work than they would during land-based exercise.[14]

There are three methods for grading deep-water running exercise intensity: heart rate, rating of perceived exertion (RPE) and cadence. Work-out programs are typically designed to reproduce the work the athlete would do on land and incorporate long runs as well as interval–speed training. The heart rate response is used primarily during long runs. RPE and cadence are most often used for interval sessions.[13]

Hydrotherapy

Hydrotherapy or pool therapy is a form of treatment widely used in the treatment of sporting injuries. It may be used in conjunction with other forms of rehabilitation or as the sole form of rehabilitation.

Specific therapeutic exercises can be performed to rehabilitate the injured part. These exercises may be aimed at relief of pain or muscle spasm, relaxation or restoration of full joint movement. Hydrotherapy exercises may result in increased muscular strength, power and endurance, as well as improvement of functional level, including coordination and balance.

Hydrotherapy may be beneficial in acute or overuse injuries. In acute injuries, the warmth and buoyancy of the water induces relaxation, reduces pain and encourages early movement. Isometric exercises can commence against the buoyancy of the water.

Range of motion exercises may be easily performed and may be assisted by buoyancy. It is also possible to use hydrotherapy wearing the appropriate splint required for treatment. Exercises may be assisted by floats to aid buoyancy.

Strength exercises may also be performed in the water. These may be isometric or isotonic (both concentric and eccentric). Graded progressive exercises can be devised utilizing buoyancy, varied speed of movement and movement patterns, varied equipment and altering the length of the lever arm creating turbulence.

Progression of rehabilitation

There are several different parameters that the therapist may manipulate to progress the athlete's program to a level at which return to sport is possible. These parameters are:

- type of activity
- duration of activity
- frequency of activity/rest
- intensity of activity
- complexity of activity.

Type of activity

In the early stages of the rehabilitation program, we recommend activities that do not directly stress the injured area. However, these exercises may still result in some mobilization or strengthening of the injured area, for example, tennis ground strokes following an ankle injury, cycling following shoulder impingement. Later in the program, activities specifically involving the injured area will test its integrity and prepare it for functional activity.

Duration of activity

Once the activity is directly stressing the injured area, the time spent performing that activity must be increased very gradually. It is advisable to slowly increase the amount of time spent performing a particular activity, for example, jogging, and then hold it constant at a particular level and vary one of the other parameters, such as frequency.

Frequency

An integral part of the rehabilitation program is recovery (Chapter 7). It allows tissues to adapt to the stress of exercise. For example, a runner with Achilles tendinopathy may initially run every third day, then every second day, then two out of every three days and ultimately six or seven days per week. On non-running days, the athlete should maintain fitness by swimming or cycling as well as performing the other elements of the rehabilitation program, for example, muscle strengthening.

Intensity

As the athlete progresses through the rehabilitation program, the intensity (speed and power) of the activity will increase. A rehabilitation program for a sprinter may involve progression from half pace to three-quarter pace to full pace. Race starts will be included later in the program.

Other variables include surfaces and shoes. Progression can be made from softer surfaces to harder surfaces or from flat running shoes to spikes once full speed is achieved.

Complexity of activity

The athlete can progress from simple activities to more complex movements. For example, a basketballer dribbles slowly in a straight line gradually increasing speed and introducing turns, or a tennis player progresses from ground strokes to incorporating overhead shots and rallying drills before playing points competitively.

Stages of rehabilitation

It is convenient to divide the process of rehabilitation into four stages according to the athlete's level of function. The initial stage is considered to be from the time of the injury to the point of almost full, pain-free range of motion. The next stage, the intermediate or pre-participation stage, corresponds with resumption of normal activities of daily living

and commencement of some sporting activity. This activity is primarily skill-related. Fitness maintenance is also included, taking care to avoid stressing the injured area. The third or advanced stage corresponds to the commencement of functional activities related to the sport. The final stage, return to sport, involves full participation in training and competition. The stages are summarized in Table 12.3.

Initial stage

Flexibility and mobilization exercises should be commenced as early as possible to improve soft tissue extensibility and joint range of motion. It is important to consider the pathophysiology of tissue healing, hence minimizing immediate inflammation, and initially restricting excessive application of force to the injured area. Frequent, gentle range of motion exercises (passive or active) can be commenced within the limits of pain. Heat, ice or electrotherapeutic modalities may be useful adjuncts before or after the exercises. Gentle passive mobilization may be appropriate to relieve pain and improve mobility.

Muscle conditioning is also commenced as early as possible within a safe, pain-free range. It is important to assess accurately the level of exercise at which the patient is able to perform the exercise correctly without pain and without exacerbation of signs and symptoms. Initially, exercises may isolate the prime mover or injured muscle. Later in the program, this muscle action will be integrated into a more functional movement.

Table 12.3 Progression of rehabilitation

Stage	Functional level	Sport	Management
Initial	Poor	Nil Substitute activities (e.g. swimming, cycling)	RICE Electrotherapeutic modalities Stretch/range of motion exercises Isometric exercises Stability program
Intermediate	Good	Isolated skills (e.g. basketball shooting)	Electrotherapy (less) Stretch/range of motion exercises Strength Neuromuscular exercises Agility exercises Stability program
Advanced	Good	Commence sport-specific agility work Skills Game drills	Strength, especially power Neuromuscular exercises Stability program Functional activity
Return to sport	Good	Full	Continue strength/power work, flexibility

In the early stages, exercises should progress from muscle activation to maximal isometric exercises, then to multiple angle exercises and short arc exercises. Isometric and short arc strength gains will transfer to the isotonic and isokinetic programs in the intermediate phase. Performing the exercises frequently will improve endurance. Initially, exercises may be performed in a non-weight-bearing or partial weight-bearing position and should progress to a functional weight-bearing position as tolerated.

Resistance may be introduced into isometric and short arc exercises by the use of light weights and elastic devices such as rubber bands or tubing. These devices can provide a wide variety of exercises in any plane of motion. Progressions should consider the tissue healing times as mentioned previously.

Stability work should be commenced soon after initial injury. After establishing deficiencies in this area (e.g. poor scapular control, inadequate lumbo-pelvic stability), motor re-education programs can be commenced early, as frequently they are distant from the injured joint or muscle and are, therefore, not painful to perform.

Agility type exercises, such as side stepping, grapevine stepping (lateral stepping with the trailing leg going over the lead leg then under the lead leg, Fig. 12.13), and stepping forward and backward over a line while moving sideways can also be utilized as pain allows.[2]

Proprioceptive and balance exercises may be commenced once the patient is allowed to weight bear. Gait re-education will enhance proprioception in the early stages. Simple standing and balancing exercises or rocker board exercises may also be introduced as tolerated.

At this stage functional activities are limited to the pool or stationary bicycle to maintain cardiovascular and muscular endurance.

Intermediate stage

The intermediate stage has been reached when the patient is able to perform activities of daily living, and has good range of motion and reasonable strength throughout that range. This should correspond to part-way through the proliferation/repair phase of tissue healing.

To reduce cross-linkages in scar collagen, flexibility exercises for the injured part and adjacent areas should be performed regularly. Any other tight structures implicated in the original injury should also be stretched. Soft tissue therapy may also be helpful. If possible, a variety of different stretching

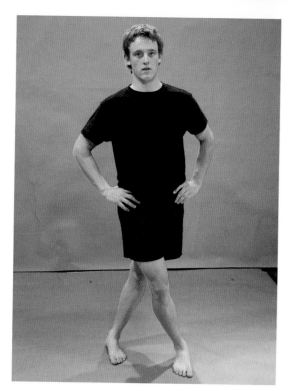

Figure 12.13 Grapevine step. Lateral stepping with the trailing leg going over the leading leg, then under the leading leg

techniques should be used on the same area. If generalized muscular tightness is present, the athlete should embark on a comprehensive general stretching program (Chapter 6).

Joints restricted in range of motion should be mobilized. Techniques include passive and active exercises performed by the patient and mobilization performed by the therapist.

In the intermediate stage, strengthening exercises are progressed according to the general principle of overload. Increased resistance and number of repetitions are used to increase strength. Increase in volume of work has a positive effect on endurance. In the later intermediate and advanced stages, power will be developed by increasing the speed of resisted exercises. Exercises should be performed through the full range of motion available. Therapists should be mindful that the tensile strength of the healing tissue is still compromised and progress is dependent on the patient's signs and symptoms.

The patient should use a variety of exercise modes depending on the availability of equipment. Free weights, machines, pulleys and rubber tubing are all effective. Pool, exercise bike, stair climber and isokinetic devices may also be used if available. The athlete should perform isotonic (concentric and eccentric) exercises through a full velocity spectrum.

The closer the positions adopted during exercise correspond to the required sporting activity, the more beneficial they will be. It is important to integrate these exercises slowly into functional exercises. This will facilitate return to full function and develop appropriate neural patterns. For example, seated quadriceps exercises, such as knee extension or seated vastus medialis obliquus exercises, can be integrated into quarter squats and step-downs. These functional exercises can be gradually progressed in speed and load. Progression to more functional, closed kinetic chain exercise (e.g. leg press, squat, climbing stairs) will better facilitate return to weight-bearing function. Proprioceptive and balance exercises are progressed by the use of more difficult tasks, for example, hopping or skipping, and the introduction of equipment (e.g. rebounder, ski simulator [Fitter], rocker board).

Functional exercises are usually introduced in the intermediate stage to prepare the athlete for return to sport. Progression through supervised walking, jogging, striding and agility work acts as a bridge back to the sport-specific activities to be undertaken in the advanced stage. Take care to ensure a gradual increase in load to the injured area to allow time for adaptation. This should initially involve alternate day activity with a gradual increase in volume with subsequent increases in frequency and intensity. Only one of these parameters should be increased at any one time.

During this stage it may be possible for the athlete to maintain some sport-specific activities but these should not involve the injured part. Examples of this may be a tennis player with a lower limb injury standing at the net hitting volleys, a hockey player hitting without running or a basketball player shooting.

Other treatment modalities may be used in the intermediate stage but usually in diminishing amounts. These include passive joint mobilization, massage therapy and electrotherapeutic modalities that may be used as a precursor to exercise.

Advanced stage

To reach the advanced stage of rehabilitation, the patient must have good strength and endurance with full flexibility and range of motion. Activities of daily living will produce little or no symptoms or signs. Proprioceptive, agility and functional exercises are performed without adverse effect and the athlete is able to tolerate a reasonable volume of work. General cardiovascular fitness has also been maintained. These patients are then ready to commence a graduated return to sporting activity while continuing to progress their muscle conditioning, flexibility work and proprioceptive and agility exercises. This should correspond to the healing tissue entering the remodeling/maturation phase.

Muscle conditioning should be specific to the activity required, for example, an emphasis on power for sprinters and lifters, and endurance for distance runners. The exercise position should be as specific as possible to the sport, such as wall sits for the skier, prone bench pulleys for the swimmer or closed kinetic chain exercises for weight-bearing sports. The athlete will continue to progress strength work with high load, low repetition exercise and maintain an endurance base with low load, high repetitions appropriate to their deficits and the needs of the particular sport. Power work is enhanced with the use of fast-speed isotonic exercises and functional plyometric exercises (e.g. hopping, bounding, depth jumps). A wide variety of exercise modes and equipment may be used. These exercises can be performed in a gymnasium as well as the clinic.

The athlete is gradually prepared for return to sport by progressing through a sequence of functional activities required for the sport. This may include progression from jogging to striding to hopping to bounding, and agility skills of increasing complexity, intensity and volume. These activities are often performed initially in isolation and then slowly integrated into a more realistic sports environment. This may involve the introduction of equipment such as a ball or racquet and then performing activities with a team mate. Further progression occurs with the introduction of team drills and increased skills practice.

Particular attention must be devoted to the athlete's biomechanics. If incorrect technique was implicated as a possible cause for the original injury (Chapter 5), the coach and therapist must ensure that the athlete relearns the correct technique. Alternatively, the athlete may develop a new fault in technique after injury. Unconscious guarding or protective mechanisms may result in altered patterns of movement or technique. Video analysis may be helpful.

The athlete is usually participating in between 70% and 90% of normal training load by the later part of the advanced stage. As well as regaining the necessary muscle conditioning, flexibility and function to facilitate return to sport, an important component at this stage of the rehabilitation program is to restore the athlete's confidence. During this stage of rehabilitation, the athlete may fear injury recurrence, lack of full return of skills or permanent residual disability. Athletes may be particularly apprehensive about performing the activity that caused the original injury. These fears will gradually subside with support from the therapist and a well-programmed return to sport.

Return to sport

The following criteria should be used when determining whether an athlete is ready to return to full sporting activity:

- time constraints for soft tissue healing have been observed
- pain-free full range of movement
- no persistent swelling
- adequate strength and endurance
- good flexibility
- good proprioception and balance
- adequate cardiovascular fitness
- skills regained
- no persistent biomechanical abnormality
- athlete psychologically ready
- coach satisfied with training form.

There are a number of relative contraindications to return to sport. These include:

- persistent recurrent swelling—indicates a joint is not ready for activity, although some minor degree of swelling may be tolerated
- joint instability—may be controlled by brace or tape and good muscle control
- loss of joint range of motion—some loss may be acceptable in certain sports
- lack of full muscle strength—strength of at least 90% of the contralateral limb is recommended (strength of 80% of the contralateral limb may be acceptable in long-term ligamentous injury as long as there are no functional deficits).

It is vital to emphasize to the athlete that rehabilitation does not stop when he or she returns to sport. Therapists should be aware that collagen maturation and remodeling may continue for up to 12 months post injury. An athlete should not be considered completely rehabilitated until he or she has completed a full season of sport successfully following injury.

Monitoring the rehabilitation program

The therapist should continually monitor the patient's progress, both subjectively and objectively, to assess its effectiveness and to determine any negative effects. A number of parameters should be monitored:

- pain
- tenderness
- range of motion
- swelling
- heat
- redness
- ability to perform exercises and functional activities.

If adverse effects occur, the program should be either reduced or continued at the same level, depending on their severity. Otherwise the patient progresses gradually through the program.

Psychology and rehabilitation of injury

When athletes are recovering from injury, their focus narrows due to pain and fear about consequences of the injury and the possibility of recurrence. This can result in a feedback loop developing between the attention of the athlete and the injury, causing increased tension in the affected area. This may aggravate pain and impede the healing process.

The factors that affect rehabilitation include:

- type of injury
- circumstances of the injury
- external pressure (e.g. fear of losing position on the team)
- pain tolerance
- psychological attributes of the player
- player–player and coach–player support system.

Players with high self-esteem and good concentration are more able to control their frustration levels, have a positive outlook and focus on the rehabilitation tasks they are required to perform. As a result they may have a more rapid recovery from injury. Players with good psychological skills tend to cope well with external sources of pressure during rehabilitation. These pressures may include pressure from team mates, the worry of missing important events or being permanently replaced, and the risk of financial loss. Injuries that result from malice from opponents, from a mistake by a team mate or from lack of professionalism, such as not warming up or not following doctor's instructions, may cause a player to develop high levels of frustration.

To enhance recovery, appropriate treatment must be delivered in an environment where the athlete feels comfortable and can relate to the practitioners. Visualization may enhance the healing process. Athletes should be taught to understand their injury and visualize it healing.

The clinician should assist players to identify and confront views they may have about their future. Goal-setting is crucial to allow a step-wise approach and to ensure that the player concentrates on intermediate treatment goals rather than becoming anxious about the long-term outcome. In this way, the player gains positive feedback during injury.

When performing functional exercises and sport-specific skills, the injured athlete has a tendency to focus on the injury rather than the task to be performed. The player can be taught psychological skills (e.g. progressive muscular relaxation, behavior modification, visualization) to change this focus (Chapter 39).

Often, full-time athletes have difficulty occupying themselves when injured. It may be useful to structure the day's activities for these athletes.

Conclusion

Rehabilitation of the injured athlete requires careful assessment and subsequent correction of the athlete's deficit. The rehabilitation program should be individualized for the athlete's need. Using a recipe approach is fraught with danger. Functional and sport-specific activities should form a major part of the program. The injured athlete should be able to return to sport without functional deficit and with any predisposing factors to injury corrected.

Recommended Reading

Chaitow L. *Muscle Energy Techniques*. New York: Churchill Livingstone, 1997.

Chaitow L. *Modern Neuromuscular Techniques*. 2nd edn. New York: Churchill Livingstone, 2003.

Chandler J. Functional reconditioning. In: Kibler WB, Herring SA, Press JM, eds. *Functional Rehabilitation of Sports and Musculoskeletal Injuries*. Gaithersburg, MD: Aspen Publishers, 1998.

Cools AM, Witvrouw EE, Danneels LA, et al. Does taping influence electromyographic muscle activity in the scapular rotators in the healthy shoulders. *Man Ther* 2002; 7(3): 154–62.

Cowan SM, Schache AG, Brukner P. Delayed onset of transversus abdominis in long-standing groin pain. *Med Sci Sports Exerc* 2004; 36(12): 2040–5.

Ellenbecker TS, Davies GJ. *Closed Kinetic Chain Exercise*. Champaign, IL: Human Kinetics, 2001.

Frontera WR. *Exercise in Rehabilitation Medicine*. Champaign, IL: Human Kinetics, 1999.

Frontera WR. *Rehabilitation of Sports Injuries. Scientific Basis*. Oxford: Blackwell Science, 2003.

Hillman S. Principles and techniques of open kinetic chain rehabilitation: the upper extremity. *J Sport Rehabil* 1994; 3: 319–30.

Kibler WB, Chandler TJ. Sport-specific conditioning. *Am J Sports Med* 1994; 22(3): 424–32.

Kibler WB, Herring SA, Press JM, eds. *Functional Rehabilitation of Sports and Musculoskeletal Injuries*. Gaithersburg, MA: Aspen Publishers, 1998.

Lieber RL, Friden J. Mechanisms of muscle injury after eccentric contraction. *J Sci Med Sport* 1999; 2: 253–65.

A review of experimental data, primarily from the animal model, indicating which factors cause injury and how this provides an approach for how muscle injury can be prevented.

Petty NJ. *Principles of Neuromuscular Treatment and Management. A Guide for Therapists*. Edinburgh: Churchill Livingstone, 2004.

Richardson C, Hodges P, Hides J. *Therapeutic Exercise for Lumbopelvic Stabilization*. 2nd edn. Edinburgh: Churchill Livingstone, 2004.

Stensdotter AK, Hodges PW, Mellor R, et al. Quadriceps activation in closed and open kinetic chain exercise. *Med Sci Sports Exerc* 2003; 35(12): 2043–7.

The Philadelphia Panel Members and Ottawa Methods Group. Philadelphia Panel evidence-based clinical practice guidelines on selected rehabilitation interventions: overview and methodology. *Phys Ther* 2001; 81: 1629–40.

Wilk KE, Meister K, Andrews JR. Current concepts in the rehabilitation of the overhead throwing athlete. *Am J Sports Med* 2002; 30(1): 136–51.

Zachazewski JE, Magee DJ, Quillen WS. *Athletic Injuries and Rehabilitation*. Philadelphia: WB Saunders, 1996.

Zuluaga M, Briggs C, Carlisle J, et al. *Sports Physiotherapy. Applied Science and Practice*. Melbourne: Churchill Livingstone, 1995.

References

1. Levin S. Early mobilization speeds recovery. *Physician Sportsmed* 1993; 21: 70–4.

2. Sherry MA, Best TM. A comparison of two rehabilitation programs in the treatment of acute hamstring strains. *J Orthop Sports Phys Ther* 2004; 34: 116–25.

3. Bergmark A. Stability of the lumbar spine. *Acta Orthop Scand Suppl* 1989; 230: 20–4.

4. Hodges PW. Is there a role for transversus abdominis in lumbo-pelvic stability? *Man Ther* 1999; 4: 74–86.

5. Richardson CA, Jull GA. Muscle control—pain control. What exercises would you prescribe? *Man Ther* 1995; 1: 2–10.

6. Clarkson PM. Exercise induced muscle damage—animal and human models. *Med Sci Sports Exerc* 1992; 24: 510–11.

7. Alfredson H, Pietila T, Jonsson P, et al. Heavy-load eccentric calf muscle training for the treatment of chronic Achilles tendinosis. *Am J Sports Med* 1998; 26: 360–6.

8. Niesen-Vertommen SL, Taunton JE, Clement DB, et al. The effect of eccentric versus concentric exercise in the management of Achilles tendonitis. *Clin J Sport Med* 1992; 2: 109–13.

9. Draganich LF, Jaeger RJ, Kralj AR. Coactivation of the hamstrings and quadriceps during extension of the knee. *J Bone Joint Surg* 1989; 71: 1075–81.

10. Shelbourne KD, Nitz P. Accelerated rehabilitation after anterior cruciate ligament reconstruction. *Am J Sports Med* 1990; 18: 292–9.

11. Sobel J, Pettrone FA, Nirschl RP. Prevention and rehabilitation of racquet sports injuries. In: Nicholas JA, Hershman EB, eds. *The Upper Extremity in Sports Medicine*. St Louis: Mosby Yearbook, 1995: 805–23.

12. Gleim GW, McHugh MP. Flexibility and its effect on sports injury and performance. *Sports Med* 1997; 24: 289–99.

13. Wilder RP, Cole AJ, Becker BE. Aquatic strategies for athletic rehabilitation. In: Kibler WB, Herring SA, Press JM, eds. *Functional Rehabilitation of Sports and Musculoskeletal Injuries*. Gaithersburg, MD: Aspen Publishers, 1998: 109–26.

14. Wilder RP, Brennan DK. Physiological responses to deep water running in athletes. *Sports Med* 1993; 16: 374–80.

Regional Problems

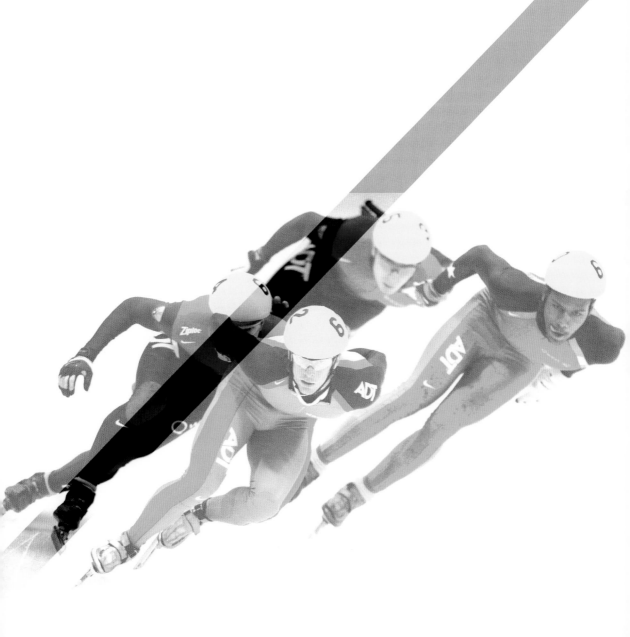

Sports Concussion

WITH PAUL McCRORY

Although head injuries are common in all contact sports, the vast majority are minor. Sports in which minor head injuries are seen include football, boxing, gymnastics, horse riding and martial arts.

Major head injuries are a medical emergency. The sports medicine practitioner's role in the management of acute head injuries is to recognize the problem, ensure immediate resuscitation and transfer the injured athlete to the appropriate facility. The immediate management of severe head injuries is considered in Chapter 44.

Definition

Concussion is the term commonly used to describe a type of minor head injury. The recent expert consensus conferences on sports concussion held in Vienna (2001) and Prague (2004) redefined sports concussion as follows: concussion is 'a complex pathophysiological process affecting the brain, induced by traumatic biomechanical forces'. Several common features that incorporate clinical, pathological, and biomechanical injury constructs that may be used in defining the nature of a concussive head injury include:

1. Concussion may be caused by direct blow to the head, face, neck or elsewhere on the body with an 'impulsive' force transmitted to the head.
2. Concussion typically results in the rapid onset of short-lived impairment of neurological function that resolves spontaneously.
3. Concussion may result in neuropathological changes but the acute clinical symptoms largely reflect a functional disturbance rather than structural injury.

4. Concussion results in a graded set of clinical syndromes that may or may not involve loss of consciousness. Resolution of the clinical and cognitive symptoms typically follows a sequential course.
5. Concussion is typically associated with grossly normal structural neuroimaging studies.[1, 2]

Many publications on concussion also refer to the Glasgow Coma Scale. The Glasgow Coma Scale has stood the test of time in distinguishing between mild, moderate and severe head injury and for the measurement of serial change in clinical status post-injury. The Scale, however, does not encompass sport concussion due to the mild nature of the symptoms involved. The terms 'mild brain injury' (MBI) and 'concussion' are not synonymous. Concussion is a subset of MBI but the converse is not true.

The recent Prague consensus conference[1, 2] also separated different subtypes of concussion based on symptom duration. While this separation remains to be validated scientifically, it nevertheless reflects the common clinical management situation and may have implications in future management and/or resource utilization. The two categories are as follows:

1. *Simple concussion*: the injury progressively resolves without complication over seven to 10 days.
2. *Complex concussion*: the athlete suffers persistent (>10 days) symptoms either at rest or with exertion.

Concussion is common in all contact sports. The incidence ranges from 0.25–5 per 1000 player hours of exposure. Professional horse jumping jockeys have the highest concussion rate of any sport, followed by Australian footballers.

Applied pathophysiology

Although neurological dysfunction in concussion is transient, the athlete has sustained significant impact to the brain. More severe forms of diffuse brain injury involve shearing forces to the brain, which cause pathological damage. In concussion, it remains controversial as to whether any pathological damage occurs. Most, if not all, of the neurological symptoms reflect a functional rather than structural injury to neurons.

The concussed athlete, although conscious and without obvious focal neurological signs, may have impaired higher cortical function, for example, impaired short-term memory. These subtle cognitive changes may only be detected by neuropsychological testing.

Following a blow to the head, the athlete's conscious state may be altered. This may vary from simply being stunned to a significant loss of consciousness. Memory is typically affected in a concussive episode. A period of retrograde amnesia, that is, loss of memory of events prior to the incident, or post-traumatic amnesia, that is, loss of memory of events after the incident, may follow minor head injury. The duration of retrograde or post-traumatic amnesia does not indicate the severity of the concussive episode.

The ability to think clearly, concentrate on tasks and process information will also be affected. Concussive symptoms such as headache, dizziness, blurred vision and nausea may also be present.

Frequently, in episodes of mild concussion ('bell ringers'), the athlete will be dazed or stunned for a period of seconds only and continue playing. The other players and coaches may be unaware that a concussive episode has occurred. Alert medical and training staff should closely observe the actions of a player who has received a knock to the head for any signs of impaired performance.

Grading of concussion

There is no reliable or scientifically validated system of grading the severity of sports-related concussion. At the present time, there are at least 28 published anecdotal severity scales. The danger is that athletes and/or their coaches may 'shop around' for a scale that is not in their best medical interests. At the end of the day, good clinical judgment should prevail over written guidelines.

At the first international conference on concussion in sport (Vienna, 2001)[3] the expert committee endorsed no specific grading system for concussion but recommended that combined measures of recovery should be used to assess injury severity and guide individual decisions on return to play. This was re-endorsed at the Prague 2004 meeting.[1, 2] Sideline evaluation such as using the SCAT (Standardized Concussion Assessment Tool) card[1, 2] or similar tool is recommended.

Complications of concussion

Impaired reaction time and delayed information processing associated with concussion may result in the athlete failing to cope with potentially injurious situations and sustaining further cerebral or musculo-skeletal injury.

In the acute situation, concussive convulsions or tonic posturing may be observed immediately after impact. These benign but dramatic phenomena are a non-epileptic manifestation of concussion.[4]

If a player recommences playing while symptomatic, post-concussive symptoms may be prolonged. This may also increase the chance of developing the 'post-concussive syndrome', in which fatigue, difficulty in concentration and headaches persist for some time, often months, following the original injury. This syndrome is uncommon in sport.

The so-called second impact syndrome is said to result in catastrophic brain swelling in response to repeated concussive injury. A recent review has cast doubt as to the existence of this syndrome.[5]

Multiple concussive episodes may result in chronic cortical dysfunction. This is most evident in boxers who suffer repetitive head injuries, often over a lengthy period, resulting in gross pathological and neuropsychological changes. This is referred to as the 'punch-drunk syndrome'.

Management of the concussed athlete

Exclude serious injury

The most important task for the clinician confronted with a concussed athlete is to exclude the presence of serious head injury or spinal injury. If the athlete is unconscious, the clinician should assume the presence of a head injury and spinal injury and manage the patient accordingly (Chapter 44).

If the patient is conscious, the first step is to exclude the presence of a spinal injury. Once this is done, the athlete needs to be removed from the field of play (Chapter 44).

Assess severity

Once the athlete has been removed from the field of play, a full neurological examination should be performed and the features of the concussion assessed according to the clinical guide shown in Table 13.1. If prolonged loss of consciousness, signs of cortical dysfunction or post-traumatic amnesia are present, a significant concussive episode has occurred.

More serious cases of concussion may require admission to hospital for observation. The criteria for admission to hospital are:

- loss of consciousness for longer than 5 minutes
- post-traumatic convulsion
- focal neurological signs
- symptoms of marked cerebral irritation persisting for more than 1 hour
- any deterioration of mental state, for example, development of drowsiness after a period of alertness
- more than one episode of moderate or severe concussion during any playing session.

In less serious cases of concussion, more subtle changes should be sought. The effectiveness of the athlete's short-term memory should be determined by asking questions relating to activity over the previous hour. If the concussive episode has occurred in a competitive match, appropriate questions to determine the presence of a memory deficit are

critical (e.g. the SCAT[1] or the Maddocks[6] questions). Other valid but less practical diagnostic tools include the Standardised Assessment of Concussion (SAC) designed for athletic trainer use.[7]

Neuropsychological testing

The major difficulty in the management of concussion has always been the lack of objective assessment of the degree of concussion and evidence of recovery. A number of neuropsychological tests have been evaluated in order to find an objective measure of cognitive function that is simple, sensitive and easy to use in sporting situations.

One example of such pen and paper tests is a test known as the Digit Symbol Substitution Test (DSST), derived from the Wechsler Adult Intelligence Scale. This tests speed of information processing and is a sensitive marker of cognitive dysfunction in concussed athletes. The test involves substituting a symbol for a random succession of numbers. The athlete is given 90 seconds to fill in as many symbols as possible and given a score (Fig. 13.1). In sports with a high potential for episodes of concussion, such as football, players are tested prior to the commencement of the season. Then, if an episode of concussion occurs, a baseline score is available for comparison.

The DSST can be used in the competition setting as it does not require elaborate equipment. This provides an advantage over many other neuropsychological tests. An example of changes in DSST scores following mild and moderate episodes of concussion is shown in Figure 13.2. The DSST may be used on the field

Table 13.1 Guide to clinical evaluation of concussion

Cognitive features	Typical symptoms	Physical signs
Unaware of period, opposition, score of game	Headache	Impaired conscious state
Confusion	Dizziness	Poor coordination, balance
Amnesia	Nausea	Concussive convulsion
Unaware of time, date, place	Unsteadiness Feeling 'dinged', stunned or dazed Having one's 'bell rung' Seeing stars or flashing lights Tinnitus Double vision Sleepiness, sleep disturbance, drowsiness, fatigue in the setting of an impact	Gait unsteadiness Slow to answer questions or follow directions Loss of consciousness Easily distracted, poor concentration Unusual or inappropriate emotions Nausea/vomiting Vacant stare, glassy eyed Slurred speech Personality changes Impaired playing ability

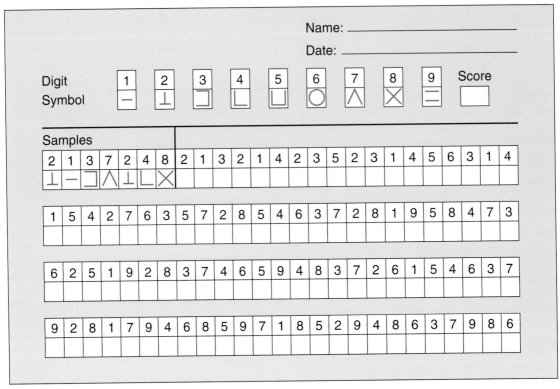

Figure 13.1 The Digit Symbol Substitution Test (DSST). The athlete completes as many boxes as possible in 90 seconds

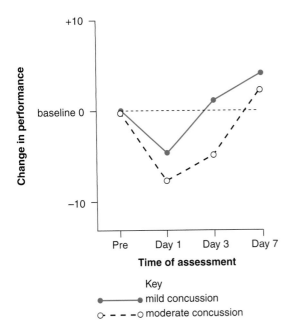

Figure 13.2 DSST changes in mild and moderate concussion ADAPTED FROM MADDOCKS ET AL. 1995[8]

immediately after the episode of concussion or a few days later to aid the clinician in deciding the timing of an athlete's return to sport.

Most of these pen and paper tools have now been superseded by the use of computerized neuropsychological screening batteries such as CogSport, Impact, Headminders and ANAM.

It must be remembered that such neuropsychological tests are only an aid to the assessment of the degree of recovery from concussion. Other, more elaborate tests, including reaction time, may be used to assess the degree of recovery. Although the most important determinants are the patient's symptoms and signs, there appears to be a marked correlation between clinical symptoms and neuropsychological test results.

Return to activity

Whether or not to allow the concussed patient to return to training and then competition is one of the most difficult decisions the sports physician must make. In minor cases of concussion, where all symptoms resolve quickly and there is no amnesia, sign of cortical dysfunction nor evidence of impairment of short-term memory or information processing, the player may be allowed to return once recovered. Neuropsychological testing may be used to confirm full recovery. A player permitted to return to play should be closely observed for any signs of impaired function.

Apart from professional sport, it is recommended that the athlete does not return to the field of play on the day of the concussive episode. The player should then be monitored clinically over several days for evidence of full recovery. The most common persisting symptoms following an episode of concussion are headache, dizziness, lack of concentration, sleep disturbance and a non-specific complaint of 'dullness' in the head. The athlete should not be permitted to resume training or playing until completely asymptomatic.

Once asymptomatic and with evidence of full short-term memory and information processing as determined by neuropsychological testing, the athlete is allowed to resume activity, initially at a reduced level, slowly increasing to full training. The athlete's performance in training, particularly performance of skills that involve hand–eye coordination, should be closely monitored for any signs of impairment. If symptoms such as headache, nausea or dizziness develop during exercise, the exercise should be ceased immediately and not resumed until symptoms resolve.

In professional sports where there is rapid access to expert neurological advice and computerized neuropsychological testing, more rapid return to play may occur providing the athlete has recovered from the injury fully. The difference between return to play in professional versus non-elite sports is not the individual recovery of the athlete but rather the access to better resources to assess recovery.

Mandatory exclusion

In a number of contact sports, such as boxing and Rugby football, authorities have legislated for a mandatory exclusion period from competition for concussed players. While the intent of such a policy is praiseworthy, an arbitrary exclusion period is hard to justify scientifically as each episode of concussion requires individual evaluation. For some players, the period of exclusion will be too long, and for other players not long enough.

Ideally, concussed players should be examined by an experienced medical practitioner with the decision about return to play based on the clinical findings and, if possible, neuropsychological testing.

Post-concussion syndrome

Athletes who suffer an episode of concussion may, rarely, have persistence of non-specific symptoms for a number of weeks. This phenomenon is known as the post-concussion syndrome.[9] Symptoms include headache and dizziness. Impaired mental capacity is revealed by poor memory, poor concentration and slow decision making and it is unclear whether these symptoms reflect an ongoing injury or recovery process or are the consequence of psychological factors.

These patients should undergo formal neuropsychological testing as well as an MRI brain scan. If these tests are normal, there is no specific treatment other than rest and reassurance. Return to sport is not advisable while symptoms are present as exercise appears to prolong the condition.

Recurrent episodes of concussion

Recurrent episodes of concussion are a cause for concern. If an athlete has more than one episode of concussion in a season, it is mandatory that he or she recovers fully and completely prior to resumption of sport. This may involve extensive neurological and neuropsychological assessment. The use of concepts such as 'three episodes means retirement' has no scientific basis and should be abandoned.

Prevention of concussion

There are a number of possible ways of reducing the likelihood and severity of the concussion, however, none of these theoretical mechanisms has been scientifically validated. The wearing of mouthguards will reduce dental and mandibular injuries although the evidence that concussions are reduced is non-existent.[10–12] All players in collision sports should wear a properly fitting mouthguard. The mouthguard should be a laminated custom-molded guard in order to fit comfortably and allow the athlete to speak and breathe during play without restriction.

The second theoretical means of reducing the severity of concussion is improved conditioning of the neck musculature. Although strengthening of the neck muscles will not prevent head injury, it is thought that properly conditioned neck muscles are able to absorb and withstand some of the force that occurs with impact. This may be particularly important in Rugby football and boxing.

Properly fitted and maintained hard-shell helmets possibly reduce the incidence of major head injury in certain sports, such as skull fractures in cycling. The effect of wearing helmets on the incidence or severity of concussion is less clear and is unlikely to be significant.[9] The commercially available soft-shell helmets have little or no protective capability against concussive forces when tested in laboratory situations, and in two randomized controlled trials in Rugby and Australian football did not reduce head injury rates.

The major concern with the recommendation for helmet use in sport is the phenomenon known as 'risk compensation', whereby helmeted athletes change their playing behavior in the misguided belief that the protective equipment will stop all injury. As a result, the rate of head injury increases rather than decreases. This is a particular concern in child and adolescent athletes.

The most effective way to reduce head injuries may well be through rule changes, rule enforcement and coaching techniques.

Recommended Reading

Aubry M, Cantu R, Dvorak J, et al. Summary and agreement statement of the First International Conference on Concussion in Sport, Vienna 2001. Recommendations for the improvement of safety and health of athletes who may suffer concussive injuries. *Br J Sports Med* 2002; 36(1): 6–10.

Johnson K, McCrory P, Mohtadi N, et al. Evidence-based review of sport-related concussion: clinical science. *Clin J Sport Med* 2001; 11: 150–60.

Lovell MR, Collins MW. New developments in the evaluation of sports-related concussion. *Curr Sports Med Rep* 2002; 1: 287–92.

McCrory PM, Johnston K, Meeuwisse W, et al. Summary and agreement statement of the 2nd international conference on concussion in sport, Prague 2004. *Clin J Sport Med* 2005; 15(2): 48–55.

McCrory P. What advice should we give to athletes postconcussion? *Br J Sports Med* 2002; 36: 316–18.

McCrory P, Johnson K. Acute clinical symptoms of concussion. Assessing prognostic significance *Physician Sportsmed* 2002; 30(8): 43–7.

McCrory P, Johnson K, Meeuwisse W, et al. Evidence-based review of sport-related concussion: basic science. *Clin J Sport Med* 2001; 11: 160–6.

Schnirring L. New recommendations for concussion management. *Physician Sportsmed* 2004; 32(12): 12–14.

References

1. McCrory P, Johnston K, Meeuwisse W, et al. Summary and agreement statement of the 2nd international conference on concussion in sport, Prague 2004. *Br J Sports Med* 2005; 39(4): 196–204.

2. McCrory PM, Johnston K, Meeuwisse W, et al. Summary and agreement statement of the 2nd international conference on concussion in sport, Prague 2004. *Clin J Sport Med* 2005; 15(2): 48–55.

3. Aubry M, Cantu R, Dvorak J, et al. Summary and agreement statement of the First International Conference on Concussion in Sport, Vienna 2001. Recommendations for the improvement of safety and health of athletes who may suffer concussive injuries. *Br J Sports Med* 2002; 36(1): 6–10.

4. McCrory PR, Berkovic SF. Concussive convulsions. Incidence in sport and treatment recommendations. *Sports Med* 1998; 25(2): 131–6.

5. McCrory P, Berkovic SF. Second impact syndrome. *Neurology* 1998; 50(3): 677–84.

6. Maddocks DL, Dicker GD, Saling MM. The assessment of orientation following concussion in athletes. *Clin J Sport Med* 1995; 5(1): 32–5.

7. McCrea M, Kelly J, Randolph C, et al. Standardised assessment of concussion (SAC): on site mental status evaluation of the athlete. *J Head Trauma Rehabil* 1998; 13: 27–36.

8. Maddocks DL, Saling MM, Dicker GD. A note on the normative data for a test sensitive to concussion in Australian rules footballers. *Aust Psychol* 1995; 30: 125–7.

9. Johnson K, McCrory P, Mohtadi N, et al. Evidence-based review of sport-related concussion: clinical science. *Clin J Sport Med* 2001; 11: 150–60.

10. McCrory P. Do mouthguards prevent concussion? *Br J Sports Med* 2001; 35: 81–2.

11. Labella CR, Smith BW, Sigurdsson A. Effect of mouthguards on dental injuries and concussions in college basketball. *Med Sci Sports Exerc* 2002; 34(1): 41–4.

12. Barbic D, Pater J, Brison RJ. Comparison of mouth guard designs and concussion prevention in contact sports. *Clin J Sport Med* 2005; 15(5): 294–8.

Headache

WITH PAUL McCRORY

Headache has been called 'the most common complaint of civilized man' affecting approximately two-thirds of the population. Athletes suffer from the same causes of headache as non-athletes. In addition, there are several causes of headache that relate directly to exercise. Numerous attempts have been made to classify the different types of headache. Headaches may be classified into seven groups, the first four of which are seen commonly and the second three less commonly:

1. headache associated with viral illness, for example, respiratory infections, sinusitis, influenza
2. vascular headaches, for example, migraine, cluster headache
3. cervical headache, for example, referred from joints, muscles and fascia of the cervical region
4. tension headache or muscle contraction headache
5. intracranial causes, for example, tumor, hemorrhage, subdural hematoma, meningitis
6. exercise-related headache, for example, benign exertional headache, 'footballers' migraine'
7. other causes, for example, drugs, psychogenic, post-spinal procedure, post-traumatic.

The first four causes listed are seen frequently in the community. Exercise-related and post-traumatic headache are of particular concern in athletes. While it is usually possible to differentiate between the groups, headaches of mixed type occur commonly.

The International Headache Society (IHS), in conjunction with the World Health Organization (WHO), has proposed an overall classification for headache.[1] While this classification system is used mainly for research purposes, it nevertheless provides a framework to assist in clinical management.

Clinical approach to the patient with headache

The majority of headaches do not require medical assessment. However, certain symptoms may indicate the presence of more serious abnormalities and require medical assessment. These symptoms are:

- new or unaccustomed headache
- atypical headache
- stiff neck or meningeal signs
- systemic symptoms, for example, fever, weight loss, malaise
- neurological symptoms, for example, drowsiness, weakness, numbness of limbs
- local extracranial symptoms, for example, ear, sinus, teeth
- changes in the pattern of headache
- headache increasing over a few days
- sudden onset of severe headache
- headaches that wake the patient up during the night or in the early morning
- chronic headache with localized pain.

The clinical approach to the athlete complaining of headache is shown in Figure 11.1. The practitioner should:

1. exclude possible intracranial causes. These include hemorrhage, tumor, infection and subdural hematoma. If an intracranial abnormality is suspected as a result of a full neurological examination, imaging of the brain with CT or MRI may be indicated.

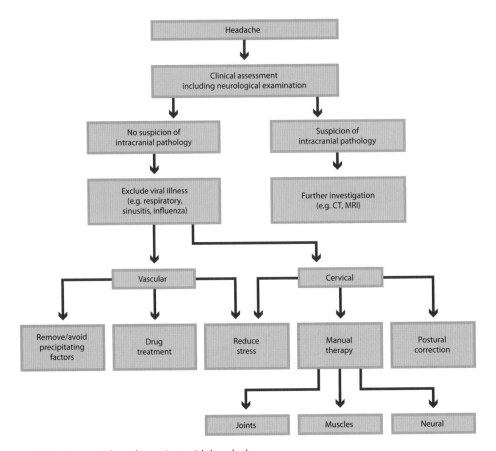

Figure 14.1 Clinical approach to the patient with headache

2. exclude headache associated with a viral illness. The presence of common illnesses that may provoke headache should be excluded. These include respiratory tract infection, sinusitis and influenza.

3. exclude drug-induced headaches. Many commonly used drugs can provoke headache. A list of these drugs is shown below:
   - alcohol
   - analgesics, such as aspirin (ASA), codeine
   - antibiotics and antifungals
   - antihypertensives, such as methyldopa
   - caffeine
   - corticosteroids
   - cyclosporin
   - dipyridamole
   - indomethacin
   - monoamine oxidase inhibitors (MAOIs)
   - nicotine
   - nitrazepam
   - nitrous oxide
   - oral contraceptives
   - sympathomimetics
   - theophylline
   - vasodilators.

4. exclude exercise-related headache.

5. differentiate between vascular, tension and cervical causes. If the above three groups are excluded, the majority of headaches are then due either to vascular causes, such as migraine, or referred from the joints and/or muscles of the neck. Classic vascular and cervical headaches each have distinctive features (Table 14.1), although frequently features of both types may be present. Tension headaches may occur unrelated to cervical injury or dysfunction and tend to be of a low-grade daily headache presentation. In some cases, external stress is important in both their genesis and continuity.

Table 14.1 Clinical features of vascular and cervical headaches

Features	Vascular headache	Cervical headache
Age of onset	10–40 years	20–60 years
Onset	Fast	Slow
Site	Frontal or temporal	Occipital (usually), retro-orbital or temporal
Side	Unilateral/bilateral	Unilateral
Type of pain	Throbbing	Dull ache
Constancy	Episodic	Constant
Time course	Hours	Days
Neurological symptoms	Common (e.g. visual disturbances, nausea)	Occasionally (e.g. paresthesia)
History of trauma	Rare	Common (e.g. 'whiplash')
Triggers	Food, drugs, stress	Trauma, posture
Treatment	Avoid precipitating factors Drugs Stress reduction	Manual therapy Stress reduction Postural correction

History

The clinical history is the most important component of the assessment of the athlete with headache. The location of the headache is typically frontal or temporal in migrainous headaches and occipital in cervical headaches. However, cervical headaches may also present as retro-orbital or temporal headaches.

Sudden onset of severe headache may indicate a cerebral hemorrhage or migraine, while cervical headaches typically have a more gradual onset. A recent history of a blow to the head may also be relevant. Recent exposure to possible precipitating factors, such as particular foods, should be noted if migraine is suspected.

Migrainous headaches are typically severe, as are headaches associated with meningeal irritation due to hemorrhage or meningitis. Cervical headaches are usually less severe. A throbbing pain is typical of a vascular headache, while a dull ache is more typical of a cervical headache.

The behavior of a headache in both the short term and long term is important. Migrainous headaches typically occur episodically. The frequency of these attacks should be noted. Migraines usually have a finite duration (hours), whereas cervical headache can last for days. The presence of any neck and arm symptoms should also be noted. Brief episodes of headache associated with exercise may indicate benign exertional headache. Whether the headache is easily irritated, for example, by neck movement, should be noted. This is particularly relevant for manual therapy treatment.

Headache aggravated by neck movements may indicate a cervical cause for the headache. Exercise usually aggravates headaches of all types. Migraine is usually relieved by sleep.

Prior to the onset of migrainous headaches, there may be associated visual or sensory symptoms (migraine with aura). Nausea and vomiting are also commonly associated with migrainous headaches and usually follow the headache episode. The presence of neurological symptoms or systemic symptoms such as weight loss and malaise may be indicative of a more serious cause of headache.

Associated upper or lower respiratory tract symptoms, symptoms of sinusitis, temporomandibular joint problems or influenza-like symptoms may indicate an association with one of these conditions. The presence of neck pain or stiffness should also be noted.

A past history of head trauma, even if relatively minor, may be significant as subdural hematoma may present some time after the trauma. Previous problems such as encephalitis or major systemic illnesses should be recorded.

Whether the athlete is taking any medications (e.g. oral contraceptive pill) or recreational drugs (e.g. nicotine, alcohol and caffeine) should also be noted.

Stress aggravates both vascular and, particularly, cervical headache. An assessment of life stresses is an important part of the history. These include personal relationships, work pressures and problems related to the athlete's sporting activity.

Examination

In all patients presenting with headache, a full neurological examination is required and the skull and cervical spine must always be particularly examined. The examination should consist of some or all of the following components depending on the presence or absence of specific symptoms in the history:

- general appearance
- mental state
- speech
- skull examination
- cervical spine examination
- gait and stance
- pupils and fundi
- special senses (e.g. smell, vision, hearing)
- other cranial nerves
- motor system
- sensory system
- general examination.

Vascular headaches

Vascular headaches include migraine, cluster headache, toxic headache, exertional headache and some types of post-traumatic headache. Vascular headaches affect at least one-fifth of the population at some time during their lives. Common to all these headaches is a tendency towards extracranial vascular dilatation manifested by the throbbing headache phase of a particular attack. Vasoconstriction may also be evident and responsible for the painless sensory phenomena prior to the onset of head pain.

Vascular headaches usually begin early in life, often at puberty or in the second decade. There may be a familial tendency (50%). The headache usually begins early in the morning and reaches high intensity within 2 hours. It may last for a number of hours. Headaches usually resolve within a day but can recur daily or several times a week. There may be an increased frequency of occurrence in certain seasons, especially during spring.

Marked variations in headache frequency are seen within individuals. After menopause, headaches are usually diminished but in some women they may become more frequent and severe. The use of medications, such as vasodilators, hormone replacement therapy or the oral contraceptive pill, may exacerbate an underlying tendency towards vascular headaches.

Migraine

Migraine with and without aura, that is, vascular headache occurring with and without neurological symptoms respectively, present a difficult management problem, particularly in athletes who develop migraine headaches after exercise. Although most people think of migraine as headache alone, the true migraine sufferer usually notices a spectrum of symptoms, including nausea, vomiting, diarrhea and weight gain. They may notice a prodromal period with evidence of endocrine disturbance (e.g. fluid retention). In the typical migraine attack with aura, painless sensory neurological symptoms such as visual disturbances (e.g. scotomas), paresthesia, vertigo, hemiplegia and ophthalmoplegia may precede the headache.

The type of neurological symptoms that develop vary depending on which part of the intracranial vascular tree is affected by the disturbance. In migraine with aura, occipital branches of the vascular tree may be affected and visual symptoms such as flashing lights and scotoma predominate. In a rare form of migraine seen in children known as vertebrobasilar migraine, brain stem abnormalities such as behavioral disturbances and even death have been described.

The IHS criteria for the diagnosis of migraine without aura are shown in Table 14.2

Table 14.2 The International Headache Society (IHS) criteria for the diagnosis of migraine without aura (IHS 1.1)[1]

A. At least five attacks fulfilling criteria B–D below
B. Headache attacks lasting 4–72 hours
C. Headache has at least two of the following characteristics:
   1. Unilateral location
   2. Pulsating quality
   3. Moderate or severe intensity (inhibits or prohibits daily activities)
   4. Aggravation by walking stairs or similar routine physical activity
D. During headache at least one of the following:
   1. Nausea and/or vomiting
   2. Photophobia and phonophobia

Clinical features

Patients describe migraine headache pain as sharp and intense. It is often throbbing, beating or pulsing, although occasionally the pain is steady. Commonly, it begins in the temple or forehead on both sides. When it starts on one side, it may spread to the other side. If the headache is intense, it may spread to the occiput and even change to a muscle contraction type of headache. Occasionally, the vascular headache begins at the back of the head and moves forward.

Many patients do not spontaneously volunteer their visual or sensory symptoms, either because they fail to link them with their headache or because they are hesitant to share the hallucinatory experiences. Occasionally, patients may suffer the sensory phenomena without the headache developing. The common neurological accompaniments to migraine with aura are visual. Patients speak of bright colored or white objects (stars, edges, angles, balls) often to one side of the visual field. These objects may shine or flicker and may move across the visual field, leaving in their wake darkness or a scotoma. The visual symptoms usually last about 20 minutes and most often clear before the sensory, cognitive or headache symptoms begin.

Sensory symptoms are usually described as tingling, pricking or pins and needles. These commonly commence in the face or fingers and gradually spread up the limb or over the same side of the body. Vertigo, dysphasia, diplopia, confusion and amnesia are less commonly reported. Headache most often follows the neurological symptoms but may precede or accompany them.

Nausea, vomiting and dizziness are common during or after the attack. After the headache, diuresis, diarrhea, euphoria or a surge of energy are commonly described. The typical features associated with migraine are:

- precipitating factors, such as tiredness, stress or release from stress (e.g. 'weekend migraine')
- character and location of headache
- periodicity
- presence of migraine accompaniments (e.g. visual, gastrointestinal symptoms)
- relief with anti-migraine therapy (e.g. sumatriptan).

Precipitating factors in migraine

A number of precipitating factors are commonly found in association with migraine headaches. These are:

- endocrine changes (e.g. premenstrual or menstrual, oral contraceptive pills, pregnancy, puberty, menopause, hyperthyroidism)
- metabolic changes (e.g. fever, anemia)
- rhinitis
- change in temperature or altitude
- change in activity
- alcohol, especially red wine
- foods (e.g. chocolates, cheese, nuts, 'hot dogs')
- drugs (e.g. glyceryl trinitrate [nitroglycerin], nitrates, indomethacin)
- blood pressure changes
- sleep—too much or too little.

Treatment

Most patients choose to lie quietly in a dark room during a migraine attack. Sleep often terminates the attack. The primary method of active treatment is pharmacological. High-dose aspirin (ASA) (900–1200 mg) is the drug of choice for the acute treatment of migraine. Other acute agents such as sumatriptan (intramuscular or intranasal[2]) or ergot preparations may be used as second-line therapy. Frequent sufferers of migraine may find prophylactic drug therapy necessary and reasonably effective. An important part of the management of the migraine sufferer is to identify and avoid precipitating factors. Traditional herbal remedies such as 'feverfew' may be helpful.

It is critical in the management of migraine and other forms of headache that the use of repeated doses of simple analgesia alone be avoided. One of the consequences of the overuse of analgesic medication is the so-called 'analgesic rebound headache', which becomes a self-generating headache requiring increasing doses of analgesia. Analgesic rebound headache, once established, is extremely difficult to treat and usually requires a specialist headache neurological clinic. For this reason, the use of simple analgesics in headache treatment should be limited to a maximum of three days per week. Treatment of the headache should be directed at the cause of the problem not simply pain management.

Cluster headache

Cluster headache is also known as histamine headache, migrainous neuralgia and Horton's headache. This form of headache may be distinguished from other vascular headaches by the typical nature of the history. The pain typically occurs in attacks and is an intense burning or 'boring' sensation. The attacks frequently begin in middle age and may be precipitated by alcohol. On the affected side there may be associated rhinorrhea, nasal obstruction, perspiration and conjunctival injection. A partial Horner's syndrome is often seen. This condition is five times more common in males than females. There is usually no family history. Patients are usually disabled during a cluster headache.

Patients with cluster headache are usually extremely sensitive to vasodilating agents. Oral glyceryl trinitrate (nitroglycerin) has been used as a provocative test for this condition.

Treatment depends on the age and health of the patient and the timing of attacks. Acute attacks may be aborted by inhalation of 100% oxygen at 7 L per minute. The mechanism of this relief is unclear. Headache prophylaxis may be necessary. Methysergide may be used in younger patients and either prednisolone or lithium or both in older patients. Generally, the use of these medications requires specialist input due to the side-effect profile. Ergot preparations may also be used.

Cervical headache

Cervical or cervicogenic headache is a term used to describe headache caused by abnormalities of the joints, muscles, fascia and neural structures of the cervical region. There are a number of classifications for cervical or cervicogenic headache with differing criteria for physical dysfunction. These criteria are summarized in Table 14.3.

Mechanism

The mechanism of production of headache from abnormalities in the cervical region is variable. It may be primarily referred pain caused by irritation of the upper cervical nerve roots. This may be due to damage to the atlantoaxial joint or compression of the nerves as they pass through the muscles. Headache emanating from the lower cervical segments probably originates from irritation of the posterior primary rami, which transmit sensation to the spinal portion of the trigeminocervical nucleus.

Commonly, pain may also be referred to the head from active trigger points (Fig. 14.2). Frontal headaches are associated with trigger points in the suboccipital muscles, while temporal headaches are associated with trigger points in the upper trapezius, splenius capitis and cervicis, and sternocleidomastoid muscles.

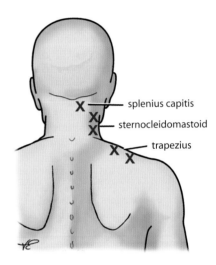

Figure 14.2 Sites of trigger points causing cervical headache

Table 14.3 Current criteria for physical dysfunction in headache classification[3]

International Headache Society[1]	International Association for the Study of Pain[4]	Sjaadstad et al.[5]
Resistance to or limitation of passive neck movements	Reduced range of motion in the neck	Restriction of range of movement in the neck
Changes in neck muscle contour, texture or tone or response to active stretching or contraction	–	–
Abnormal tenderness in neck muscles	–	Pressure over the ipsilateral upper cervical or occipital region reproduces headache

Clinical features

History

A cervical headache is typically described as a constant, steady, dull ache, often unilateral but sometimes bilateral. The patient describes a pulling or gripping feeling or, alternatively, may describe a tight band around the head. The headache is usually in the suboccipital region and is commonly referred to the frontal, retro-orbital or temporal regions.

Cervical headache is usually of gradual onset. The patient often wakes with a headache that may improve during the day. Cervical headaches may be present for days, weeks or even months. There may be a history of acute trauma, such as a 'whiplash' injury sustained in a motor accident, or repetitive trauma associated with work or a sporting activity.

Cervical headache is often associated with neck pain or stiffness and may be aggravated by neck or head movements, such as repetitive jolting when traveling in a car or bus. It is often associated with a feeling of light-headedness, dizziness and tinnitus. Nausea may be present but vomiting is rare. The patient often complains of impaired concentration, an inability to function normally and depression. Poor posture is often associated with a cervical headache. This may be either a contributory factor or an effect of a headache. The abnormal posture typically seen with cervical headache is rounded shoulders, extended neck and protruded chin. This results in tightness of the upper cervical extensor muscles and weakness of the cervical flexor muscles (Chapter 16).

Stress is often associated with cervical headache. It may be an important contributory factor to the development of the soft tissue abnormalities causing the headache or may aggravate abnormalities already present. Thus, it is important to elicit sources of stress in the clinical history.

Examination

Examination of the patient with suspected cervical headache involves systematic examination of the joints, muscles and neural structures of the cervical region as well as assessment of cervical posture. As with any musculoskeletal examination, one of the aims of the examination is to reproduce the patient's symptoms. It is important to remember that abnormalities of a number of different structures may contribute to the patient's pain.

Common joint abnormalities found on examination of the patient with cervical headache include stiffness and tenderness over the upper cervical (C1–2, C2–3) joints. Tenderness may be maximal centrally, especially where bilateral pain is present, or unilaterally over the apophyseal joints if unilateral pain is present. It is not uncommon for abnormalities of the lower cervical joints to be present as well.

On examination of the muscles of the cervical region, it is common to find tightness in the suboccipital and erector spinae muscles. This is often associated with weakness in the cervical flexors. Active trigger points are frequently present, particularly in the suboccipital, sternocleidomastoid and trapezius muscles.

Deficits in cervical flexor and extensor muscle strength have been documented in patients with cervicogenic headache. Jull and others have developed the craniocervical flexion test (C-CFT) to assess deficits in the endurance of the deep flexor muscles.[6]

A neural component of the patient's headache is suspected if movements that increase neural tension increase the patient's pain (Chapter 3). Neural tension may be increased by adding cervical flexion to the upper limb tension test and slump test (Chapter 8).

Treatment

Treatment of the patient with cervical headache requires correction of the abnormalities of joints, muscles and neural structures found on examination as well as correction of any possible precipitating factors such as postural abnormalities or emotional stress.

Treatment of cervical intervertebral joint abnormalities involves mobilization or manipulation of the C1–2 and C2–3 joints. Stretching of the cervical extensor muscles and strengthening of the cervical flexor muscles are important.

Soft tissue therapy to the muscles and the fascia of the cervical region is aimed at releasing generally tight muscles and fascia (commonly the cervical extensors). Active trigger points should be treated with spray and stretch techniques or dry needling (Chapter 10).

Cervical muscle retraining has been shown to be beneficial by itself and in combination with manipulative therapy in reducing the incidence of cervicogenic headache.[7] This includes retraining of the deep cervical flexors (Fig. 14.3), extensors and scapular stabilizers.

Postural retraining is an essential part of treatment. The patient must learn to reduce the amount of cervical extension by retracting the chin (Chapter 16). Identification and reduction of sources of stress to the patient should be incorporated in the treatment program.

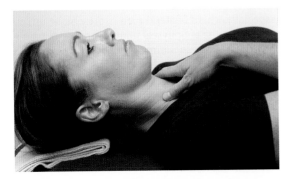

Figure 14.3 Retraining of the deep cervical flexors (see also Fig. 16.7, p. 239). *[Photo courtesy of Professor Gwendolen Jull.]*

Exercise-related causes of headache

Benign exertional headache

Benign exertional headache (BEH) has been reported in association with weightlifting, running and other sporting activities. The IHS criteria include that the headache:

- is specifically brought on by physical exercise
- is bilateral, throbbing in nature at onset and may develop migrainous features in those patients susceptible to migraine
- lasts from 5 minutes to 24 hours
- is prevented by avoiding excessive exertion
- is not associated with any systemic or intracranial disorder.

The onset of the headache is with straining and Valsalva maneuvers such as those seen in weightlifting and competitive swimming. The major differential diagnosis is subarachnoid hemorrhage, which needs to be excluded by the appropriate investigations.

It has been postulated that exertional headache is due to dilatation of the pain-sensitive venous sinuses at the base of the brain as a result of increased cerebral arterial pressure due to exertion. Studies of weightlifters have shown that systolic blood pressure may reach levels above 400 mmHg and diastolic pressures above 300 mmHg with maximal lifts.

A similar type of headache is described in relation to sexual activity and has been termed benign sex headache or orgasmic cephalalgia (IHS 4.6).

The management of this condition involves either avoiding the precipitating activity or drug treatment, for example, indomethacin (25 mg three times a day). In practise, the headaches tend to recur over weeks to months and then slowly resolve, although in some cases they may be lifelong.

Exertional migraine

Exertional migraine shows the typical pattern of migraine with exertion as the precipitating factor. Most patients with this condition describe the migraine beginning immediately after exercise, more frequently when the exercise has been vigorous. Exertional migraine is often severe and may be worse in hot weather. Treatment is based on standard migraine treatment.

Post-traumatic headache

Trauma to the head and neck in sport may lead to the development of headache. The initiating traumatic event may not necessarily be severe. The IHS diagnostic criteria for post-traumatic headache are shown in Table 14.4.

There are a number of specific subtypes of post-traumatic headaches and these are outlined below.

Post-traumatic migraine

This may be seen in sports such as soccer, where repetitive heading of the ball gives rise to the term 'footballer's migraine'.[8] Even mild head trauma can induce migraine. One particular syndrome that is recognized in the setting of minor head blows is migrainous cortical blindness. This disturbing condition often raises fear of serious cerebral injury but tends to resolve over 1–2 hours.

Extra-cranial vascular headache

There is a tendency to develop periodic headaches at the site of head or scalp trauma. These headaches may share a number of migrainous features, although at times they can be described as 'jabbing' pains.

Table 14.4 The International Headache Society (IHS) criteria for the diagnosis of acute post-traumatic headache (IHS 5.1–5.2)

A. Significant head trauma as documented by:
   1. Loss of consciousness
   2. Post-traumatic amnesia >10 minutes
   3. At least two abnormalities of the following: clinical examination, skull X-ray, neuroimaging, evoked potentials, cerebrospinal fluid examination, vestibular function test, neuropsychological testing
B. Headache onset <14 days post-trauma
C. Headache disappears within 8 weeks after trauma

Dysautonomic cephalalgia

Dysautonomic cephalalgia occurs in association with trauma to the anterior triangle of the neck, resulting in injury to the sympathetic fibers alongside the carotid artery. This results in autonomic symptoms such as Horner's syndrome and excessive sweating associated with a unilateral headache. Propranolol has been used with some success in the management of this condition.

External compression headache

External compression headache (IHS 4.2), formerly known as 'swim goggle headache', presents with pain in the facial and temporal areas produced from wearing excessively tight face masks or swimming goggles. It is commonly seen in swimmers and divers. In divers, this may be referred to as 'mask squeeze', and is seen on descent to depth as the effects of pressure reduce the air space inside the mask. The etiology is believed to be due to continuous stimulation of cutaneous nerves by the application of pressure.

High-altitude headache

High-altitude headache (IHS 10.1.1) is a well-recognized accompaniment of acute mountain sickness, which occurs within 24 hours of ascent to altitudes above 23 000 m. The headaches are vascular in nature and are seen in unacclimatized individuals. Typically these are associated with other physiological effects of altitude or may be an early manifestation of acute mountain sickness. The treatment is to descend to lower altitude, although pharmacological interventions such as acetazolamide, ibuprofen and sumatriptan may be used.

Hypercapnia headache

Hypercapnia headache (IHS 10.2) or 'diver's headache' is a vascular type of headache thought to be due to carbon dioxide accumulation during 'skip' breathing. The arterial P_{CO_2} level is usually increased above 50 mmHg in the absence of hypoxia. Divers are also prone to headaches from other causes such as cold exposure, muscular or temporomandibular joint pain from gripping the mouthpiece too tightly,

cervicogenic headaches from incorrect buoyancy technique, middle ear and sinus barotrauma, and cerebral decompression illness.

Recommended Reading

Boyling JD, Jull GA, eds. *Grieve's Modern Manual Therapy*. 3rd edn. Edinburgh: Churchill Livingstone, 2004.

Jensen S. Neck related causes of headache. *Aust Fam Physician* 2005; 34(8): 635–9.

McCrory P. Headaches and exercise. *Sports Med* 2000; 30: 221–9.

Sallis RE, Jones K. Prevalence of headaches in footballers. *Med Sci Sports Exerc* 2000; 32(11): 1820–4.

Turner J. Exercise-related headache. *Curr Sports Med Rep* 2003; 2: 15–17.

References

1. International Headache Society Headache Classification Committee. Classification and diagnostic criteria for headache disorders, cranial neuralgias and facial pain. *Cephalalgia* 1988; 8(7S): 1–96.

2. McCrory P, Heywood J, Ugoni A. Open label study of intranasal sumatriptan (Imigran) for footballer's headache. *Br J Sports Med* 2005; 39: 552–4.

3. Merskey H, Bogduk N. *Classification of Chronic Pain*. Seattle, WA: IASP Press, 1994: 94–5.

4. Sjaastad O, Fredriksen TA, Pfaffenrath V. Cervicogenic headache: diagnostic criteria. *Headache* 1998; 38: 442–5.

5. Jull GA, Niere KR. The cervical spine and headache. In: Boyling JD, Jull GA, eds. *Grieve's Modern Manual Therapy*. 3rd edn. Edinburgh: Churchill Livingstone, 2004: 291–310.

6. Jull GA, Falla D, Treleaven J, et al. A therapeutic exercise approach for cervical disorders. In: Boyling JD, Jull GA, eds. *Grieve's Modern Manual Therapy*. 3rd edn. Edinburgh: Churchill Livingstone, 2004: 451–70.

7. Jull GA, Trott P, Potter H, et al. A randomized controlled trial of exercise and manipulative therapy for cervicogenic headache. *Spine* 2002; 27(17): 1835–43.

8. Matthews W. Footballer's migraine. *BMJ* 1972; 2: 326–7.

Facial Injuries

Injuries to the face in sport usually result from direct trauma. This chapter outlines management of injuries to the nose, ears, eyes, teeth and facial bones.

Functional anatomy

The bones of the face are shown in Figure 15.1. As most of these bones are subcutaneous, they are easily

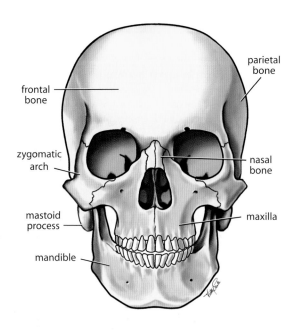

Figure 15.1 Facial bones

examined. Examination should include palpation of the forehead and supraorbital rims for irregularities and contour deformities.

The orbit is a cone-shaped cavity formed by the union of seven cranial and facial bones. The orbital margin consists of the supraorbital ridge above, the infraorbital margin below, the zygomatic arch laterally and the nasal bone medially. The recess formed protects the eye from a blow from a large object. A smaller, deformable object such as a squash ball may, nevertheless, compress the eyeball and cause a 'blow-out' fracture of the orbit.

The zygomatic arch of the malar bone creates the prominence of the cheek. Fractures in this region may cause flattening of the cheek and a palpable irregularity in the inferior orbital margin.

The maxilla forms the upper jaw. Its superior surface helps create the floor of the orbit and the inferior surface forms the major part of the hard palate. Mobility of the hard palate, determined by grasping the central incisors, indicates a maxillary fracture.

The lower jaw consists of the horseshoe-shaped mandible. The mandible is made up of body, angle and ramus, which are easily palpated. The coronoid process can be palpated by a direct intraoral approach. The gingiva overlying the alveolar ridge may be lacerated in mandibular body fractures.

Assessment

Facial injuries[1] are frequently associated with profuse bleeding, however, while it is important to control the bleeding, it is also vital to assess the underlying structures fully. All head and neck injuries should be considered closed head injuries. Cervical spine precautions should be taken if the patient is unconscious or has neurological deficits or cervical spine tenderness. The airway is particularly vulnerable to obstruction because of bleeding, structural compromise of bony structures (e.g. mandible), or dislodged teeth, tooth fragments or dental appliances.

The mechanism of injury should be ascertained and the source of the patient's pain located. Signs or symptoms of blurred vision, diplopia, concussion or cerebrospinal compromise should be evaluated. Immediate attention should focus on:

1. identifying areas of bruising or active bleeding
2. inspecting the nasal septum and external ear for hematomas and nasal obstruction
3. observing facial asymmetry or structural depressions
4. looking for a sunken eye globe suggestive of a blow-out fracture
5. observing lacerations or deep abrasions overlying suspected fractures.

Systematic palpation of the facial bones (orbital rims, nasal bones, temporomandibular joints) will reveal significant tenderness, crepitus, numbness or contour irregularities. Midface instability or crepitus may be demonstrated by stabilizing the forehead with one hand while gently pulling on the maxillary incisors with the other gloved hand. Bimanual palpation along the mandible and maxilla (one gloved hand palpating intraorally) will uncover instability, irregularity or tenderness.

Extraocular eye movements and cranial nerves III, IV and VI can be assessed by having the patient keep his or her chin in a fixed position while tracking the examiner's finger movements in all four quadrants. If the patient is able to track the movements without reporting diplopia, acute extraocular nerve entrapment caused by an orbital blow-out fracture can be ruled out. An inability to raise the eyebrow or wrinkle the forehead following laceration to the eyebrow suggests injury to the temporal branch of the facial nerve on that side. Reduced sensation over the skin below the eye in the distribution of the infraorbital nerve may be associated with a blow-out fracture of the orbit. The nerve distribution includes the upper gum and lip.

If the patient is unable to open his or her mouth or exhibits severe pain along the lateral aspect of the cheek or jaw when attempting to open, a fracture of the mandible or zygoma must be considered. With the mouth open, the oral cavity should be assessed to rule out damage to the teeth and lacerations in the intraoral mucosa or tongue. Locate fractured or missing teeth, when possible, to avoid accidental

aspiration. When asked to close the mouth, the patient's sense of malocclusion suggests a significant fracture of the mandible, maxilla or palate.

Leakage of cerebrospinal fluid (CSF) following a blow to the nose (CSF rhinorrhea) may indicate a fracture of the base of the anterior cranial fossa. CSF is a clear discharge and the patient may report a salty taste in the mouth. If there is doubt about the origin of a nasal discharge associated with trauma, the discharge should be tested with a urinary dipstick for glucose. CSF is positive for glucose.

A list of common conditions and conditions not to be missed is shown in Table 15.1.

Soft tissue injuries

Contusions and lacerations to the face and scalp are a common occurrence, particularly in sports such as football, ice hockey, martial arts and racquet sports.[1] Examination should include palpation of the underlying bone to detect bony tenderness. Neurological examination is required if there is a history of loss of consciousness or suspected skull fracture.

Begin immediate management with ice and pressure to reduce local swelling. Control bleeding with direct pressure over the wound using sterile gauze. A player with a bleeding wound must be removed from the field of play immediately as there is concern that the presence of blood may increase the risk of hepatitis B or human immunodeficiency virus (HIV) infection for other players (Chapter 51).

After removing the athlete from the field of play, examine the laceration closely under good light. Further cleaning and removal of foreign bodies may be required. If necessary, infiltrate a local anesthetic agent to clean the wound adequately. The local anesthetic used should be 1% or 2% lignocaine (lidocaine) containing adrenalin (epinephrine) 1:100 000 to provide some vasoconstriction as well as analgesia.

Lacerations greater than 0.25–0.5 cm (0.1–0.2 in.) long should be closed if they appear clean. Closure may be obtained by suturing or by taping with adhesive strips (Steristrips). Steristrips are ideal for small wounds; however, persistent bleeding or excessive sweating may prevent adhesion. To overcome this, tincture of benzoin (friar's balsam) may be applied to increase adhesiveness. Adequate dressings will be required to keep the adhesive strips in place, especially if the player is returning to the field. Scalp wounds often bleed profusely. Small wounds can be controlled with local pressure but larger ones require suturing.

If facial lacerations require suturing, use 5/0 or 6/0 nylon. It is important that the skin edges are

Table 15.1 Facial injuries in sport

Category	Common	Less common	Not to be missed
Facial soft tissue	Contusion Laceration		
Nose	Fracture of nasal bones Epistaxis	Fracture of nasal septum Septal hematoma	

Ear	Contusion ('cauliflower ear')
	Otitis media
	Otitis externa
		Laceration
		Ruptured tympanic
		  membrane
			Fractured petrous temporal
			  bone
			Torn auditory nerve

Eye	Corneal abrasion Corneal foreign body Conjunctival foreign body Subconjunctival hemorrhage Eyelid laceration	Chemical burns Vitreous hemorrhage Retinal hemorrhage Retinal edema Hyphema	Corneal laceration Retinal detachment Lens dislocation Blow-out fracture of the orbit Optic nerve injury Injury to lacrimal system
Teeth	Enamel chip fracture Luxated tooth Avulsed tooth	Crown fracture	
Facial bones	Temporomandibular joint sprain or malalignment	Fractured maxilla Fractured mandible	

healthy. Pieces of devitalized skin should be debrided. Take care to approximate the skin edges carefully while suturing. Remove sutures after five days and place adhesive strips over the wound for a further week. The wound should be kept dry for at least 48 hours.

An alternative to suturing is skin staples, particularly as these can be inserted more quickly than sutures. If the player is returning to the field of play, staples must be covered. This prevents them from being accidentally torn out or from injuring another player in a collision. Another alternative is the use of histoacryl glue.

Deep wounds require closure in appropriate layers. Deep forehead and scalp lacerations involve damage to the galea aponeurotica. This layer should be closed with interrupted 5/0 absorbable sutures prior to skin closure.

Lacerations of the eyebrow and lip require strict anatomical approximation. Eyebrow hair should not be shaved. In lacerations involving the vermilion border of the lip, accurate alignment is obtained by placing the first suture at the mucocutaneous junction.

Full thickness lacerations of the lip require a three layer closure, preferably performed by a plastic surgeon. The oral mucosa is closed first, then the orbicularis oris layer and finally skin. Deep intraoral lacerations should be closed with 3/0 silk sutures that should remain in place for one week.

All patients with potentially contaminated wounds should receive tetanus prophylaxis and a short course of oral antibiotic therapy, for example, cephalexin (250–500 mg, 6 hourly) or flucloxacillin (250–500 mg, 6 hourly). Wounds that may be contaminated by another player's saliva, such as bite wounds, should not be closed but should be cleaned meticulously. The player should be treated with oral metronidazole (400 mg, 8 hourly) in addition to penicillin and observed very closely for the development of cellulitis. If signs of infection appear, treat with intravenous antibiotics.

Nose

Nasal injuries are common in contact sports such as football and boxing.

Epistaxis (nosebleed)

Nasal hemorrhage occurs frequently in association with nasal injuries. It usually arises from the nasal septum, which receives its blood supply from branches of the internal and external carotid arteries. In most cases, the bleeding arises from a rich plexus of vessels in the anterior part of the septum, known as Little's or Kiesselbach's area (Fig. 15.2).

Initial management consists of prolonged direct digital pressure on the lower nose for up to 20 minutes,

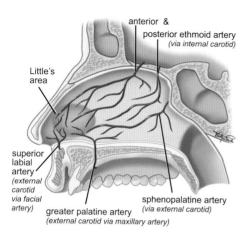

anterior &
posterior ethmoid artery
(via internal carotid)

Little's
area

superior
labial
artery
*(external
carotid
via facial
artery)*

greater palatine artery
(external carotid via maxillary artery)

sphenopalatine artery
(via external carotid)

Figure 15.2 Little's (Kiesselbach's) area

compressing the vessels on the nasal septum with the patient sitting upright. Cold compresses over the bridge of the nose promote vasoconstriction. If bleeding continues, apply cotton wool soaked in adrenalin (epinephrine) 1:1000 to the nasal septum. If the bleeding site can be located, it may be cauterized with silver nitrate applicators (cotton swabs soaked in 4% trichloracetic acid).

If bleeding persists, specialist referral is indicated. The nose will usually be packed with 1 cm (0.5 in.) ribbon gauze impregnated with bismuth iodoform petroleum paste (BIPP) and left for 48 hours. Post-nasal packing may be required if the bleeding originates from the back of the nose. In the rare cases that bleeding persists despite these local measures, maxillary artery or anterior ethmoidal artery ligation may be indicated.

Nasal fractures

Fractures of the nose are usually caused by a direct blow. Symptoms and signs of nasal fracture include pain, epistaxis, swelling, crepitus, deformity and mobility of the nose. Nasal distortion may not be obvious once soft tissue swelling develops. Initial management is directed towards controlling the nasal hemorrhage. An associated laceration should be sutured with 6/0 nylon and requires prophylactic antibiotic therapy. The nasal passages should be examined to exclude a septal hematoma and patients should be advised to return if they notice increased pain or develop a fever (see below).

X-rays are probably not required as undisplaced fractures require no treatment and displaced fractures are clinically obvious. Displaced nasal fractures may

require reduction. There are two indications for reduction of fractures. The first is obstruction of the nasal passages and the second is cosmetic deformity.

In young athletes, displaced fractures are almost always reduced because of a tendency towards increased sinus infections and a decrease in the size of the nasal passage. Attempts at immediate reduction of nasal fractures are associated with a risk of arterial damage and severe acute hemorrhage. Thus, it is preferable to delay fracture reduction and refer the patient to a surgeon within seven days of the injury. When the soft tissue swelling has settled sufficiently, reduction, if necessary, can be carried out under general anesthesia.

Many sportspeople decide to delay reduction of their nasal fracture, provided there is no obstruction to the nasal passages, until a more convenient time such as the end of a season or at the time of retirement from contact sports.

Septal hematoma

This important condition can complicate what seems to be a trivial nosebleed. A septal hematoma is caused by hemorrhage between the two layers of mucosa covering the septum. The presenting complaint is either nasal obstruction or nasal pain. The patient may be febrile and nasal examination reveals a cherry-like structure (the dull, red swollen septum) that occludes the nasal passages. Treatment of a large septal hematoma involves evacuation of the clot using a wide-bore needle or through a small incision followed by nasal packing to prevent recurrence of the hematoma. Antibiotic prophylaxis should be given to prevent development of a septal abscess and subsequent cartilage necrosis.

Ear

Ear injuries in sport are not common. The most frequent injury is a contusion to the ear known as an auricular hematoma.

Auricular hematoma

This injury occurs mainly in Rugby scrums, boxing or wrestling as a result of a shearing blow. Recurrent contusions result in hemorrhage between the perichondrium and the cartilage. This may eventually develop into a chronic swelling, commonly known as 'cauliflower ear'. An acute hematoma (Fig. 15.3) should be treated initially with ice and firm compression, but may need to be drained by aspiration under strict aseptic conditions. A pressure dressing (cotton wool soaked in collodion) is then applied and is carefully

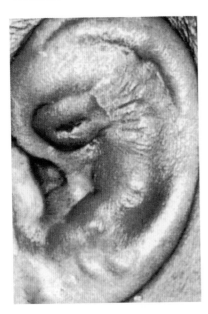

Figure 15.3 Acute auricular hematoma

packed against the ear to follow the contours of the outer ear. This is bandaged firmly. The ear must be examined daily to assess progress. Return to non-contact sports can be immediate, but headgear or a helmet is required for return to contact sport. Rugby forwards frequently wear headgear which protects their ears as a preventive measure.

Lacerations to the ear require careful cleansing and suture. As lacerations located between the scalp and the ear are easily missed, this area should always be examined, especially if there is a history of the ear being pulled forwards. Tears of the auricular cartilage should be carefully aligned and sutured with absorbable 5/0 sutures. The perichondrium should be closed as a separate layer. Prophylactic oral antibiotic therapy is recommended.

Perforated eardrum

A blow across the side of the head may occasionally injure the eardrum. Pain, bleeding from the ear or impaired hearing suggest tympanic membrane rupture. These ruptures usually heal spontaneously. Prophylactic antibiotic therapy (amoxycillin [amoxicillin] 250–500 mg 8 hourly if not allergic to penicillin) should be administered. It is important to keep the ear dry while a perforation is present. In sports where significant pressure changes occur, such as platform diving, scuba diving and high-altitude mountain climbing, athletes should not return to play until the tympanic membrane has healed. Athletes participating in water sports, such as swimming and water polo, should use custom-fabricated ear plugs to maintain a dry ear canal. Dry land athletes may return to play as soon as any vertigo has resolved.[1]

A severe blow across the head may fracture the skull and cause inner ear bleeding. Discharge from the ear (otorrhea) may signal a neurosurgical emergency and, thus, patients should be referred immediately for specialist treatment.

Otitis externa

Otitis externa is the most common ear condition affecting competitive swimmers. It is generally caused by bacteria, although fungal infection can also contribute. Symptoms include earache, pruritus, discharge and impaired hearing. On examination, there may be discharge in the ear and local redness along the external auditory meatus. There may be tragal tenderness and pain on tragal pull.

Management involves careful aural toilet combined with topical antibiotic and corticosteroid ear drops. The patient should, preferably, abstain from swimming until fully recovered and avoid rubbing or drying the ear until after the infection has cleared. The use of earplugs in this condition is controversial. They may traumatize the ear canal and predispose the swimmer to infection. Recurrent attacks of otitis externa may be prevented by instillation of alcohol ear drops, for example, 5% acetic acid in isopropyl alcohol (Aquaear), after each swimming session.

Eye

Eye injuries are seen most commonly in stick sports, racquet sports, especially squash, and contact sports.[2] All eye injuries, even those that appear to be minor, require thorough examination. All serious eye injuries should be referred immediately to an ophthalmologist. The most difficult dilemma for the clinician in dealing with eye injuries is determining which injury is serious and requires immediate referral. The indications for immediate referral to an ophthalmologist are shown in the box opposite.

Athletes with a previous history of impaired vision in one or both eyes or previous eye trauma or surgery should be evaluated by an ophthalmologist prior to participating in a high-risk sport.

Assessment of the injured eye

To assess the injured eye properly, it is important to understand the relevant anatomy. The anatomy of the eye is shown in Figure 15.4.

Indications for immediate referral to a specialist ophthalmologist

Symptoms

Severe eye pain
Persistent blurred or double vision
Persistent photophobia

Signs

Suspected penetrating injury (corneal laceration, pear-shaped pupil)
Hyphema
Embedded foreign body
No view of fundus (suspected vitreous hemorrhage or retinal detachment)
Markedly impaired visual acuity: 6/12 or less
Loss of part of visual field

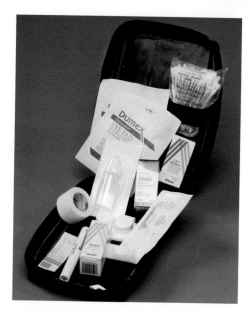

Figure 15.5 Eye injuries kit

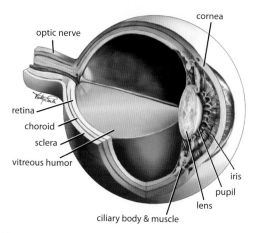

Figure 15.4 Anatomy of the eye

For a thorough assessment of the injured eye, an 'eye injuries kit' (Fig. 15.5) is very useful and can be carried as part of the 'physician's bag' (Chapter 58). The kit includes a small mirror, a pencil torch, an ophthalmoscope, a sterile solution for irrigation, local anesthetic eye drops (e.g. amethocaine), fluorescein, antibiotic drops and ointments, cotton buds, contact lens lubricant and case, eye patches, tape and a Snellen chart to assess visual acuity.

The history of the eye injury provides useful diagnostic information. Seek to discover the history of the mechanism of injury. Were glasses, contact lenses or a protective device being worn at the time of injury? Note any previous eye injury or problems. Ask about

symptoms such as pain, blurred vision, loss of vision, flashing lights and diplopia (double vision).

Test the visual acuity of each eye using a Snellen chart, with and without glasses or contact lenses. If a Snellen chart is not available, use pages of a newspaper with variable print sizes as an approximate assessment of visual acuity. On the sporting arena, a scoreboard can be used to test distant vision.

Inspect the eyelids for bruising, swelling or laceration. Note any obvious foreign body, hemorrhage or change in pupil size.

If pain or photophobia due to the injury prevent examination of the eye, instil a drop of a sterile topical anesthetic agent, such as amethocaine, to assist examination.

Inspect the cornea for foreign material and abrasions. Fluorescein staining will help reveal areas of corneal ulceration or foreign bodies. Evert the upper lid to exclude the presence of a subtarsal foreign body.

Test eye movements in all directions. A restriction in any direction or the presence of diplopia may indicate orbital fracture. Compare the size, shape and light reaction of the pupil with the uninjured eye. An enlarged, poorly reacting pupil may be present after injury to the iris. A pear-shaped pupil suggests the presence of a full thickness corneal or scleral laceration (penetrating injury).

Inspect the anterior chamber for the presence of blood. Blood in the anterior chamber is known as hyphema (Fig. 15.6).

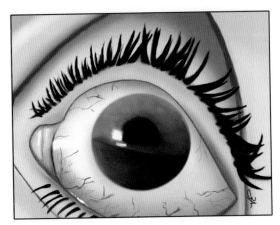

Figure 15.6 Hyphema—note the fluid level in the anterior chamber

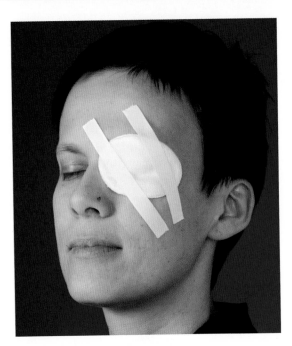

Figure 15.7 Eye padding

Ophthalmoscopic examination should routinely be performed to inspect the lens, vitreous humor and retina. The absence of a red reflex on ophthalmoscopic examination may be due to a corneal opacity, a lens opacity (cataract), intraocular bleeding or a retinal detachment. Failure to visualize the fundus may be a sign of vitreous hemorrhage, which can result from a retinal tear. Contusion of the retina may produce retinal edema, seen as areas of pallor (and thickening) as well as retinal hemorrhage.

Radiological examination of the orbit is indicated in all cases of traumatic eye injury with diplopia and in cases where an intraocular or intraorbital foreign body is suspected.

Corneal injuries: abrasions and foreign body

Corneal injuries in sport include abrasion, foreign body and, less commonly, alkali burn. Corneal abrasion, one of the most frequent injuries to the eye during sport, occurs as a result of a scratch from either a fingernail or foreign body. The patient complains of pain, a sensation of a foreign body being present in the eye and blurred vision if the central cornea is involved.

A topical anesthetic drop should be instilled to assist in corneal examination. Fluorescein staining will help locate corneal abrasions or foreign bodies. Evert the upper lid to exclude a subtarsal foreign body.

Treatment of corneal abrasions includes the instillation of antibiotic eye drops, for example, chloramphenicol, and padding of the eye (Fig. 15.7). If pain and photophobia are severe, add a topical mydriatic, for example, 2% homatropine. A local anesthetic agent should never be used for pain relief as it can delay healing and result in further damage.

Corneal foreign bodies can be removed with a cotton tip applicator by an appropriately trained practitioner. If they are more deeply embedded, patients should be referred to an ophthalmologist for removal of the foreign body. Rust rings, which occasionally remain after metallic foreign bodies have been embedded in the cornea, require removal by an ophthalmologist. Antibiotic eye ointment should be administered following foreign body removal and the eye padded for 24 hours until the corneal epithelium has healed.

If an athlete has sustained an alkali burn (from line markings), irrigate the eye copiously for 20 minutes with sterile saline or tap water and instil a local anesthetic agent to assist this. The player should be seen as soon as possible by an ophthalmologist.

Subconjunctival hemorrhage

Trauma to the conjunctiva may cause subconjunctival hemorrhage—a bright red area in the white conjunctiva. Unless the hemorrhage is extensive or visual symptoms or photophobia are present, it is not clinically important. Blood pressure should be measured to exclude hypertension. It may, however, obscure a perforation of the globe. If this is suspected, the patient should be referred to an ophthalmologist. In most cases, however, the athlete merely requires reassurance.

Eyelid injuries

In all injuries to the eyelids, the eye also needs to be examined to exclude ocular injury. Direct trauma to the eyelids may cause a large amount of bruising, which should be treated with cold compresses in the first 24 hours. Hemorrhage may spread subcutaneously across the midline to the other eye. A coexisting orbital fracture needs to be excluded in these patients.

Lacerations of the eyelid require meticulous primary repair. Each anatomical layer (conjunctiva, tarsal plate and skin) should be repaired separately by an ophthalmic surgeon.

Trauma near the medial canthus may lacerate the upper or lower lacrimal canaliculus (tear duct). If this is not repaired, the patient may have permanent watering of the eye. Such injuries require ophthalmological referral for microscopic suturing of the cut ends of the canaliculus.

Hyphema

Bleeding into the anterior chamber of the eye results from ruptured iris vessels and may only be visible with slit lamp examination. More significant bleeds will present with a clear layer in the anterior chamber, visible after the blood settles (Fig. 15.6). In hyphemas of small volume, visual acuity may be unaffected. Associated injuries may occur and all patients with a hyphema should be referred to an ophthalmologist.

The aim of treatment of this condition is to prevent further bleeding, which may, in turn, result in uncontrollable glaucoma or blood staining of the cornea. The patient needs to rest in bed while the hemorrhage clears, usually over three to five days. Aspirin and other anti-inflammatory medications should be avoided as these may provoke further bleeding.

Lens dislocation

Blunt trauma may result in varying degrees of lens displacement. Partial dislocation causes few symptoms. Complete lens dislocation results in blurred vision. A common sign of lens dislocation is a quivering of the iris when the patient moves the eye. Iritis and glaucoma are possible sequelae of lens dislocation. Immediate ophthalmological referral is required. Surgical removal of the displaced lens may be indicated.

Vitreous hemorrhage

Bleeding into the vitreous humor signifies damage to the retina, choroid or ciliary body. Ophthalmoscopic examination reveals loss of the red reflex and a hazy appearance. Treatment generally consists of bed rest but more severe cases may require removal of the blood and vitreous humor.

Retinal hemorrhage

Injury to the retina can result from a direct blow to the eye or a blow to the back of the head. Valsalva maneuvers (e.g. in weightlifting) may also produce retinal edema and hemorrhage. The patient may remain asymptomatic if peripheral areas of the retina are affected. Central retinal damage, however, blurs vision. On ophthalmoscopic examination, central retinal edema appears as a white opacity that partially obscures the retinal vessels. Boxers may develop atrophic macular holes and loss of central vision as a result of recurrent contusive injuries.

Retinal detachment

Retinal detachment may result from any blunt or perforating trauma and may occur months or even years after the initial injury. The patient complains of flashes of light or the appearance of a 'curtain' spreading across the field of vision. Ophthalmoscopic examination reveals elevation and folding of the detached retina, which trembles with each eye movement. Immediate referral for surgical treatment is indicated. An unusual case of retinal detachment in sport occurred in a swimmer who received an accidental blow to the goggles.[3]

Orbital injuries

'Blow-out' fracture of the orbit results from direct trauma such as a fist, cricket ball, baseball[4] or squash ball (Fig. 15.8). Compression of the globe and orbital contents produces a fracture in the weakest part of the orbit, the orbital floor. Contents of the orbit may herniate through the defect. The patient typically presents with a periorbital hematoma, protruding or sunken eye, double vision on upward gaze and numbness of the cheek. Double vision on upward gaze is due to the entrapment of the inferior rectus muscle in the fracture.

A detailed examination of the eye must be performed to exclude intraocular injuries such as hyphema, lens dislocation or ruptured globe. If an orbital fracture is suspected, X-ray should be performed. The X-ray may not show the fracture but may demonstrate some clouding of the maxillary sinus. CT examination is used to confirm the fracture.

Antibiotic therapy should be commenced immediately and the patient referred to an ophthalmologist.

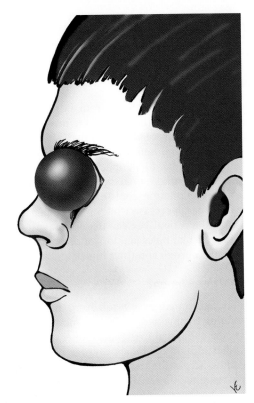

Figure 15.8 A squash ball fits precisely into the eye socket

Surgery may be required to release the trapped muscle and repair the bony defect.

Prevention of eye injuries

Athletes with certain eye problems should avoid contact sports altogether. These problems include:

- functionally only one eye
- severe myopia
- Marfan's syndrome
- previous retinal detachment.

For squash, protective eye wear must be worn by people who have either only one good eye, amblyopia (lazy eye), recent eye surgery, history of preretinal detachment conditions or diabetic retinopathy. Protective eye wear should meet the Australian Standard AS4066 1992 or the US Standard ASTM F803.

Contact lenses offer no protection against eye trauma. Hard contact lenses are not suitable for sporting activity and should never be used in contact sport. Soft lenses appear to be reasonably safe in contact sport. One of the most common 'crises' in

injury management is a lost contact lens. The athlete will complain that the contact lens is no longer in its correct position and cannot be located. Usually the lens has been displaced and with careful examination can be located elsewhere on the eye, often at the lower lid. Occasionally, the lens is displaced completely from the eye and lost on the playing surface. Those who wear contact lenses during sport should always carry a spare pair of contact lenses or a pair of protective spectacles as a back-up.

Those athletes who cannot or do not like to wear contact lenses can use protective goggles made of polycarbonate, which are available for most prescriptions. These polycarbonate goggles are also used as eye protection in sports with a high risk for eye injuries. The most obvious examples of these are squash and racquetball, where the size of the ball enables it to enter the orbit and compress the globe. The routine use of closed goggles is strongly recommended (Fig. 15.9).

Certain sports require protection not only of the eye but of the other facial structures. In sports such as American football, ice hockey, cricket and lacrosse, protective helmets and faceguards should also provide adequate eye protection. Because of the profound effect of major eye injury, we encourage athletes and sport-governing bodies to be proactive in promoting and enforcing the use of eye protection where indicated.[5]

Teeth

Collisions with opponents during contact sports are the most common cause of dental injuries. Direct blows from equipment such as hockey sticks and bats may also injure teeth.

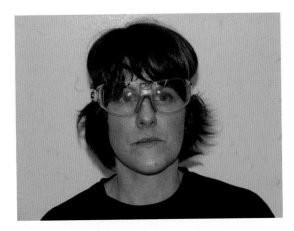

Figure 15.9 Protective goggles

Thorough examination of the oral cavity should be carried out in all cases of facial trauma to detect injuries to the teeth. If a chipped or avulsed tooth cannot be found, chest and abdominal X-ray may be required to locate the missing fragment.

Enamel chip fractures are not painful and require non-urgent dental referral. Crown fractures that expose the dentine are painful when exposed to air, heat or cold and require urgent dental referral. A severe crown injury exposing the dental pulp requires immediate dental referral. The fractured tooth fragment should be retained in milk.

Occasionally, a forceful blow causes a tooth or teeth to be luxated or moved. These teeth should be repositioned to their original site using firm finger pressure and subsequently splinted with aluminium foil prior to dental referral.

Tooth avulsion may also occur as a result of a direct blow. The tooth may be saved by quick and appropriate action.[6] The critical time is in the first 15 minutes following the injury. An avulsed tooth should be retrieved and handled by the crown. If dirty, it should be irrigated with sterile saline solution or milk, or sucked clean under the tongue. Debris should not be scraped off the root. If the patient is conscious and alert, the tooth should then be reimplanted and splinted. It is essential to confirm that the labial and lingual surfaces of the tooth are in proper position by comparison with the adjacent teeth. When the tooth has been implanted into the proper position the patient should be asked to bite on sterile gauze and be transported immediately for dental treatment. If the patient is not fully alert, the tooth can be stored in a suitable medium such as a glass jar, paper cup or sealable plastic bag containing sterile saline or fresh milk, preferably skim milk, for transport and the patient immediately referred to a dentist. With suitable storage, the tooth may be successfully reimplanted by the dentist within 2 hours of the injury.

Prevention of dental injuries

Most dental injuries can be prevented or reduced in severity by the wearing of an effective mouthguard. The standard 'one size fits all' mouthguard has limited effectiveness and a custom-made mouthguard fitted by a dentist should be worn in sports where the risk of dental injury is high. In youth sports, parents, as well as coaches, should take responsibility for ensuring that competitors wear mouthguards.[7] Sports such as basketball, baseball and soccer have a higher rate of dental injuries than many parents and athletes realize. Medical personnel should encourage mouthguard use

in these sports, in addition to the traditional contact sports such as American football, Rugby, ice hockey and wrestling.

Bimaxillary mouthguards are also available to cover both the upper and lower teeth. These tend to make breathing and speech difficult and are not popular with sportspeople.

Mouthguards should be kept in a plastic box and regularly rinsed with an antiseptic mouthwash. They should not be allowed to overheat as they will deform.

Fractures of facial bones

In sport, facial fractures may result from blows by implements such as bats or sticks, equipment such as skis[8] and from collision injuries. Mountain biking is a sport that causes a significant proportion of facial injuries. It appears that eye wear can protect against facial injuries.[9]

Symptoms and signs range from pain, swelling, laceration and bruising to gross deformity. Examination may reveal facial asymmetry, discoloration or obvious deformity. The bite should be examined for malocclusion. Bimanual examination of the facial bones may show areas of discontinuity and mobility. If maxillary fracture is suspected, the upper teeth can be grasped to determine evidence of excessive movement of the upper jaw and midface. Opening and closing the jaw may reveal pain, limitation or deviation with mandibular injuries.

Initial management of facial fractures is directed towards maintenance of the patient's airway. In mandibular body fractures or maxillary fractures, this may require emergency manual reduction. Associated head and cervical spine injuries should be excluded. The oral cavity requires inspection for bleeding or dental damage.

Fractures of the zygomaticomaxillary complex

Zygomaticomaxillary complex fractures (Fig. 15.10) occur from a direct blow to the cheek such as from a fist, hockey stick or baseball. Signs include swelling and bruising, flatness of the cheek and mandibular function disturbance. If associated with an orbital fracture, there may be concomitant diplopia, numbness of the affected cheek, limitation of ocular movement and asymmetry of the eyes.

Surgical treatment consists of closed or open reduction under general anesthesia. Unstable fractures require fixation. Associated orbital fractures

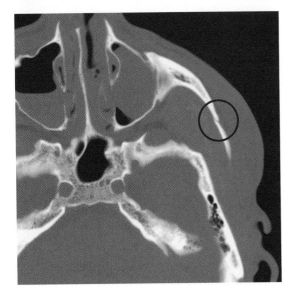

Figure 15.10 CT scan confirming a fractured zygomatic arch; plain radiography did not detect the fracture

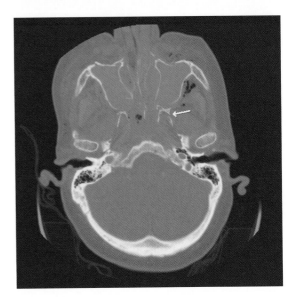

Figure 15.11 CT scan of Le Fort III fracture

are treated by open reduction and reconstruction of the orbital floor.

Maxillary fractures

Maxillary fractures usually result from a direct crushing blow to the middle portion of the face such as from a hockey stick, a baseball or collision. They are classified as Le Fort I, II and III fractures depending on whether the nasal or cheek bones are involved. Le Fort I fractures result in the separation of the maxilla from the nasal–septal structures and the pterygoid plates. Clinically, Le Fort I fractures are identified when the entire maxilla moves as a separate unit. Le Fort II fractures separate the maxilla and the nasal complex from the orbital–zygomatic structures. On clinical examination the maxilla and nose move together as one unit. Le Fort III fractures separate the maxillary, zygomatic, nasal and orbital structures from the cranial base (Fig. 15.11).[10]

Maxillary fractures are often accompanied by cranial damage, obstruction of the nasal airway, edema of the soft palate, hemorrhage into the sinuses and disturbance of the contents of the orbit. CSF rhinorrhea may occur, indicating fracture of the cribriform plate. Reduced sensation in the infraorbital region is common.

Examination findings include lengthening of the face, midface mobility, malocclusion of the bite and periorbital bruising. Initial treatment is aimed at protecting the airway—the conscious patient should

sit leaning forward. This should be followed by rapid transfer for definitive diagnosis and treatment. Surgical treatment involves reduction and fixation with wires, screws or a plate.

Mandibular fractures

Fracture of the mandible is one of the most common facial fractures in sport and usually results from a direct blow. The most common fracture sites are the mandibular angle and the condyle. The mandible usually breaks in more than one place as a result of the trauma and these fractures usually occur on opposite sides of the midline. Fractures may be displaced or undisplaced.

Undisplaced fractures

Minor mandibular fractures are painful, tender and swollen. These are managed conservatively with analgesia and rest. The patient should eat soft food only for up to four weeks as symptoms resolve.

Displaced mandibular fractures

Displaced mandibular fractures are severe injuries that result from considerable force. Alveolar (tooth-bearing) fractures are the most common type. These fractures range from single tooth fractures or avulsions to complete segment mobility. The clinical diagnosis is obvious when two or more teeth move as a unit.

Inspection may reveal malalignment of teeth and bruising to the floor of the mouth. Palpation reveals malocclusion, tenderness and defects along the lower border of the mandible. Paresthesia or anesthesia of the lower lip and chin suggest damage to the inferior alveolar nerve.

Initial treatment includes maintenance of the airway in a forward sitting position with the patient's hands supporting the lower jaw. A jaw bandage can be used in comminuted or badly displaced fractures but needs to be applied with caution as it may compromise the airway by causing backward displacement of the mandible. A cervical collar can be used as an alternative. A concussed or unconscious patient should be placed in a lateral position with head tilt and jaw support after the mouth has been cleared of any dislodged teeth or tooth fragments. Occasionally, the tongue may need to be held forward to maintain an open airway.

Most displaced mandibular fractures require closed reduction and intermaxillary fixation for four to six weeks. If adequate closed reduction cannot be achieved, then open reduction and internal fixation is required. A fracture of one condyle usually does not require immobilization except to control pain. Active jaw exercises should be commenced as soon as pain permits.

During the period of intermaxillary fixation, the athlete may perform mild exercises such as stationary bike riding and light weightlifting. Resumption of contact sport should be delayed until at least one to two months after the jaws are unwired. Earlier resumption is possible when internal fixation has been used. The use of a protective polycarbonate facial shield may offer some protection if early return to play is contemplated.

Patients with mandibular fractures who are eating soft food or have their jaws wired must be referred to a dietitian for dietary advice. It is important to maintain weight and strength during the period of wiring. A dietitian will advise on suitable liquid meals and foods suitable for vitamizing.

Temporomandibular injuries

Blows to the mandible can produce a variety of temporomandibular joint (TMJ) injuries. Trauma to the jaw while the mouth is open occasionally produces TMJ dislocation. Other injuries include hemarthrosis, meniscal displacement and intracapsular fracture of the head of the condyle.

Examination of the injured TMJ may reveal limitation of opening, pain and malocclusion. Dislocation of the TMJ causes inability to close the mouth. A dislocated TMJ may be reduced by placing both thumbs along the line of the lower teeth as far posteriorly as possible and applying downward and backward pressure. Longstanding dislocations may require general anesthesia for reduction. Management of TMJ dislocation includes rest with limitation of mouth opening for up to seven to 10 days, a soft diet and analgesics such as aspirin. Contact sport should be avoided for up to two weeks depending on the symptoms. Boxers should not attempt sparring for at least six weeks.

Chronic TMJ problems are sometimes referred to as 'temporomandibular joint dysfunction' or 'myofascial pain dysfunction syndrome'. This syndrome appears to affect males more than females with a peak incidence in the early twenties. Patients complain of pain, limitation of movement, clicking and locking of the TMJ. Treatment is difficult but should include assessment by a dentist to exclude any malocclusion problem, as well as exercise therapy.

Prevention of facial injuries

Protective equipment has been designed for sports where facial injury is a risk (Chapter 6). Properly designed helmets have reduced the incidence of faciomaxillary injuries. Ideally, helmets should be individually fitted for each athlete. Helmets are designed for a single impact or multiple impact. Single-impact helmets such as most pushbike and motorbike helmets must be discarded after the user has had a fall.

Recommended Reading

Echlin P, McKeag DB. Maxillofacial injuries in sport. *Curr Sports Med Rep* 2004; 3: 25–32.

Echlin PS, Upshur REG, Peck DM, et al. Craniomaxillofacial injury in sport: a review of prevention research. *Br J Sports Med* 2005; 39: 254–63.

Gassner R, Hackl W, Tuli T, et al. Facial injuries in skiing. A retrospective study of 549 cases. *Sports Med* 1999; 27: 127–34.

Harrison A, Telander DG. Eye injuries in the young athlete: a case-based report. *Pediatr Ann* 2002; 31: 33–4.

Kaufman BR, Heckler FR. Sports-related facial injuries. *Clin Sports Med* 1997; 16: 543–62.

Newsome PRH, Tran DC, Cooke MS. The role of the mouthguard in the prevention of sports related dental injuries: a review. *Int J Paediatr Dent* 2001; 11: 396–404.

Petrigliano FA, Williams RJ. Orbital fractures in sport: a review. *Sports Med* 2003; 33: 317–22.

Ranalli DN. Dental injuries in sports. *Curr Sports Med Rep* 2005; 4: 12–17.

Ranalli DN, Demas PN. Orofacial injuries from sport: preventative measures for sports medicine. *Sports Med* 2002; 32: 409–18.

Romeo SJ, Hawley CJ, Romeo MW, et al. Facial injuries in sports. *Physician Sportsmed* 2005; 33(4): 000–00.

Sports Medicine Australia. *Squash as a Safe Sport. Guidelines.* Canberra: Sports Medicine Australia, 1991.

Vinger PF. A practical guide for sports eye protection. *Physician Sportsmed* 2000; 28: 49–69.

References

1. Romeo SJ, Hawley CJ, Romeo MW et al. Facial injuries in sports: a team physician's guide to diagnosis. *Physician Sportsmed* 2005; 33(4): 45–53.

2. Drolsum L. Eye injuries in sports. *Scand J Med Sci Sports* 1999; 9: 53–6.

3. Killer HE, Blumer BK, Rust ON. Avulsion of the optic disc after a blow to swimming goggles. *J Pediatr Ophthalmol Strabismus* 1999; 36: 92–3.

4. Vinger PF, Duma SM, Crandall J. Baseball hardness as a risk factor for eye injuries. *Arch Ophthalmol* 1999; 117: 354–8.

5. Jones NP. Eye injuries in sport: where next? *Br J Sports Med* 1998; 32: 197–8.

6. Ranalli DN. Dental injuries in sports. *Curr Sports Med Rep* 2005; 4: 12–17.

7. Diab N, Mourino AP. Parental attitudes towards mouthguards. *Pediatr Dent* 1997; 19: 455–60.

8. Gassner R, Ulmer H, Tuli T, et al. Incidence of oral and maxillofacial skiing injuries due to different injury mechanisms. *Br J Oral Maxillofac Surg* 1999; 57: 1068–73.

9. Webster DA, Bayliss GV, Spadaro JA. Head and face injuries in scholastic women's lacrosse with and without eyewear. *Med Sci Sports Exerc* 1999; 31: 938–41.

10. Ranalli DN, Demas PN. Orofacial injuries from sport: preventative measures for sports medicine. *Sports Med* 2002; 32: 409–18.

Neck Pain

WITH MEENA SRAN

This chapter will consider those acute and chronic soft tissue conditions that cause neck pain. Severe neck injuries are considered in Chapter 44.

The surface anatomy of the neck is shown in Figure 16.1. Structures that are likely to cause pain are the cervical disks, apophyseal joints, the ligaments and muscles of the neck, and neural structures.

Clinical perspective

Patients with neck pain may present with articular, muscular and neural system dysfunction and appropriate examination and clinical reasoning can often elucidate the primary source of the problem. Although selective local anesthesia block of each individual spinal structure may be the only way to precisely determine which structure is causing the patient's pain, manual examination accurately identifies the segmental level responsible for a patient's complaint when compared against a spinal block.[1,2] Multimodal treatment, including specific therapeutic exercise and manual therapy, is effective in the treatment of neck pain.[3,4]

The management of neck pain, therefore, requires a thorough history, assessment of the joints, muscles

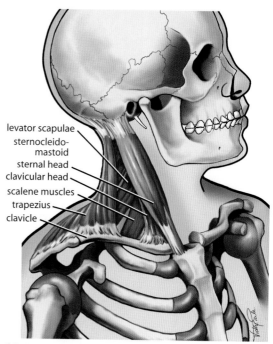

Figure 16.1 Anatomy of the neck

(a) Surface anatomy of the neck from in front

sternocleidomastoid (sternal head)

clavicle

trapezius

levator scapulae
sternocleido-
mastoid
sternal head
clavicular head
scalene muscles
trapezius
clavicle

(b) Anatomy of the anterior neck

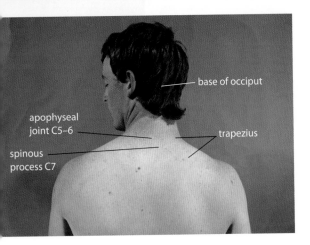

(c) Surface anatomy of the neck from behind

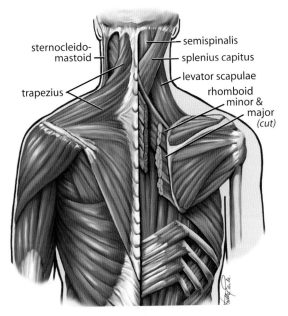

(d) Anatomy of the posterior neck

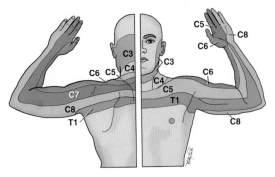

(e) Dermatomal distribution of the neck region

and neural structures, sound clinical reasoning and appropriate treatment to correct the abnormalities found on examination. There are, however, a number of recognizable syndromes associated with neck pain.

The acute wry neck is a well-recognized syndrome causing neck pain. Another is the acute acceleration/deceleration injury commonly known as 'whiplash' injury. Occasionally, patients present with an insidious onset of symptoms associated with nerve root compression, often as the result of a local or general degenerative process.

Patients with mechanical neck pain typically also have a postural component to their condition. In some patients, pain is caused by posture alone—the 'cervical postural syndrome'. Common postural faults seen in the neck region include chin protrusion, usually as a result of prolonged forward head posture (e.g. working at a computer screen). Excessive lordosis of the upper cervical spine can develop with subsequent irritation of the posterior structures (e.g. the apophyseal joints). Abnormalities and deficits in the muscular system are common with this posture.

In the older patient, osteoarthritis may particularly affect the apophyseal joints. Cervical headaches (Chapter 14) constitute 14–18% of all chronic headaches[5, 6] and are often accompanied by neck pain and stiffness.[7] The other common site of referral of pain from the neck is to the shoulder and upper arm (Chapter 17).

History

The location of the symptoms must be determined: whether upper or lower cervical and/or referred to the head, whether primarily central, right-sided or left-sided, or whether there is a generalized ache. The onset of the patient's symptoms is another important feature. It may have been sudden, either due to external trauma or an abnormal movement, or delayed following trauma (e.g. following acute acceleration/deceleration injury [whiplash]). Alternatively, the onset may have been insidious as a result of repetitive movement or prolonged abnormal posture.

The irritability of the pain is assessed by determining how easily the pain is aggravated. If the condition is irritable, the pain may be aggravated by relatively minor movements and may take several minutes to hours to ease. The degree of irritability will influence the examination (limited or full) and the intensity of treatment.

The nature of the pain may give an indication of the likely cause. Severe, lancinating pain referred in a dermatomal distribution (Fig. 16.1e) suggests nerve root compression.

The time relationship of the symptoms may be important if the condition is primarily inflammatory in nature, in which case it is often worse in the morning. If it is due to a mechanical problem, it is often worse with movement. Whether the condition improves during the day, whether it is related to any particular activity, and whether it wakes the patient at night are all important aspects of the history.

Any radiation of the pain to the head, shoulder, interscapular area, upper arm, forearm, hand or fingers should be noted.

Factors that appear to increase the pain give a guide to the possible source of the pain. For example, if reading aggravates pain, it may indicate that prolonged flexion is aggravating a disk problem. If looking up (extension) aggravates the pain, it is more suggestive of an apophyseal joint problem. If talking on the telephone (lateral flexion) produces ipsilateral pain, it may indicate compression of structures exiting the foramen or apophyseal compression. Pain reproduced or aggravated by a combined movement position should also be noted. The effect of lying down, the position of maximum comfort and the number and organization of pillows used to sleep at night should all be considered.

Similarly, any movement or position that reduces the patient's pain should be noted. Such a position may be an indication of a possible initial treatment position. If the pain is not relieved at all, then more serious pathology should be suspected.

Any associated symptoms in the upper arm such as pins and needles, numbness or weakness may be an indication of nerve root involvement. Any symptoms of vertebral artery insufficiency, such as dizziness or syncope with turning, looking up or a sustained position, should be determined.

Previous treatment and the patient's response to that treatment should be noted. General health questions, a recent history of unexplained weight loss and the use of medications may also be relevant.

Examination

The history will give the clinician a guide to the structures that may be producing the patient's symptoms and thus influence the physical examination. The practitioner must determine whether the pain is primarily coming from joints (including ligaments), muscles or neural structures in order to provide appropriate treatment. As with any soft tissue injury, all three components may be involved to some extent. Neurological examination is required if symptoms exist below the level of shoulder. Examination involves:

1. Observation
   (a) from behind
   (b) from in front
   (c) from each side
2. Active movements
   (a) upper cervical flexion (Fig. 16.2a)
   (b) lower cervical flexion (Fig. 16.2b)
   (c) upper cervical extension (Fig. 16.2c)
   (d) lower cervical extension (Fig. 16.2d)
   (e) lateral flexion
   (f) rotation
   (g) combined movements (Fig. 16.2e)
3. Passive movements
   (a) as above (if active limited)
   (b) muscle length tests (if not acute and no suggestion of mechanosensitive neural tissue): levator scapulae, upper trapezius, scalenes, pectoralis major, upper cervical extensors

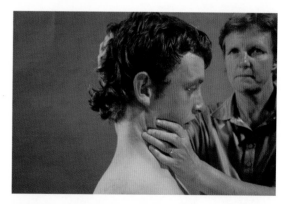

Figure 16.2 Examination of the patient with neck pain

(a) Active movement—upper cervical flexion

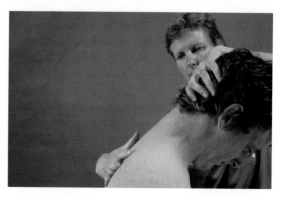

(b) Active movement—lower cervical flexion

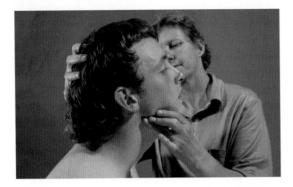

(c) Active movement—upper cervical extension with chin protruding

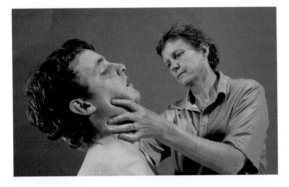

(d) Active movement—lower cervical extension with upper cervical spine in neutral or flexion

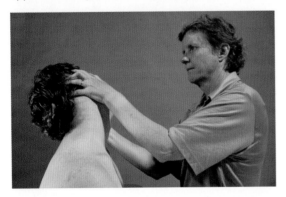

(e) Combined movements, using a combination of flexion or extension and lateral flexion or rotation, may reproduce pain or other symptoms. The movements can be adapted to be more specific for the upper cervical spine with upper cervical flexion or extension. Overpressure may be applied as shown.

4. Palpation
   (a) occiput
   (b) spinous processes (Fig. 16.2f)

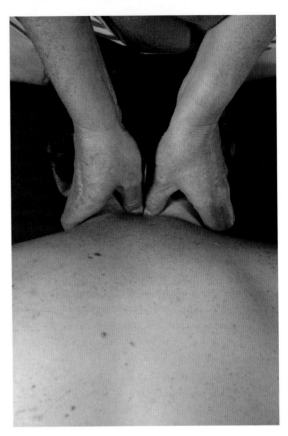

(f) Palpation—spinous process: assessing vertebral position

    (c) apophyseal joints
    (d) paraspinal muscles
    (e) levator scapulae, upper trapezius
    (f) anterior neck muscles (scalenes, sternocleidomastoid)
5. Special tests
    (a) neurological examination
    (b) neural tension tests (upper limb tension tests) (Chapter 8)
    (c) craniovertebral ligament/instability tests

Investigations

Most patients presenting with neck pain do not require further medical investigation. However, X-rays should be performed if there has been trauma to the neck, acute acceleration/deceleration injury, or the patient has nerve root symptoms. CT scans and MRI may show further detail in patients with nerve root symptoms, especially if surgery is being considered.

Treatment of the athlete with neck pain

The management of the athlete with neck pain depends on careful assessment of the muscles, joints and neural structures. Technique selection will depend on the diagnosis and the irritability of the condition.

There are a number of different techniques available for the correction of these abnormalities (Chapter 10). These include manual therapy techniques applied to the joints (e.g. mobilization, manipulation), muscles (e.g. hold–relax, soft tissue therapy and dry needling) and neural structures (e.g. neural tissue mobilization), as well as therapeutic exercise. As there is often more than one structure involved (e.g. joint and muscle), a combination of treatment methods is commonly required (e.g. joint mobilization and specific therapeutic exercise).

The general principles of treatment should be followed. These include trialing one technique at a time and assessing the effect of that technique by comparing pre-treatment and post-treatment clinical findings. If one technique is not effective, then a different technique should be attempted.

Muscles and fascia

The common soft tissue abnormalities found in patients with neck pain are focal areas of increased muscle tone, trigger points, muscle tightness and shortening, and deficits in motor activity and control (e.g. proprioception).[8]

Treatment should be aimed at restoring normal muscle length, tone, timing, strength, endurance and control, with the overall aim of restoring normal movement. Soft tissue techniques aimed at reducing pain and improving muscle length and tone are shown in Figure 16.3. Dry needling of trigger points in the suboccipital muscles, sternocleidomastoid, scalenes, trapezius and levator scapulae can restore normal muscle length and eliminate trigger points. Specific therapeutic exercise, such as training of the deep neck flexors, is discussed in further detail on page 238.

Joint abnormalities

The joints of the cervical spine frequently make a significant contribution to the patient's pain. The most common abnormality found on examination is hypomobility of one or more intervertebral segments. Manual therapy techniques can be used to treat stiff or painful intervertebral joints. The aim when treating joint dysfunction is to restore full, pain-free range of

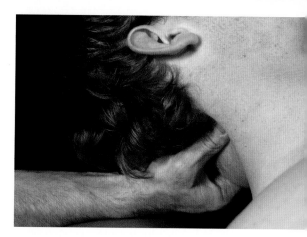

Figure 16.3 Soft tissue therapy

(a) Transverse friction to extensors with segmental rotation

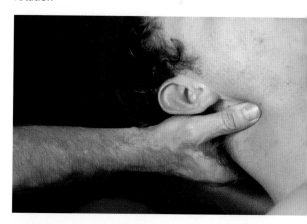

(b) Sustained myofascial tension to sternocleidomastoid with ipsilateral passive rotations

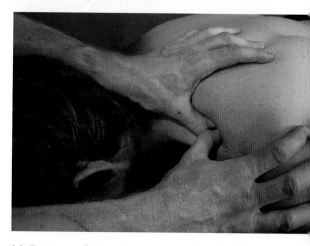

(c) Transverse friction to levator scapulae distally

motion. The two major types of manual therapy used in the treatment of joint abnormalities are mobilization and manipulation (Chapter 10). The choice of which manual therapy techniques to use depends on the diagnosis, the clinician's knowledge of trauma, pathology and the repair process, and the irritability of the condition.

Mobilization

A number of different mobilization techniques are used in the treatment of neck pain. There are three commonly used techniques for upper cervical spine (occiput–C2) problems and six techniques for the lower cervical spine.

The basic techniques for the upper cervical spine are:

1. longitudinal movement (e.g. manual traction) (Fig. 16.4a)
2. posteroanterior (PA) central pressure (Fig. 16.4b)
3. PA unilateral pressure (Fig. 16.4c)

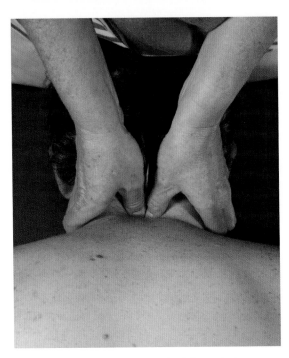

(b) PA central—pressure is applied through the therapist's thumbs in a posteroanterior direction over the spinous processes

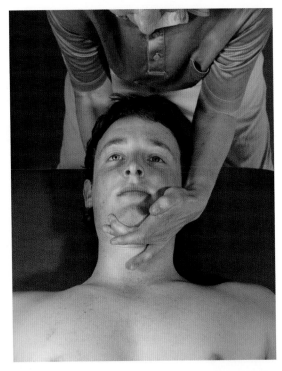

Figure 16.4 Mobilization techniques for the cervical spine

(a) Longitudinal movement (e.g. manual traction)— oscillatory or sustained longitudinal pulling is performed gently

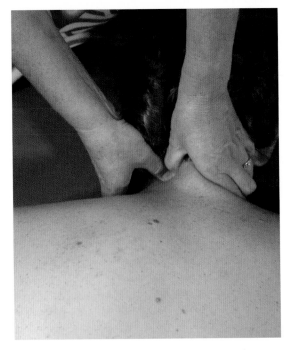

(c) PA unilateral—pressure is applied through the therapist's thumbs in a posteroanterior direction over the apophyseal joints

The basic techniques used in the middle and lower cervical spine are:

1. the above three
2. lateral flexion (Fig. 16.4d)
3. rotation (Fig. 16.4e)
4. anteroposterior (AP) unilateral pressure (Fig. 16.4f).

The choice of which manual therapy techniques to use depends on: the severity, irritability and nature of the pain; the direction of movement dysfunction gained from movement tests and manual examination; and knowledge of the underlying pathology. The application of the technique is influenced by pain (may need to alter the joint position), the relationship between pain and resistance, whether the pain is influenced by weight-bearing, and the clinician's ability to control the technique. When to progress a technique and the rate of progression depends on the results of continuous reassessment. Possible progressions include the grade of mobilization, the position of the joint, the speed of the technique, the amount of compression and the use of combined movements.

A highly irritable condition should be treated with techniques that do not aggravate the condition. It is

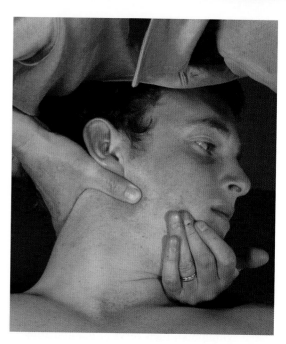

(e) Segmental rotation (non-locking)—hand contact is with the cephalad vertebra of the level to be mobilized; the other hand grips the chin to assist with rotation

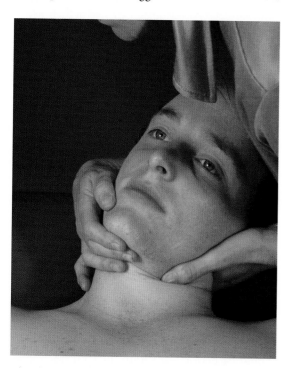

(d) Lateral flexion—the oscillating movement is produced by the therapist using a pivoting movement at the pelvis to produce the lateral flexion movement

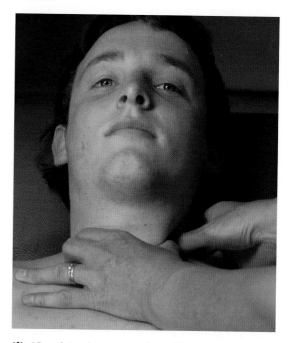

(f) AP unilateral—very gentle oscillating movements are performed with the therapist's thumb over the transverse process. This movement should be performed with great care

often helpful to begin with accessory movements performed in a neutral position or a position of ease, short of discomfort. Higher grades of mobilization or manipulation can be used in non-irritable conditions if loss of motion and increased tissue resistance are the primary problems.

Manipulation

Manipulation of the cervical spine may be an extremely effective technique but it is also potentially dangerous due to the location of the vertebral artery relative to the spine as well as possible congenital anomalies and pathology that may cause instability of the upper cervical spine. It should, therefore, only be performed carefully by those appropriately trained in manipulative techniques.

Prior to manipulation of the cervical spine, tests for vertebrobasilar insufficiency should be performed, including a pre-manipulative hold.[9, 10] If any vertebrobasilar insufficiency tests are positive (e.g. tests produce or reproduce dizziness or any associated symptoms), then cervical manipulation is contraindicated.

Traction

Traction can be a useful technique, particularly for the treatment of a patient with cervical diskogenic or radicular pain. Traction can be performed manually by the therapist or by machine. The traction applied may be constant or intermittent. The clinician should attempt manual traction first and, if it relieves the pain, then mechanical traction may be trialed. In lower cervical problems, traction should be applied with the neck in slight flexion. In the case of an acute nerve root problem, sustained traction is typically more helpful, whereas intermittent traction is typically better in the case of chronic degenerative cervical conditions.

The amount of traction applied can be varied by altering the weight or duration. The amount of weight to be used depends on the size and weight of the patient and the irritability of the condition. The therapist should palpate at the interspinous space to determine whether movement is occurring at the intended spinal level. The patient's response to treatment should also guide the intensity.

Traction should be commenced with light weights (e.g. 5 kg [12 lb]) for short duration (e.g. 5 minutes). The patient should be reassessed to determine whether there is a change post treatment. Based on this reassessment the therapist can decide whether to increase the duration or weight. Traction should not be used if it increases the pain.

Neural tissue mobilization

Increased neural tissue sensitivity may be detected by neural tension tests, such as the upper limb tension tests, passive neck flexion and the slump test (Chapter 8). These tests apply a longitudinal mechanical stimulus to test the compliance of the nerve trunks to changes in their anatomical course.[11] If neural tension is contributing to the patient's condition, then movement can be achieved using direct mobilization of the nervous system, typically with tension tests (and their derivatives) and/or palpation techniques, and treatment of the interfacing structures (i.e. joints, muscles, fascia and skin).[12] The clinician should think about moving neural tissue, as opposed to stretching it. The patient must be relaxed and comfortable and symptoms must be monitored repeatedly. If the condition is not irritable, the initial technique will typically move into some resistance, whereas with an irritable condition it is best to start with a technique some distance from the symptomatic area (e.g. opposite limb or lower limbs).[12] Neural mobilization (Chapter 10), including home mobilizing exercises, can help reduce neural tissue sensitivity and restore neural tissue mobility. Neural tension tests and neural mobilization techniques should only be applied by clinicians who are adequately trained in their use.

Exercise therapy

Exercise therapy is an important component of the treatment of the patient with neck pain. The different types of exercise therapy used include stretching, range of motion, strength, endurance and motor control exercises.

Stretching

A number of different stretching exercises can be performed by the patient. Muscles that can benefit from stretching include:

- lateral flexors (Fig. 16.5a)
- levator scapulae (Fig. 16.5b)
- trapezius (Fig. 16.5c)
- pectoralis major (Fig. 16.5d)
- upper cervical extensors.

Range of motion exercises

Active flexion, rotation and side flexion exercises should be performed within the pain-free range. Caution is required with extension exercises as they may irritate the condition. Circular combined movements should not be performed.

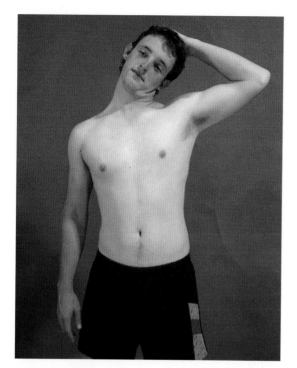

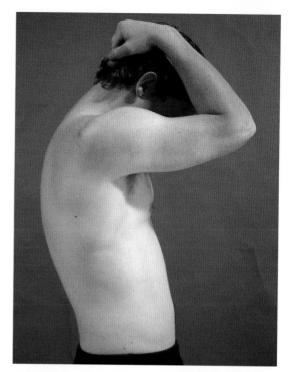

Figure 16.5 Stretching exercises

(a) Lateral flexors

(c) Trapezius

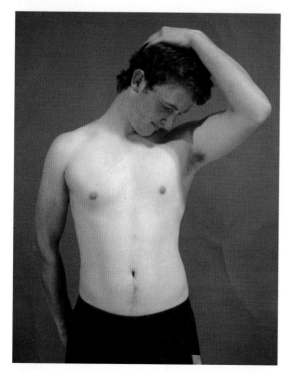

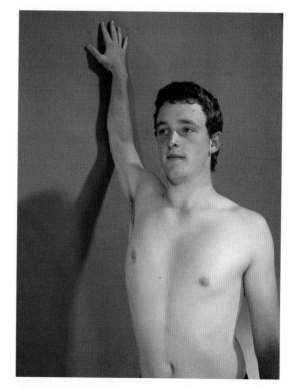

(b) Levator scapulae

(d) Pectoralis major

Endurance and motor control

Individuals with neck pain, both traumatic and non-traumatic, have a reduced ability to hold inner range positions of upper cervical flexion.[13, 14] The deep neck flexor muscles (longus colli and longus capitis) are thought to be critical for controlling intervertebral motion and cervical lordosis.[15] Patients with neck pain displayed signs of motor dysfunction, including delayed onset of the deep neck flexors and contralateral sternocleidomastoid and anterior scalene muscles during unilateral shoulder flexion/extension[16] and a trend for greater sternocleidomastoid and anterior scalene activity than controls.[17]

The craniocervical flexion test was devised as a staged test of deep neck flexor action. This test (Fig. 16.6) should be conducted on patients with neck pain to detect deficits in endurance (holding capacity) of the deep neck flexors and the degree of coactivation of the superficial neck flexors (sternocleidomastoid, anterior scalenes).[13, 17] Greater superficial neck muscle fatigue (both sternocleidomastoid and anterior scalenes) found on the side of the patient's pain (in patient's with chronic unilateral neck pain) suggests the need for exercise training to be specific.[18] It is important to train cervical muscle control in patients with neck pain. The clinician must pay particular attention to compensation strategies such as cervical retraction or excessive superficial muscle activity.

Strengthening

Self-resisted isometric strengthening exercises can be performed in lateral flexion, rotation, flexion (Fig. 16.7) and extension.

Posture

In those patients with a forward head posture and increased upper cervical lordosis, postural retraining is aimed at reducing the amount of cervical extension and chin protrusion. It may also be necessary to improve thoracic and shoulder girdle posture with mobilization, manipulation and scapular exercises, including the lower trapezius. The position of the pelvis should also be addressed as it can dramatically influence thoracic and cervical posture. Taping can be useful in providing proprioceptive feedback for patients with postural problems (Fig. 16.8).

Appropriate soft tissue therapy can facilitate postural training, and stretches to the pectoral muscles may also help to improve posture.

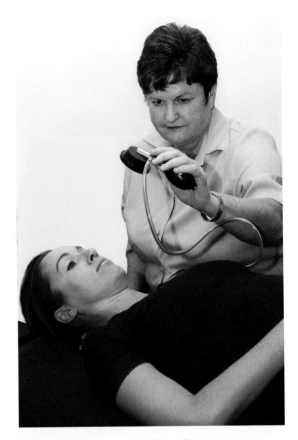

Figure 16.6 Endurance testing using pressure biofeedback suboccipitally to detect increases in pressure with the gentle nodding action of craniocervical flexion. The pressure sensor is inflated to 20 mmHg and then the patient is instructed to keep the superficial muscles relaxed and flex the upper cervical spine very slowly with a gentle nodding action and to hold the position steady for 10 seconds. Patients receive visual feedback of the pressure level. Ideally, the patient will increase the pressure by 10 mmHg but most patients who present with neck pain can only increase the pressure by 2–4 mmHg at first and they are unable to hold the position steady[17]. *[Photo courtesy of Professor Gwendolen Jull.]*

Stress management

Increased stress may lead to increased muscle tension and postural abnormalities. Stress management may play an important role in the treatment of some patients with neck pain. Widely used relaxation techniques include breathing exercises, yoga, meditation and relaxation massage.

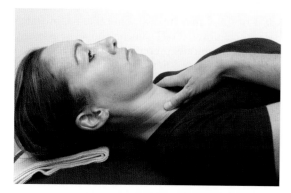

Figure 16.7 Deep cervical flexor strengthening exercises. Using a towel behind the head as shown to place the neck in a neutral position, the patient nods as if saying 'yes' (not losing contact with the towel). The patient is trained to palpate the superficial neck muscles (between the fingers) to ensure the superficial muscles remain relaxed and the movement is being made by the deep cervical flexors

Neck pain syndromes

As mentioned previously, most neck pain is non-specific. However, commonly recognized 'syndromes' causing neck pain include the cervical postural syndrome, acute wry neck, acceleration/deceleration injury, acute nerve root pain, as well as stingers/burners.

Cervical postural syndromes

These syndromes are characterized by a typical posture of protruding chin and increased upper cervical lordosis (Fig. 16.9). The patient typically has reduced thoracic extension, rounded shoulders, tight pectoral muscles, restricted shoulder movements and forward carriage of the head. It may be seen in athletes whose sport requires them to adopt prolonged postures. This includes cyclists, baseball catchers and hockey players. Similar problems occur in the workplace among people working at a computer screen, painters and production line workers. Problems arising in the

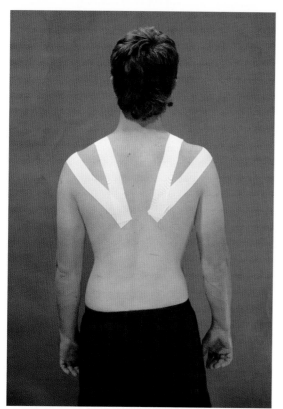

Figure 16.8 Taping. Rigid sports tape is applied across the scapular region to encourage correct posture. Taping is varied according to which correction is required

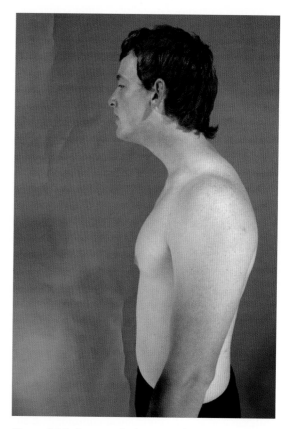

Figure 16.9 Poor cervical posture showing the chin protruding and increased upper cervical lordosis

workplace may benefit from ergonomic assessment. Individuals with osteoporotic vertebral compression fractures also frequently present with a similar thoracic, shoulder and cervical posture and reduced mobility.

The patient may complain of a burning or aching pain across the shoulders and neck or of suboccipital pain around the attachment of the trapezius and the upper cervical extensors. Pain is aggravated by prolonged static posture and is typically relieved by movement.

Examination usually reveals hypomobility of the lower cervical and upper thoracic spine with tightness and the presence of trigger points in the suboccipital muscles. There is weakness of the deep neck flexors and serratus anterior as well as the mid and lower trapezius and/or rhomboids. There may be evidence of adverse neural tension, such as reduced mobility in the upper limb tension test.

Treatment includes a multimodal approach, with therapeutic exercise, manual therapy, ergonomic advice and postural retraining. Joint mobilization should be performed to improve mobility of stiffer spinal segments. Postural retraining is an essential component of the treatment program and should include education and correction of not only cervical, thoracic and scapular position, but also the pelvis and lumbar spine, which influence head and thorax position.

Release of tight structures, for example, the suboccipital muscles, with sustained myofascial tension techniques or dry needling of trigger points may improve cervical and shoulder mobility and facilitate postural retraining. Stretching the pectoral muscles may also be indicated. Taping may be helpful in postural retraining (Fig. 16.8).

Acute wry neck

The acute wry neck is characterized by a sudden onset of sharp neck pain with deformity and limitation of movement. It typically occurs either after a sudden, quick movement or on waking. There may have been unusual movements or prolonged abnormal postures prior to the onset of pain but not necessarily. The apophyseal joint and the diskogenic wry neck are the two most common types. They can be differentiated based on the history and examination.

Apophyseal wry neck

The apophyseal wry neck occurs more frequently in children and young adults, most commonly at the C2–3 level.[19] It is commonly associated with a sudden movement resulting in sharp pain. Locking of

C0–1 or C1–2 may involve some trauma, in which case the craniovertebral ligaments should be assessed. The patient typically presents with an antalgic posture—usually lateral flexion away from the side of the damaged joint and slight flexion. The patient is unable to correct the abnormal posture due to pain and muscle spasm.

Active movements in sitting are difficult to assess due to muscle spasm. Joint mobilization and/or manipulation can be effective in treating this condition. Lateral flexion (Fig. 16.4d) or manual traction in the line of the deformity are often the first techniques employed. Manual treatment should be followed by range of motion and motor control exercises (e.g. of lower trapezius, deep neck flexors). Range of motion may not be fully restored immediately post manual therapy, possibly due to the presence of swelling. Ice, ultrasound or electrotherapeutic modalities may be an effective adjunct to treatment. Mobilization and manipulation techniques should only be performed by therapists with appropriate training.

Diskogenic wry neck

The diskogenic wry neck, on the other hand, usually has a more gradual onset and classically occurs when waking after a long sleep in an awkward posture. This tends to occur in an older age group (e.g. middle-aged adults) and pain is often felt in the lower cervical or upper thoracic region. This condition usually occurs in the lower cervical spine (C4–7), pain often feels deeper and the patient typically presents with a lateral flexion deformity with a bit of rotation and possibly flexion. There may be some radiation of pain to the medial scapular region[20] and the patient may have a history of degenerative joint disease in the lower cervical spine. It is important to differentiate this condition from a locked apophyseal joint as treatment that is appropriate for the apophyseal wry neck (such as manipulation) may seriously aggravate the diskogenic wry neck.

Treatment often begins in a position of ease with AP (Fig. 16.4f) or PA (Fig. 16.4c) mobilization, rotation (Fig. 16.4e) and/or cervical traction. Temporary use of a soft collar may provide some relief, as may analgesic medication. Postural retraining and motor control exercises should begin as soon as possible.

Acceleration/deceleration injury

Acute acceleration/deceleration injury to the cervical spine is a common injury in motor vehicle accidents. It can also occur in sports when the cervical spine is suddenly extended in contact with the ground or by a direct blow from an opponent. This syndrome is commonly known as 'whiplash'. In motor vehicle accidents it may result from rear end or side impact collisions. The most common symptoms of whiplash include neck pain, headache and decreased neck mobility.[21, 22] Occasionally, this mechanism of injury may result in cervical spine fracture (Chapter 44).

The patient may not feel pain immediately post injury but symptoms may increase gradually in the 48 hours following injury. Muscles, joints (including ligaments) and neural tissue may all be affected. Early mobilization is essential in the management of acute whiplash, including education and spinal range of motion exercises within a comfortable range. After the acute phase, treatment should focus on increasing function and return to normal activity as soon as possible. Therapeutic exercise, ergonomic advice and manual therapy should be used.

Acute nerve root pain

Acute cervical nerve root pain is characterized by moderate-to-severe arm pain which is very irritable. Neck pain may or may not be a feature. The pain is aggravated by movements of the cervical spine that reduce the intervertebral foramen (extension, rotation) or any movement or posture that increases tension on the nerve root (cervical lateral flexion, shoulder depression, arm movements such as shoulder abduction or elbow extension). The pain is eased by cervical flexion or positions that decrease tension on the nerve root (e.g. arm cradled or overhead). There may be associated sensory symptoms, such as pins and needles, paresthesia and muscle weakness, and possibly reduced reflexes. Nerve root pain may be insidious in onset, especially following prolonged abnormal posture. This condition usually affects older adults and results from compromise of the intervertebral foramen due to the presence of osteophytes (zygapophyseal or uncovertebral joints), disk changes, spondylosis and/or inflammation of a nearby structure.

Neural tension tests should not be performed but nerve palpation may be used to assess sensitivity. High-velocity manipulation is contraindicated. Treatment consists of techniques that open up the foramen (e.g. rotation away, AP mobilization); however, care must be taken as this condition is usually irritable. Sustained traction in the position of ease can be very effective in some cases. Indirect neural tissue techniques (e.g. opposite arm) may be helpful. Treatment should include discussion of sleeping positions and a full explanation of the problem. Muscular deficits should be treated as soon as possible (e.g. deep neck

flexors) using modified positions. This should be accompanied by local measures to reduce pain and inflammation, for example, ice, heat, TENS, interferential stimulation and analgesic medication.

'Stingers' or 'burners'

The 'stinger' or 'burner' phenomenon is seen relatively frequently in American footballers but rarely in other sports. The player experiences transient upper extremity burning type pain, paresthesia and weakness. Symptoms may radiate to the hand on the affected side or be localized to the neck. The mechanism of injury frequently involves downward displacement of the shoulder with concomitant lateral flexion of the neck towards the contralateral shoulder. The symptoms are usually transient but persistent neurological dysfunction may occur.

Proposed mechanisms include brachial plexus stretch or traction injury, nerve root compression in the intervertebral foramen or injury from a direct blow to the brachial plexus. Most cases are thought to involve the upper trunk (C5, C6) of the brachial plexus. Footballers with recurrent or chronic burner syndromes were shown to have nerve root compression in the intervertebral foramina secondary to disk disease. A high incidence of cervical canal stenosis was found in this group.[23]

There does not appear to be any helpful treatment for this condition. Usually symptoms resolve over a varying period of time from minutes to days. The athlete should be removed from all sport until the symptoms fully resolve.[24]

Recommended Reading

Beazell JR, Magrum EM. Rehabilitation of head and neck injuries in the athlete. *Clin Sports Med* 2003; 22(3): 523–57.

Butler D. *The Sensitive Nervous System*. Adelaide: Noigroup Publications, 2000. Available online: <http://www.noigroup.com/sns.html>.

Drake DF, Nadler SF, Chou LH, Toledo SD, Akuthota V. Sports and performing arts medicine. 4. Traumatic injuries in sports. *Arch Phys Med Rehabil* 2004; 85(3 suppl. 1): S67–S71.

Eddy D, Congeni J, Loud K. A review of spine injuries and return to play. *Clin J Sport Med* 2005; 15(6): 453–8.

Shannon B, Klimkiewicz JJ. Cervical burners in the athlete. *Clin Sports Med* 2002; 21(1): 29–35, vi.

Vaccaro AR, Watkins B, Albert TJ, et al. Cervical spine injuries in athletes: current return-to-play criteria. *Orthopedics* 2001; 24: 699–703.

References

1. Jull G, Bogduk N, Marsland A. The accuracy of manual diagnosis for cervical zygapophysial joint pain syndromes. *Med J Aust* 1988; 148: 233–6.

2. Phillips DR, Twomey LT. A comparison of manual diagnosis with a diagnosis established by a uni-level lumbar spinal block procedure. *Man Ther* 2000; 1: 82–7.

3. Gross AR, Hoving JL, Haines TA, et al. A Cochrane review of manipulation and mobilization for mechanical neck disorders. *Spine* 2004; 29: 1541–8.

4. Hoving JL, Koes BW, de Vet HC, et al. Manual therapy, physical therapy, or continued care by a general practitioner for patients with neck pain. A randomized, controlled trial. *Ann Intern Med* 2002; 166: 716–22.

5. Nilsson N. The prevalence of cervicogenic headache in a random population sample of 20–59 year olds. *Spine* 1995; 20: 1884–8.

6. Pfaffenrath V, Kaube H. Diagnostics of cervicogenic headache. *Funct Neurol* 1990; 5: 159–64.

7. Zito G, Jull G, Story I. Clinical tests of musculoskeletal dysfunction in the diagnosis of cervicogenic headache. *Man Ther* 2006; 11(2): 118–29.

8. Sterling M, Jull G, Wright A. The effect of musculoskeletal pain on motor activity and control. *J Pain* 2001; 2: 135–45.

9. Arnold C, Bourassa R, Langer T, Stoneham G. Doppler studies evaluating the effect of a physical therapy screening protocol on vertebral artery blood flow. *Man Ther* 2004; 9: 16–21.

10. Grant R. Vertebral artery concerns: premanipulative testing of the cervical spine. In: Grant R, ed. *Physical Therapy of the Cervical and Thoracic Spine*. New York: Churchill Livingstone, 1994: 145–65.

11. Elvey R, Hall T. Neural tissue evaluation and treatment. In: Donatelli R, ed. *Physical Therapy of the Shoulder*. New York: Churchill Livingstone, 1997: 131–52.

12. Butler DS. *Mobilisation of the Nervous System*. Melbourne: Churchill Livingstone, 1994.

13. Jull GA. Deep cervical flexor muscle dysfunction in whiplash. *J Musculoskelet Pain* 2000; 8: 143–54.

14. Jull G, Barrett C, Magee R, Ho P. Further clinical clarification of the muscle dysfunction in cervical headache. *Cephalalgia* 1999; 19: 179–85.

15. Mayoux-Benhamou MA, Revel M, Vallee C, et al. Longus colli has a postural function on cervical curvature. *Surg Radiol Anat* 1994; 16: 367–71.

16. Falla D, Jull G, Hodges PW. Feedforward activity of the cervical flexor muscles during voluntary arm movements is delayed in chronic neck pain. *Exp Brain Res* 2004; 157: 43–8.

17. Falla DL, Jull GA, Hodges PW. Patients with neck pain demonstrate reduced electromyographic activity of the deep cervical flexor muscles during performance of the craniocervical flexion test. *Spine* 2004; 29: 2108–14.

18. Falla D, Jull G, Rainoldi A, Merletti R. Neck flexor muscle fatigue is side specific in patients with unilateral neck pain. *Eur J Pain* 2004; 8: 71–7.

19. Grieve G. *Common Vertebral Joint Problems*. New York: Churchill Livingstone, 1988.

20. Cloward RB. Cervical diskography. A contribution to the etiology and mechanism of neck, shoulder and arm pain. *Ann Surg* 1959; 150: 1052–64.

21. Balla J, Iansek R. Headaches arising from disorders of the cervical spine. In: Hopkins A, ed. *Headache. Problems in Diagnosis and Management*. London: Saunders, 1988: 241–67.

22. Stovner LJ. The nosologic status of the whiplash syndrome: a critical review based on a methodological approach. *Spine* 1996; 21: 2735–46.

23. Levitz CL, Reilly PJ, Torg JS. The pathomechanics of chronic, recurrent cervical nerve root neuropraxia. The chronic burner syndrome. *Am J Sports Med* 1997; 25: 73–6.

24. Weinberg J, Rokito S, Silber JS. Etiology, treatment, and prevention of athletic 'stingers'. *Clin Sports Med* 2003; 22: 493–500, viii.

Shoulder Pain

WITH W. BEN KIBLER AND GEORGE A. C. MURRELL

CHAPTER

17

Normal shoulder function is essential for many popular sports and shoulder dysfunction causes significant impairment of everyday quality of life. In recent years, there have been many advances in understanding the abnormalities underpinning shoulder pain and in new treatments for shoulder problems. However, the shoulder remains one of the most challenging regions for all sports medicine practitioners.

The aim of this chapter is to provide a sound background in the functional anatomy and dynamic forces acting around the shoulder joint so that the pathological processes around the shoulder can be understood. After describing the key features of the clinical history and illustrating how to conduct a physical examination for this region, we detail the treatment of the various shoulder abnormalities. The chapter concludes with a prescription for practical shoulder rehabilitation, which is designed to aid the practitioner managing shoulder problems in the office.

Functional anatomy

The glenohumeral joint is a ball and socket joint. Unlike the hip joint, which has a deep socket, the glenoid cavity is a shallow socket and is inherently unstable. The relationship between the humeral head and the glenoid cavity has been likened to a seal balancing a ball on its nose. This implies that shoulder stability arises from a dynamic ball and socket stability that involves other structures. This additional stability is provided by static constraints—the glenohumeral ligaments, glenoid labrum and capsule—and dynamic constraints, predominantly the rotator cuff and scapular stabilizing muscles (Fig. 17.1).

The main static stabilizers of the shoulder in the abducted or functional position are the anterior and posterior bands of the inferior glenohumeral ligament. They are attached to the labrum, which, in turn, attaches directly to the margin of the glenoid fossa. The anterior band of the inferior glenohumeral ligament prevents anterior translation and the posterior band prevents posterior translation of the humeral head. The superior margin of the anterior band of this ligament attaches to the glenoid fossa anteriorly at the two o'clock position. When the arm is placed into abduction and external rotation, this broad ligamentous band rotates anteriorly to prevent subluxation of the joint.[1] Shoulder stability is also enhanced by the glenoid labrum, a ring of fibrous tissue attached to the rim of the glenoid, which expands the size and depth of the glenoid cavity. It increases the superior–inferior diameter of the glenoid by 75% and the anterior–posterior diameter by 50%.

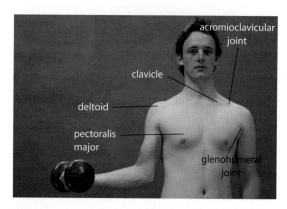

Figure 17.1 Anatomy of the shoulder region

(a) Surface anatomy from the front

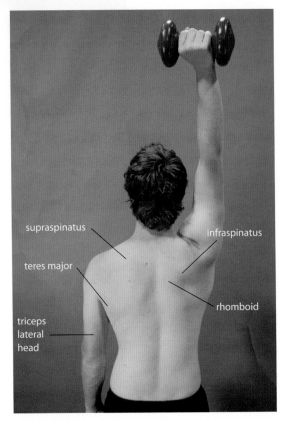

(b) Surface anatomy from behind

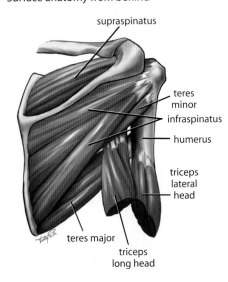

(c) Rotator cuff musculature from behind

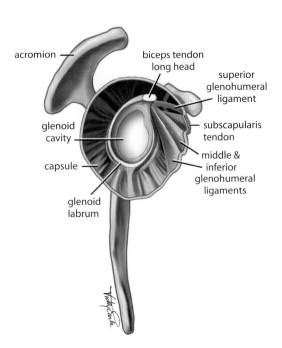

(d) Ligaments and muscles of the glenoid

rotator cuff musculature, by acting as a humeral head depressor, balances the forces of the deltoid muscle, which acts to elevate the arm and force the humeral head superiorly towards the acromion and coraco-acromial arch. The rotator cuff muscles, principally the supraspinatus and, to a lesser extent, infraspinatus, teres minor and subscapularis, counteract the action of the deltoid by preventing the head of the humerus from moving superiorly when the arm is raised. An imbalance between the deltoid and the rotator cuff muscle strength may result in excessive superior movement of the humeral head, causing impingement of subacromial structures.

The scapular stabilizers also play an important role in shoulder joint movement. Glenohumeral movement requires the scapulothoracic, acromio-clavicular (AC) and sternoclavicular joints to also move. Normal shoulder function requires smooth integration of movement of these joints. This inte-grated movement is referred to as 'scapulohumeral rhythm'.

Adequate scapulohumeral rhythm is required to achieve full upper limb elevation. Scapular movement ensures that the coracoacromial arch is removed from the path of the upwardly elevating humerus, in par-ticular its greater tuberosity, via upward rotation of the scapula, thus avoiding potential impingement.

The dynamic stabilizers of the glenohumeral joint are the rotator cuff muscles, which serve to control the position of the humeral head in the glenoid fossa. The

Correct scapulohumeral rhythm also enhances joint stability at greater than 90° of abduction by placing the glenoid fossa under the humeral head, where stability is assisted by the action of the deltoid muscle. A stable scapula provides a base for the muscles arising from the scapula and acting on the humerus, allowing them to maintain their optimal length–tension relationship. Scapulohumeral rhythm should be smooth, coordinated and symmetrical.

Disturbed scapulohumeral rhythm may be detected clinically by altered, jerky patterns of scapulohumeral movement. This may indicate injury to the shoulder girdle. Abnormal scapulohumeral rhythm may predispose to the development of a shoulder injury. Abnormalities of scapulohumeral rhythm are most commonly due to weakness of the scapular stabilizers (with or without weakness of the rotator cuff muscles), tightness and shortening of the scapulohumeral muscles (infraspinatus, teres minor and subscapularis) or involuntary adaptation to avoid a painful arc.

The muscles controlling scapular rotation are the trapezius (all three portions), serratus anterior (upper and lower portions), rhomboids, levator scapulae and pectoralis minor. For full upper limb extension, upward rotation of the glenoid is required. These muscles work in coordinated patterns called force couples to control three-dimensional scapular motion as part of scapulohumeral rhythm. The main upward rotation force couple involves the upper trapezius coordinating with the lower trapezius/serratus anterior. Anterior/posterior tilt and rotation involves the upper trapezius/pectoralis minor force coupled with the serratus anterior/lower trapezius. Following shoulder injury, adequate strengthening and retraining of the scapula stabilizers facilitates rotator cuff muscle strengthening.

Clinical perspective

A practical approach to shoulder pain

Because there are numerous structures that can cause shoulder pain, it is helpful if the clinician can narrow the problem down into one or more of the following five 'categories' of shoulder pain:

1. rotator cuff musculature
2. instability
3. stiffness
4. AC joint
5. referred pain.

Furthermore, the clinician must seek predisposing factors for the injury that is diagnosed. Careful clinical assessment can often go a long way to achieving both of these goals. Before explaining the key features of the history and physical examination, we provide a brief overview of the five common categories of shoulder pain listed above.

Injuries to the rotator cuff muscles and tendons may be acute, chronic or acute on chronic. Acute injuries include muscle strains and partial or complete tendon tears. Overuse injuries include tendinopathy. An example of an acute on chronic injury is a complete rotator cuff tendon tear in a previously degenerative tendon. Athletes with rotator cuff tendon injuries frequently present with shoulder impingement.

Shoulder instability is another common cause of shoulder pain. Pain resulting from instability may arise from the anterior, posterior or superior shoulder capsule and labrum and from the periscapular muscles. Glenoid labral lesions may occur either as an acute injury or from repetitive injury. Instability may be obvious clinically in patients with recurrent episodes of dislocation or subluxation. In many cases, however, instability may initially cause relatively minor symptoms, such as impingement or joint pain.

It is important to assess the AC joint in an athlete presenting with shoulder pain. The athlete may complain of shoulder pain and assume that the pain is from the glenohumeral joint itself. The AC joint is one area of the shoulder where pain is localized.[2]

Shoulder stiffness may be secondary to trauma, including surgery, or from injury to the cervical nerve roots and brachial plexus. It may occur spontaneously in middle age for no apparent reason—a condition often termed idiopathic adhesive capsulitis.

The shoulder is a common site for referral of pain from the cervical spine, the upper thoracic spine and associated soft tissues, especially the trapezius, levator scapulae and rotator cuff muscles. In the patient with chronic shoulder problems, there are usually a number of factors contributing to the pain. Cervical and thoracic joint dysfunction, soft tissue tightness, fatigue and trigger points are often present, in addition to primary shoulder joint abnormalities such as rotator cuff tendinopathy and/or instability.

As with any sporting injury it is important to identify, and subsequently correct, any predisposing factors. Predisposing factors to the development of shoulder injuries include abnormal biomechanics (Chapter 5), such as poor throwing technique or faulty swimming style, stiffness of the lower cervical and upper thoracic spines, or muscle imbalance and weakness, especially rotator cuff weakness and weakness of the scapular stabilizing muscles. It is essential to consider the whole kinetic chain, as any deficiency in the chain (e.g. stiff lumbar spine) puts additional stress on distal parts of the chain (e.g. rotator cuff).

Diagnosis of shoulder pain in the athlete requires taking a thorough history, examination and investigation. A list of possible causes of shoulder pain is shown in Table 17.1.

History

Endeavour to determine the exact site of the patient's pain; this can be difficult. Although AC joint pain is well localized and bicipital pain reasonably well localized, the pain of most other shoulder pathologies is poorly localized. The onset of shoulder pain may be either acute, for example, a dislocation, subluxation or rotator cuff tear, or insidious, such as rotator cuff tendinopathy.

The position of the shoulder at the time of an acute injury provides useful information. If the arm was wrenched backwards while in a vulnerable position, it suggests anterior dislocation or subluxation. The history of a fall onto the point of the shoulder can cause AC joint injury. In chronic shoulder pain, the activity or position that precipitates the patient's pain should be noted, such as the cocking phase of throwing or the pull-through phase of swimming.

Note the severity of the pain and the effect of the pain on activities of daily living and sporting activity. Although night pain is very common in complete tear of the rotator cuff, serious abnormalities such as malignancy should be excluded.

Shoulder pain may radiate proximally into the neck, the upper arm or, less commonly, the forearm, wrist and hand. The activities that aggravate and relieve pain should also be noted. In particular, the position of the shoulder that relieves the pain or symptoms is of great clinical assistance as it helps determine when stresses on the tissue are minimized. Periscapular and trapezial pain is common when the glenohumeral joint is malfunctioning.

Sensory symptoms such as numbness or pins and needles should be noted as should any muscle weakness in the upper limb. Any episodes of 'dead arm' are significant.

To assess whether there are any deficiencies in the kinetic chain, inquire as to past or present spinal or lower limb problems such as knee or ankle sprains or lower back pain. Also, it is important to know the exact previous physiotherapy for prior local or distant problems. Attempts should be made to determine the existence of any predisposing factors. A training diary may indicate excessive load on the structures around the shoulders.

Examination

A complete examination involves:

1. Observation
   (a) from the front
   (b) from behind (Fig. 17.2a)
   (c) lateral slide test
2. Active movements
   (a) arm elevation—watch scapular motion and position (Fig. 17.2b)
   (b) external rotation with elbows at side (Fig. 17.2c)

Table 17.1 Causes of shoulder pain

Common	Less common	Not to be missed
Rotator cuff	Rotator cuff	Tumor (bone tumors in the young)
Strain	Tear	Referred pain from:
Tendinopathy	Calcific tendinopathy	Diaphragm
Glenohumeral dislocation	Adhesive capsulitis	Gall bladder
Glenohumeral instability	Biceps tendinitis	Perforated duodenal ulcer
Glenoid labral tears	Nerve entrapment	Heart
Referred pain from:	Suprascapular	Spleen (left shoulder pain)
Cervical spine	Long thoracic	Apex of lungs
Thoracic spine	Fracture	Thoracic outlet syndrome
Myofascial structures	Scapula	Axillary vein thrombosis
Fracture of clavicle	Neck of humerus	
AC joint sprain	Stress fracture of coracoid process	
Other muscle tear	Levator scapulae syndrome	
Pectoralis major	Glenohumeral joint arthritis	
Long head of biceps	Brachial plexus	
	Neuropraxia ('burner')	
	Neuritis (viral)	

(c) external rotation at 90° of abduction
(Fig. 17.2d)

(d) internal rotation (Fig. 17.2e)

(e) horizontal flexion (Fig. 17.2f)

3. Passive movements
(a) as above
(b) accessory movements

4. Resisted movements
(a) external rotation (Fig. 17.2g)
(b) subscapularis lift-off test—Gerber's test
(Fig. 17.2h)
(c) deltoid (Fig. 17.2i)
(d) supraspinatus (Fig. 17.2j)
(e) biceps—Speed's test (Fig. 17.2k)
(not validated)
(f) biceps—Yergason's test (Fig. 17.2l)
(not validated)

5. Palpation
(a) AC joint
(b) shoulder joint
(c) rotator cuff tendon
(d) bicipital groove
(e) rotator cuff muscles
(f) periscapular muscles and anterior coracoid
muscles
(g) cervicobrachial muscles

6. Special tests
(a) AC joint compression using the Paxinos test
(Fig. 17.2m)
(b) scapular tests—scapular assistance test (SAT)
(Fig. 17.2n)
(c) impingement—Neer test (Fig. 17.2o)
(d) impingement—Hawkins/Kennedy test
(Fig. 17.2p)
(e) instability—load and shift test (Fig. 17.2q)
(f) instability—apprehension, augmentation,
relocation test (Fig. 17.2r)
(g) inferior—sulcus sign (Fig. 17.2s)
(h) SLAP lesion—anterior slide (Fig. 17.2t)
(i) SLAP lesion—O'Brien test (Fig. 17.2u)
(j) SLAP lesion—crank test (Fig. 17.2v)
(k) specific palpation for trigger points
(Fig. 17.2w)
(l) neural tension—upper limb tension test
(Chapter 8)
(m) cervical spine (Chapter 16)

 A rapid screening examination may consist
of:
1. observation from the front and back
(Fig. 17.2a)
2. palpation and the Paxinos test for AC
joint pain (Fig. 17.2m)

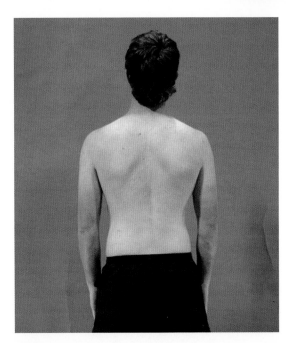

Figure 17.2 Examination of the patient with shoulder pain

(a) Observation from behind. Look for wasting or asymmetry of shoulder height, scapular position and muscle bulk

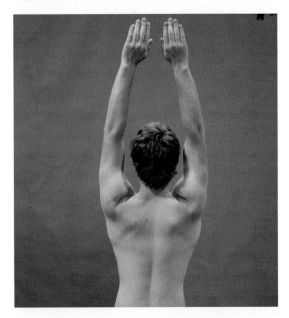

(b) Active movements—elevation. Watch for prominence of the medial scapular border. This indicates loss of scapular control, which is called scapular dyskinesis

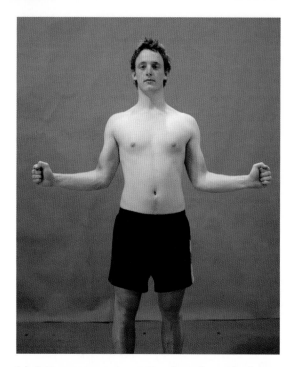

(c) Active movements—external rotation with elbows at side

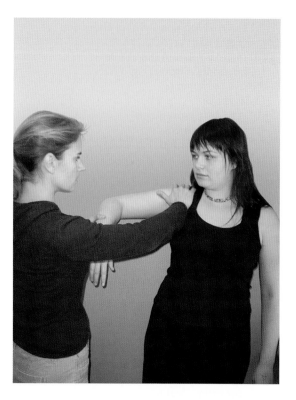

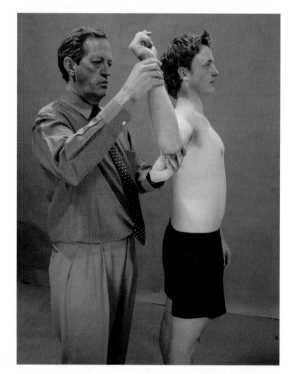

(d) Active movements—external rotation at 90° of abduction

 (e) Active movements—internal rotation. With the arm at 90° abduction, stabilize the scapula and rotate the arm in internal/external rotation to tightness. This test is superior to the traditional 'reach up behind the back test', which has 7° of freedom, only one of which is glenohumeral rotation

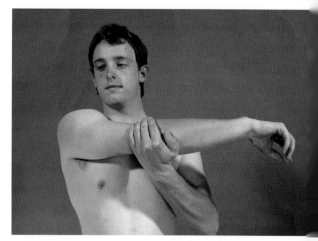

(f) Active movements—horizontal flexion. AC joint injury may be painful with this movement

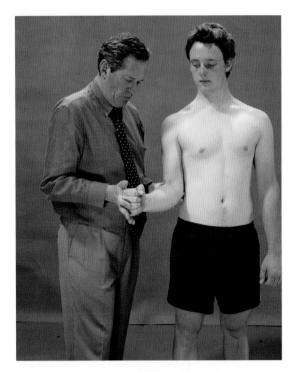

(g) Resisted movements—external rotation. Commence in the modified neutral position to isolate muscles

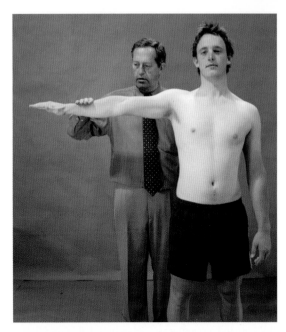

(i) Resisted movements—deltoid. Resisted abduction at 90° with the arm in neutral rotation

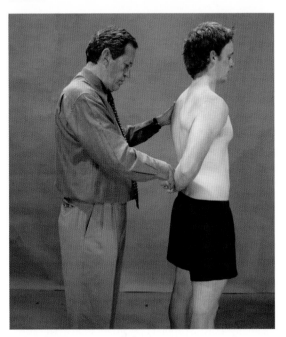

(h) Resisted movements—subscapularis lift-off test (Gerber's test). Push away from the spine against resistance

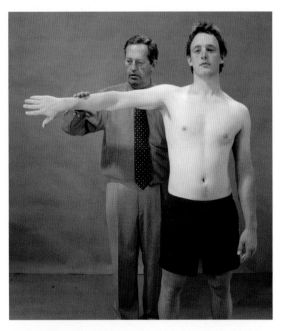

(j) Resisted movements—'empty can' position (90° of abduction, 30° of horizontal flexion and full internal rotation). This test may indicate supraspinatus abnormalities. Repeat with a retracted scapula. Improved strength with scapular retraction indicates that the rotator cuff is not injured but is weak due to scapular dyskinesis

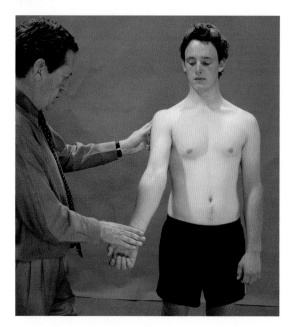

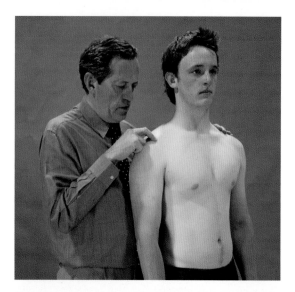

(m) Special tests—AC joint compression using the Paxinos test

(k) Resisted movements—Speed's test. Forward flex the shoulder against resistance while maintaining the elbow in extension and the forearm in supination. Pain or tenderness in the bicipital groove indicates bicipital tendinopathy

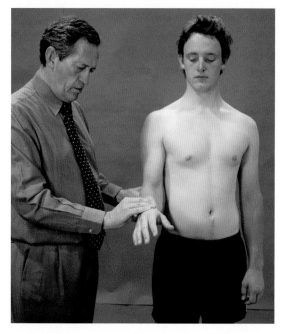

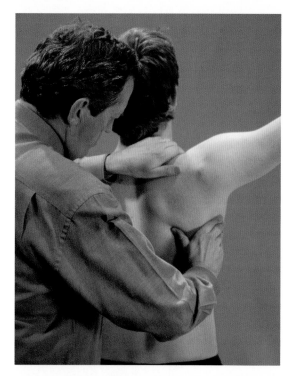

(l) Resisted movements—Yergason's test. Elbow flexed to 90° and the forearm pronated. Examiner holds the patient's wrist to resist active supination. Pain in the bicipital groove is a positive test for biceps injury

(n) Special tests—scapular tests (scapular assistance test). One hand is placed on the upper trapezius, the other on the inferior medial scapular border. The examiner assists scapular upward rotation as the arm is elevated. A positive test reduces impingement signs and symptoms and indicates that scapular control is required as part of rehabilitation

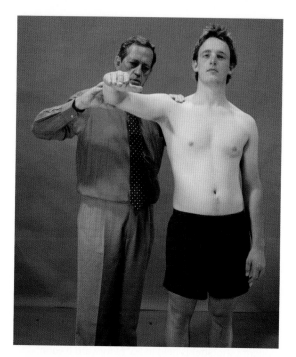

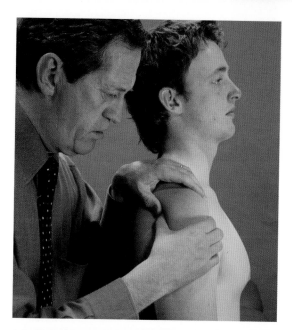

(q) Special tests—instability (load and shift test, or 'drawer test'). The right humeral head is grasped with the right hand, while the left hand stabilizes the scapula. The right hand loads the joint to ensure concentric reduction and then applies anterior and posterior shearing forces. The direction and translation can be graded using a scale of 0–3

(o) Special tests—impingement. The aim is to elicit pain while moving the greater tuberosity under the acromion

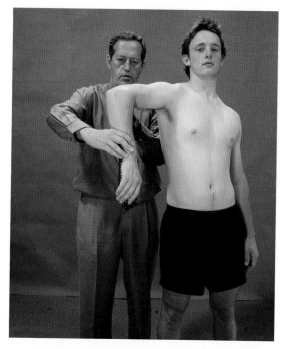

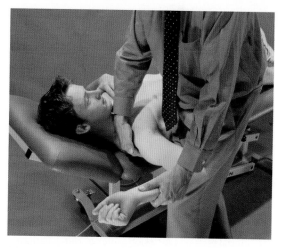

(r) Special tests—instability (apprehension and relocation test). With the patient supine, the arm is taken into abduction and external rotation. The test can be augmented by pushing the humeral head anteriorly from behind. The relocation test is performed by pushing posteriorly on the upper part of the humerus. The relocation test is positive if the apprehension or pain is relieved

(p) Special tests—impingement (Hawkins/Kennedy test). The shoulder is placed in 90° of forward flexion and then forcibly internally rotated

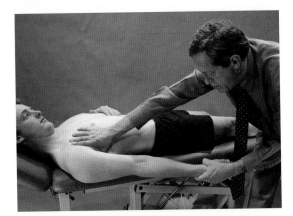

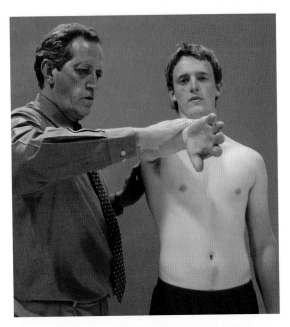

(s) Special tests—instability (inferior). Inferior instability is tested with the examiner placing inferior traction onto the shoulder joint. A positive test is when the humeral head is translated inferiorly such that a visible sulcus appears between the acromion and the humeral head (the 'sulcus sign')

(u) Special tests—SLAP lesion (O'Brien test). The patient's shoulder is held in 90° of forward flexion, 10° of horizontal adduction and maximal internal rotation. The examiner holds the patient's wrist and resists the patient's attempt to horizontally adduct and forward flex the shoulder

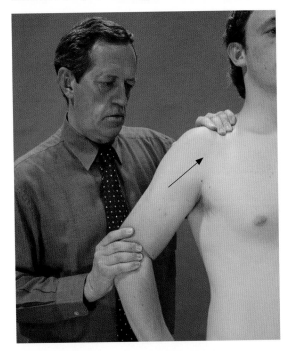

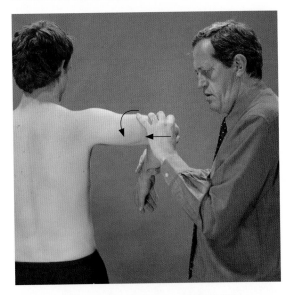

(t) Special tests—SLAP lesion (anterior slide). Patient stands with hands on hips. One of the examiner's hands is placed over the shoulder and the other hand behind the elbow. A force is then applied anteriorly and superiorly, and the patient is asked to push back against the force. The test is positive if pain is localized to the anterosuperior aspect of the shoulder, if there is a pop or a click in that region, or if the maneuver reproduces that patient's symptoms

(v) Special tests—SLAP lesion (crank test). The patient's shoulder is abducted 90° and slowly internally rotated while a gentle axial load is applied through the glenohumeral joint. The test is considered positive if the patient reports pain, catching or grinding in the shoulder

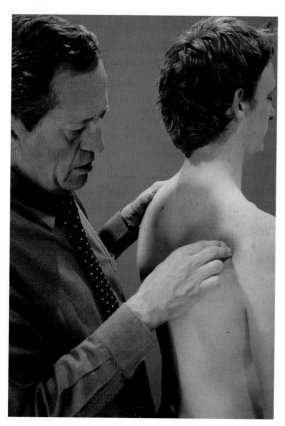

(w) Assessment of trigger points (e.g. infraspinatus)

3. palpation of the bicipital groove
4. passive external rotation (restriction may indicate frozen shoulder or arthritis)
5. impingement signs in internal and external rotation (for impingement and rotator cuff pathology) and with the scapular assistance test (SAT)
6. power of external rotation and of the supraspinatus (for rotator cuff tear)[3]
7. crank test for SLAP lesion—scapula-stabilized glenohumeral internal/external rotation for evaluation of glenohumeral internal rotation deficit (Fig. 17.2v)
8. apprehension, augmentation, relocation signs if suspected instability (Fig. 17.2r).

Investigations

Plain X-rays are important in the diagnosis of shoulder abnormalities. Routine views (AP with internal and external rotation and axillary lateral) provide a good overview of the region. In cases of trauma, an adequate axillary view may not be possible and it is mandatory to obtain a true lateral film to exclude dislocation. The following can be identified on plain films: calcific tendinopathy, glenohumeral joint arthritis, impingement (sclerosis of anterior and/or lateral acromion, sclerosis of greater tuberosity), proximal humeral head migration (severe rotator cuff dysfunction) and fractures.

Special views have been described to evaluate instability and impingement. Supraspinatus outlet views and down-tilted acromial films are obtained to evaluate impingement. In cases of instability, special views such as the West Point view or the Stryker notch view are used to better detect Bankart and Hill-Sachs' lesions.

In the past, double contrast arthrography was used to evaluate instability and rotator cuff damage. Today, far more detailed anatomical information is obtained when arthrography is combined with CT of the shoulder (CT arthrogram) or with MRI (see below). This examination gives excellent detail of capsular attachments and of the labrum. Small avulsion fractures of the glenoid rim (Bankart lesion) and the humeral head (Hill-Sachs' lesion) are clearly defined.

High-resolution ultrasound, in the hands of an experienced operator, is a reliable non-invasive technique for imaging the rotator cuff and adjacent muscles, the bursae and the long head of the biceps muscle. The examination may be performed as a static or dynamic investigation. Tendon swelling, thickening of the bursa or abnormal fluid collection may be detected, as may a partial or complete rotator cuff tear. The size of the defect and the thickness of the intact tissue can be measured. A dynamic examination performed while the patient is actively abducting the shoulder may confirm the presence of impingement.

MRI allows multiplanar, non-invasive examination of the shoulder and is used to detect a rotator cuff tear. Bone detail is not defined as well as with CT and examination with shoulder movement is not possible. MRI with contrast (MR arthrogram) is well suited to evaluate labral tears or instability. The examination under anesthesia (EUA) performed in conjunction with arthroscopy may sometimes be helpful to assess the presence, direction and severity of shoulder laxity, and to assess shoulder range of motion.

Arthroscopy of the shoulder can be either a diagnostic procedure, a therapeutic procedure or both. Shoulder arthroscopy permits inspection of the glenohumeral joint and the subacromial space in turn. Arthroscopy of the glenohumeral joint cavity is particularly useful as it:

- enables inspection of the glenoid labrum for evidence of a Bankart lesion or a SLAP lesion
- permits assessment of the state of the articular cartilage
- will demonstrate the presence of a Hill-Sachs' lesion
- allows inspection of the shoulder capsule and synovium (a red synovium and thickened capsule are characteristic of adhesive capsulitis)
- will identify a drive-through sign for laxity
- permits inspection of the under surface of the rotator cuff tendons, the biceps tendon and the subacromial bursa
- enables inspection and probing of the bursal surface of the rotator cuff.

Arthroscopy of the subacromial space allows assessment of:

- bursitis
- coracoacromial ligament ossification (spur formation)
- lateral spurs
- os acromionale
- bursal side rotator cuff tears
- full thickness rotator cuff tears.

It is important to remember that these sophisticated investigations are only an adjunct to the clinical findings. In many cases of shoulder pain, the clinical findings provide sufficient information to diagnose the cause of the shoulder pain.

Impingement

Before discussing the commonly diagnosed shoulder conditions in detail, it is important to understand the concept of rotator cuff impingement. Despite the popularity of the label 'impingement' as a diagnostic entity in patient charts, rotator cuff impingement is a clinical sign, not a diagnosis. The exact pathophysiology of impingement is not completely clear but current opinion suggests that shoulder impingement occurs when the rotator cuff tendons are impinged as they pass through the subacromial space formed between the acromion, coracoacromial arch and AC joint above and the glenohumeral joint below. The impingement causes mechanical irritation of the rotator cuff tendons and may result in swelling and damage to the tendons. The exact reason for the change in the tendon or the space is not known.

At least nine specific diagnoses may be associated with the signs and symptoms of impingement.[4–6] These are outlined in the box.

> ## Diagnoses associated with rotator cuff impingement
>
> 1. Subacromial bone spurs and/or bursal hypertrophy
> 2. AC joint arthrosis and/or bone spurs
> 3. Rotator cuff disease
> 4. Superior labral injury
> 5. Glenohumeral internal rotation deficit (GIRD)
> 6. Glenohumeral instability
> 7. Biceps tendinopathy
> 8. Scapular dyskinesis
> 9. Cervical radiculopathy

Shoulder impingement may be (Fig. 17.3):

1. external
   (a) primary
   (b) secondary
2. internal

Primary external impingement

Abnormalities of the superior structures may lead to encroachment into the subacromial space from above. The undersurface of the acromion may be abnormally beaked, curved or hooked (Fig. 17.4). These abnormalities result from either a congenital abnormality (os acromiale) or osteophyte formation. Other abnormalities that tend to occur in older age groups include thickening of the coracoacromial arch or osteophyte formation on the inferior surface of the AC joint.

Secondary external impingement

Encroachment into the subacromial space from above in younger athletes may also occur as a result of excessive angulation of the acromion due to inadequate muscular stabilization of the scapula. The muscles attached to the medial border of the scapula, such as the serratus anterior, become relatively weak and fail to control protraction and rotation of the scapula with glenohumeral movement. This results in antero-inferior movement of the acromion encroaching into the subacromial space (Fig. 17.5). This is exacerbated by excessive tightness of the pectoralis minor, which pulls the scapula into a protracted position.

The rotator cuff tendons are also liable to be weakened following large volumes of load (e.g. through resistance in swimming or throwing).

Excessive elevation of the humeral head may also occur as a result of imbalance between the elevators

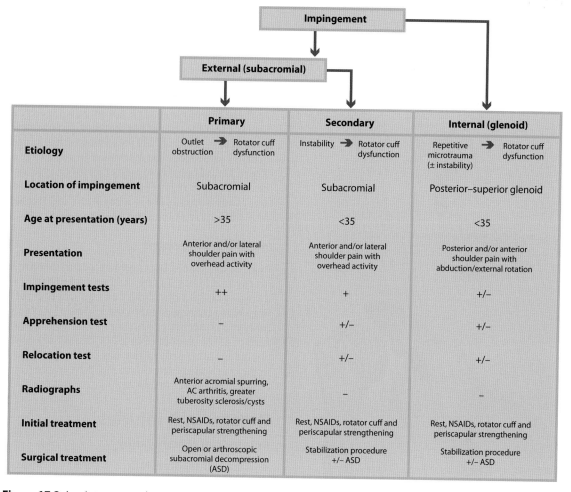

	Primary	**Secondary**	**Internal (glenoid)**
		External (subacromial)	
Etiology	Outlet obstruction ➡ Rotator cuff dysfunction	Instability ➡ Rotator cuff dysfunction	Repetitive microtrauma (± instability) ➡ Rotator cuff dysfunction
Location of impingement	Subacromial	Subacromial	Posterior–superior glenoid
Age at presentation (years)	>35	<35	<35
Presentation	Anterior and/or lateral shoulder pain with overhead activity	Anterior and/or lateral shoulder pain with overhead activity	Posterior and/or anterior shoulder pain with abduction/external rotation
Impingement tests	++	+	+/–
Apprehension test	–	+/–	+/–
Relocation test	–	+/–	+/–
Radiographs	Anterior acromial spurring, AC arthritis, greater tuberosity sclerosis/cysts	–	–
Initial treatment	Rest, NSAIDs, rotator cuff and periscapular strengthening	Rest, NSAIDs, rotator cuff and periscapular strengthening	Rest, NSAIDs, rotator cuff and periscapular strengthening
Surgical treatment	Open or arthroscopic subacromial decompression (ASD)	Stabilization procedure +/– ASD	Stabilization procedure +/– ASD

Figure 17.3 Impingement subtypes

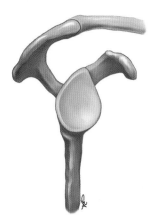

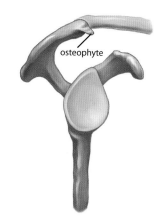

Figure 17.4 Acromial shapes. Abnormalities are not necessarily associated with clinical symptoms

(a) Normal acromion

(b) Acromion with anterior osteophyte

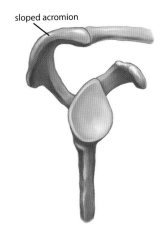

(c) Congenital sloped acromion

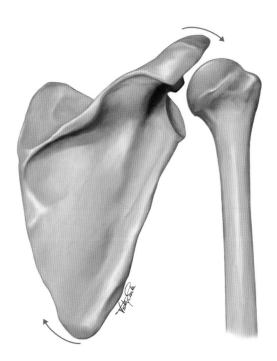

Figure 17.5 Lack of scapular stabilization results in excessive rotation and protraction of the scapula with glenohumeral movement. This causes inferior movement of the acromion

of the humeral head (deltoid) and the humeral head stabilizers (rotator cuff muscles). This imbalance may lead to the humeral head moving superiorly with deltoid contraction, thereby narrowing the space through which the rotator cuff tendons pass. This movement forces the humeral head up against the undersurface of the rotator cuff tendons, leading to further damage.

There are, therefore, numerous factors that may combine to cause external impingement (Fig. 17.6). To treat the cause of shoulder pain effectively, it is essential to recognize which factor(s) are contributing to the impingement. It is not sufficient merely to diagnose that the patient has shoulder impingement. In particular, in any athlete presenting with impingement, the presence of instability must be considered as expert clinical opinion suggests that this may lead to the development of impingement via several mechanisms. Unless instability is recognized and treated, impingement symptoms are likely to persist.

Internal impingement

Internal or glenoid impingement occurs mainly in overhead athletes during the late cocking stage of throwing (extension, abduction and external rotation) when impingement of the undersurface of the rotator cuff occurs against the posterior–superior surface of the glenoid (Fig. 17.7). This is normally a physiological occurrence but may become pathologic in the overhead athlete due to repetitive trauma, and injury to the superior labrum.

Rotator cuff injuries

Rotator cuff tendinopathy

Rotator cuff tendinopathy is a common cause of shoulder pain and impingement in athletes. In this condition, the rotator cuff tendons become swollen and hypercellular, the collagen matrix is disorganized and the tendon weaker. Studies in running rats and in human swimmers suggest the major determinant of the onset of tendinopathy is the volume (e.g. distance swum, time running) of work. Apoptosis (programmed cell death) and associated pathways are increased in overuse tendinopathy and may play a role in the pathogenesis of tendinopathy (Fig. 17.8).[7]

Clinical features

The athlete with rotator cuff tendinopathy complains of pain with overhead activity such as throwing, swimming and overhead shots in racquet sports. Activities undertaken at less than 90° of abduction are usually pain-free. There may also be a history of associated symptoms of instability, such as recurrent subluxation or episodes of 'dead arm'.

On examination, there may be tenderness over the supraspinatus tendon proximal to or at its insertion

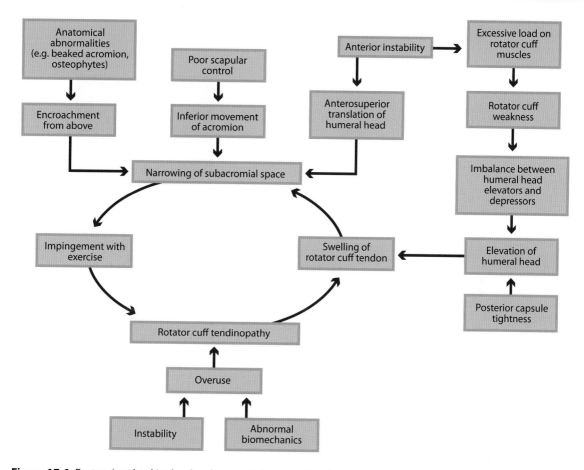

Figure 17.6 Factors involved in the development of external impingement

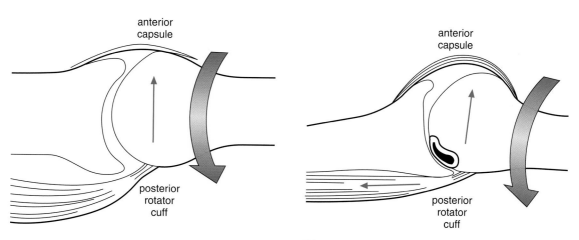

Figure 17.7 Internal impingement

(a) Superior view of an abducted, externally rotated shoulder demonstrates anterior displacement of the humeral head with anterior capsular laxity

(b) Impingement of the supraspinatus and infraspinatus tendons on the posterosuperior glenoid rim occurs with further anterior translation and posterior angulation (horizontal extension) of the humerus

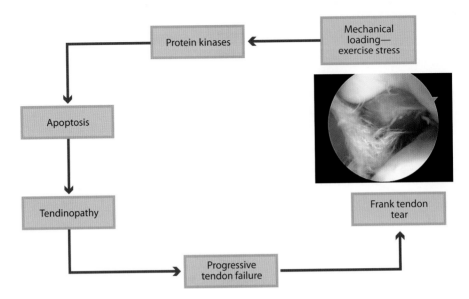

Figure 17.8 box diagram with text boxes: "Protein kinases", "Mechanical loading— exercise stress", "Apoptosis", "Tendinopathy", "Frank tendon tear", "Progressive tendon failure"

Figure 17.8 A schematic representation of how tendinopathies may arise. An increase in the load that a tendon cell experiences may activate protein kinases, which, when persistently activated, cause the tendon cells to undergo apoptosis (programmed cell death). Increased cell death results in poor collagen synthesis and matrix remodelling and a collagenous matrix that is weaker and more prone to tearing. With time, this tendon may rupture[7]

ADAPTED FROM MURRELL GA. UNDERSTANDING TENDINOPATHIES. *BR J SPORTS MED* 2002; 36: 392–3.

into the greater tuberosity of the humerus. Active movement may reveal a painful arc on abduction between approximately 70° and 120°. Internal rotation is commonly reduced. The most accurate method to clinically assess rotator cuff strength is to measure developed resistance when the scapula is stabilized in a retracted position.

For the athlete with rotator cuff tendinopathy, symptoms can be reproduced with impingement tests (Figs 17.2o, p), as well as pain at the extremes of passive flexion. Pain will also occur with resisted contraction of the supraspinatus, which is best performed with resisted upward movement with the shoulder joint in 90° of abduction, 30° of horizontal flexion and internal rotation (Fig. 17.2j).

The investigation of choice in rotator cuff tendinopathy is MRI. These examinations may also demonstrate the presence of a partial tear of the rotator cuff (Fig. 17.9).

Treatment of rotator cuff tendinopathy

The treatment of rotator cuff tendinopathy should be considered in two parts. The first part is to treat the tendinopathy itself. The patient should avoid the aggravating activity and apply ice locally. There is no level 2 evidence to support NSAIDs, ultrasound,

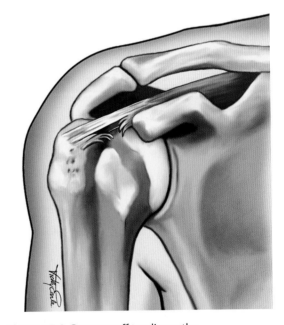

Figure 17.9 Rotator cuff tendinopathy

(a) Pathology generally begins on the inferior surface of the tendon

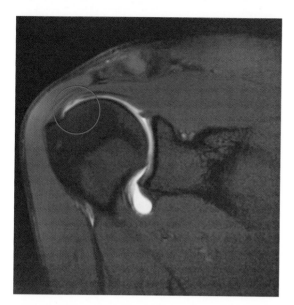

(b) MR arthrogram shows high signal contrast (white) corresponding to a partial supraspinatus tendon tear

interferential stimulation, laser, magnetic field therapy or local massage. There is level 2 evidence to support nitric oxide donor therapy (glyceryl trinitrate [GTN] patches applied locally at 1.25 mg/day)[8] and for a single corticosteroid injection.[9] Glyceryl trinitrate patches come in varying doses: a 0.5 mg patch should be cut in quarters and applied for 24 hours at a time and then replaced (Fig. 17.10); a 0.2 mg patch would best be cut in half and applied similarly. Successful

outcomes occurred at three to six months, so patients need to have this explained. A corticosteroid injection into the subacromial space (Fig. 17.11) may reduce the athlete's symptoms sufficiently to allow commencement of an appropriate rehabilitation program.

It has been reported that the second part of the treatment of rotator cuff tendinopathy should be the correction of associated abnormalities. These include glenohumeral instability, muscle weakness or incoordination, soft tissue tightness, impaired scapulohumeral rhythm and training errors. Impaired scapulohumeral rhythm may predispose to rotator cuff tendinopathy and must be assessed and treated. The treatment of scapulohumeral rhythm abnormalities is considered on page 276.

Decreased rotator cuff strength or an imbalance between the internal and external rotators of the shoulder also predisposes to the development of rotator cuff tendinopathy. Treatment involves strengthening of the external rotators as they are usually relatively weak compared with the internal rotators. An exercise program to strengthen the rotator cuff muscles is described on pages 282–3.

Posterior capsular tightness is commonly associated with decreased internal rotation and reduced rotator cuff strength. Stretching of the posterior capsule is helpful (Fig. 17.12). Instability is a common cause of rotator cuff tendinopathy and must be considered in any patient who presents with symptoms typical of rotator cuff tendon problems. If the presence of instability is not recognized, rotator cuff tendinopathy is likely to recur upon return to sport.

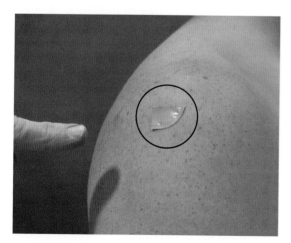

Figure 17.10 Nitric oxide donor therapy: glyceryl trinitrate (GTN) patches applied locally at 1.25 mg/day to the site of maximal tenderness. Patches remain on the skin for 24 hours and are then replaced[8]

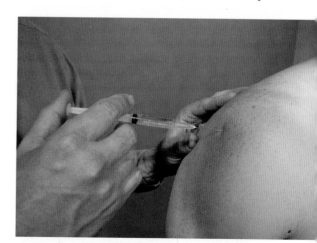

Figure 17.11 Subacromial injection. One technique is to insert the needle from the posterolateral aspect of the acromion in an anterior and superior direction towards the coracoid process.

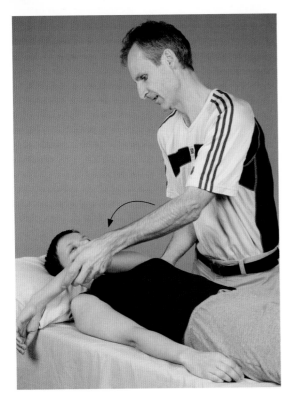

Figure 17.12 Posterior shoulder capsular stretching

(a) Motion is mainly between the scapular and thoracic wall, which exacerbates scapular slide

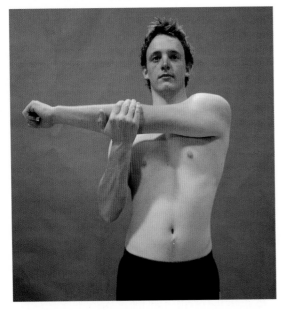

(b) Exercise with the scapula stabilized allows stretch at an appropriate location

The treatment of shoulder instability is discussed on pages 264–6.

While it is possible that correction of any of these disorders may improve tendinopathy, there is no level 2 evidence to support any particular rehabilitation strategy or regimen for managing supraspinatus tendinopathy. This provides fertile ground for novel clinical research trials.

Tightness and focal muscle thickening of the rotator cuff muscle bellies may also predispose to the development of rotator cuff tendinopathy. These changes reduce the ability of the musculotendinous complex to elongate and absorb shock. They may also alter biomechanics by reducing the full range of motion and impairing scapular control. These soft tissue abnormalities should be corrected. Abnormalities along the kinetic chain must be identified and corrected. Technique faults, for example, in throwing or swimming (Chapter 5), should be corrected with the aid of a coach. Training errors (Chapter 6) need to be corrected. Overuse should be avoided.

Rotator cuff strains/tears

Minor rotator cuff muscle strains occur commonly in athletes. They usually present with sudden onset of pain or a 'twinge' felt in the shoulder area. There is usually some limitation of function. These minor strains respond quickly to rest from aggravating activity, stretching and soft tissue therapy.

Complete and partial tears of the rotator cuff tendon are commonly seen in older athletes who present with shoulder pain during activity. These patients often complain of an inability to sleep on the affected shoulder. Examination reveals positive impingement signs and sometimes weakness on supraspinatus testing. Diagnosis is confirmed on ultrasound or by MRI. If the tear is small and of partial thickness, treatment may be conservative. Full thickness rotator cuff tears in young athletes require surgical repair.

Calcific tendinopathy

Calcification may occur in any of the rotator cuff tendons but it is most often seen in the supraspinatus tendon.[10] The cause of this calcification is undetermined. Pain is often severe at rest, with movements and at night. Deposits of calcium may be seen on plain X-ray and on ultrasound.

Management of this condition is difficult. If there is a defined calcific lesion that is still fluid in nature, instant relief may be obtained by aspiration under ultrasound guidance. Mature calcific lesions may be disrupted by extracorporeal shock wave therapy (also called 'lithotripsy') (Chapter 10).[11-14] Surgery is rarely indicated unless the calcific lesion is external to the tendon—for instance, in the subacromial bursa.

Glenoid labrum injuries

The glenoid labrum is a ring of fibrous tissue attached to the rim of the glenoid. It expands the size and depth of the glenoid cavity, thus increasing the stability of the glenohumeral joint. The labrum varies in size and shape and has a wedge-shaped appearance in cross-section. The labral attachment is generally continuous with the edge of the glenoid and blends directly into the articular surface. Occasionally, the attachment is meniscoid with the free edge extending over the rim of the glenoid onto the articular surface. This can sometimes be mistaken for a tear but is a normal anatomical variant.

The labrum is the primary attachment site for the shoulder capsule and glenohumeral ligaments. The superior aspect of the glenoid labrum also serves as the attachment site for the tendon of the long head of the biceps muscle. Injuries to the glenoid labrum are divided into superior labrum anterior to posterior (SLAP) or non-SLAP lesions, and further into stable or unstable lesions.[15, 16] SLAP lesions are injuries to the labrum that extend from anterior to the biceps tendon to posterior to the tendon. Snyder et al.[17] have divided these injuries into four types (Fig. 17.13).

SLAP lesions are either stable or unstable depending on whether the majority of the superior labrum and the biceps tendon are firmly attached to the glenoid margin. Non-SLAP lesions include degenerative, flap and vertical labral tears,[17] as well as unstable lesions such as Bankart lesions.

The most common mechanisms of injury to the superior glenoid labrum are repetitive overhead throwing and excessive inferior traction (e.g. carrying or dropping and catching a heavy object). Throwing injuries occur due to a combination of peel-back traction of the biceps on the labrum in shoulder cocking, abnormal posterosuperior humeral head translation in cocking due to glenohumeral internal rotation deficit, and excessive scapular protraction.[4-6] Patients complain of poorly localized pain in the shoulder exacerbated by overhead and behind-the-back arm motions. Popping, catching or grinding may also be present.

On examination, there may be tenderness over the anterior aspect of the shoulder and pain on resisted biceps contraction. A number of specific tests have been described for SLAP lesions.

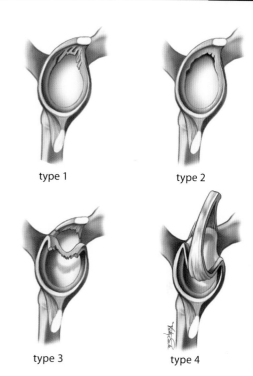

type 1   type 2

type 3   type 4

Figure 17.13 Four types of SLAP lesions have been described. In type 1, the attachment of the labrum to the glenoid is intact but there is evidence of fraying and degeneration. Type 2 lesions involve detachment of the superior labrum and tendon of the long head of biceps from the glenoid rim. In type 3 injuries, the meniscoid superior labrum is torn away and displaced into the joint but the tendon and its labral rim attachment are intact. In type 4 lesions, the tear of the superior labrum extends into the tendon, part of which is displaced into the joint along with the superior labrum

None of the tests are 100% sensitive or specific but they are reasonably reliable when used in combination. The three tests shown are the anterior slide (Fig. 17.2t), the O'Brien (Fig. 17.2u) and the crank tests (Fig. 17.2v).

Plain radiography is usually unremarkable in this condition. MR arthrography, a further refinement of MRI by injection of contrast agent into the shoulder, yields greater detail of intra-articular shoulder structures than does conventional MRI (Fig. 17.14).[18] MR arthrography is particularly useful for the detection and assessment of not only glenoid labral tears, but also small loose bodies, or cartilage flaps. Nevertheless, interpretation of MR arthrograms of the shoulder is best performed by a radiologist with particular

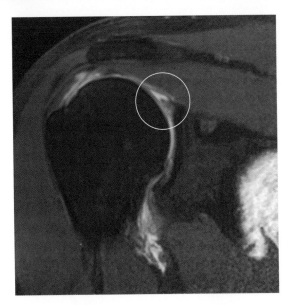

Figure 17.14 Glenoid labral tear. The MR arthrogram reveals the torn labral tissue (circle) surrounded by the high-signal arthrographic contrast medium

anterior dislocations damage the attachment of the labrum to the anterior glenoid margin (Bankart lesion). There may also be an associated fracture of the anterior glenoid rim (bony Bankart lesion) or disruption of the glenohumeral ligaments. A compression fracture of the humeral head posteriorly (Hill-Sachs' lesion) or tearing of the posterior or superior labrum may also be present.

The history is usually one of acute trauma, either direct or indirect, associated with sudden onset of acute shoulder pain. A patient may describe a feeling of the shoulder 'popping out'.

On examination, the dislocated shoulder has a characteristic appearance with a prominent humeral head and a hollow below the acromion. There is a loss of the normal smooth contour compared with the uninjured side. Anterior dislocations of the glenohumeral joint are occasionally associated with damage to the axillary nerve, resulting in impaired sensation on the lateral aspect of the shoulder. This should be assessed in any acute dislocation.

Ideally, the dislocated shoulder should be X-rayed (Fig. 17.15b) prior to reduction as a fracture may be

expertise in the area as interpretation is complicated by a wide range of normal anatomical variants. Interestingly, a comparison of MRI and clinical findings found a combination of clinical tests to be more sensitive than MRI.[19] Often a clear obvious history is sufficient and MRI examination unnecessary.

Conservative management of all but the most minor SLAP lesions is usually unsuccessful. Unstable SLAP lesions (types 2 and 4) should be repaired arthroscopically by reattaching the labrum to the glenoid. For stable SLAP lesions (types 1 and 3) and stable non-SLAP lesions, arthroscopic debridement to eliminate mechanical irritation is usually adequate. Unstable non-SLAP lesions, such as Bankart lesion, should be treated with arthroscopic fixation.[20]

Labral lesions are frequently associated with shoulder instability and this must be addressed as part of the management.

Dislocation of the glenohumeral joint

Anterior dislocation

One of the most common traumatic sports injuries is acute dislocation of the glenohumeral joint (Fig. 17.15a). In almost all cases, this is an anterior dislocation and it results from the arm being forced into excessive abduction and external rotation. Most

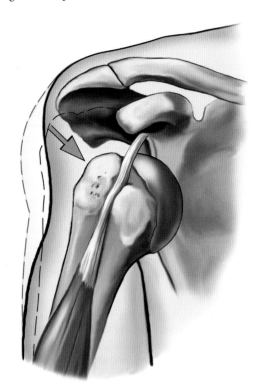

Figure 17.15 (a) Anterior dislocation of the shoulder disrupts the joint capsule plus/minus the stabilizing ligaments.

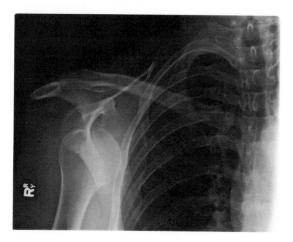

(b) Typical radiographic appearance—the humeral head sits medially over the scapula

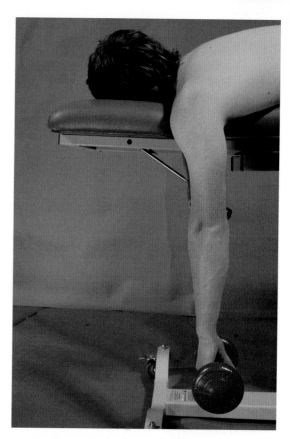

Figure 17.16 Position of patient with anterior dislocation of the shoulder to allow reduction of the shoulder. A small weight may be held in the hand to facilitate reduction

present. In most cases, however, this is not practical as the dislocation should be reduced as soon as possible. In these cases, a post-reduction film should be obtained.

The sooner the dislocated shoulder is reduced, the easier it usually is to reduce. There are a number of methods to relocate the humeral head onto the glenoid cavity. One method is demonstrated in Figure 17.16. Injection of 10–15 mL of xylocaine into the joint can reduce pain and muscle spasm and aid reduction.

Once the shoulder has been reduced, it is usually stable unless placed in gross abduction and external rotation. A sling should not be used. Several studies have shown that when the arm is internally rotated, the Bankart lesion worsens by becoming detached from bone.[21, 22] The Bankart lesion can be restored by placing the arm in external rotation (i.e. an external rotation pillow or splint). Non-operative treatment in such a brace for three weeks day and night has been shown to reduce the incidence of recurrent dislocation.[23]

Arthroscopic repair of a Bankart lesion has little morbidity and can reduce the rate of redislocation to 10%. The most effective post-operative regimen is undetermined. However, most surgeons initiate an intensive isometric exercise program to strengthen the internal rotators so as to reduce the incidence of recurrent dislocation. After three weeks, the patient is allowed to start active external rotation in addition to the strengthening exercises. However, combined abduction and external rotation must be avoided for six weeks.

Shoulder dislocations in young athletes have a high rate of recurrence, leading to chronic shoulder instability. Because of this high incidence of recurrent dislocation, an arthroscopy should be considered after shoulder dislocation in the younger athlete.

 PRACTISE PEARL If a Bankart lesion is found at arthroscopy, this should be repaired, either arthroscopically or as an open surgical procedure.

Following a Bankart repair, the patient may commence pendular movements with the arm within 24 hours, and maintain the arm in a sling for three to four weeks. Once the initial pain from the procedure has subsided, active external rotation movements, to just short of the limit of rotation achieved on the operating table, are commenced. It may be helpful to place the arm in a splint in some abduction and external rotation to limit the amount of anterior capsular shortening. Active internal rotation exercises can be gradually introduced as pain subsides. By six weeks, active strengthening can commence. Return to full sport is often achieved at three to four months.

Posterior dislocation of the glenohumeral joint

Acute traumatic posterior dislocation is far less common than anterior dislocation. It occurs either as a result of direct trauma or due to a fall on the outstretched arm that is in some degree of internal rotation or adduction. It may also be caused by a fit of any cause (e.g. electric shock or epileptic fit).

Inspection of the patient's shoulder may reveal loss of the normal rounded appearance at the front of the shoulder. The arm is held in internal rotation and adduction. The cardinal sign is limitation of external rotation. Suspicion of a posterior dislocation should be based on the mechanism of injury and the presence of pain and impaired function.

 Posterior dislocation can easily be overlooked in the AP X-ray.

X-ray must include a true lateral or, if possible, axillary view. The shoulder is reduced by applying traction forward with forward pressure on the humerus.

Shoulder instability

Shoulder instability may be anterior, posterior, inferior or multidirectional.

Anterior instability

Anterior glenohumeral instability may be post-traumatic, as a result of an acute episode of trauma causing anterior dislocation or subluxation, or atraumatic, or a combination—for instance, an acute traumatic episode in a lax shoulder.

In differentiating between the two types of anterior instability, the history is the most useful factor. In post-traumatic instability, the patient usually reports a specific incident that precipitated the problem. This is commonly a moderately forceful abduction and external rotation injury. Following this episode, however, the patient reports that the shoulder has never returned to normal. In many post-traumatic types of instability, a true dislocation may not have occurred and the symptoms are related to recurrent subluxation.

The atraumatic type of abnormality is common in people with capsular laxity, including sportspeople, especially those involved in repeated overhead activities such as baseball pitchers, javelin throwers, swimmers and tennis players.

Clinical features

The symptoms of anterior instability include recurrent dislocation or subluxation, shoulder pain and episodes of 'dead arm' syndrome. Pain usually arises from impingement of the rotator cuff tendons with recurrent anterior translation of the humeral head and recurrent 'silent subluxation'. This is aggravated by the eventual weakening of the rotator cuff muscles which, in turn, fail to depress the humeral head adequately. The recurrent episodes of impingement result in a rotator cuff tendinopathy.

Anterior shoulder pain in association with post-traumatic anterior instability may be due to 'catching' of a labral detachment. This pain and sensation of 'catching' may be reproduced on anterior drawer or load and shift testing.

The 'dead arm' effect is thought to arise from traction or impingement on the neurovascular structures, causing transient numbness and weakness of the arm. This usually resolves after a few minutes.

The episodes of subluxation and dislocation usually increase in frequency. Occasionally, a stage is reached where relatively minor activities such as yawning or rolling over in bed may result in a subluxation or dislocation.

On examination, it is important to note the presence of any generalized ligamentous laxity. A sulcus sign upon downward traction on the arm points to the diagnosis of generalized ligamentous laxity. The amount of external rotation at the shoulder should also be noted. Full assessment of the power of all the primary and secondary muscles controlling the shoulder should be performed to exclude any neurological deficit. Tenderness may be present anteriorly, related to damage to the anterior structures, or posteriorly, if there has been significant traction injury.

The patient is then asked which position causes the shoulder to dislocate. With anterior instability, this is usually in abduction and external rotation. The degree of anterior shoulder laxity can then be assessed with the load and shift drawer test (Fig. 17.2q). The apprehension–augmentation–relocation test (Fig. 17.2r) is also an indicator of anterior instability and has greater inter- and intra-observer reliability than all other tests for shoulder instability.[24] If instability is present, these positions will cause either pain or apprehension that the shoulder may dislocate. The presence of apprehension is a more specific indicator of traumatic anterior instability than pain.[24, 25] If the examiner pushes the humeral head forward, this may aggravate the athlete's apprehension and confirm the diagnosis of anterior instability (augmentation test). Conversely, posterior pressure on the humeral head may reduce apprehension (relocation test). If the degree of instability is relatively minor and apprehension is not perceived in this position, then an alternative method of examination is firstly to perform the anterior drawer test and then, while maintaining the humeral head subluxated anteriorly, bring the arm into abduction and external rotation.

Investigations may be useful in demonstrating some of the associated features of instability, such as the Hill-Sachs' lesion (Fig. 17.17) or the Bankart lesion (Fig. 17.18). Appropriate plain X-rays (Fig. 17.17b) or CT scans (Fig. 17.18b) may demonstrate

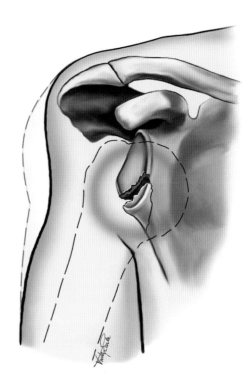

Figure 17.18 (a) Bankart lesion showing a fragment of bone separated from the glenoid rim.

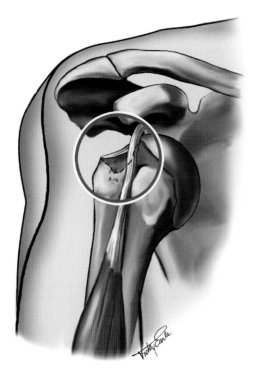

Figure 17.17 (a) Hill-Sachs' lesion showing where the humeral head has impacted on the glenoid rim.

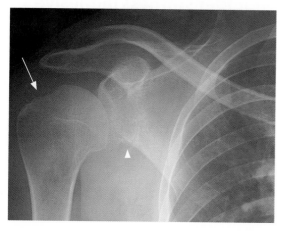

(b) A radiograph showing a Hill-Sachs' lesion (arrow) and a Bankart lesion (arrowhead)

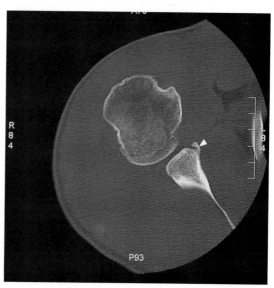

(b) CT scan of a bony Bankart lesion (arrowhead). CT may show this pathology where it is undetected by plain radiography

these lesions. MRI will reliably demonstrate the presence of bony lesions as well as soft tissue abnormalities of the labrum, the capsule and the associated tendons, however, an X-ray is usually all that is necessary to demonstrate traumatic anterior instability.

Treatment

As outlined earlier, a traditional sling should not be used to manage instability. If aggressive non-operative treatment is to be pursued, then the arm should be placed in external rotation of 30° for three weeks night and day to reduce the Bankart lesion.

There are a large number of different procedures used to treat shoulder instability. In athletes, particularly those whose dominant throwing arm is involved, the underlying mechanical lesion should be corrected. In most cases, this involves repair of the Bankart lesion, which may be performed either as an open or arthroscopic procedure. Other mechanical problems such as a tear in the rotator cuff may also be corrected. If an extremely large Hill-Sachs' lesion is present, then a procedure such as bone grafting may be necessary. Tendon transfer and other non-anatomical procedures, such as the Magnusson-Stack and Putti-Platt procedures, are not recommended for athletes as they invariably lead to a loss of external rotation and reduced shoulder power.

In treating atraumatic instability, intensive rehabilitation involves strengthening of the dynamic stabilizers (rotator cuff muscles) and scapular stabilizing muscles, with particular emphasis on the muscles opposing the direction of the instability (see pp. 276–83). Modification of sporting activity may also be helpful. If conservative measures fail, then surgery should be considered. This usually involves a capsular shift procedure.

Posterior instability

The most common type of posterior instability seen in athletes is an atraumatic type that is part of a multidirectional instability. Often, in these patients, the shoulder may be voluntarily posteriorly subluxated. In this group of patients, there is usually a marked posterior drawer (Fig. 17.2q).

Most cases of atraumatic posterior instability can be treated by strengthening of the posterior stabilizing muscles. If these measures fail, then surgery should be considered.

As a result of dislocation or subluxation, the posterior labrum may be torn, resulting in a type of post-traumatic posterior instability. If this is symptomatic,

then surgical correction of the underlying damage may be indicated.

Multidirectional instability

Multidirectional instability of the glenohumeral joint involves a combination of two or three instabilities—anterior, posterior or inferior. Most commonly, multidirectional instability is an atraumatic type of instability, often associated with generalized ligamentous laxity throughout the body. However, it may also result from repetitive trauma, especially at the extremes of motion or, rarely, from a direct blow.

Generalized ligamentous laxity can be assessed by examination of the wrists, thumbs, elbows and knees to determine the presence of hyperextensibility. On examination of the shoulder, the presence of instability in the anterior or posterior direction may be assessed by the anterior and posterior drawer tests (Fig. 17.2q). Inferior laxity is determined by inferior traction on the arm as it is held by the side. An inferior subluxation of the glenohumeral joint will be shown by the presence of a 'sulcus sign' under the acromion, as shown in Figure 17.2s.

The treatment of multidirectional instability involves strengthening exercises of the shoulder stabilizers. Stretching of the muscles around the shoulder joint should be avoided. If multidirectional instability fails to respond to conservative measures, then surgical treatment may be attempted. However, the results of surgical treatment, particularly in those patients with generalized ligamentous laxity, are not as good as in post-traumatic instability.

Shoulder stiffness (adhesive capsulitis, 'frozen shoulder')

Glenohumeral joint stiffness is not uncommon after significant trauma, for instance, a fracture or surgery. It may follow an injury to the neural structures in the neck or it may occur spontaneously.

The age group in which spontaneous shoulder stiffness, commonly referred to as adhesive capsulitis, occurs is between 40 and 60 years of age. Idiopathic adhesive capsulitis more commonly affects the left shoulder (1.3:1) and is more prevalent in women than men (1.3:1). Adhesive capsulitis is more common in patients with diabetes and there is an association with thyroid disorders and drugs that involve inhibition of matrix degradation.

The diagnosis of shoulder stiffness is relatively easy to make, for instance, when evaluating passive external rotation with the elbow at the side. Care should be taken to stabilize the scapula when examining for shoulder stiffness as significant range of motion can occur at the scapulothoracic articulation. Surgical or post-traumatic surgical stiffness usually resolves within 12 months and surgical intervention is rarely necessary. Symptomatic physiotherapy may be valuable.

Idiopathic adhesive capsulitis is a self-limiting condition that resolves, on average, over 2.5 years. One management option, therefore, is to wait for it to resolve on its own. There is no evidence that physiotherapy, injections or any drugs change the outcome of idiopathic adhesive capsulitis. Arthroscopic capsular release to divide the thickened shoulder capsule and an early aggressive supervised range of motion program is effective at restoring motion and relieving pain in patients with idiopathic adhesive capsulitis.[26, 27] The results from this procedure are not as good in patients with diabetes.

Fracture of the clavicle

Fracture of the clavicle is one of the most common fractures seen in sporting activities. It is usually caused by either a fall onto the point of the shoulder, for example, in horse riding or cycling, or by direct contact with opponents in sports such as football. The clavicle usually fractures in its middle third with the outer fragment displacing inferiorly and the medial fragment superiorly. It is extremely painful. On examination, there is localized tenderness and swelling and the bony deformity may be palpated. X-ray reveals the fracture.

The principles of treatment are to provide pain relief. Clavicle fractures almost always heal in four to six weeks. However, often the ends overlap and the clavicle is foreshortened. A foreshortened clavicle is associated with significant functional deficits. A figure-of-eight bandage is designed to prevent foreshortening and has significant theoretical advantages over a sling or collar and cuff. During this time the patient should perform self-assisted shoulder flexion to a maximum of 90° to prevent stiffness of the glenohumeral joint.

These fractures are best managed conservatively and usually heal surprisingly well. The main indicator for early surgical fixation is compromise of the skin by bony fragments or foreshortening of greater than 1–2 cm (0.5–1 in.). Occasionally, non-union of a fracture of the clavicle may occur with a fibrous pseudoarthrosis forming. This is treated surgically by

open reduction and internal fixation with a dynamic compression plate and bone chips,[28] ensuring that the length of the clavicle is maintained.

Distal clavicle fractures

Distal clavicle fractures comprise 12–15% of all clavicle fractures. Many of these fractures involve disruption of the AC and/or coracoclavicular ligaments. These fractures are more prone to non-union and delayed union. Classification for these fractures, proposed by the American Shoulder and Elbow Society, is shown in Table 17.2.

Generally, fractures medial to the ligament attachments tend to have greater displacement of fracture fragments and this is associated with increased risk of delayed or non-union if treated non-operatively.

Minimally displaced fractures distal to the coracoclavicular ligament attachments (type I) may be treated with a sling for comfort and early range of motion and isometric strengthening exercises. If displacement is present, then rehabilitation should progress slowly, with active range of motion exercises only introduced when pain resolves and healing has begun radiographically.

Treatment of the more medial (type II) fractures is more controversial. As there is a high rate of non-union, surgical treatment is often recommended. Distal intra-articular fractures (type III), if stable, should be treated non-surgically as they tend to heal with minimal dysfunction.

The treatment of distal clavicle fractures in the immature adult is different from that in the adult. Even fractures that present with significant displacement are stable and will eventually heal in an anatomical position. This is due to the fact that, although the fracture is medial to the coracoclavicular ligament attachment, the periosteal envelope remains attached to the coracoclavicular ligaments. The hematoma and subsequent new bone formation stimulated by the periosteum results in remodeling and complete union.

Table 17.2 Classification of distal clavicle fractures

Type	Pathology
I	Fracture distal to coracoclavicular ligaments with little displacement
IIa	Fracture medial to coracoclavicular ligaments
IIb	Fracture between coracoclavicular ligaments
III	Intra-articular fracture without ligament disruption

Acromioclavicular joint injuries

The AC joint is another common site of injury in athletes who fall onto the point of the shoulder.

Stability of the AC joint is provided by a number of structures. These are, in order of increasing importance, the joint capsule, the AC ligaments and the coracoclavicular ligament comprising the conoid and trapezoid ligaments (Fig. 17.19).

The most commonly used classification system for AC joint injuries is that modified by Rockwood, which recognizes six different types of injury (Fig. 17.20).[29] Type I injury corresponds to sprain of the capsule of the joint and is characterized clinically by localized tenderness and pain on movement, especially horizontal flexion. Type II injuries correspond to a complete tear of the AC ligaments with sprain of the coracoclavicular ligaments. On examination, as well as localized tenderness, there is a palpable step deformity. Type III and V injuries consist of complete tears of the coracoclavicular ligaments, the conoid and trapezoid. In type III and V injuries, a marked step deformity is present (Fig. 17.21).

Type V injuries can be distinguished from type III injuries radiographically by the amount of displacement. A type V injury has between three and five times greater coracoclavicular space than normal, whereas a type III injury has 25–100% greater coraco-clavicular distance than the uninjured side. Type V injury typically involves much greater soft tissue injury and includes damage to the muscle fascia and occasionally the skin. Type IV injuries are characterized by posterior displacement of the clavicle and type VI injuries have an inferiorly displaced clavicle into either a subacromial or subcoracoid position. Types IV, V and VI injuries also have complete rupture of all the ligament complexes and are much rarer injuries than types I, II and III.[30]

Management is based on the general principles of management of ligamentous injuries. Initially, ice is applied to minimize the degree of damage and the injured part is immobilized in a sling for pain relief. This may be for two to three days in the case of type I injuries or up to six weeks in severe type II or type III injuries. Isometric strengthening exercises should be commenced once pain permits. Return to sport is possible when there is no further localized tenderness and full range of pain-free movement has been regained. Protection on return to sport can be provided by tape applied to the AC joint (Fig. 17.22).

The treatment of type III injuries is controversial. Historically, most of these injuries have been treated surgically. However, recently most clinicians consider that results with conservative management are at least as good. Surgery should then be reserved for type IV, V and VI injuries and those type III injuries that fail to respond adequately to conservative management.[30]

The surgical treatment of AC joint injuries has been hampered by the large forces distracting the arm inferiorly from the clavicle and the paucity of techniques available to anatomically restore the coracoclavicular ligaments while holding the arm in the reduced position.

Chronic acromioclavicular joint pain

Chronic AC joint pain may occur as a result of repeated minor injuries to the AC joint or following a type II or type III injury. The fibrocartilaginous meniscus situated within the AC joint may be damaged. Osteolysis of the outer end of the clavicle is seen occasionally, especially in weightlifters performing large numbers of bench presses. X-ray in this condition shows marked osteoporosis of the distal end of the clavicle (Fig. 17.23). Movements such as horizontal flexion are painful. Another symptom is rotator cuff impingement due to the abnormal scapular position that results from loss of the clavicle strut. Treatment consists of local physiotherapy, including electrotherapeutic modalities and mobilization, combined with muscle strengthening. A corticosteroid injection

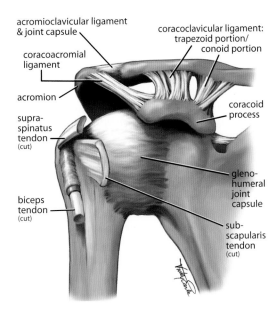

acromioclavicular ligament & joint capsule

coracoclavicular ligament: trapezoid portion/ conoid portion

coracoacromial ligament

acromion

coracoid process

supraspinatus tendon (cut)

glenohumeral joint capsule

biceps tendon (cut)

subscapularis tendon (cut)

Figure 17.19 The AC joint

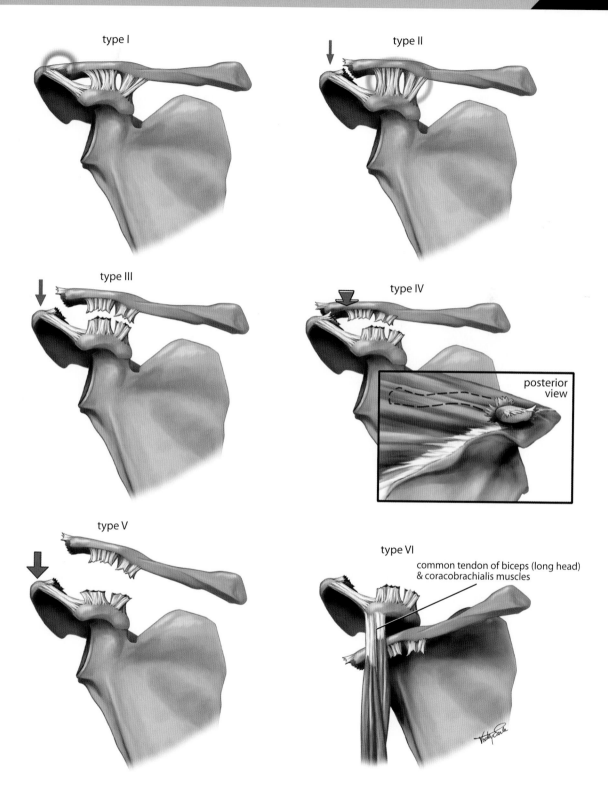

type I

type II

type III

type IV

posterior view

type V

type VI

common tendon of biceps (long head) & coracobrachialis muscles

Figure 17.20 Classification of AC joint injuries

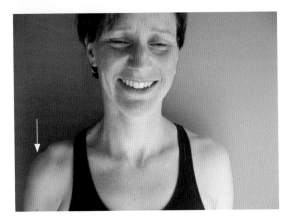

Figure 17.21 Marked step deformity at the AC joint in type III injury

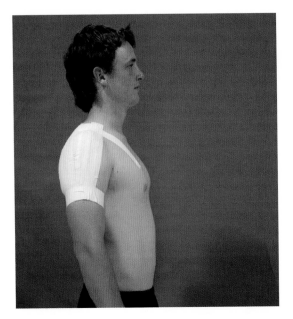

Figure 17.22 Protective taping after AC joint injury

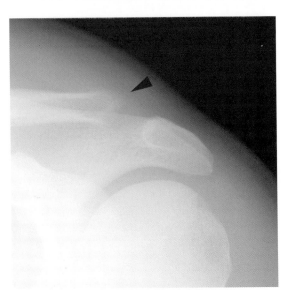

Figure 17.23 Osteolysis of the outer end of the clavicle

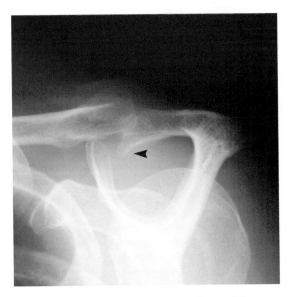

Figure 17.24 Post-traumatic osteoarthritis of the AC joint showing a spur and bony irregularity on the acromion

into the AC joint may relieve pain. Persistent cases require resection of the distal clavicle.[31]

Osteoarthritis of the AC joint may occur as a result of recurrent injuries. This is characterized by a typical X-ray appearance with sclerosis and osteophyte formation (Fig. 17.24).

 AC joint pain is usually localized to the AC joint. Symptoms may be reproduced by AC joint compression using the Paxinos test[2] (Fig. 17.2m) or cross-arm adduction.

The diagnosis can be confirmed and treatment initiated with an injection of local anesthetic and corticosteroid into the AC joint. Persistent AC joint pain may be managed by distal clavicle excision. This procedure can be carried out arthroscopically.

While this procedure is technically reasonably easy to perform, the procedure aims to replace half a joint with scar tissue. From a biological perspective this makes little sense, which may be why there are very few publications reporting the outcomes of this procedure.

Referred pain

The shoulder and upper arm are common sites of referred pain. The pain perceived by the athlete may result from local abnormalities, referred pain or both. The joints of the cervical and upper thoracic spine frequently refer pain to the shoulder region. It is important to ascertain in the history whether the patient experiences pain or stiffness of the neck. It must be remembered that the neck or upper thoracic spine may refer pain even when there is little or no local neck pain present. Similarly, a malfunctioning shoulder often has associated periscapular and trapezial (i.e. neck) pain.

Examination of the shoulder must include an examination of the cervical and upper thoracic spine. Often, cervical lateral flexion or rotation away from the side of the shoulder pain may be reduced or painful. Palpation of the spine, both centrally over the spinous processes and disk spaces and laterally over the apophyseal joints, may reveal stiffness or tenderness. If the cervical or upper thoracic spine is suspected of being a possible cause of shoulder pain, it is useful to treat the hypomobile segment(s) and reassess shoulder movements following treatment to see if there is any reduction in pain. This may indicate that there is a contribution to shoulder pain from the intervertebral joints.

Muscles and fascia in the neck, upper thoracic and scapular regions may also contribute to shoulder pain. Active trigger points can be found in any of the muscles of the neck and shoulder but those that commonly contribute to shoulder pain are in the trapezius, infraspinatus, levator scapulae and rhomboids (Fig. 17.25). Soft tissue techniques (Fig. 17.26) and dry needling can be used to treat trigger points.

The contribution of neural structures to the patient's shoulder pain can be assessed by the upper limb tension test (Chapter 8). Reproduction of the patient's shoulder pain with this test or restriction of stretch compared with the non-painful side may indicate a neural component to the patient's pain. This may be improved by correction of the intervertebral abnormalities if present. Neural stretching (Chapter 10) may help restore normal movement of neural tissues.

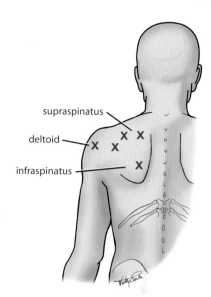

Figure 17.25 Site of trigger points that may refer pain to the shoulder

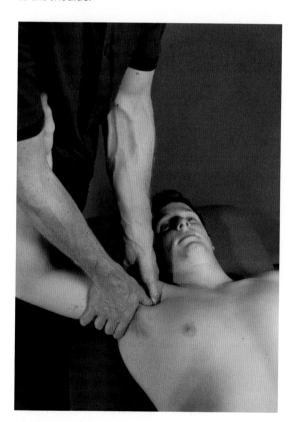

Figure 17.26 Several soft tissue techniques are used in clinical practice to treat shoulder pain

(a) Ischemic pressure to the pectoralis major

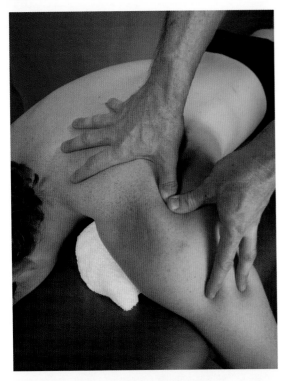

(b) Ischemic pressure to the infraspinatus

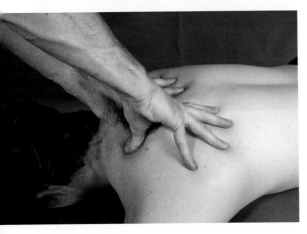

(c) Ischemic pressure to the lower fibers of the trapezius

Less common causes of shoulder pain

Biceps tendinopathy

The long head of the biceps tendon that passes from the superior lip of the glenoid through the bicipital groove in the humerus is susceptible to overuse injury. This occurs particularly in athletes performing a large volume of weight training, such as bench presses and 'dips'. This injury is not common but it is often incorrectly diagnosed when, in fact, referred pain or rotator cuff tendinopathy are producing pain in the biceps region.

Palpation of the region may show local tenderness of the biceps tendon, either in the bicipital groove close to its attachment to the glenoid or at the musculo-tendinous junction. Pain may be reproduced by passive stretching of the biceps or resisted active contraction of the biceps in Speed's test (Fig. 17.2k) or Yergason's test (Fig. 17.2l). No form of treatment has been shown to be of benefit for biceps tendinopathy/fraying.

Rupture of the long head of the biceps

Rupture of the long head of the biceps muscle may occur in the older athlete. Occasionally, there is a previous history of injury to the biceps tendon. The tendon may rupture with any activity involving the biceps muscle and is usually accompanied by sharp pain and a tearing sensation.

The deformity is obvious, with the muscle becoming detached from its proximal attachment and bunching up in the distal arm. The deformity is accentuated by contraction of the biceps. Often there is little pain. Surprisingly, biceps strength is almost fully maintained. Imaging is via MRI.[32] Those who do not rely on their upper arm in sport are generally satisfied with reassurance and require no definitive treatment. In those who perform power sports, surgery may be indicated.

Pectoralis major tears

Pectoralis major tears may be partial ruptures (grades I–II) or complete (grade III). Complete rupture occurs at the site of its insertion in the humerus. This is usually seen in weight training, especially when performing a bench press. The typical history is of sudden onset of pain on the medial aspect of the upper arm. On examination, localized tenderness and swelling are found. Resisted contraction of the pectoralis major is weak and may be painful.

A partial tear is treated conservatively with ice, electrotherapeutic modalities and a strengthening program over a period of four to six weeks. A complete tear of the pectoralis major should be treated by surgical repair of the muscle.[33] It is usually possible to differentiate between a partial and a complete tear clinically. Ultrasound or MRI examination may assist in this differentiation.

Subscapularis muscle tears

Tears of the subscapularis muscle can occur with sudden forceful external rotation or extension applied to the abducted arm. There is usually no associated instability. The main complaint is pain and range of motion may be maintained. On examination, the patient will have increased passive external rotation with the shoulder adducted at the side, weakness of internal rotation and a positive lift-off sign (Fig. 17.2h). Ultrasound and MRI will confirm the diagnosis. Treatment should be acute surgical repair.

Levator scapulae syndrome

The levator scapulae muscle is a site of pain and source of referred pain. In this particular syndrome, there is chronic inflammation indicated by tenderness at the site of the levator scapulae insertion onto the scapula. Accurate palpation of the levator scapulae should be carried out to detect any abnormalities.

Local soft tissue therapy should be applied at the site of attachment with distal ischemic pressure progressing to transverse friction as pain settles. Treatment of local areas of muscle thickening in the muscle belly is also necessary. This should be performed with myofascial soft tissue release techniques or dry needling. Occasionally, corticosteroid injection at the site of maximal tenderness is necessary. Patients should be encouraged to avoid habitual postures involving shoulder elevation and to stretch the muscle regularly.

Nerve entrapments

A number of nerve entrapments around the shoulder may produce shoulder pain.

Suprascapular nerve

The most common is entrapment of the suprascapular nerve.[34] The suprascapular nerve is derived from the upper trunk of the brachial plexus formed by the roots of the C5 and C6 nerves. The course of the nerve is shown in Figure 17.27. The nerve passes downwards beneath the trapezius to the superior border of the scapula. Here it passes through the suprascapular notch. The roof of this notch is formed by the transverse scapular ligament. After passing through the notch, the nerve supplies the supraspinatus muscle as well as articular branches to both the glenohumeral and AC joints. The nerve then turns around the lateral edge of the base of the spine of the scapula (the spinoglenoid notch) to innervate the infraspinatus muscle. Entrapment of the suprascapular nerve

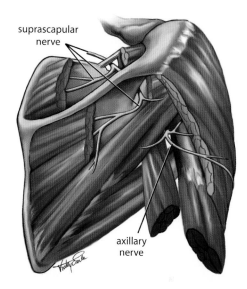

Figure 17.27 Course of the suprascapular nerve

may occur at either the suprascapular notch or the spinoglenoid notch.

The patient usually complains of pain that is deep and poorly localized. It is often felt posteriorly and laterally in the shoulder, or referred to the arm, neck or upper anterior chest wall. The patient may describe shoulder weakness. On examination, there may be wasting of the supraspinatus and/or infraspinatus muscles accompanied by weakness on abduction and external rotation. Tenderness over the suprascapular notch may also be present.

The site of entrapment in cases of combined supraspinatus and infraspinatus weakness is the suprascapular notch. The nerve may be stretched and kinked in this position by extremes of scapular motion associated with the throwing action. It may also occur in tennis players who complain of a weakness and lack of control over backhand volleys. Diagnosis is made on the clinical symptoms and confirmed by an abnormal electromyogram (Chapter 9). Surgical decompression of the nerve at the site of entrapment is occasionally required.

Isolated infraspinatus weakness and wasting may occur when the suprascapular nerve is trapped at the spinoglenoid notch. This condition has been seen in volleyball players who use the 'float' serve[35] and in weight-lifters. It can also arise due to a cyst that results from superior glenoid labral tears compressing the nerve. Treatment is generally non-operative but occasionally surgical decompression is required, particularly if a cyst is present.

Long thoracic nerve

The long thoracic nerve is formed from the roots of the C5, C6 and C7 nerves. The nerve passes behind the brachial plexus to perforate the fascia of the proximal serratus anterior, passing medial to the coracoid with branches throughout the length of the serratus anterior. Long thoracic nerve palsy causes paralysis of the serratus anterior, with winging of the scapula. The nerve may be injured by traction on the neck or shoulder or by blunt trauma. Isolated long thoracic nerve palsy may also follow viral illnesses.

Clinical features include pain and limited shoulder elevation. Patients may complain of difficulty in lifting weights or an uncomfortable feeling of pressure from a chair against a winged scapula while sitting. They may also develop secondary impingement due to poor scapular control. The most striking feature on examination is winging of the scapula when pushing against a wall with both hands. Electromyographic studies will confirm the diagnosis. Initial treatment is conservative and most patients will recover fully. Surgical tendon transfer may occasionally be required.

Axillary nerve compression

Axillary nerve compression or quadrilateral space syndrome is an uncommon condition caused by compression of the posterior humeral circumflex artery and axillary nerve or one of its major branches in the quadrilateral space. The quadrilateral or quadrangular space is located over the posterior scapula in the subdeltoid region and consists of the teres minor superiorly, teres major inferiorly, the long head of triceps medially and the surgical neck of the humerus laterally. The axillary nerve and the posterior humeral circumflex artery pass through the space at a level inferior to the glenohumeral joint capsule.[36]

Quadrilateral space syndrome is seen in throwing athletes and is characterized by poorly localized posterior shoulder pain, paresthesia over the lateral aspect of the shoulder and arm, and deltoid and teres minor weakness. The condition may occur secondary to abnormal fibrous bands, although traumatic causes have been described. Diagnosis is by electromyography or subclavian arteriogram, although this is associated with some risk. Treatment is initially conservative. Occasionally, surgical exploration is required.

Axillary nerve injuries can also occur with anterior dislocation of the shoulder and by blunt trauma to the anterior lateral deltoid muscle.[37]

Thoracic outlet syndrome

The term thoracic outlet syndrome (TOS) refers to a group of conditions that results from compression of the neurovascular structures that course from the neck to the axilla through the thoracic outlet (Fig. 17.28). The brachial plexus and subclavian vessels are especially susceptible to compression because of their proximity to one another in the thoracic outlet. The most common site of compression is the costoclavicular space between the clavicle and the first rib (costoclavicular syndrome).[38, 39] Other sites of compression are the triangle between the anterior scalene muscle, the middle scalene muscle and the upper border of the first rib (anterior scalene syndrome); and the angle between the coracoid process and the pectoralis minor insertion (hyperabduction syndrome or pectoralis minor syndrome).

Among athletes, this condition occurs most commonly in overhead sportspeople.[40] Poor posture with drooping shoulders can decrease the diameter of the cervicoaxillary canal, causing TOS symptoms. Congenital anatomical abnormalities that can compress the neurovascular structures include a complete cervical rib, incomplete cervical ribs with fibrous bands, fibrous bands from the transverse process of C7, and clavicular abnormalities. Complete cervical

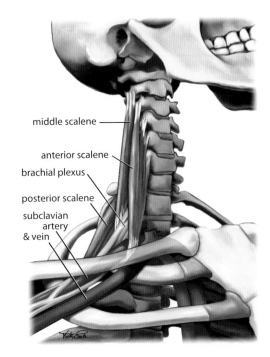

middle scalene

anterior scalene

brachial plexus

posterior scalene

subclavian
artery
& vein

Figure 17.28 Anatomy of the thoracic outlet

ribs are rare but, if present, are often bilateral. However, only 10% of patients with cervical ribs have TOS symptoms. TOS symptoms may be caused by shortening of the scalene muscles secondary to active trigger points. Traumatic structural changes that can cause TOS include fractures of the clavicle and/or first rib, pseudoarthrosis of the clavicle, malunion of clavicle fractures, exuberant callus formation or a crush injury of the upper thorax. TOS symptoms are common in patients with chronic scapular dyskinesis. They have tight pectoralis minor, scalene and upper trapezius muscles, with weak serratus anterior and lower trapezius muscles; this causes excessive anterior tilt and protraction.

While patients with TOS occasionally present with a pure arterial, venous or neurogenic picture, most often the picture is mixed. The patient may complain of pain in the neck or shoulder, or numbness or tingling involving either the entire upper limb or the forearm and hand. The patient may state that the arm feels weak or easily fatigued. There may be venous engorgement or coolness of the involved arm.

Physical signs may be absent. Various clinical tests have been proposed to assist in the diagnosis of this condition. A patient with arterial compression may have a positive Adson's test. The patient begins the test with the head laterally rotated to the side of the symptoms and extended. The patient then abducts the involved arm and inspires deeply. A positive test obliterates the radial pulse and reproduces symptoms. The sensitivity of this test can be greatly increased by the use of Doppler flow patterns during the maneuver. The most sensitive provocation test is the Roos hyperabduction/external rotation test, in which the patient opens and closes his or her hands for 1–3 minutes with elbows bent and arms abducted to 90° and externally rotated in an attempt to reproduce the symptoms. Evaluation of scapular motion and position can help to rule scapular dyskinesis in or out.

Treatment for any subset of TOS focuses on the specific area compromised.[40] However, certain treatments apply to all forms of TOS. Correction of drooping shoulders, poor posture and poor body mechanics is vital. The patient should be taught proper positioning while sitting, standing and lying down. Physiotherapy should address pectoral and scalene stretching and trigger point treatment, soft tissue mobilization of restricted tissues, scapular mobilization and scapulo-thoracic mobility. Joint mobilization of the first rib can restore accessory motion of the sternoclavicular and AC joints. Side-bending and cervical retraction exercises can correct forward head posture by stretching the soft tissues of the lateral cervical spine. Thoracic extension and brachial plexus stretching exercises are added as tolerated.

Surgical consultation and treatment is warranted for patients who have neurogenic TOS that does not respond to aggressive non-surgical management and for patients who have vascular compromise or thrombus formation. Arterial compression caused by a complete cervical rib is usually treated by first rib resection.

Axillary vein thrombosis ('effort' thrombosis)

Axillary vein thrombosis is also known as 'effort' thrombosis because of its frequent association with repetitive, vigorous activities or with blunt trauma that results in direct or indirect injury to the vein. The eponymous name, Paget-von Schrötter syndrome, is falling out of favor. The axillary vein can be compressed at various sites along its path, most significantly in the costoclavicular space. Compression most often occurs when the patient hyperextends the neck and hyperabducts the arm simultaneously, or when the patient assumes a military brace position with a backward thrust of the shoulders. Compression can also occur between the clavicle and the first rib, the costocoracoid ligament and first rib, or the subclavian muscles and first rib.

Patients complain of dull, aching pain, numbness or tightness, and heaviness of the upper arm and shoulder, along with fatigue after activities involving the extremity. The entire upper extremity will be swollen, the skin may be mottled and cold, and superficial veins may be prominent. The diagnosis is confirmed on venography. Treatment involves rest and anticoagulant therapy. Most patients make a full recovery and are able to resume sporting activities.[41]

Fractures around the shoulder joint

Stress fractures around the shoulder joint are uncommon. Stress fracture of the coracoid process is associated with the sport of trapshooting. Patients with this stress fracture have localized tenderness over the coracoid process and a focal area of increased uptake on isotopic bone scan.

Scapular fractures are usually due to a crushing force, either a fall on the shoulder or direct violence. Examination reveals marked tenderness and swelling. X-rays should be taken to exclude other associated injuries, such as a rib fracture, dislocated shoulder or dislocated sternoclavicular joint. Scapular fractures usually heal well, even if displaced. A broad arm sling is worn for comfort and active movements are commenced as soon as pain permits.

Fracture of the neck of the humerus is caused by a fall on the outstretched hand or direct violence. It is seen in adolescents, young adults and the elderly. Fractures involving more than two fragments displaced by more than 1 cm (0.5 in.) or associated with shoulder dislocation require surgical assessment. Minimally displaced or angulated fractures may be treated conservatively. Impacted fractures heal rapidly and can be supported in a broad arm sling. Displaced fractures are best treated in a collar and cuff that allows gravity to correct any angulation. For the first two weeks the arm should be kept in a sling under a shirt. After two weeks, pendular movement exercises of the shoulder joint should be commenced. From four weeks, a collar and cuff may be worn outside the clothes and gradually removed in stages over the following two weeks.

An unusual fracture is seen among throwing athletes.[42] These athletes sustain a closed external rotation spiral fracture of their humerus immediately below the insertion of the deltoid muscle at the junction of the middle and lower thirds of the humerus or along the radial groove. Many, but not all, patients with this fracture give a history of pain at the site of the fracture so it may be regarded as an acute stress fracture. The fracture heals well in a cast or functional brace.

Guidelines for shoulder rehabilitation

There are no definitive studies on the most effective rehabilitation protocols for the shoulder. However, in our practise, certain guidelines based on physiology and biomechanics have provided very good outcomes in terms of return to play. There are probably several protocols that can be used to optimize rehabilitation of the shoulder as long as they conform to the guidelines.

Make a complete and accurate diagnosis

Principle

The rehabilitation program can only be as good as the diagnosis. Too often, diagnosis of shoulder injuries is incomplete due to the number of factors that combine to influence shoulder function.

Practise

The diagnosis must not only include the local anatomical deficit, such as rotator cuff tear, Bankart lesion,

labral injury or fracture, but also the local biomechanical deficits that exist either as a result of the injury or of treatment. These would include inflexibility of internal or external rotation or adduction, force couple imbalance either of the internal and external rotators or of the supraspinatus in relationship to the deltoid, or acquired alterations in shoulder position, such as dropping the arm in the throwing position because of impingement. In addition, the regional deficits that may occur in the AC joint can also inhibit some of the muscle firing patterns. The scapula is a very important link in shoulder joint function. The position, motion and strength of the scapula and its muscles should be considered in the diagnosis.[43]

Finally, distant deficits should be evaluated as well. Back and hip inflexibility, injuries or strength imbalances should be evaluated. Inflexibilities of hip rotation, hamstrings or the back often commonly contribute to shoulder abnormalities. In addition, alterations in mechanics, whether it be hyperlordosis of the back, lack of rotation of the hip or trunk, or alteration of the plant leg in throwing, need evaluation. A complete diagnosis identifies not only the clinical symptoms and the tissues that are injured but also the tissues that are overloaded, the functional biomechanical deficits that exist and the subclinical adaptations that the athlete uses to try to maintain performance.[44] Rehabilitation should address all components of the complete and accurate diagnosis.

Early pain reduction

Principle

Pain is a major cause of altered shoulder function. Avoidance of painful positions causes the athlete to assume abnormal positions of the arm or back. Pain also creates a high degree of muscle inhibition, which alters muscle firing patterns.

Practise

Pain should be controlled early in rehabilitation. Strategies to decrease pain include relative rest of the area, with decreased throwing activities, avoidance of painful arcs of motion, cryotherapy, ultrasound, galvanic stimulation and medications.[45] This also may include judicious injection into the subacromial space if there are true signs of inflammation, non-steroidal medications and analgesia as needed. Exercises should be kept within pain-free arcs; these arcs become progressively greater as pain is controlled.

Integration of the kinetic chain into rehabilitation

Principle

It is important to re-establish the kinetic chain early in the rehabilitation process. In ground-based sports, all of the activities of the shoulder work within a kinetic chain linkage from the ground through to the trunk. While the shoulder is recovering from the injury or surgery, leg and trunk exercises can be prescribed so that when the shoulder is ready for rehabilitation, the base of the kinetic chain is also ready for link activity. After the shoulder is ready for rehabilitation, activation of the kinetic chain patterns from the legs through the back to the shoulder restores the force-dependent motor activation patterns and normal biomechanical positions. This then allows normal link sequencing to generate velocity and force.

Practise

Before starting formal strength rehabilitation, it is important to correct any inflexibilities of the hamstrings, hip and trunk; weakness or imbalances of the rotators of the trunk, flexors and extensors of the trunk and hip; and any subclinical adaptations of stance patterns or gait pattern.

Rehabilitation of the legs and hips should be concerned with generating appropriate sport-specific force and velocity from the lower extremity and should be done in a closed chain fashion. This pattern, which is done with the foot on the ground, simulates the patterns that exist in the throwing or hitting activities. Eccentric patterns should also be emphasized to absorb the load from jumping forward movement or stopping of the plant leg in the baseball throw. Combined patterns of hip and trunk rotation in both directions, hip and shoulder diagonal patterns from the left hip to the right shoulder and from the right hip to the left shoulder, should also be emphasized as most shoulder activities involve rotation and diagonal patterns (Fig. 17.29).[44] An excellent exercise involves jumping on a mini-trampoline and simultaneously extending the hips and scapula upon landing (Fig. 17.30). This extensor pattern allows for hip extension, trunk extension and scapular retraction in the same pattern that exists in the cocking phase of throwing activities. Integration of the scapular retraction muscles to the hip is very important because these reactions tend to be coupled in the cocking phases of throwing. Aim to correct abnormal reversal of the thoracic kyphosis and neck lordosis in this preliminary phase to allow normal positioning of the scapula.

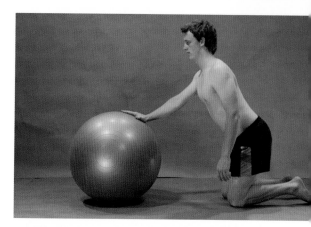

Figure 17.29 Integration of hip and trunk with the scapula

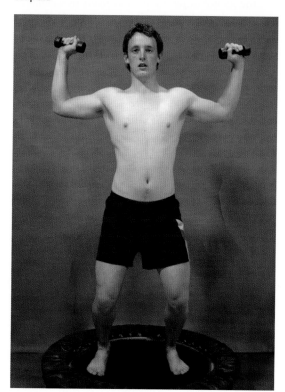

Figure 17.30 Minitrampoline exercise for coordinating extensor activity of the hip, trunk and shoulder

Endurance activities in the legs should also be emphasized, as should aerobic endurance for recovery from exercise bouts and anaerobic endurance for agility and power work. Examples include mini-trampoline exercises, agility drills with running and jumping, jumping jacks and slider or fitter boards.

Scapular stabilization

Principle

The scapula is the base upon which all shoulder activities rest. The four main roles of the scapula include:

1. retraction and protraction in the different phases of throwing motion
2. elevation of the acromion in abduction of the arm
3. acting as a socket for the glenohumeral joint
4. acting as a base of origin for all of the intrinsic muscles of the rotator cuff and the extrinsic muscles of the deltoid, biceps and triceps.

In addition, the scapula acts as a platform for shoulder rotation and arm activities. In biomechanics, the glenohumeral joint has been described as the equivalent of a golf ball on a tee due to the size relationships. A more accurate biomechanical description would be of a ball on a seal's nose. As the ball or humeral socket moves, the seal's nose or the scapula needs to move to maintain the position of the ball on the glenoid.

Acromial elevation and scapular stabilization is often jeopardized early in the injury process due to pain inhibiting the serratus anterior and lower trapezius, and to subclinical alterations of the position of the scapula to accommodate injury patterns in subluxation or impingement.[46]

Practise

Evaluation of the scapula is a high priority. Evaluate the motion and position of the scapula in various phases of the throwing motion and also assess muscular strength and scapular stabilization.[46] Appropriate exercises early in the rehabilitation process for scapular control include scapular pinch, an isometric activity in which the scapulae are retracted towards the midline. Integration of scapular retraction with rotator cuff co-contractions allows a more normal physiological pattern to redevelop. Most of the scapular control exercises are done through the method of closed chain rehabilitation (see below). Recent studies have shown that four specific exercises selectively activate the scapular stabilizing muscles: the scapular clock, low row, lawn mower and inferior glide (see Fig. 17.33).

Early achievement of 90° of abduction and improved glenohumeral rotation

Principle

Most throwing activities in sports demand 90° of shoulder abduction, as throwing activities occur between 85° and 110° of abduction, and require a large arc of glenohumeral rotation. Skilled length-dependent motor patterns and force-dependent patterns are based upon the achievement of 90° of abduction. Alteration of the joint position by 15° changes the motor activation patterns. Therefore, the thrower's shoulder should be rehabilitated at the 90° position to allow for the normal motor patterns to be recreated. This is the physiological angle for length-dependent motor patterns. Furthermore, at 90° of abduction, the inferior glenohumeral ligamentous constraints become taut in this position and, thus, contribute maximally to control of the instant center of rotation.

Practise

Aim to achieve 90° of abduction early in the rehabilitation process by reducing pain from impingement or other sources as quickly as possible. Maintain scapular stabilizer strength so that acromial elevation clears the acromion from the rotator cuff. Tendinopathy should be minimized to allow the tendons to slide under the coracoacromial arch. In operative cases, the subacromial space should be cleared of impediments to abduction, such as calcific deposits, bone spurs or excessively thick bursal tissue. When performing surgical reconstruction for shoulder stability, the surgeon must ensure that 90° of abduction can be obtained on the operating table. This will allow early achievement of 90° of abduction without undue stress on the ligaments. This is analogous to ensuring full extension of the knee in anterior cruciate ligament reconstructions. Specific exercises to achieve 90° of abduction include active-assisted wand maneuvers (Fig. 17.31), gentle joint mobilizations, proprioceptive neuromuscular facilitation patterns and passive stretching. The pace of progression should be relatively slow in the healing phases but may be more vigorous after three to six weeks. Sleeper stretches are very effective in achieving and maintaining glenohumeral rotation.

Closed chain rehabilitation

Principle

The predominant method of muscle activation around the shoulder articulation is a closed chain activity emphasizing co-contraction force couples at the scapulothoracic and glenohumeral joint. This results in proper scapular position and stability and allows the rotator cuff to work as a 'compressor cuff', conferring concavity–compression and a stable instant center of rotation. Closed chain activity also simulates the normal proprioceptive pathways that exist in the

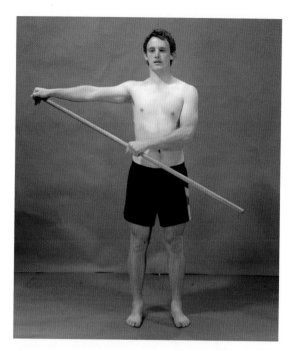

Figure 17.31 Wand exercise for active-assisted range of motion

throwing motion and allows feedback from the muscle spindles and Golgi tendon organs in their proper anatomical positions. Closed chain activity replicates the normal ball and socket kinematics, minimizing translation in the mid ranges of motion. Finally, by decreasing deltoid activation, these activities decrease the tendency for superior humeral migration if the rotator cuff is weak.

Open chain activities, which involve agonist–antagonist force couples and generate force for the shoulder and the kinetic chain, also are seen around the shoulder articulation but are of secondary importance. They require deltoid and other extrinsic muscle activation, create shear forces at the glenohumeral joint and require large ranges of motion. Exercises to simulate these activities should be instituted later in rehabilitation as they produce larger forces and require greater motions than the shoulder can tolerate early in rehabilitation. Closed chain rehabilitation provides a stable scapular base and early rotator cuff strength, which allows open chain activities.

Practise

The exercises are started at levels below 90° of abduction in the early phases of rehabilitation to allow for healing of the tissues.[44, 46] They may be started at 45° of abduction and 60° of flexion and then proceed to 90° of

abduction as tolerated. The hand is placed against some object, such as a table, a ball or the wall, and resistance is generated through the activities of the scapula and shoulder. When the arm can be safely positioned at 90° of abduction, it is placed in either abduction or flexion and a specific progression is started.

The closed chain activities are first started with scapular stabilization. Patterns of retraction and protraction of the scapula are started in single planes and then progress to elevation and depression of the entire scapula and then selective elevation of the acromion (Fig. 17.32).

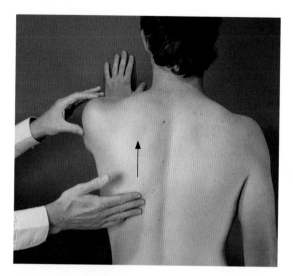

Figure 17.32 Scapular exercises

(a) Scapular elevation

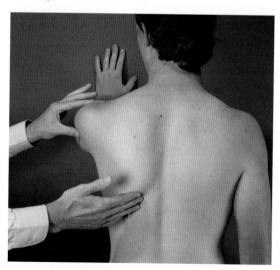

(b) Scapular retraction

The next progression is on to rotator cuff activity. Joint compression with contraction into the shoulder joint is followed by 'clock' exercises, in which the hand is moved to the various positions on the clock face, ranging from eight o'clock to four o'clock (Fig. 17.33a). This allows for rotation of the humerus with the arm at 90° of abduction, which replicates rotator cuff activity throughout all components of the rotator cuff. These activities are first done against fixed resistance, such as a wall, and then can be moved to movable resistance, such as a ball or some other movable implement. These exercises may be done early in the rehabilitation phase as they do not put shear on the joint and allow rotator cuff muscles to be activated without being inhibited by pain or deltoid overactivity.

Closed chain progressions may be used in later phases of rehabilitation. They include various types of push-ups (wall leans, knee push-ups and regular push-ups; Fig. 17.34) and scaption exercises (Fig. 17.35).

Plyometric exercises

Principle

Most athletic activities involve development of power. Power is the rate of doing work and, therefore, has a

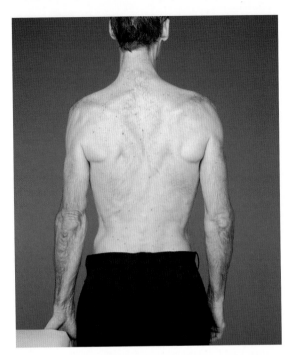

(b) Low row—the patient pushes back isometrically with the arm in no more than 10° of extension. The patient is instructed to 'push back with your entire arm and slide your scapula down at the same time'

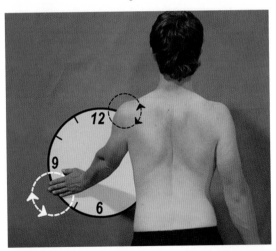

Figure 17.33 Scapular exercises

(a) Scapular clock—the patient envisions a clock tattooed on the injured shoulder then places the arm against a wall (as shown) or on a ball which may be rolled against the wall or on a table/couch. The patient then moves the shoulder in the direction of 12 o'clock, 3 o'clock or 6 o'clock which facilitates scapula elevation, retraction, and depression, respectively.

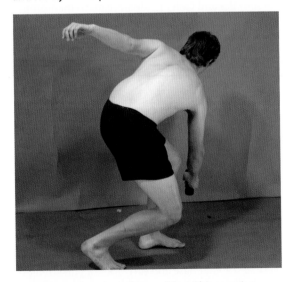

(c) Lawn mower—starting position. This exercise simulates pulling the starting cord of a lawn mower. It can be commenced with large amounts of trunk rotation and lower limb extension to guide shoulder motion. Early in rehabilitation it is done without weights; dumbbells (shown) and tubing can be used to progress the exercise

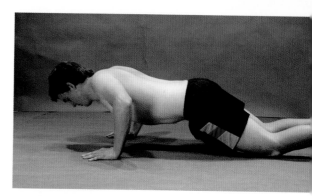

(d) Lawn mower—finishing position

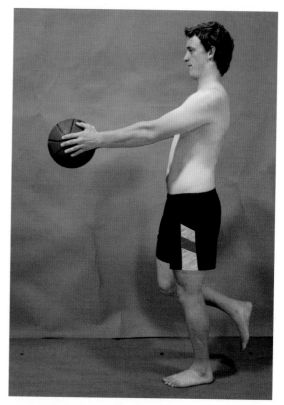

(b) Knee push-ups

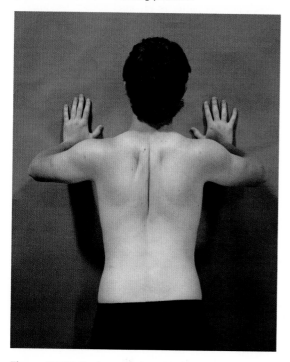

Figure 17.34 Push-up progressions

(a) Wall push-ups

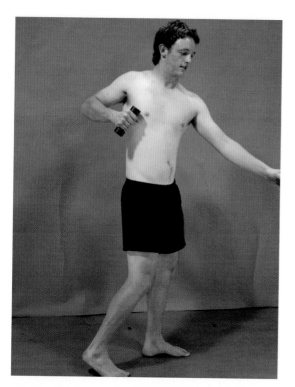

Figure 17.35 Scaption exercises

time component. For most sports, this time component is relatively rapid. Plyometric activities develop the athlete's ability to generate power by producing a stretch-shortening cycle in which the muscle is eccentrically stretched and slowly loaded. This pretensioning phase is followed by a rapid concentric contraction to develop a large amount of momentum and force. Because these exercises develop a large amount of strain in the eccentric phase of the activity and force in the concentric phase of the activity, they should be done when complete anatomical healing has occurred. Similarly, because large ranges of motion are required, full range of motion should be obtained before the plyometric activities are started. These stretch-shortening activation sequences are part of the normal force-dependent patterns that are present in skilled athletes.

Practise

Plyometrics should be done for all body segments involved in the activity and not just the shoulder. Hip rotation, knee flexion/extension and trunk rotation are all power activities that require plyometric activation. Plyometric activities for the lower extremity can be done in the early phases of rehabilitation but plyometric exercises for the upper extremity should be instituted in later phases. Many different activities and devices can be utilized in plyometric exercises.

Rubber tubing is a very effective plyometric device (Fig. 17.36). The arm or leg can be positioned exactly in the position of the athletic activity and then the motion can be replicated by use of the rubber tubing. Balls are also excellent plyometric devices. The weight of the ball creates a prestretch as the ball is caught and creates resistance for contraction forces (Fig. 17.37). Light weights can also be used for plyometric activities but caution must be used in using

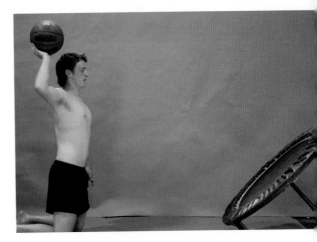

Figure 17.37 Throwing and catching basketball against minitrampoline

heavier weights in a plyometric fashion due to the forces applied on the joint. Plyometric activities with larger weights can be done more easily in the lower extremity than the upper extremity. By reproducing these stretch-shortening cycles at positions of physiological function, these plyometric activities also stimulate proprioceptive feedback to fine tune the muscle activity patterns. Plyometric exercises are the most appropriate open chain exercises for functional shoulder rehabilitation.

Rotator cuff exercises

Principle

The rotator cuff muscles are very important in creating concavity compression to maintain the humeral head in the glenoid socket. They do this by participating with the deltoid in the abduction force couple and with themselves in a rotation force couple. Because of their relatively small size, they are frequently overpowered and inhibited by deltoid activity. For these reasons, they are often the site of overload abnormalities around the shoulder. Rotator cuff weakness is often the final common pathway that leads to clinical symptoms and dysfunction around the shoulder. However, because many pathological conditions contribute to rotator cuff overload, selective isolated rotator cuff exercises are frequently not successful in relieving the clinical symptoms. The rotator cuff muscles act as a unit in functional shoulder activities.

Practise

Rotator cuff muscles should be rehabilitated as an integrated unit, rather than as individual muscles.

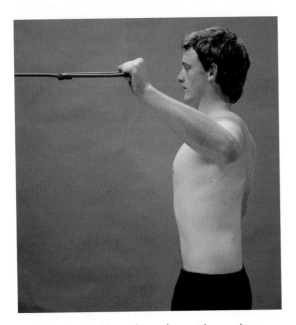

Figure 17.36 Rubber tubing plyometric exercises. The tubing creates an eccentric stretch and offers resistance to concentric contraction

They do not work in isolation in shoulder function, and the anatomical positions and motions that are used for testing are not seen in shoulder function. Because they require a stabilized scapula to provide a stable base of muscle origin, and because individual rotator cuff activity creates shear across the glenohumeral joint, early rotator cuff exercises should be done in a closed chain fashion. This allows rotator cuff strengthening without inducing shear on the joint nor allowing deltoid overactivity to create impingement. We have found that closed chain rotator cuff strengthening exercises redevelop the composite rotator cuff effectively and that isolated rotator cuff exercises are increasingly less commonly needed in later stages of rehabilitation. If rotator cuff deficits are still observed in the later phases of rehabilitation, isolated rotator cuff exercises can be prescribed.

Isolated rotator cuff exercises may be very effective as part of a preparticipation conditioning program. The exercises strengthen the individual rotator cuff muscles as part of a spectrum of isolated and integrated conditioning exercises.

A useful clinical sign for deficiencies in rotator cuff rehabilitation is exacerbation of clinical symptoms when rotator cuff exercises are started. If rotator cuff exercises increase clinical symptoms, this can be traced to abnormalities in other parts of the kinetic chain. Further evaluation of the kinetic chain should be done and the exercises should be directed to the source of weakness. This source is most commonly the scapular stabilizers.

Summary of the principles

These guidelines are very effective in clinical practise. They emphasize a sequence of rehabilitation and address all the functional deficits that may occur in association with shoulder abnormalities. Many different therapeutic exercises can be used to fulfil each of the guidelines. The exact protocol may be based on the patient's presentation, the clinical examination, the therapist's skill and the therapist's imagination. Adherence to this program requires patient education and guidance from the physician and physiotherapist on the techniques of rehabilitation. However, most of the physiotherapy can be done by home programs once the exercises have been taught appropriately. Physiotherapy office visits are used for assessment of achievement of the individual goals for the rehabilitation sequence, instruction in the exercises to be done in the next phase and specific guidance as to goals to achieve for the next rehabilitation phase. Modalities such as ice, electrogalvanic stimulation, ultrasound or heat are very rarely needed after the initial stages of pain reduction.

Putting it all together: specific rehabilitation protocols

The general rehabilitation protocol listed is the basic protocol. Deviations from this protocol may be based on the individual needs of the patient and his or her progression.

This protocol assumes, if surgery has been performed, stable repair of the labrum, capsule or rotator cuff and ability to achieve 90° of abduction without impingement or excessive capsular stretch at the time of the operation. The time frame depends on the severity of the injury or extent of the surgical procedure(s). The rehabilitation goal is to progress post-operative labral repairs, shoulder reconstructions and acromioplasties to 90° of passive or active-assisted abduction by three weeks and rotator cuff repairs to 90° of passive or active-assisted abduction by four to six weeks.

Acute phase

The goals of the acute phase are:

- tissue healing
- reduction of pain and inflammation
- re-establishment of non-painful range of motion below 90° of abduction
- retardation of muscle atrophy
- scapular control
- maintenance of fitness in other components of the kinetic chain.

Tissue healing

Tissue healing is the combination of:

- rest
- short-term immobilization
- modalities
- surgery.

Reduce pain and inflammation

Aggressive treatment is used to control pain to decrease inhibition-based muscle atrophy and scapular instability due to serratus and/or trapezius inhibition. This is done through:

- medications, either non-steroidal or judicious use of corticosteroids orally or by injection
- modalities, usually ultrasound (two per week every two weeks)
- cold compression devices.

Re-establish range of motion

The range of motion should be started in pain-free arcs, kept below 90° of abduction, and may be passive or active-assisted. The degree of movement is guided by the stability of the operative repair. Range of motion should be re-established by:

- pendulum exercises
- manual capsular stretching and cross-fiber massage
- T-bar or ropes and pulleys.

Retard muscle atrophy

Isometric exercises, with the arm below 90° of abduction and 90° of flexion, should be done in patients with labral or capsular repair but not in those with rotator cuff repairs.

Scapular control

The exercises to maintain scapular control include:

- isometric scapular pinches and scapular elevation
- low row (Fig. 17.33b)
- closed chain weight shifts, with hands on table and the shoulders flexed less than 60° and abducted less than 45°
- tilt board or circular board weight shifts with the same limitations (Fig. 17.38).

Maintain fitness in rest of kinetic chain

Exercises to maintain fitness in the rest of the kinetic chain include:

- aerobic exercises such as running, bicycling or stepping

- anaerobic agility drills
- lower extremity strengthening by machines, squat exercises or open chain leg lifts
- elbow and wrist strengthening by isometric exercises or rubber tubing
- flexibility exercises, especially for areas that are shown to be tight on evaluation
- integration of the kinetic chain by leg and trunk stabilization on a ball, employing rotational and oblique patterns of contraction (Fig. 17.39).

Criteria for movement out of the acute phase

The criteria for movement out of the acute phase include:

- progression of tissue healing (healed or sufficiently stabilized for active motion and tissue loading)
- passive range of motion at 66–75% of opposite side
- minimal pain
- manual muscle strength in non-pathological areas of 4+/5
- achievement of scapular asymmetry of less than 1.5 cm (0.6 in.)
- kinetic chain function and integration.

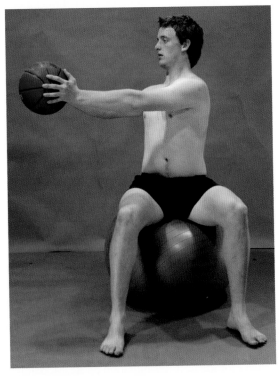

Figure 17.39 Plyoball hip and trunk rotation exercise

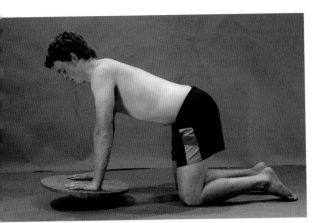

Figure 17.38 Closed chain weight shift using tilt board

Recovery phase

The goals of the recovery phase are:

- normal active and passive shoulder and glenohumeral range of motion
- improved scapular control
- normal upper extremity strength and strength balance
- normal shoulder arthrokinetics in single and then multiple planes of motion
- normal kinetic chain and force generation patterns.

Normal range of motion

Normal active and passive shoulder and glenohumeral range of motion is achieved by:

- active-assisted motion above 90° of abduction with wand
- active-assisted, then active, motion in internal and external rotation with scapula stabilized so that glenohumeral rotation is normalized without substitution movements from the scapula.

Scapular control

Scapular control is improved by:

- scapular proprioceptive neuromuscular facilitation patterns
- closed chain exercises at 90° of flexion, 90° of abduction, scapular retraction/protraction and scapular elevation/depression (Fig. 17.32)
- modified push-ups (Fig. 17.34b)
- regular push-ups
- ball catch and push exercises (Fig. 17.37)
- dips
  — clock
  — low row
  — lawn mower

Upper extremity strength and strength balance

Normal upper extremity strength and strength balance is achieved by:

- glenohumeral proprioceptive neuromuscular facilitation patterns
- closed chain exercises at 90° of flexion then 90° of abduction, using the glenohumeral depressors and glenohumeral internal/external rotators
- forearm curls
- isolated rotator cuff exercises

- machines or weights for light bench presses, military presses and pull-downs. The resistance should initially be light, then progress as strength improves. Emphasis is placed on proper mechanics, proper technique and joint stabilization.

Normal shoulder arthrokinetics

Normal shoulder arthrokinetics is achieved by:

- range of motion exercises with arm at 90° of abduction—this is the position where most throwing and serving activities occur; the periarticular soft tissues must be completely loose and balanced at this position
- muscle activity at 90° of abduction—normal muscle firing patterns must be re-established at this position, both in organization of force generation and force regulation patterns, and in proprioceptive sensory feedback; closed chain patterns are an excellent method to re-establish the normal neurological patterns for joint stabilization
- open chain exercises, including mild plyometric exercises, which may be built upon the base of the closed chain stabilization to allow normal control of joint mobility.

Normal kinetic chain and force generation

Normal kinetic chain and force generation patterns are achieved by:

- normalization of all inflexibilities throughout the kinetic chain
- normal agonist–antagonist force couples in the legs using squats, plyometric depth jumps, lunges and hip extensions
- trunk rotation exercises with medicine ball or tubing
- integrated exercises with leg and trunk stabilization, rotations, diagonal patterns from hip to shoulder, and medicine ball throws
- rotator cuff strength of 4+/5 or higher
- normal kinetic chain function.

Functional phase

The goals of the functional phase are:

- to increase power and endurance in the upper extremity
- to increase normal multiple-plane neuromuscular control—locally, regionally and in the entire kinetic chain
- instruction in rehabilitation activities
- sport-specific activity.

Power and endurance in upper extremity

Power is the rate of doing work. Work may be done to move the joint and the extremity or it may be done to absorb a load and stabilize the joint or extremity. Power has a time component and, for shoulder activity, quick movements and quick reactions are the dominant ways of doing work. These exercises should, therefore, be done with relatively rapid movements in planes that approximate normal shoulder function (i.e. 90° of abduction in shoulder, trunk rotation and diagonal arm motions, rapid external/internal rotation). The exercises include:

- diagonal and multiplanar motions with rubber tubing (Fig. 17.36), light weights, small medicine balls and isokinetic machines
- plyometrics—wall push-ups (Fig. 17.34a), corner push-ups, weighted ball throws and tubing. Tubing exercises may be used to mimic any of the needed motions in throwing or serving. Medicine balls are very effective plyometric devices. The weight of the ball creates a prestretch and an eccentric load as it is caught. It also creates a resistance for contraction forces, demanding a powerful agonist contraction to propel it forward.

Increase multiple-plane neuromuscular control

The force-dependent motor firing patterns should be re-established. No subclinical adaptations, such as 'opening up' (trunk rotation too far in front of shoulder rotation), three-quarter arm positioning on throwing or excessive wrist snap should be allowed. Help in this area can be obtained by watching pre-injury videos or by using a knowledgeable coach in the particular sport. Special care must be taken to integrate all of the components of the kinetic chain completely to generate and funnel the proper forces to and through the shoulder.

Rehabilitation

The athlete who is injured while playing a sport will most often return to the sport with the same sports demands. The body should be healed from the symptomatic standpoint and should be prepared for resuming the stresses inherent in playing the sport. The aim of rehabilitation is to improve:

- flexibility—general body flexibility, with an emphasis on sport-specific problems (shoulder internal rotation and elbow extension in the arm, low back, hip rotation and hamstrings in the legs)

- strength—appropriate amounts and locations of strength for force generation, trunk rotation strength for sport-specific activities (quadriceps/hamstring strength for force generation, trunk rotation strength, strength balance for the shoulder)
- power—rapid movements in appropriate planes with light weights
- endurance—mainly anaerobic exercises due to short duration, explosive and ballistic activities seen in throwing and serving. These exercises should be based on the periodization principle of conditioning.

Sport-specific activity

Functional progressions of throwing or serving must be completed before full completion is allowed. These progressions will gradually test all of the mechanical parts of the throwing or serving motion. Very few deviations from normal parameters of arm motion, arm position, force generation, smoothness of all of the kinetic chain and pre-injury form should be allowed as most of these adaptations will be biomechanically inefficient. The athlete may move through the progressions as rapidly as possible.

Criteria for return to play

The criteria for return to play include:

- normal clinical examination
- normal shoulder arthrokinetics
- normal kinetic chain integration
- completed progressions.

Recommended Reading

Burkhart SS, Morgan CD, Kibler WB. The disabled throwing shoulder: spectrum of pathology. Part I: pathoanatomy and biomechanics. *Arthroscopy* 2003; 19(4): 404–20.

Burkhart SS, Morgan CD, Kibler WB. The disabled throwing shoulder: spectrum of pathology. Part II: evaluation and treatment of SLAP lesions in throwers. *Arthroscopy* 2003; 19(5): 531–9.

Burkhart SS, Morgan CD, Kibler WB. The disabled throwing shoulder: spectrum of pathology. Part III: The SICK scapula, scapular dyskinesis, the kinetic chain, and rehabilitation. *Arthroscopy* 2003; 19(6): 641–61.

Kibler WB. The role of the scapula in athletic shoulder function. *Am J Sports Med* 1998; 26: 325–37.

Kibler WB. Shoulder rehabilitation: principles and practice. *Med Sci Sports Exerc* 1998; 30: S40–S50.

Tzannes A, Murrell GAC. Clinical examination of the unstable shoulder. *Sports Med* 2002; 32: 1–11.

References

1. Pagnani M, Warren R. Stabilisers of the glenohumeral joint. *J Shoulder Elbow Surg* 1994; 3: 173–90.
2. Walton J, Mahajan S, Paxinos A, et al. Diagnostic values of tests for acromioclavicular joint pain. *J Bone Joint Surg Am* 2004; 86A(4): 807–12.
3. Murrell GA, Walton JR. Diagnosis of rotator cuff tears. *Lancet* 2001; 357(9258): 769–70.
4. Burkhart SS, Morgan CD, Kibler WB. The disabled throwing shoulder: spectrum of pathology. Part I: pathoanatomy and biomechanics. *Arthroscopy* 2003; 19(4): 404–20.
5. Burkhart SS, Morgan CD, Kibler WB. The disabled throwing shoulder: spectrum of pathology. Part III: The SICK scapula, scapular dyskinesis, the kinetic chain, and rehabilitation. *Arthroscopy* 2003; 19(6): 641–61.
6. Burkhart SS, Morgan CD, Kibler WB. The disabled throwing shoulder: spectrum of pathology. Part II: evaluation and treatment of SLAP lesions in throwers. *Arthroscopy* 2003; 19(5): 531–9.
7. Yuan J, Murrell GA, Wei AQ, Wang MX. Apoptosis in rotator cuff tendonopathy. *J Orthop Res* 2002; 20(6): 1372–9.
8. Paoloni JA, Appleyard RC, Nelson J, et al. Topical glyceryl trinitrate application in the treatment of chronic supraspinatus tendinopathy: a randomized, double-blinded, placebo-controlled clinical trial. *Am J Sports Med* 2005; 33(6): 806–13.
9. Blair B, Rokito AS, Cuomo F, et al. Efficacy of injections of corticosteroids for subacromial impingement syndrome. *J Bone Joint Surg Am* 1996; 78(11): 1685–9.
10. Uhthoff HK, Loehr JW. Calcific tendinopathy of the rotator cuff: pathogenesis, diagnosis, and management. *J Am Acad Orthop Surg* 1997; 5(4): 183–91.
11. Gerdesmeyer L, Wagenpfeil S, Haake M, et al. Extracorporeal shock wave therapy for the treatment of chronic calcifying tendonitis of the rotator cuff: a randomized controlled trial. *JAMA* 2003; 290(19): 2573–80.
12. Harniman E, Carette S, Kennedy C, Beaton D. Extracorporeal shock wave therapy for calcific and noncalcific tendonitis of the rotator cuff: a systematic review. *J Hand Ther* 2004; 17(2): 132–51.
13. Moretti B, Garofalo R, Genco S, et al. Medium-energy shock wave therapy in the treatment of rotator cuff calcifying tendinitis. *Knee Surg Sports Traumatol Arthrosc* 2005; 13(5): 405–10.
14. Peters J, Luboldt W, Schwarz W, et al. Extracorporeal shock wave therapy in calcific tendinitis of the shoulder. *Skeletal Radiol* 2004; 33(12): 712–18.
15. Wilk KE, Reinold MM, Dugas JR, et al. Current concepts in the recognition and treatment of superior labral (SLAP) lesions. *J Orthop Sports Phys Ther* 2005; 35(5): 273–91.
16. Rhee YG, Lee DH, Lim CT. Unstable isolated SLAP lesion: clinical presentation and outcome of arthroscopic fixation. *Arthroscopy* 2005; 21(9): 1099.
17. Snyder SJ, Banas MP, Karzel RP. An analysis of 140 injuries to the superior glenoid labrum. *J Shoulder Elbow Surg* 1995; 4(4): 243–8.
18. Applegate GR, Hewitt M, Snyder SJ, et al. Chronic labral tears: value of magnetic resonance arthrography in evaluating the glenoid labrum and labral-bicipital complex. *Arthroscopy* 2004; 20(9): 959–63.
19. Liu SH, Henry MH, Nuccion S, et al. Diagnosis of glenoid labral tears. A comparison between magnetic resonance imaging and clinical examinations. *Am J Sports Med* 1996; 24(2): 149–54.
20. Fabbriciani C, Milano G, Demontis A, et al. Arthroscopic versus open treatment of Bankart lesion of the shoulder: a prospective randomized study. *Arthroscopy* 2004; 20(5): 456–62.
21. Itoi E, Sashi R, Minagawa H, et al. Position of immobilization after dislocation of the glenohumeral joint. A study with use of magnetic resonance imaging. *J Bone Joint Surg Am* 2001; 83A(5): 661–7.
22. Miller BS, Sonnabend DH, Hatrick C, et al. Should acute anterior dislocations of the shoulder be immobilized in external rotation? A cadaveric study. *J Shoulder Elbow Surg* 2004; 13(6): 589–92.
23. Itoi E, Hatakeyama Y, Kido T, et al. A new method of immobilization after traumatic anterior dislocation of the shoulder: a preliminary study. *J Shoulder Elbow Surg* 2003; 12(5): 413–15.
24. Tzannes A, Paxinos A, Callanan M, et al. An assessment of the interexaminer reliability of tests for shoulder instability. *J Shoulder Elbow Surg* 2004; 13(1): 18–23.
25. Speer KP, Hannafin JA, Altchek DW, et al. An evaluation of the shoulder relocation test. *Am J Sports Med* 1994; 22(2): 177–83.
26. Warner JJ, Allen A, Marks PH, et al. Arthroscopic release for chronic, refractory adhesive capsulitis of the shoulder. *J Bone Joint Surg Am* 1996; 78(12): 1808–16.
27. Diwan DB, Murrell GA. An evaluation of the effects of the extent of capsular release and of postoperative therapy on the temporal outcomes of adhesive capsulitis. *Arthroscopy* 2005; 21(9): 1105–13.
28. Kabak S, Halici M, Tuncel M, et al. Treatment of midclavicular nonunion: comparison of dynamic compression plating and low-contact dynamic

compression plating techniques. *J Shoulder Elbow Surg* 2004; 13(4): 396–403.

29. Bradley JP, Elkousy H. Decision making: operative versus nonoperative treatment of acromioclavicular joint injuries. *Clin Sports Med* 2003; 22(2): 277–90.

30. Turnbull JR. Acromioclavicular joint disorders. *Med Sci Sports Exerc* 1998; 35(suppl.): S26–S32.

31. Kay SP, Dragoo JL, Lee R. Long-term results of arthroscopic resection of the distal clavicle with concomitant subacromial decompression. *Arthroscopy* 2003; 19(8): 805–9.

32. Zanetti M, Weishaupt D, Gerber C, et al. Tendinopathy and rupture of the tendon of the long head of the biceps brachii muscle: evaluation with MR arthrography. *AJR Am J Roentgenol* 1998; 170(6): 1557–61.

33. Petilon J, Carr DR, Sekiya JK, et al. Pectoralis major muscle injuries: evaluation and management. *J Am Acad Orthop Surg* 2005; 13(1): 59–68.

34. Bayramoglu A, Demiryurek D, Tuccar E, et al. Variations in anatomy at the suprascapular notch possibly causing suprascapular nerve entrapment: an anatomical study. *Knee Surg Sports Traumatol Arthrosc* 2003; 11(6): 393–8.

35. Ferretti A, De Carli A, Fontana M. Injury of the suprascapular nerve at the spinoglenoid notch. The natural history of infraspinatus atrophy in volleyball players. *Am J Sports Med* 1998; 26: 759–63.

36. Feinberg JH, Nadler SF, Krivickas LS. Peripheral nerve injuries in the athlete. *Sports Med* 1997; 24(6): 385–408.

37. Krivickas LS, Wilbourn AJ. Peripheral nerve injuries in athletes: a case series of over 200 injuries. *Semin Neurol* 2000; 20(2): 225–32.

38. Atasoy E. Thoracic outlet syndrome: anatomy. *Hand Clin* 2004; 20(1): 7–14, v.

39. Brantigan CO, Roos DB. Etiology of neurogenic thoracic outlet syndrome. *Hand Clin* 2004; 20(1): 17–22.

40. Richardson AB. Thoracic outlet syndrome in aquatic athletes. *Clin Sports Med* 1999; 18(2): 361–78.

41. Chaudhry MA, Hajarnavis J. Paget-von Schrotter syndrome: primary subclavian-axillary vein thrombosis in sport activities. *Clin J Sport Med* 2003; 13(4): 269–71.

42. Ogawa K, Yoshida A. Throwing fracture of the humeral shaft. An analysis of 90 patients. *Am J Sports Med* 1998; 26(2): 242–6.

43. Kibler BW. The role of the scapula in athletic shoulder function. *Am J Sports Med* 1998; 26: 325–7.

44. Kibler WB. Rehabilitation of rotator cuff tendinopathy. *Clin Sports Med* 2003; 22(4): 837–47.

45. Kibler WB, McMullen J, Uhl T. Shoulder rehabilitation strategies, guidelines, and practice. *Orthop Clin North Am* 2001; 32(3): 527–38.

46. Kibler WB, McMullen J. Scapular dyskinesis and its relation to shoulder pain. *J Am Acad Orthop Surg* 2003; 11(2): 142–51.

Elbow and Arm Pain

WITH SIMON BELL

Use of the upper limb in sport demands a well-functioning elbow. In addition, injuries in this region may interfere with the patient's everyday activities. The clinical approach to elbow pain is considered under the following headings:

- lateral elbow pain, with a particular focus on extensor tendinopathy
- medial elbow pain
- posterior elbow pain
- acute elbow injuries
- forearm pain
- upper arm pain.

Lateral elbow pain

Lateral elbow pain is an extremely common presentation among sportspeople and manual workers. The most common cause is an overuse syndrome related to excessive wrist extension. This condition has traditionally been known as 'tennis elbow'. This is an unsatisfactory term as it gives little indication of the pathological processes involved. In fact, the condition is more common in non-tennis players than in tennis players. It has also been referred to as 'lateral epicondylitis'. This is also inappropriate as the site of the abnormality is usually just below the lateral epicondyle (Fig. 18.1) and the primary pathology is due to collagen disarray rather than inflammation (Chapter 2).

The primary pathological process involved in this condition is tendinosis (Chapter 2) of the extensor carpi radialis brevis (ECRB) tendon, usually within 1–2 cm (0.5–1 in.) of its attachment to the common extensor origin at the lateral epicondyle. This condition will be referred to as extensor tendinopathy.

Other conditions that may cause lateral elbow pain include synovitis of the radiohumeral joint, radiohumeral bursitis and entrapment of the posterior interosseous branch of the radial nerve (radial tunnel syndrome). These conditions may exist by themselves or in conjunction with extensor tendinopathy.

There is often a contribution to lateral elbow pain from the cervical and upper thoracic spines and neural structures (Chapter 3). This may be a relatively minor contribution or, in some cases, the main cause of the patient's elbow pain. A full assessment of the cervical spine (Chapter 16) and neural structures (Chapter 8) is essential in examination of the patient with lateral elbow pain. The causes of lateral elbow pain are summarized in Table 18.1.

History

The characteristics of the patient's lateral elbow pain should be elicited. The diffuse pain of extensor tendinopathy typically radiates from the lateral epicondyle into the proximal forearm extensor muscle mass. Occasionally the pain may be more localized. The onset of pain may be either acute or insidious. There may have been recent changes in training or technique, note-taking or equipment used in sport or work.

The severity of pain ranges from relatively trivial pain to an almost incapacitating pain that may keep the patient awake at night. It is important to note whether the pain is aggravated by relatively minor everyday activities, such as picking up a cup, or whether it requires repeated activity, such as playing tennis or bricklaying, to become painful.

Pain may radiate into the lateral aspect of the forearm. This may be consistent with posterior

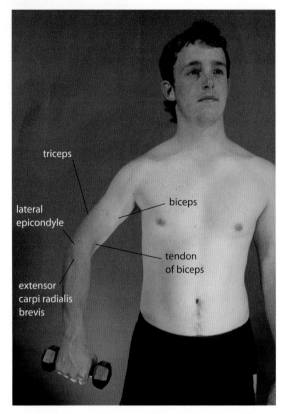

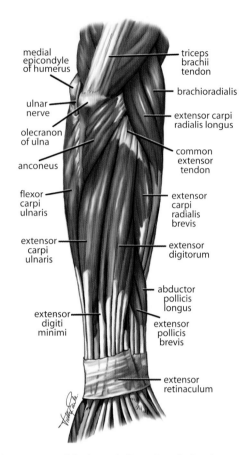

Figure 18.1 Anatomy of the lateral elbow

(a) Surface anatomy of the lateral elbow

(b) Anatomy of the lateral elbow from behind

interosseous nerve entrapment or irritation of other neural structures. If pain is closely related to the activity level, it is more likely to be of a mechanical origin. If pain is persistent, unpredictable or related to posture, referred pain should be considered.

Certain movements, usually those involving wrist extension or gripping, will aggravate mechanical pain. Referred pain is affected by prolonged posture, such as lengthy periods seated at a desk or in a car. Associated sensory symptoms, such as pins and needles, may indicate a neural component. Presence

of neck, upper thoracic or shoulder pain should also be noted.

Often by the time the patient presents to the sports medicine clinician, he or she will already have undergone a variety of treatments. It is important to note the response to each of these treatments.

An activity history should also be taken, noting any recent change in the level of activity. In tennis players, note any change in racquet size, grip size or string tension and whether or not any comment has been made regarding his or her technique.

Table 18.1 Causes of lateral elbow pain

Common	Less common	Not to be missed
Extensor tendinopathy	Synovitis of the radiohumeral joint	Osteochondritis dissecans
Referred pain	Radiohumeral bursitis	Capitellum
Cervical spine	Posterior interosseous nerve	Radius (in adolescents)
Upper thoracic spine	entrapment (radial tunnel	
Neuro-myofascial	syndrome)	

Examination

Examination involves:

1. Observation from the front
2. Active movements
   (a) elbow flexion/extension
   (b) supination/pronation
   (c) wrist flexion (forearm pronated) (Fig. 18.2a)
   (d) wrist extension
3. Passive movements
   (a) as above
4. Resisted movements
   (a) wrist extension (Fig. 18.2b)
   (b) extension at the third metacarpophalangeal joint (Fig. 18.2c)
   (c) grip test (Fig. 18.2d)
5. Palpation
   (a) lateral epicondyle (Fig. 18.2e)
   (b) extensor muscles (Fig. 18.2f)
6. Special tests
   (a) neural tension
   (b) cervical spine examination (Chapter 16)
   (c) thoracic spine examination (Chapter 20)
   (d) periscapular soft tissues (Fig. 18.2g)

Investigations

Investigations are usually not performed in the straightforward case of lateral elbow pain. However,

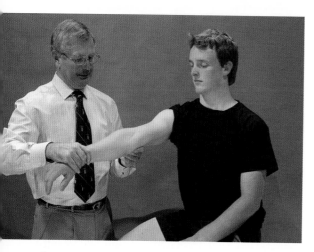

Figure 18.2 Examination of the patient with lateral elbow pain

(a) Active movement—wrist flexion with forearm fully pronated

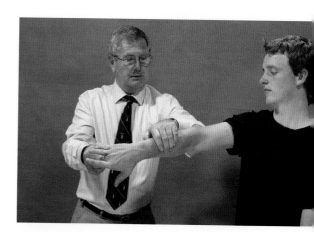

(c) Resisted muscle testing—extension at third metacarpophalangeal joint

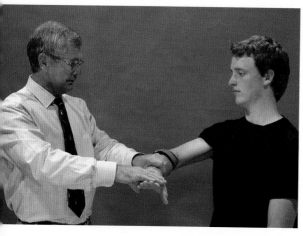

(b) Resisted muscle testing—wrist extension

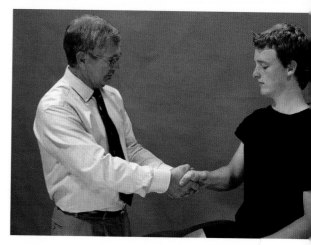

(d) Resisted muscle testing—grip strength. Attempt to reproduce pain

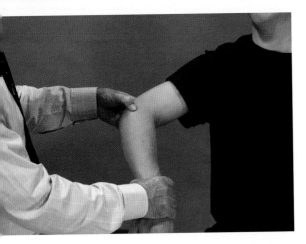

(e) Palpation—lateral epicondyle. Attempt to locate painful site distal to lateral epicondyle. Degenerative tissue has a distinctive 'glassy' feel

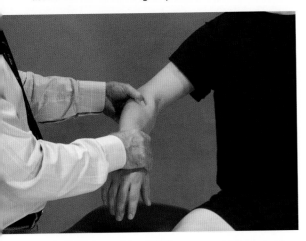

(f) Palpation—extensor muscles. Pincer grip is used with passive flexion and extension to provide exact feel of damaged tissue

in longstanding cases, plain X-ray (AP and lateral views) of the elbow may show osteochondritis dissecans, degenerative joint changes or evidence of heterotopic calcification.

Ultrasound examination may prove to be a useful diagnostic tool in the investigation of patients with lateral elbow pain. Ultrasound may demonstrate the degree of tendon damage as well as the presence of a bursa.

Extensor tendinopathy

For this major sports medicine condition, we review the pathology, outline the clinical presentation, and

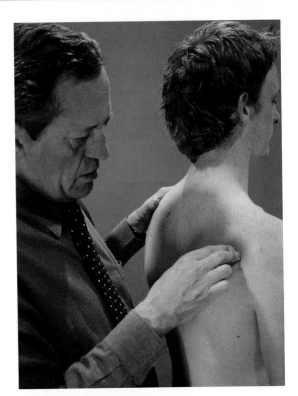

(g) Periscapular soft tissues—palpation of active trigger points and changes in muscle tone and length in the periscapular soft tissues

then discuss evidence-based and clinically founded treatment.

Clinically relevant pathology

The primary pathological process in extensor tendinopathy tendinosis[1] (Chapter 2) of the ECRB tendon is in the first 1–2 cm (0.5–1 in.) distal to its attachment to the extensor origin at the lateral epicondyle. Light microscopy reveals an excess of both fibroblasts and blood vessels.[2-4] The vessels appear consistent with what Alfredson calls 'neovessels'[5] and pathologists call 'angiogenesis'. This abnormal tissue has a large number of nociceptive fibers, which may explain why the lesion is so painful. With continued use, tendinosis may extend into microscopic partial tears.[6] Conversely, a tear may be the primary abnormality with degenerative change being secondary. A summary of the processes leading to the development of extensor tendinopathy is shown in Figure 18.3.

With wrist movements, especially wrist extension, a considerable shearing stress is placed on the ECRB tendon. The ECRB muscle crosses both the elbow and the wrist and, therefore, contracts eccentrically

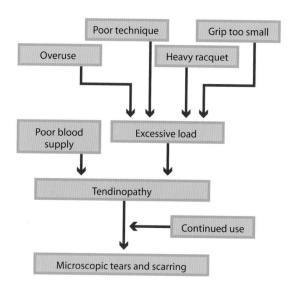

Figure 18.3 Processes leading to the development of ECRB tendinopathy

at both ends during certain maneuvers. Additional stress is applied by the head of the radius, which rotates anteriorly, compressing the ECRB tendon during pronation of the forearm. This may further compromise the blood supply or excessively stretch the tendon.

Neural structures may contribute to the patient's lateral elbow pain. Lateral elbow pain is often associated with cervical and upper thoracic abnormalities, particularly of the C5–6 region.

Clinical features

Extensor tendinopathy occurs in association with any activity involving repeated wrist extension against resistance. This includes sporting activities, such as tennis, squash and badminton, as well as occupational and leisure activities, such as carpentry, bricklaying, sewing and knitting. Computer use has been shown to be associated with the development of this condition.[7] The peak incidence is between the ages of 40 and 50 years but this condition may affect any age group.

There are two distinct clinical presentations of this condition. The most common is an insidious onset of pain, which occurs 24–72 hours after unaccustomed activity involving repeated wrist extension. This occurs typically after a person spends the weekend laying bricks or using a screwdriver. It is also seen after prolonged sewing or knitting. In the tennis player, it may occur after the use of a new racquet, playing with wet, heavy balls or overhitting, especially hitting into the wind. It also occurs when the player is hitting 'late'

(getting into position slowly), so that body weight is not transferred correctly and the player relies on the forearm muscles exclusively for power.

The other clinical presentation is a sudden onset of lateral elbow pain associated with a single instance of exertion involving the wrist extensors, for example, lifting a heavy object, or in tennis players attempting a hard backhand with too much reliance on the forearm and not enough on the trunk and legs. The insidious onset is thought to correspond to microscopic tears within the tendon, whereas the acute onset may correspond to a macroscopic tear of the tendon.

On examination, the maximal area of tenderness is usually approximately 1–2 cm (0.5–1 in.) distal to the lateral epicondyle in the ECRB tendon. The experienced clinician may palpate irregularities within the tendon at this site. The rest of the ECRB muscle should be palpated for areas of excessive tightness and hypersensitivity.

Typically, the pain is reproduced by resisted wrist extension, especially with the wrist pronated and radially deviated (Mills' test). Resisted extension of the middle finger is also painful (Fig. 18.2c). The ECRB tendon is preferentially stressed in this position as it must contract synergistically to anchor the third metacarpal to allow extension to take place at the digits.

The upper limb tension test, especially the radial nerve variation, may reproduce lateral elbow pain or show restriction of movement compared with the other side. In either situation, this indicates a possible neural component to the pain. Examination of the cervical spine will frequently detect decreased range of movement, especially lateral flexion. Palpation of the cervical and upper thoracic spine may show stiffness and tenderness both centrally and over the apophyseal joint on the side of the pain, usually around the C5–6 level. Active trigger points may be found in the periscapular soft tissues (Fig. 18.2g).

Treatment

No single treatment has proven to be totally effective in the treatment of this condition. A combination of the different treatments mentioned below will result in resolution of the symptoms in nearly all cases.

The basic principles of treatment of soft tissue injuries apply. There must be control of pain, encouragement of the healing process, restoration of flexibility and strength, treatment of associated factors (e.g. increased neural tension, referred pain), gradual return to activity with added support and correction of the predisposing factors.

Control of pain

It remains unclear as to how much pain is 'ideal' in the treatment of tendinopathies. Clinical experience suggests that a low level of pain, which does not worsen with training, is likely to not be harmful for tendon healing. However, some patients require relative rest, application of ice and analgesia for comfort.

Electrotherapeutic modalities

The application of electrotherapeutic modalities such as ultrasound, laser and high voltage galvanic stimulation may encourage the healing process. A summary of clinical trials investigating the efficacy of ultrasound therapy in 'lateral epicondylitis' found the advantage in success rate between ultrasound and sham ultrasound to be 15%.[8] The use of low-level laser treatment was not found to be helpful.[9] Heat may also be helpful and a heat-retaining brace such as a neoprene sleeve may be worn during the rehabilitation process.

Soft tissue therapy

Soft tissue therapy is performed at the site of the lesion and to adjacent tight or thickened tissues. Transverse friction to the site of the lesion should be performed with the tissue held in tension by having the wrist in passive flexion (Fig. 18.4a). Sustained myofascial tension at the site of the lesion may also be performed (Fig. 18.4b). The symptoms must be reassessed after treatment. Areas of hypersensitivity and palpable bands in the ECRB muscle should be treated in active wrist flexion with sustained myofascial tension and digital ischemic pressure (Fig. 18.4c).

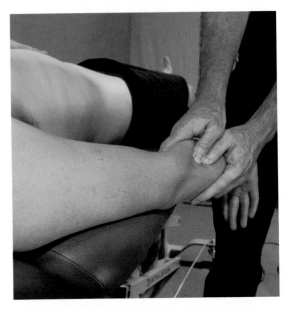

(b) Sustained longitudinal pressure to the ECRB muscle in the position of maximum elbow extension and wrist flexion

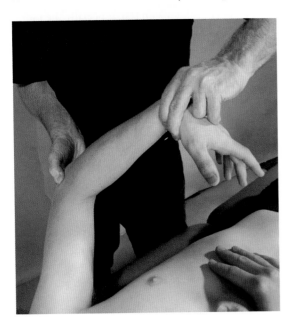

Figure 18.4 Soft tissue techniques

(a) Transverse friction with extensor tissue under tension—wrist and hand flexion

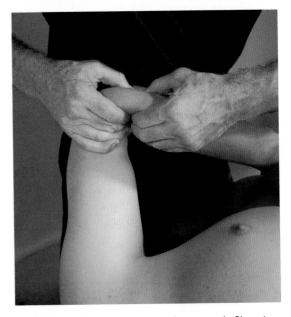

(c) Digital ischemic pressure to deep muscle fibers in the shortened position

Manual therapy

There is evidence of positive short-term effects with elbow manipulation, but no long-term studies have been performed.[10, 11] Cervical manipulation was also found to be helpful in the short term,[12] but manipulation of the wrist was not found to be helpful.[13] Cervical mobilization (Fig. 18.5), thoracic mobilization and neural stretching (Fig. 18.6) are commonly used as adjuncts to other forms of treatment.

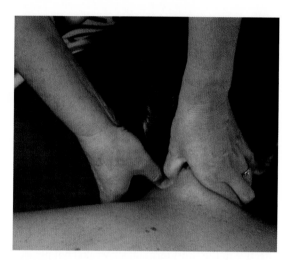

Figure 18.5 Cervical mobilization

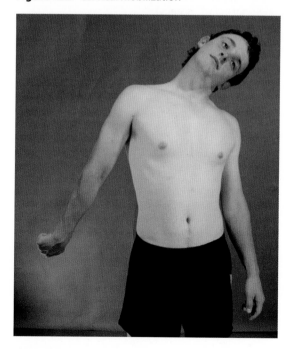

Figure 18.6 Neural stretch

Trigger points

In patients with lateral elbow pain, active trigger points associated with muscle shortening are frequently found in the forearm extensor muscles—brachioradialis, extensor carpi radialis longus, ECRB, extensor digitorum, extensor carpi ulnaris, extensor digiti minimi and anconeus, as well as the periscapular area. Digital ischemic pressure or dry needling of these trigger points will help restore normal muscle length and reduce forces at the lateral epicondyle.

Stretching

Stretching of the ECRB muscle and associated wrist extensors should be performed (Fig. 18.7).

Muscle strengthening

A muscle strengthening program should be commenced as soon as pain permits. This should commence with isometric contraction of the wrist extensors. When this can be performed without pain, gradual progression to concentric and then eccentric exercises should occur (Fig. 18.8). Studies support the use of muscle strengthening.[14, 15]

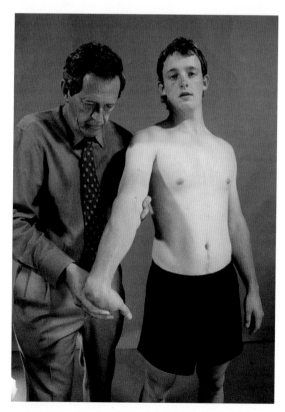

Figure 18.7 Stretching the ERCB tendon

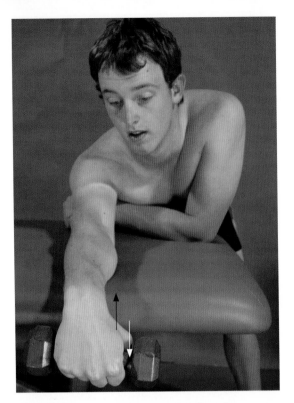

Figure 18.8 Strengthening exercises for wrist extensors. Exercises can be isometric, concentric (black arrow), eccentric (white arrow) or functional

Counterforce bracing

Counterforce bracing (Fig. 18.9) appears to reduce the forces on the extensor tendons although studies of its efficacy show conflicting results.[9] One study showed a reduction in 'inconvenience during daily activities'.[16] The brace should be applied during the rehabilitation process and on return to the aggravating activity, such as tennis. Many patients mistakenly assume that the brace should be applied over the painful area itself but the correct site is in the upper forearm, approximately 10 cm (4 in.) below the elbow joint. The brace should be applied firmly.

Taping

One study showed that the application of a diamond-shaped taping technique resulted in an improvement of symptoms.[17]

Iontophoresis

The application of a corticosteroid agent by the process of iontophoresis is not supported by controlled trial evidence.[18, 19]

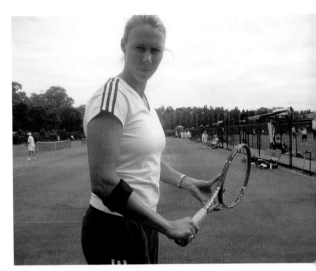

Figure 18.9 Counterforce brace

Corticosteroid injection

The use of corticosteroid injection in the treatment of this condition is controversial. Corticosteroid injection was compared to physiotherapy (ultrasound, deep friction massage, exercise program) and a 'wait and see' group and found to be significantly more effective in the short term (at six weeks) but physiotherapy appeared a more effective treatment in the longer term (>12 weeks).[20]

The indications for corticosteroid injection in this condition include failure of an appropriate rehabilitation program after three months or localization of pain to the lateral epicondyle probably due to periostitis. Corticosteroid and local anesthetic agents should be injected around the ECRB tendon, directly over the point of maximal tenderness but not into the tendon substance itself (Fig. 18.10). If used, corticosteroid

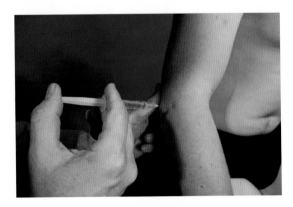

Figure 18.10 Corticosteroid injection

injections should be regarded as just one component of the treatment program and followed by appropriate rehabilitation.

Nitric oxide donor therapy

An Australian study provided level 2 evidence that nitric oxide donor therapy (glyceryl trinitrate [GTN] patches applied locally 1.25 mg/day) improved pain and function within three to six months.[21] Glyceryl trinitrate patches come in varying doses; a 0.5 mg patch should be cut in quarters and applied for 24 hours at a time and then replaced (Fig. 18.11). A 0.2 mg patch would best be cut in half and applied similarly. Successful outcomes occurred at three to six months, so patients need to have this explained. Although further studies are needed, this treatment has also proven effective in the management of Achilles and supraspinatus tendinopathies (Chapter 10).

Botulinum toxin

Initial reports suggested that botulinum toxin (Botox) injection was an effective treatment,[22, 23] however, a double-blind, randomized controlled study failed to show any improvement in pain although there was a small non-significant improvement in grip strength.[24]

Acupuncture

There is some evidence of short-term (two to eight weeks) benefit with the use of acupuncture for lateral elbow pain.[25]

Extracorporeal shock wave therapy

There have been a number of studies assessing the effectiveness of extracorporeal shock wave therapy

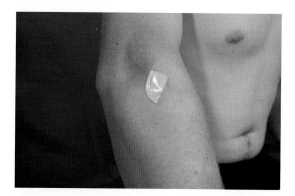

Figure 18.11 Nitric oxide donor therapy: one-quarter of a 0.5 mg/24 hour glyceryl trinitrate (GTN) patch in place over the most tender site of extensor tendinopathy

for lateral elbow pain, again with conflicting results. The few well-designed studies have failed to demonstrate any significant effect and show a relatively high incidence of minor side-effects.[9]

Autologous blood injection

It has been suggested that the introduction of autologous blood in a relatively atraumatic manner may initiate an inflammatory cascade and promote healing in an otherwise degenerative process. A preliminary study using this modality demonstrated a good clinical result in 79% of cases.[26] It has now been used for some time in our clinic and we have begun a randomized trial.

Correct predisposing factors

Probably the most important factor to be avoided is excessive or unaccustomed activity. In tennis players, a major cause is a faulty backhand technique with the elbow leading (Fig. 18.12a). Other technique faults that may predispose to the development of extensor tendinopathy include excessive forearm pronation while attempting to hit top spin forehands and excessive wrist flick (flexion) movement while serving. Correction of these faults requires assistance of a qualified tennis coach. Other factors, such as racquet type, grip size, string tension, court surface and ball weight, may influence the amount of shock imparted to the elbow (Chapter 6). A mid-sized, graphite racquet with a large 'sweet spot' and a grip size that feels comfortable should be used. Care should be taken to avoid using racquets with excessively large or, especially, small grips.

Surgery

Very occasionally, particularly in cases with a long history of lateral elbow pain, the treatment program mentioned above fails to resolve the patient's symptoms. Failure of conservative treatment after 12 months is a reasonable indication for surgery. Surgery involves excision of the degenerative tissue within the ECRB tendon and release of the tendon from the lateral epicondyle. There is some evidence that percutaneous surgery may lead to greater improvements in function, quicker return to work and greater patient satisfaction.[27]

Combination therapy

It is clear from both our clinical experience and the relatively few well-designed studies that no one treatment is effective in the management of lateral elbow tendinosis. We recommend a combination of therapies, as shown in Table 18.2.

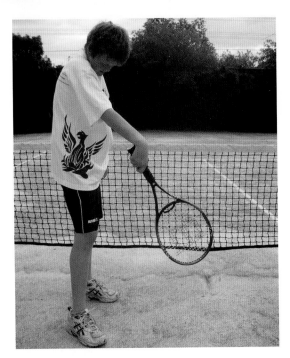

Figure 18.12 Backhand technique

(a) Incorrect

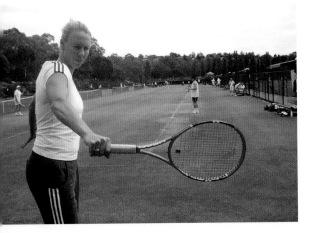

(b) Correct

Graduated return to activity

As with all soft tissue injuries, it is important to return gradually to activity following treatment. The tennis player should initially practice backhand technique without a ball, then progress slowly from gentle hitting from the service line to eventually hitting full length shots (Chapter 12). Depending on the severity of the condition and the length of the rehabilitation

Table 18.2 Recommended treatment regimen for lateral extensor tendinosis of the elbow

Ice and simple analgesics (in acute phase)
Counterforce brace
Stretching of wrist extensors
Soft tissue techniques to local area of pain, forearm muscles and periscapular soft tissues
Concentric/eccentric strengthening program for wrist extensors
Nitric oxide donor therapy
Mobilization of lower cervical and thoracic spine
Neural stretches
Identify and correct any predisposing factors (e.g. technique)
Corticosteroid injection (only if severe pain prevents above measures)
Surgery (only after failure of high-quality conservative program)

program, this graduated return should take place over a period of three to six weeks.

Entrapment of the posterior interosseous nerve (radial tunnel syndrome)

The radial nerve divides into the superficial radial and the posterior interosseous nerve at the level of the radiocapitellar joint. The posterior interosseous nerve (PIN) passes distal to the origin of the ECRB and enters the arcade of Frohse. Prior to entering the arcade of Frohse, it gives off branches to the ECRB and supinator muscles. The arcade is a semicircular fibrous arch at the proximal head of the supinator muscle, which begins at the tip of the lateral epicondyle and extends downwards, attaching to the medial aspect of the lateral epicondyle. The PIN then emerges from the supinator muscle distally, where it divides into terminal branches that innervate the medial extensors. Compression of the PIN may occur at one of four sites, as shown in Figure 18.13.[28]

It is often difficult to differentiate between extensor tendinopathy and the early stages of PIN entrapment. PIN entrapment is seen in patients who repetitively pronate and supinate the forearm, whereas extensor tendinopathy is more frequently associated with repetitive wrist extension. Symptoms of PIN entrapment include paresthesia in the hand and lateral forearm, pain over the forearm extensor mass, wrist aching and middle or upper third humeral pain.

Maximal tenderness is over the supinator muscle, four finger breadths below the lateral epicondyle (distal to the area of maximal tenderness in extensor tendinopathy). Nerve entrapment also causes marked pain on resisted supination of the forearm with the

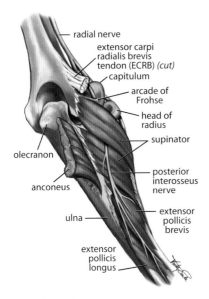

Figure 18.13 Posterior interosseous nerve entrapment
Possible entrapment at:
1. fibrous bands in front of the radial head
2. recurrent radial vessels
3. arcade of Frohse
4. tendinous margin of the extensor carpi radialis brevis muscle.

elbow flexed to 90° and the forearm fully pronated. The third sign is pain with resisted extension of the middle finger with the elbow extended, although this can be positive in extensor tendinopathy as well. Neural tension tests may reproduce the patient's symptoms and nerve conduction studies may be performed to confirm the diagnosis.

Treatment consists of soft tissue therapy over the supinator muscle at the site of entrapment and neural stretching. If this is unsuccessful, decompression surgery may be required and is almost uniformly successful.[28]

Other causes of lateral elbow pain

Other causes of lateral elbow pain may occur in isolation or in conjunction with the previously mentioned conditions. Radiohumeral bursitis is occasionally seen in athletes. This may be distinguished from extensor tendinopathy by the site of tenderness that is anterior and distal to the lateral epicondyle, maximally over the anterolateral aspect of the head of the radius. The presence of this bursitis may be confirmed on ultrasound examination. Injection with a corticosteroid agent is the most effective form of treatment.

Osteochondritis of the capitellum or radial head may occur in younger athletes (Chapter 40) involved in throwing sports. This is a significant condition as it can cause an enlarged, deformed capitellum that may predispose to the development of osteoarthritis. The treatment of this condition involves avoidance of aggravating activities.

The lateral elbow is a common site of referred pain, especially from the cervical and upper thoracic spine and periscapular soft tissues. Most patients with chronic lateral elbow pain have some component of their pain emanating from the cervical and thoracic spine (Chapter 16). Any associated abnormalities of the cervical and thoracic spine should be treated and the patient's signs reassessed immediately after treatment. If there is a noticeable difference, this may indicate a significant component of referred pain.

Medial elbow pain

Patients who present with medial elbow pain can be considered in two main groups. One group has pain associated with excessive activity of the wrist flexors. This is the medial equivalent of extensor tendinopathy with a similar pathological process occurring in the tendons of pronator teres and the flexor group. This condition will be referred to as 'flexor/pronator tendinopathy'.

The second group of patients have medial elbow pain related to excessive throwing activities. Throwing produces a valgus stress on the elbow that is resisted primarily by the anterior oblique portion of the medial collateral ligament (MCL) of the elbow and secondarily by the stability of the radiocapitellar joint. Repetitive throwing, especially if throwing technique is poor (Chapter 6), leads to stretching of the MCL and a degree of valgus instability. A fixed flexion deformity of the elbow may develop as a result of scarring of the MCL. Subsequently, there may be some secondary impingement of the medial tip of the olecranon onto the olecranon fossa, producing a synovitis or loose body formation. With valgus stress, the compressive forces may also damage the radiocapitellar joint. Several of these pathological entities may be present in combination.

In children, repetitive valgus stress may result in damage to the medial epicondylar epiphysis with pain and tenderness in this region. This usually responds to a period of rest but may progress to avulsion with continued activity. This condition, commonly known as 'little leaguer's elbow', is considered in Chapter 40. The causes of medial elbow pain are shown in Table 18.3.

Table 18.3 Causes of medial elbow pain

Common	Less common	Not to be missed
Flexor/pronator tendinopathy	Ulnar nerve compression	Referred pain
Medial collateral ligament sprain	Avulsion fracture of the medial	
Acute	epicondyle (adolescents)	
Chronic	Apophysitis (adolescents)	

Flexor/pronator tendinopathy

This condition is not as common as its lateral equivalent but is seen especially in golfers ('golfer's elbow') and in tennis players who impart a lot of top spin on their forehand shot. The primary pathology exists in the tendinous origin of the forearm flexor muscles, particularly in the pronator teres tendon.

On examination, there is usually localized tenderness just at or below the medial epicondyle with pain on resisted wrist flexion and resisted forearm pronation, especially when passive stretch is placed on the tendon (reverse Mills' test) (Fig. 18.14).

Treatment is along the same lines as treatment of extensor tendinopathy. Particular attention should be paid to the tennis forehand or the golf swing technique. Due to its close proximity to the medial epicondyle, the ulnar nerve may become trapped in scar tissue. This should be treated with neural stretching.

Medial collateral ligament sprain

Sprain of the MCL of the elbow may occur as an acute injury, which is discussed on page 305, or as the result of chronic excessive valgus stress due to throwing. This occurs particularly in baseball pitchers

and javelin throwers. The repeated valgus stress, especially in throwers who 'open up too soon' (i.e. become front-on too early in the throwing motion), leads initially to inflammation of the ligament, then scarring and calcification and occasionally ligament rupture. The biomechanics of throwing is discussed in Chapter 5.

On examination, there will be localized tenderness over the ligament and mild instability on valgus stress (Fig. 18.15a). There will often be associated abnormalities such as a flexion contracture of the forearm muscles, synovitis and loose body formation around the tip of the olecranon, as well as damage to the radiocapitellar joint.

Treatment in the early stages of the disease involves modification of activity, correction of faulty technique, local electrotherapeutic modalities and soft tissue therapy to the medial ligament. Medial strapping of the elbow may offer additional protection (Fig. 18.15b). Specific muscle strengthening should be commenced, concentrating on the forearm flexors and pronators (Fig. 18.16). Advanced pathology may require arthroscopic removal of loose bodies and bony spurs. Occasionally, significant instability develops and requires ligament reconstruction. This

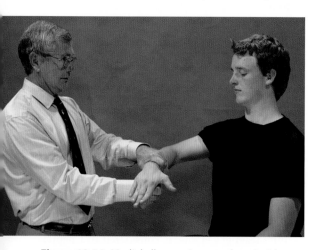

Figure 18.14 Medial elbow pain reproduced with resisted wrist flexion and forearm pronation

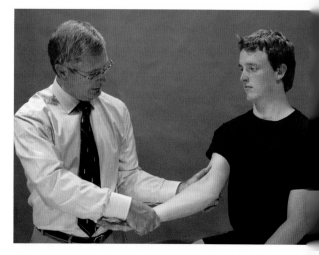

Figure 18.15 (a) Assessment of integrity of the medial collateral ligament

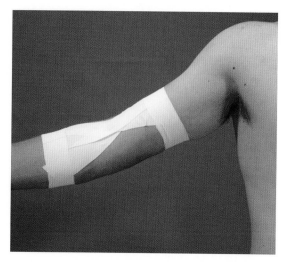

(b) Elbow stability taping

should be avoided if possible as the results of surgery are often disappointing.

Ulnar nerve compression

The ulnar nerve pierces the intermuscular septum in the middle of the arm and then passes deep to the medial head of the triceps muscle to locate in a superficial groove (the ulnar sulcus) between the olecranon and the medial epicondyle. It then enters the forearm between the humerus and the ulnar heads of the flexor carpi ulnaris muscle.

Entrapment of the ulnar nerve can occur as a result of a combination of any of four factors:[29]

1. traction injuries to the nerve may occur because of the dynamic valgus forces of throwing, especially when combined with valgus instability of the elbow
2. progressive compression can occur at the cubital tunnel secondary to inflammation and adhesions from repetitive stresses, or where the nerve passes between the two heads of the flexor carpi ulnaris due to muscle overdevelopment secondary to resistance weight-training exercises
3. recurrent subluxation of the nerve due to acquired laxity from repetitive stress or direct trauma, leading to ulnar neuritis
4. irregularities within the ulnar groove, such as spurs commonly seen from overuse injuries in throwers.

The patient presents with posteromedial elbow pain and sensory symptoms such as pins and needles or

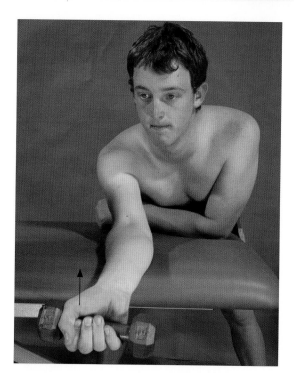

Figure 18.16 Strengthening exercises for the forearm flexors and pronators

numbness along the ulnar nerve distribution on the ulnar border of the forearm and the ulnar one and a half fingers. The nerve may be tender behind the medial epicondyle (Fig. 18.17) and tapping over the nerve may reproduce symptoms. Patients with clinical features of ulnar nerve compression should undergo nerve conduction studies.

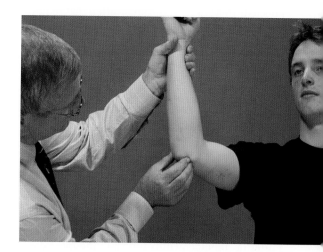

Figure 18.17 Palpation of the ulnar nerve

Treatment of this condition initially consists of local soft tissue therapy to the nerve in the ulnar groove in order to break down adhesions that may be compressing the nerve and restricting its free movement. Neural stretching should also be performed. Surgical transposition of the nerve may be required if symptoms persist or if conduction studies show deteriorating nerve function.

Posterior elbow pain

The main causes of posterior elbow pain are olecranon bursitis, triceps tendinitis and posterior impingement. Gout should always be considered.

Olecranon bursitis

Olecranon bursitis may present after a single episode of trauma or, more commonly, after repeated trauma, such as falls onto a hard surface affecting the posterior aspect of the elbow. This is commonly seen in basketballers 'taking a charge'. It is also seen in individuals who rest their elbow on a hard surface for long periods of time and is known as 'student's elbow'. The olecranon bursa is a subcutaneous bursa that may become filled with blood and serous fluid (Fig. 18.18).

Treatment consists initially of NSAIDs, rest and firm compression. If this fails, then aspiration of the contents of the bursa and injection with a mixture of corticosteroid and local anesthetic agents will usually be effective. The needle should be inserted at an oblique angle to reduce the risk of sinus formation. If recurrent bursitis does not respond to aspiration and injection, surgical excision of the bursa is required.

Occasionally, olecranon bursitis can become infected. This is a serious complication that requires immediate drainage, strict immobilization and antibiotic therapy. Osteomyelitis and septic arthritis can follow. Excision of the bursa is occasionally required.

Triceps tendinopathy

Tendinopathy at the insertion of the triceps onto the olecranon is occasionally seen. Standard conservative measures for treatment of tendinopathy should be used. Soft tissue therapy and dry needling to reduce excessive tightness of the triceps musculotendinous complex are often helpful.

Posterior impingement

Posterior impingement is probably the most common cause of posterior elbow pain. It occurs in

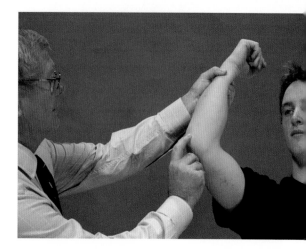

Figure 18.18 Olecranon bursa

(a) Palpation at site of bursa

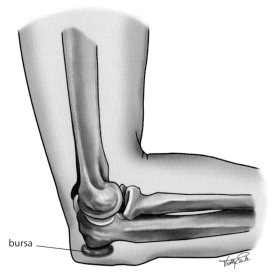

bursa

(b) Olecranon bursitis

two situations. In the younger athlete there is the 'hyperextension valgus overload syndrome'. Repetitive hyperextension valgus stress to the elbow results in impingement of the posterior medial corner of the olecranon tip on the olecranon fossa. Over time this causes osteophyte formation, exacerbating the impingement and leading to a fixed flexion deformity.

In the older patient the most common cause is early osteoarthritis, which often predominantly affects the radiocapitellar joint. Generalized osteophytes form through the elbow. Impingement of these osteophytes posteriorly results in posterior pain. The main clinical feature in athletes with posterior impingement is a fixed flexion deformity of some degree and posterior pain with forced extension (Fig. 18.19).

If conservative measures fail, then arthroscopic removal of the impinging posterior bone and soft tissue is very effective in relieving symptoms and improving extension.

Acute elbow injuries

Acute elbow injuries include fractures, dislocations and ligament or tendon ruptures.

Fractures

As the complication rate for elbow fractures is higher than with fractures near other joints, it is essential that fractures in this region are recognized and treated early and aggressively. Unstable fractures, usually those associated with displacement, should be referred early for orthopedic management. When the articular or cortical surface has less than 2 mm (0.1 in.) of vertical or horizontal displacement, the fracture can be regarded as stable and treated conservatively.[30]

The most common complication of elbow fractures is stiffness, particularly loss of terminal extension. Prompt diagnosis and treatment that includes an early rehabilitation program can help avoid this outcome. Thus, treatment of elbow fractures must be aggressive. Surgically stabilizing an adult elbow fracture allows early commencement of a post-operative range of motion program.

A stable fracture that involves no significant comminution, displacement or angulation may be treated

conservatively. In adults, immobilizing the arm for a few days, even up to a week, is generally well tolerated. Then the arm should be placed in a removal splint and early motion commenced. The fracture should then be protected for six to eight weeks, with early and frequent radiographic checks to ensure the reduction stays anatomical.

The other main complication of elbow fractures, particularly in high energy injuries, is heterotopic ossification. Traumatized elbows that are forcefully or passively manipulated may also be at greater risk of this complication. Therefore, gentle, active assisted range of motion exercises are preferred. Heterotopic bone formation has also been associated with elbow fractures treated surgically between one and five days after injury or treated with multiple surgical procedures. Thus, surgery should be performed in the first 24 hours after injury or after five to seven days.

Supracondylar fractures

Supracondylar fractures are more common around the age of 12 than in adults. They often occur from a fall on an outstretched arm, either from a height or a bicycle. Because they are rotationally unstable and have a high rate of neurovascular complications, these fractures should be regarded as an orthopedic emergency.

For fractures that are unstable, displaced or cannot be reduced without jeopardizing the blood supply, the treatment of choice is closed reduction in the operating room under general anesthesia. Percutaneous pins placed across the fracture maintain the reduction and prevent late slippage. The arm is initially placed in a splint and then several days later in a cast. The pins are removed after four to six weeks. Stiffness is typically not a problem in children recovering from fractures.

Olecranon fractures

Olecranon fractures occur from a fall onto an outstretched hand or from direct trauma to the elbow. If the fracture is non-displaced and stable, the patient should be able to extend the arm against gravity. Treatment consists of immobilizing the arm for two to three weeks in a posterior splint, and then in a removable splint and a range of motion program commenced. If the patient is unable to extend the elbow against gravity or if radiographs show significant displacement, open reduction with internal fixation by tension-band wiring is preferred. Early motion is started within one week of surgery.

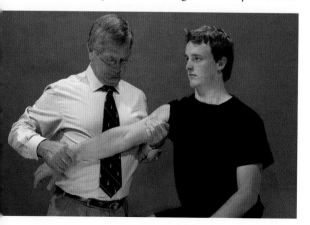

Figure 18.19 Posterior impingement. The elbow is forced into end-range extension. If posterior pain is produced, then posterior impingement is present

Radial head fracture

The most common fracture around the elbow in athletes is the radial head fracture, almost always resulting from a fall onto an outstretched hand. Most radial head fractures are minimally displaced or non-displaced (type 1) and are very difficult to see on radiographs. Sometimes the only clue is the fat pad sign, which appears as a triangular radiolucency just in front of the elbow joint. Early aspiration, splinting with an easily removable device and early commencement of a range of motion program will yield excellent results. Complete healing can be expected within six to eight weeks. For displaced radial head fractures (type 2), surgical intervention with operative fixation or excision is preferred. Comminuted fractures (type 3) are treated by excision. Type 4 fractures occur in the presence of a dislocation and can be very unstable. They always require surgical treatment.

Posterior dislocation

The most serious acute injury to the elbow is posterior dislocation of the elbow. This can occur either in contact sports or when falling from a height such as while pole vaulting. There is often an associated fracture of the coronoid process or radial head. The usual mechanism is a posterolateral rotatory force resulting from a fall on an outstretched hand with the shoulder abducted, axial compression, forearm in supination and then forced flexion of the elbow.[31]

The major complication of posterior dislocation of the elbow is impairment of the vascular supply to the forearm. Assessment of pulses distal to the dislocation is essential. If pulses are absent, reduction of the dislocation is required urgently. Reduction is usually relatively easy. With the elbow held at 45°, the clinician grips the anterior aspect of the humerus and traction is placed longitudinally along the forearm (Fig. 18.20). The elbow usually reduces with a pronounced clunk. If vascular impairment persists after reduction, urgent surgical intervention is required.

Following reduction, the stability of the collateral ligaments should be assessed (Fig. 18.15a). A post-reduction X-ray should also be performed. Small fractures of the coronoid process or undisplaced fractures of the radial head only require conservative treatment with support in a sling for two to three weeks. Large coronoid fractures, however, may result in chronic instability and should be reduced and fixed surgically. Large fractures of the radial head may be difficult to manage but in most cases can be internally fixed. Occasionally, a large fracture of the capitellum may occur. This also requires internal fixation.

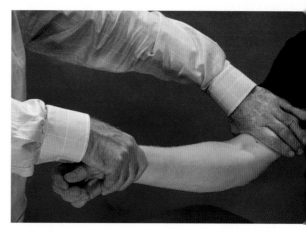

Figure 18.20 Technique for reduction of posterior dislocation of the elbow

Sometimes a piece of bone becomes trapped in the joint after reduction. This needs to be excluded with good quality post-reduction X-rays.

Long-term loss of extension is frequently a problem following elbow dislocation. Immediate active mobilization under supervision has been shown to result in less restriction of elbow extension with no apparent increase in instability.[32] Professional sportspeople with a simple dislocation with no associated fracture or instability are able to return to sport relatively quickly after an accelerated rehabilitation program. Verrall described three cases of stable dislocations in professional footballers who returned to sport after 13, 21 and seven days respectively with no further complications.[33] Joint mobilization (Fig. 18.21) may

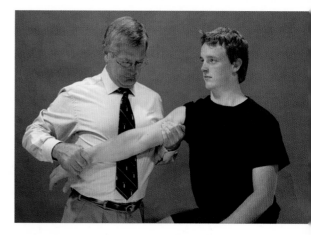

Figure 18.21 Elbow mobilization. Gentle oscillations at end range of elbow extension to restore full range of motion

be required as part of the treatment. Surrounding muscles should also be strengthened. Elbow stability taping should be applied on return to sport (Fig. 18.15b).

Heterotopic ossification occasionally occurs following elbow dislocation. The use of NSAIDs for a period of three months following the injury may reduce the incidence of this complication.

Elbow dislocations in directions other than posterior occur occasionally. These are often associated with severe ligamentous disruption and patients should be referred to an orthopedic surgeon immediately.

Some patients may develop chronic instability of the elbow following an acute dislocation. This is classically posterior lateral instability with a positive pivot shift test. If symptoms are unacceptable, then a reconstruction of the lateral ulnar collateral ligament may be indicated.

Acute rupture of the medial collateral ligament

Acute rupture of the MCL may occur in a previously damaged ligament or in a normal ligament subjected to extreme valgus stress, for example, elbow dislocation. The degree of instability should be assessed by applying valgus stress to the elbow at 30° of flexion (Fig. 18.15a). If complete disruption is present with associated instability, surgical repair of the ligament is required. Incomplete tears should be treated with protection in a brace and muscle strengthening for a period of three to six weeks.

Tendon ruptures

Acute avulsion of the biceps or triceps tendons from their insertions is a rare condition. Rupture of the biceps tendon insertion occurs predominantly in strength activities (e.g. weightlifting). Rupture of the triceps tendon occurs most commonly with excessive deceleration force, such as occurs during a fall or by a direct blow to the posterior aspect of the elbow. Partial and complete triceps ruptures are seen in American National Football League linemen.[34] Partial tears tend to heal well without surgery. Acute complete ruptures at the insertion of either of these tendons should be treated surgically.

Forearm pain

Fracture of the radius and ulna

The bones of the forearm are commonly injured by a fall on the back or front of the outstretched hand.

It is usual for both bones to break, although a single bone may be fractured in cases of direct violence or in fractures of the distal third where there is no shortening.

A displaced fracture is usually clinically obvious. X-rays should be taken for post-reduction comparison and for exclusion of a concurrent dislocation. Two types of dislocation occur—the Monteggia injury (fractured ulna with dislocated head of the radius at the elbow joint) and the Galeazzi injury (fractured radius with dislocated head of the ulna at the wrist joint).

In the child, angulation of less than 10° is acceptable. Other fractures should be reduced under local or general anesthesia depending on the age of the child. The usual position for immobilization is in pronation, although in proximal radial fractures and in Smith's fracture at the wrist the forearm should be held in supination. The plaster should extend above the elbow and leave the metacarpophalangeal joints free. Depending on the age of the child, immobilization should last four to six weeks. The position should be checked by X-ray every one to two weeks depending on stability.

In the adult, perfect reduction of radial and ulnar fractures is necessary to ensure future sporting function. Most of these fractures are significantly displaced and require internal fixation by plate and screw. Depending on the accuracy of reduction, either a cast or crepe bandage support is required post-operatively for eight to 10 weeks. Isolated fracture of the ulna is treated conservatively by an above-elbow cast in mid pronation for eight weeks. Monteggia and Galeazzi injuries are usually displaced and should be referred to an orthopedic surgeon for reduction.

Stress fractures

Stress fractures of the forearm bones occur occasionally in sportspeople involved in upper limb sports, such as baseball, tennis or swimming.[35] Treatment involves rest and correction of the possible predisposing factors, such as faulty technique.

Forearm compartment pressure syndrome

Forearm compartment pressure syndromes have been described in kayakers, canoeists, motor cyclists and weight-training athletes. The flexor compartment is most usually affected. Symptoms include activity-related pain that is relieved by rest. Diagnosis requires compartment pressure testing (Chapter 8). Treatment consists of local soft tissue therapy. Surgical fasciotomy may be required.

Upper arm pain

An aching pain in the upper arm is a common complaint, especially among manual workers (e.g. bricklayers, carpenters) and sportspeople. The most common cause is myofascial pain, but stress fracture of the humerus needs to be considered.

Myofascial pain

A dull non-specific pain in the upper arm is most likely to be myofascial in nature. The most common source of the upper arm pain is trigger points in the infraspinatus muscle (Fig. 18.22). Firm palpation of these trigger points will often reproduce the patient's pain.

Treatment consists of digital ischemic pressure or dry needling to the trigger points. Attention should also be paid to the lower cervical and upper to mid thoracic spine. Increased muscle tone and trigger points may be found in the paraspinal muscles and hypomobility of the intervertebral segments may be present. These abnormalities must also be treated.

Stress fracture of the humerus

Stress fracture of the humerus has been described in baseball pitchers, a tennis player, javelin thrower, bodybuilder and weightlifter. Most of the fractures occurred in adolescents and were associated with a recent increase in activity. In a number of cases the diagnosis was made retrospectively when an acute fracture occurred and the patient admitted symptoms leading up to the acute episode.

Recommended treatment follows the general principles of management of simple stress fractures, involving avoidance of the aggravating activity until symptom-free and no local tenderness, then gradual resumption of the activity.

Recommended Reading

Bisset L, Paungmail A, Vicenzino B, et al. A systematic review and meta-analysis of clinical trials on physical interventions for lateral epicondylalgia. *Br J Sports Med* 2005; 39: 411–22.

Cain EL, Dugas JR, Wolf RS, et al. Elbow injuries in throwing athletes: a current concepts review. *Am J Sports Med* 2003; 31(4): 621–35.

Chen AL, Youm T, Ong BC, et al. Imaging of the elbow in the overhead throwing athlete. *Am J Sports Med* 2003; 31(3): 466–73.

Frostick SP, Mohammad M, Ritchie DA. Sport injuries of the elbow. *Br J Sports Med* 1999; 33: 301–11.

Salyapongse A, Hatch JD. Advances in the management of medial elbow pain in baseball pitchers. *Curr Sports Med Rep* 2003; 2: 276–80.

Sevier TL, Wilson JK. Methods utilized in treating lateral epicondylitis. *Phys Ther Rev* 2000; 5: 117–24.

References

1. Nirschl RP. Elbow tendinosis/tennis elbow. *Clin Sports Med* 1992; 11: 851–70.

2. Coonrad RW, Hooper WR. Tennis elbow: its course, natural history, conservative and surgical management. *J Bone Joint Surg Am* 1973; 55: 1177–82.

3. Nirschl RP, Pettrone FA. Tennis elbow. The surgical treatment of lateral epicondylitis. *J Bone Joint Surg Am* 1979; 61: 832–9.

4. Kraushaar BS, Nirschl RP. Tendinosis of the elbow (tennis elbow). Clinical features and findings of histological, immunohistochemical, and electron microscopy studies. *J Bone Joint Surg Am* 1999; 81A: 269–78.

5. Alfredson H, Ohberg L, Forsgren S. Is vasculo-neural ingrowth the cause of pain in chronic Achilles tendinosis? An investigation using ultrasonography and colour Doppler, immunohistochemistry, and diagnostic injections. *Knee Surg Sports Traumatol Arthrosc* 2003; 11(5): 334–8.

6. Regan WD, Wold LE, Coonrad R, et al. Microscopic histopathology of chronic refractory lateral epicondylitis. *Am J Sports Med* 1992; 20: 746–9.

7. Waugh EJ, Jaglal SB, Davis AM. Computer use associated with poor long-term prognosis of conservatively managed lateral epicondylalgia. *J Orthop Sports Phys Ther* 2004; 34(12): 770–80.

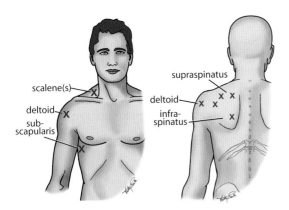

Figure 18.22 Myofascial trigger points in the infraspinatus referring pain to the upper arm

8. van der Windt D, van der Heidjen GJ, van den Berg SG, et al. Ultrasound therapy for musculoskeletal disorders: a systematic review. *Pain* 1999; 81: 257–71.

9. Bisset L, Paungmali A, Vicenzino B, et al. A systematic review and meta-analysis of clinical trials on physical interventions for lateral epicondylalgia. *Br J Sports Med* 2005; 39(7): 411–22.

10. Paungmali A, O'Leary S, Souvlis T, et al. Hypoalgesic and sympathoexcitatory effects of mobilization with movement for lateral epicondylalgia. *Phys Ther* 2003; 83(4): 374–83.

11. Vicenzino B, Paungmali A, Buratowski S, et al. Specific manipulative therapy treatment for chronic lateral epicondylalgia produces uniquely characteristic hypoalgesia. *Man Ther* 2001; 6(4): 205–12.

12. Vicenzino B, Collins D, Wright A. The initial effects of a cervical spine manipulative physiotherapy treatment on the pain and dysfunction of lateral epicondylalgia. *Pain* 1996; 68: 69–74.

13. Struijs PAA, Kerkhoffs GMMJ, Assendelft WJJ, et al. Conservative treatment of lateral epicondylitis: brace versus physical therapy or a combination of both—a randomized clinical trial. *Am J Sports Med* 2004; 32(2): 462–9.

14. Pienimaki T, Tarvainen T, Sira P, et al. Progressive strengthening and stretching exercises and ultrasound for chronic lateral epicondylitis. *Physiotherapy* 1996; 82: 522.

15. Svernlov B, Adolfsson L. Non-operative treatment regime including eccentric training for lateral humeral epicondylalgia. *Scand J Med Sci Sports* 2001; 11: 328–34.

16. Struijs PAA, Kerkoffs GMMJ, Assendelft WJJ, et al. Conservative treatment of lateral epicondylitis. *Am J Sports Med* 2004; 32(2): 462–9.

17. Vicenzino B, Brooksbank J, Minto J, et al. Initial effects of elbow taping on pain-free grip strength and pressure pain threshold. *J Orthop Sports Phys Ther* 2003; 33: 400–7.

18. Nirschl RP, Rodin DM, Ochiai DH, et al. Iontophoretic administration of dexamethasone sodium phosphate for acute epicondylitis. *Am J Sports Med* 2003; 31(2): 189–95.

19. Runeson L, Haker E. Iontophoresis with cortisone in the treatment of lateral epicondylalgia (tennis elbow)—a double-blind study. *Scand J Med Sci Sports* 2002; 12(3): 136–42.

20. Smidt N, van der Windt D, Assendelft W, et al. Corticosteroid injections, a physiotherapy, or wait-and-see policy for lateral epicondylitis: a randomised controlled trial. *Lancet* 2002; 359: 657–62.

21. Paoloni JA, Appleyard RC, Nelson J, et al. Topical nitric oxide application in the treatment of chronic extensor tendinosis at the elbow: a randomized, double-blinded, placebo-controlled clinical trial. *Am J Sports Med* 2003; 31(6): 915–20.

22. Keizer SB, Rutten HP, Pilot P, et al. Botulinum toxin injection versus surgical management for tennis elbow: a randomised pilot study. *Clin Orthop* 2002; 401: 125–31.

23. Morre HH, Keizer SB, van Os JJ. Treatment of chronic tennis elbow with botulinum toxin. *Lancet* 1997; 349: 1746.

24. Hayton MJ, Santini AJA, Hughes PJ, et al. Botulinum toxin injection in the treatment of tennis elbow. A double-blind, randomized, controlled, pilot study. *J Bone Joint Surg Am* 2005; 87(3): 503–7.

25. Green S, Buchbinder R, Barnsley L, et al. Acupuncture for lateral elbow pain. *Cochrane Database Syst Rev* 2002; 1: CD003527.

26. Edwards S, Calandruccio J. Autologous blood injections for refractory lateral epicondylitis. *J Hand Surg [Am]* 2003; 28A: 272–8.

27. Dunkow PD, Jatti M, Muddu BN, et al. Functional outcome was better after percutaneous surgery than after open formal release for tennis elbow. *J Bone Joint Surg Br* 2004; 86: 701–4.

28. Lutz FR Jr. Radial tunnel syndrome: an etiology of chronic lateral elbow pain. *J Orthop Sports Phys Ther* 1991; 14: 14–17.

29. Frostick S, Mohammad M, Ritchie D. Sports injuries of the elbow. *Br J Sports Med* 1999; 33: 301–11.

30. Shapiro MS, Wang JC. Elbow fractures. Treating to avoid complications. *Physician Sportsmed* 1995; 23(4): 39–50.

31. O'Driscoll SW, Morrey BF, Korinek S, et al. Elbow subluxation and dislocation. *Clin Orthop* 1992; 280: 186–97.

32. Ross G, McDevitt ER, Chronister R, et al. Treatment of simple elbow dislocation using an immediate motion protocol. *Am J Sports Med* 1999; 27(3): 308–11.

33. Verrall GM. Return to Australian rules football after acute elbow dislocation: a report of three cases and review of the literature. *J Sci Med Sport* 2001; 4(2): 245–50.

34. Mair SD, Isbell WM, Gill TJ, et al. Triceps tendon ruptures in professional football players. *Am J Sports Med* 2004; 32(2): 431–4.

35. Brukner PD, Bennell KL, Matheson GO. *Stress Fractures.* Melbourne: Blackwell Scientific, 1999.

Wrist, Hand and Finger Injuries

WITH ANDREW GARNHAM, MAUREEN ASHE AND PETER GROPPER

The wrist and hand are frequently injured during sport.[1] Sport-related injuries account for up to 15% of all hand injuries seen in accident and emergency departments.[2] Upper extremity injuries are frequent; distal radial fractures are the most common fracture seen in emergency departments,[3] and scaphoid fractures are the most common carpal fracture.[4] Men are more likely to sustain a hand or wrist injury[2] and children/adolescents are more likely to have a wrist injury compared with adults.[5] Injuries to the hand and wrist range from acute traumatic fractures, such as occur during football, hockey and snowboarding, to overuse conditions, which occur in racquet sports, golf and gymnastics. Finger trauma is common in ball-handling sports and rock climbing. If wrist, hand and finger injuries are not treated appropriately at the time of injury, they can lead to future impairments that can affect not only sporting endeavors but also activities of daily living.[6]

In clinical practise, patients can present with either an acute wrist injury (usually as a result of a fall onto the outstretched hand) or because of longer-term (chronic, or subacute) wrist pain. When pain has been ongoing, it may have developed gradually, or there may be a clear history of a past injury. We address each of those presentations in major sections. We then discuss conditions that affect the hand and fingers.

Acute wrist injuries

The wrist joint has multiple axes of movement: flexion–extension and radial–ulnar deviation occur at the radiocarpal joints, and pronation–supination occurs at the distal and proximal radioulnar joints. These movements provide mobility for hand function.

Injuries to the wrist often occur due to a *fall on the outstretched hand* (FOOSH). In sportspeople, the most common acute injuries are fractures of the distal radius or scaphoid, or damage to an intercarpal ligament. Intercarpal ligament injuries are becoming more frequently recognized and, if they are not treated appropriately (e.g. including surgical repair where indicated), may result in long-term disability. The causes of acute pain in this region are shown in Table 19.1.

The anatomy of the wrist and hand is complex and therefore a thorough knowledge of this region is essential to diagnose and treat sports injuries

Table 19.1 Causes of acute wrist pain

Common	Less common	Not to be missed
Distal radius fracture (often intra-articular in the athlete)	Fracture of hook of hamate	Carpal dislocation
	Triangular fibrocartilage complex tear	Anterior dislocation of lunate
Scaphoid fracture	Distal radioulnar joint instability	Perilunar dislocation
Wrist ligament sprain/tear	Scapholunate dissociation	Traumatic ulnar artery aneurysm or thrombosis (karate)
Intercarpal ligament		
Scapholunate ligament		
Lunotriquetral ligament		

accurately (Fig. 19.1). It is helpful to know the surface anatomy of the scaphoid tubercle, hook of hamate, pisiform, Lister's tubercle and anatomical snuffbox. The bony anatomy consists of a proximal row (lunate, triquetrum, pisiform) and a distal row (trapezium, trapezoid, capitate, hamate), which are bridged by the scaphoid bone. Normally, the distal carpal row should be stable; thus, a ligamentous injury here can greatly impair the integrity of the wrist. The proximal row permits more intercarpal movement to allow wrist flexion/extension and radial and ulnar deviation. Here a ligamentous injury disrupts important kinematics between the scaphoid, lunate and triquetrum, resulting in carpal instability with potential weakness and impairment of hand function.

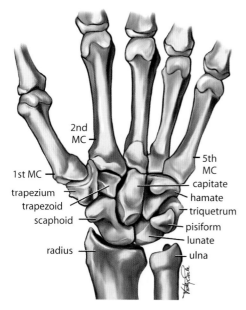

Figure 19.1 Anatomy of the wrist

(a) Carpal bones (MC = metacarpal)

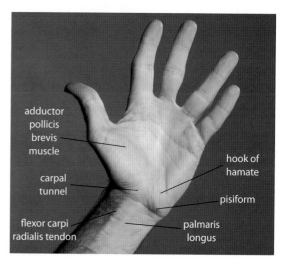

(c) Surface anatomy, volar view

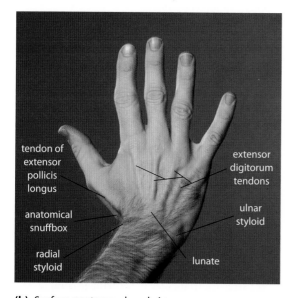

(b) Surface anatomy, dorsal view

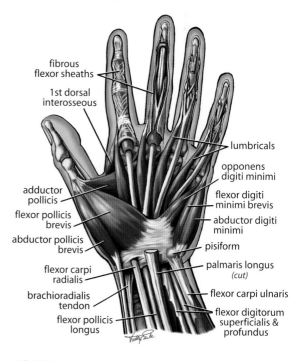

(d) Volar aspect

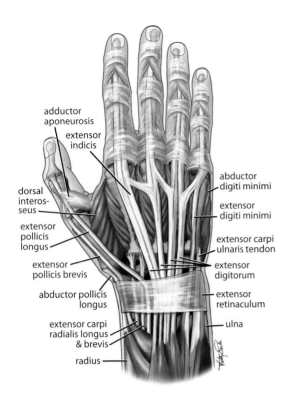

adductor aponeurosis

extensor indicis

dorsal interosseus

extensor pollicis longus

extensor pollicis brevis

abductor pollicis longus

extensor carpi radialis longus & brevis

radius

abductor digiti minimi

extensor digiti minimi

extensor carpi ulnaris tendon

extensor digitorum

extensor retinaculum

ulna

(e) Dorsal aspect

Table 19.2 Clinical distinction between dorsal and volar pain in acute wrist pain

Causes of dorsal wrist pain	Causes of volar wrist pain
Scaphoid fracture	Carpal instability
Scaphoid impaction syndrome	Hook of hamate
Fracture dislocation of carpus	fracture
Lunate fracture	
Distal radius fracture	
Scapholunate ligament tear	
Kienböck's disease (acute onset)	
Lunotriquetral ligament tear	
Distal radioulnar joint injury	
Carpometacarpal dislocation	

- history of past upper extremity fractures including childhood fractures/injuries
- history of osteoarthritis, rheumatoid arthritis, thyroid dysfunction, diabetes
- any unusual sounds (e.g. clicks, clunks, snaps, etc.)
- recurrent wrist swelling raises the suspicion of wrist instability
- musician (number of years playing, hours of practise per week, change in playing, complex piece, etc.)
- gardening, crafts, hobbies.

History

It is essential to determine the mechanism of the injury causing wrist pain. A fall on the outstretched hand may be severe enough to fracture the scaphoid or distal radius or damage the intercarpal ligaments and/or triangular fibrocartilage complex. These injuries are commonly encountered in high-velocity activities such as snowboarding,[7] rollerblading[8, 9] or falling off a bike. A patient may fracture the hook of hamate while swinging a golf club,[10] tennis racquet or bat and striking a hard object (e.g. the ground). Rotational stress to the distal radioulnar joint and forced ulnar deviation and rotation may tear the triangular fibrocartilage complex. It is very useful to determine the site of the pain; the causes of volar pain are different from those of dorsal wrist pain (Table 19.2). Other important aspects of the history may include:

- hand dominance
- occupation (computer related, manual labor, food service industry)
- degree of reliance upon hands in occupation/recreation

Examination

Examination involves:

1. Observation (Fig. 19.2a)
2. Active movements
   (a) flexion/extension
   (b) supination/pronation
   (c) radial/ulnar deviation (Fig. 19.2b)
3. Passive movements
   (a) extension (Fig. 19.2c)
   (b) flexion (Fig. 19.2d)
4. Palpation
   (a) distal forearm (Fig. 19.2e)
   (b) radial snuffbox (Fig. 19.2f)
   (c) base of metacarpals
   (d) lunate (Fig. 19.2g)
   (e) head of ulna (Fig. 19.2h)
   (f) radioulnar joint
5. Special tests
   (a) hamate/pisiform (Fig. 19.2i)
   (b) Watson's test for scapholunate injury (Fig. 19.2j)
   (c) stress of triangular fibrocartilage complex (Fig. 19.2k)

(d) grip—Jamar dynamometer (may be contraindicated if a maximal effort is not permitted, e.g. after tendon repair)
(e) dexterity—Purdue pegboard (19.2l)
(f) dexterity—Moberg pick-up test
(g) sensation—Semmes Weinstein monofilament testing
(h) sensation—temperature
(i) nerve entrapment—Tinel's sign

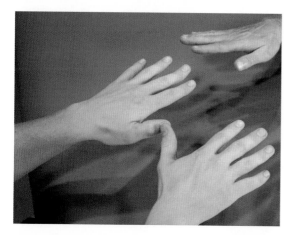

Figure 19.2 Examination of the patient with an acute wrist injury

(a) Observation. The wrist is inspected for obvious deformity suggesting a distal radial fracture. Swelling in the region of the radial snuffbox may indicate a scaphoid fracture. Inspect the hand and wrist posture, temperature, color, muscular wasting, scars, normal arches of the hand

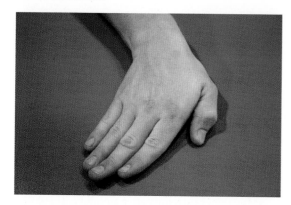

(b) Active movement—radial/ulnar deviation. Normal range is radial 20° and ulnar 60°. Pain and restriction of movement should be noted. Always compare motion with that of the other hand

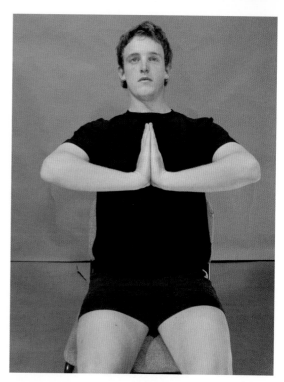

(c) Range of motion—the 'prayer position'. Normal range of motion in wrist extension is 70°

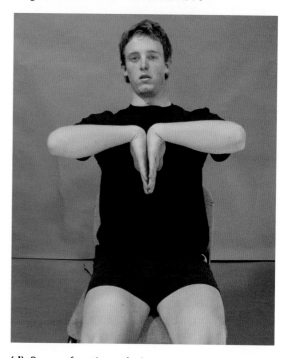

(d) Range of motion—the 'reverse prayer position'. Normal range of motion in wrist flexion is 80°

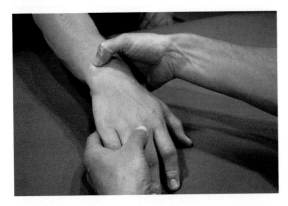

(e) Palpation—the distal forearm is palpated for bony tenderness or deformity

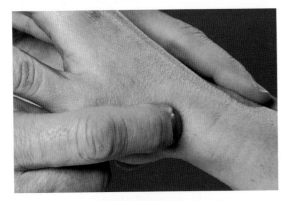

(f) Palpation—radial snuffbox. The proximal snuffbox is the site of the radial styloid, the middle snuffbox is the site of the scaphoid bone, while the distal snuffbox is over the scaphotrapezial joint

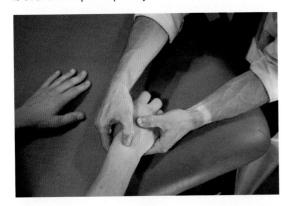

(g) Palpation—the lunate is palpated as a bony prominence proximal to the capitate sulcus. Lunate tenderness may correspond to a fracture. On the radial side of the lunate lies the scapholunate joint, which may be tender in scapholunate ligament sprain. This is a site of ganglion formation

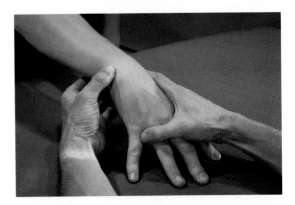

(h) Palpation—head of ulna and ulnar snuffbox. Swelling and tenderness over the dorsal ulnar aspect of the wrist is present with fractures of the ulnar styloid. Distal to the ulnar head is the ulnar snuffbox. The triquetrum lies in this sulcus and can be palpated with the wrist in radial deviation. Tenderness may indicate triquetral fracture or triquetrolunate injury. The triquetrohamate joint is located more distally. Pain here may represent triquetrohamate ligament injury

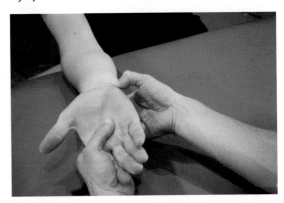

(i) Palpation—the pisiform is palpated at the flexor crease of the wrist on the ulnar side. Tenderness in this region may occur with pisiform or triquetral fracture. The hook of hamate is 1 cm (0.5 in.) distal and radial to the pisiform. Examination may show tenderness over the hook or on the dorsal ulnar surface

6. Standardized rating scales
   Several valid and reliable assessment scales can quantify function of the wrist specifically or the upper extremity after an injury. These include the Patient Rated Wrist Evaluation (PRWE)[11, 12] and the Disability of the Arm, Shoulder and Hand (DASH and Quick DASH)[13, 14] measurements.

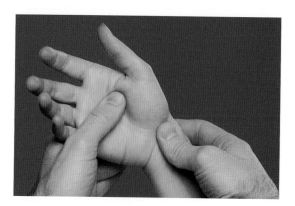

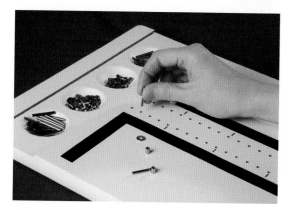

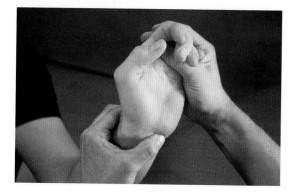

(j) Special test—Watson's test for scapholunate instability. The examiner places the thumb on the scaphoid tuberosity as shown with the wrist in ulnar deviation. The wrist is then deviated radially with the examiner placing pressure on the scaphoid. If the athlete feels pain dorsally (over the scapholunate ligament) or the examiner feels the scaphoid move dorsally, then scapholunate dissociation is present

(l) Special test—Purdue pegboard dexterity test. This measures dexterity for activities that involve gross movements of the hands, fingers and arms, and also those that require 'fingertip' dexterity

(k) Special test—triangular fibrocartilage complex integrity. The wrist is placed into dorsiflexion and ulnar deviation and then rotated. Overpressure causes pain and occasionally clicking in patients with a tear of the triangular fibrocartilage complex

Investigations

Plain radiography

Following trauma, routine radiograph views should include PA and PA with both radial and ulnar deviation. If ligament injury is suspected, also obtain a PA view with clenched fist. A straight lateral view of the wrist, with the dorsum of the distal forearm and the hand forming a straight line, permits assessment of the distal radius, the lunate, the scaphoid and the capitate and may reveal subtle instability. Undisplaced distal radial and scaphoid fractures, however, are often difficult to see on initial radiographs; clinical suspicion of fracture warrants investigation with other modalities (see 'special imaging studies' below).

The normal PA view is shown in Figure 19.3a. Inspect each bone in turn. Note the line joining the proximal ends of the proximal row of the carpus and the C-shape of the midcarpal joint (Gilula's arcs). If these lines are not smooth, a major abnormality is present. Assess the size of the scapholunate gap and look for scaphoid flexion (the signet ring sign) as these are signs of scapholunate instability.

The lateral radiograph of the normal wrist can be seen in Figure 19.3b. The proximal pole of the lunate fits into the concavity of the distal radius and the convex head of the capitate fits into the distal concavity of the lunate. These bones should be aligned with each other and with the base of the third metacarpal. A clenched fist PA view should be taken if scapholunate instability is suspected. This is indicated by a widened gap of 3 mm (0.1 in.) or greater between the scaphoid and lunate on the PA view but this may not present until some time after a scapholunate tear.

 Scapholunate instability cannot be ruled out on initial plain radiographs as it may take some months for the scaphoid and lunate to separate significantly radiographically.

Special imaging studies

The combination of the complex anatomy of the wrist and subtle wrist injuries that can cause substantial morbidity has led to development of specialized wrist imaging techniques. Special scaphoid views should

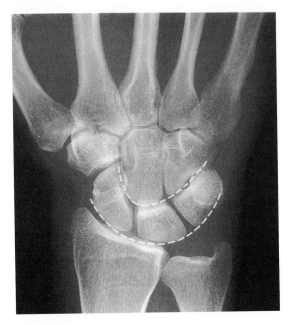

Figure 19.3 Radiograph of the wrist

(a) PA view—Gilula's arcs

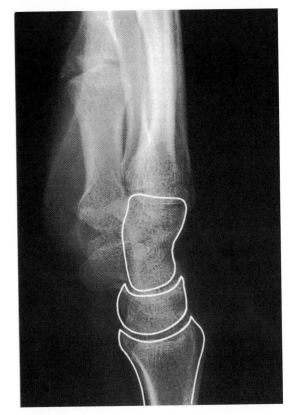

(b) Lateral view

be requested if a scaphoid fracture is suspected. A carpal tunnel view with the wrist in dorsiflexion allows inspection of the hook of hamate and ridge of the trapezium. For suspected mechanical pathology, such as an occult ganglion, an occult fracture, non-union or bone necrosis, several modalities are useful (e.g. ultrasonography, radionuclide bone scan, CT scan or MRI). Ultrasonography is a quick and accessible way to assess soft tissue abnormalities such as tendon injury, synovial thickening, ganglions and synovial cysts. Bone scans have high sensitivity and low specificity; thus, they can effectively rule out subtle fractures. MRI may be equally sensitive and more specific than a bone scan. CT scanning is particularly useful for evaluating fractures that are difficult to evaluate fully on plain films but MRI can also provide information about soft tissue injuries. Thus, a complete scapholunate ligament tear is more effectively identified with MRI than with CT. Arthrography of the wrist, criticized for low sensitivity and specificity, is no longer used as an investigative tool. If all imaging results are negative but clinically significant wrist pain persists, the clinician should refer the patient to a specialist for further evaluation, which may include arthroscopy, an increasingly used diagnostic and therapeutic procedure. Arthroscopy is excellent for detecting early scapholunate ligament tears in patients; also, it is the investigation of choice for patients with ulnar side wrist pain persisting after an acute injury.

Fracture of the distal radius and ulna

Distal radius fractures (Fig. 19.4) are very common peripheral fractures.[3] As the force required to fracture young adults' bones is great, athletes may simultaneously incur an intra-articular fracture and ligamentous strain or rupture. The higher the forces involved (e.g. in high-velocity sports), the greater the likelihood of a complex injury involving articular structures. Thus, thorough assessment of ligamentous injury is essential when fractures occur. Initial treatment of the fracture is anatomical reduction and immobilization for up to six weeks in a cast that covers the distal half of the forearm, the wrist and the hand, leaving the metacarpophalangeal (MCP) joints free. Radiographs are required every two weeks during healing to ensure that satisfactory reduction is maintained.

Inaccurate reduction, articular surface angulation, radial inclination, or inadequate restoration of length all require early internal fixation with fixed angle-volar plating. While it is sometimes not possible to achieve perfect reduction because of dorsal comminution,

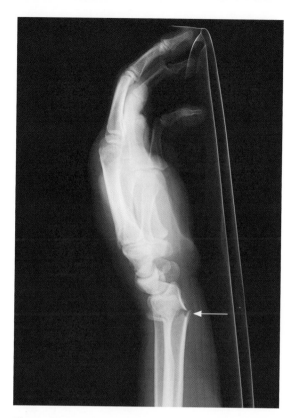

Figure 19.4 Colles' fracture, a specific type of distal radial fracture

every effort should be made to restore anatomical alignment to avoid ongoing functional impairment. Overall, there is a trend to more aggressive treatment using volar plating and this has led to improved functional outcomes.

Fracture of the scaphoid

Carpal fractures account for many hand/wrist fractures. The most common carpal fracture involves the scaphoid[4] and the usual mechanism is a fall on the outstretched hand. As the patient's pain may settle soon after the fall, he or she may not present to a clinician until some time after the injury. The key examination finding is tenderness in the anatomical snuffbox. This may be accompanied by swelling and loss of grip strength. Snuffbox tenderness should be compared with the other wrist, as some degree of tenderness is normal. Swelling in the snuffbox should also be sought. A more specific clinical test for scaphoid fracture is pain on axial compression of the thumb towards the radius or direct pressure on the scaphoid tuberosity with radial deviation of the

wrist. Plain radiographs with special scaphoid views will usually demonstrate the fracture (Fig. 19.5).

 If a scaphoid fracture is suspected clinically but the radiograph is normal, a fracture cannot be ruled out. MRI is an ideal, and increasingly used, diagnostic test for an acute injury; it may be a cost-effective routine investigation for scaphoid fractures in some settings.[15] Bone scan also has excellent sensitivity for scaphoid fracture. Note that it can take 24 hours for the injury to be revealed on MRI or bone scan. If these imaging modalities are not available, the wrist should be immobilized for 12 days as if a fracture were present, and then the radiograph should be repeated.

Note that scaphoid fracture is the most commonly missed fracture leading to litigation. If there is no bony damage, scapholunate instability should also be considered (see below).

Treatment of stable and unstable scaphoid fractures

A stable scaphoid fracture should be immobilized for eight weeks in a scaphoid cast extending from the proximal forearm to, but not including, the interphalangeal joint of the thumb (Fig. 19.6a). Upon removing the cast, re-evaluate the fracture clinically and radiologically. As with all fractures, clinical union precedes radiological union and determines readiness

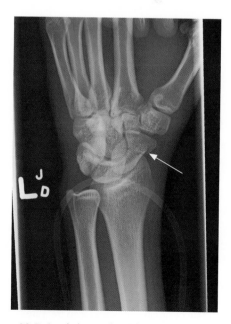

Figure 19.5 A subtle scaphoid fracture

to return to sport. Radiological union of the scaphoid should occur before finally discharging the patient.

Unstable or significantly displaced fractures require immediate percutaneous fixation (Fig. 19.6b) or open reduction and internal fixation.

Complications of scaphoid fracture

Because the blood supply to the scaphoid originates distally, flow to the proximal pole can be diminished, which can then be at risk of necrosis after a fracture. Scaphoid fractures have a risk of delayed union or non-union and, if there is clinical evidence of incomplete union when the cast is removed, the fracture should be immobilized for a further four to six weeks. Further immobilization beyond this time is unlikely to prove beneficial. CT scan is the investigation of choice to detect non-union, but MRI can be used if CT is not available. Contemporary treatment of non-union is with compression screw fixation.[16]

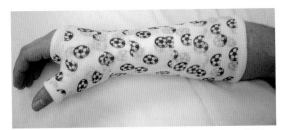

(a)

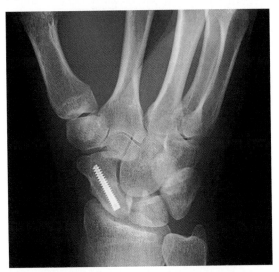

(b)

Figure 19.6 Treatment of two types of scaphoid fractures **(a)** Stable fracture—cast immobilization **(b)** Unstable or significantly displaced fracture—surgical fixation

Post-immobilization rehabilitation

Following successful treatment of a scaphoid fracture, the patient is invariably left with a stiff wrist joint and wasted muscles. Mobilization and strengthening of the wrist and other stiff structures should begin immediately after cast removal. Post-fracture, it is prudent to ensure there has been no ligamentous involvement by using the clenched-fist radiograph or MR plus/minus arthroscopy if clinical suspicion is high. If the wrist is intact, the athlete may be able to return to certain activities using a protective device. Compression tubing (Fig. 19.7a) worn under the protective splint reduces edema and improves comfort. Different sports have different rules about what constitutes an 'allowable' protective cast (Fig. 19.7b).

Fracture of the hook of hamate

Fracture of the hook of hamate may occur while swinging a golf club,[10, 17, 18] tennis racquet or baseball bat. The fracture is especially likely to occur when

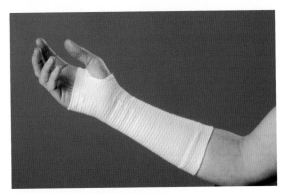

(a)

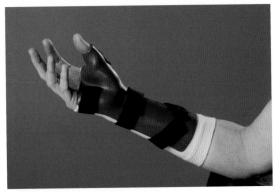

(b)

Figure 19.7 Following a scaphoid fracture the athlete may wear **(a)** Compression tubing underneath **(b)** A protective cast

the golf club strikes the ground instead of the ball, forcing the top of the handle of the club against the hook of the hamate of the top hand (Fig. 19.8a). This mechanism may compress the superficial and deep terminal branches of the ulnar nerve, producing both sensory and motor changes. Symptoms include reduced grip strength and ulnar wrist pain. Examination reveals volar wrist tenderness over the hook of hamate. Routine radiographs of the wrist do not image the fracture and even the classic 'carpal tunnel view' with the wrist in dorsiflexion is an insensitive test. CT scan (Fig. 19.8b) and MRI (Fig. 19.8c) are the best imaging tools.

This fracture often fails to heal with immobilization; most sports medicine cases of the fracture are actually stress fractures that present late. In some sportspeople (e.g. baseball players) the hook of hamate fracture is likely to be a completed stress fracture not due to acute trauma. If diagnosis is delayed, or the fracture fails to heal clinically within four weeks of immobilization, current surgical practice is excision of the fractured hook followed by three weeks' wrist immobilization, (in preference to open reduction

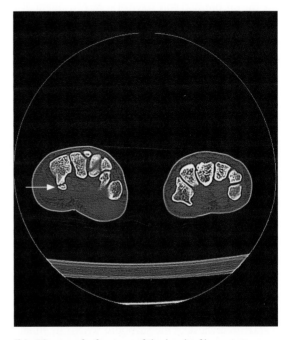

(b) CT scan of a fracture of the hook of hamate

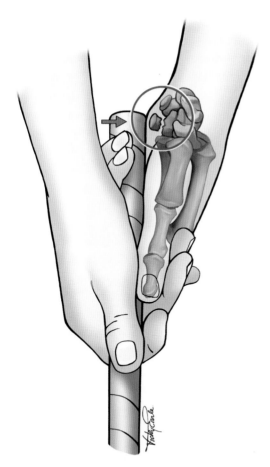

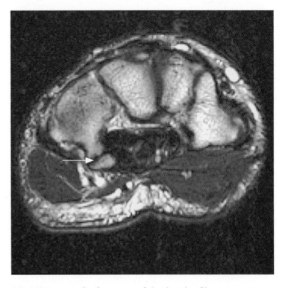

Figure 19.8 Fracture of the hook of hamate

(a) Possible mechanism—when the golf club is suddenly decelerated (e.g. hitting the ground), the grip is forced against the hook of hamate

(c) MRI scan of a fracture of the hook of hamate

and internal fixation).[10, 19, 20] The pain only dissipates slowly, but the patient can usually resume sport six weeks after surgery. How this affects treatment is not yet known.

Dislocation of the carpal bones

There are a number of different types of dislocation of the carpal bones, mostly involving the lunate. They are the uncommon end-stage of severe ligament disruption. Failure to recognize them generally results in disastrous consequences.

Anterior dislocation of the lunate

The lunate may dislocate anteriorly because of forced dorsiflexion when the athlete falls onto the outstretched hand, or the carpus and hand may dislocate dorsally on the lunate, leading to perilunar dislocation. Pain is usually severe and deformity obvious. Plain radiograph reveals the dislocation best in the lateral view with the lunate tilted volarly and not articulating with the capitate. Treatment is open reduction and primary ligament repair followed by eight weeks' cast immobilization. Anterior lunate dislocation may be associated with median nerve compression and paresthesia in the radial three and a half digits. This requires surgical decompression and repair of the ligament.

Perilunar dislocation of the lunate

Perilunar dislocation is occasionally associated with a fractured waist of the scaphoid when the lunate remains with the radius and the capitate is dislocated dorsally. This complex injury requires treatment by a hand and wrist surgeon.

Scapholunate dissociation

Pain and dysfunction at the wrist can be disabling. A complex composition of different joint surfaces with multiple ligamentous attachments contributes to the challenges faced when trying to understand wrist pain and dysfunction. Thus, a thorough assessment of range of motion and ligamentous stability is essential to rule out serious threats to the architectural integrity of the wrist and hand. Fortunately, most wrist traumatic events do not lead to significant capsuloligamentous or bony structural failure, which means the injury can be treated conservatively. However, a minor ligamentous structural injury or failure can progress; if not identified and managed correctly in the early stages there is the potential for significant structural failure leading to a chronic impairment. A predynamic injury can progress to a dynamic or static carpal instability, and

may lead to a chronic regional wrist joint synovitis or overlying tendinosis.[21]

Scapholunate dissociation is due to scapholunate ligament tear and loss of secondary restraints (Fig. 19.9a). Rotatory subluxation of the scaphoid may occur as a result of disruption of its ligamentous attachments due to acute trauma (e.g. a fall on the dorsiflexed hand). Examination reveals tenderness 2 cm (1 in.) distal to Lister's tubercle on the radial side of the lunate. There may be little, or no, swelling. The key examination maneuver is Watson's test (Fig. 19.2j). If the test causes pain or reveals dorsal movement of the scaphoid, scapholunate instability is present.

Conventional radiographic views may not show any abnormality but stress films such as the clenched fist PA view may reveal a gap greater than 3 mm (0.1 in.) between the scaphoid and lunate (Fig. 19.9b). A lateral radiograph may show an increased volar flexion of the distal pole of the scaphoid and dorsiflexion of the lunate. If these tests are negative but the injury is suspected clinically, MRI is indicated (Fig. 19.9c).

Treatment of scapholunate dissociation is open reduction and repair of the ligaments and internal fixation. The patient must accept that any surgical repair will result in permanent reduction in wrist

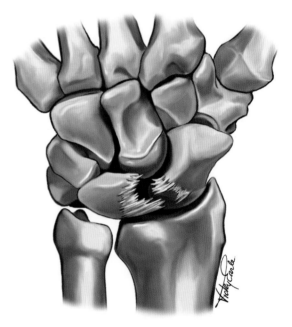

Figure 19.9 Scapholunate dissociation.

(a) Coronal graphic shows a tear of the dorsal component of the scapholunate ligament

motion. Hence, minor dissociations in the presence of normal movement probably should not be repaired.

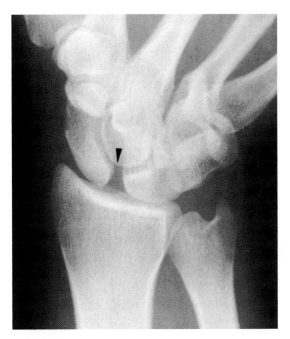

(b) In a classic case, radiograph reveals separation of the scaphoid and lunate. This can be a late sign, so normal radiography does not rule out this condition

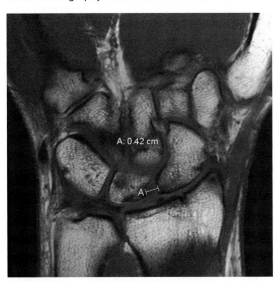

(c) MRI shows that the scapholunate interval diastasis (A) is 4.2 mm (0.14 in.). The upper limit of normal is 3 mm (0.1 in.)

Subacute onset and chronic wrist pain

When a patient presents with subacute onset or chronic wrist pain, the clinician should consider whether the pain may be a manifestation of a systemic condition (e.g. metabolic disorder or spondyloarthopathy [Chapter 50]). Also, the clinician should rule out an uncommon presentation of radiating pain from a more proximal problem such as a herniated cervical disk.

A detailed history will reveal whether the problem stems from an overuse condition (e.g. tenosynovitis) or, rather, from an acute injury that has not been correctly diagnosed or treated. Some patients suffer only minor discomfort at the time of an initial injury and fail to seek attention at that time. Acute injuries are discussed above.

The location of wrist pain narrows down the diagnosis of subacute onset wrist pain. Determine whether the wrist pain is essentially dorsal, volar, radial or ulnar (Table 19.3), as this is the first step to determining the differential diagnosis.

History

A thorough history of the onset of pain and the circumstances surrounding the onset will provide the best clues to a previous acute injury. Factors that aggravate the pain provide useful information as to which structures are involved in chronic wrist pain.

Pain after repeated movement, with stiffness after a period of rest, suggests an inflammatory condition such as tenosynovitis. Pain aggravated by weightbearing activities, such as gymnastics or diving, suggests bone or joint involvement. A history of joint clicking may be associated with carpal instability, triangular fibrocartilage tears or extensor carpi ulnaris subluxation. Characteristic night pain, with or without paresthesia, is found in carpal tunnel syndrome. Associated neck or elbow symptoms suggest referred pain.

Examination

Inspection may reveal a ganglion on the dorsum of the wrist. Swelling over the radial styloid may indicate de Quervain's tenosynovitis. Muscle wasting of the thenar or hypothenar eminence is found in the late stages of median or ulnar nerve compression respectively. Palpate the wrist to detect tenderness and to determine whether the pathology appears to be extra-articular (i.e. soft tissue) or articular. Examine the

Table 19.3 Causes of subacute onset wrist pain according to location of pain. More common causes are listed first

Dorsal	Volar	Ulnar	Radial
Ganglion	Scaphoid aseptic necrosis	Triangular fibrocartilage complex tears	Scaphoid fracture (missed)
Intersection syndrome	Stenosing tendinopathies	Ulnar impaction syndrome	Non-union of scaphoid fracture
Kienböck's disease	Flexor carpi ulnaris tendinopathy	Distal radioulnar joint instability	de Quervain's tenosynovitis
Dorsal pole of lunate and distal radius impingement (gymnasts)	Flexor carpi radialis tendinopathy	Carpal instability	Scaphoid impaction syndrome
Posterior interosseous nerve entrapment	Carpal tunnel syndrome	Scapholunate dissociation	Intersection syndrome
Inflammatory arthropathy	Ulnar tunnel syndrome	Ulnar nerve compression (cyclists, golfers)	Flexor carpi radialis tendinopathy
Degenerative joint disease	Pisotriquetral degenerative joint disease	Flexor carpi ulnaris tendinopathy	Dorsal pole of lunate impingement on distal radius (gymnasts)
Extensor carpi ulnaris tendinopathy	Avascular necrosis of the capitate (weightlifters)	Extensor carpi ulnaris tendinopathy	Scapholunate dissociation
Extensor carpi ulnaris subluxation	Extensor pollicis longus impingement/rupture (gymnasts)	Extensor carpi ulnaris subluxation	
Injuries to distal radial epiphysis (children)		Distal radioulnar joint impaction syndromes (golfers)	
Extensor pollicis longus impingement on Lister's tubercle (occasional rupture)		Scaphoid impaction syndrome	

radial side of the lunate closely (Fig. 19.2g). Tenderness is present in scapholunate ligament sprain. On the ulnar side of the lunate lies the triquetrolunate ligament. Tenderness and an associated click on radial and ulnar deviation of the wrist may occur with partial or complete tears of this ligament. On the volar aspect of the wrist, palpate the tuberosity of the trapezium as a bony prominence at the base of the thenar eminence (Fig. 19.10a).

Additional tests may be performed to diagnose overuse injuries. Restricted wrist movements and pain on passive stretching of the tendons is associated with tenosynovitis. Tenosynovitis of the abductor pollicis longus and extensor pollicis brevis (de Quervain's disease) may be confirmed by Finkelstein's test (Fig. 19.10b). Tinel's sign is positive if carpal tunnel syndrome is present (Fig. 19.10c). Tears of the triangular fibrocartilage complex can be detected using the 'press test' (Fig. 19.10d).[22]

Extra-articular conditions

Many conditions can cause subacute and chronic wrist pain; clinical assessment can provide insight into whether this is due to extra-articular (soft tissue) conditions, or articular (bone/joint) conditions. Common extra-articular conditions include de Quervain's tenosynovitis, intersection syndrome, ganglia, impingement syndromes and tendinopathies.

de Quervain's tenosynovitis

de Quervain's tenosynovitis is an inflammation of the synovium of the abductor pollicis longus and extensor pollicis brevis tendons as they pass in their synovial sheath in a fibro-osseous tunnel at the level of the radial styloid (Fig. 19.11). This is the most common radial-sided tendinopathy in athletes and occurs particularly with racquet sports, ten pin bowlers, rowers and canoeists. The left thumb of a

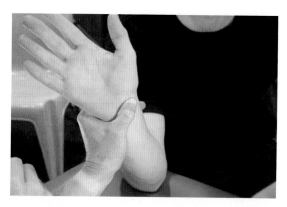

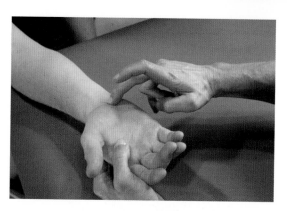

Figure 19.10 Additional examination of the patient with wrist pain of gradual onset

(a) Palpation—tuberosity of the trapezium at the base of the thenar eminence. Tenderness proximal to the tuberosity may be associated with flexor carpi radialis tendinopathy. Tenderness distal may indicate injury to the carpometacarpal ligament of the thumb

(c) Special tests—Tinel's test. Tapping over the median nerve at the wrist produces tingling and altered sensation in the distribution of the median nerve in carpal tunnel syndrome

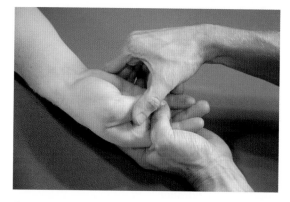

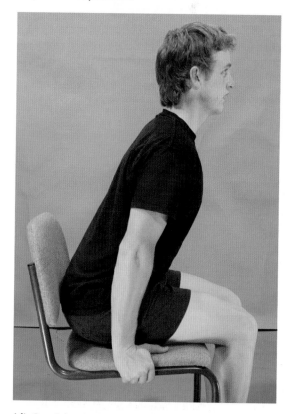

(b) Special test—Finkelstein's test to detect de Quervain's disease. The thumb is placed in the palm of the hand with flexion of the MCP and interphalangeal joints while the examiner deviates the wrist in the ulnar direction

right-handed golfer is particularly at risk because of the hyperabduction required during a golf swing. There is local tenderness and swelling, which may extend proximally and distally along the course of the tendons. In severe cases, crepitus may be felt. A positive Finkelstein's test is diagnostic (Fig. 19.10b) but not pathognomonic because flexor carpi radialis tendinopathy also causes a positive test.

Treatment includes splinting, local electrotherapeutic modalities, stretches and graduated strengthening. Patients often find a pen build-up (a rubber addition to enlarge the diameter of the pen) useful

(d) Special tests—press test (or 'sitting hands' test). Attempting to raise body weight from a chair reproduces the pain of the triangular fibrocartilage complex injury

as this reduces the stretch on the extensor tendons. An injection of corticosteroid and local anesthetic into the tendon sheath will usually prove helpful.

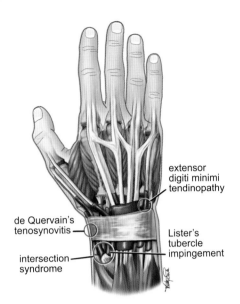

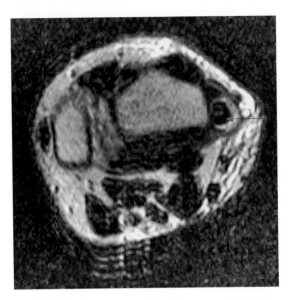

(c) MRI of the region reveals increased signal and a thickened tendon

Figure 19.11 Some extra-articular causes of pain around the wrist

(a) Sites of pain where tendons pass through fibro-osseous tunnels

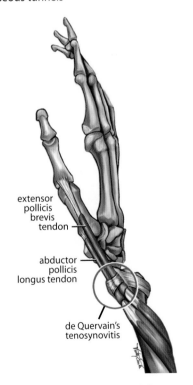

(b) Graphic view of the radial styloid showing the thickening and edema of the first extensor compartment tendons in de Quervain's tenosynovitis

In rare cases, surgical release is necessary. A recent study that pooled the results of seven investigations concluded that cortisone alone cured 83% of cases, injection and splinting cured 61%, and splinting alone cured 14%. It is noteworthy that no patients gained symptom reduction from rest and NSAIDS.[23] Unfortunately, the original studies did not compare injection to another form of treatment; thus, further studies are needed to determine the most effective treatment for this condition.

Intersection syndrome

Intersection syndrome is a bursitis that occurs at the site where the abductor pollicis longus and extensor pollicis brevis tendons cross over the extensor carpi radialis tendons (Fig. 19.12) just proximal to the extensor retinaculum. It may be due to friction at the site of crossing or it may also arise from teno-synovitis of the two extensor tendons within their synovial sheath. Tenderness is found dorsally on the radial side, with swelling and crepitus a short distance proximal to the site of maximal tenderness in de Quervain's disease (Fig. 19.11). This condition is sometimes called 'oarsmen's wrist' because of its common occurrence in rowers,[24] but it is also seen in canoeists, and in weight-training and racquet sports. Treatment involves relative rest and early intervention with corticosteroid injection into the bursa if there is no response. Surgical decompression is rarely necessary. For rowers, other considerations

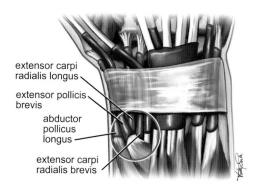

extensor carpi
radialis longus

extensor pollicis
brevis

abductor
pollicus
longus

extensor carpi
radialis brevis

Figure 19.12 Sites of pain and mechanisms of intersection syndrome. Causes of intersection syndrome include inflammation at the site where the abductor pollicis longus and extensor pollicis brevis cross the wrist extensors (extensor carpi radialis brevis and longus) and tenosynovitis of the wrist extensors themselves

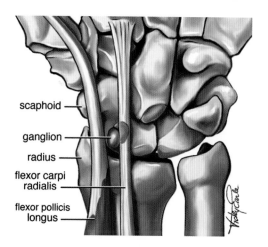

scaphoid

ganglion

radius

flexor carpi
radialis

flexor pollicis
longus

Figure 19.13 Ganglion cyst

(a) Graphic view of the dorsum of the wrist showing the ganglion arising from the joint

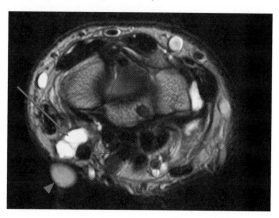

(b) MRI shows the bilobed high-signal ganglion (larger arrow) surrounding the tendon of flexor carpi radialis (small arrow) and very close to the patient's site of pain (the MR-compatible marker placed over the skin, arrowhead)

include reducing the amount of rowing, and changing the size of the oar and/or rowing technique.[24] Windy conditions commonly provoke this condition in canoeists.

Ganglions

Ganglions occur in athletes of any age. They are a synovial cyst communicating with the joint space (Fig. 19.13). They most often present as a relatively painless swelling. They occur in several common sites on both the dorsal and volar aspects of the wrist, most commonly the scapholunate space, presumably as a result of previous ligamentous trauma. They may also be intracapsular, or even intra-osseous. The patient's main complaint is of intermittent wrist pain and reduced movement. Swelling may be visible intermittently or not at all and so should not be relied upon to make the diagnosis. Ultrasonography is a useful investigation; however, T2-weighted MRI highlights ganglion cysts (Fig. 19.13b) and is the investigation of choice. The athlete must be reassured that the ganglion is benign. Treatment is only indicated for a symptomatic ganglion. When symptoms persist, aspiration and/or corticosteroid infiltration are at least temporarily effective and can be performed under ultrasound guidance where this is feasible. Some persistent symptomatic ganglions require surgery. Without complete removal, the lesion returns rapidly.

Impingement syndromes

A number of impingement syndromes may cause wrist pain. Scaphoid impaction syndrome may occur because of repetitive hyperextension stresses (e.g. in weightlifting, gymnastics). This mechanism is also responsible for avascular necrosis of the capitate in weightlifters. Impaction of the dorsal pole of the lunate on the distal radius is seen in gymnasts. The extensor pollicis longus may impinge on Lister's tubercle and occasionally ruptures. Triquetrohamate impingement syndrome may result from forced wrist extension and ulnar deviation (e.g. in racquet sports, gymnastics). Radial styloid impaction syndrome can result from repeated forced radial deviation, especially among golfers. Patients with these syndromes present with localized tenderness and are treated with rest and a protective brace. Occasionally, corticosteroid injection or surgical exploration may be helpful.

Tendinopathies around the wrist

Any of the flexor and extensor tendons around the wrist may become painful with excessive activity. On examination, there is tenderness and occasionally swelling and crepitus. The principles of treating tendinopathies apply; management should include attention to biomechanics (ergonomics), relative rest, ice, progressive strengthening and functional rehabilitation.[25]

Injuries to the distal radial epiphysis

Injuries to the distal radial epiphysis occur in elite young gymnasts. Fractures may occur but overuse injury to the epiphysis is more common. The gymnast complains of pain and limitation of dorsiflexion. Examination reveals minimal swelling and tenderness about the distal radial epiphysis with no signs of tendinopathy, synovial cysts or joint dysfunction. Common radiographic findings include widening of the growth plate, cystic changes (usually of the metaphyseal aspect of the epiphyseal plate) and haziness in the normal radiolucent area of the epiphyseal plate when compared with the asymptomatic side. If there is narrowing of the growth plate, the possibility of a Salter Harris V stress fracture must be considered (Chapter 40). Prevention by alteration of the training program is the best means of managing this condition. Once pain is present, avoidance of aggravating activities is required but the condition can take months to settle. There should be particular attention to strengthening of the forearm flexors as incorrect weight-bearing through an excessively extended wrist is a major causative factor.

Articular causes of subacute and chronic wrist pain

Common articular causes of subacute and chronic wrist pain include triangular fibrocartilage complex (TFCC) tears, Kienboch's disease and injuries to the distal radial epiphysis.

Triangular fibrocartilage complex tear

The triangular fibrocartilage complex (TFCC) lies between the ulna and the carpus. It is the major stabilizer of the distal radioulnar joint. The 'complex' consists of the triangular fibrocartilage, ulnar meniscus homolog, ulnar collateral ligament, numerous carpal ligaments and the extensor carpi ulnaris

tendon sheath. The TFCC is a common site of ulnar wrist pain. Compressive loads to the wrist, especially if accompanied by ulnar deviation (e.g. in gymnastics, diving, golf and racquet sports), may tear the central portion of the cartilage. It can also be disrupted after a distal radial–ulnar fracture or potential with disruption to the distal radioulnar joint.

Examination reveals tenderness and swelling over the dorsal ulnar aspect of the wrist, pain on resisted wrist dorsiflexion and ulnar deviation, a clicking sensation on wrist movement and reduced grip strength. The 'press test'[26] may be helpful (Fig. 19.10d). The patient creates an axial ulnar load by attempting to lift his/her weight up off a chair using the affected wrist. A positive test replicates the presenting symptom. High-quality MRI can image the TFCC and this is an increasingly popular investigation for ulnar-sided wrist pain. Estimates of sensitivity and specificity are about 60% and 90% respectively,[27] which suggests that a negative MRI should not be used to rule out the condition if it is clinically suspected. Interestingly, ultrasonography shows promise for matching MRI in the detection of TFCC lesions.[28]

Treatment may include protective bracing, strengthening when able, heat and/or electrotherapy modalities for pain. Arthroscopy permits accurate diagnosis and excision of any torn cartilage if required. If the ulna is longer than the radius (positive ulnar variance), it impinges on the triangular fibrocartilage and predisposes it to tearing. It may be necessary to shorten the ulna as well as excising the torn fibrocartilage.[29]

Distal radioulnar joint instability

The thickened dorsal and volar aspects of the triangular fibrocartilage act as the dorsal and volar ligaments of the distal radioulnar joint. Subluxation of the ulnar head occurs because of avulsion of these ligaments. It may be either volar or dorsal. Dorsal subluxation of the ulnar head associated with a tear of the volar radioulnar ligament is more common and may be due to repetitive or forceful pronation in contact sports, tennis or gymnastics. Dorsal displacement of the ulnar styloid process during pronation may be detected on true lateral radiograph. Treatment requires repair of the TFCC.

Kienböck's disease

Kienböck's disease is avascular necrosis of the lunate, possibly because of repeated trauma. This can present as chronic dorsal or volar wrist pain in an athlete who has repeated impact to the wrist. It is most common in those aged in their twenties. There is localized tenderness over the lunate and loss of grip strength.

Radiographs may show a smaller lunate of increased radio-opacity but false negatives can occur, so clinical suspicion warrants further investigation with isotopic bone scan or MRI. In the acute stage, immobilization may be therapeutic, whereas in chronic cases surgery is required, although results are not superior to conservative management.

Missed acute injuries presenting with articular chronic wrist pain

Conditions that may mimic gradual onset wrist pain include scaphoid fracture and scapholunate dissociation (see above). Chronic scapholunate dissociation should always be considered in patients with persistent pain and/or clicking (p. 318).

Numbness and hand pain

Another type of clinical presentation is that characterized by numbness or paresthesia. This suggests a neurological pathology and the commonest such problems at the wrist are carpal tunnel syndrome and ulnar nerve compression.

Carpal tunnel syndrome

The median nerve may be compressed as it passes through the carpal tunnel along with the flexor digitorum profundus, flexor digitorum superficialis and flexor pollicis longus tendons (Fig. 19.14). This condition is characterized by burning volar wrist pain with numbness or paresthesia in the distribution of the median nerve (thumb, index finger, middle

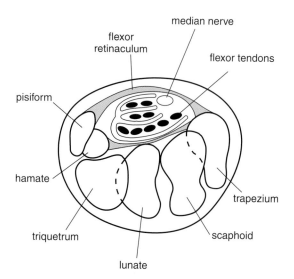

Figure 19.14 Axial view of the median nerve trapped in the carpal tunnel

finger and radial side of the ring finger). Nocturnal paresthesiae are characteristic. The pain can radiate to the forearm, elbow and shoulder. Tinel's sign may be elicited by tapping over the volar aspect of the wrist (Fig. 19.10c). The most important aspects in diagnosis are the history and physical examination but nerve conduction studies can help confirm the diagnosis and may predict how the patient will respond to surgery.[30] Diabetes mellitus should be excluded as it is a risk factor for carpal tunnel syndrome. Mild cases may be treated conservatively with NSAIDs and splinting. A single corticosteroid injection may provide relief[31] but persistent cases require surgical treatment.[32] Surgery may be either open or endoscopic and systematic reviews to date show no difference between the two techniques for symptom relief.[33]

Ulnar nerve compression

The ulnar nerve may be compressed at the wrist as it passes through Guyon's canal. This injury is most commonly seen in cyclists due to supporting body weight over a long duration ride[34] because of poor bike fit or a failure to use several relaxed handlebar grip positions. It also occurs in karate players, and a recent study highlighted the risk of hand neurovascular changes in baseball players, especially catchers, from repeated trauma associated with catching a ball.[35] Within Guyon's canal, the nerve lies with the ulnar artery between the pisiform bone on the ulnar side and the hamate radially. Symptoms include pain and paresthesia to the little finger and ulnar side of the fourth finger. Weakness usually develops later. Conservative treatment involves splinting, NSAIDs and changes in the cyclist's grip on the handlebars (Chapter 5). Surgical exploration of Guyon's canal may be required.

Hand and finger injuries

Hand and finger injuries are extremely common in sport and, although the majority require minimal treatment, some are potentially serious and require immobilization, precise splinting or even surgery. Finger injuries are often neglected by athletes in the expectation that they will resolve spontaneously. Many present too late for effective treatment. The importance of early assessment and management must be stressed so that long-term deformity and functional impairment can be avoided. Many hand and finger injuries require specific rehabilitation and appropriate protection upon resumption of sport. Joints in this region do not respond well to immobilization, therefore, full immobilization should be minimized.

The causes of pain in this region are shown in Table 19.4. The anatomy of this area is demonstrated in Figure 19.15.

History

The mechanism of injury is the most important component of the history of acute hand injuries. A direct, severe blow to the fingers may result in a fracture, whereas a blow to the point of the finger may produce an interphalangeal dislocation, joint sprain or long flexor or extensor tendon avulsion. A punching injury often results in a fracture at the base of the first metacarpal or to the neck of one of the other metacarpals, usually the fifth. An avulsion of the flexor digitorum profundus tendon, usually to the fourth finger, is suggested by a history of a patient grabbing an opponent's clothing while attempting a tackle. Associated features such as an audible crack, degree of pain, swelling, bruising and loss of function should also be noted.

Examination

Carefully palpate the bones and soft tissues of the hand and fingers, looking for tenderness. The examiner should always be conscious of what structure is being palpated at any particular time. The joints should be examined to determine active and passive range of movement and stability. Stability should be tested both in an anteroposterior direction and with ulnar and radial deviation to assess the collateral ligaments. The cause of any loss of active range of movement should be carefully assessed and not presumed to be due to swelling. Normal range of motion for the second to fifth digits is approximately 80° of flexion at the DIP, 100° of flexion at the PIP and 90° of flexion at the MCP joint. A common injury site that can be overlooked is the volar plate, a thick fibrocartilagenous tissue

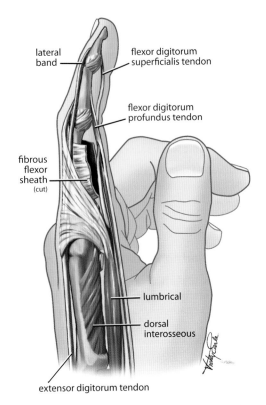

Figure 19.15 Anatomy of the metacarpals and fingers

(a) Metacarpals and fingers

that reinforces the phalangeal joints on the palmar or volar surface (Figs 19.15b, c).

The extensor tendons of the hand are often divided into six compartments. At the wrist on the dorsal side of the hand, the tendons are encased in synovial sheaths as they pass under the extensor retinaculum (Fig. 19.11). When palpating in the most radial

Table 19.4 Causes of hand and finger pain

Common	Less common	Not to be missed
Metacarpal fracture	Bennett's fracture	Potential infection (e.g. human bite)
Phalanx fracture	Dislocation of the MCP joint	Avulsion of long flexor tendons
Dislocation of the PIP joint	Dislocation of the DIP joint	
Ulnar collateral ligament sprain/ tear, first MCP joint	Radial collateral ligament sprain, first MCP joint	
Sprain of the PIP joint	Sprain of the DIP joint	
Laceration	Mallet finger	
Infections	Stress fractures	
Subungual hematoma	Glomus tumor	

PIP = proximal interphalangeal. DIP = distal interphalangeal. MCP = metacarpophalangeal.

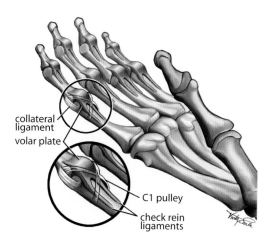

(b) The volar plate

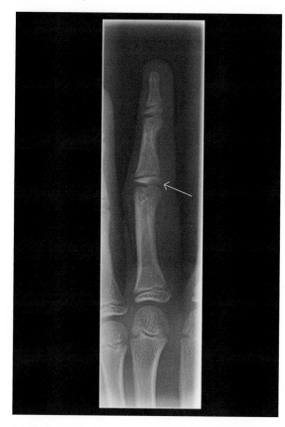

(c) Radiograph confirms the subtle nature of a volar plate avulsion

of the distal end of the radius. The extensor pollicis longus angles sharply around the bony prominence and can damage or even rupture the tendon after a serious wrist fracture. The anatomical snuffbox is composed of the extensor pollicis longus and brevis and abductor pollicis longus. The floor of the snuffbox is the carpometacarpal joint of the thumb. Clinically this is a significant region for several reasons. Tenderness may suggest scaphoid fracture. The deep branch of the radial arterial passes through as well as the superficial branch of the radial nerve; consequently, if a cast or splint is applied too tightly, it can lead to numbness in the thumb.

Examination involves:

1. Observation and sensation testing as per the wrist. Special note should be made of the hand arches and any deformities at the proximal or distal interphalangeal joints.
   (a) hand at rest (Fig. 19.16a)
   (b) hand with clenched fist (Fig. 19.16b)
2. Active movements—fingers (all joints)
   (a) flexion
   (b) extension
   (c) abduction
   (d) adduction
3. Active movements—thumb
   (a) flexion
   (b) extension
   (c) palmar abduction (Fig. 19.16c)
   (d) palmar adduction (Fig. 19.16d)
   (e) opposition (Fig. 19.16e)
4. Resisted movements (tendons)
   (a) flexor digitorum profundus (Fig. 19.16f)
   (b) flexor digitorum superficialis (Fig. 19.16g)
   (c) extensor tendon (Fig. 19.16h)
5. Special test
   (a) ulnar collateral ligament of the first MCP joint (Fig. 19.16i)
   (b) IP joint collateral ligaments

Investigations

Routine radiographs of the hand include the PA, oblique and lateral views. All traumatic finger injuries should be X-rayed. Ideally, 'dislocations' need to be radiographed before reduction to exclude fracture and after reduction to confirm relocation. Even when pre-reduction radiographs are not performed because reduction has occurred on the field, post-reduction films should be obtained after the game. Care should be taken with lateral views to isolate the affected finger to avoid bony overlap. The use of more sophisticated investigation techniques is usually not required.

compartment—compartment one—the examiner identifies abductor pollicis longus and extensor pollicis brevis, the tissues involved in de Quervain's tenosynovitis. Lister's tubercle is located on the dorsal surface

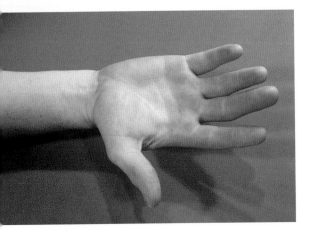

Figure 19.16 Examination of fingers

(a) Attitude of hand at rest

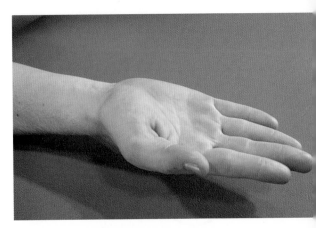

(d) Thumb movement—palmar adduction

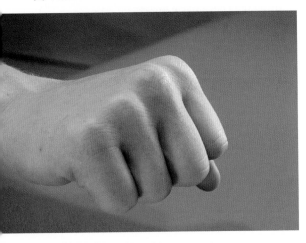

(b) Attitude of hand with clenched fist

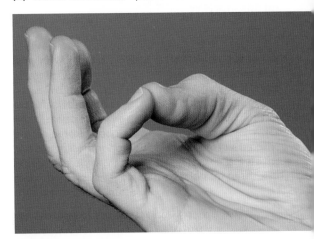

(e) Thumb movement—opposition

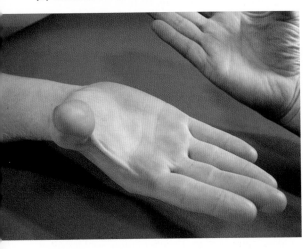

(c) Thumb movement—palmar abduction

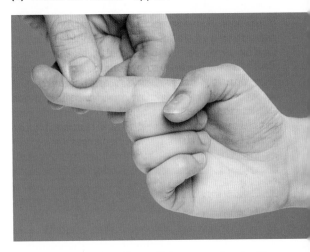

(f) Tendon integrity—flexor digitorum profundus. The patient flexes the DIP joint with the PIP joint held in extension

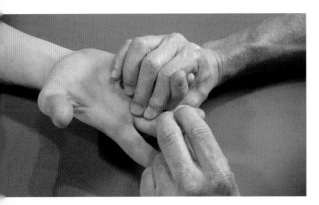

(g) Tendon integrity—flexor digitorum superficialis. The patient flexes the PIP joint with the other DIP joint held in extension

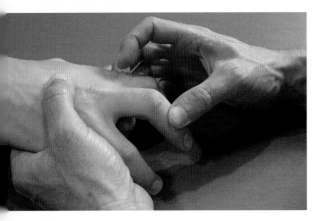

(h) Tendon integrity—extensor tendon. The patient extends the PIP joint with the MCP joint in extension

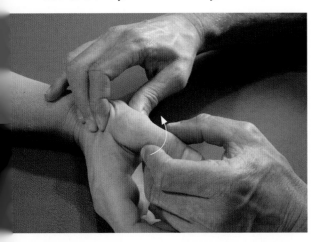

(i) Special test—the ulnar collateral ligament of the thumb is tested with 10° of flexion at the first MCP joint

Principles of treatment of hand injuries

The functional hand requires mobility, stability, sensitivity and freedom from pain. It may be necessary to obtain stability by surgical methods. However, conservative rehabilitation is essential to regain mobility and long-term freedom from pain. Treatment and rehabilitation of hand injuries is complex. As the hand is unforgiving of mismanagement, practitioners who do not see hand injuries regularly should ideally refer patients to an experienced hand therapist, or at least obtain advice while managing the patient.

Inflammation and swelling are obvious in the hand and fingers. During the inflammatory phase, the therapist must aim to reduce edema and monitor progress by signs of redness, heat and increased pain. During the regenerative phase (characterized by proliferation of scar tissue), the therapist can use supportive splints and active exercises to maintain range of motion. During remodeling, it is appropriate to use dynamic and serial splints, and active and active assisted exercises, in addition to heat, stretching and electrotherapeutic modalities.

Control of edema

Control of edema can be achieved through splinting, compression, ice, elevation and electrotherapeutic modalities. Splinting needs to be in the intrinsic plus position, with the wrist in 30° of dorsiflexion, the MCP joints flexed to 70° and the PIP joint extended to 0° with the thumb abducted (Fig. 19.17). Splints are periodically removed to allow exercise. Fist-making exercises are used to maintain joint movement and to help remove edema. During exercise, the hand should be elevated. Short frequent exercise periods are optimum.

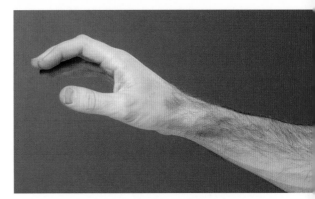

Figure 19.17 The 'intrinsic plus' position for splinting of hand injuries: 30° of wrist dorsiflexion, 70° of MCP flexion and minimal PIP flexion

Compression in the hand can be achieved with a number of compression gloves and by using a Coban elastic bandage: a 2.5 cm (1 in.) size is appropriate for fingers. If appropriate, active tendon gliding and range of motion exercises in combination with elevation can assist in the reduction of swelling. Electrotherapeutic modalities can be useful in the control of edema.

Exercises

Exercises may be active, active assisted or resisted. Tendon lacerations or ruptures are generally treated by protocols determined by the surgical technique and preferences of the treating surgeon. A full description of the protocols is beyond the scope of this chapter and the reader is referred elsewhere. Exercise prescription for other injuries includes:

- blocking exercises, which isolate the muscle being used by immobilizing appropriate joints with the other hand
- composite flexion exercises (e.g. tendon gliding exercises)
- extension exercises
- active assisted exercises in which the patient takes a joint through the full range of motion and then the therapist assists in gaining slightly greater range with overpressure.

Taping and splinting

The most commonly used method of taping is 'buddy taping' (Fig. 19.18). Its role is to provide a vehicle for active assisted exercise. The uninjured digit provides additional stability and encourages full range of motion.

In the acute phase of injury, static splints are used to reduce edema. Dynamic splints can also be used in the repair phase of injury to provide some force along joints and encourage increased range of motion (Fig. 19.19). With dynamic splinting, the splint should be worn with less tension for a longer period.

Fractures of the metacarpals

Fracture of the base of the first metacarpal

Fractures of the base of the first metacarpal commonly occur because of a punch connecting with a hard object, such as an opponent's head, or a fall on the abducted thumb. There are two main types of fracture: the extra-articular transverse fracture of the base of the first metacarpal about 1 cm (0.5 in.) distal to the joint (Fig. 19.20a) and a Bennett's fracture dislocation of the first carpometacarpal joint (Fig. 19.20b).

The transverse fracture near the base of the first metacarpal results in the thumb lying flexed across the palm. Reduction of this fracture involves extension of the distal segment of the metacarpal. This fracture can usually be immobilized in a short arm spica cast.

A Bennett's fracture dislocation of the first carpometacarpal joint occurs as a result of axial compression when the first metacarpal is driven proximally, shearing off its base. A small medial fragment of the metacarpal remains attached to the strong volar ligament and the main shaft of the metacarpal is pulled proximally by the unopposed pull of the abductor pollicis longus muscle. This injury should be referred to a hand surgeon. Treatment requires closed reduction and percutaneous Kirschner wire

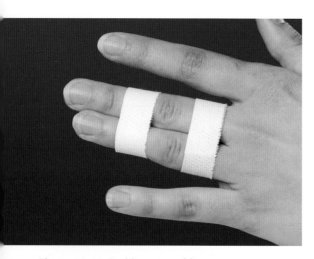

Figure 19.18 Buddy taping of fingers

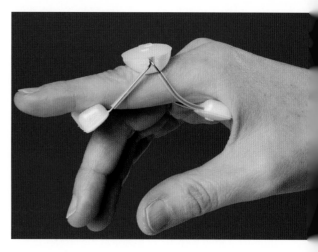

Figure 19.19 Dynamic finger extension splint

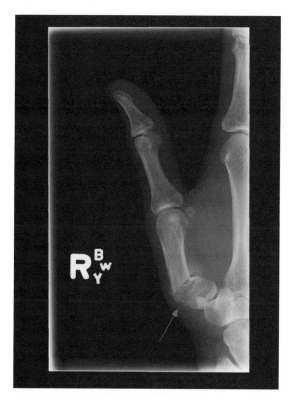

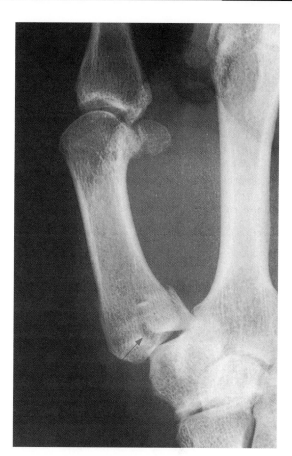

Figure 19.20 Fractures of the base of the first metacarpal

(a) Healing transverse fracture

(b) Bennett's fracture

fixation together with cast immobilization for four to six weeks. Upon removal of the cast, mobilization of the surrounding joints is required and, if early return to sport is required, a protective device should be worn. Persons not engaging in contact sport find soft neoprene braces (Fig. 19.21) supportive and comfortable after a Bennett's fracture and other common hand injuries. These are not replacements for firmer splints and braces that might be needed when trauma can be anticipated.

Fractures of the other metacarpals

Fractures of the second to fifth metacarpals may also occur as the result of a punch. These fractures are most commonly seen in the fourth and fifth metacarpals, and have been referred to as 'boxer's fracture'. The fracture is usually accompanied by considerable flexion deformity of the distal fragment, however, this deformity results in surprisingly little functional disability (Figs 19.22, 19.23). The acceptable angulation for fractures of the neck of the fourth and

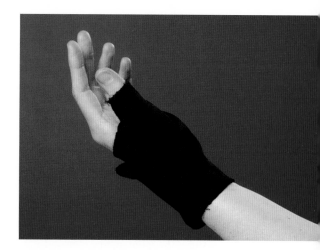

Figure 19.21 Soft neoprene splints can provide support during rehabilitation after a hand injury

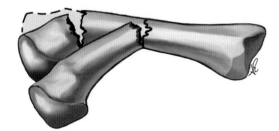

Figure 19.22 In metacarpal fractures, the more proximal the fracture, the more the knuckle will drop

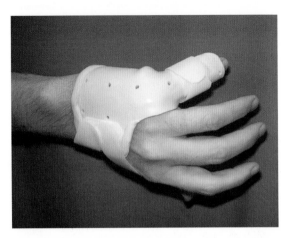

Figure 19.24 Treatment splint for fracture of the fifth metacarpal

Intra-articular fractures of the metacarpals require anatomical correction. In displaced fractures, this usually involves Kirschner wiring. Long spiral fractures of the metacarpal shaft may require internal fixation or percutaneous pinning if they are angulated or rotated. Check for rotation of finger fractures clinically and not by using radiographs. If fractures are undisplaced, they can be immobilized in a gutter splint with flexion of the MCP joint.

Fractures of phalanges

Proximal phalanx fractures

Fractures of the proximal phalanx may lead to functional impairment due to the extensor and flexor tendons coming into contact with callus and exposed bone.

To control and reduce the fracture under ring block, the MCP joint should be flexed to 70°. The PIP joint is then flexed and longitudinal traction applied in line with the shaft of the distal fragment to oppose the fracture. However, this is often difficult. The fracture is immobilized with the wrist slightly extended and at 70° of flexion of the MCP joints. These fractures require weekly radiographs to ensure movement has not occurred. If further stability is needed, the adjacent finger can be buddy taped. The splint is removed after three to four weeks and buddy taping continued. Motion is essential at three to four weeks. Unstable fractures require urgent surgical referral.

Rotational deformity of phalangeal fractures may not be obvious in extension so the fingers should be examined end on with PIP and DIP flexion to reveal

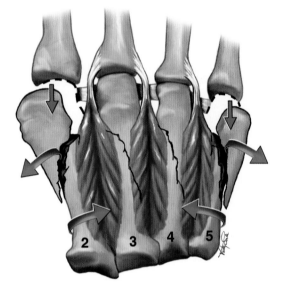

Figure 19.23 Spiral fractures of the second and fifth metacarpals (border digits) are more unstable than those of the third and fourth metacarpals as only one side of the border metacarpals is supported by the strong, deep transverse intercarpal ligaments

fifth metacarpals is up to 30° as long as there is little rotational deformity. Up to 10° angulation is acceptable in the second and third metacarpals. However, prominence of the metacarpal head in the palm of the hand may be a problem for tennis players and athletes who require a firm grip.

Treatment involves splinting or casting in a position of 90° of flexion of the MCP joints to prevent shortening of the collateral ligament and subsequent stiffness (Fig. 19.24). Check that this position does not displace the fracture. The splint may be removed after two to three weeks and sport resumed immediately with protection.

any deformity present. All malrotated fractures need open reduction and possibly internal fixation.

Middle phalanx fractures

Fractures of the middle phalanx involve hard cortical bone. Generally oblique or transverse, these fractures heal slowly. The central slip of the extensor tendon attaches dorsally to the base of the bone and the flexor digitorum inserts on the volar surface more distally. Thus, fractures distal to the flexor tendon attachment show flexion of the proximal fragment and extension of the distal fragment.

Stable fractures are immobilized in a splint for three weeks in 70° of MCP joint flexion and 0° of PIP joint flexion. When the splint is removed, range of motion exercises are begun.

Unstable fractures, or intra-articular fractures involving more than 25% of the PIP joint surface, require open reduction and internal fixation. Small-caliber Kirschner wires are used and range of motion exercises are begun as soon as fixation is considered to be stable. Volar plate avulsion fracture can occur at the PIP joint following a hyperextension injury. This injury is very common, and usually ignored owing to an unawareness of the potential consequences. The typical anatomy and radiographic appearance are shown in Figure 19.15. At present, non-randomized controlled trials have compared early mobilization with splinting and found that mobilization has led to good functional outcomes.[36] As a result, the recommendations are to follow 'local guidelines' (i.e. the expertise available in the setting of the injury).

Distal phalanx fractures

Fractures of the distal phalanx are usually caused by crushing injuries, such as fingers being jammed between a fast-moving ball and a stick or a bat. They are usually non-displaced.

Often a splint and compression dressing will provide adequate treatment for non-displaced fractures. Much of the pain associated with these fractures can be due to subungual hematoma. Significant subungual hematoma requires nail bed exploration and excision as the nail bed is often disrupted. In this case surgical repair may be required to prevent future nail deformity. This represents a compound fracture and should be treated as such. Perforation of the nail to drain a subungual hematoma is contraindicated in this instance as it converts a closed fracture to a compound fracture.

 PRACTISE PEARL Most distal phalangeal fractures heal in four to six weeks.

Dislocation of the metacarpophalangeal joints

Dorsal dislocation of the MCP joints of the fingers is uncommon and usually occurs in the index finger or thumb. It has been called the 'irreducible dislocation' because the metacarpal head is pushed through the volar plate of the MCP joint and caught between the lumbrical and long flexor tendons with a buttonholing effect. Suspect this injury when examination reveals hyperextension of the involved MCP joint with ulnar deviation of the finger overlapping the adjacent finger.

An attempt to reduce the dislocation may be made by increasing the deformity and pushing the proximal phalanx through the tear in the volar plate. However, open reduction is usually required. The MCP joint is usually stable after reduction in 30° of MCP flexion and early movement can be commenced in a dorsal splint allowing full flexion but preventing the last 30° of MCP joint extension. The immobilization is maintained for five to six weeks. Associated osteochondral fractures require open reduction and internal fixation.

Dislocations of the finger joints

Dislocations of the PIP joint

Dorsal PIP joint dislocations are the most common hand dislocation. They usually result from a hyperextension stress with some degree of longitudinal compression such as may occur in ball sports. This may produce disruption of both the volar plate and at least one collateral ligament. Ideally, radiographs should precede treatment to confirm the diagnosis and exclude an associated fracture. In practise, reduction often occurs on or beside the playing area. Reduction is maintained in a splint that allows full PIP flexion but blocks the final 30° of PIP extension for three weeks (Fig. 19.25). If left untreated, a hyperextension deformity and instability may develop. Radiography must be performed after reduction. As discussed above in the section on middle phalanx fractures, all of these fractures must be tested for instability into hyperextension.

If there is no tendency to hyperextension following reduction, the finger can be splinted as above for several days and then buddy taped to an adjacent finger to allow motion. Swelling should be managed using an elastic pressure bandage, soft tissue treatment and electrotherapeutic modalities. If radiographs reveal a fracture of the volar lip of the middle phalanx involving more than one-third of the joint surface,

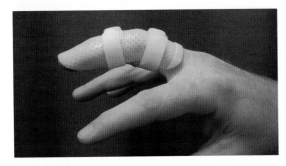

Figure 19.25 Splinting following a PIP joint dislocation. This dorsal block splint allows flexion but stops full extension at the PIP joint

open reduction and internal fixation is required to restore stability.

Volar dislocations of the PIP joint are uncommon and are often resistant to closed reduction.

There is almost always an associated rupture of one or more collateral ligaments along with disruption of the extensor central slip insertion. This injury predisposes to the development of a boutonnière (buttonhole) deformity and should be treated with a splint, holding the PIP joint of the affected finger in extension for six weeks while encouraging DIP movement, or with surgical repair.

Dislocations of the DIP joint

Dislocations of the DIP joint usually occur dorsally and are commonly associated with a volar skin laceration. The injury is most often due to a ball hitting the finger and causing hyperextension. Reduction is achieved by traction and flexion. The joint should be splinted for three weeks in 10° of flexion. Collateral ligament injuries are rare. Flexor tendon function must be assessed as avulsion can occur with this injury.

The less common volar dislocation occurs in association with a fracture and usually involves damage to the extensor tendon. This presents with the mallet finger deformity. Thus, all mallet fingers must be radiographed to exclude fracture. If volar dislocation has occurred, open repair is indicated.

Ligament and tendon injuries

Sprain of the ulnar collateral ligament of the first MCP joint

Injury to the ulnar collateral ligament of the thumb is one of the most common hand injuries seen in athletes. It is known colloquially as 'skier's thumb' and usually results from forced abduction and hyperextension of the MCP joint. The mechanism of injury is

characteristic. The patient may complain of weakness of thumb–index (tip) pinch grip (Fig. 19.26a).

Examination reveals swelling and tenderness over the ulnar aspect of the first MCP joint. Before testing stability, radiography should be performed to exclude an avulsion fracture. Stability of the ligament is tested by stressing the joint in a radial direction (Fig. 19.16i). Pain occurs with both complete and partial tears of the ulnar collateral ligament.

 PRACTISE PEARL If the injured thumb deviates 10–20° greater than the non-injured side and there is no clear end feel, then complete disruption of the ligament is likely.

Deviation within 10–20° of the non-injured side indicates a partial tear of the ulnar collateral ligament. This should be treated with immobilization in a splint with the MCP joint in slight flexion for six weeks. Further protective splinting is required during return to sport and may be required for up to 12 months (Fig. 19.26b). The thumb may also be taped with the index finger, which acts as a less secure check rein to prevent hyperabduction (Fig. 19.26c).

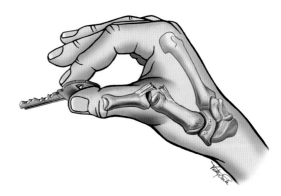

Figure 19.26 Complete ligament tear causes pain on pinch grip

(a) Pinching is affected

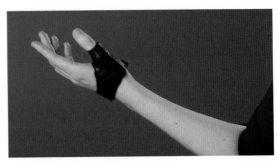

(b) Protective splint worn during return to sport

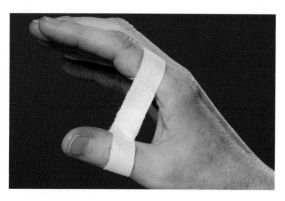

(c) Check rein to prevent hyperabduction of thumb

A complete tear of the ulnar collateral ligament (Stener lesion) requires surgical repair because of interposition of the extensor hood (Fig. 19.27). A displaced avulsion fracture of the base of the proximal phalanx also requires open reduction and internal fixation with

Kirschner wires. Residual volar or lateral subluxation of the proximal phalanx on the metacarpal head is also an indication for surgery, as is a chronic injury to the ulnar collateral ligament with functional instability, pain and weakness of thumb–index pinch grip. After surgery, the thumb is placed in a thumb spica cast for four to six weeks followed by protective splinting during sporting activity for a further three months.

Injuries to the radial collateral ligament of the first MCP joint

Injuries to the radial collateral ligament of the thumb are not as common as those to the ulnar collateral ligament but complete ruptures can be as disabling as those of the ulnar collateral ligament. Deviation of greater than 10–20° more than on the non-injured side with ulnar stress indicates a complete tear. As there is no soft tissue caught between the two ends of the ligament, six weeks' cast immobilization is the treatment of choice.

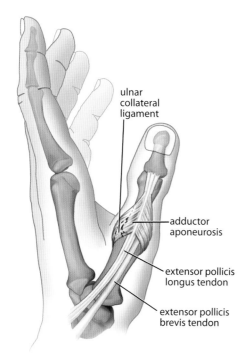

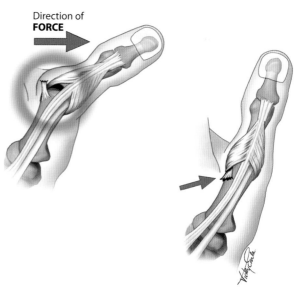

(b) Valgus stress opens up the joint and the adductor aponeurosis slips past the distal end of the proximal portion of the ruptured ulnar collateral ligament

ulnar collateral ligament

Direction of
FORCE

adductor aponeurosis

extensor pollicis longus tendon

extensor pollicis brevis tendon

Figure 19.27 Mechanism of formation of a Stener lesion of the thumb

(a) Anatomy

(c) As alignment returns to normal, the adductor aponeurosis catches the proximal portion of the ulnar collateral ligament and flips it back proximally to form the Stener lesion

Capsular sprain of the first MCP joint

Capsular sprains of the first MCP joint are an extremely common injury in ball-handling sports. They result from a hyperextension injury and are prone to recurrence. Treatment involves active rehabilitation and protection of the joint from hyperextension. This is achieved with the use of a thermoplastic brace over the dorsal aspect of the MCP joint.

PIP joint sprains

The collateral ligaments of the PIP joints are commonly injured as a result of a sideways force. Partial tears of the collateral ligament are painful but remain stable on lateral stress. Complete tears show marked instability with lateral stress. This injury also includes hyperextension stress to the volar plate, which may avulse its insertion from the base of the metacarpal.

Partial tears should be treated by buddy taping and active exercises. Complete tears of the collateral ligament should ideally be treated with surgical repair, although in most cases conservative management provides an adequate result.

Mallet finger

Mallet finger is a flexion deformity resulting from avulsion of the extensor mechanism from the DIP joint. It commonly results from a ball striking the extended fingertip, forcing the DIP joint into flexion while the extensor mechanism is actively contracting. This produces disruption or stretching of the extensor mechanism over the DIP joint. This is seen in baseball catchers, fielders, football receivers, cricketers and basketball players.

Examination reveals tenderness over the dorsal aspect of the distal phalanx and an inability to actively extend the DIP joint from its resting flexed position. If left untreated, a chronic mallet finger type deformity develops (Fig. 19.28a). This flexion deformity is caused by the unopposed action of the flexor digitorum profundus tendon.

Radiography must be performed to exclude an avulsion fracture of the distal phalanx or injury and subluxation to the DIP joint. The avulsion fracture is considered significant if greater than one-third of the joint surface is involved, in which case open reduction and internal fixation is required. Any subluxation requires open reduction and internal fixation. A fracture dislocation of the epiphyseal plate may occur in children. This injury requires open or closed reduction.

Treatment of uncomplicated mallet finger involves splinting the DIP joint in slight hyperextension for a

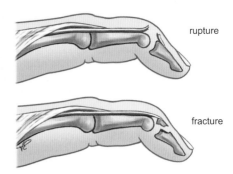

Figure 19.28 Mallet finger

(a) Mechanism of deformity—rupture or avulsion

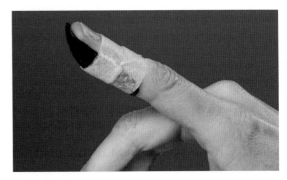

(b) 'Stack' splint. A dorsal splint can also be used

period of up to eight weeks, with regular monitoring. The splint is then worn for an additional six to eight weeks while engaging in sporting activity and at night. Treatment is reinstituted at any sign of recurrence of a lag. The splint may be made of metal or plastic and applied to either the volar or dorsal surface (Fig. 19.28b); patients with dorsal splints maintain pulp sensation. The finger should be kept dry and examined regularly for skin slough and maceration.

When treating mallet finger, emphasize to the patient that the joint must be kept in hyperextension at all times during the eight weeks, even when the splint is removed for cleaning. If a patient is not prepared to do this, then the joint should not be splinted. The consequences of not splinting are a chronic mallet finger type flexion deformity with osteophyte formation and degeneration of the DIP surface.

Boutonnière deformity

The boutonnière deformity results from disruption of the central slip of the extensor digitorum communis tendon at its insertion at the base of the middle phalanx, which allows migration of the lateral bands in a volar and proximal direction. This disruption allows the middle phalanx to be pulled into flexion by the flexor digitorum superficialis. It may arise from blunt trauma over the dorsal aspect of the PIP joint or acute flexion of the joint against active resistance, such as occurs in ball sports. The PIP joint herniates through the central slip tear. The deformity is often absent at initial presentation but develops some time later in the untreated case. The classic deformity consists of hyperextension of the DIP joints with a flexion deformity of the PIP joint (Fig. 19.29).

Early examination findings may include flexion deformity of the PIP joint and point tenderness over the dorsal slip of the middle phalanx. The patient will lack full extension of the PIP joint. Radiography may occasionally reveal an avulsion fracture from the middle phalanx. The patient can often extend the PIP joint initially. Boutonnière deformity always follows a volar PIP dislocation.

Any acute PIP joint injury showing any lag of extension in conjunction with point tenderness over the base of the middle phalanx should be regarded as an acute extensor tendon rupture. Treatment of choice, even if the lag is less than 30°, is to splint the finger with the PIP joint in full extension while allowing active flexion of the DIP joint for six weeks. On return to sport, protective splinting is continued for a further six to eight weeks or until a full pain-free range of flexion and extension is present. Associated avulsion fractures of the middle phalanx involving greater than one-third of the joint surface require open reduction and internal fixation if displaced.

In longstanding injuries, there may already be a fixed flexion deformity of the PIP joint. This may be treated with a dynamic splint (Fig. 19.19) that gradually extends the joint to a neutral position or a 'joint jack'. Surgery may be indicated if this is unsuccessful.

Avulsion of the flexor digitorum profundus tendon

This injury is most commonly seen in the ring finger and may be caused by the sportsperson grabbing an opponent's clothing, resulting in the distal phalanx being forcibly extended while the athlete is actively flexing. The patient often feels a 'snap'. The condition is often referred to as Jersey finger.

Examination may reveal the finger assuming a position of extension relative to the other fingers. There is an inability to actively flex the DIP joint of the affected finger. Radiography should be performed to exclude an associated avulsion fracture of the distal phalanx. The bone fragment may be seen volar to the middle phalanx or PIP joint. A lump may be palpated more proximally in the finger corresponding to the avulsed tendon. Treatment is urgent surgical repair with reattachment of the profundus tendon to the distal phalanx. This must take place within 10 days of the injury as tendon ischemia occurs when the tendon has retracted into the palm.

Lacerations and infections of the hand

Lacerations to the fingers and hand occur frequently in sport as a result of contact with equipment such as the undersurface of a football boot. All lacerations have the potential to become infected and should, therefore, be thoroughly cleaned with an antiseptic solution and observed closely for signs of infection. Tetanus toxoid should also be administered where appropriate (Chapter 51).

A particular concern is a laceration of the hand, often over the MCP/PIP joint, caused by teeth, usually from a punch to the mouth. These injuries should always be assumed to be contaminated and an immediate course of a broad-spectrum antibiotic should be commenced. The wound should not be closed.

Lacerations over volar DIP or PIP joints may represent compound dislocations. If this has occurred, the joint has been contaminated and the patient requires hospital admission for surgical debridement and repair. Otherwise septic arthritis may follow.

Overuse conditions of the hand and fingers

Important but sometimes overlooked are the overuse problems associated with the hand. These include trigger finger and other small joint injuries that are commonly seen in rock climbers.[37–39] Trigger finger is caused by a tenosynovitis in the flexor tendon that

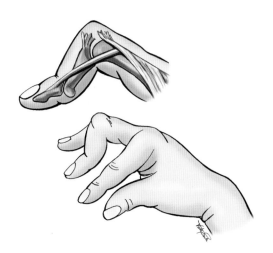

Figure 19.29 Boutonnière deformity

is large enough to be impeded by the proximal A1 (annular) pulley located at the base of the finger. Conservative treatment involves splinting and local treatment to reduce the enlarged tendon. Corticosteroid injection is often advocated first, and then surgical release of the impeded A1 pulley.[40, 41]

Recommended Reading

Cooney WP, Linscheid RL, Dobyns JH. *The Wrist: Diagnosis and Operative Treatment*. 2 volume set. Philadelphia: Mosby, 1998.

Forman TA, Forman SK, Rose NE. A clinical approach to diagnosing wrist pain. *Am Fam Physician* 2005; 72(9): 1753–8. Available online: <http://www.aafp.org/afp/20051101/1753.html>.

Hunter JM, Mackin EJ, Callahan AD. *Rehabilitation of the Hand and Upper Extremity*. 5th edn. 2 volume set. Philadelphia: Mosby, 2002.

Lichtman D, Alexander AH. *The Wrist and its Disorders*. 2nd edn. Toronto: Elsevier, 1998.

Orbay JL, Fernandez DL. Volar fixed-angle plate fixation for unstable distal radius fractures in the elderly patient. *J Hand Surg [Am]* 2004; 29(1): 96–102.

Rettig AC. Athletic injuries of the wrist and hand. Part I: traumatic injuries of the wrist. *Am J Sports Med* 2003; 31: 1038–48.

Rettig AC. Athletic injuries of the wrist and hand. Part II: overuse injuries of the wrist and traumatic injuries to the hand. *Am J Sports Med* 2004; 32: 262–73.

Stoller DW, Tirman PFJ, Bredella MA, et al. *Diagnostic Imaging: Orthopaedics*. Salt Lake City, UT: Amirsys, 2004.

References

1. Rettig AC. Athletic injuries of the wrist and hand. Part I: traumatic injuries of the wrist. *Am J Sports Med* 2003; 31: 1038–48.

2. Hill C, Riaz M, Mozzam A, Brennen MD. A regional audit of hand and wrist injuries. A study of 4873 injuries. *J Hand Surg* 1998; 23(2): 196–200.

3. Vendittoli PA, Major D, Simpson A, Jean S, Brown JP. Descriptive study of osteoporotic fractures and hip fracture risk evaluation of subjects with past minor fractures [abstract]. *Osteoporosis Int* 2000; 11(suppl. 2): S109.

4. Phillips TG, Reibach AM, Slomiany WP. Diagnosis and management of scaphoid fractures. *Am Fam Physician* 2004; 70(5): 879–84.

5. Parmelee-Peters K, Eathorne SW. The wrist: common injuries and management. *Prim Care* 2005; 32(1): 35–70.

6. Dekker R, Groothoff JW, van der Sluis CK, Eisma WH, Ten Duis HJ. Long-term disabilities and handicaps following sports injuries: outcome after outpatient treatment. *Disabil Rehabil* 2003; 25(20): 1153–7.

7. Chow TK, Corbett SW, Farstad DJ. Spectrum of injuries from snowboarding. *J Trauma* 1996; 41(2): 321–5.

8. Heller DR, Routley V, Chambers S. Rollerblading injuries in young people. *J Paediatr Child Health* 1996; 32(1): 35–8.

9. Ellis JA, Kierulf JC, Klassen TP. Injuries associated with in-line skating from the Canadian hospitals injury reporting and prevention program database. *Can J Public Health* 1995; 86(2): 133–6.

10. Aldridge JM 3rd, Mallon WJ. Hook of the hamate fractures in competitive golfers: results of treatment by excision of the fractured hook of the hamate. *Orthopedics* 2003; 26(7): 717–19.

11. MacDermid J, Richards R, Donner A, Bellamy N, Roth J. Responsiveness of the Short Form-36, Disability of the Arm, Shoulder and Hand Questionnaire, Patient Rated Wrist Evaluation, and Physical Impairment Measurements in Evaluating recovery after a distal radius fractures. *J Hand Surg [Am]* 2000; 25A(2): 330–40.

12. MacDermid JC, Turgeon T, Richards RS, Beadle M, Roth JH. Patient rating of wrist pain and disability: a reliable and valid measurement tool. *J Orthop Trauma* 1998; 12(8): 577–86.

13. Beaton DE, Katz JN, Fossel AH, et al. Measuring the whole or the parts? Validity, reliability, and responsiveness of the Disabilities of the Arm, Shoulder and Hand outcome measure in different regions of the upper extremity. *J Hand Ther* 2001; 14(2): 128–46.

14. The DASH Outcome Measure. Toronto: Institute for Work and Health, 2004. Available online: <http://www.dash.iwh.on.ca/index.htm>.

15. Brooks S, Cicuttini FM, Lim S, et al. Cost effectiveness of adding magnetic resonance imaging to the usual management of suspected scaphoid fractures. *Br J Sports Med* 2005; 39(2): 75–9.

16. Dias JJ, Wildin CJ, Bhowal B, Thompson JR. Should acute scaphoid fractures be fixed? A randomized controlled trial. *J Bone Joint Surg Am* 2005; 87(10): 2160–8.

17. Jacobson JA, Miller BS, Morag Y. Golf and racquet sports injuries. *Semin Musculoskelet Radiol* 2005; 9(4): 346–59.

18. Theriault G, Lachance P. Golf injuries. An overview. *Sports Med* 1998; 26(1): 43–57.

19. Scheufler O, Radmer S, Erdmann D, et al. Therapeutic alternatives in nonunion of hamate hook fractures: personal experience in 8 patients and review of literature. *Ann Plast Surg* 2005; 55(2): 149–54.

20. Scheufler O, Andresen R, Radmer S, et al. Hook of hamate fractures: critical evaluation of different therapeutic procedures. *Plast Reconstr Surg* 2005; 115(2): 488–97.

21. Watson HK, Weinzweig J. Physical examination of the wrist. *Hand Clin* 1997; 13(1): 17–34.

22. Skirven T. Clinical examination of the wrist. *J Hand Ther* 1996; 9(2): 96–107.

23. Richie CA 3rd, Briner WW Jr. Corticosteroid injection for treatment of de Quervain's tenosynovitis: a pooled quantitative literature evaluation. *J Am Board Fam Pract* 2003; 16(2): 102–6.

24. McNally E, Wilson D, Seiler S. Rowing injuries. *Semin Musculoskelet Radiol* 2005; 9(4): 379–96.

25. Ashe MC, McCauley T, Khan KM. Tendinopathies in the upper extremity: a paradigm shift. *J Hand Ther* 2004; 17(3): 329–34.

26. Lester B, Halbrecht J, Levy IM, Gaudinez R. 'Press test' for office diagnosis of triangular fibrocartilage complex tears of the wrist. *Ann Plast Surg* 1995; 35(1): 41–5.

27. De Smet L. Magnetic resonance imaging for diagnosing lesions of the triangular fibrocartilage complex. *Acta Orthop Belg* 2005; 71(4): 396–8.

28. Keogh CF, Wong AD, Wells NJ, Barbarie JE, Cooperberg PL. High-resolution sonography of the triangular fibrocartilage: initial experience and correlation with MRI and arthroscopic findings. *AJR Am J Roentgenol* 2004; 182(2): 333–6.

29. Tomaino MM, Weiser RW. Combined arthroscopic TFCC debridement and wafer resection of the distal ulna in wrists with triangular fibrocartilage complex tears and positive ulnar variance. *J Hand Surg [Am]* 2001; 26(6): 1047–52.

30. Schrijver HM, Gerritsen AA, Strijers RL, et al. Correlating nerve conduction studies and clinical outcome measures on carpal tunnel syndrome: lessons from a randomized controlled trial. *J Clin Neurophysiol* 2005; 22(3): 216–21.

31. Wong SM, Hui AC, Lo SK, et al. Single vs. two steroid injections for carpal tunnel syndrome: a randomised clinical trial. *Int J Clin Pract* 2005; 59(12): 1417–21.

32. Hui AC, Wong S, Leung CH, et al. A randomized controlled trial of surgery vs steroid injection for carpal tunnel syndrome. *Neurology* 2005; 64(12): 2074–8.

33. Thoma A, Veltri K, Haines T, Duku E. A systematic review of reviews comparing the effectiveness of endoscopic and open carpal tunnel decompression. *Plast Reconstr Surg* 2004; 113(4): 1184–91.

34. Capitani D, Beer S. Handlebar palsy—a compression syndrome of the deep terminal (motor) branch of the ulnar nerve in biking. *J Neurol* 2002; 249(10): 1441–5.

35. Ginn TA, Smith AM, Snyder JR, et al. Vascular changes of the hand in professional baseball players with emphasis on digital ischemia in catchers. *J Bone Joint Surg Am* 2005; 87A(7): 1464–9.

36. Body R, Ferguson CJ. Best evidence topic report. Early mobilisation for volar plate avulsion fractures. *Emerg Med J* 2005; 22(7): 505.

37. Schoffl V, Hochholzer T, Winkelmann HP, Strecker W. Pulley injuries in rock climbers. *Wilderness Environ Med* 2003; 14(2): 94–100.

38. Schweizer A. Lumbrical tears in rock climbers. *J Hand Surg* 2003; 28(2): 187–9.

39. Klauser A, Frauscher F, Hochholzer T, et al. Diagnosis of climbing related overuse injuries. *Der Radiologe* 2002; 42(10): 788–98.

40. Nimigan AS, Ross DC, Gan BS. Steroid injections in the management of trigger fingers. *Am J Phys Med Rehabil* 2006; 85(1): 36–43.

41. Rohrbough JT, Mudge MK, Schilling RC. Overuse injuries in the elite rock climber. *Med Sci Sports Exerc* 2000; 32: 1369–72.

Thoracic and Chest Pain

WITH KEVIN SINGER

Thoracic pain

As with neck pain (Chapter 16) and low back pain (Chapter 21), it is often not possible for the clinician to make a precise pathological diagnosis in patients with pain in the region of the thoracic spine. The most common musculoskeletal problems are disorders of the thoracic intervertebral joints and the numerous rib articulations. Injury to the intervertebral disk, the zygapophyseal (also spelled as zygoapophyseal and zygapophysial in various countries) joints or other nociceptive structures of the thoracic spine may contribute local or referred pain. A typical presentation of these intervertebral joint problems is hypomobility of one or more intervertebral segments, given that this region of the spine is primarily required to contribute stability to the axial skeleton. There may be associated abnormalities of the paraspinal and periscapular muscles as well as adverse neural tension (Chapter 3). Thoracic intervertebral joint problems frequently refer pain to the lateral or anterior chest wall. Prolapse of a thoracic intervertebral disk is rare in sportspeople, however, it may be under-reported given the often diffuse symptoms that arise.[1, 2]

While costovertebral joints are less commonly injured, problems may exist in isolation or in conjunction with an intervertebral joint problem.

In adolescents, the most common cause of pain in the area of the thoracic spine is Scheuermann's disease, a disorder of the growth plates of the thoracic vertebra. A list of the causes of pain in the region of the thoracic spine is shown in Table 20.1. The surface, muscle and cross-sectional anatomy of this area is shown in Figure 20.1.

History

The patient often complains of pain between or around the shoulder blades. The pain may be central, unilateral or bilateral. The pain may have commenced suddenly as a result of a sudden movement or may have been of more gradual onset. Thoracic spine pain is commonly aggravated by rotation (Fig. 20.2) or lateral flexion. Any associated sensory symptoms such as pins and needles or numbness should be noted. Although dermatomal patterns are more predictable in the thoracic region, symptoms may depart from such conventions. Vague pain noted in the region of

Table 20.1 Causes of thoracic pain

Common	Less common	Not to be missed
Intervertebral joint sprain	Fracture of the rib posteriorly	Cardiac causes
Disk	Thoracic disk prolapse	Peptic ulcer
Zygapophyseal joints	T4 syndrome	Tumor (e.g. carcinoma of the breast,
Paraspinal muscle strain		secondary deposits)
Costovertebral joint sprain		
Scheuermann's disease (adolescents)		

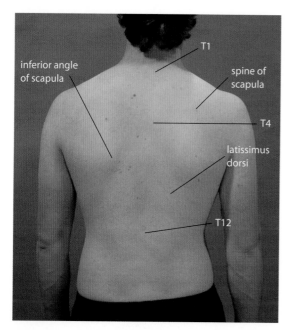

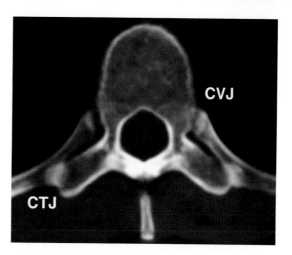

(c) Axial CT image of the typical motion segment from the lower thoracic region. The most accessible rib articulation for palpation and mobilization is the costotransverse joint (CTJ), with the costovertebral joint (CVJ) attached firmly to the lateral margin of the vertebral body

Figure 20.1 Anatomy of the thoracic spine region

(a) Surface anatomy

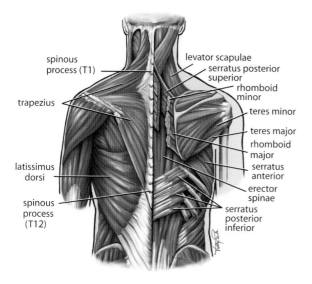

(b) Muscles of the thoracic spine region

the shoulder may relate to disturbance of the cervicothoracic junction and, similarly, buttock, hip or inguinal region symptoms may have a low thoracic origin.[3] The astute clinician should maintain an index of suspicion when examining the thoracic region given the close proximity between the internal organs and structural elements of the thoracic spine.[4]

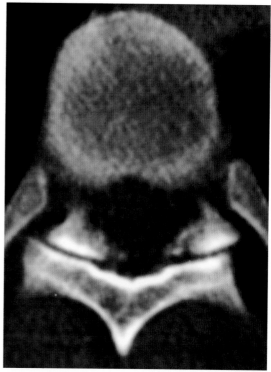

Figure 20.2 Axial CT depicting the nature of zygapophyseal joint translation in response to induced segmental rotation

Examination

Examination of the thoracic spine region involves an assessment of range of motion and mobility of each intervertebral segment as well as careful palpation of the paraspinal and periscapular soft tissue. Examination of the lower cervical and upper lumbar spine should also be included. Neurological examination should be included as should assessment of neural structures.

1. Observation (Fig. 20.3a)
2. Active movements
   (a) flexion
   (b) extension
   (c) rotation (Fig. 20.3b)
   (d) cervical movements
3. Palpation
   (a) spinous processes (Fig. 20.3c)
   (b) zygapophyseal joints
   (c) costotransverse joints and, indirectly, the costovertebral joints
   (d) paraspinal muscles (Fig. 20.3d)
   (e) sternal, chondral and clavicular joints
4. Special tests
   (a) springing of the ribs (Fig. 20.3e)
   (b) maximal inspiration
   (c) cough/sneeze
   (d) neural tension test (upper limb tension test, slump test)
   (e) cervical spine examination (Chapter 16)
   (f) lumbar spine examination (Chapter 21)

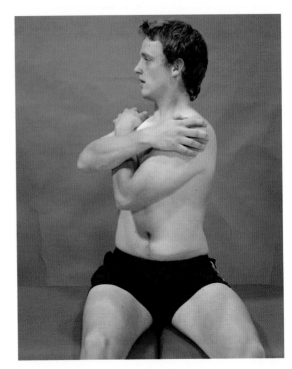

(b) Active movement—rotation

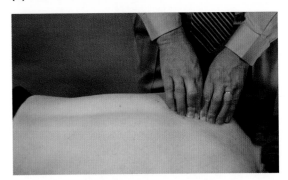

(c) Palpation—spinous processes

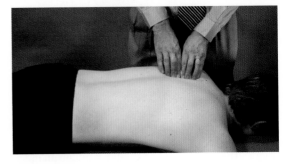

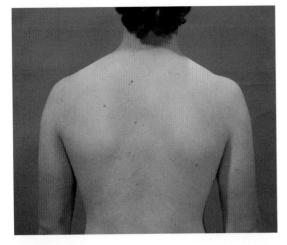

Figure 20.3 Examination of the patient with thoracic pain

(a) Observation—any scoliosis or kyphosis should be noted

(d) Palpation—paraspinal muscles. Palpate for tightness and the presence of taut bands and active trigger points

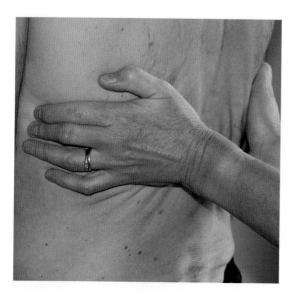

(e) Springing of the ribs adjacent to the costotransverse joints and costochondral junction

Investigations

X-ray of the thoracic spine is not routinely indicated as it usually adds little to the clinical picture. It may, however, demonstrate the presence of intervertebral growth plate abnormalities indicative of Scheuermann's disease. X-ray may show the presence of a secondary neoplastic disorder affecting the thoracic spine. CT and MRI scans are rarely indicated in the investigation of mechanical thoracic spine pain. They may, however, confirm the presence of a thoracic intervertebral disk prolapse and highlight neoplastic changes, which are important in staging the disease. Noting weight loss and recording pain patterns, such as night pain versus activity-related pain, will assist in determining the role of imaging investigations. Atypical pain patterns unresponsive to routine management should signal the need for investigation, even in the young sportsperson.

Thoracic intervertebral joint disorders

Intervertebral joint injuries, especially abnormalities of the intervertebral disks, rib articulations and zygapophyseal joints, are the most common cause of pain in this region. They may be of sudden or gradual onset. Examination reveals hypomobility of one or more intervertebral segments associated with local tenderness over the spinous processes, the zygapophyseal joints, the transverse processes or the surrounding paravertebral muscles.

Treatment aims to restore full mobility by mobilization or manipulation techniques (Fig. 20.4). Soft tissue therapy may be required to correct abnormalities in the paravertebral and periscapular muscles. Techniques used include digital ischemic pressure and sustained myofascial tension. Trigger points in the paraspinal muscles are common and should be treated with dry needling. Stretching and strengthening exercises should also be included, as shown in Figure 20.5.

It is worth noting that considerable variation in joint anatomy often presents at the transitional junctions of the spine and, particularly at the thoracolumbar junction,[5] variations may contribute to subtle differences in segmental mechanics and injury patterns. While some zygapophyseal joints depict remarkable asymmetry, others may show a morphology that acts to severely constrain motion (Fig. 20.6).

Costovertebral and costotransverse joint disorders

Disorders of the rib articulations include inflammation, such as ankylosing spondylitis, degenerative change, such as osteoarthritis, and mechanical joint sprains. Costotransverse joint problems are associated with localized tenderness and restricted mobility of the joints. Treatment may include posteroanterior mobilization of the costotransverse joints, which will have a modest influence also on the deeper costovertebral articulations. On rare occasions, a corticosteroid injection into the involved joint(s) may be required. This procedure should only be undertaken by a practitioner experienced in this

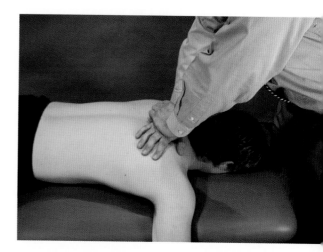

Figure 20.4 Posteroanterior mobilization (central) of the thoracic spine

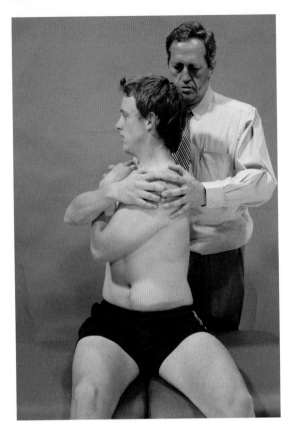

Figure 20.5 Stretching exercises

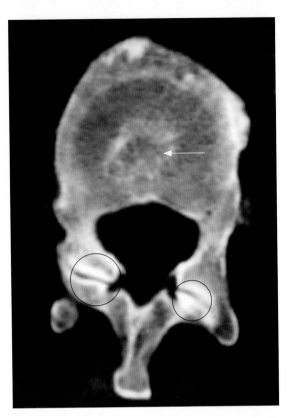

(b) Axial CT scan highlighting marked zygapophyseal joint tropism (circled). Evidence of a central Schmorl's node is noted within the end plate (arrow)

technique and, for specificity, should be performed under radiological control. A common problem of these small synovial joints may be the entrapment of small synovial fold inclusions which occupy the

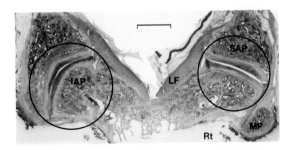

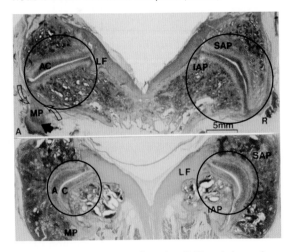

Figure 20.6 Zygapophyseal joint abnormalities

(a) Horizontal section (100 µm) through the region of the thoracolumbar junction (T11–12) to demonstrate marked asymmetry of the zygapophyseal joints, which is a common feature of these transitional joints (circled)

(c) Horizontal histological section (100 µm) through the zygapophyseal joints of the thoracolumbar junction to demonstrate variations in articular morphology from asymmetric (top image) to an enclosing morphology which constrains motion (lower image)

fringes of the joint cavity (Fig. 20.7). These joints are amenable to manipulation.

Scheuermann's disease

Scheuermann's disease is the most common cause of pain in the thoracic spine region in adolescents and is characterized by an accentuated thoracic kyphosis arising from multiple vertebral end-plate irregularities involving four or more vertebral bodies (Fig. 20.8). This condition is described in Chapter 40. Accentuated kyphosis may also arise from habitual training postures which involve loading into flexion.[6] Extended training periods in one posture (e.g. cycling) tend to

be associated with adaptive changes and modification to training postures may need to be considered when recommending long-term management.

Thoracic intervertebral disk prolapse

Prolapse of a thoracic intervertebral disk is a rare condition that may be under-reported in the community.[7] The segments that tend to be most commonly involved are the larger disks of the lower thoracic segments (Fig. 20.9). The clinical presentation involves local back pain with radicular pain radiating in the distribution of the affected thoracic spinal nerve(s). However, it must be noted that referral of symptoms arising from a thoracic disk prolapse often does not follow a characteristic referral pattern.[8]

T4 syndrome

Occasionally, patients present with diffuse arm pain and sensory symptoms such as pins and needles or

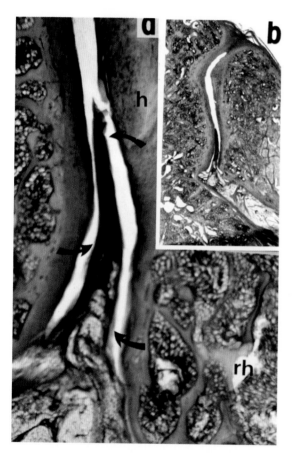

Figure 20.7 Costovertebral joint synovial inclusions

(a) Horizontal histological section (100 μm) through the dorsal region of a costovertebral joint to demonstrate a long fibro-fatty synovial inclusion within the joint cavity. Entrapment of these innervated inclusions may contribute to localized thoracic pain relieved through manipulation

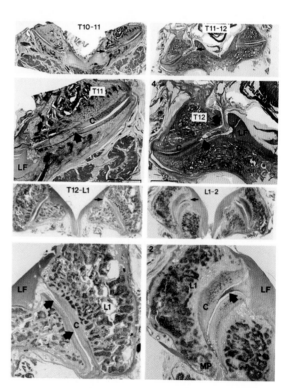

(b) Horizontal histological sections (100 μm) through lower thoracic zygapophyseal joints to demonstrate different patterns and disposition of intra-articular synovial folds which occupy space within the articular cavity

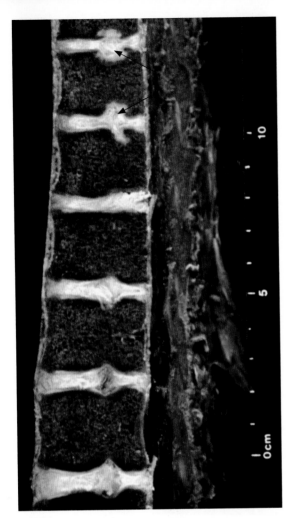

Figure 20.8 Multiple end-plate lesions (Schmorl's nodes) evident within the lower thoracic vertebral bodies (arrows) typical of Scheuermann's disease

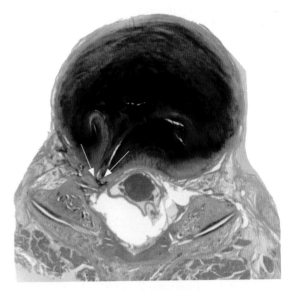

Figure 20.9 Thoracic disk prolapse

(a) Hematoxylin and eosin (H&E) stained horizontal section at T10–11 depicting a posterolateral prolapse of the intervertebral disk (arrows). Such prolapses are most common in the lower thoracic segments given the greater volume and height of these disks

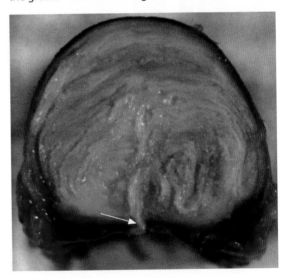

(b) Macroscopic horizontal section of a T11–12 disk to demonstrate a midline annular fissure and small central prolapse (arrow), which is a common presentation for thoracic disk lesions

numbness in the upper arm due to intervertebral joint problems around the upper thoracic region. This vague constellation of symptoms has been labeled the T4 syndrome. Although not verified clinically, it may be speculated that symptoms arise from the autonomic nervous system due to the close proximity of the sympathetic trunk to the thoracic spine. Examination often reveals hypomobility of the upper to middle thoracic segments. Restoration of full mobility to these joints by mobilization or manipulation may relieve the symptoms. Another associated feature is the tendency for patterns of specific muscle tightness, which accentuate the forward head and shoulder posture. Selective strengthening of shoulder girdle retractors, particularly the inferior trapezius, with stretching of tight muscles may contribute to the management of this problem.

Chest pain

Chest pain occurs not infrequently in athletes, usually due to musculoskeletal causes. In mature athletes, the possibility that pain is of cardiac origin must be considered. This possibility is increased in the presence of associated symptoms such as palpitations or shortness of breath or when there is a family history of cardiac disease. Other causes of chest pain include peptic ulceration, gastroesophageal reflux, chest infection and malignancy.

The most common cause of chest pain in the young athlete under 35 years is referred pain from the thoracic spine. This may or may not be associated with thoracic pain. Thus, patients presenting with anterior or lateral chest wall pain require a thorough examination of the thoracic spine.

A list of the possible causes of chest pain in athletes is presented in Table 20.2. The surface anatomy of this region is shown in Figure 20.10.

It may be difficult to distinguish between chest pain of cardiac origin and pain referred from the thoracic spine. They may both be unilateral and related to exercise. The clinical features of these two causes of chest pain in the athlete are considered in Table 20.3.

Major trauma to the chest wall is a medical emergency (Chapter 44). Injuries sustained in contact sport commonly affect the ribs, resulting in either bruised or fractured ribs. These may lead to secondary dysfunction of the thoracic zygapophyseal joints, which can cause persistence of pain. Sternoclavicular joint injuries are not uncommon. Intercostal muscle strains have been considered a cause of chest wall pain but, on close clinical examination, many patients with this presentation are actually suffering referred pain from the thoracic spine. Stress fractures of the ribs are uncommon but seen in sports such as rowing, tennis, golf, gymnastics and baseball pitching.

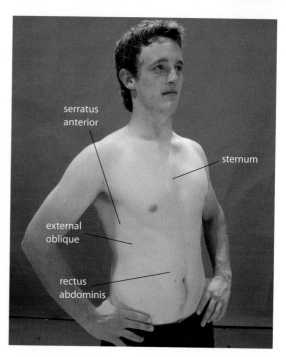

Figure 20.10 Surface anatomy of the anterior chest

History

A history of trauma to the chest wall will lead the clinician to suspect a rib injury. In the absence of trauma, the history should distinguish between musculoskeletal conditions and other cardiac, gastrointestinal and respiratory causes. It is important to elicit the type of pain and the location of the pain. Associated symptoms such as palpitations, shortness of breath and sweating may indicate that the pain is cardiac in nature. A history of productive cough may suggest pain is of respiratory origin, while symptoms of reflux and relief of pain with antacid medication may indicate that gastroesophageal reflux or peptic ulceration may be the cause of pain.

Table 20.2 Causes of chest pain in the athlete

Common	Less common	Not to be missed
Rib trauma	Costochondritis	Cardiac causes
Fracture	Sternocostal joint sprain	Peptic ulceration
Contusion	Intercostal muscle strain	Gastroesophageal reflux
Referred pain from the thoracic spine	Rib stress fracture	Pneumothorax
Sternoclavicular joint disorders	Fractured sternum	Herpes zoster
		Pulmonary embolism

Table 20.3 Comparison of clinical features of chest pain of cardiac origin and chest pain referred from the thoracic spine

Feature	Referred pain from thoracic spine	Myocardial ischemia
Age	Any age, especially 20–40 years	Older, with increased possibility with increased age
History of injury	Sometimes	No
Site and radiation	Spinal and paraspinal, arms, lateral chest, anterior chest, substernal, iliac crest	Retrosternal, parasternal, jaw, neck, inner arms, epigastrium, interscapular
Type of pain	Dull, aching, occasionally sharp, severity related to activity, site and posture, sudden onset and offset	Constricting, vice-like ('clenched-fist' sign), may be burning, gradual onset and offset
Aggravation	Deep inspiration, postural movement of thorax, certain activities (e.g. slumping or bending, walking upstairs, lifting, sleeping or sitting for long periods)	Exercise, activity, heavy meals, cold, stress, emotion
Relief	Maintaining erect spine, lying down, firm pressure on back (e.g. leaning against wall)	Rest Glyceryl trinitrate (GTN)
Associations	Chronic poor posture, employment requiring constant posture such as at a keyboard or computer	Cardiac risk factors such as family history, obesity, smoking, dyspnea, nausea, tiredness, pallor, sweating, vomiting

Pain aggravated by deep inspiration or coughing may be musculoskeletal in nature or indicative of a respiratory problem. Associated thoracic and, to a lesser extent, cervical or lumbar pain may suggest the thoracic spine as a possible source of the patient's chest pain. An increase in pain with trunk rotation might add to this suspicion.

Examination

Examination of the patient with chest wall pain should include palpation of the painful area and of possible sites of referral, especially the thoracic spine. Examination of the thoracic spine has been described earlier in this chapter. The cardiovascular and respiratory systems must always be examined. The abdomen should be examined for sources of referred pain.

Investigations

If there has been significant rib trauma, a chest X-ray should be performed to exclude the presence of a pneumothorax. Specific rib views may be necessary to detect rib fractures. Chest X-ray will indicate cardiac size and may reveal evidence of respiratory infection.

Electrocardiography and other cardiac investigations including a stress ECG/EKG and an echocardiograph may be performed if there is clinical suspicion of cardiac dysfunction. Gastroscopy may be indicated if peptic ulceration or reflux is suspected.

Rib trauma

A direct blow to the chest may result in trauma to the ribs. This may range from bruising to an undisplaced or displaced rib fracture. Typically, the patient complains of pain aggravated by deep inspiration or coughing. Examination reveals local tenderness over one or more ribs.

A pneumothorax, or rarely, a hemopneumothorax, may occur as a result of a rib fracture. Any athlete with rib trauma must undergo a respiratory examination to exclude these conditions. It is also important to consider trauma to underlying structures such as the liver, spleen and kidneys. Injuries to these organs are considered in Chapter 44.

X-ray may be performed to confirm the presence of a rib fracture, although it is not essential as treatment is symptomatic. Injury to the upper four ribs is unusual as they are somewhat protected. The lower two ribs are likewise rarely fractured as they are not attached to the sternum.

Treatment consists of analgesia and encouragement of deep breathing to prevent localized lung collapse. A fractured rib can be extremely painful. It will continue to be painful and tender to palpation for at least three weeks. Bruised ribs may also be painful and tender for up to three weeks.

Return to sport for athletes with an undisplaced rib fracture is appropriate when pain settles. Protective padding may be used in contact sports after a rib injury. The use of local anesthesia, either at the site of injury or as an intercostal nerve block, is usually not particularly effective and has the risk of causing pneumothorax. Contusion of the costochondral joints can be painful with local treatment consisting of cold therapy, strapping to splint the region, or corticosteroid injection.

Referred pain from the thoracic spine

Referred pain from the thoracic spine is probably the most common cause of chest wall pain in the young athlete. There may or may not be a history of associated thoracic spine pain. On examination there will usually be marked tenderness and stiffness, either centrally over the spinous processes of the thoracic vertebrae or, more commonly, on the same side as the chest pain over the thoracic zygapophyseal or costovertebral joints. There is often also associated areas of tenderness in the soft tissues surrounding the thoracic spine, especially the paravertebral muscles. Active trigger points may develop and contribute to the referred pain. Referred pain, however, may not follow predictable patterns, which requires the clinician to explore symptoms and to rule out visceral disorders and, conversely, unusual symptom patterns.[3, 8]

Local treatment aims to restore full range of motion of the involved thoracic intervertebral segments by mobilization or manipulation (Fig. 20.4). Soft tissue therapy to surrounding areas may be helpful. This includes digital ischemic pressure to painful sites and sustained myofascial tension where chronic muscle and soft-tissue tightness is established.

Sternoclavicular joint problems

The sternoclavicular (SC) joint is the sole articulation between the upper extremity and the axial skeleton. The joint itself is diarthrodial, with an articular disk interposed between the two bones. The articular surface of the medial clavicle is much greater than the sternal articulation. Only about 25% of the distal clavicle's surface articulates with the sternum at any one time, making the SC joint the joint with the least bony stability in the body.

The integrity of the joint comes from the strong surrounding ligaments, including the anterior, posterior, superior and inferior SC ligaments, and the interclavicular, costoclavicular and intra-articular disk ligaments (Fig. 20.11). The epiphysis of the medial clavicle is the last to ossify and fuse, at around 18 and 25 years of age respectively. Another feature of this joint is the number of vital structures located directly posterior to the joint. These include the subclavian veins and artery, the trachea, the esophagus and the mediastinum.

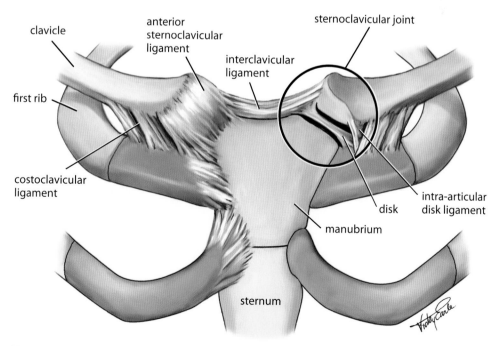

Figure 20.11 Anatomy of the sternoclavicular joint

The SC joint can be injured by a direct blow or, more commonly, indirectly from a blow to the shoulder. Simultaneous injuries of the AC and SC joints are reasonably common.[9–11]

Traumatic injuries of the SC joint can be divided into first- and second-degree sprains involving the joint capsule, subluxations and dislocations involving rupture of the SC and/or costoclavicular ligaments, and fractures of the medial clavicle. Subluxations and dislocations are further divided into anterior (more common; Fig. 20.12) and posterior (more dangerous).

Patients present with local pain and swelling depending on the severity of the injury. Anterior subluxations can be treated symptomatically by a figure of eight bandage for one to two weeks. Anterior dislocations can be reduced with lateral traction on the abducted arm and direct pressure over the medial clavicle. Dislocations are immobilized for three to four weeks in a clavicular strap. If, after closed reduction, the joint redislocates, a period of observation is appropriate. Many patients remain asymptomatic.

Posterior dislocations are potentially dangerous because of the close proximity of vital structures behind the joint.[12–14] Closed reduction should be performed under general anesthesia as soon as possible after the injury. Traction is applied to the patient's abducted arm and the medial clavicle is brought forward manually or with a towel clip. Reductions are generally stable and are held with a figure of eight strap for four weeks.

Costochondritis

Costochondritis occurs at the plane joints between the sternum and ribs. It is characterized by activity-related pain and tenderness localized to the costochondral junction. This condition is sometimes known as Tietze's syndrome.

Treatment consists of NSAIDs, local physiotherapy and mobilization of the costochondral joints. This can prove an extremely difficult condition to treat. Corticosteroid injection to the costochondral junction may be of some assistance in refractory cases.

Stress fracture of the ribs

Stress fracture of the ribs has been reported with a number of sports and is due to excessive muscle traction at the muscular attachments to the ribs.[15] Stress fracture of the first rib is seen in baseball pitchers and appears to occur at the site of maximal distraction between the upward and downward muscular forces on the rib. This stress fracture tends to heal poorly.

Anterolateral stress fractures of the ribs (Fig. 20.13), mainly the fourth and fifth ribs, are seen in rowers. This stress fracture is thought to be due to excessive action of the serratus anterior muscle. The biomechanics of the pitching or rowing action should

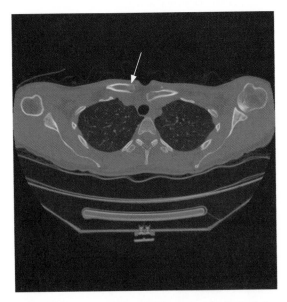

Figure 20.12 CT scan of anterior sternoclavicular joint dislocation showing clear asymmetry between the dislocated side (arrow) and the normal articulation

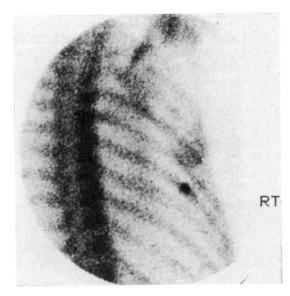

Figure 20.13 Isotopic bone scan of a stress fracture of the ribs

be assessed and discussed with the coach and athlete to determine the possible cause(s).

Recommended Reading

Ashton-Miller JA. Thoracic hyperkyphosis in the young athlete: a review of the biomechanical issues. *Curr Sports Med Rep* 2004; 3(1): 47–52.

Rockwood CAJ. Disorders of the sternoclavicular joint. In: Rockwood CAJ, Matsens FAI. *Disorders of the Sternoclavicular Joint.* Philadelphia: WB Saunders, 1990: 477–525.

Singer KP, Giles LGF. *Clinical Anatomy and Management of Thoracic Spine Pain.* Oxford: Butterworth-Heinemann, 2000.

Stahlman GC, Hanley EN Jr. Thoracic disk disease. *Orthop Int Ed* 1997; 5(3): 185–91.

References

1. Benson MK, Byrnes DP. The clinical syndromes and surgical treatment of thoracic intervertebral disc prolapse. *J Bone Joint Surg Br* 1975; 57B(4): 471–7.

2. Singer KP, Edmondston J. Introduction. The enigma of the thoracic spine. In: Singer KP, Giles LGF, eds. *Clinical Anatomy and Management of Thoracic Spine Pain.* Oxford: Butterworth-Heinemann, 2000: 3–13.

3. Maigne JY. Cervicothoracic and thoracolumbar spinal pain syndromes. In: Singer KP, Giles LGF, eds. *Clinical Anatomy and Management of Thoracic Spine Pain.* Oxford: Butterworth-Heinemann, 2000: 157–68.

4. Groen GJ, Stolker RJ. Thoracic neural anatomy. In: Singer KP, Giles LGF, eds. *Clinical Anatomy and Management of Thoracic Spine Pain.* Oxford: Butterworth-Heinemann, 2000: 114–41.

5. Singer KP, Malmivaara A. Pathoanatomical characteristics of the thoracolumbar junction region. In: Singer KP, Giles LGF, eds. *Clinical Anatomy and Management of Thoracic Spine Pain.* Oxford: Butterworth-Heinemann, 2000: 100–13.

6. Ashton-Miller JA. Thoracic hyperkyphosis in the young athlete: a review of the biomechanical issues. *Curr Sports Med Rep* 2004; 3(1): 47–52.

7. Wood KB, Garvey TA, Gundry C, et al. Magnetic resonance imaging of the thoracic spine. Evaluation of asymptomatic individuals. *J Bone Joint Surg Am* 1995; 77A: 1631–8.

8. Whitcomb DC, Martin SP, Schoen RE, et al. Chronic abdominal pain caused by thoracic disc herniation. *Am J Gastroenterol* 1995; 90: 835–7.

9. Bicos J, Nicholson GP. Treatment and results of sternoclavicular joint injuries. *Clin Sports Med* 2003; 22: 359–70.

10. Garretson RB III, Williams GR Jr. Clinical evaluation of injuries to the acromioclavicular and sternoclavicular joints. *Clin Sports Med* 2003; 22: 239–54.

11. Wroble RR. Sternoclavicular injuries. Managing damage to an overlooked joint. *Physician Sportsmed* 1995; 23(9): 19–24, 26.

12. Williams CC. Posterior sternoclavicular joint dislocation. *Physician Sportsmed* 1999; 27(2): 105–13.

13. Kiroff GK, McClure DN, Skelley JW. Delayed diagnosis of posterior sternoclavicular joint dislocation. *Med J Aust* 1996; 164: 242–3.

14. Mirza AH, Alam K, Ali A. Posterior sternoclavicular dislocation in a rugby player as a cause of silent vascular compromise: a case report. *Br J Sports Med* 2005; 39(5): e28.

15. Brukner PD, Bennell KL, Matheson GO. *Stress Fractures.* Melbourne: Blackwell Scientific, 1999.

Low Back Pain

WITH JOEL PRESS

L ow back pain is an extremely common symptom in the general population and among athletes. In this chapter we outline some salient epidemiological data and detail a clinical perspective of managing low back pain before discussing the evaluation and treatment of back pain.

Epidemiology

Back pain affects up to 85% of the population at some time in their lives. The vast majority (90%) improve over a three-month period, but nearly 50% will have at least one recurrent episode. The estimated annual cost of low back pain in the United States is over US$40 billion. Low back pain is the most common disability in those under the age of 45, and the most expensive health care problem in those between the ages of 20 and 50. Back problems account for a significant percentage (25% in United States) of workers compensation claims, although the incidence of work-related low back pain varies considerably among countries (e.g. much less in Scandinavia than the United States).

Considerable research has been undertaken investigating the risk factors for low back pain, which are summarized in Table 21.1.

Clinical perspective

As with neck pain, it is often not possible to make a precise anatomical and pathological diagnosis. However, this does not prevent management and treatment. In the majority of cases of low back pain, the principles of management depend on careful assessment to detect any abnormality and then appropriate treatment to correct that abnormality. The anatomy

of the low back is shown in Figure 21.1. The lumbar spine pain generators are listed in Table 21.2.

There are a small number of conditions causing low back pain in which a definitive diagnosis can be made. Fractures related to direct trauma, such as a transverse process fracture or compression fracture of

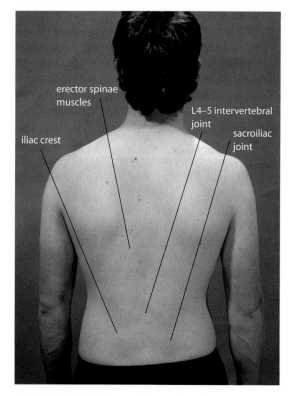

Figure 21.1 Anatomy of the low back

(a) Surface anatomy

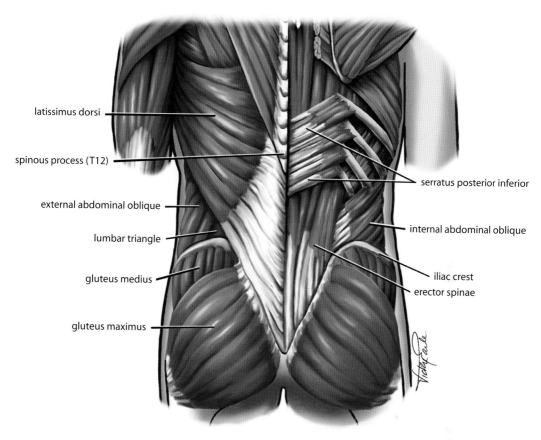

latissimus dorsi

spinous process (T12)

external abdominal oblique

lumbar triangle

gluteus medius

gluteus maximus

serratus posterior inferior

internal abdominal oblique

iliac crest

erector spinae

(b) Muscles of the lower back from behind

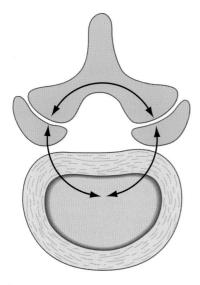

(c) The three joint complex consisting of the intervertebral disk and the two zygapophyseal (facet) joints

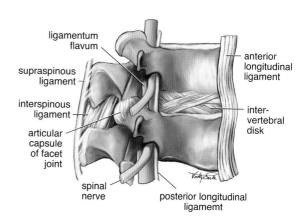

ligamentum flavum

supraspinous ligament

interspinous ligament

articular capsule of facet joint

spinal nerve

anterior longitudinal ligament

inter-vertebral disk

posterior longitudinal ligamemt

(d) The intervertebral segment

the vertebra, occur infrequently in the lumbar spine. Significant soft tissue injury is usually associated with these fractures. It is usually also possible to make a definitive diagnosis in those patients presenting with nerve root compression who have typical lancinating

Table 21.1 Risk factors associated with low back pain (LBP)

Risk factor	Evidence
Age	Increased risk until age 50, then relative risk decreases in men but increases in women
Gender	Multiparous women: three times risk
Obesity	Unclear
Height	Unclear
Posture	No association with lordosis or leg length discrepancy
Smoking	Strong association with LBP and sciatica
Physical work	Increased risk in those whose work involves bending, twisting or heavy physical labor Increased risk of LBP and sciatica with exposure to vibration Coal miners have fewer disk protrusions than other occupations Low risk of LBP in farmers
Sedentary occupation	Increased risk when seated Driving a motor car may cause LBP or herniated disk Jobs involving all standing or all sitting show higher incidence of LBP than those with changing positions
Increased fitness	Some evidence that good isometric endurance of back muscles may be associated with reduced LBP
Psychological factors	Stress, anxiety, depression associated with work-related LBP

Table 21.2 Lumbar spine pain generators

- Nucleus pulposus
- Anulus fibrosus
- Facet joints
- Ligaments
- Muscles
- Nerve
- Synovium

pain radiating to the leg in a narrow band, with or without accompanying back pain. Sensory symptoms or muscle weakness (or both) are also present. Reflexes are often abnormal. Nerve root compression in the athlete is usually due to herniation of disk material from the nucleus pulposus of the intervertebral disk.

Spondylolysis or stress fracture of the pars inter-articularis is seen in sports involving repeated hyper-extension plus or minus rotation, such as gymnastics, fast bowling (cricket), throwing sports and tennis. A spondylolisthesis or slipping of one vertebra on another may occur in athletes with bilateral pars defects. Spinal canal stenosis is rare in young and middle-aged athletes but may occasionally be seen in older athletes. It is characterized by pain aggravated by walking and relieved by rest.

Abnormalities of the hip joint such as labral tears and rim lesions may present as low back pain, and a thorough examination of the hip joint should be included in the assessment of the patient with low back pain.

The above conditions constitute considerably less than 10% of patients presenting with low back pain. The rest of the patients presenting with low back pain may be grouped together as having 'somatic' low back pain.

Somatic low back pain

Any of the nociceptive (pain-producing) structures of the lumbar spine may cause low back pain. These structures include the vertebral venous plexus, dura mater, ligaments of the vertebral arches, muscles and their fascia, vertebral bodies, laminae, apophyseal joints and the anulus fibrosus of the intervertebral disk.

Provocation techniques have demonstrated that damage to the intervertebral disks and the apophyseal joints are the most common causes of low back pain. With low back pain of lengthy duration, a number of factors will contribute to the overall clinical picture. These may include abnormalities of the ligaments of the intervertebral joints, muscles and fascia, as well as neural structures.

For many years, the disk was thought to have no sensory innervation. However, it is now recognized that the outer one-third to one-half of the posterior anulus fibrosus has a nerve supply. Previously, only two types of disk injury were recognized. One was herniation or rupture, in which the contents of the nucleus pulposus are extruded through a tear in the anulus fibrosus into the spinal canal to impinge on structures such as the nerve root. The other was disk degeneration identified on X-ray as a narrowing of the disk space accompanied by osteophyte formation.

The disks may, however, be a source of pain without rupture or degeneration. There are two specific entities that may cause disk pain—torsional injury of the anulus fibrosus and compression injury.

Excessive rotational or torsional stress (Fig. 21.2) may damage the apophyseal joint, the anulus fibrosus or both. The anulus fibrosus is most vulnerable to a combination of axial rotation and forward flexion, which corresponds to the clinical situation of lifting in a bent and rotated position. Repeated torsional injuries to the anulus fibrosus may produce radial fissures as seen on diskography. The location of these fissures corresponds to the tracks along which nuclear material is found to herniate. This suggests that previous torsional injuries of the anulus fibrosus may predispose to nuclear herniation. A tear in the anulus is thought to provoke an inflammatory response with chemical stimulation of the nociceptors. This pathological process explains the common presentation of a patient with poorly localized back pain that may be referred to the lower limb and which is aggravated by any movement of the lumbar spine, especially rotation and flexion.

Compression injuries arise as a result of excessive weight-bearing and are initiated by fractures of the vertebral end plate. As a result of this end-plate fracture, the matrix of the nucleus pulposus may be exposed to the circulation of the vertebral body. This may lead to degradation of the nucleus and increased load on the anulus. If the degradation process of the nucleus reaches the outer third of the anulus fibrosus, it is likely to produce pain. There may be both chemical and mechanical irritation of the pain receptors. These disk injuries may cause local, deep-seated low back pain as well as referred somatic pain (Chapter 3) to the buttock and lower leg.

The other common site of damage is the apophyseal joint. Possible causes of pain from the apophyseal joint include subchondral fractures, capsular tears, capsular avulsions and hemorrhage into the joint space.

It may be possible to differentiate clinically between disk and apophyseal joint injury. Differences in pain-provoking activities (flexion with disk injuries and extension in apophyseal joint injuries) and differences

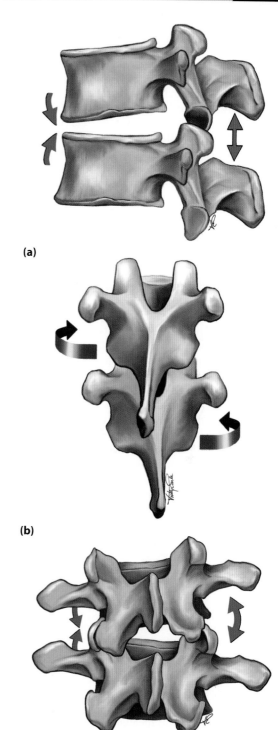

(a)

(b)

(c)

Figure 21.2 Segmental motion: **(a)** flexion/extension (sagittal plane motion); **(b)** torsion (transverse plane motion); **(c)** side-bending (frontal plane motion)

in the sites of maximal tenderness (centrally with disk injuries and unilaterally with apophyseal joint injuries) may assist. However, this clinical differentiation is not always reliable and may be used only as a guide. Frequently the two conditions coexist.

Disk and apophyseal joint injuries may be associated with hypomobility of one or more intervertebral segments (Fig. 21.1d). The assessment of the mobility of each intervertebral segment is a major component of the examination of the athlete with low back pain. Correction of segmental hypomobility forms an important part of the treatment program.

Less commonly, low back pain may be associated with hypermobility. Generalized hypermobility is usually not symptomatic but an isolated hypermobile segment may be significant clinically as an indicator of the presence of structural lumbar instability.

Trigger points frequently make a significant contribution to a patient's back pain. These may not have been the original problem but they can become the main source of pain. Trigger points thought to be commonly associated with low back pain include quadratus lumborum, erector spinae and gluteal. As a result of the associated muscle tightness, it may be impossible to treat the underlying joints adequately until the trigger points are eliminated and the shortened muscles returned to their normal length.

Abnormalities of joints, muscles and neural structures may contribute significantly to the pain. In low back pain of relatively recent onset, the greatest contribution to the pain is usually from the joints. In longstanding cases of low back pain, there may be considerable contributions from the muscles and neural structures. Each of these components must be assessed clinically and abnormalities treated. Following treatment, the signs need to be reassessed to determine the effectiveness of each treatment. A list of the causes of low back pain is shown in Table 21.3.

Functional (clinical) instability in low back pain

Stability of the lumbar intervertebral segments is principally provided by osseous and ligamentous restraints. However, without the influence of neuromuscular control, the segments are inherently unstable upon movement. Therefore, a combination of muscle forces and passive structures are utilized to dynamically stabilize the ligamentous spine under various demands of daily living and athletic activity.

It is important that the definition of stability includes the concept of control, rather than just hypermobility or increased displacement and range of movement, as it has been historically, although this will be the case in some conditions such as spondylolisthesis.

The concept of core stability is discussed in Chapter 11. It is important to remember the difference between local and global muscles. Global (dynamic, phasic) muscles are the large, torque-producing muscles, such as rectus abdominis, external oblique and the thoracic part of lumbar iliocostalis, which link the pelvis to the thoracic cage and provide general trunk stabilization as well as movement.

Local (postural, tonic) muscles are those that attach directly to the lumbar vertebrae and are responsible for providing segmental stability and directly controlling the lumbar segments during movement. These muscles include lumbar multifidus, psoas major, quadratus lumborum, the lumbar parts of iliocostalis and longissimus, transversus abdominis, the diaphragm and the posterior fibers of internal oblique (see Fig. 11.2).

There is now considerable evidence to show that the function of at least two of these local muscles, lumbar multifidus and transversus abdominis, is impaired in patients with low back pain. Research has shown a significant reduction in segmental lumbar

Table 21.3 Causes of low back pain

Common	Less common	Not to be missed
Non-osseous injury	Intervertebral disk prolapse	Malignancy
Intervertebral disk	Spondylolisthesis	Primary
Apophyseal joint	Lumbar instability	Metastatic
Stress fracture of the pars interarticularis (spondylolysis)	Spinal canal stenosis	Osteoid osteoma
Sacroiliac joint injury/inflammation	Vertebral crush fracture	Multiple myeloma
Paravertebral and gluteal muscle trigger points	Fibromyalgia	Severe osteoporosis
Hip joint pathology	Rheumatological	
	Gynecological	
	Gastrointestinal	
	Genitourinary	

multifidus cross-sectional area in patients with acute, first episode, unilateral back pain.[1] It has also been shown that lumbar multifidus demonstrated greater fatigability relative to other parts of the erector spinae in patients with chronic low back pain compared with a normal population. Additionally, lumbar multifidus will not spontaneously increase its cross-sectional size post acute injury, perhaps giving an insight into one of the reasons for recurring low back pain. The work of Hides et al.,[1] however, demonstrated that a localized lumbar multifidus exercise program will significantly increase the cross-sectional area of the muscle.

The timing of onset of activity of transversus abdominis has been shown to be delayed in sufferers of chronic low back pain compared with individuals who have never experienced back pain.[2,3] No significant change was detected between the two groups in any other muscle of the abdominal wall, suggesting that the local stabilizing abdominal muscles have a 'feed-forward mechanism' to protect the lumbar spine during loading. This is not dissimilar to the hypothesized role of the vastus medialis obliquus on the patella (Chapter 28).

Other muscles are also affected in patients with low back pain. Seventy-five per cent of patients with radiating low back pain were shown to have abnormal EMG findings in the medial spine extensor muscles.[4] McGill and colleagues found deficiencies in spinal extensor muscle endurance, as well as flexion/extension and lateral/extensor ratios.[5]

What is not clear is whether these deficiencies in muscle strength, endurance and activation are the cause or effect of low back pain. What is clear is that these deficits need to be addressed as part of any comprehensive rehabilitation program in those with low back pain.

History

The aim of the history in a patient with low back pain is to determine the location of the pain, its mechanism of onset, its degree of irritability, any radiation to the buttocks or legs, the aggravating and relieving factors, the presence of any associated features including sensory and motor symptoms, and any previous history of back problems and response to treatment in the past. Factors that aggravate and relieve the pain, such as flexion/extension and how easily the pain is aggravated, are important in determining the type and intensity of treatment. Potentially serious symptoms that must be noted include:

- cauda equina symptoms, for example, bladder or bowel dysfunction
- spinal cord symptoms, for example, difficulty walking, tripping over objects
- sensory symptoms, for example, pins and needles, paresthesia
- motor symptoms, for example, muscle weakness
- systemic symptoms, for example, weight loss, malaise
- night pain.

The use of standardized outcome self-reporting measures, such as the Oswestry or Roland-Morris questionnaires, are also recommended as a way of quantifying the effects of low back pain.

Examination

Examination of the patient with low back pain includes assessment of pattern, timing and range of movement, detection of stiffness and tenderness in muscles and joints, and detection of neurological abnormalities or evidence of neural irritation.

1. Observation
   (a) from behind (Fig. 21.3a)
   (b) from the side (Fig. 21.3b)
2. Active movements
   (a) flexion (Fig. 21.3c)
   (b) extension (Fig. 21.3d)
   (c) lateral flexion (Fig. 21.3e)
   (d) combined movements—quadrant position (Fig. 21.3f)
   (e) single leg extension (Fig. 21.3g)
3. Passive movements
   (a) overpressure may be applied at the end of range of active movements
   (b) muscle length (e.g. psoas, hamstring, gluteals)
   (c) hip quadrant (Chapter 23)
4. Palpation
   (a) spinous processes (Fig. 21.3h)
   (b) transverse processes
   (c) apophyseal joints
   (d) sacroiliac joint (Fig. 21.3i)
   (e) iliolumbar ligament
   (f) paraspinal muscles (Fig. 21.3j)
   (g) quadratus lumborum (Fig. 21.3k)
   (h) gluteal muscles
5. Special tests
   (a) straight leg raise/slump test (Chapter 8)
   (b) prone knee bend/femoral slump (Chapter 8)
   (c) sacroiliac joint test
   (d) neurological examination

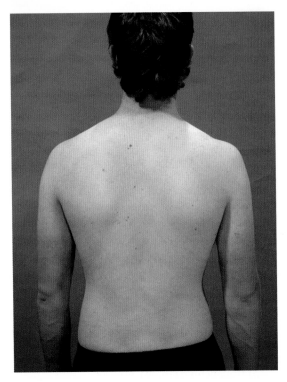

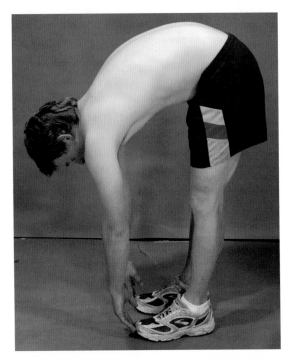

(c) Active movement—flexion. Look at symmetry of movement on both sides of the back, range of movement and, if restricted, whether it is due to pain or stiffness

Figure 21.3 Examination of the patient with low back pain

(a) Observation from behind. Look for scoliosis, tilt, rotation or asymmetrical muscle development. View the position of the spinous processes

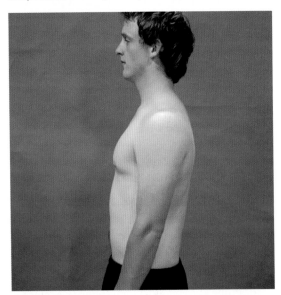

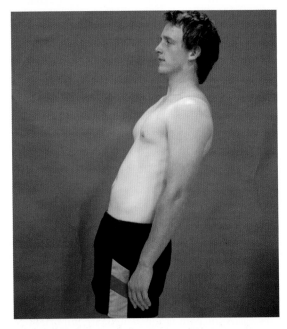

(b) Observation from the side. Assess degree of lumbar lordosis

(d) Active movement—extension. Assess degree of lumbar extension and any symptoms provoked. Patient should maintain pelvis in neutral

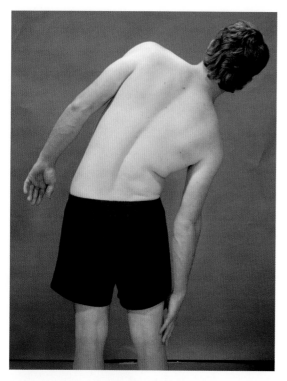

(e) Active movement—lateral flexion

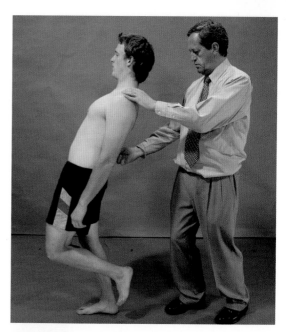

(g) Single leg extension

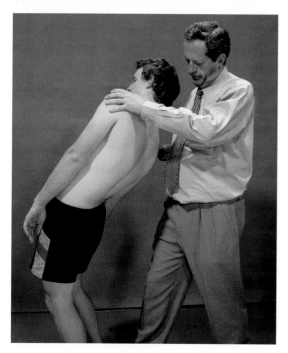

(f) Active movement—combined movement (quadrant position—extension, lateral flexion, rotation)

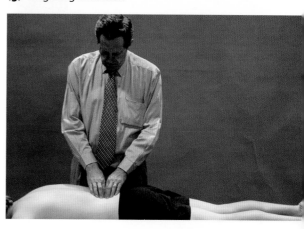

(h) Palpation—intervertebral joints. Palpate over spinous processes, apophyseal joints and transverse processes. Assess degree of tenderness and amount of accessory posteroanterior movements

Investigations

In the management of most cases of low back pain, investigations are not required. However, there are certain clinical indications for further investigation. X-ray should be performed if traumatic fracture, stress fracture, spondylolisthesis or structural lumbar instability are suspected. It is also advisable to X-ray those patients whose low back pain is not responding to treatment or where sinister abnormality may

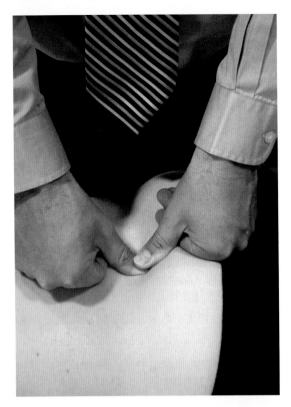

(i) Palpation—sacroiliac region. Palpate over the sacroiliac joints and iliolumbar ligaments

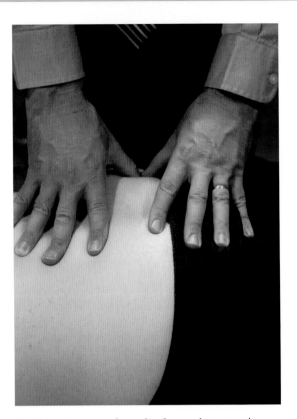

(k) Palpation—quadratus lumborum between the iliac crest and the rib cage

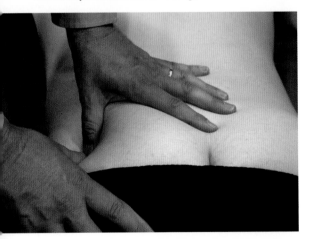

(j) Palpation—muscles and fascia. Palpate paraspinal and gluteal muscles for generalized increase in muscle tone and focal areas of tissue abnormality, including active trigger points

be suspected. Radioisotopic bone scan may be helpful in cases of suspected stress fracture of the pars interarticularis (spondylolysis).

CT scanning is commonly performed in cases of suspected nerve root compression but usually adds little to the clinical picture unless specific neurological signs are present. Disk protrusions and disk bulges are commonly seen in asymptomatic patients and the CT scan, unlike MRI, is unable to provide any further information on the internal structure of the intervertebral disk. However, spinal canal stenosis and facet joint arthropathy are well defined on CT scanning. The presence of a pars interarticularis defect may also be confirmed on CT scanning.

In the investigation of patients with low back pain, MRI can be used to image the internal structure of the disk. Degenerated disks that have lost fluid have a characteristic appearance on MRI (Fig. 21.4). MRI may confirm the presence of an anular tear in the disk and provide information about the vertebral end plate. The clinician must be wary, however, of placing too much emphasis on this investigation, as an abnormality shown on MRI may not necessarily be responsible for all or any of the patient's pain. It has been shown that a centralizing or peripheralizing pain pattern is

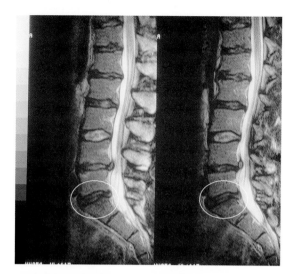

Figure 21.4 MRI of an intervertebral disk showing decreased fluid (shown as dark coloration) in the disk

a better indicator of internal disk disruption than an abnormality on MRI.[6]

Myelography is performed by infusing contrast medium into the spinal fluid to demonstrate encroachment into the spinal canal. It is used most commonly when surgery is planned for the treatment of an acute or chronic disk herniation. Diskography is performed by injecting dye into the nucleus pulposus of the intervertebral disk. Reproduction of the patient's symptoms confirms the disk as the source of pain. It will also give an indication of the internal structure of the disk and is the only true diagnostic indicator of diskogenic pain. Although diskography is the only imaging test for diskogenic pain, psychological factors can significantly alter the result of these tests.

Severe low back pain

The majority of patients with low back pain present with mild-to-moderate pain. A small group of patients present with acute onset of severe low back pain. The aim of initial management of these patients is to reduce the pain and inflammation as rapidly as possible. When this is done, the management of these patients relies on the same principles as those with mild-to-moderate low back pain.

Acute onset of severe low back pain in the absence of nerve root signs may be due either to an acute tear of the anulus fibrosus of the disk or to an acute locked apophyseal joint. A locked apophyseal joint is thought to be due to entrapment of an intra-articular meniscus.

Clinical features of severe acute low back pain

Acute low back pain is usually of sudden onset and is often triggered by a relatively minor movement such as bending to pick up an object. This minor incident may be more indicative of fatigue or lack of control, rather than tissue overload. The pain may increase over a period of hours due to the development of inflammation. Patients with chronic low back pain may also have acute exacerbations that may become more frequent and require less initiation over time.

The pain is usually in the lower lumbar area and may be central, bilateral or unilateral. It may radiate to the buttocks, hamstrings or lower leg. Sharp, lancinating pain in a narrow band down the leg is radicular pain and is associated with nerve root irritation, commonly as a result of intervertebral disk prolapse. More commonly, the pain referred to the buttock and hamstring is somatic in nature, with the patient complaining of a deep-seated ache.

The patient with acute, sudden onset of low back pain often adopts a fixed position and movements are severely restricted in all directions. Palpation of the lumbar spine reveals areas of marked tenderness with associated muscle spasm.

Management of severe acute low back pain

- Encourage the patient to adopt the position of most comfort. This position varies considerably and may be lying prone, supine or, commonly, side-lying with a degree of lumbar flexion.
- Movements that aggravate pain should be avoided, whereas movements that reduce or have no effect on pain should be encouraged.
- Bed rest in the position of most comfort may be continued for up to 48 hours depending on the amount of pain. Bed rest longer than 48 hours has been shown to be detrimental.[7]
- Taping of the low back (Fig. 21.5) can markedly reduce acute back pain and allow quicker functional restoration.
- Analgesics may control the pain and reflex muscle spasm. NSAIDs may help reduce inflammation.
- Electrotherapeutic modalities, for example, TENS, interferential stimulation and magnetic field therapy, may be helpful in reducing pain and muscle spasm in the acute stage. However, if access to these modalities in the acute stage requires any degree of travel, then bed rest alone may be preferable.

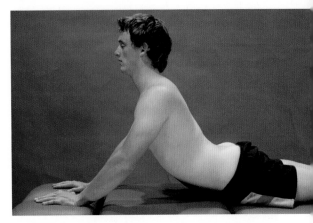

Figure 21.6 Extension exercises—the amount of extension varies according to pain

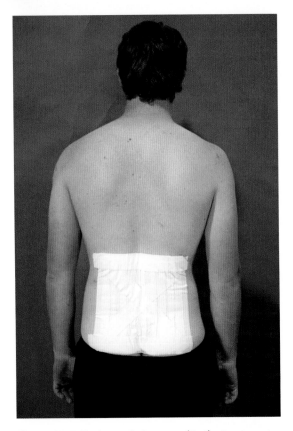

Figure 21.5 Taping technique used in the treatment of severe acute low back pain

- Exercise in a direction away from the movement that aggravates the patient's symptoms should be commenced as early as possible. For those patients in whom flexion aggravates their symptoms, extension exercises should be performed (Fig. 21.6).
- The degree of extension should be determined by the level of pain. Initially, lying prone may be sufficient. Later, extension of the lumbar spine by pushing up onto the elbows may be possible. Eventually, further extension with straight arms can be achieved.
- Exercises should be immediately discontinued if peripheral symptoms develop.
- Prolonged posture involving flexion, such as sitting, should be avoided.

In patients for whom extension movements aggravate their pain, flexion exercises (Fig. 21.7) or rotation (away from pain) exercises should be performed. For these patients, prolonged posture

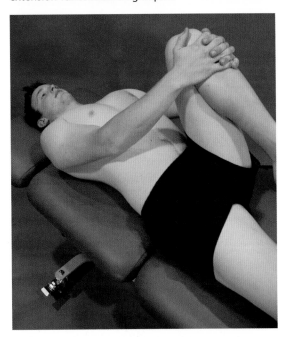

Figure 21.7 Flexion exercises—single knee to chest

involving extension, such as standing with excessive lumbar lordosis, should be avoided.

Manual therapy has only a limited role in treating severe low back pain. Gentle mobilization techniques, for example, posteroanterior (PA) mobilization, may be performed and the patient's response closely monitored. If there is any deterioration of symptoms, mobilization should be immediately ceased. The mobilization should be performed in the position of comfort adopted by the patient. Manipulation should not be attempted in the presence of marked muscle spasm. Similarly, gentle (grade I) soft tissue massage may be helpful in relieving pain and muscle spasm. Traction has not been found to be helpful in patients with acute low back pain.

Mild-to-moderate low back pain

Once the acute phase (up to 48 hours) of severe low back pain has passed with reduction in pain and muscle spasm, more intensive therapy can be commenced. Those patients whose initial presentation is with mild-to-moderate low back pain do not require such a period of rest and treatment can commence immediately.

 Intervertebral joints, paraspinal muscles and local nerves may all contribute to the patient's low back pain and must be identified and corrected.

The initial injury is most likely to be joint-related, for example, a disk or apophyseal joint. However, in response to the injury, there may be associated muscle irritation and spasm as well as neural irritation. Altered movement patterns, secondary to the initial injury, may result in the development of focal areas of increased muscle tone and trigger points. Various neural structures (nerve root or peripheral nerve) may be damaged at the initial injury. As a result, increased neural tension may develop. The longer the duration of the injury, the greater the contribution to the pain from muscle and neural structures.

Clinical features

Patients with mild low back pain complain of an aching pain that may be constant or intermittent. The pain may be central, unilateral or bilateral and is often described by the patient as a 'band across the lower back'. The pain may be aggravated by certain movements, such as flexion, extension or combined movements. There may be associated somatic pain in the buttock and/or hamstring.

On examination, there is usually reduced range of motion of the lumbar spine, commonly flexion or extension. In patients with unilateral pain, there is often reduced lateral flexion. Any increased neural tension can be demonstrated by aggravation of the pain or reduction of range of motion with the slump test or straight leg raise (Chapter 8).

On palpation, there may be marked tenderness over the spinous processes or laterally over the apophyseal joints and transverse processes. The most typical finding in these patients is of hypomobility of one or more intervertebral segments. Depending on the severity and duration of the pain, there will be associated muscle spasm as well as focal areas of increased muscle tone and trigger points in the paravertebral and gluteal muscles.

If the muscles are very taut, palpation of the region is best performed with the patient side-lying. The muscles can be palpated using landmarks such as the transverse processes and spinous processes to identify specific muscles and ligaments. Focal areas of muscle abnormality that on palpation reproduce the patient's pain (rather than a region of diffuse muscle spasm) are likely to respond well to soft tissue therapy. These lesions feel tight but are compressible, unlike the lesions of chronic tissue thickening that have a more solid feel.

Treatment of mild-to-moderate low back pain

The treatment of non-osseous lesions causing low back pain is based on the same principles as the treatment of soft tissue injuries elsewhere in the body.

1. Identify and eliminate possible causes, for example, poor posture, abnormal biomechanics.
2. Reduce pain and inflammation.
3. Restore full range of pain-free movement.
4. Achieve optimal flexibility and strength.
5. Maintain fitness.

There is no one treatment that is appropriate for all cases of low back pain. The ideal treatment regimen requires an integrated approach. To monitor the effectiveness of each type of treatment, it is necessary to reassess the objective clinical signs following treatment. This will reveal which treatment is most appropriate. The type of treatment depends, to a certain extent, on the degree of low back pain present and its irritability. Irritable lesions must be treated carefully so as not to aggravate pain. Lesions of low irritability, however, may be treated more aggressively with little risk of aggravating the symptoms.

Correction of predisposing factors

Correction of the factors causing low back pain is the most important component of the treatment program. This may be sufficient to alleviate current symptoms and prevent recurrence. If the cause is not identified and eliminated, symptoms may persist and the likelihood of recurrence is high.

In athletes, correction of abnormal biomechanics that may predispose to low back pain, such as running with an excessive lordosis or lack of pelvic stability, is required. Correction of these factors is discussed in the rehabilitation section later in this chapter. Other possible causative factors include poor posture while sitting or standing, poor lifting techniques, working in stooped positions or sleeping on a bed with poor support.

Pharmacological treatment

There is some evidence that NSAIDs are effective for short-term symptomatic relief in patients with low back pain. However, it is unclear whether NSAIDs are more effective than simple analgesics such as paracetamol (acetaminophen). There is no evidence that any one type of NSAID is more effective than another. There is no place for the long-term use of NSAIDs, both in relation to their lack of effectiveness and their significant incidence of side-effects.

Mobilization and manipulation

Mobilization and manipulation may have two advantageous effects on the patient with a soft tissue injury to the lumbar spine. They act to reduce pain (Chapter 10) and also to restore movement to the hypomobile intervertebral segments detected on examination. This will often involve joints at more than one level and, commonly, maximal stiffness is actually found in the level above or below the joint producing the patient's symptoms. Mobilization techniques used in the treatment of low back pain include:

- PA central (Fig. 21.8a)
- PA unilateral (Fig. 21.8b)
- rotations
- transverse vertebral pressure.

PA central mobilization and rotations are used in patients with central or bilateral pain. PA unilateral mobilization, rotations and, occasionally, transverse techniques are used if the pain is unilateral. The grade of mobilization technique used will depend on the irritability of the condition and the amount of tenderness and stiffness. The most commonly used manipulation technique in the treatment of low back pain is rotation (Fig. 21.9).

Soft tissue therapy

Abnormalities of the muscles and fascia are found in association with low back pain. The longer the low back pain has been present, the more widespread and severe are these abnormalities. Tender focal areas of abnormal tissue may be palpated.

Treatment of these areas consists of grade I transverse gliding, grade II sustained longitudinal pressure

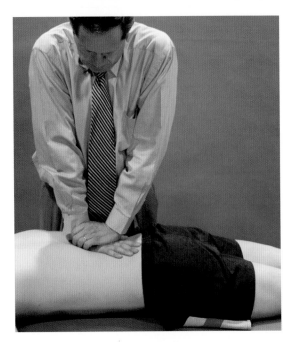

Figure 21.8 Mobilization techniques

(a) PA central. The therapist performs an oscillating movement over the spinous processes using thumbs or heels of the hands. Elbows are extended and pressure is exerted through the shoulders and arms

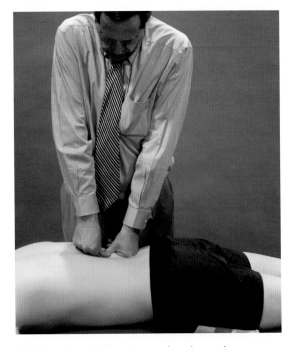

(b) PA unilateral. Thumbs are placed over the apophyseal joints

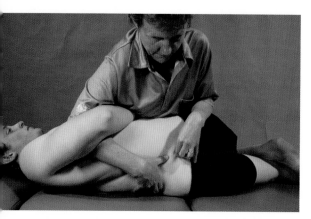

Figure 21.9 Manipulation—rotation. With the patient positioned as shown, the therapist exerts a short sudden forward thrust on the ilium while maintaining strong counterpressure on the shoulder. This position can be used for manipulation or mobilization

on the taut bands emanating away from the focal lesion and sustained ischemic pressure (grade III) on the painful focal lesion (Fig. 21.10). After each treatment, the patient should be taken through the full range of pain-free motion for assessment and muscle stretch.

In more chronic cases, structural thickening in the fibers of lumbar multifidus and longissimus are seen. Less commonly involved are the intertransverserii and the quadratus lumborum. Palpation may reveal taut bands up to 1 cm (0.5 in.) in diameter about the L4–5 apophyseal joint within the lumbar multifidus muscle. In lean athletes, these bands may be rope-like. In stocky athletes, there may be gross muscle thickening that is palpable even through the thick fascial layers of the region.

Treatment is aimed at eliminating these abnormal areas of muscle tissue and, therefore, restoring normal function. Techniques used include grade II to III digital ischemic pressure to the focal lesions and grade III transverse gliding. Sustained myofascial tension techniques may also be helpful.

In addition to assessment and treatment of the extensor muscles, attention should be paid to the flexor muscles. Tightness in the flexor muscles, commonly associated with hyperlordosis, may result in the antagonist extensors becoming excessively tight.

Dry needling

Longstanding cases of low back pain are characterized by the presence of multiple active trigger points. The most common sites are the paraspinal muscles from

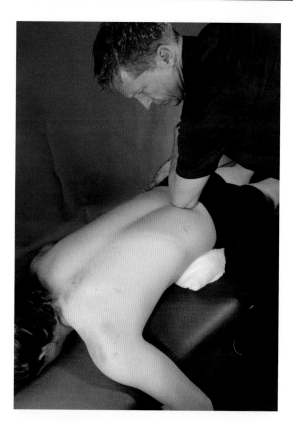

Figure 21.10 Soft tissue techniques

(a) Sustained ischemic pressure at each segmental level

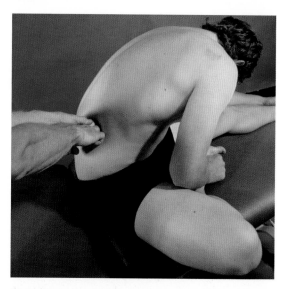

(b) Sustained ischemic pressure using the knuckles to the quadratus lumborum in the position of sustained stretch

the mid thoracic to the sacrum, quadratus lumborum and the gluteal muscles, especially gluteus medius. Dry needling to inactivate these trigger points (Fig. 21.11) will reduce pain and muscle tightness, thus facilitating mobilization and manipulation of the underlying joints and, ultimately, exercise rehabilitation.

Neural mobilization

Abnormal neural tension is often found in patients with low back pain. Neural tension tests such as the slump test and straight leg raise are often restricted and may aggravate the patient's symptoms.

Correction of joint and soft tissue abnormalities frequently results in an improvement in neural tension and in neural range of motion. This can be further improved by incorporating neural mobilizing techniques, such as slump mobilizing (Fig. 21.12), into the treatment program. Neural mobilizing should be performed with considerable caution under close supervision of an experienced clinician. Excessive use may aggravate the patient's symptoms.

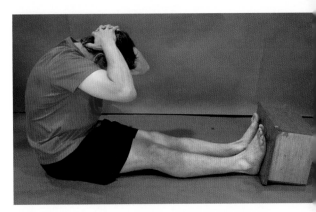

Figure 21.12 Neural stretch—slump stretch. Patient adopts the position illustrated. To increase the degree of the stretch, the trunk is flexed at the hips until discomfort is felt. This position should be held for at least 10 seconds and then further trunk flexion may be performed, again to the point of onset of discomfort

Other treatment methods

Intermittent traction, performed manually or with the aid of weights or a machine, may be an effective pain-relieving technique in patients with nerve root irritation or radicular signs and symptoms but does not play a major role in the treatment of mild-to-moderate low back pain. No good studies on the efficacy of traction for low back pain exist. Muscle energy techniques may be helpful in the treatment of patients with low back pain.

Exercise therapy

Exercise therapy is an essential component of the treatment of the patient with low back pain. Exercise therapy acts to help restore and maintain full range of motion as well as providing additional mechanical support to the low back. Exercises include stretching, range of motion, strengthening and stability exercises. Exercise therapy is discussed further in the section on rehabilitation later in this chapter.

Intervention techniques

Occasionally, patients with low back pain due to soft tissue abnormalities fail to respond to treatment methods as outlined. For those patients who fail to respond, it is important to consider alternative diagnoses, such as lumbar instability or stress fracture. The presence of undetected predisposing factors, such as abnormal biomechanics, should be considered.

There are a number of interventional techniques available for the treatment of the patient with

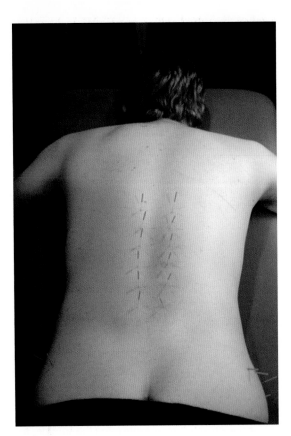

Figure 21.11 Dry needling of trigger points in the paraspinal and gluteal muscles

persistent low back pain who fails to respond to an appropriate, correctly administered treatment program. Some clinicians argue that this should occur once the pain has become chronic (i.e. of three months' duration). There is some reasonable evidence which shows that the chance of conservative management helping patients with chronic low back pain is less than 10%.

When compared to target-specific diagnoses achieved through accurate local anesthetic injections done under image intensifier, our ability to make a specific joint or disk diagnosis using clinical skill or imaging is very limited. Numerous studies have shown that findings on examination, traditionally found to have significance, lack reliability and validity.

Interventional pain management in chronic back pain follows a logical process:

1. Obtain a target-specific diagnosis.
2. Treat the diagnosis according to evidence-based medicine.
3. If the diagnosis is:
   (a) neuropathic pain
   (b) unable to be made
   (c) fails the treatment
   then block the pain pathway at the spinal cord level with spinal cord stimulation by intrathecal pump.

The identifiable causes of chronic low back pain are:

1. facet joints
2. sacroiliac joints
3. internal disk disruption (not disk bulges/prolapses etc.).

These areas can be diagnosed by the use of specific blocks, which are outlined below.

Facet joint pain can be diagnosed with medial branch blocks. These involve using an image intensifier to place a needle onto the medial branch that supplies a facet joint and injecting local anesthetic onto the nerve. To block one joint, two nerves must be blocked; to block two joints, three nerves must be blocked. The patient then completes a pain chart and if the pain goes away for several hours, the clinician can be approximately 60% sure of the diagnosis. A control block with a different local anesthetic is then done. If there is concordant pain relief, then the diagnostic confidence is approaching 90%.[8] Note that facet joint injections lack diagnostic and therapeutic validity.

Sacroiliac joint pain can be diagnosed with a sacroiliac joint injection, which some clinicians would combine with a deep interosseous joint injection. The data here are not as rigorous as for medial branch blocks but, with a control block, diagnostic confidence approaching 90% can again be achieved.

Disk pain is diagnosed differently. The most accurate test available is a pain provocation test, called provocative diskography. When performed according to the International Spine Intervention Society's guidelines, this is a relatively comfortable procedure. The posterior column (facet and sacroiliac joints) should first have been excluded as the cause of pain by the above methods. An MRI is then performed. If the disks are pristine, it is inappropriate to do a diskogram and one should look elsewhere for a diagnosis. If there is evidence of disk disease, especially high-intensity zones of type one or type two modic changes, then proceeding with diskography is reasonable if the patient's pain warrants the risk of infection.

Once a diagnosis has been made, then appropriate treatment can be undertaken. Facet joint or sacroiliac joint pain can be treated by radiofrequency neurotomy. This technique has a 90% chance of 60% pain relief and a 60% chance of 90% pain relief for lumbar facet pain.[9, 10] In the sacroiliac joint, there is evidence for a 60% chance of more than 50% pain relief, with a 30% chance of 90% pain relief.[11] Some people advocate prolotherapy for sacroiliac joint problems. Evidence for this is currently inconclusive.

There are various percutaneous treatment options for diskogenic pain. The best data support the use of intradiskal electrothermal therapy (IDET),[12] however, the data that support IDET are mixed and even the best study shows it may be effective for only very selected patients with low back pain. There is level two evidence for nucleoplasty in disk pain.

Epidural injections with a long-acting local anesthetic plus/minus a corticosteroid are a treatment for radicular leg pain and not a treatment for low back pain.

Despite the fact that over 250 000 lumbar fusions are performed annually in the United States, there is no level one evidence to support this operation for diskogenic back pain.[13, 14]

Spinal surgery should only be performed when there is a specific indication. These indications are:

- nerve root compression resulting in persistent:
  — bladder or bowel symptoms
  — radicular pain
  — sensory or motor abnormalities despite adequate conservative management
- persistent pain due to instability of a single intervertebral segment.

Acute nerve root compression

Acute nerve root compression is usually the result of an acute disk prolapse when the contents of the nucleus pulposus of the intervertebral disk are extruded through a defect in the anulus fibrosus into the spinal canal. There they may irritate the nerve root (Fig. 21.13). The irritation of the nerve root may be due to direct mechanical compression by the nuclear

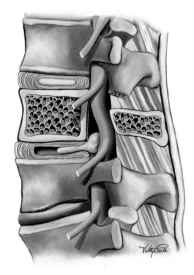

Figure 21.13 Disk extrusion compressing nerve root

(a) Spinal cord compression from severe disk prolapse

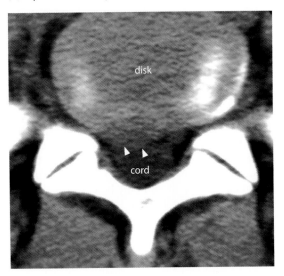

(b) Axial CT scan. Arrowheads point to the border between the bulging disk (anterior) and the compressed cord (posterior)

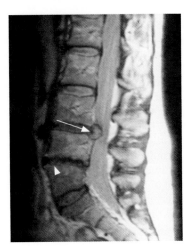

(c) Sagittal MRI showing prominent posterior L3–4 disk bulging (arrow) and cauda equina compression. The L4–5 disk (arrowhead) is also abnormal but not protruding

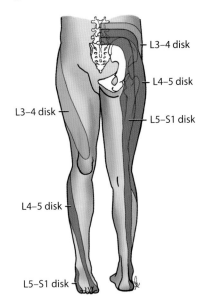

(d) Common areas of pain radiation with disk prolapse at the L3–4, L4–5 and L5–S1 levels

material or as a result of the chemical irritation caused by the extrusion. In the older athlete, nerve roots may be compressed by osteophytes formed as part of a degenerative process.

Prolapse usually occurs in disks that have been previously damaged by one of the processes mentioned already. This explains why frequently a minor movement, such as bending over to pick up an object off the floor, may cause such an apparently severe injury. Disk prolapse usually occurs between the ages of 20 and 50 years and is more common in males than females. The L5–S1 disk is the most commonly prolapsed disk and L4–5 the next most common.

Clinical features

Typically, a patient with a disk prolapse presents with acute low back pain or radicular leg pain (or both) following a relatively trivial movement usually involving flexion. On occasions, the presentation may be painless, with weakness or sensory symptoms only. The symptoms depend on the direction of the extrusion. Posterior protrusions are more likely to cause low back pain with later development of leg pain, whereas posterolateral protrusions may cause radicular symptoms without low back pain. Typical radicular symptoms include sharp shooting pain in a narrow band accompanied by pins and needles, numbness and weakness. Pain is often aggravated by sitting, bending, lifting, coughing or sneezing. Pain is usually eased by lying down, particularly on the asymptomatic side, and is often less after a night's rest.

On examination, the patient often demonstrates a list to one side, usually, although not always, away from the side of pain. This is a protective scoliosis. Examination may be difficult if there is severe pain and irritability. Straight leg raise is usually limited (less than 30° in severe cases) and all active movements, particularly flexion, are usually restricted. Palpation usually reveals acute muscle spasm with marked tenderness but occasionally it may be unremarkable. A neurological examination should always be performed when pain extends past the buttock fold or there are subjective sensory/motor changes.

Treatment

In the acute phase, the most appropriate treatment is rest in bed in a position of maximum comfort with administration of analgesics and NSAIDs. The patient should lie as much as possible and avoid sitting. Extension exercises (Fig. 21.6) should be commenced as soon as possible. However, if exercises cause an increase in peripheral symptoms, they should be ceased.

Mobilization techniques should be performed with great care. Rotations may be effective but should be performed gently as patients with disk prolapse may be made considerably worse with aggressive mobilization. Manipulation is contraindicated in conditions with acute neurological signs and symptoms.

Traction is often helpful in the treatment of acute disk prolapse with distal symptoms. However, it is not uncommon for the patient to experience considerable pain relief while undergoing traction, only to have increased symptoms after treatment. A transforaminal epidural injection of corticosteroid may help if there is no significant improvement in symptoms and signs with rest.

Surgery may be required if neurological signs persist or worsen. If bowel or bladder symptoms are present, emergency surgery may be necessary. An open laminectomy or percutaneous diskectomy using a needle aspiration technique may be performed. Chymopapain injection may be helpful when a unilateral disk bulge is present.

As the acute episode settles, it is important to restore normal pain-free movement to the area with localized mobilization and stretching. Following restoration of range of movement, active stabilization exercises should be performed. This is discussed later in this chapter. Postural advice, including correction of poor lifting techniques and adjustment of sporting technique, where necessary, is most important.

Stress fracture of the pars interarticularis

Stress fractures of the pars interarticularis (spondylolysis) occur in young athletes involved in sports that require episodes of hyperextension, especially if combined with rotation.[15] This condition was initially thought to be congenital but is probably an acquired overuse injury.

Sports in which this injury is commonly seen include gymnastics, fast bowling (cricket), tennis, rowing, dance, weightlifting, wrestling, pole vaulting and high jump, as well as throwing activities such as baseball pitching, javelin, discus and hammer throw. The fracture usually occurs on the side opposite to the one performing the activity, that is, left-sided fractures in right-handed tennis players (Fig. 21.14a).

Clinical features

The patient complains of:

- unilateral low back ache, occasionally associated with somatic buttock pain
- pain that is aggravated by movements involving lumbar extension—the athlete may describe a single episode of hyperextension that precipitated the pain.

Occasionally, stress fractures to the pars interarticularis are asymptomatic.

On examination:

- pain is produced on extension with rotation and on extension while standing on the affected leg (Fig. 21.3g)
- the athlete may often have an excessive lordotic posture with associated spasm of the hamstring muscles
- palpation reveals unilateral tenderness over the site of the fracture.

In cases with recent onset of pain, X-ray may not demonstrate the fracture. In longer standing cases, the typical 'Scotty dog' appearance of a pars defect is demonstrated on the 45° oblique X-ray. When a pars defect is suspected clinically but plain X-ray is normal, an isotopic bone scan, or preferably a single photon emission computed tomography (SPECT) scan, should be performed. The bone scan will demonstrate a focal area of increased uptake (Fig. 21.14b). Even when the X-ray demonstrates a pars defect, a SPECT scan should be performed to confirm the presence of an active stress fracture.

Patients with a positive SPECT scan result should then undergo reverse gantry CT scanning to image the fracture (Fig. 21.14c). The patient should be monitored during the healing process, both clinically and by repeat CT scan of the fracture. MRI (Fig. 21.14d) is also capable of demonstrating a pars fracture but may not be as sensitive as a combination of a SPECT and CT scan.

Treatment

There is considerable variation in the recommended treatment for pars stress fractures. Almost all clinicians agree on the need for restricting the athletic activity responsible for the pain, stretching the hamstring and gluteal muscles, and strengthening the abdominal and back extensor muscles as soon as these can be

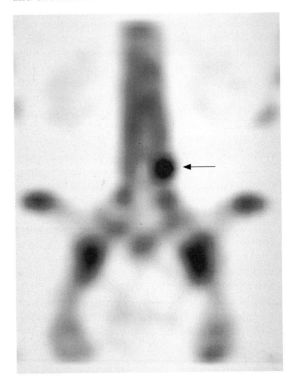

(b) SPECT scan showing increased uptake

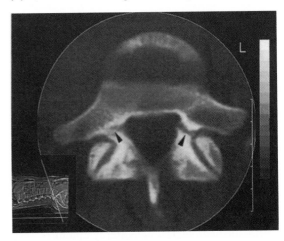

(c) CT scan showing previous (left arrow) and recent (right arrow) fractures

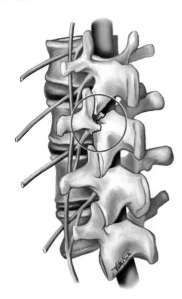

Figure 21.14 Stress fracture of the pars interarticularis

(a) Side view

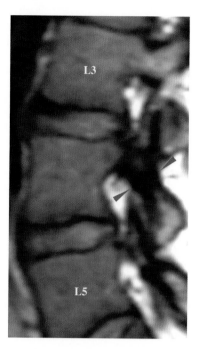

(d) MRI scan showing pars interarticularis stress fracture (COURTESY DR CRAIG ENGSTROM)

performed pain-free. However, the use of rigid anti-lordotic bracing is debated.

It would seem from studies[15] that it is the stage and site of the defect rather than the type of treatment that determines healing of the bony defect. Pars defects can be divided into early, progressive and terminal stages. The early stage is characterized by focal bony absorption or a hairline defect on radiographic appearance. In the progressive stage, the defect is wide and small fragments are present. Sclerotic change indicates the terminal stage of development. In most cases of early stage defects, radiographic union will be achieved, but this will only be achieved in approximately half the progressive stage cases and virtually none of the cases with sclerotic changes.

A unilateral defect is more likely to heal than bilateral defects. There is also an improved rate of union in defects at L4 compared with at L5 and in lesions closer to the vertebral body.

Therefore, it is important to make an early diagnosis and commence a treatment program consisting of rest from sport and rehabilitation.

We believe that there should not be a set period of time but that the patient should undergo a rehabilitation program initially involving pain-free progressive exercises but not aggravating activity (i.e. lumbar extension and rotation). When the aggravating maneuvers are pain-free and there is no local tenderness, a gradual progressive resumption of the aggravating activity over a period of four to six weeks should be conducted using pain as a guide.

O'Sullivan et al.'s landmark study[16] of the effectiveness of a specific exercise program emphasizing training of the transversus abdominis and multifidus in adults with spondylolysis and spondylolisthesis showed dramatic differences in pain scores and improved function that was maintained for 30 months compared to a control group who were treated with general fitness training, supervised exercise, modalities and trunk flexion exercises. A core stability training program (Chapter 11) should be included in the treatment program.

As with any overuse injury, it is important to identify the cause or causes and to correct them if possible. Technique adjustments should be made to limit the amount of hyperextension and, if necessary, a brace can be used during sporting activity.

This injury is extremely common among young fast bowlers in cricket. Fast bowlers use one of three techniques—side-on, front-on or a mixed technique where the lower half of the body is front-on and the upper half side-on. It is this latter combined technique that appears to be associated with the development of stress fractures of the pars interarticularis.[17] The bowler and coach should be advised to change to either a side-on or front-on technique.

Spondylolisthesis

Spondylolisthesis refers to the slipping of part or all of one vertebra forward on another. The term is derived from the Greek *spondylos*, meaning vertebra, and *olisthanein*, meaning to slip or slide down a slippery path.

It is often associated with bilateral pars defects that usually develop in early childhood and have a definite family predisposition. Pars defects that develop due to athletic activity (stress fractures) rarely result in spondylolisthesis.

Spondylolisthesis is most commonly seen in children between the ages of 9 and 14. In the vast majority of cases it is the L5 vertebra that slips forward on the S1. The spondylolisthesis is graded according to the degree of slip of the vertebra. A grade I slip denotes that a vertebra has slipped up to 25% over the body of the vertebra underlying it; in a grade II slip the displacement is greater than 25%; in a grade III slip, greater than 50%; and in a grade IV slip, greater than 75%. Lateral X-rays best demonstrate the extent of vertebral slippage (Fig. 21.15).

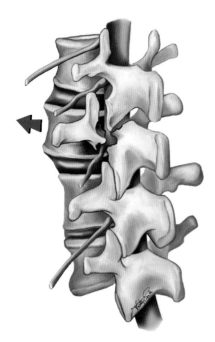

Figure 21.15 Grade I spondylolisthesis and pars defect

(a) Side view

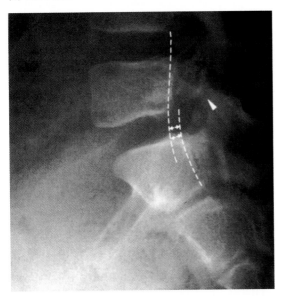

(b) X-ray (single arrow shows the defect, dotted lines show the method of measuring slippage)

Clinical features

Grade I spondylolisthesis is often asymptomatic and the patients may be unaware of the defect. Patients with grade II or higher slips may complain of low back pain, with or without leg pain. The back pain is aggravated by extension activities.

On examination, there may be a palpable dip corresponding to the slip. Associated soft tissue abnormalities may be present. In considering the treatment of this condition, it is important to remember that the patient's low back pain is not necessarily being caused by the spondylolisthesis.

Treatment

Treatment of athletes with grade I or grade II symptomatic spondylolisthesis involves:

- rest from aggravating activities combined with abdominal and extensor stabilizing exercises and hamstring stretching
- antilordotic bracing, which may also be helpful
- mobilization of stiff joints above or below the slip on clinical assessment; gentle rotations may be helpful in reducing pain; manipulation should not be performed at the level of the slip.

Athletes with grade I or grade II spondylolisthesis may return to sport after treatment when they are pain-free on extension and have good spinal stabilization. If the symptoms recur, activity must be ceased.

Athletes with grade III or grade IV spondylolisthesis should avoid high speed or contact sports. Treatment is symptomatic. It is rare for a slip to progress; however, if there is evidence of progression, spinal fusion should be performed.

Lumbar hypermobility

The majority of cases of low back pain are associated with hypomobility of one or more intervertebral segments. However, occasionally, hypermobility of an intervertebral segment may be detected on clinical assessment.

This hypermobility may be associated with a general hypermobility syndrome affecting all vertebral and peripheral joints. It is important to recognize this hypermobility syndrome because an isolated segment of reduced mobility in a generally hypermobile spine may have clinical significance.

Structural lumbar instability

The finding of an isolated hypermobile intervertebral segment may be indicative of lumbar instability. Recognition of this condition is important as it will not respond to the mobilization and manipulation techniques used to restore pain-free movement in most patients with low back pain. Treatment of lumbar instability involves retraining and strengthening of the spinal extensors and the abdominal muscles to increase stability. Any hypomobility of surrounding intervertebral segments causing pain should be treated with mobilization to ease this.

Sacroiliac joint disorders

Sacroiliac joint disorders are an important cause of low back and buttock pain and are discussed fully in Chapter 22.

Rehabilitation following low back pain

Low back pain is usually mechanical in nature. Therefore, to eliminate and prevent recurrence of low back pain, biomechanical modification is required to reduce or eliminate the stress or stresses that are responsible for, or aggravating, the back pain. This may be a sustained mechanical stress, for example, prolonged sitting with poor posture, or an intermittent stress, such as running with excessive lumbar lordosis.

Rehabilitation of the athlete with low back pain involves two main principles.

1. Modify activities to reduce stress to the lumbar spine. These activities include posture, activities of daily living and sporting technique.
2. Correct predisposing biomechanical abnormalities that may be due to:
   (a) generalized muscle weakness
   (b) tight muscles
   (c) poor muscle control.

The best results in the management of low back pain appear to come with a combination of therapies.[18] It is important to remember that spinal exercises should not be done in the first hour after awakening due to the increased hydrostatic pressures in the disk during that time.[19]

Posture

Prolonged poor posture places excessive strain on pain-provoking structures of the lumbar spine. Poor posture can occur while sitting, standing or lying.

Adopting a slouched position while sitting (Fig. 21.16a) is extremely common. The correct position is shown in Figure 21.16b. A firm, straight-backed chair will provide more support than sitting in a soft armchair or couch. The use of a lumbar roll encourages correct posture by increasing the

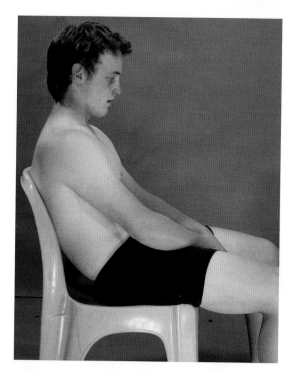

Figure 21.16 Sitting posture

(a) Slouched

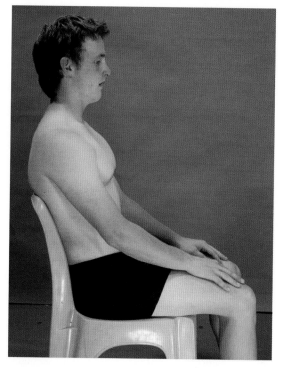

(b) Correct

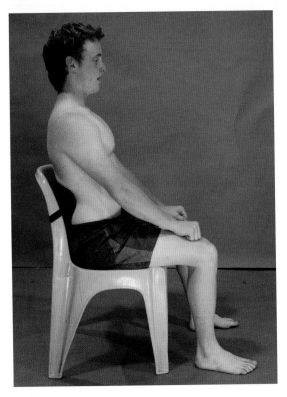

(c) Sitting with lumbar roll

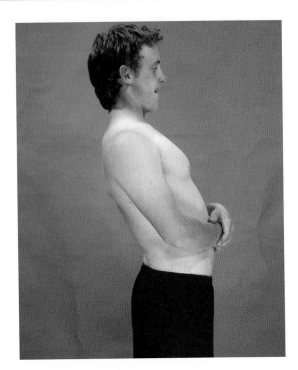

Figure 21.17 Standing posture

(a) Hyperlordotic

lumbar lordosis. The lumbar roll should be placed just above the belt line in the hollow of the back (Fig. 21.16c).

Standing with a hyperlordotic posture (Fig. 21.17a) will also place excessive strain on the structures of the lumbar spine. The correct standing position should be adopted (Fig. 21.17b). When lying, the patient needs a firm, comfortable mattress. If the bed has a tendency to sag, the mattress should be placed on the floor.

Daily activities

For those people for whom excessive or prolonged lumbar flexion aggravates their low back pain, care must be taken to avoid such activities. Patients required to perform a task low down should lower themselves to the level required while maintaining the back as vertical as possible. The patient should be advised to avoid lifting as much as possible but, when unavoidable, correct technique should be used (Fig. 21.18). There is some evidence that the key factor is the distance the object is from the body, rather than an absolutely correct technique.[5] Care should be taken when the patient is required to pick up a relatively

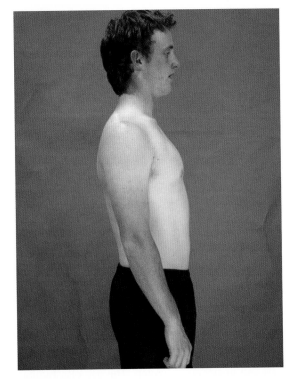

(b) Correct

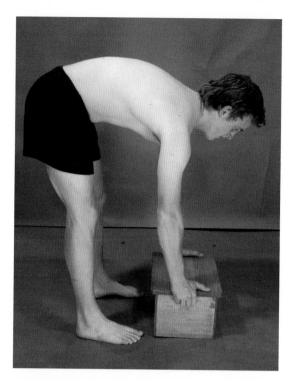

Figure 21.18 Lifting technique

(a) Incorrect

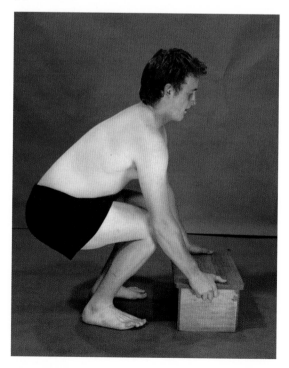

(b) Correct

light object. Often patients with low back pain take great care when lifting heavy objects but fail to brace their lumbar spine while picking up light objects. Activities that require prolonged bending and twisting, such as vacuuming, are best avoided or modified if producing low back pain.

Sporting technique

Poor technique in sporting activities may increase stress on the structures of the lumbar spine. The technique should be assessed with the aid of a coach and any necessary corrections made under supervision. Poor muscle control or weakness may contribute to the technique fault and will be discussed in the next section.

Biomechanical abnormalities, such as excessive anterior or lateral pelvic tilt with running, are common predisposing factors to the development of low back pain. These factors may increase stress on the lumbar spine. Unless corrected, recurrence of the athlete's low back pain is likely.

Core stability

 Impaired core stability with delayed onset of action of the transversus abdominis muscle has been shown to be associated with low back pain.

An important component of rehabilitation of patients with low back pain is to correct this deficiency. A core stability program is described in Chapter 11.

Once activation of the spine stabilizers (transversus abdominis and lumbar multifidus) has been achieved, global muscle strengthening should commence. In patients with low back pain, particular emphasis should be placed on strengthening the gluteal and hamstring muscles.

Adequate gluteal strength is required for pelvic control. Lack of pelvic control may lead to anterior tilting of the pelvis and increased stress on the lumbar spine. It is important that the gluteal muscles are activated during lifting and bending. Gluteal strengthening exercises should be performed while controlling pelvic movement (Fig. 21.19). The single-leg squat (Fig. 21.20) is an excellent rehabilitation exercise combining motor control and strengthening.

Specific muscle tightness

Specific muscle tightness or shortening is commonly found in association with low back pain. Commonly shortened muscles include erector spinae, psoas, iliotibial band, hip external rotators, hamstrings,

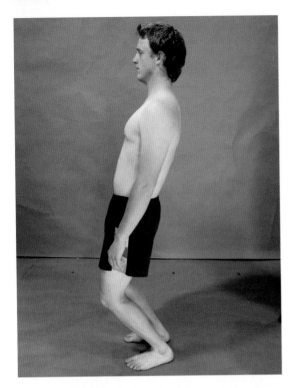

Figure 21.19 Gluteal strengthening exercises

(a) Bending without using gluteals

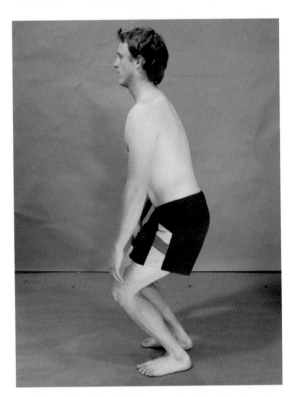

(c) Bending with gluteals and braced lumbar spine

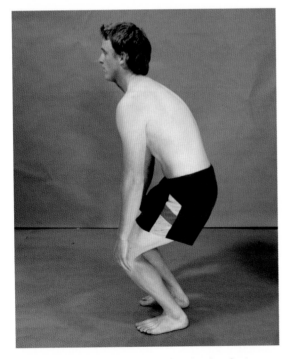

(b) Bending with gluteals but using lumbar flexion

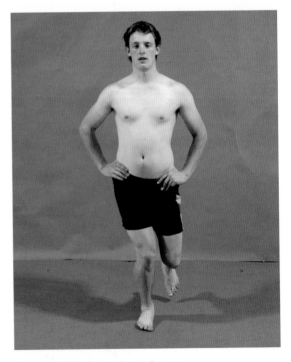

Figure 21.20 Single-legged squat

rectus femoris and gastrocnemius. Tightness of these muscles affects the biomechanics of the lumbar spine. These tight muscles should be corrected as part of the rehabilitation program. The various techniques are shown in Figure 21.21.

Muscle tightness may be corrected by the use of therapist-assisted exercises, home exercises, soft tissue therapy to the muscles and dry needling of trigger points.

Conclusion

The clinical approach to the athlete with low back pain is relatively straightforward. It involves initial assessment of abnormalities of the joints, muscles and neural structures. These abnormalities are then systematically corrected by the use of manual therapy techniques. Associated with this correction of abnormalities, a comprehensive rehabilitation program must be performed, including correction of any biomechanical factors that place increased stress on the lumbar spine in the particular athlete. This requires individual assessment of abnormalities of technique, muscle weakness, muscle tightness or poor muscle control. There is now considerable evidence that inability to use the stabilizing muscles, transversus abdominis and lumbar multifidus, are important features of patients with low back pain, and a specific rehabilitation program must be instituted to correct these deficits. Low back pain provides another example of the integrated approach required in the management of sporting injuries.

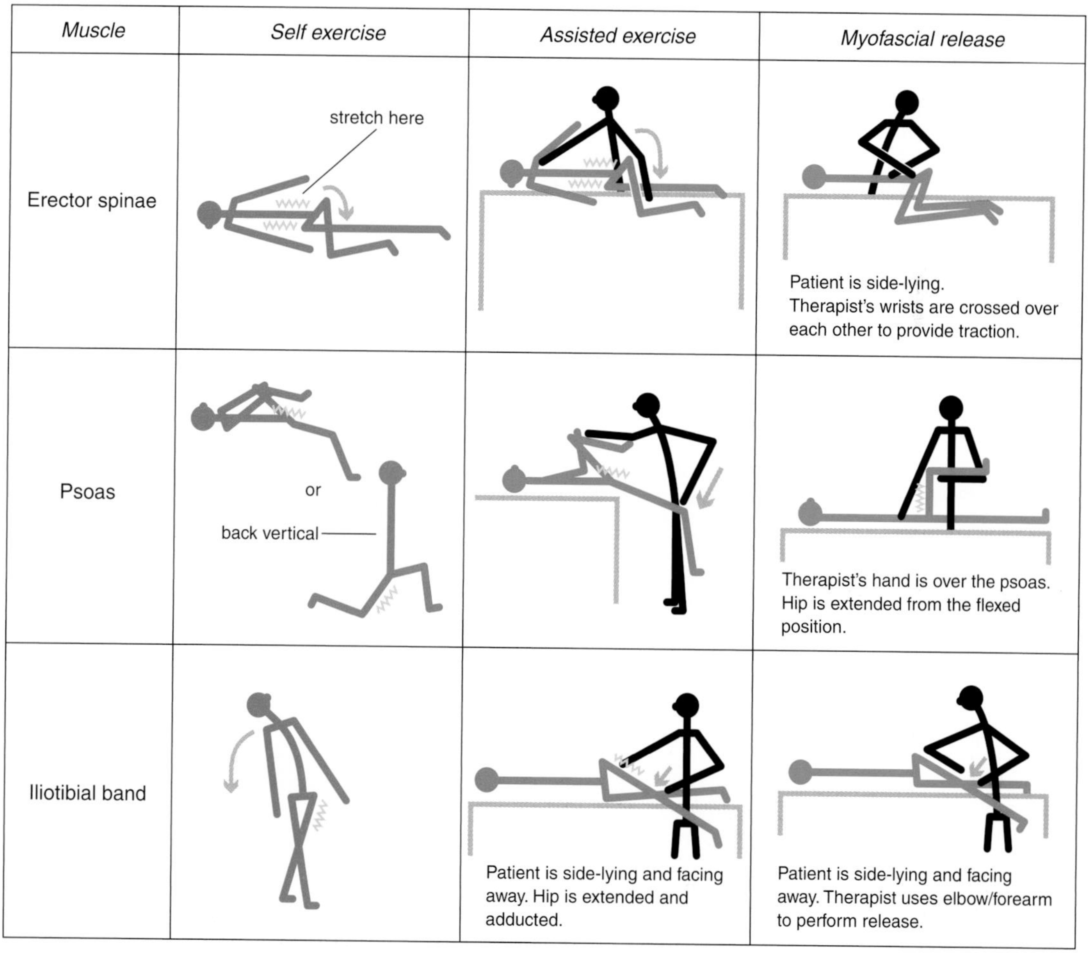

Muscle	Self exercise	Assisted exercise	Myofascial release
Erector spinae	stretch here		Patient is side-lying. Therapist's wrists are crossed over each other to provide traction.
Psoas	or back vertical		Therapist's hand is over the psoas. Hip is extended from the flexed position.
Iliotibial band		Patient is side-lying and facing away. Hip is extended and adducted.	Patient is side-lying and facing away. Therapist uses elbow/forearm to perform release.

Figure 21.21 Techniques used to treat tightness of individual muscles

Muscle	Self exercise	Assisted exercise	Myofascial release
Hip external rotators	side view front view	Hip into adduction with treatment leg crossed over opposite leg.	Patient is side-lying. Therapist stands behind and takes the top leg backward.
Hamstrings			Patient is prone. The elbow or forearm is kept stationary and the knee passively extended.
Rectus femoris		Keep pelvis down while extending hip and flexing knee.	Therapist uses forearm to massage up the thigh of the leg which is hanging off the table.
Gastrocnemius	Pressure on back leg.		Therapist uses thigh to obtain passive ankle dorsiflexion.
Soleus	Pressure on front leg.		Therapist uses chest to assist ankle dorsiflexion.

Recommended Reading

Bogduk N. *Clinical Anatomy of the Lumbar Spine and Sacrum*. 4th edn. Edinburgh: Churchill Livingstone, 2005.

Earl JE. Mechanical aetiology, recognition, and treatment of spondylolisthesis. *Phys Ther Sport* 2002; 3: 79–87.

George SZ, Delitto A. Management of the athlete with low back pain. *Clin Sports Med* 2002; 21: 105–20.

Hilde G, Bo K. Effect of exercise in the treatment of chronic low back pain: a systemic review, emphasising type and dose of exercise. *Phys Ther Rev* 1998; 3: 107–17.

Licciardone JC, Brimhall AK, King LN. Osteopathic manipulative treatment for low back pain: a systematic review and meta-analysis of randomized controlled trials. *BMC Musculoskelet Disord* 2005; 6: 43–54.

Lively MW, Bailes JE. Acute lumbar disk injuries in active patients. *Physician Sportsmed* 2005; 33: 000–00.

Maitland GD. *Vertebral Manipulation*. 5th edn. London: Butterworths, 1986.

McTimoney CAM, Micheli LJ. Current evaluation and management of spondylolysis and spondylolisthesis. *Curr Sports Med Rep* 2003; 2: 41–6.

Nadler SF, Malanga GA, DePrince M, et al. The relationship between lower extremity injury, low back pain, and hip muscle strength in male and female collegiate athletes. *Clin J Sport Med* 2000; 10(2): 89–97.

Richardson C, Jull G, Hodges P, et al. *Therapeutic Exercise for Spinal Segmental Stabilization in Low Back Pain*. 2nd edn. Edinburgh: Churchill Livingstone, 2004.

Standaert CJ. New strategies in the management of low back injuries in gymnasts. *Curr Sports Med Rep* 2002; 1: 293–300.

Standaert CJ, Herring SA, Pratt TW. Rehabilitation of the athlete with low back pain. *Curr Sports Med Rep* 2004; 3: 35–40.

Trainor TJ, Trainor MA. Etiology of low back pain in athletes. *Curr Sports Med Rep* 2004; 3: 41–6.

Urban J. Back to the future: what have we learned from 25 years of research into intervertebral disc biology? *J Back Musculoskel Rehabil* 1997; 9: 23–7.

Watkins RG. Lumbar disc injury in the athlete. *Clin Sports Med* 2002; 21: 147–65.

Recommended Website

An educational tool about low back pain can be found at: <http://www.lowbackpain.tv>.

References

1. Hides JA, Stokes MJ, Saide M, et al. Evidence of lumbar multifidus muscle wasting ipsilateral to symptoms in patients with acute/subacute low back pain. *Spine* 1994; 19: 165–72.

2. Hodges PW, Richardson CA. Inefficient muscular stabilisation of the lumbar spine associated with low back pain: a motor control evaluation of transversus abdominis. *Spine* 1996; 21: 2640–50.

3. Hodges PW, Richardson CA. Delayed postural contraction of transversus abdominis in low back pain associated with movement of the lower limbs. *J Spinal Disord Tech* 1998; 11: 46–56.

4. Sihvonen T, Lindgren K, Airaksinen O, et al. Movement disturbances of the lumbar spine and abnormal back muscle electromyographic findings in recurrent low back pain. *Spine* 1997; 22: 289–95.

5. McGill S. *Low Back Disorders: Evidence-based Prevention and Rehabilitation*. Champaign, IL: Human Kinetics, 2002.

6. Donelson R, Aprill C, Medcalf R, et al. A prospective study of centralization of lumbar and referred pain. A predictor of symptomatic discs and annular competence. *Spine* 1997; 23: 2003–13.

7. Deyo RA, Diehl AK, et al. How many days of bed rest for acute low back pain? *N Engl J Med* 1986; 315: 1064–70.

8. Lord SM, Barnsley L, Bogduk N. The utility of comparative local anesthetic blocks versus placebo-controlled blocks for the diagnosis of cervical zygapophysial joint pain. *Clin J Pain* 1995; 11(3): 208–13.

9. Dreyfuss P, Halbrook B, Pauza K, et al. Efficacy and validity of radiofrequency neurotomy for chronic lumbar zygapophyseal joint pain. *Spine* 2000; 25: 1270–7.

10. Van Kleef M, Barendse GAM, Kessels A, et al. Randomised trial of radiofrequency lumbar facet joint denervation for chronic low back pain. *Spine* 1999; 24: 1937–42.

11. Yin W, Willard F, Carreiro J, et al. Sensory stimulation-guided sacroiliac joint radiofrequency neurotomy: technique based on neuroanatomy of the dorsal sacral plexus. *Spine* 2003; 28(20): 2419–25.

12. Pauza KJ, Howell S, Dreyfuss P, et al. A randomized, placebo-controlled trial of intradiscal electrothermal therapy for the treatment of discogenic low back pain. *Spine* 2004; 4(1): 27–35.

13. Carragee EJ. The surgical treatment of disc degeneration: is the race not to be swift? *Spine* 2005; 5: 587–8.

14. Deyo RA, Nachemson A, Mirza SK. Spinal-fusion surgery: the case for restraint. *N Engl J Med* 2004; 350: 643–4.

15. Brukner PD, Bennell KL, Matheson GO. *Stress Fractures*. Melbourne: Blackwell Scientific, 1999.

16. O'Sullivan PB, Twomey LT, Allison GT. Evaluation of specific stabilizing exercises in the treatment of chronic low back pain with radiological diagnosis of spondylolysis and spondylolisthesis. *Spine* 1997; 22: 2959–67.

17. Elliot BC, Hardcastle PH, Burnett AF, et al. The influence of fast bowling and physical factors on radiologic features in high performance young fast bowlers. *Sports Train Med Rehabil* 1992; 3: 113–30.

18. Geisser ME, Wiggert EA, Haig AJ, et al. A randomized, controlled trial of manual therapy and specific adjuvant exercise for chronic low back pain. *Clin J Pain* 2005; 21: 463–70.

19. Green JP, Grenier SG, McGill SM. Low back stiffness is altered with warm up and bench rest: implications for athletes. *Med Sci Sports Exerc* 2002; 34: 1076–81.

Buttock Pain

Buttock pain is most commonly seen in athletes involved in kicking or sprinting sports. It can occur in isolation or it may be associated with low back or posterior thigh pain. Diagnosis of buttock pain can be difficult as pain may arise from a number of local structures in the buttock or can be referred from the lumbar spine or sacroiliac joint (SIJ). The causes of buttock pain are shown in Table 22.1. The anatomy of the buttock region is shown in Figure 22.1.

Clinical approach

When assessing a patient with buttock pain, the clinician should attempt to determine whether the pain is local or referred. Clues can be obtained from the nature and location of the athlete's pain. Examination may then identify which of the local or the potential pain-referring structures are causing the buttock pain. Investigation is of limited usefulness in the assessment of the patient with buttock pain.

History

A deep, aching, diffuse pain, which is variable in site, is an indication of referred pain. Buttock pain associated with low back pain suggests lumbar spine abnormality. Buttock pain associated with groin pain may suggest SIJ involvement.

When the patient is easily able to localize pain of a fairly constant nature, the source is more likely to be in the buttock region itself. Pain constantly localized to the ischial tuberosity is usually due to either tendinopathy at the origin of the hamstring muscles or ischiogluteal bursitis. Pain and tenderness more proximally situated and medial to the greater trochanter may be from the piriformis muscle.

Pain aggravated by running, especially sprinting, is not diagnostic, as most conditions causing buttock pain may be aggravated by sprinting. Increased local pain on prolonged sitting may be an indication that ischiogluteal bursitis is the cause of the problem, although lumbar spine problems can be aggravated by sitting.

Table 22.1 Causes of buttock pain

Common	Less common	Not to be missed

Referred pain
  Lumbar spine
  Sacroiliac joint
Hamstring origin
  tendinopathy
Ischiogluteal bursitis
Myofascial pain
	Piriformis conditions
	  Impingement
	  Muscle strain
	Fibrous adhesions around sciatic nerve
	Prolapsed intervertebral disk
	Chronic compartment syndrome of the
	  posterior thigh
	Stress fracture of the sacrum
	Apophysitis/avulsion fracture
	  Ischial tuberosity (children)
		Spondyloarthropathies
		  Ankylosing spondylitis
		  Reiter's syndrome (reactive arthritis)
		  Psoriatic arthritis
		  Arthritis associated with inflammatory
		    bowel disease
		Malignancy
		Bone and joint infection

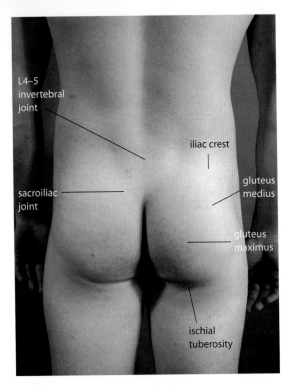

The timing of the buttock pain is of importance in establishing the nature of the diagnosis. Inflammatory pains such as that experienced in sacroiliitis as part of a spondyloarthropathy are typically worst in the morning and improve with light exercise. Such 'morning stiffness' lasts at least 30 minutes. Other features that strongly suggest the presence of spondyloarthropathy include associated enthesopathy such as Achilles tendinopathy or plantar fasciitis and multiple joint problems.

Examination

The slump test is an important part of the examination in attempting to differentiate between local and referred pain. However, not all cases of referred pain will have a positive slump test result. The lumbar spine should always be carefully examined, particularly for evidence of hypomobility of one or more intervertebral segments.

1. Observation
   (a) from behind (Fig. 22.2a)
   (b) from the side
2. Active movements—lumbar spine (Chapter 21)
   (a) flexion
   (b) extension
   (c) lateral flexion

Figure 22.1 Anatomy of the buttocks

(a) Surface anatomy

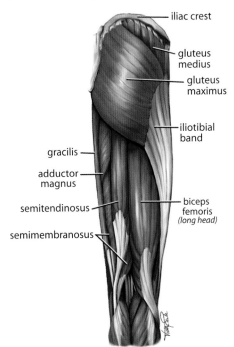

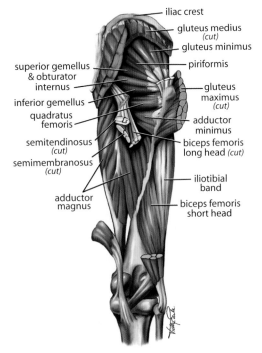

(b) Muscles of the buttock: superficial (left) and deep (right)

    (d) combined movements
3. Active movements—hip joint
    (a) flexion/extension (Fig. 22.2b)
    (b) abduction/adduction
    (c) internal/external rotation
4. Passive movements
    (a) hip movements
    (b) hip quadrant (Fig. 22.2c)
    (c) external rotator stretch (Fig. 22.2d)
5. Resisted movements
    (a) hip extension (Fig. 22.2e)
    (b) hip internal rotation (Fig. 22.2f)
    (c) hip external rotation (Fig. 22.2g)
    (d) knee flexion (Fig. 22.2h)
6. Palpation
    (a) sacroiliac joint (Fig. 22.2i)
    (b) gluteal muscles (Fig. 22.2j)
    (c) ischial tuberosity
    (d) sacrotuberous ligament
    (e) iliolumbar ligament
    (f) anterior superior iliac spines
7. Special tests
    (a) slump test (Fig. 22.2k)
    (b) lumbar spine examination (Chapter 21)
    (c) sacroiliac tests

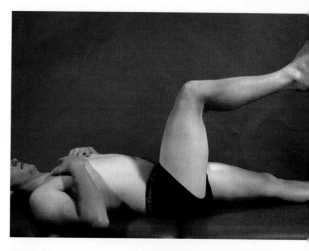

(b) Active movement—hip flexion/extension

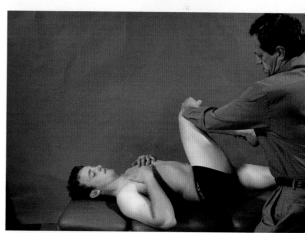

(c) Passive movement—hip quadrant. The hip joint is placed into the quadrant position, which consists of flexion, adduction and internal rotation

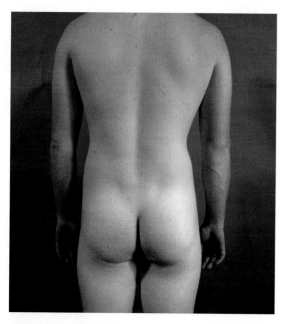

Figure 22.2 Examination of the patient with buttock pain

(a) Observation from behind may detect asymmetrical muscle wasting. Observation from the side may detect the presence of a lumbar lordosis or anterior pelvic tilt

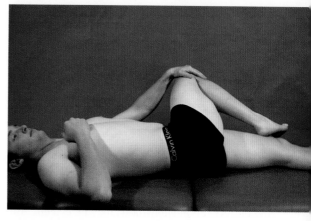

(d) Muscle stretch—external rotators

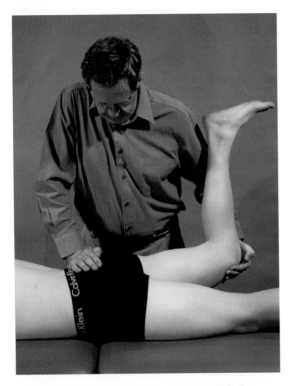

(e) Resisted movement—hip extension. With the knee flexed, this may reproduce pain arising from the gluteal muscles

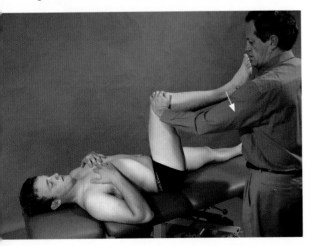

(f) Resisted movement—internal rotation

Investigations

A plain X-ray may demonstrate a stress fracture of the pars interarticularis, which may refer pain to the buttock. Spondylolisthesis may be evident. The presence of spondylolisthesis does not necessarily

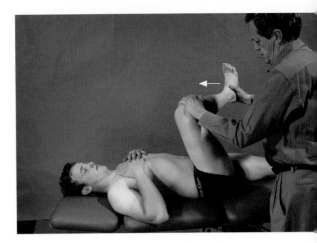

(g) Resisted movement—external rotation. Resisted external rotation from a position of internal rotation is used to isolate the piriformis muscle

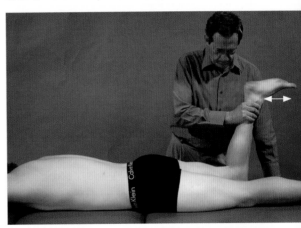

(h) Resisted movement—knee flexion. This should be performed both concentrically and eccentrically to reproduce hamstring origin pain

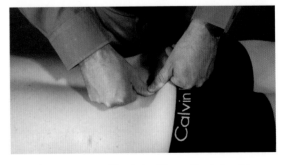

(i) Palpation—sacroiliac joint. The patient should be palpated in a posteroanterior direction over the region of the SIJ. This area also includes the iliolumbar ligament

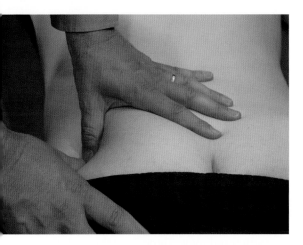

(j) Palpation—buttock. The patient should be lying prone with a pillow under the knee to place the hip into slight passive extension and relax the hip extensor muscles. Palpate from the hamstring origin across to the greater trochanter. Palpation of the gluteus medius, piriformis and the external rotators should be performed in varying degrees of hip rotation

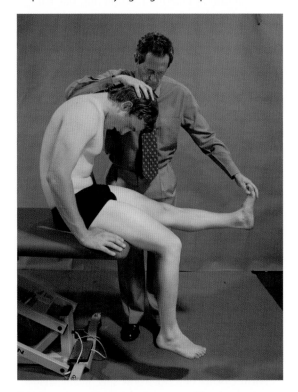

(k) Neural tension test—slump test. The slump test should be performed. Reproduction of the patient's buttock pain and alteration of the pain by alteration of neural tension is regarded as a positive slump test

mean, however, that the slip is causing the patient's pain (Chapter 21).

X-ray may also show degenerative changes in the SIJ in the older athlete. Inflammatory sacroiliitis with loss of definition of the SIJ strongly suggests a spondyloarthopathy. X-rays of the ischial tuberosity in cases of chronic hamstring origin tendinopathy are usually normal; however, occasionally erosions can be demonstrated. In the adolescent, apophysitis or avulsion of the ischial tuberosity may be demonstrated.

Isotopic bone scan may show increased uptake in the region of the SIJ or identify a stress fracture of the ischium or pubic ramus. Soft tissue ultrasound examination or MRI may image an ischiogluteal bursa or show evidence of chronic scarring at the hamstring origin.

Blood tests may indicate the presence of systemic disease. Useful screening tests are a full blood examination looking for a raised white cell count, suggesting possible infection, and erythrocyte sedimentation rate, which may be elevated in the presence of an inflammatory condition (Chapter 50).

Referred pain from the lumbar spine

Buttock pain may be referred from the lumbar spine in the presence or absence of low back pain. Any of the somatic, innervated structures of the lumbar spine may refer pain to the buttock. Abnormalities are found most often in the intervertebral disks and the apophyseal joints. Spondylolysis and spondylolisthesis may also cause buttock pain.

The patient usually gives a history of a diffuse ache in the buttock that may vary in severity. The slump test (Fig. 22.2k) may reproduce the buttock pain with relief of pain on cervical spine extension. A positive slump test result indicates increased neural tension. This may be due to damage to the nerve itself or may be secondary to lumbar spine abnormalities. Failure of the slump test to reproduce the patient's buttock pain does not necessarily rule out the possibility of referred pain as the cause of pain.

Palpation of the lumbar spine may reveal areas of tenderness and hypomobility of intervertebral segments. The best means of assessing whether a lumbar spine abnormality is the cause of buttock pain is to improve mobility of the stiff segments by mobilization or manipulation and to reassess the symptoms and signs, both immediately after treatment and prior to the next treatment.

Local areas of buttock tenderness may occur with referred pain. In cases of longstanding referred pain, soft tissue abnormalities are usually found, especially in the gluteal muscles, external rotators and lumbar multifidus. These include taut fibrous bands within muscles and general muscle tightness. Active trigger points may refer pain in a characteristic distribution.

The treatment of lumbar disorders has been described in Chapter 21 and requires an integrated approach. Local electrotherapy can reduce pain and inflammation. Mobilization or manipulation is required to restore full mobility to stiff intervertebral segments. Soft tissue therapy and dry needling may be used to treat chronic muscle thickening both around the lumbar vertebrae and in the gluteal region. Specific stretching of the gluteal muscles and hip external rotators should be commenced if there is any evidence of tightness. Neural stretches such as the slump stretch should be included if there is evidence of restriction. The patient should be shown an exercise program involving stretching and strengthening of the muscles supporting the lumbar spine (Chapter 21).

Sacroiliac joint disorders

The concept of the sacroiliac joint (SIJ) as a pain generator is now well established.[1] However, the evaluation and treatment of SIJ dysfunction remains controversial. One issue is the broad categorization and terminology utilized for the anatomical etiologies of the pain by various health professionals. Controversy also exists because of the complex anatomy and biomechanics of the SIJ.

There is no specific symptom or cluster of symptoms, nor any specific examination technique that is both sensitive and specific for the diagnosis of SIJ abnormalities. There are no imaging studies that distinguish the asymptomatic from the symptomatic patient.[1] It can only be diagnosed using local anesthetic blocks.[2] There is currently no gold standard for treatment.[1]

In patients with low back pain, the prevalence of sacroiliac pain, diagnosed by local anesthetic blocks, is 15%.[3,4] The incidence may be even higher in high level sportspeople. One study showed an incidence of over 50% in elite rowers.[5]

Functional anatomy

The SIJ is diarthrodial (synovial anterior and fibrous posterior). Its joint surfaces are reciprocally shaped but not congruent, have a high friction coefficient and have two large elevations allowing interdigitation with

the reciprocal surface. Age changes begin to occur on the iliac side of the joint as early as the third decade. The joint surface irregularities increase with age and seem to be weight-bearing related. The capsule becomes more thickened and fibrous with age.

SIJ motion is best described as a combination of flexion and extension, superior and inferior glide, and anterior and posterior translation. SIJ motion is minimal, with approximately 2.5° of rotation and 0.7 mm (0.3 in.) of translation,[2] and it is best regarded as a stress-relieving joint in conjunction with its counterpart and the pubic symphysis.

In the normal gait cycle, there are combined activities that occur conversely in the right and left innominate bones, and function in connection with the sacrum and spine. Throughout this cycle there is also rotatory motion at the pubic symphysis, which is essential to all normal motion through the joint. In static stance, when one bends forward and the lumbar spine regionally extends, the sacrum regionally flexes, with the base moving forward and the apex moving posterior. During this motion, both innominates go into a motion of external rotation and out-flaring. This combination of motion during forward flexion is referred to as nutation of the pelvis. The opposite occurs in extension and is called counternutation.

SIJ dysfunction refers to an abnormal function (e.g. hypo- or hypermobility) at the joint, which places stresses on structures in or around it. Therefore, SIJ dysfunction may contribute to lumbar, buttock, hamstring or groin pain.

The precise etiology of sacroiliac dysfunction is uncertain. Osteopaths describe a number of dysfunctions associated with hypomobility:

1. innominate shears, superior and inferior
2. innominate rotations, anterior and posterior
3. innominate in-flare and out-flare
4. sacral torsions, flexion and extension
5. unilateral sacral lesions, flexion and extension.

Vleeming and colleagues[6] have described their integrated model of joint dysfunction. It integrates structure (form and anatomy), function (forces and motor control) and the mind (emotions and awareness). Integral to the biomechanics of SIJ stability is the concept of a self-locking mechanism. The ability of the SIJ to self-lock occurs through two types of closure: form and force.

Form closure describes how specifically shaped, closely fitting contacts provide inherent stability independent of external load. Force closure describes how external compression forces add additional stability. The fascia and muscles within the region provide significant self-bracing and self-locking to the SIJ and its ligaments through their cross-like anatomical configuration.

As shown in Figure 22.3, this is formed ventrally by the external abdominal obliques, linea alba, internal abdominal obliques, and transverse abdominals; dorsally the latissimus dorsi, thoracolumbar fascia, gluteus maximus and iliotibial tract contribute significantly. Vleeming et al. further proposed that the posterior layer of the thoracolumbar fascia acted to transfer load from the ipsilateral latissimus dorsi to the contralateral gluteus maximus.[6] This load transfer is thought to be critical during rotation of the trunk, helping to stabilize the lower lumbar spine and pelvis. A connection has also been shown between the biceps femoris muscle and the sacrotuberous ligament allowing the hamstring to play an integral role in the intrinsic stability of the SIJ. The biceps femoris, which is frequently found to be shortened on the side of the SIJ dysfunction, may act to compensate to help stabilize the joint.

Clinical features

The patient with SIJ pain classically describes low back pain below L5. The pain is usually restricted to one side but may occasionally be bilateral. SIJ disorders commonly refer to the buttock, groin and posterolateral thigh. Occasionally, SIJ pain refers to the scrotum or labia.

Broadhurst[7] describes a clinically useful description of pelvic/SIJ dysfunction. Clinically, the patient has deep-seated buttock pain, difficulty in negotiating stairs and problems rolling over in bed, with a triad of signs—pain over the SIJ, tenderness over the sacrospinous and sacrotuberous ligaments, and pain reproduction over the pubic symphysis.

The physical examination[1] should begin by observation of the athlete both statically and dynamically. The patient should be evaluated in standing, supine and prone positions, and symmetry assessed in the heights of the iliac spines, anterior superior iliac spines, posterior superior iliac spines, ischial tuberosities, gluteal folds, and greater trochanters, as well as symmetry of the sacral sulci, inferior lateral angles and pubic tubercles.

Leg length discrepancy should be assessed. True leg length discrepancies will generally cause asymmetry and pain, whereas a functional leg length discrepancy is usually the result of SIJ and/or pelvic dysfunction. Dynamic observation may reveal a decrease in stride length with walking, leading to a limp, or a Trendelenburg gait due to reflex inhibition of the gluteus medius.

Muscle strength and flexibility should be assessed. Full assessment of the hips and lumbar spine should also be performed. The presence of trigger points in surrounding muscles, particularly gluteus medius, should be noted. Palpation over the SIJ may reveal local tenderness.

Numerous clinical tests have been described to assess SIJ function, but none have proven reliable. Some of the more popular tests include standing and seated flexion tests, the stork test and Patrick (Faber) test.

There is no specific gold standard imaging test to diagnose SIJ dysfunction due to the location of the joint and overlying structures that make visualization difficult.[1]

Treatment

Due to the complex nature of the SIJ and its surrounding structures, treatment must focus on the entire abdomino–lumbo–sacro–pelvic–hip complex, addressing articular, muscular, neural and fascial restrictions, inhibitions and deficiencies.[1]

Core stability training (Chapter 11) should be included. A recent study has suggested that the

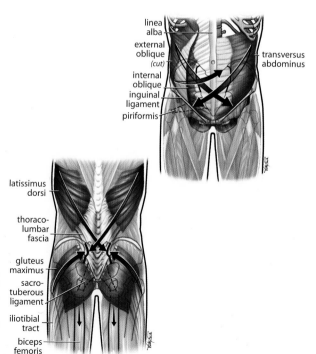

linea alba
external oblique (cut)
internal oblique
inguinal ligament
piriformis
transversus abdominus

latissimus dorsi
thoraco-lumbar fascia
gluteus maximus
sacro-tuberous ligament
iliotibial tract
biceps femoris

Figure 22.3 The cross-like configuration demonstrating the force closure of the sacroiliac joint

clinical benefits incurred with training the transversus abdominis muscle may be due to significantly reduced laxity in the SIJ.[8] Exercise rehabilitation is an integral part of recovery from SIJ dysfunction. Pelvic or SIJ dysfunction should be considered with the lumbar spine in any program designed to improve the overall control of the lumbopelvic area.

Stretching and soft tissue therapy are useful in correcting pelvic/SIJ imbalance. The most common soft tissue abnormalities found with unilateral anterior tilt are tight psoas and rectus femoris muscles. A technique to reduce psoas tightness is shown in Figure 22.4. Muscle energy techniques (Chapter 10) may also be helpful, as may osteopathic manipulation. Sacroiliac belts have not been shown to be particularly helpful.

If these manual techniques fail to control the sacroiliac pain, injection therapy may prove useful.

A combination of local anesthetic and corticosteroid agents may be injected into the region of the SIJ, as shown in Figure 22.5, either with or without fluoroscopic guidance. Sclerosants are occasionally used when hypermobility is present, sometimes referred to as prolotherapy.

Precipitating factors for the development of SIJ disorders may include muscle imbalance between the hip flexors and extensors or between the external and internal rotators of the hip, leg length imbalance and biomechanical abnormalities, such as excessive subtalar pronation.

Iliolumbar ligament sprain

The iliolumbar ligament extends from the transverse process of the fifth lumbar vertebrae to the posterior part of the iliac crest. Sprain of this ligament may cause sacroiliac pain, particularly at its iliac attachment. It is almost impossible, however, to differentiate clinically between pain from this ligament and pain from the SIJ and its associated ligaments.

Useful techniques to mobilize the soft tissues and joints of the region are shown in Figures 22.6 and 22.7. This should be combined with passive hip extension (Fig. 22.6). Injection of a mixture of local anesthetic and corticosteroid agents to the insertion of the iliolumbar ligament at the iliac crest may also be effective.

Hamstring origin tendinopathy

Tendinopathy of the hamstring origin may occur near the ischial tuberosity after an acute tear that is

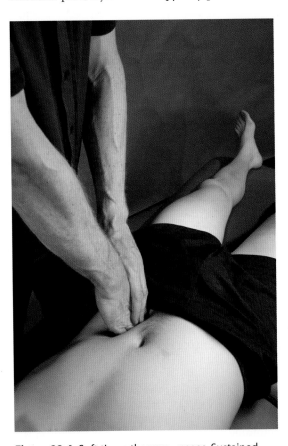

Figure 22.4 Soft tissue therapy—psoas. Sustained longitudinal pressure is applied to the psoas muscle fibers superior to the inguinal ligament with the hip initially flexed and slowly moved into increased extension

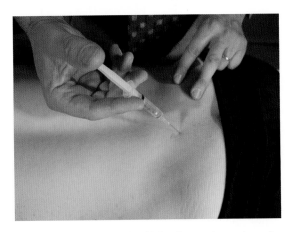

Figure 22.5 Corticosteroid injection to the region of the SIJ. Injection is directed inferolaterally

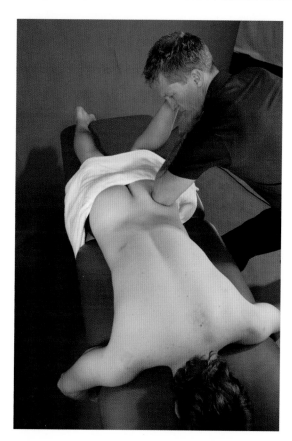

Figure 22.6 Ischemic pressure with the elbow to the origin of the hip external rotators and associated passive internal and external rotation of the hip

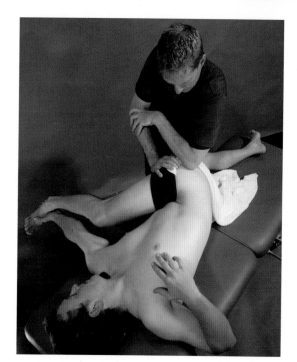

Figure 22.7 Ischemic pressure with the elbow to the hip abductors in the position of increased neural tension

inadequately treated or, more commonly, as a result of overuse.[9] It is frequently seen in sprinters.

There may be a sudden onset of sharp pain but, more often, there is an insidious onset after a session of sprinting. On examination, there is local tenderness with pain on hamstring stretch and resisted contraction. The lesion may be found at the attachment site, within the tendon or at the musculotendinous junction. The slump test may reproduce the pain but cervical extension makes little or no difference to the degree of pain.

Initial treatment of this condition should include manual therapy (Fig. 22.8), specifically deep transverse friction to the area of palpable abnormality after reduction of inflammation with ice and NSAIDs. Initial friction treatment should be relatively light. As the inflammation settles, treatment can be more vigorous. Abnormalities within the musculotendinous unit can be treated with stretching, sustained myofascial tension, and dry needling if trigger points are present.

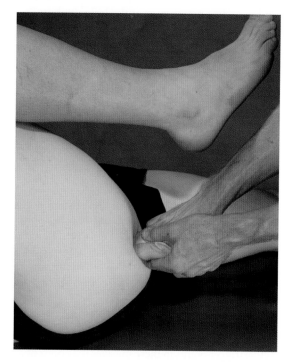

Figure 22.8 Ischemic pressure with the knuckles to the hamstring origin in the position of increased length

In longstanding cases of hamstring origin tendinopathy, there will be marked muscle tightness and weakness of the hamstring muscles, which can be corrected by stretching and progressive strengthening (Chapter 26). Successful rehabilitation also requires stretching of the shortened antagonist muscles such as psoas and rectus femoris. Recalcitrant cases may benefit from a course of shock wave treatment to the region (Chapter 10) or injection of autologous blood.

Fibrous adhesions

Occasionally, in cases of chronic tendinopathy of hamstring origin, fibrous adhesions develop and irritate the sciatic nerve as it descends from medial to lateral just above the ischial tuberosity and then passes under the biceps femoris muscle. These adhesions may fail to respond to manual therapy, particularly if they have been present for some time. On these occasions, exploration of the sciatic nerve may be required with division of the adhesions and bands of fibrous tissue. This condition has been termed the 'hamstring syndrome'.[10]

Ischiogluteal bursitis

The ischiogluteal bursa lies between the hamstring tendon and its bony origin at the ischial tuberosity. This bursa occasionally becomes inflamed. It may exist in isolation or in conjunction with hamstring origin tendinopathy.

Clinically, it is almost impossible to differentiate between ischiogluteal bursitis and hamstring origin tendinopathy as both may present as pain aggravated by sitting or sprinting, and both are associated with local tenderness with pain on muscle contraction. One indication that ischiogluteal bursitis may be the diagnosis is that deep friction therapy fails to relieve the pain.

Ultrasound examination may reveal a fluid-filled bursa. In this case, an injection of corticosteroid and local anesthetic agents into the bursa may be appropriate. As a result of pain-induced muscle inhibition, there is usually associated hamstring muscle weakness that requires comprehensive rehabilitation.

Myofascial pain

The gluteus medius and piriformis muscles are two of the most common sites at which trigger points develop. Active trigger points in these muscles may present as buttock and/or posterior thigh pain (Fig. 22.9). These muscles will be shortened (Fig. 22.2d).

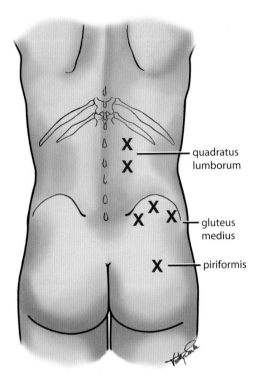

Figure 22.9 Site of trigger points which commonly refer pain to the buttock

Careful palpation of these muscles should be performed, palpating for taut bands and exquisitely tender points that may be just tender locally or may refer pain distally into the posterior thigh. Recommended treatment is dry needling, which will result in immediate lengthening of the muscles with increased hip rotation and hamstring stretch on assessment.

It is important to remember that trigger points are a secondary phenomenon. The clinician needs to be aware of the possible underlying causes, which include lumbar spine disorders and reduced lumbo-pelvic stability.

Less common causes

Stress fracture of the sacrum

Sacral stress fractures occur most frequently in female distance runners. They may be associated with osteopenia secondary to menstrual and/or eating disorders. Athletes describe unilateral, non-specific, low back, buttock or hip pain exacerbated by weight-bearing activity. The diagnosis of stress fracture may be confirmed with bone scan or MRI. Treatment consists of non-weight-bearing until free of pain (one to two weeks), then a gradual increase in activity, initially non-weight-bearing (e.g. swimming, cycling, water running), and then graduated weight-bearing. Average return to sport is eight to 12 weeks. Attention should be paid to possible causative factors.[11, 12]

Piriformis conditions

The piriformis muscle arises from the anterior surface of the sacrum and passes posterolaterally through the sciatic notch to insert into the upper border of the greater trochanter. The sciatic nerve exits the pelvis through the sciatic notch and descends immediately in front of the piriformis muscle. In 10% of the population, anatomical variations result in the sciatic nerve passing through the piriformis muscle (Fig. 22.10).[13]

In addition to the myofascial condition described above, there are two other piriformis conditions seen in athletes. One results from pressure on the sciatic nerve, usually as a result of its aberrant course through the piriformis muscle. This presents with local and referred pain and abnormal neurological symptoms in the posterior thigh and calf. Although known as the 'piriformis syndrome', this would be better referred to as 'piriformis impingement'.[14] Treatment consists of stretching and massage therapy. Surgery may be required.

The second condition is piriformis muscle strain. This may be acute or chronic and may be associated with chronic muscle shortening. It may present as deep buttock pain aggravated by sitting, climbing stairs and squats.

On examination, there is tenderness either in the belly of the piriformis or more distally near its insertion into the greater trochanter. Passive internal hip rotation is reduced and resisted abduction with the hip adducted and flexed may reproduce the pain over the piriformis. Pain may also be reproduced by resisted external rotation with the hip and knee flexed, beginning from a position of internal rotation so that end range is tested (Fig. 22.2d).

Treatment involves stretching of the external rotators (Figs 22.11a, b), electrotherapeutic modalities (e.g. ultrasound, laser, high voltage galvanic stimulation), and soft tissue therapy to the tender area in the piriformis muscle. Longitudinal gliding combined with passive internal hip rotation (Fig. 22.11c) is an effective technique, as is transverse gliding and sustained longitudinal release with the patient side-lying.

Posterior thigh compartment syndrome

This is an unusual condition that presents with the typical symptoms of a compartment syndrome, that

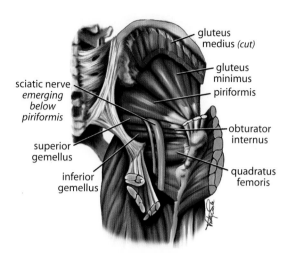

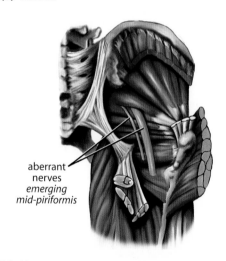

Figure 22.10 Course of the sciatic nerve in the buttock

(a) Normal

(b) Aberrant

is, pain increasing with exercise and a feeling of tightness. Pain is typically in the buttock and posterior thigh and treatment involves massage therapy and, occasionally, surgery. Limited fasciectomy involving the ischial tuberosity and upper 5 cm (2 in.) of the posterior fascia is performed.

Apophysitis/avulsion fracture of the ischial tuberosity

In adolescents, apophysitis may occur at the attachment of the hamstring muscles to the ischial tuberosity apophysis. This is frequently associated with overuse. Treatment consists of ice, restriction of activity, gentle

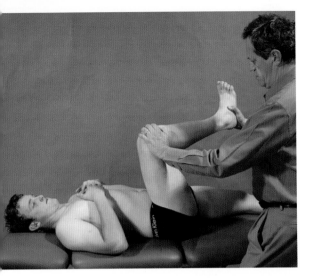

Figure 22.11 Treatment of tight piriformis muscle

(a) Muscle stretch—hip external rotators. The hip is placed into flexion, adduction and then alternated into external and internal rotation

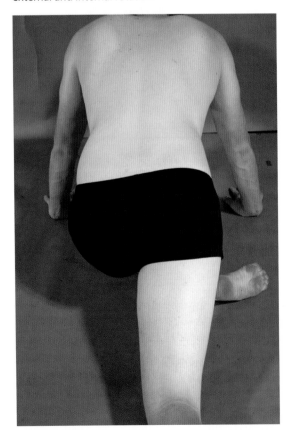

(b) Muscle stretch—external rotators

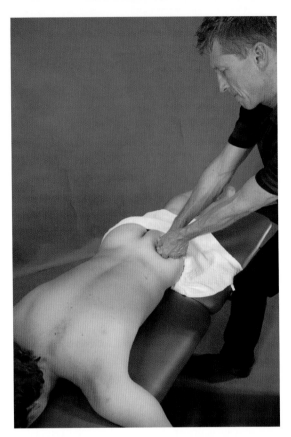

(c) Soft tissue therapy—piriformis. Sustained longitudinal pressure to the belly of the piriformis muscle, initially in passive external rotation and then moving into internal rotation (illustrated)

stretching and soft tissue therapy to overcome muscle tightness. This is a self-limiting condition.

Avulsion fracture of the ischial tuberosity is seen in adolescents where, instead of the hamstring muscle tearing, muscle traction separates a fragment of bone from its origin at the ischial tuberosity. This fragment of bone is clearly demonstrated on plain X-ray (Fig. 22.12). Management of this condition is generally conservative. The patient should be treated as for a severe (grade III) tear of the hamstring muscle (Chapter 26). However, if there is marked separation (greater than 2.5 cm [1 in.]) of the fragment, then surgery is indicated. There have been a number of reports of this injury in adults. The results of late surgical repair have been good.[15, 16]

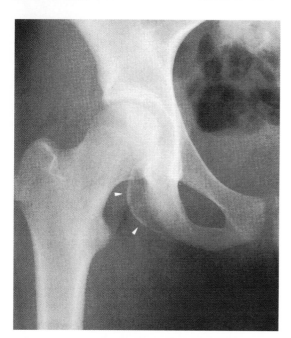

Figure 22.12 Avulsion of the ischial tuberosity

Conditions not to be missed

It should also be remembered that buttock pain may be the presenting symptom of systemic disorders, most commonly, sacroiliitis associated with spondylo-arthropathies, such as ankylosing spondylitis.

Recommended Reading

Bogduk N. *Clinical Anatomy of the Lumbar Spine and Sacrum.* 4th edn. Edinburgh: Churchill Livingstone, 2004.

Brolinson PG, Kozar AJ. Sacroiliac joint dysfunction in athletes. *Curr Sports Med Rep* 2003; 2(1): 47–56.

Vleeming A, Mooney V, Dorman T, et al. *Movement, Stability and Low Back Pain: the Essential Role of the Pelvis.* Edinburgh: Churchill Livingstone, 1997.

References

1. Brolinson PG, Kozar AJ. Sacroiliac joint dysfunction in athletes. *Curr Sports Med Rep* 2003; 2(1): 47–56.
2. Bogduk N. *Clinical Anatomy of the Lumbar Spine and Sacrum.* 4th edn. Edinburgh: Churchill Livingstone, 2004.
3. Maigne JY, Aivaliklis A, Pfeffer F. Results of sacroiliac joint double block and value of sacroiliac joint pain provocation tests in 54 patients with low back pain. *Spine* 1996; 21: 1889–92.
4. Schwartzer AC, April CD, Bogduk N. The sacroiliac joint in chronic low back pain. *Spine* 1992; 20(1): 31–7.
5. Timm KE. Sacroiliac joint dysfunction in elite rowers. *J Orthop Sports Phys Ther* 1999; 29: 288–93.
6. Vleeming A, Mooney V, Dorman T, et al. *Movement, Stability and Low Back Pain: the Essential Role of the Pelvis.* Edinburgh: Churchill Livingstone, 1997.
7. Broadhurst NA. Sacroiliac dysfunction as a cause of low back pain. *Aust Fam Physician* 1989; 18(6): 623–8.
8. Richardson CA, Snijders CJ, Hides JA, et al. The relation between the transversus abdominis muscles, sacroiliac joint mechanics, and low back pain. *Spine* 2002; 27: 399–405.
9. Fredericson M, Moore W, Guillet M, et al. High hamstring tendinopathy in runners. *Physician Sportsmed* 2005; 33(5): 32–43.
10. Puranen J, Orava S. The hamstring syndrome. A new diagnosis of gluteal sciatic pain. *Am J Sports Med* 1988; 16(5): 517–21.
11. Brukner PD, Bennell KL, Matheson GO. *Stress Fractures.* Melbourne: Blackwell Scientific, 1999.
12. Fredericson M, Salamancha L, Beaulieu C. Sacral stress fractures. Tracking down non-specific pain in distance runners. *Physician Sportsmed* 2003; 31(2): 31–42.
13. Beaton LE, Anson BJ. The relation of the sciatic nerve and its subdivision to the piriformis muscle. *Anat Rec* 1937; 70(suppl. 1): 1–5.
14. Rich BSE, McKeag D. When sciatica is not disk disease. Detecting piriformis syndrome in active patients. *Physician Sportsmed* 1992; 20(10): 105–15.
15. Cross MJ, Vandersluis R, Wood D, et al. Surgical repair of chronic complete hamstring tendon rupture in the adult patient. *Am J Sports Med* 1998; 26(6): 785–8.
16. Servant CTJ, Jones CB. Displaced avulsion of the ischial apophysis: a hamstring injury requiring internal fixation. *Br J Sports Med* 1998; 32: 255–7.

Acute Hip and Groin Pain

WITH CHRIS BRADSHAW AND PER HOLMICH

Acute hip and groin pain occurs frequently in sports involving twisting and turning and kicking such as the various football codes, especially soccer and Australian football. Symptoms can arise from various structures including the adductor muscles and tendons, the hip joint and associated muscles and bursae. Careful clinical assessment usually permits an accurate diagnosis. Appropriate treatment and respect for the conditions that cause acute pain in the groin and hip region generally lead to a rapid functional recovery. Attempting to ignore symptoms or rush return to sport can lead to longstanding exercise-related hip and groin pain, which is a diagnostic and therapeutic challenge that is the subject of Chapter 24.

Clinical approach

In patients with acute hip and groin pain it is vital to localize the area of abnormality to make an anatomical diagnosis (Fig. 23.1). The most common causes of acute hip/groin pain are strains of the adductor or, less commonly, the iliopsoas muscles, or injuries to the hip joint itself, such as a labral tear and/or chondral injury.

The clinician must not overlook the less common but important causes of pain in this region, such as an intra-abdominal abnormality (e.g. appendicitis), urinary tract abnormality, gynecological abnormality and rheumatological disorders (e.g. ankylosing spondylitis). Infections such as osteomyelitis should also be considered. A list of causes of pain in this region is shown in Table 23.1.

History

The major goals of history taking in the sportsperson presenting with acute pain in the groin and hip region

are to localize the anatomical region from which pain may be arising and identify 'red-flag' conditions when they exist. The acute onset of pain strongly suggests a muscle strain. The adductor longus is the most commonly affected muscle. The localization of the pain is also important to determine which structure may be causing the pain. Hip joint trauma can cause the athlete to present soon after injury, and skeletal conditions such as stress fractures may present with either acute or insidious onset of pain.

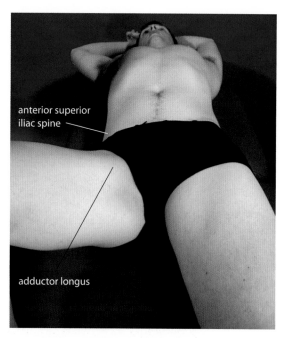

anterior superior iliac spine

adductor longus

Figure 23.1 Anatomy of the hip and groin area

(a) Surface anatomy

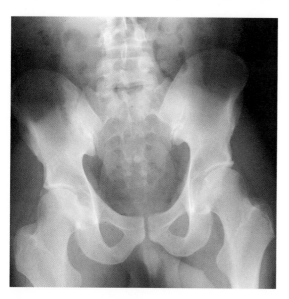

(b) Plain X-ray of the pelvis

iliacus

psoas

iliopsoas

inguinal ligament

pubic tubercle

tensor fascia latae

pectineus

rectus femoris

adductor longus

gracilis

(c) Muscles of the hip and groin region

Examination

Each region of the hip and groin that has the potential to produce pain must be examined. This includes the adductor muscles, the hip flexors and the hip joint.

Examination involves:

1. Observation
   (a) standing
   (b) walking (Fig. 23.2a)
   (c) supine

2. Active movements
   (a) hip flexion/extension
   (b) hip abduction/adduction
   (c) hip internal/external rotation
   (d) circumduction test

Table 23.1 Causes of acute hip and groin pain

Common	Less common	Not to be missed
Adductor muscles	Iliopsoas strain	Slipped capital femoral epiphysis[a]
Muscle strain	Trochanteric bursitis	Intra-abdominal abnormality
Tendinopathy[a]	Stress fracture[a]	Appendicitis
Hip joint	Neck of femur	Prostatitis
Synovitis	Pubic ramus	Urinary tract infections
Labral tear	Acetabulum	Gynecological conditions
Chondral lesion	Referred pain[a]	
	Lumbar spine	
	Sacroiliac joint	
	Infection	
	Osteomyelitis	
	'Snapping' hip	
	Rectus femoris muscle strain (upper third)	
	Avulsion apophysitis/fracture	
	Anterior superior iliac spine	
	Anterior inferior iliac spine (adolescents)	

(a) Conditions that more commonly present as hip and groin pain of gradual onset but may have an acute presentation. These conditions are described more fully in Chapter 24.

3. Passive movements
   (a) adductor muscle stretch (Fig. 23.2b)
   (b) hip quadrant—flexion, adduction, internal
       rotation (Fig. 23.2c)
   (c) internal rotation, then with added adduction
   (d) flexion, abduction and external rotation
       (FABER or Patrick's test) (Fig. 23.2d)
   (e) quadriceps muscle stretch
   (f) psoas muscle stretch/impingement (Thomas
       position) (Fig. 23.2e)
4. Resisted movements
   (a) hip flexion (Fig. 23.2f)
   (b) hip adduction
5. Palpation
   (a) adductor muscles/tendons (Fig. 23.2g)
   (b) iliopsoas
6. Functional movements
   (a) hopping (to reproduce pain)
7. Special tests
   (a) standing Trendelenberg test

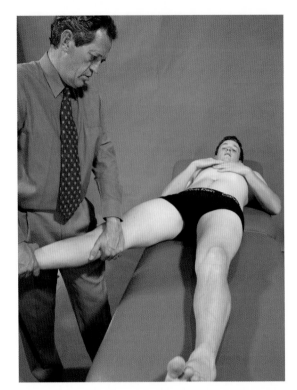

(b) Passive movement—adductor muscle stretch

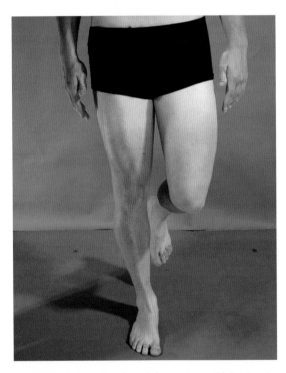

Figure 23.2 Examination of the patient with hip/groin pain

(a) Observation—patient walking. Assess lower limb alignment from in front, particularly for evidence of excessive internal or external hip rotation and muscle wasting. Assess lumbar postural abnormalities from the side

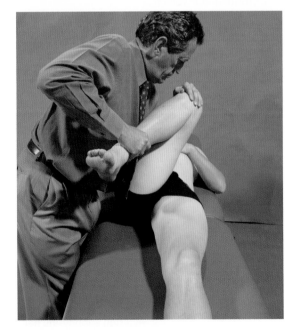

(c) Passive movement—hip quadrant (flexion, adduction and internal rotation). This is a combined movement that is performed if hip range of motion is normal in single planes

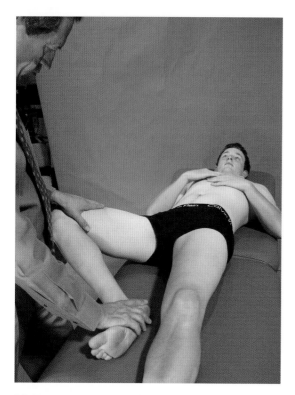

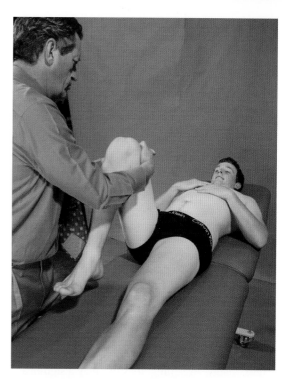

(f) Resisted movement—hip flexion

(d) Passive movement—flexion, abduction and external rotation (FABER or Patrick's) test. Range of motion, apart from extreme stiffness/laxity, is not that relevant. Some caution needs to be exercised, as it is possible to sublux an unstable hip in this position. Pain felt in the groin is very non-specific. Pain in the buttock is more likely to be due to sacroiliac joint problems. However, pain felt over the greater trochanter suggests hip joint pathology

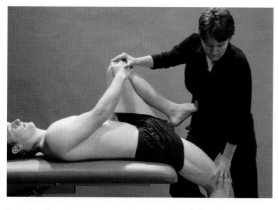

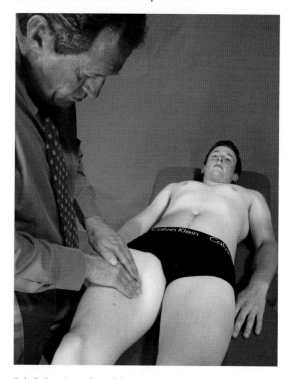

(e) Passive movement—psoas stretch (Thomas position). Pain in the hip being stretched suggests psoas abnormality. Pain in the hip being compressed can be significant for anterior impingement of the hip joint

(g) Palpation. The adductor muscles and tendons are carefully palpated

Investigations

X-ray of the pelvis has a limited role in investigation of acute hip and groin pain. Ultrasound may be useful in imaging muscle tears. MRI is used to image the hip joint, especially to detect labral tears, as well as soft tissue changes in the adductor muscles and tendons.

Adductor muscle strains

Adductor muscle strains are a common injury in sports that involve sudden changes of direction. The onset is acute and pain is usually well localized, either to the belly of the adductor longus, the proximal musculotendinous junction or the tendon near its origin on the inferior pubic ramus. Examination findings are localized tenderness, pain on passive abduction and pain on resisted adduction or combined flexion/adduction.

Treatment commences with initial reduction of bleeding and swelling using the RICE regimen (Chapter 10). Due to concerns that early stretching may predispose to the development of chronic tendinopathy, stretching does not play a significant role in the management of adductor muscle strains. Progressive strengthening exercises should not be commenced until at least 48 hours after injury. It is not until passive range of motion returns to normal, with full strength, that activities involving rapid change of direction can be recommended. The treatment regimen is summarized below.

1. 0–48 hours
   (a) RICE
   (b) active pain-free exercises
2. After first 48 hours
   (a) gradually increase strengthening
      (i) active abduction/adduction
      (ii) adduction/flexion against resistance (e.g. rubber tube, pulleys, light weights)
      (iii) stabilizing exercises (e.g. pulleys with other leg, one-leg squats)
   (b) functional strengthening
      (i) bike
      (ii) pool running
      (iii) jogging
      (iv) swimming
   (c) sport-specific skills
      (i) running—straight line
      (ii) running—figure of eight
      (iii) rapid changes of direction
      (iv) kicking—gradually increase

Recurrent adductor muscle strain

Recurrent adductor muscle strains are common. This may be due to inadequate rehabilitation of the initial injury, resuming sport too quickly or not resolving associated problems such as lumbar spine stiffness or pelvic imbalance. If untreated, these injuries can lead to chronic exercise-related groin pain.

In order to find the cause of adductor abnormalities in running athletes, it may be necessary to analyze running technique. The adductors play a major role in dampening the contraction of the gluteus medius after the propulsion phase of running. They also work synergistically with the hip abductors to maintain the stability of the pelvis during the stance phase. Thus, pelvic stability is required to prevent excessive eccentric load on the adductors.

Acute presentation of adductor tendinopathy

Adductor tendinopathy may begin as a primary condition or, alternatively, may occur secondary to an adductor muscle strain. It is believed in some centers that the treatment of an acute adductor muscle strain should include ice and rest, but that stretching the muscle should not begin until at least four days after the injury. It may be that premature stretching of these muscles can lead to a tendinopathy.

Adductor tendinopathy causes proximal groin pain, which has a tendency to develop with increasing activity. If the condition remains untreated, the pain tends to persist during activity and may migrate either to the contralateral groin or to the suprapubic region. Examination findings include local tenderness over the adductor origin and over the pubic tubercle, with pain on passive hip abduction and resisted hip adduction.

Treatment of an acute presentation includes a few days relative rest from the aggravating activity, followed by a gradual progression of adductor strengthening.

Iliopsoas strains

The iliopsoas muscle is the strongest flexor of the hip joint. The iliopsoas muscle is shown in Figure 23.3. It arises from the five lumbar vertebrae and the ilium and inserts into the lesser trochanter of the femur. It is occasionally injured acutely but frequently becomes tight with neural restriction.

Iliopsoas problems may occur as an overuse injury resulting from excessive hip flexion, such as kicking.

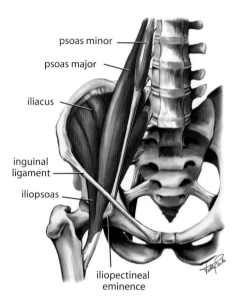

- psoas minor
- psoas major
- iliacus
- inguinal ligament
- iliopsoas
- iliopectineal eminence

Figure 23.3 The iliopsoas muscle

They present as a poorly localized ache that patients usually describe as being a deep ache in one side of the groin. They are also a common injury in sprinters.

Direct palpation of the iliopsoas muscle is difficult in its proximal portion as it lies deep within the pelvis. The skilled examiner may detect tenderness in thin athletes by palpating carefully with the muscle positioned appropriately in passive hip flexion. Pain on iliopsoas stretch (Fig. 23.2e) that is exacerbated on resisted hip flexion in the stretch position suggests the iliopsoas as the source of the pain. It is important to examine the lumbar spine as there is frequently an association between iliopsoas tightness and hypomobility of the upper lumbar spine from which the muscle originates.

Treatment consists of avoiding aggravating activity, stretching of the psoas muscle (Fig. 23.2e) and strengthening involving resisted hip flexion exercises. Often, mobilization of the lumbar intervertebral joints at the origin of the iliopsoas muscles will result in an increase in muscle length.

Hip joint injuries

WITH BRUCE MITCHELL

Hip joint injuries can be difficult to diagnose as they often present in association with other painful pathologies generating problems. The patient may present with a confusing pain pattern; pain may derive from the pelvis and back, as well as from the soft tissues surrounding the hip.

Mechanisms of hip injuries include high-velocity trauma (e.g. motor racing accident, equestrian) and overuse injuries in which altered biomechanics affect energy transference between the lower limb and trunk.

Clinical features

Pain from the hip joint may be felt in a number of areas. Colson et al. recorded the areas of pain in 81 patients awaiting hip arthroscopy and found that the most common areas of significant (Visual Analog Scale >4) pain were deep inside the hip (58%), groin (51%), outside of hip (45%) and low back (42%).[1] The pain is commonly a dull ache, although it may be associated with a clicking or catching sensation. The pain may be referred to the anterior aspect of the knee.

The hip may be inflamed as part of a generalized rheumatological disorder. Primary idiopathic osteoarthritis of the hip may be seen in the older athlete. The pain of an osteoarthritic hip may be worse in the mornings or after activity. Septic arthritis of the hip is rare.

In children between 5 and 12 years, Perthes' disease should be considered, while in older adolescents between the ages of 12 and 16 years, a slipped capital femoral epiphysis may cause hip pain. A young patient with a slipped capital femoral epiphysis may present with very little pain and may simply present with a painless limp. These conditions are fully described in Chapter 40.

Examination

No one test is definitive for hip joint pathology. However, there are a number of tests used to assess irritation and restriction of the hip joint itself. These include: the circumduction test; hip quadrant flexion, adduction and internal rotation (Fig. 23.2c); internal rotation with added adduction; flexion, abduction and external rotation (FABER or Patrick's test) (Fig. 23.2d); and the impingement test (Fig. 23.2e).

It is unusual to find a case of an injured hip that does not have coexisting iliopsoas dysfunction. The reason for this is not known, but possible causes include direct irritation of the iliopsoas as it crosses the anterior aspect of the hip joint; the iliopsoas being recruited as a secondary stabilizer; and the iliopsoas being overloaded as a hip flexor due to restriction in hip movement.

Findings on examination due to iliopsoas dysfunction include:

1. myofascial tightness in the iliopsoas muscle on abdominal palpation

2. tenderness and thickening of the mid-lumbar facets (L3–4) on lumbar palpation
3. restricted extension on modified Thomas testing.

There is usually inhibition of the ipsilateral transversus abdominis in cases of hip joint pathology. This causes a loss of force closure across the ipsilateral SIJ, resulting in ipsilateral innominate instability. This is evidenced on examination by a positive pelvic stabilization assessment test (PSAT). This is performed with the patient supine. The patient is asked to actively raise their contralateral leg as far as possible; the degree of flexion is recorded. This procedure is repeated with the ipsilateral leg. Once these two readings have been recorded, a compression force is applied to the ilia by the examiner and the patient repeats the straight leg raises. The side with the unstable innominate will usually be raised further when the examiner locks the pelvis. Further, the patient may state that it was easier to raise the leg, or they feel less pain. A positive 'Trendelenberg stability test' (TST) may also be present.

There is frequently evidence of peripelvic instability. This is evidenced by weakness in the ipsilateral gluteus medius muscle, weakness and timing deficit (late onset) of the ipsilateral gluteus maximus muscle, tenderness and a 'sharpness' to palpation of the L5–S1 facet on lumbar palpation, and an inability to shunt weight onto the affected leg while walking (leans with shoulders).

Neural pathologies can contribute to hip pain. The cause for this can be multifactorial. The piriformis syndrome (Chapter 22) may be a factor as the piriformis abuts the posterior aspect of the hip. A classic radiculopathy with minimal straight leg raise suggests lumbar disk disease. If there is confusion between a disk and the hip joint as the source of the patient's pain, one approach is to undertake soft tissue treatment to the piriformis, gluteus minimus and gluteus medius muscles, and then to reassess for effectiveness. If the neurological signs are eased, they are much more likely to be due to piriformis problems secondary to a hip injury.

Signs of neurological compromise are weakness of the L4, L5 or S1 nerve roots, decreased sensation of the L4, L5 or S1 nerve roots, decreased distal reflexes, restricted straight leg raise, and positive slump test.

Investigations

Investigations include plain radiographs of the pelvis and lateral views of the hip. A full pelvis view is necessary to be able to assess the hip joint for the presence of dysplasia and to compare the two sides. Pathology seen on plain X-ray of the hip is often missed or referred to as a normal variant.

Evidence of dysplasia (Fig. 23.4) includes a short or angled roof, and signs of acute/chronic impingement, such as an os acetabulae (often mistakenly called a normal variant), femoral bossing, Ganz lesions and impingement cysts (often called synovial pits).

A 'Ganz' lesion is a thickening or bump on the superior femoral neck in response to chronic impingement in this area. The thickening of the bone then causes worsening impingement and a vicious cycle develops. The thickened bone often needs to be surgically resected in the elite athlete.

Low postural tone or a torn ligamentum teres may be diagnosed with traction views. If a slipped capital femoral epiphysis is suspected but not confirmed on plain X-ray, or if a stress fracture is suspected, a bone scan or MRI is indicated.

The reliability of MRI in diagnosing intra-articular pathology is controversial. Several early studies claimed more than 90% accuracy for MRI arthrography with injection of the contrast medium gadolinium, however, these studies had major methodological flaws. More recent papers have cast doubt on this accuracy.[2] High-quality, narrow-slice proton density scans in the plane of the hip joint may improve accuracy, but these still have an accuracy below 80% in detecting any pathology, and 50% at best for making the right diagnosis.

Injection of the hip joint with local anesthetic with post-injection assessment of pain using a pain

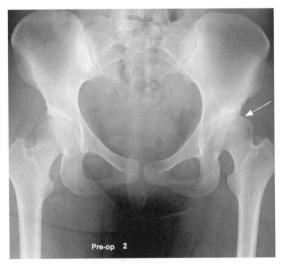

Pre-op 2

Figure 23.4 X-ray of hip showing acetabular dysplasia (arrow)

chart is probably about 70% accurate. This accuracy can be improved by examining the hip pre- and post-injection.

Arthroscopy of the hip joint remains the most sensitive and specific investigation. In patients presenting with pain in the areas described and hip joint signs on examination, the clinician should maintain a high index of suspicion for labral injury, irrespective of the results of imaging.

Thus, if the clinician has a high index of suspicion of hip joint pathology, examination of the hip under local anesthetic or early arthroscopy is warranted.

Synovitis

Synovitis is a complication of most hip injuries but can present as the primary problem, particularly when associated with rheumatological conditions. It usually responds well to X-ray guided injections of corticosteroid.

Labral tears

With the increasing use of MRI and hip arthroscopy (Fig. 23.5), labral tears of the hip joint are being increasingly recognized as a cause of hip pain. The mechanism of injury can be due to extrinsic or intrinsic mechanisms.

Extrinsic mechanisms include:

- motor vehicle accidents
- lateral impact syndrome (landing on the side of the hip)
- lifting/twisting incidents
- squatting/loading
- twisting on a weight-bearing hip (athletes)
- passive impingement (e.g. in cyclists, horse riders, truck drivers, builders up ladders)
- active impingement (e.g. in dancers, martial arts, water polo).

Intrinsic mechanisms include:

- instability:
  — dysplasia (congenital and acquired)
  — low postural tone
  — torn ligamentum teres
  — incongruity of femoral head
- structural impingement:
  — pistol grip deformity (old slipped capital femoral epiphysis)
  — femoral bossing
  — Ganz lesions.

The natural history of an untreated acetabular labral tear is slow but progressive degeneration to

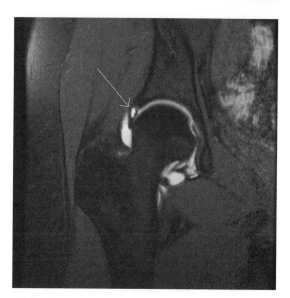

Figure 23.5 Labral tear

(a) Arthrogram

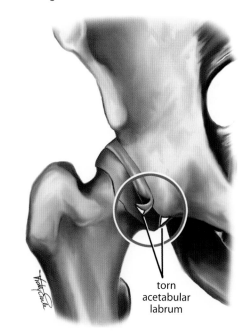

torn acetabular labrum

(b) Pathology

degenerative hip joint disease. Treatment of these injuries involves arthroscopic debridement of the torn part of the labrum. Generally the results of arthroscopic surgery have been good, especially in those with minimal or no associated chondral damage (see below).[3–6]

Chondral lesions

Chondral injuries (Fig. 23.6a) may occur in association with labral tears but also with a number of other hip conditions such as loose bodies, posterior dislocation, osteonecrosis, slipped capital femoral epiphysis, dysplasia and osteoarthritis. The common initiating site for labral as well as chondral injuries has been termed 'the watershed zone'. The watershed lesion, which occurs at the labrochondral junction, may destabilize adjacent articular cartilage. It is postulated that when the damaged labral cartilage is subjected to repetitive loading conditions, joint fluid is pumped beneath the acetabular chondral cartilage causing delamination of the articular cartilage. By this same mechanism, the fluid eventually burrows beneath subchondral bone to form a subchondral cyst.[7] This cyst is the result, not the cause, of the symptoms (Fig. 23.6b).[8]

Outcomes of surgical treatment are directly dependent on the degree and extent of the labral and chondral lesions.[4, 8]

Other hip injuries

Loose bodies

Loose bodies in the hip are relatively rare but can present with catching and locking of the hip joint. Occasionally they are associated with synovial chondromatosis. Loose bodies may not appear on X-ray and usually need to be removed arthroscopically.

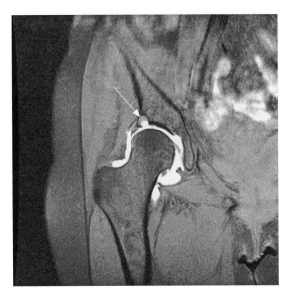

(b) Subchondral cyst (arrow)

Tears of the ligamentum teres

Tears of the ligamentum teres[9] can occur in major trauma, but also occur in athletes trying to achieve more hip abduction, such as in gymnastics, dance and aerobics. This can lead to some instability of the hip joint. Scarring after the tear can cause a 'cyclops' lesion and catching/clunking of the hip. These scars usually need arthroscopic debridement if rehabilitation does not ease the symptoms.

Trochanteric bursitis/gluteus medius tendinopathy

Long-distance runners can present with fairly acute onset of pain in the lateral hip region about the greater trochanter that may radiate down the lateral aspect of the thigh. This can be due to bursitis in one of several bursae around the hip (Fig. 23.7) and it is aggravated by activities involving hip movements, such as climbing stairs and getting out of a car.

The anatomy of the greater trochanter and its associated tendons and bursae is shown in Figure 23.7. There are two bursae around the greater trochanter. The gluteus medius bursa lies beneath the tendon of the gluteus medius and medial to the greater trochanter. The trochanteric bursa is lateral to the greater trochanter.

Gluteus medius tendinopathy/enthesopathy and bursitis often exist together. The site of tenderness in these conditions is typically immediately above

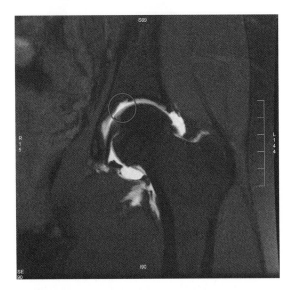

Figure 23.6 MRI scans of chrondral lesions

(a) Chondral lesion (acetabular side)

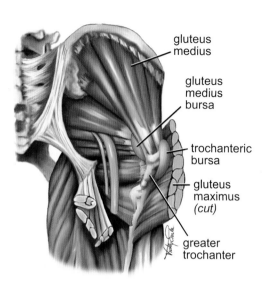

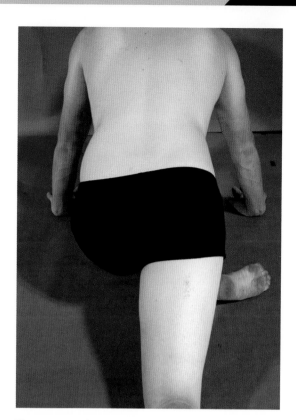

Figure 23.7 Anatomy of the greater trochanter and surrounds

the greater trochanter and pain can be reproduced on stretching the gluteus medius.

Treatment for these conditions involves initial rest from aggravating activities, stretching (Fig. 23.8) and strengthening of the gluteus medius. Corticosteroid injection may be required and should be placed into the area of maximal tenderness above and behind the greater trochanter. As the conditions are often associated with biomechanical abnormality, muscle tightness or excessive lateral tilt of the pelvis, pelvic stability exercises may play an important role in treatment.

Specific concerns for adolescents

A number of specific conditions may cause acute hip and groin pain in adolescents. Conditions of the hip joint such as Perthes' disease and a slipped capital femoral epiphysis have already been mentioned and are described more fully in Chapter 40. Epiphyseal fractures may also occur.

Acute avulsion fractures and chronic apophysitis occur in adolescents as a result of excessive muscle contraction. The most common site is the attachment of the long head of the rectus femoris from the anterior inferior iliac spine.

Avulsion fractures present as an acute onset of anterior hip pain with marked loss of function. On

Figure 23.8 Gluteus medius stretch

examination, there is considerable localized tenderness and restriction of movement. In most cases, these should be treated as for a severe rectus femoris strain. Surgical reattachment of the avulsed fragment is usually not necessary but may be required when the fragment is separated from the bone by greater than 3 cm (1.5 in.). Rehabilitation is required for up to three months.

Recommended Reading

Ekstrand J, Hilding J. The incidence and differential diagnosis of acute groin injuries in male soccer players. *Scand J Med Sci Sports* 1999; 9(2): 98–103.

Larson CM, Swaringen J, Morrison G. Evaluation and management of hip pain. *Physician Sportsmed* 2005; 33(10): 26–32.

McCarthy JC, Lee J. Hip arthroscopy: indications, outcomes, and complications. *J Bone Joint Surg Am* 2005; 87A: 1138–44.

Narvani AA, Tsiridis E, Tai CC, et al. Acetabular labrum and its tears. *Br J Sports Med* 2003; 37: 207–11.

References

1. Colson E, Mitchell B, Brukner P, et al. The area of pain of patients undergoing hip arthroscopic surgery. *Clin J Sport Med* 2006; in press.

2. Mitchell B, Lee B, Brukner PD, et al. Correlation of hip arthroscopy findings and different MRI techniques. A review of 99 cases. *J Sci Med Sport* 2003; 6(4 suppl.): 48.

3. Byrd JW, Jones KS. Prospective analysis of hip arthroscopy with 2-year follow-up. *Arthroscopy* 2000; 16(6): 578–87.

4. Farjo LA, Glick JM, Sampson TG. Hip arthroscopy for acetabular labral tears. *Arthroscopy* 1999; 15(2): 132–7.

5. O'Leary JA, Berend K, Vail TP. The relationship between diagnosis and outcome in arthroscopy of the hip. *Arthroscopy* 2001; 17(2): 181–8.

6. Santori N, Willar RN. Acetabular labral tears: result of arthroscopic partial limbectomy. *Arthroscopy* 2000; 16(1): 11–15.

7. McCarthy JC, Noble PC, Schuck MR, et al. The role of labral lesions to development of early degenerative hip disease. *Clin Orthop* 2001; 393: 25–7.

8. McCarthy JC, Lee J. Hip arthroscopy: indications, outcomes, and complications. *J Bone Joint Surg Am* 2005; 87A: 1138–45.

9. Byrd JW, Jones KS. Traumatic rupture of the ligamentum teres as a source of hip pain. *Arthroscopy* 2004; 20(4): 385–91.

Longstanding Groin Pain

WITH CHRIS BRADSHAW AND PER HOLMICH

Acute injuries to the hip and groin region have been discussed in Chapter 23. In this chapter we discuss the common presentation of exercise-related groin pain, frequently of a longstanding nature.

The anatomy of the groin area is shown in Figures 23.1 and 24.1.

Epidemiology, terminology and pathogenesis

Longstanding groin pain in athletes has been recognized in activities that combine high running loads, rapid changes of direction, and kicking.[1] The two most common sports associated with this syndrome are soccer and Australian football, which both require players to run fast and kick across the body. Longstanding groin pain is also a major concern in basketball, American football, Rugby and field hockey.

'Osteitis pubis' and other popular diagnoses

Non-specific exercise-related groin pain has been given many different 'diagnostic' labels; by far the most popular have been osteitis pubis (UK, Europe and Australia) and athletic pubalgia (North America). The term osteitis pubis was originally used to describe an infectious or inflammatory complication of suprapubic surgery.[2] It was subsequently used to describe the syndrome of exercise-related groin pain associated with radiographic bony changes at the symphysis pubis and/or increased uptake on radionuclide bone scan in the pubic symphysis. More recently, 'osteitis pubis' has become an umbrella term for all exercise-related groin pain in athletes. However, as longstanding groin pain is rarely inflammatory in nature, and the finding of increased uptake on bone

scan is not universal, the term osteitis pubis seems inappropriate. Thus, we, and an increasing number of clinicians who work with sportspeople, are avoiding the term 'osteitis pubis' when diagnosing longstanding groin pain. The term is both inaccurate with regard to pathology and confusing as it means different things to different people.

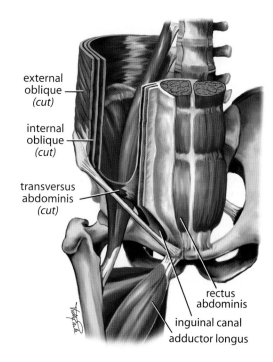

external oblique *(cut)*

internal oblique *(cut)*

transversus abdominis *(cut)*

rectus abdominis

inguinal canal

adductor longus

Figure 24.1 Anatomy of the groin area

(a) Muscles of the abdominal wall

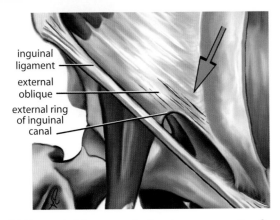

inguinal ligament

external oblique

external ring of inguinal canal

(b) External oblique muscle showing common site of tears

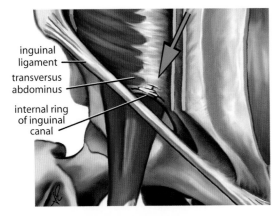

inguinal ligament

transversus abdominus

internal ring of inguinal canal

(c) Transversus abdominis muscle showing common site of tears

Other 'diagnoses' of longstanding exercise-related groin pain include adductor tendinopathy/enthesopathy, iliopsoas dysfunction, posterior inguinal wall deficiency, sportsperson's hernia, sports hernia, tear of external oblique aponeurosis, Gilmore's groin and chronic adductor muscle strain. However, even though some clinicians believe that all longstanding groin pain in athletes has a single specific diagnosis, this is unlikely.

Local overload causing failure of various structures

Our clinical experience suggests that longstanding groin pain can be the end result of a number of different pathologies. By the time pain has been experienced for months, several pathologies may be present. The fundamental etiology is that mechanical *overload* of the pelvic region (i.e. due to sport) causes

failure of local tissue—muscle, tendon or bone alone or in combination.

 PEARL Expanding on Holmich et al.'s concept of three 'diagnostic entities,'[3] we assess the patient for evidence of one or more of four clinical entities (Table 24.1).

In our experience, usually more than one entity is present by the time the problem is recognized (Fig. 24.2). This is because they may have a common cause, or because the condition may commence as a single entity which then progresses to involve other areas. An example of how this develops is shown in the box.

Table 24.1 Four clinical entities that may be involved in longstanding groin pain

Clinical entity	Pathological elements likely to underpin the entity
Adductor related[3]	Musculotendinous injuries, enthesopathy, neuromyofascial
Iliopsoas related[3]	Neuromyofascial tightness, iliopsoas tendinopathy, lumbar spine abnormalities, iliopsoas bursitis (uncommon)
Abdominal wall related[4]	Posterior inguinal wall weakness, conjoint tendon tear, external oblique aponeurosis tear
Pubic bone stress related[5]	Stress reaction or stress fracture of the pubic bone

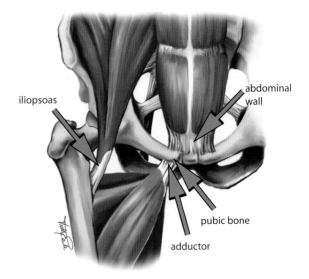

iliopsoas

abdominal wall

pubic bone

adductor

Figure 24.2 Overlapping clinical entities in longstanding groin pain in athletes

How multiple clinical entities may develop

A soccer player develops an overuse problem in the adductor region and gradually the pain is concentrated at the adductor longus insertion at the inferior pubic bone. After a period of continued soccer playing the iliopsoas muscle becomes painful as well. It becomes a little tight and develops tender points. The tendon insertion is thicker on ultrasound examination. The athlete now has two causes of pain in the groin region.

Late in a match, as a result of not being able to control the pelvis properly because of the painful adductors and the iliopsoas not working properly, the athlete develops a small avulsion/lesion of the conjoint tendon affecting the inguinal canal, leading to signs of an 'incipient hernia'.

The original cause of overuse of the adductors (or iliopsoas, lower abdominals, etc.) could be a range of problems, such as muscular pelvic instability, decreased range of motion in the hip joint for a number of reasons, generalized poor physical condition compared to the level of physical activity, pain/injury elsewhere leading to compensatory movements affecting the pelvis, and so on. The athlete also might have some dysfunction related to the low back/thoracolumbar region or the SIJ.

What role does bone stress play?

Whether pubic bone stress causing groin pain is an entity that arises de novo or whether it must be preceded by failure of the local stabilizing structures (e.g. adductors, iliopsoas, abdominal wall) is a current area of debate and research. Australian sports physician Geoff Verrall[5] found MRI evidence of bone marrow edema in a large percentage (77%) of footballers presenting with longstanding groin pain and associated pubic symphysis tenderness. He proposed that pubic bone stress was a possible cause of the symptoms. Danish surgeon Per Holmich believes that pubic bone stress arises because bending and/or torsional forces acting through the pelvis have become unbalanced.[3] He contends that at least one of his three 'primary' diagnostic entities generally precedes pubic bone stress, and thus, suggests that clinical assessment and treatment focus on those entities.

It is possible that pubic bone stress is the result of one or more of the other three clinical entities listed in Table 24.1. To use Kibler's terms in relation to shoulder injuries, the pubic bone may be a 'victim' rather than the 'culprit' in longstanding groin pain. A number of factors lead to stress on the pubic bones and an excess of one or more of these stressors, or an imbalance between them, may lead to pubic bone stress.

Factors that increase local bone stress

A number of abnormalities in joints and muscles around the groin may increase the mechanical stress placed on the pubic region (Fig. 24.3):

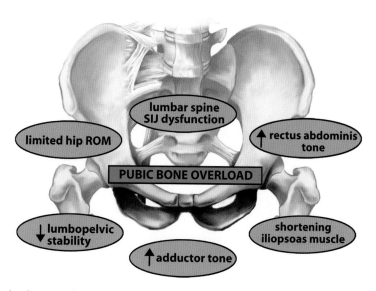

Figure 24.3 Factors leading to pubic bone overload

1. Limited hip range of motion[6–8]—this may be due to:
   (a) intra-articular hip pathology (e.g. dysplasia, labral tear, chondral lesion)
   (b) joint capsule tightness[8]
   (c) extra-articular myofascial tightness (e.g. gluteal muscle tightness associated with trigger points)
2. Increased adductor muscle tone
   (a) after an acute adductor strain
   (b) due to chronic tightness (associated with adductor muscle trigger points)
3. Increased rectus abdominis tone
4. Iliopsoas muscle shortening often associated with hypomobility of upper lumbar intervertebral joints
5. Lumbar spine/SIJ dysfunction
   (a) hypomobile intervertebral joint(s)
   (b) SIJ stiffness[9, 10]
6. Decreased lumbopelvic stability
   (a) reduced transversus abdominis (TA) activation[11]—TA provides compression of the pelvic ring anteriorly, contributing to the mechanical stability of the joint[12]
   (b) impaired pelvic floor muscle function—the pelvic floor muscles contribute to tension of the pelvic ring[13]

Clinical approach

The aim of the clinical examination is to assess the various components of the athlete's pain, particularly the clinical entities (Table 24.1). Also, it is important to consider stress fractures, hip joint pathology (Chapter 23), and referred pain from the lumbar spine (Chapter 21) or SIJ (Chapter 22). As always, a thorough examination includes attention to possible contributing factors that have led to the longstanding groin pain.

In addition, longstanding groin pain can arise from intra-abdominal, urinary tract or gynecological abnormalities, as well as rheumatological disorders (e.g. ankylosing spondylitis). Patients with tumors, such as testicular tumors, occasionally present with groin pain. A list of causes of longstanding groin pain is shown in Table 24.2.

History

The athlete experiences an insidious onset of groin pain, which is usually felt in one or both proximal pubic bones, and/or one or both proximal adductors, but may be centered on the lower abdomen or inguinal regions. The pain frequently starts in one region and is unilateral and then spreads to other regions and can

Table 24.2 Causes of longstanding groin pain

Common	Less common	Not to be missed
Adductor related	Hip joint	Slipped capital femoral epiphysis
Tendinopathy	Osteoarthritis	Perthes' disease (adolescents)
Neuromyofascial tightness	Chondral lesion	Intra-abdominal abnormality
Iliopsoas related	Labral tear	Prostatitis
Neuromyofascial tightness	'Snapping' hip	Urinary tract infections
Tendinopathy	Stress fracture	Gynecological conditions
Bursitis[a]	Neck of femur	Spondyloarthropathies
Abdominal wall related	Pubic ramus	Ankylosing spondylitis
Posterior inguinal wall weakness	Acetabulum	Avascular necrosis of the head of the femur
Tear of external oblique	Nerve entrapment	Tumors
aponeurosis	Obturator	Testicular
'Gilmore's groin'	Ilioinguinal	Osteoid osteoma
Rectus abdominis tendinopathy	Genitofemoral	
Pubic-bone related	Referred pain	
Pubic bone stress	Lumbar spine	
	Sacroiliac joint	
	Apophysitis	
	Anterior superior iliac spine	
	Anterior inferior iliac spine	
	(adolescents)	

(a) Iliopsoas bursitis as an isolated condition is probably relatively uncommon in sports medicine. It is retained here as part of the iliopsoas clinical entity, which is common.

become bilateral. The pain is aggravated by exercise, with running, twisting/turning and kicking being the most challenging activities. The athlete and coach usually notice a decrease in sports performance.

The pain in athletes with longstanding groin pain typically presents initially following activity and is accompanied by stiffness, particularly the next morning. The pain and stiffness then gradually lessens with daily activities and warm-up for the next training session or match. When the condition becomes worse, pain is present immediately upon exercise.

NSAIDs tend to decrease pain but provide no cure. Short periods of rest reduce the severity of the symptoms but on resumption of normal sporting activities the pain returns to its original intensity and severity. The natural history is one of progressive deterioration with continued activity until symptoms prevent participation in the activity.

The localization of the pain is important to determine which structure may be causing the pain. Adductor-related pain is located medially in the groin—centered primarily at the attachment of the adductor longus tendon to the pubic bone. Iliopsoas-related pain is located more centrally in the groin and proximal thigh.

The type of activity that aggravates the pain may be a clue to the primary site of the problem. Side-to-side movements, twisting and turning activities which aggravate the pain suggest adductor-related pain. Straight line running or kicking suggest iliopsoas problems. Pain with sit-ups may suggest an inguinal-related pain. Note that these clinical observations are guidelines rather than hard-and-fast rules.

Pain that becomes progressively worse with exercise may suggest a stress fracture, bursitis or nerve entrapment. A history of associated pain such as low back or buttock pain indicates that the groin pain may be referred from another site, such as the lumbar spine, the SIJ or the thoracolumbar junction.

A full training history should be taken to determine if any recent changes in training, such as a generalized increase in volume or intensity, or the introduction of a new exercise or increase in a particular component of training, may have led to the development of the groin pain.

Examination

Each region of the groin that has the potential to produce groin pain must be examined. This includes the adductor muscles, the pelvic bones, the hip joint and its surrounds, the hip flexors (including tensor fascia lata and sartorius) and the lower abdominal muscles. The lumbar spine and SIJ are also examined. Pelvic alignment must be assessed and any leg length discrepancy noted. Some figures are shown in Chapter 23. Examination involves:

1. Observation
   (a) standing
   (b) walking (Fig. 23.2a)
   (c) supine
2. Active movements
   (a) hip flexion/extension
   (b) hip abduction/adduction*
   (c) hip internal/external rotation
   (d) lumbar spine movements (Chapter 21)
   (e) abdominal flexion*
3. Passive movements
   (a) hip quadrant—flexion, adduction, internal rotation (Fig. 23.2c)
   (b) internal rotation, then with added adduction
   (c) adductor muscle stretch* (Fig. 23.2b)

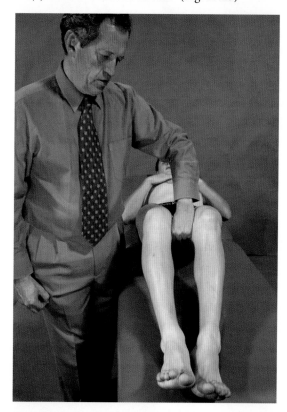

Figure 24.4 Examination of the patient with hip/groin pain

(a) Resisted movement—squeeze test. Examiner places fist between knees as shown. Patient then adducts bilaterally against the fist

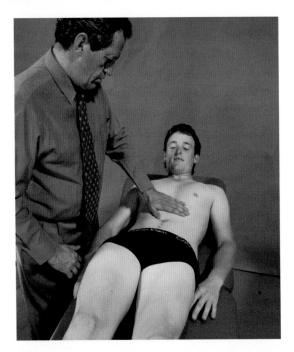

(b) Resisted movement—rectus abdominis. Resisted sit-up is performed

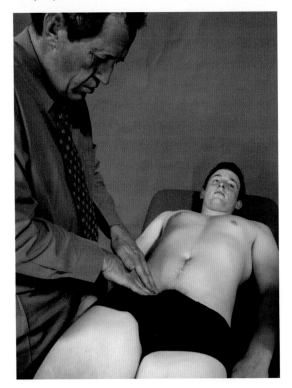

(c) Palpation—pubic and inguinal regions are carefully palpated

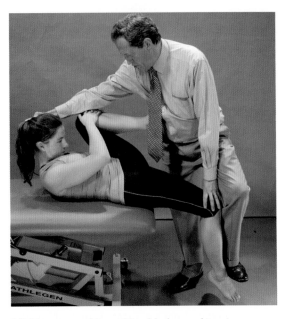

(d) Thomas position with added neural tension. Patient is initially placed in the iliopsoas stretch position. The neural tension is slowly increased by addition of cervical and upper thoracic flexion, then passive knee flexion. This test will always cause some discomfort and tightness. It is clinically significant if the patient's pain is reproduced, then reduced when the tension is taken off

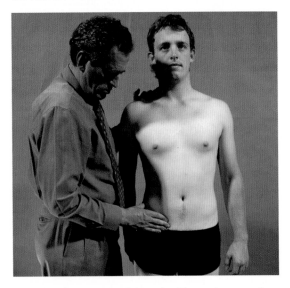

(e) Special tests—cough impulse. The patient stands and the examiner feels for a cough impulse at the sites of direct and indirect inguinal hernias. The examiner should then invaginate the scrotum and ask the patient to cough. Note dilation of the ring and discomfort

(d) quadriceps muscle stretch

(e) iliopsoas muscle stretch—Thomas position (Fig. 23.2e)

4. Resisted movements
  (a) hip flexion—Thomas position (Fig. 23.2f)
  (b) hip flexion in adduction
  (c) hip adduction
  (d) 'squeeze test' (bilateral hip adduction) (Fig. 24.4a)
  (e) adduction/abduction
  (f) abdominal flexion (Fig. 24.4b)

5. Palpation
  (a) adductor muscles/tendons* (Fig. 23.2g)
  (b) pubic symphysis/ramus* (Fig. 24.4c)
  (c) rectus abdominis*
  (d) iliopsoas*

6. Special tests
  (a) pelvic symmetry
  (b) lumbar spine (Chapter 21)
  (c) sacroiliac joint (Chapter 22)
  (d) Thomas position with added neural tension (Fig. 24.4d)
  (e) FABER test (Fig. 23.2d)
  (f) cough impulse (Fig. 24.4e)
  (g) Trendelenberg test

Note: Those physical examination tests that Holmich et al. advocate in the 'quick groin examination' are marked with an asterisk; they proved reliable when tested within and among examiners.[14]

A sign that helps clinicians assess severity of the condition is the 'crossover sign'. A positive crossover sign means that the patient's typical groin pain is reproduced when one of the provocation tests (e.g. passive hip abduction, resisted hip adduction, resisted hip flexion in Thomas position) is performed on the *contralateral* side to the symptoms. A positive crossover sign suggests substantial functional impairment and the clinical implication is that the player is very unlikely to be able to run, train or play.

Investigations

Investigations, an important part of the management of groin pain, should be conducted after clinical examination has provided a working diagnosis. Pelvic radiography may reveal characteristic changes of pubic-related groin pain, hip joint abnormality (e.g. osteoarthritis) or stress fracture of the neck of the femur or pubic ramus. Sclerosis or osteophyte formation around the SIJ indicate that this joint may be a cause of referred pain, although frequently X-ray does not reveal SIJ abnormalities. In cases of chronic ankylosing spondylitis, there will be obliteration of the joint space of the SIJ. Lumbar spine X-ray may show degenerative changes or spondylolisthesis.

Radionuclide bone scan shows a characteristic pattern of increased uptake in pubic-related groin pain and may confirm a suspected stress fracture in those cases where an X-ray fails to demonstrate the fracture. Ultrasound has been used to detect inguinal hernias.[15]

MRI is used to image the hip joint, especially to detect labral tears (+/– arthrogram), and is also advocated by some as being the investigation of choice in pubic-related groin pain and stress fracture of the neck of the femur. It can provide evidence of soft tissue changes in the adductor muscles and tendons, as well as showing hernias.[16]

Adductor-related longstanding groin pain

Longstanding adductor-related groin pain is localized medially in the groin and may radiate down along the adductor muscles. The key examination features that distinguish this clinical entity from others are maximal tenderness at the adductor tendon insertion and pain with resisted adduction ('squeeze test') (Figs 23.2g, 24.4a). Weakness of the adductor muscles is common and palpation of the adductors reveals generally increased muscle tone with trigger points along the adductor longus. The pubic symphysis is frequently tender but this does not help to differentiate the four clinical entities (Table 24.1).

Occasionally there may be an obvious adductor tendinopathy or enthesopathy (see below) with localized tenderness, pain and weakness on contraction, especially eccentric contraction, and a typical appearance of tendinopathy on ultrasound or MRI examination. More frequently there is no specific tendinopathy present.

Early warning signs: overlooked at peril!

Unfortunately most patients with adductor-related groin pain continue to train and play until pain prevents them from running. When the condition has reached that stage, a lengthy period of rest and rehabilitation is usually required. However, if early warning signs are heeded, appropriate measures may prevent the development of the full blown syndrome. These early clinical warning signs are (from most common to least):

- tightness/stiffness during or after activity with nil (or temporary only) relief from stretching
- loss of acceleration

- loss of maximal sprinting speed
- loss of distance with long kick on run
- vague discomfort with deceleration.

Treatment

Traditional treatment for most types of groin pain was 'rest' but this most often resulted in a return of symptoms on resumption of activity. Compared with rest and passive electrotherapy, active rehabilitation provides more than 10 times the likelihood of pain-free successful return to sport.[17] Thus, we outline a treatment protocol that combines experience and evidence from leading clinical centers.[17, 18]

Five basic principles underpin a treatment regimen:

1. Ensure that exercise is performed without pain.
2. Identify and reduce the sources of increased load on the pelvis.
3. Improve lumbopelvic stability.
4. Strengthen local musculature using proven protocols.
5. Progress the patient's level of activity on the basis of regular clinical assessment.

These are outlined below.

Ensure that exercise is performed without pain

The first and most important step is for the patient to cease training and playing in pain. *Pain-free exercise* is absolutely crucial for this rehabilitation program. If pain is experienced during any of the rehabilitation activities, or after them, that activity should be reduced or ceased altogether. Experienced clinicians use absence of pain on the key provocation tests (e.g. squeeze test and Thomas test) as a guide to progress the rehabilitation program and minimize the mechanical stress on injured tissues (see progression of program below).

Identify and reduce the sources of increased load on the pelvis

As discussed previously, it is essential to identify and reduce the sources of increased load on the pubic bones. This may involve:

- reducing adductor muscle tone and guarding with soft tissue treatment (Fig. 24.5a) and/or dry needling
- correcting iliopsoas muscle shortening with local soft tissue treatment (Fig. 24.5b), neural stretching (Fig. 24.5c) and mobilization of upper lumbar intervertebral joints (Chapter 21)

- reducing gluteus medius muscle tone and myofascial shortening with soft tissue treatment and/or dry needling
- identifying and correcting any hip joint abnormality (Chapter 23)
- mobilizing stiff intervertebral segments (Chapter 21)
- improving core stability (Chapter 11), especially activation of transversus abdominis and anterior pelvic floor muscles.

Improve lumbopelvic stability

Research has demonstrated a delayed onset of action of transversus abdominis activity in patients with longstanding groin pain,[11] suggesting that impaired core or lumbopelvic stability (Chapter 11) plays a role in the development of this condition.

Pain on resisted adduction (the 'squeeze test') was significantly reduced by the application of a pelvic

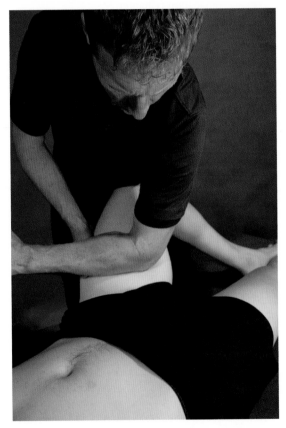

Figure 24.5 Treatment techniques used in adductor-related pain

(a) Soft tissue therapy—sustained myofascial tension to the adductor muscle group

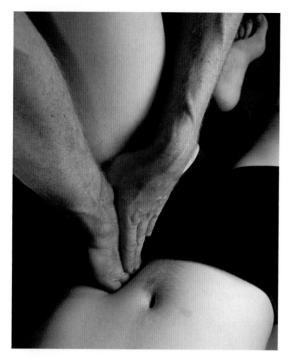

(b) Soft tissue therapy—sustained myofascial tension to the iliopsoas muscle. The hip should be slowly passively extended from the flexed position shown to increase the tension

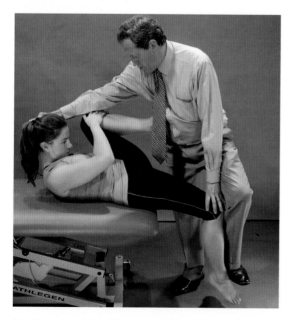

(c) Neural stretch—Thomas position. Commence in the iliopsoas stretch position, then add passive cervical/upper thoracic tension, and then passive knee flexion to elicit a stretch

belt,[19] which suggests that reduced stability of the pelvis may be the cause of the groin pain. The authors suggested using the terminology 'adduction-related groin pain' rather than 'adductor-related'.

In our clinical experience, a core stability program has proven to be an important component of the rehabilitation program for longstanding groin pain. This program has been described in Chapter 11.

Strengthen local musculature using proven protocols

Once pain has settled and muscle shortening has been corrected in the adductor, iliopsoas and gluteal muscles, then a graduated pain-free muscle strengthening program can be commenced. A randomized clinical trial comparing an active training program aimed at improving muscle strength and coordination of the muscles acting on the pelvis, in particular the adductor muscles, was more effective in the treatment of a group of athletes with longstanding groin pain than a physiotherapy program consisting of laser, TENS, friction massage and stretching without active training.[17] This program is described in the box on page 414. A similar pre-season adductor muscle strengthening program reduced the incidence of adductor muscle strains in ice hockey players who were identified as at risk.[20]

Progress the patient's level of activity on the basis of regular clinical assessment

The aim of the graded exercise program is to gradually increase the load on the pubic bones and surrounding tissues. Once the patient is pain-free (see above), pain-free walking can begin and be gradually increased in speed and distance.

The criteria for when the patient may return to running are when:

- brisk walking is pain-free
- resisted hip flexion in the Thomas position is pain-free
- there is no 'crossover' sign (p. 411)
- there is minimal adductor guarding.

Various progressive running regimens can be used. One effective program is described here:[18]

- 100 m run-throughs with 10 m acceleration and deceleration phases with walk recovery. Patient should commence with six to eight repetitions on alternate days. Key criteria (adductor guarding, squeeze test) should be assessed immediately after each session and again the next morning. The running program can be progressed further by replacing walk recovery

Exercise rehabilitation program for longstanding groin pain in athletes[17]

This program consists of static and dynamic exercises aimed at improving the muscles stabilizing the pelvis and the hip joints, in particular the adductor muscles. The program consists of two parts:

- Module 1: Two-week familiarization program—adductor activation
- Module 2: More demanding exercises with heavier resistance training and balance and coordination. The training program is performed three times a week and the exercises from module 1 are performed on the days in between the treatment days. The total length of the training period is 8–12 weeks. Sport activities are not allowed in the treatment period. Pain-free bike riding is allowed. After 6 weeks, pain-free jogging is allowed. Return to sport is allowed when neither treatment nor jogging causes any pain.

Stretching of the adductor muscles is not advised, but stretching of the other lower extremity muscles, particularly the iliopsoas, is recommended.

Module 1: Static and dynamic exercises (2 week base training program)

Static

1. (a) Adduction for 30 seconds against a soccer ball placed between the feet when lying in the supine position with the knees fully extended and the first toe pointing straight upwards (Fig. 24.6a).
1. (b) Adduction for 30 seconds against a soccer ball placed between the knees when lying in the supine position with the knees and the hips flexed at 45° and the feet flat on the floor pointing straight ahead (Fig. 24.6b).

Exercises 1(a) and (b) should be repeated 10 times with 15 second recovery periods between each contraction. The force of the adduction should be just sufficient to reach the point where pain begins.

Dynamic

1. (c) Sit-ups from the supine position with the hip and knee joints flexed at 45° and the feet against the floor. The sit-ups are performed as a straight abdominal curl and also with a quarter twist towards the opposite knee. Five sets of 10 with 15 second recovery periods.
1. (d) In the same starting position as for the sit-ups but clamping a soccer ball between the knees, the player does a combination of a sit-ups while pulling the ball towards the head. The exercise is performed rhythmically and with accuracy to gain balance and coordination. Five sets of 10 with 15 second recovery periods.
1. (e) Wobble board training for 5 minutes.
1. (f) Adductor lateral slide. Using a sliding board with an extremely smooth surface (or a very smooth floor) and wearing a low friction sock on the sliding foot, one foot is positioned next to the sliding board and the other foot on the board parallel to the first one. The foot on the board slides out laterally and is then pulled back to the starting position. The foot should be pressed against the surface through the whole exercise with as much force as tolerated within the patient's threshold of pain (Fig. 24.6c).
1. (g) Forward slide. The same procedure is also done with the foot on the board placed in a 90° angle to the foot outside the board. Both exercises 1(f) and (g) are performed continuously for 1 minute with each leg in turn.

All the above exercises should be commenced carefully and the number of sets and range of motion gradually increased respecting pain and exhaustion.

Module 2: Dynamic exercises

This entire module is done twice at each training session for three training sessions per week with a day in between. *Note*: Module 1 is done on alternate days, so players are training a total of six days per week. Exercises 2(a) to (e) are done as five sets of 10 repetitions.

2. (a) Lying on one side with the lower leg stretched and the upper leg bent and placed in front of the lower leg, the lower leg is moved up and down, pointing the heel upwards.
2. (b) Lying on one side with the lower leg bent and the upper leg stretched, the upper leg is moved up and down, pointing the heel upwards.
2. (c) Begin by standing at the end of a high couch and then lie prone so that the torso is supported by the couch. The hips are at the edge of the couch at 90° of flexion and the feet are on the floor. From this position, both hips are slowly extended so both legs are lifted to the greatest possible extension of hips and spine; legs are then lowered together.
2. (d) Standing abduction/adduction using ankle pulleys. Begin with a low weight and gradually increase the weight but keep it submaximal.

2. (e) Standing on one leg, the knee of the supporting leg is flexed and extended rhythmically and in the same rhythm swinging both arms back and forth independently ('cross-country skiing on one leg') (Fig. 24.6d). The non-weight-bearing leg is not moved. The balance and position is kept accurately, and the exercise is stopped when this is no longer possible.

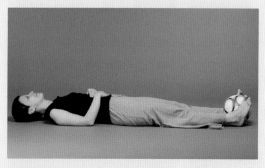

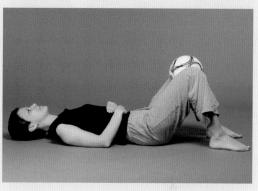

Figure 24.6 Static and dynamic exercises to improve the muscles stabilizing the pelvis and the hip joints

(a) Static exercise—adduction for 30 seconds against a soccer ball placed between the feet

(b) Static exercise—adduction for 30 seconds against a soccer ball placed between the knees when lying in the supine position with the knees and the hips flexed at 45°

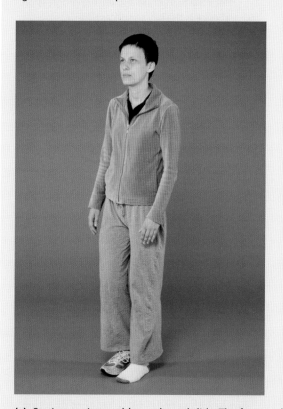

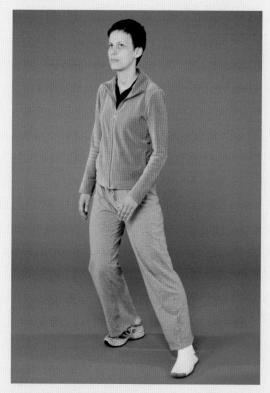

(c) Static exercise—adductor lateral slide. The foot on the slippery surface slides out laterally and is then pulled back to the starting position in contact with the surface and with as much force as tolerable

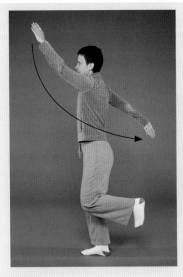 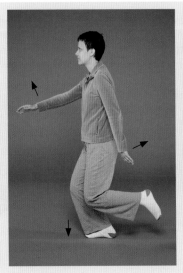 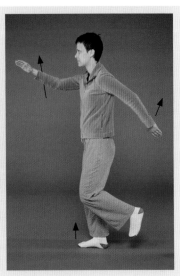

(d) Dynamic exercise—cross-country skiing on one leg. Note that the non-weight-bearing leg is not moved

Progression of the exercise is obtained by holding a 1 kg (2.2 lb) weight in each hand.

2. (f) 'Fitter' training for 5 minutes.
2. (g) Standing on the sliding board, side-to-side skating movements on the sliding board are done as five sets of 1 minute training periods with 15 second recovery.

Practical tips

- Supervision is important—the patient should be instructed by a physiotherapist, a physician, an athletic trainer or another qualified person who has been trained in the details of the program.
- Exercises such as 1(d) and 2(e) are very important, especially at the end of the training period, but they are technically difficult.
- The athletes can do the program at home or at the 'gym' or the fitness club, but we recommend physiotherapist supervision for three to four times within the first 2 weeks

and after that a visit every 10–14 days to check the technique and ensure progression.

- Patience is the key to success.
- Patients often make good progress in the first few weeks, but symptoms can plateau from that period until the 6–9 week period, when there is a positive 'breakthrough'.
- It is important to use pain as a guide to how much to do. Muscle soreness similar to that after a regular practise in the sports field is not a problem, but if the patient experiences pain from the injury, the intensity of the exercises should be adjusted.
- Pain medication including NSAIDs should be avoided.
- Athletes should continue with some of the exercises on a regular basis (1–2 times a week) for at least a year after total recovery and return to sport.
- The athlete must appreciate that successful rehabilitation of chronic groin pain takes a minimum of 8–12 weeks.

with jog recovery. The aim should be to build up to 20 × 100 m run-throughs and jog back.
- Lateral running (gradual change of direction such as figure eight) can be commenced when the above running program is completed pain-free, the hip flexion test is still pain-free with no

crossover sign, there is no adductor guarding and, in addition, the squeeze test is pain-free. Figure of eight running should commence slowly with very gradual change of direction, then gradually increase both speed and sharpness of changes of direction.

In kicking sports, short stationary kicking can be commenced when hip flexion tests are pain-free without crossover. The player may gradually increase the kicking distance and then start shorter kicking on the run. The last stage in the kicking program is long kicks at full pace and kicking around the body.

Key clinical signs suggestive of 'excessive loading' during rehabilitation

As the therapist must continually guard against the player 'overdoing' rehabilitation, we share the following signs that appear to suggest excessive loading and deterioration during rehabilitation:

* pain on passive hip abduction
* adductor muscle 'guarding' with increased muscle tone on passive combined hip external rotation and abduction
* pain and weakness with resisted adductor contraction
* pain on the 'squeeze test' (Fig. 24.4a)
* pain on resisted hip flexion (Fig. 23.2e)
* pain on resisted hip flexion and adduction in the Thomas test position
* positive crossover sign.

Other non-surgical treatments

Compression shorts have been advocated for those with mild pain who insist on continuing to train and play, and for those returning to sport after rehabilitation.[7, 21, 22] The shorts substantially reduced pain when worn during exercise.[23] The mechanism of action of compression shorts remains unclear, but Dutch researchers have reported that groin pain on resisted adduction (the 'squeeze test') was significantly reduced by the application of a pelvic belt.[19] They speculated that relative pelvic instability may contribute to the groin pain typically attributed to tendinopathy.

Failure of conservative management

Conservative management as outlined above might fail for a number of reasons. These include:

* incorrect diagnosis (hip joint pathology, hernia, stress fracture, referred pain)
* inadequate period of rest
* poor compliance
* exercising into pain
* inappropriate progressions
* inadequate core stability
* persistent lumbar intervertebral hypomobility
* persistent adductor guarding.

Surgery

If persistent adductor shortening/guarding is a problem that does not respond to soft tissue treatment and/or dry needling, then a partial adductor tendon release may be helpful.[24, 25] Abolition of the patient's symptoms and signs with a trial injection of local anesthetic is advocated by some as an indication that the release will be successful in alleviating symptoms. One technique advocated is to release the superficial section of the normal adductor longus tendon at a point distal to the insertion. It is postulated that this may have the effect of transferring stress from the superficial section of the tendon to the stress-shielded deeper portion.[26] Anecdotally, these patients often make a quick recovery and return to high-level sport after four to six weeks.

Iliopsoas-related longstanding groin pain

The iliopsoas muscles may be the sole cause of the athlete's longstanding groin pain, but this component is frequently present in conjunction with adductor abnormalities. The iliopsoas component needs to be recognized and subsequently treated.

The iliopsoas muscle (Fig. 23.3) is the strongest flexor of the hip joint. It arises from the five lumbar vertebrae and the ilium and inserts into the lesser trochanter of the femur. It is occasionally injured acutely (Chapter 23) but frequently becomes tight with neural restriction.

Whether or not iliopsoas tendinopathy and bursitis contribute substantially to exercise-related groin pain remains unclear. Most case reports associate these conditions with hip surgery and with rheumatological conditions (e.g. polymyalgia rheumatica). The thin-walled iliopsoas bursa commonly communicates with the hip joint. Experienced clinicians feel that muscular and neuromyofascial elements are likely to contribute far more commonly than do iliopsoas bursitis and tendinopathy.

Iliopsoas problems may occur as an overuse injury resulting from excessive hip flexion, such as kicking. They present as a poorly localized ache that patients usually describe as being a deep ache in one side of the groin.

There are two key clinical signs that point to the iliopsoas as the source of groin pain. The first, tenderness of the muscle in the lower abdomen, relies on palpation of the iliopsoas muscle, which is difficult in its proximal portion, deep within the pelvis. Nevertheless, the skilled examiner may detect tenderness more distally, particularly in thin athletes, by palpating carefully just below the inguinal ligament, lateral to the femoral artery and medial to the sartorius muscles. Passive hip flexion facilitates this palpation.

The second key clinical sign that helps distinguish the iliopsoas from other sources of groin pain is pain and tightness on iliopsoas stretch that is exacerbated on resisted hip flexion in the stretch position (Fig. 23.2e). Frequently, the further addition of passive cervical flexion and knee flexion (Fig. 24.4d) will aggravate the pain, indicating a degree of neural restriction through the muscle. It is important to examine the lumbar spine as there is frequently an association between iliopsoas tightness and hypomobility of the upper lumbar spine from which the muscle originates.

Treatment

Treatment of iliopsoas-related groin pain is similar to that of adductor-related groin pain (above) but with an increased emphasis on soft tissue treatment of the iliopsoas (Fig. 24.5b) and iliopsoas stretching (Fig. 23.2e) with the addition of a neural component (Fig. 24.5c). Often, mobilization of the lumbar intervertebral joints (Chapter 21) at the origin of the iliopsoas muscles will markedly decrease the patient's pain.

Abdominal-wall-related longstanding groin pain

The subject of 'hernias' as a common cause of groin pain in athletes is controversial. While true inguinal hernias are relatively rare in this population, other conditions similar to hernias have been described and have come in and out of favor as common causes of groin pain. These include terms such as 'sportsman's hernia', 'footballer's hernia', 'inguinal insufficiency', 'conjoint tendon tear', 'hockey player's groin' and 'Gilmore's groin'. Many of these entities are probably describing the same or similar clinical conditions and all seem to respond to similar surgical treatment.

Posterior inguinal wall weakness ('sports hernia', 'sportsman's hernia')

A significant group of patients with groin pain, usually male football players, present with a long history of gradually worsening, poorly localized pain aggravated by activity, especially kicking. These patients have been classified as having 'inguinal insufficiency', 'footballer's hernia' or 'sportsman's hernia'. This diagnosis is popular in soccer players in the United Kingdom and Europe. It is important to note that this presentation is uncommon in women; other diagnoses should be thoroughly explored.[25]

Various authors have described slightly different pathologies including a tear in the transversalis or external oblique fascia, a tear in the external oblique aponeurosis, a tear in the conjoined tendon, a separation of the inguinal ligament from the conjoined tendon or tearing of the conjoined tendon from the pubic tubercle.[27–33] Some or all of these pathologies may lead to dilation of the external inguinal ring.

A number of contributing factors have been suggested. The condition is commonly bilateral, suggesting that a congenital posterior inguinal wall deficiency may be present.[34] Intense sporting activity particularly involving kicking places increased downward stress on the conjoined tendon, and causes muscle fatigue.[35] An increase in intra-abdominal pressure during sport increases stress on the transversalis fascia fibers of the posterior inguinal wall.[36]

The onset of pain is usually insidious, but it may also present as an acute injury followed by chronic pain. The pain initially tends to occur after or near the end of activity. As the condition progresses, the pain worsens and occurs earlier in activity. The pain is usually located in the posterior inguinal floor inside the external ring. It may also radiate to the testicle, adductors or laterally in the upper thigh. The pain is usually aggravated by sudden movement and is aggravated by sneezing, coughing, sexual activity and the Valsalva maneuver. Symptoms have a tendency to settle after prolonged absence from sporting activity, only to recur when high-intensity exercise is resumed.

On examination, maximal tenderness is usually over the pubic tubercle. The most helpful diagnostic sign is dilation and/or discomfort to palpation of the external inguinal ring after invagination of the scrotum (Fig. 24.4e). Peritoneograms are used, particularly in Scandinavia, to confirm the diagnosis in some cases but have generally gone out of favor elsewhere. There is some evidence that ultrasound examination[15] and MRI[16] may be able to detect these hernias.

Surgery is the most popular treatment for this condition. The most common procedure is a Bassini hernia repair, paying added attention to identification and repair of tears in the transversalis fascia or other structures. Most surgeons also insert a polypropylene mesh. This procedure can be performed as an open operation or laparoscopically.[33, 37, 38]

Taylor et al.[39] and Meyers et al.[25] in the United States, and Biedert et al.[40] in Switzerland have reported a procedure in which they performed a broad surgical reattachment of the inferolateral edge of the rectus abdominis muscle with its fascial investment to the pubis and adjacent anterior ligaments.[39] The operation is similar to a Bassini hernia repair with the main difference being a focus on attachment of the rectus abdominis muscle fascia to the pubis, rather than protection of the inguinal floor near the internal ring.[25] A number of the patients in these studies also had an adductor release.

If tenderness at the attachment of the inguinal ligament is present, laparoscopic release of the ligament may be effective. This procedure is currently common in the United Kingdom.

Reports of results of surgery are generally very positive, but in our experience there is a relatively high rate of recurrence of symptoms. It is unclear whether this is because of an incorrect diagnosis or recurrence of the problem.

Theoretically, a rehabilitation program consisting of strengthening of the abdominal obliques, transversus abdominis, adductors and hip flexors should help in this condition, and a trial of such a program may be worthwhile before resorting to surgery.[41] No scientific evidence exists as to the efficacy of such a program.

'Gilmore's groin'

A similar condition has been described by Gilmore and is known as 'Gilmore's groin'.[42–44] Gilmore describes an injury involving a torn external oblique aponeurosis, causing dilatation of the superficial inguinal ring, a torn conjoint tendon (common tendon of insertion of the internal oblique and transversus abdominis muscles), and a dehiscence between the inguinal ligament and the conjoint tendon. Gilmore advocates surgical repair of the defect described above with a reported 96% of his patients returning to sport within 15 weeks.[42]

Tear of the external oblique aponeurosis ('hockey groin')

An unusual condition involving a tear of the external oblique aponeurosis and superficial inguinal ring has been described in elite ice hockey players.[44, 45] These players all complained of a muscular type of pain of gradual onset, exacerbated by ipsilateral hip extension and contralateral torso rotation. The discomfort is often worse in the morning, specifically during hip extension from a sitting position, as in getting up from a bed or chair. Pain is felt mostly during the propulsion phase of skating (the first few strides) and during the slapshot motion. It is consistently located on the opposite side to the player's forehand shot. The dull ache may radiate to the scrotum, hip and back.

On examination there are no consistent findings, although the superficial inguinal ring may be tender and/or dilated. Imaging studies are consistently negative. Various conservative therapies have been attempted without success and the definitive treatment is surgery involving repair of the torn external oblique aponeurosis. The ilioinguinal nerve is often trapped in scar tissue. If so, neurectomy is performed. Postoperatively, the patients are advised to avoid skating for four weeks, then slowly allowed to return to activity over the next six to eight weeks.

Inguinal hernia

Inguinal hernias occur in athletes as in the general population. They can be either direct or indirect. Small hernias may become painful as a result of exertion. Symptoms may include a characteristic dragging sensation to one side of the lower abdomen aggravated by increased intra-abdominal pressure, such as coughing. On examination, there is occasionally an obvious swelling and there may be a palpable cough impulse. Treatment consists of surgical correction of the defect.

Rectus abdominis tendinopathy

Rectus abdominis abnormalities occur at its tendinous insertion into the superior ramus of the pubis. These may occur as the result of an acute strain while lifting or, more commonly, as an overuse injury associated with excessive abdominal contractions (e.g. sit-ups).

On examination, there is tenderness at the insertion of the rectus abdominis into the superior pubic ramus. Pain is aggravated by active contraction, such as a sit-up. Treatment consists of correction of soft tissue dysfunction and a gradual strengthening program. Some clinicians advocate an injection of corticosteroid and local anesthetic agents into the area of attachment in recalcitrant cases, but this approach is losing favor in tendinopathies in general. If injection is tried, it should be accompanied by active rehabilitation. Rarely, surgery is required. This is performed in a similar way to an adductor tenotomy, where the tendon is released from its attachment.

Pubic-bone-stress-related longstanding groin pain

It has been well accepted that athletic groin pain can arise from bony stress around the pubic symphysis, hence the term 'osteitis pubis'. That 'diagnosis' is confirmed by typical radiographic and radionuclide imaging appearances. The radiographic features are the typical 'moth-eaten' appearance along the margins of the pubic symphysis (Fig. 24.7b) with asymmetrical bony erosions, osteophytes, sclerotic bony margins and subchondral bone cysts. The radionuclide bone scan shows increased uptake on the delayed static images over the pubic tubercle (Fig. 24.7a).

CT scanning is also a sensitive investigation for displaying abnormalities of the bony architecture, such as cystic changes and perisymphysis erosions (Fig. 24.7c). In more recent times, MRI has shown bone marrow edema in the body of the pubis (Fig. 24.7d).[5]

The significance of the bone marrow edema in sportspeople (mainly men) with longstanding groin pain is presently a topic of great interest and vigorous debate. As mentioned previously, Verrall et al.[5] have shown that bone marrow edema is present on MRI in a large percentage (77%) of footballers presenting with longstanding groin pain that is associated with

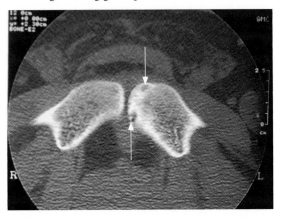

(c) Appearance on CT scan, showing degenerative cyst formation and erosions, with widening of the anterior margins of the symphysis

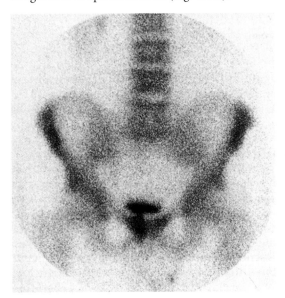

Figure 24.7 Imaging appearance of pubic-bone-stress-related longstanding groin pain (traditionally described as 'osteitis pubis')

(a) Appearance on radionuclide bone scan

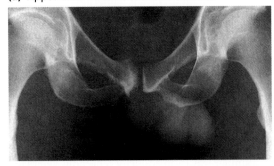

(b) X-ray showing the characteristic moth-eaten appearance

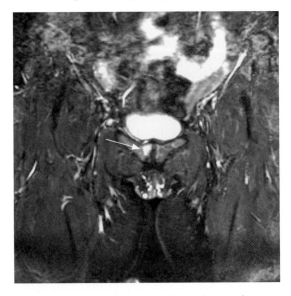

(d) Appearance on T2-weighted MRI, showing bony edema (arrow) in the body of the pubis

pubic symphysis tenderness and a positive squeeze test. They proposed that pubic bone stress was a possible cause of the symptoms and signs such as the squeeze test but their subsequent research showed only moderate levels of sensitivity[46] of the squeeze test when correlated with clinical and MRI criteria.

Abnormalities in all imaging modalities are seen in athletes who have no history of groin pain; nevertheless, the presence of bone marrow edema elsewhere in the body is considered significant. For example, on MRI it is characteristic of the bone bruises associated with serious knee injuries (Chapter 27).

The pubic bones are subjected to considerable forces by the various pelvic structures mentioned above. It may be that pubic bone abnormalities are the cause of pain in a small group of patients or they may simply be a sign of increased bone stress when the other clinical entities (e.g. adductor related) are affected.

Treatment

A variety of treatments have focused on the symphysis pubis and bony abnormalities.

The use of corticosteroids both as a local injection into the symphysis pubis[47] and in oral form (25–50 mg/day for 7 days) has been anecdotally helpful, but no controlled trial has been reported. We have found a short (5–7 days) course of oral prednisolone (50 mg/day) to be helpful in settling pain, thus enabling the patient to commence the rehabilitation program earlier.

Dextrose prolotherapy injections have been shown to be helpful in one study.[48] Monthly injections of 12.5% dextrose and 0.5% lignocaine (lidocaine) into the adductor origins, suprapubic abdominal insertions and symphysis pubis were given until resolution of symptoms. An average of 2.8 treatments were required.

Three- to six-monthly courses of intravenous injection of the bisphosphonate pamidronate were found to be helpful in one report of three cases.[49] Some physicians are advocating the use of extracorporeal shock wave therapy but there is no evidence to support this.

Surgery has been advocated by some clinicians. In the chronic stage of the condition, where imaging shows erosions and cystic changes in the pubic symphysis (Fig. 24.7c), surgical exploration and debridement of the symphysis may be indicated.[50] Symphyseal wedge resection[51] is out of favor as it can give rise to progressive sacroiliac arthrosis and ultimately posterior pelvic instability requiring

major pelvic stabilization.[52] Arthrodesis of the pubic symphysis by bone grafting and a compression plate has been used successfully in patients with proven pubic instability.[53]

Less common causes

Obturator neuropathy

Obturator neuropathy is a fascial entrapment of the obturator nerve as it enters the adductor compartment and accounts for approximately 4% of the patients with groin pain seen at our clinic. It has distinct clinical features that separate it from other causes of groin pain.[54, 55]

Obturator neuropathy presents as exercise-related groin pain, which initially is concentrated on the proximal groin but with increasing exercise radiates towards the distal medial thigh. There may be associated weakness or a feeling of a lack of propulsion of the limb during running but numbness is very rarely reported. At rest, examination findings can be non-specific, with pain on passive abduction of the hip, and pain and weakness on resisted hip adduction. The ipsilateral pubic tubercle is often tender. The essential component of the physical examination is to exercise the patient to a level that reproduces his or her symptoms followed by immediate examination of the patient. This examination will reveal weakness of resisted adduction and numbness over the distal medial thigh.

Bone scan in this condition often shows increased uptake over the ipsilateral pubic tubercle, frequently called osteitis pubis by the reporting radiologist. The diagnosis is confirmed by needle EMG, which shows chronic denervation patterns of the adductor muscle group.

Conservative treatment of this condition, including sustained myofascial tension massage over the adductor compartment, neural stretches, spinal mobilization and iliopsoas soft tissue techniques, is generally unsuccessful.

The definitive treatment of this condition is surgical. An oblique incision is made in the proximal groin. The plane between the adductor longus and pectineus is identified and dissected, revealing the obturator nerve under the fascia over the adductor brevis. This fascia is divided and the nerve is freed up to the level of the obturator foramen. The fascial anatomy (Fig. 24.8) here is very important, with the fascia of the adductor longus curving around the muscle medially and passing back deep to the muscle to become the fascia over the adductor brevis, which

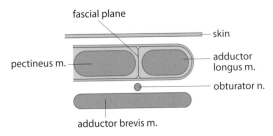

Figure 24.8 Obturator neuropathy—fascial arrangements

is thought to be responsible for the fascial entrapment of the obturator nerve. Post-surgical management includes wound management, soft tissue techniques and a graduated return to full activity over a period of four to six weeks.

Other nerve entrapments

A number of superficial nerves in the groin may become entrapped and should be considered as possible causes of groin pain. The ilioinguinal nerve supplies the skin around the genitalia and inside of the thigh and may produce pain as a result of entrapment. The genitofemoral nerve innervates an area of skin just above the groin fold. The lateral cutaneous nerve of the thigh is the most common nerve affected. This nerve supplies the outside of the thigh. This condition is known as 'meralgia paresthetica'.

Treatment of these conditions is usually not necessary as they often spontaneously resolve. Meralgia paresthetica is sometimes treated with a corticosteroid injection at the site where the nerve exits the pelvis, 1 cm (0.5 in.) medial to the anterior superior iliac spine. Occasionally, the nerve needs to be explored surgically and the area of entrapment released.

Stress fractures of the neck of the femur

Stress fracture of the neck of the femur is another cause of groin pain.[56] The usual history is one of gradual onset of groin pain, poorly localized and aggravated by activity. Examination may show some localized tenderness but often there is relatively little to find other than pain at the extremes of hip joint movement, especially internal rotation. X-ray may demonstrate the fracture if it has been present for a number of weeks but this investigation should not be relied on to rule out the condition; isotopic bone scan and MRI (Fig. 24.9) are the most sensitive tests.

Stress fractures of the neck of the femur occur on either the superior or tension side of the bone or on

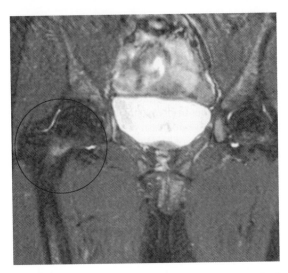

Figure 24.9 MRI showing stress fracture of the neck of the femur

the inferior or compression side (Fig. 24.10). Stress fractures of the superior aspect of the femoral neck should be regarded as a surgical emergency and treated with either urgent internal fixation or strict bed rest. The concern is that such stress fractures have a tendency to go on to full fracture, which compromises the blood supply to the femoral head.

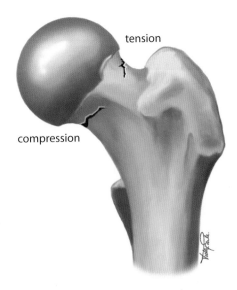

Figure 24.10 Stress fractures of the neck of the femur—superior or tension fracture on the superior aspect of the femoral neck and inferior or compression fracture on the inferior side

Stress fractures of the inferior surface of the femoral neck are more benign and can be treated with an initial period of non-weight-bearing rest followed by a period of weight-bearing without running. They require at least six weeks of rest and usually considerably longer. Following the period of rest, a further six weeks of progressive loading will take the patient back to full training. Biomechanical (Chapter 5), nutritional and endocrine risk factors (Chapter 41) should be assessed and treated as appropriate.

Stress fracture of the pubic ramus

Stress fracture of the inferior pubic ramus occurs occasionally, especially in distance runners, and is an important differential diagnosis of adductor tendinopathy. There is usually a history of overuse and localized tenderness, which is not aggravated by passive abduction or resisted adduction. In this condition, pain is often referred to the buttock.

A stress fracture may not be visible on plain X-ray for several weeks, whereas a radionuclide bone scan will demonstrate a focal area of increased activity within hours (Fig. 24.11). As with any stress fracture, etiological factors must be considered. Stress fractures of the inferior pubic ramus in females may be associated with reduced bone density; nutritional insufficiency is a key risk factor for the prolonged amenorrhea often associated with this stress fracture (Chapter 41).

Treatment consists of relative rest from aggravating activities, such as running, until there is no longer any local tenderness. Fitness should be maintained with swimming or cycling with gradual return to

weight-bearing over a number of weeks. Predisposing factors such as a negative energy intake, muscular imbalance or biomechanical abnormality also require correction.

Hip injuries

Synovitis, labral tears, ligamentum teres tears, loose bodies and chondral lesions of the hip usually present as acute injuries but may also present with long-standing pain. These conditions are fully described in Chapter 23.

Osteoarthritis

Because people in their sixth decade and beyond often remain active, it is increasingly common for clinicians to see patients present to the sports medicine clinic with groin pain and be diagnosed with primary osteoarthritis of the hip joint. Also, patients diagnosed with osteoarthritis by a family physician or physiotherapist might attend a sports medicine clinic for exercise prescription (Chapter 55).

It seems most unlikely that sporting activities (e.g. long distance running) that do not involve collisions contribute to the development of osteoarthritis of the hip. A systematic review determined that there was moderate evidence for a positive relationship when traumatic events were included in the analysis.[57]

This condition is a degenerative joint process often preceded by an injury. Treatment includes activity modification initially, but when pain is unremitting joint replacement surgery should be considered. Interim measures, which may be helpful in reducing pain, include intra-articular corticosteroid injection, NSAIDs and a course of intra-articular injections with hyalin G-F 20. This is a joint lubricating substance, biochemically related to healthy joint fluid, which may delay the need for joint replacement surgery.

Avascular necrosis (osteonecrosis) of the head of the femur

The blood supply to the head of the femur can be compromised in a number of different circumstances, leading to death of the femoral head. Fractures of the neck of the femur, surgery around the hip joint, corticosteroid administration and intra-articular injection have all been implicated in the etiology of avascular necrosis.

The condition is diagnosed clinically and is confirmed with progressive plain X-rays. Bone scan can be useful in making an early diagnosis. The focus of most efforts to diagnose and treat this condition has been on preventing collapse of the subchondral bone.

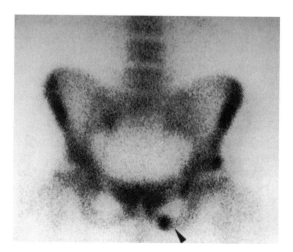

Figure 24.11 Radionuclide bone scan demonstrating stress fracture of the inferior pubic ramus

Revascularization, especially with free vascularized fibular grafting, is done in an attempt to alter the natural history of the disease.[58]

Transient osteoporosis

This is a poorly understood condition, more common in females, where a flame-shaped area of bone edema becomes visible in the femoral neck on MRI. A bone scan will be hot in the delayed phase. It can be very painful, but non-weight-bearing rest on crutches is usually sufficient for pain control. The condition is usually self-limiting, but orthopedic involvement in care is mandatory.

'Snapping' hip

'Snapping' hip, a condition seen in ballet dancers, refers to a snapping noise in the hip region. There are two forms of snapping hip. Lateral (or external) snapping hip is localized at the lateral aspect of the hip and is produced by the tensor fascia lata or the abducting fibers of gluteus maximus sliding over the greater trochanter and producing a characteristic sound. It is usually not painful.

The young dancer (and usually the parent) requires reassurance that this does not signify any bony abnormality. Although the condition may resolve with rest, attention to ballet technique, sustained myofascial tension to excessively tight soft tissue structures, pelvic stability exercises and stretching of the involved tissues may hasten recovery.

A second form of snapping hip (internal snapping hip) is caused by the iliopsoas tendon as it flips over the iliopectineal eminence (Fig. 24.12). The patient complains of pain with hip flexion. Treatment consists of iliopsoas stretches and soft tissue therapy to the iliopsoas muscle. Occasionally surgical release may be required.[59]

Referred pain to the groin

The possibility of referred pain to the groin should always be considered, especially when there is little to find on local examination. A common site of referral to the groin is the SIJ and this should always be assessed in any examination of a patient with groin pain. The SIJ may also refer pain to the scrotum in males and labia in females. The assessment and treatment of sacroiliac problems have been discussed in Chapter 22.

The lumbar spine may refer pain to the groin. The lumbar spine and thoracolumbar junction should always be examined in a patient with groin pain. Neural tension tests, such as the slump and neural

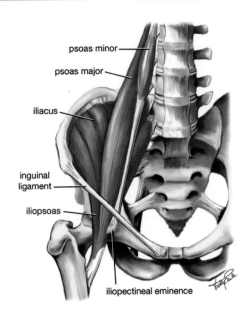

Figure 24.12 Internal snapping hip refers to the iliopsoas tendon flipping over the iliopectineal eminence

Thomas tests, should be performed as part of the assessment (Chapter 8). Variations such as the addition of adduction or hip rotation may reproduce the patient's pain.

A positive neural tension test result requires further evaluation to determine the site of the abnormality. The position of reproduction of pain can be used to correct neural tightness by stretching. Active trigger points may also refer to the groin and should be treated with soft tissue therapy.

Recommended Reading

Holmich P. Adductor-related groin pain in athletes. *Sports Med Arthrosc Rev* 1997; 5: 285–91.

Holmich P, Renstrom PAFH, Saartok T. Hip, groin and pelvis. In: Kjaer M, Krogsgaard M, Magnusson P, et al., eds. *Textbook of Sports Medicine*. Malden, MA: Blackwell Scientific, 2003: 616–37.

Holmich P, Uhrskow P, Ulnits L, et al. Effectiveness of active physical training for longstanding adductor-related groin pain in athletes. *Lancet* 1999; 353: 439–53.

Joesting DR. Diagnosis and treatment of sportsman's hernia. *Curr Sports Med Rep* 2002; 1: 121–4.

Johnson JD, Briner WW. Primary care of the sports hernia. *Physician Sportsmed* 2005; 33(2): 35–9.

Johnson R. Osteitis pubis. *Curr Sports Med Rep* 2003; 2: 98–102.

References

1. Renstrom P, Peterson L. Groin injuries in athletes. *Br J Sports Med* 1980; 14: 30–6.

2. Adams RJ, Chandler FA. Osteitis pubis of traumatic etiology. *J Bone Joint Surg* 1953; 35: 685–96.

3. Holmich P, Renstrom PAFH, Saartok T. Hip, groin and pelvis. In: Kjaer M, Krogsgaard M, Magnusson P, et al., eds. *Textbook of Sports Medicine*. Malden, MA: Blackwell Scientific, 2003: 616–37.

4. Taylor DC, Meyers WC, Moylan JA, et al. Abdominal musculature abnormalities as a cause of groin pain in athletes. Inguinal hernias and pubalgia. *Am J Sports Med* 1991; 19(3): 239–42.

5. Verrall GM, Slavotinek JP, Fon GT. Incidence of pubic bone marrow oedema in Australian Rules football players: relation to groin pain. *Br J Sports Med* 2001; 35: 28–33.

6. Williams JPG. Limitation of hip joint movement as a factor in traumatic osteitis pubis. *Br J Sports Med* 1978; 12: 129–33.

7. Fricker PA, Taunton JE, Ammann W. Osteitis pubis in athletes. *Sports Med* 1991; 12(4): 266–79.

8. Verrall GM, Hamilton IA, Slavotinek JP, et al. Hip joint range of motion reduction in sports-related chronic groin injury diagnosed as pubic bone stress injury. *J Sci Med Sport* 2005; 8(1): 77–84.

9. Major NM, Helms CA. Pelvic stress injuries: the relationship between osteitis pubis (symphysis stress injury) and sacroiliac abnormalities in athletes. *Skeletal Radiol* 1997; 26: 711–17.

10. Miller J, Schultz A, Anderson G. Load-displacement behavior of the sacro-iliac joint. *J Orthop Res* 1987; 5: 92–101.

11. Cowan SM, Schache AG, Brukner P, et al. Delayed onset of transversus abdominis in long-standing groin pain. *Med Sci Sports Exerc* 2004; 36(12): 2040–5.

12. Snijders CA, Vleeming R, Stoeckart J, et al. Biomechanical modeling of the sacroiliac stability in different postures. *Spine* 1995; 9: 419–32.

13. Pool-Goudzwaard A, Hoek van Dijke G, van Gurp M, et al. Contribution of pelvic floor muscles to stiffness of the pelvic ring. *Clin Biomech* 2004; 19: 564–71.

14. Holmich P, Holmich LR, Bjerg AM. Clinical examination of athletes with groin pain: an intraobserver and interobserver reliability study. *Br J Sports Med* 2004; 38: 446–51.

15. Orchard JW, Read JW, Neophyton J, et al. Groin pain associated with ultrasound finding of inguinal canal posterior wall deficiency in Australian Rules footballers. *Br J Sports Med* 1998; 32: 134–9.

16. van den Berg JC, de Valois JC, Go PM, et al. Detection of groin hernia with physical examination, ultrasound, and MRI compared with laparoscopic findings. *Invest Radiol* 1999; 34(12): 739–43.

17. Holmich P, Uhrskou P, Ulnits L, et al. Effectiveness of active physical training as treatment for long-standing adductor-related groin pain in athletes: a randomised trial. *Lancet* 1999; 353: 439–43.

18. Hogan A. *A Rehabilitation Program for Osteitis Pubis in Football*. Adelaide: OP Publications, 2006.

19. Mens J, Inklaar HK, Koes BW, et al. A new view on adduction-related groin pain. *Clin J Sport Med* 2006; 16(1): 15–19.

20. Tyler TF, Nicholas SJ, Campbell RJ, et al. The effectiveness of a preseason exercise program to prevent adductor muscle strains in professional ice hockey players. *Am J Sports Med* 2002; 30(5): 680–3.

21. Batt ME, McShane JM, Dillingham MF. Osteitis pubis in collegiate football players. *Med Sci Sports Exerc* 1995; 27: 629–33.

22. Ruane JJ, Rossi TA. When groin pain is more than 'just a strain': navigating a broad differential. *Physician Sportsmed* 1998; 26: 78.

23. McKim K, Taunton JE. The effectiveness of compression shorts in the treatment of athletes with osteitis pubis. *NZ J Sports Med* 2001; 29(4): 70–3.

24. Akemark C, Johansson C. Tenotomy of the adductor longus tendon in the treatment of chronic groin pain in athletes. *Am J Sports Med* 1992; 20: 640–3.

25. Meyers WC, Foley DP, Garrett WE, et al. Management of severe lower abdominal or inguinal pain in high-performance athletes. *Am J Sports Med* 2000; 28(1): 2–8.

26. Orchard JW, Cook JL, Halpin N. Stress-shielding as a cause of insertional tendinopathy: the operative technique of limited adductor tenotomy supports this theory. *J Sci Med Sport* 2004; 7(4): 424–8.

27. Fredberg U, Kissmeyer-Nielsen P. The sportsman's hernia—fact or fiction? *Scand J Med Sci Sports* 1996; 6: 201–4.

28. Hackney RG. The sports hernia: a cause of chronic groin pain. *Br J Sports Med* 1993; 27(1): 58–62.

29. Kemp S, Batt ME. The 'sports hernia'. A common cause of groin pain. *Physician Sportsmed* 1998; 26(1): 36–44.

30. Lovell G. The diagnosis of chronic groin pain in athletes: a review of 189 cases. *Aust J Sci Med Sport* 1995; 27(3): 76–9.

31. Malycha P, Lovell G. Inguinal surgery in athletes with chronic groin pain: the 'sportsman's' hernia. *Aust NZ J Surg* 1992; 62: 123–5.

32. Kumar A, Doran J, Batt ME. Results of inguinal canal repair in athletes with sports hernia. *J R Coll Surg Edinb* 2002; 47(3): 561–5.

33. Srinivasan A, Schuricht A. Long-term follow-up of laparoscopic preperitoneal hernia repair in professional athletes. *J Laparoendosc Adv Surg Tech A* 2002; 12(2): 101–6.

34. Simonet WT, Saylor HL, Sim L. Abdominal wall muscle tears in hockey players. *Int J Sports Med* 1995; 16: 126–8.

35. Hemmingway AE, Herrington L, Blower AL. Changes in muscle strength and pain in response to surgical repair of posterior abdominal wall disruption followed by rehabilitation. *Br J Sports Med* 2003; 37(1): 54–8.

36. Polglase AL, Frydman GM, Farmer KC. Inguinal surgery for debilitating chronic groin pain in athletes. *Med J Aust* 1991; 155: 674–7.

37. Susmallian S, Ezri T, Elis M, et al. Laparoscopic repair of 'sportsman's hernia' in soccer players as treatment of chronic inguinal pain. *Med Sci Monit* 2004; 10(2): CR52–54.

38. Genitsaris M, Goulimaris I, Sikas N. Laparoscopic repair of groin pain in athletes. *Am J Sports Med* 2004; 32(5): 1238–42.

39. Taylor DC, Meyers WC, Moylan JA, et al. Abdominal musculature abnormalities as a cause of groin pain in athletes. Inguinal hernias and pubalgia. *Am J Sports Med* 1991; 19: 239–42.

40. Biedert RM, Warnke K, Meyer S. Symphysis syndrome in athletes. Surgical treatment for chronic lower abdominal, groin, and adductor pain in athletes. *Clin J Sports Med* 2003; 13: 278–84.

41. Johnson JD, Briner WW Jr. Primary care of sports hernia. *Physician Sportsmed* 2005; 33(2): 35–39.

42. Brannigan AE, Kerin MJ, McEntee GP. Gilmore's groin repair in athletes. *J Orthop Sports Phys Ther* 2000; 30(6): 329–32.

43. Gilmore J. Groin pain in the soccer athlete: fact, fiction, and treatment. *Clin J Sport Med* 1998; 17: 787–93.

44. Lacroix VJ, Kinnear DG, Mulder DS, et al. Lower abdominal pain syndrome in national hockey league players: a report of 11 cases. *Clin J Sport Med* 1998; 8(1): 5–9.

45. Irshad K, Feldman LS, Lavoie C, et al. Operative management of 'hockey groin syndrome': 12 years of experience in national hockey league players (a). *Surgery* 2001; 130(4): 764–6.

46. Verrall GM, Slavotinek JP, Barnes PG, et al. Description of pain provocation tests used for the diagnosis of sports-related chronic groin pain: relationship of tests to defined clinical (pain and tenderness) and MRI (pubic bone marrow oedema) criteria. *Scand J Med Sci Sports* 2005; 15(1): 36–42.

47. Holt MA, Keene JS, Graf BK, et al. Treatment of osteitis pubis in athletes. Results of corticosteroid injections. *Am J Sports Med* 1995; 23(5): 601–6.

48. Topol GA, Reeves KD, Hassanein KM. Efficacy of dextrose prolotherapy in elite male kicking-sport athletes with groin pain. *Arch Phys Med Rehabil* 2005; 86: 697–702.

49. Maksymowych WP, Aaron SL, Russell AS. Treatment of refractory symphysis pubis with intravenous pamidronate. *J Rheumatol* 2001; 28(12): 2754–7.

50. Mulhall KJ. Osteitis pubis in professional soccer players: a report of outcome with symphyseal curettage in cases refractory to conservative management. *Clin J Sport Med* 2002; 12: 179–81.

51. Grace JN, Sim FH, Shives TC, et al. Wedge resection of the symphysis pubis for the treatment of osteitis pubis. *J Bone Joint Surg Am* 1989; 71A: 358–64.

52. Moore RSJ, Stover MD, Matta JM. Late posterior instability of the pelvis after resection of the symphysis pubis for the treatment of osteitis pubis. A report of two cases. *J Bone Joint Surg Am* 1998; 80A: 1043–8.

53. Williams PR, Thomas DP, Downes EM. Osteitis pubis and instability of the pubic symphysis: when nonoperative measures fail. *Am J Sports Med* 2000; 28(3): 350–5.

54. Bradshaw C, McCrory P, Bell S, et al. Obturator nerve entrapment: a cause of groin pain in athletes. *Am J Sports Med* 1997; 25(3): 402–8.

55. Brukner P, Bradshaw C, McCrory P. Obturator neuropathy. A cause of exercise-related groin pain. *Physician Sportsmed* 1999; 27(5): 62–73.

56. Brukner PD, Bennell KL, Matheson GO. *Stress Fractures.* Melbourne: Blackwell Scientific, 1999.

57. Lievense AM, Bierma-Zeinstra SMA, Verhagen AP, et al. Influence of sporting activities on the development of osteoarthritis of the hip: a systematic review. *Arthritis Rheum* 2003; 49(2): 228–36.

58. McCarthy JC, Lee J. Hip arthroscopy: indications, outcomes, and complications. *J Bone Joint Surg Am* 2005; 87A: 1138–45.

59. Ilizaliturri VMJ, Villalobos FEJ, Chaidez PA, et al. Internal snapping hip syndrome: treatment by endoscopic release of the iliopsoas tendon. *Arthroscopy* 2005; 21(11): 1375–80.

Anterior Thigh Pain

The anterior thigh (Fig. 25.1) is the site of common sporting injuries such as quadriceps muscle contusion and strain of the quadriceps muscle. Referred pain from the hip, sacroiliac joint (SIJ) or lumbar spine may also cause anterior thigh pain. Stress fracture of the femur is an uncommon, but important, diagnosis. The causes of anterior thigh pain are shown in Table 25.1.

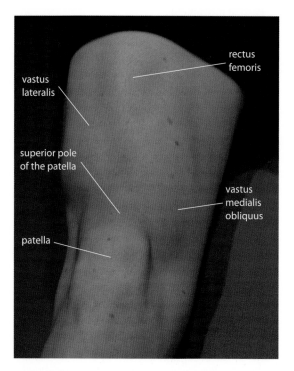

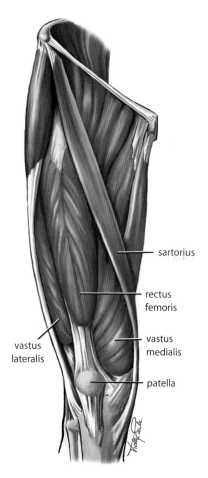

Figure 25.1 Anatomy of the anterior thigh

(a) Surface anatomy

(b) Muscles of the anterior thigh

Table 25.1 Causes of anterior thigh pain

Common	Less common	Not to be missed
Quadriceps muscle contusion (cork thigh, charley horse)	Referred pain (upper lumbar spine, sacroiliac joint, hip joint)	Slipped capital femoral epiphysis
Quadriceps muscle strain (rectus femoris)	Stress fracture of the femur	Perthes' disease
Myositis ossificans	Sartorius muscle strain	Tumor (e.g. osteosarcoma of the femur)
	Gracilis strain	
	Avulsion of the apophysis of rectus femoris	

Clinical approach

History

The two most important aspects of the history of a patient with anterior thigh pain are the exact site of the pain and the mechanism of injury. The site of the pain is usually well localized in cases of contusion or muscle strain. Muscle strains occur in the mid belly. Contusions can occur anywhere in the quadriceps muscle but they are most common anterolaterally or in the vastus medialis obliquus.

The mechanism of injury may help differentiate between the two conditions. A contusion is likely to be the result of a direct blow, whereas a muscle strain usually occurs when an athlete is striving for extra speed running or extra distance kicking. In contact sports, however, the athlete may have difficulty recalling the exact mechanism of injury.

Whether the athlete was able to continue activity, the present level of function and the degree of swelling are all guides to the severity of the condition. Determine whether the RICE regimen was implemented initially and whether any aggravating factors, such as a hot shower, heat rub, excessive activity or alcohol ingestion were present. Gradual onset of poorly localized anterior thigh pain in a distance runner worsening with activity may indicate stress fracture of the femur. If the pain is variable and not clearly localized and if specific aggravating factors are lacking, consider referred pain. Bilateral pain suggests the pain is referred from the lumbar spine.

Examination

In anterior thigh pain of acute onset, the diagnosis is usually straightforward and examination is confined primarily to local structures. In anterior thigh pain of insidious onset, diagnosis is more difficult. Examination should include sites that refer pain to the thigh, such as the lumbar spine, SIJ and hip.

The aim of the examination is to determine the exact site of the abnormality and to assess range of motion and muscle strength. Functional testing may be necessary to reproduce the symptoms.

1. Observation
   (a) standing
   (b) walking
   (c) supine
2. Active movements
   (a) hip flexion
   (b) knee flexion
   (c) knee extension
3. Passive movements
   (a) hip and knee (e.g. hip quadrant)
   (b) muscle stretch (e.g. quadriceps) (Fig. 25.2a)

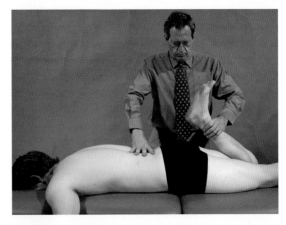

Figure 25.2 Examination of the patient with anterior thigh pain

(a) Passive movement—quadriceps stretch. A passive stretch of the quadriceps muscles is performed with full knee flexion. Passive hip extension may be added to increase the stretch on the rectus femoris, which may reproduce the patient's pain

4. Resisted movements
    (a) knee extension (Fig. 25.2b)
    (b) straight leg raise
    (c) hip flexion (Fig. 25.2c)

5. Functional tests
    (a) squat (Fig. 25.2d)
    (b) jump
    (c) hop
    (d) kick
6. Palpation
    (a) quadriceps muscle (Fig. 25.2e)
7. Special tests
    (a) femoral stress fracture (Fig. 25.2f)
    (b) neural tension (Fig. 25.2g)
    (c) lumbar spine (Chapter 21)
    (d) SIJ (Chapter 22)

Investigations

Investigations are usually not required in athletes with anterior thigh pain. If a quadriceps contusion fails to respond to treatment, X-ray may demonstrate myositis ossificans. This is usually not evident until at least three weeks after the injury. Ultrasound examination will confirm the presence of a hematoma and may demonstrate early evidence of calcification.

If a stress fracture of the femur is suspected, plain X-ray is indicated. If this is normal, an isotopic bone scan or MRI is required.

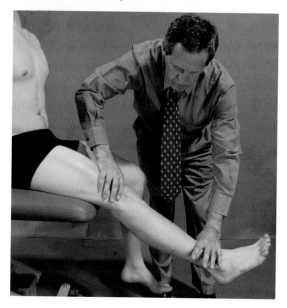

(b) Resisted movement—knee extension. With the hip and knee flexed to 90°, the knee is extended against resistance

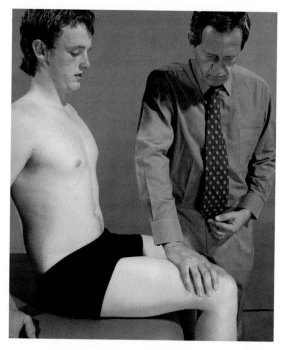

(c) Resisted movement—hip flexion

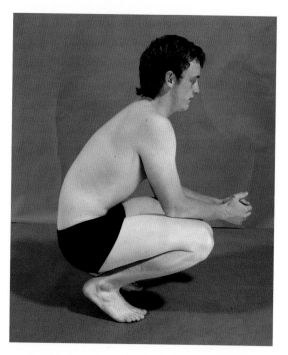

(d) Functional movements—squat. If the previous activities have failed to reproduce the patient's pain, functional movements should be used to reproduce the pain. These may include squat, hop or jump

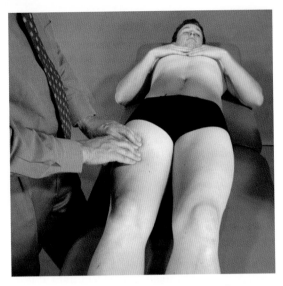

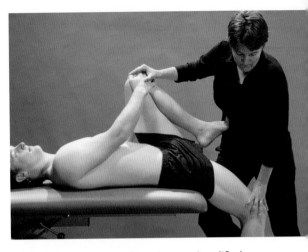

(e) Palpation. The anterior thigh is palpated for tenderness, swelling and areas of focal muscle thickening. A focal defect in the muscle belly may be palpated, especially with active muscle contraction

(g) Special tests—neural tension test (modified Thomas's test). The patient is placed in the psoas stretch position. Cervical and upper thoracic flexion is added and then the clinician passively bends the patient's knee (using his or her own leg). Reproduction of the patient's symptoms when the extra neural tension is added indicates a neural contribution

An X-ray of the hip joint should be performed if thigh pain is associated with restricted or painful hip motion. Although hip pathology most often refers to the groin (Chapter 23), it can refer to the anterior, and occasionally lateral, thigh. In adults, the most likely abnormality is degenerative, while in adolescents, a slipped capital femoral epiphysis or avulsion fracture must be considered.

Quadriceps contusion

If the patient suffered a direct blow to the anterior thigh and examination confirms an area of tenderness and swelling with worsening pain on active contraction and passive stretch, thigh contusion with resultant hematoma is the most likely diagnosis. In severe cases with extensive swelling, pain may be severe enough to interfere with sleep.

Quadriceps contusion is an extremely common injury and is known colloquially as a 'charley horse' or 'cork thigh'. It is common in contact sports such as football and basketball. In sports such as hockey, lacrosse and cricket, a ball traveling at high speed may cause a contusion.

Trauma to the muscle will cause primary damage to myofibrils, fascia and blood vessels. Localized bleeding may increase tissue pressure and cause relative regional anoxia that can result in secondary tissue

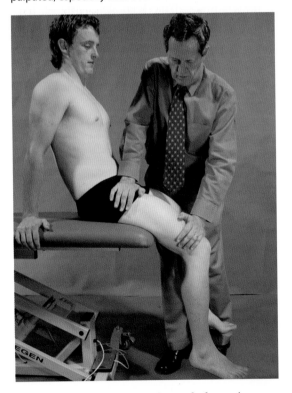

(f) Special tests—for the presence of a femoral stress fracture. This is performed with pressure over the distal end of the femur. Reproduction of the patient's pain may be indicative of a femoral stress fracture

damage. The contusion may be either intramuscular or intermuscular. In the intermuscular hematoma, the blood escapes through the fascia and is distributed between the compartments of the thigh. The intramuscular hematoma is confined to the muscle compartment which fills up with blood. The intramuscular hematoma is more painful and restrictive of range of motion. Usually only a single quadriceps muscle will be affected.

It is important to assess the severity of the contusion to determine prognosis (this can vary from several days to a number of weeks off sport) and plan appropriate treatment. The degree of passive knee flexion after 24 hours is an indicator of the severity of the hematoma. For optimal treatment and accurate monitoring of progress, it is important to identify the exact muscle involved. MRI will show significant edema throughout the involved muscle (Fig. 25.3). Blood from contusions of the lower third of the thigh may track down to the knee joint and irritate the patellofemoral joint.

Treatment

The treatment of a thigh contusion can be divided into four stages: stage 1—control of hemorrhage;

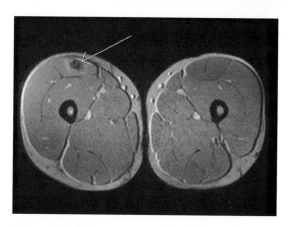

Figure 25.3 MRI appearance of severe hematoma (arrow) of the vastus intermedius muscle

stage 2—restoration of pain-free range of motion; stage 3—functional rehabilitation; stage 4—graduated return to activity.

A summary of the types of treatment appropriate for each stage is shown in Tables 25.2 and 25.3. Progression within each stage, and from one stage to the next, depends on the severity of the contusion and the rate of recovery.

Table 25.2 Grading and treatment of quadriceps contusion

Grading	Clinical features	Treatment
Mild	May or may not remember incident Usually can continue activity Sore after cooling down or next morning May restrict full ROM (stretch) 5–20% Tender to palpation Minimal loss of strength	Ice, magnetic field therapy, stretch and bandage for first 24–48 hours Then should regain full ROM and start functional strengthening—bike, running, swimming Strengthening may be required Soft tissue therapy and electrotherapy are effective
Moderate	Usually remembers incident but can continue activity although may stiffen up with rest (e.g. half-time or full-time) Moderate restriction of ROM 20–50% Some pain on restricted contraction Tender to palpation May have tracking Usually FWB, but often limp	See Table 25.3
Severe	Usually remembers incident May not be able to control rapid onset of swelling/bleeding Severe loss of movement (50%) Difficulty with FWB Tender over large area (tracking) Obvious bleeding Functional loss of strength	Ice regularly over 2–3 days Stretches (active after 2–3 days) No massage/ultrasound No overpressure with passive stretching for 7–10 days

ROM = range of motion; FWB = full weight-bearing.

Table 25.3 Treatment of moderate quadriceps contusion or grade II muscle strain

Stage	Aim	Weight-bearing	RICE	Electrotherapy	Soft tissue therapy	Stretching	Strengthening
1	Control of hemorrhage	Crutches if unable to FWB	RICE, compression to include knee joint if lower third of thigh (Fig. 25.4)	Electrical stimulation Magnetic field therapy Laser if superficial Pulsed ultrasound	Contraindicated	Gentle stretch to onset of pain (Fig. 25.5a)	Static muscle contraction if possible
2	Restore and maintain pain-free ROM and muscle strength	Progress to PWB and FWB as tolerated	Maintain compression bandage when limb is dependent. Ice after exercise	As for stage 1 Higher dosages for thermal effect (ultrasound)	Grade I–II longitudinal gliding away from site of injury Grade II transverse gliding away from site of injury	Increase stretches	Static muscle contraction inner range through range (Fig. 25.6a) Stationary exercise: bike Pool (walk/swim/kick) Concentric and eccentric exercise (Fig. 25.6b)
3	Functional rehabilitation	FWB		Usually not required	Longitudinal gliding Transverse gliding	Maintain stretch (Fig. 25.5b)	All stage 2 exercises gradually increasing repetitions, speed and resistance Include pulleys, rebounder, profitter, wall squats, step-downs (Fig. 25.6c) Hop/jumping, running Increase eccentric exercises
4	Gradual return to sports				Myofascial tension in knee flexion (Fig. 25.7)		Kicking action with pulleys Multidirectional activities Figure of eight Jumping Plyometrics Graduated specific sporting activities Must complete full training before return to sport Heat-retaining brace may be helpful

PWB = partial weight-bearing; FWB = full weight-bearing; ROM = range of motion.

The most important period in the treatment of a thigh contusion is in the first 24 hours following the injury. Upon suffering a thigh contusion, the player should be removed from the field of play and the RICE regimen (Chapter 10) instituted immediately. The importance of rest and elevation of the affected leg must be emphasized. The use of crutches ensures adequate rest if full weight-bearing is painful and encourages the athlete to recognize the serious nature of the condition.

 In the acute management of a thigh contusion, ice should be applied in a position of maximal pain-free quadriceps stretch (Fig. 25.4).

The patient must be careful not to aggravate the bleeding by excessive activity, alcohol ingestion or the application of heat.

Loss of range of motion is the most significant finding after thigh contusion and range of movement must be regained in a gradual, pain-free progression.

After a moderate-to-severe contusion there is a considerable risk of rebleed in the first seven to 10 days. Therefore, care must be taken with stretching, electrotherapy, heat and massage. The patient must be careful not to overstretch. Stretching should be pain-free.

Soft tissue therapy is contraindicated for 48 hours following contusion. Subsequently, soft tissue therapy may be used but great care must be taken not to aggravate the condition. Treatment must be light and it must produce absolutely no pain (Fig. 25.7). The aim of soft tissue therapy in the first few days after a thigh contusion is to promote lymphatic drainage.

Excessively painful soft tissue therapy will cause bleeding to recur and is never indicated in the treatment of contusion.

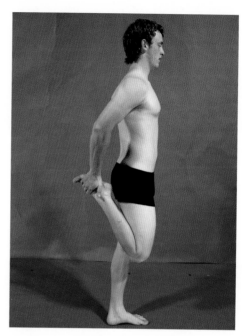

Figure 25.5 Quadriceps stretching exercises

(a) Standard quadriceps stretch while standing. It is important to have good pelvic control and not to lean forward while performing the stretch

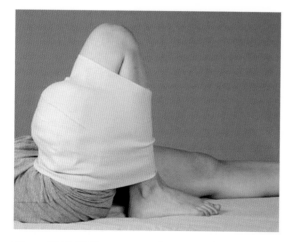

Figure 25.4 RICE treatment of an acute thigh contusion in a position of maximal pain-free stretch

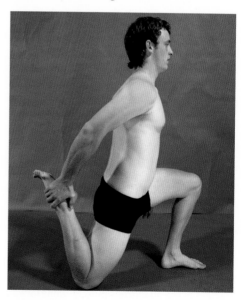

(b) Passive stretch. The tension of the stretch can be altered by adding hip extension

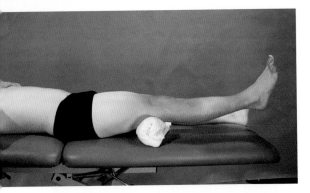

Figure 25.6 Quadriceps strengthening exercises

(a) Active quadriceps exercises. Initially inner range quadriceps strengthening is performed with a rolled towel under the knee as shown. The range is slowly increased, depending on symptoms, until through-range quadriceps contraction can be performed pain-free

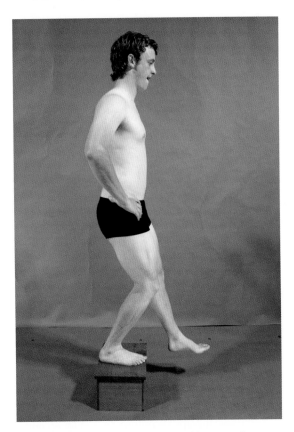

(c) Functional exercises. A variety of functional exercises can be performed in the late stage of rehabilitation: squats, wall squats, step-downs (illustrated), shuttle. Most of these involve both eccentric and concentric contraction of the quadriceps

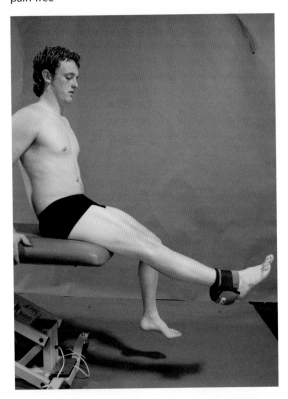

(b) Resisted quadriceps. Concentric and eccentric exercises are performed against gradually increased resistance. Knee extension involves concentric contraction of the quadriceps muscle, while lowering the foot from extension involves eccentric quadriceps contraction

Quadriceps contusion is a condition that can be prevented. Patients who are recovering from a previous contusion may benefit from thigh protection. Athletes in high-risk sports should consider wearing thigh protection routinely.[1]

Players such as ruckmen in Australian football, forwards in basketball and running backs in American football may sustain a series of minor contusions during the course of a game. These appear to have a cumulative effect and may impair performance later in the game. Protective padding helps to minimize this effect.

Compartment syndrome of the thigh

Intramuscular hematoma of the thigh after a blunt contusion may result in high intracompartment pressures and a diagnosis of compartment syndrome of

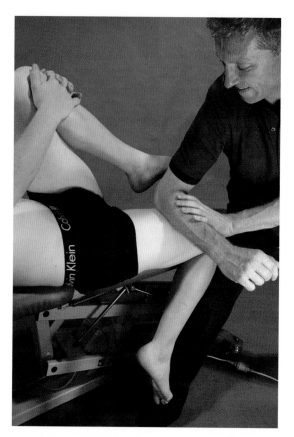

Figure 25.7 Soft tissue therapy—sustained myofascial tension in the position of maximal hip extension and knee flexion

following the injury and lay down new bone over a number of weeks. After approximately six or seven weeks, this bone growth ceases. At this stage, a lump is often palpable. Slow resorption of the bone then occurs but a small amount of bone may remain.

Why some contusions develop calcification is not known. The more severe the contusion the more likely is the development of myositis ossificans. Inappropriate treatment such as heat or massage may increase the risk of the complication arising.[5] The risk of myositis ossificans is especially high if the contusion results in prone knee flexion of less than 45° two to three days after the injury. Thus, particular care should be taken when managing these severe contusions. A significant rebleed may also result in the development of myositis ossificans. The incidence of myositis ossificans appears to be increased when a knee effusion is present.

Symptoms of developing myositis ossificans include an increase in morning pain and pain with activity. Patients often complain of night pain. On palpation, the developing myositis ossificans has a characteristic 'woody' feel. Initial improvement in range of motion ceases with subsequent deterioration.

Once myositis ossificans is established, there is very little that can be done to accelerate the resorptive process. Treatment may include local electrotherapy to reduce muscle spasm and gentle, painless range of motion exercises. Corticosteroid injection is absolutely contraindicated in this condition and anecdotal reports suggest that surgery is unhelpful and at times appears to accelerate progress of the condition.

the thigh. However, unlike other compartment syndromes, there is no evidence that this condition needs to be treated by surgical decompression. A number of cases of surgery have been reported but none have reported evidence of necrotic muscle or subsequent clinical evidence of muscle fibrosis, restriction of knee motion or loss of function.[2] Treatment of this condition should be conservative as described above.[2, 3]

Myositis ossificans

Occasionally after a thigh contusion, the hematoma calcifies. This condition is known as myositis ossificans and can usually be seen on a plain X-ray a minimum of three weeks after the injury. If there is no convincing history of recent trauma, the practitioner must rule out the differential diagnosis of the X-ray—bone tumor (Chapter 4).[4]

In myositis ossificans, osteoblasts replace some of the fibroblasts in the healing hematoma one week

Quadriceps muscle strain

Strains of the quadriceps muscle usually occur during sprinting, jumping or kicking. Strains are seen in all the quadriceps muscles but are most common in the rectus femoris, which is more vulnerable to strain as it passes over two joints: the hip and the knee. The most common site of strain is the distal musculotendinous junction of the rectus femoris. Management of this type of rectus femoris strain and of strains of the vasti muscles is relatively straightforward; rehabilitation time is short. Strains of the proximal rectus are not as straightforward and considered separately below.

Like all muscle strains, quadriceps strains may be graded into mild (grade I), moderate (grade II) or severe, complete tears (grade III). The athlete feels the injury as a sudden pain in the anterior thigh during an activity requiring explosive muscle contraction. There is local pain and tenderness and, if the strain is severe, swelling and bruising.

Grade I strain is a minor injury with pain on resisted active contraction and on passive stretching. An area of local spasm is palpable at the site of pain. An athlete with such a strain may not cease activity at the time of the pain but will usually notice the injury after cooling down or the following day.

Moderate or grade II strains cause significant pain on passive stretching as well as on unopposed active contraction. There is usually a moderate area of inflammation surrounding a tender palpable lesion. The athlete with a grade II strain is generally unable to continue the activity.

Complete tears of the rectus femoris occur with sudden onset of pain and disability during intense activity. A muscle fiber defect is usually palpable when the muscle is contracted. In the long term, they resolve with conservative management, often with surprisingly little disability.

Treatment

The principles of treatment of a quadriceps muscle strain are similar to those of a thigh contusion. The various treatment techniques shown in Table 25.3 are also appropriate for the treatment of quadriceps strain; however, depending on the severity of the strain, progression through the various stages may be slower.

Although loss of range of motion may be less obvious than with a contusion, it is important that the athlete regain pain-free range of movement as soon as possible. Loss of strength may be more marked than with a thigh contusion and strength retraining requires emphasis in the rehabilitation program. As with the general principles of muscle rehabilitation, the program should commence with low resistance, high repetition exercise. Concentric and eccentric exercises should begin with very low weights. General fitness can be maintained by activities such as swimming (initially with a pool buoy) and upper body training. Functional retraining should be incorporated as soon as possible. Full training must be completed prior to return to sport. Unfortunately, quadriceps strains often recur, either in the same season, or even a year to two later.[6]

Proximal rectus femoris strains

With the advent of MRI, a second type of rectus femoris strain injury was recognized occurring proximally, apparently within the belly of the muscle. This has been termed a *bull's eye* lesion[7] and seemed to contradict the basic tenet that muscle strain occurs at

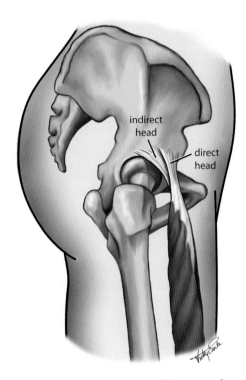

Figure 25.8 Schematic drawing of the rectus femoris muscle–tendon unit ADAPTED FROM HASSELMAN ET AL. P. 495

the muscle–tendon junction. In subsequent cadaveric studies[8] it was shown that the proximal tendon of the rectus femoris muscle actually has two components: the direct and indirect heads (Fig. 25.8). The tendon of the indirect head arises from the superior acetabular ridge and travels distally initially deep to the direct head. As it progresses along the muscle it flattens out, laterally rotates, and migrates to the middle of the muscle belly. This has been termed the *central tendon*.

In three series of these injuries,[7, 9, 10] the average time to presentation was five to seven months and the patients complained of a tender anterior thigh mass and/or weakness and pain with activities such as running and kicking. Hughes et al.[7] hypothesized that this was due to the indirect (central tendon) and direct heads of the proximal tendon acting independently, creating a shearing phenomenon in contrast to what occurs in the normal rectus femoris. A more recent series diagnosed on MRI[11] showed an average return to full training in professional footballers after a comprehensive rehabilitation program of 27 days for central tendon lesions compared to nine days for peripheral rectus femoris strains and 4.5 days for strains of the vasti muscles.

Differentiating between a mild quadriceps strain and a quadriceps contusion

Occasionally, it may be difficult to distinguish between a minor contusion and a minor muscle strain but the distinction needs to be made as an athlete with a thigh strain should progress more slowly through a rehabilitation program (Table 25.3) than should the athlete with quadriceps contusion. The athlete with thigh strain should avoid sharp acceleration and deceleration movements in the early stages of injury. Some of the features that may assist the clinician in differentiating these conditions are shown in Table 25.4. Diagnostic ultrasound examination may be helpful in differentiating between the two conditions.

Less common causes

Stress fracture of the femur

Stress fracture of the shaft of the femur, although uncommon, should be suspected in an athlete, especially a distance runner, who complains of a dull ache, poorly localized in the anterior thigh. Pain may be referred to the knee. There may be tenderness over the shaft of the femur that can be aggravated if the patient sits with the leg hanging over the edge of a bench, particularly if there is downward pressure placed on the distal femur, the so-called *hang test* or *fulcrum test* (Fig. 25.2f).

 A positive 'hang test' is strongly suggestive of stress fracture of the femur.

X-ray may show a stress fracture but more commonly an isotopic bone scan or MRI (Fig. 25.9) is required.

Treatment involves rest from painful activities and maintenance of fitness by cycling or swimming. Predisposing factors such as excessive training,

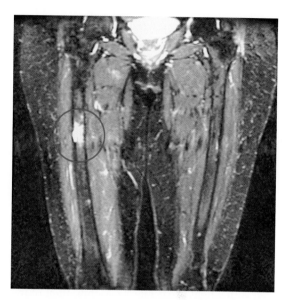

Figure 25.9 MRI of a stress fracture of the shaft of the femur

Table 25.4 Distinguishing features of minor quadriceps contusion and grade I quadriceps muscle strain

Diagnostic features	Quadriceps contusion	Grade I rectus femoris muscle strain
Mechanism	Contact injury	Non-contact
Pain onset	Immediate or soon after	After cool-down (next day)
Behavior of pain (24 hours post trauma)	Improves with gentle activity	Painful with use
Location	Usually lateral or distal	Rectus femoris muscle belly (proximal or middle third)
Bruising/swelling	May be obvious early	May be absent or delayed
Palpation findings	Tenderness more obvious, lump may feel ovoid or spherical, becomes progressively harder	May be difficult to find or small area of focal tenderness with a characteristic ring of inflammation surrounding it Muscle spasm in adjacent fibers proximally and distally
Effect of gentle stretch	May initially aggravate pain	Not associated with pain
Strength testing	No loss of strength except pain inhibition	Loss of strength (may need eccentric or functional testing to reproduce pain)

biomechanical abnormality and, in females, menstrual disturbance should be sought, and corrected where possible. When the hang test is completely negative, on average after seven weeks, it is thought to be safe to return to sport gradually.[12]

Referred pain

Referred pain may arise from the hip joint, the SIJ, the lumbar spine (especially upper lumbar) and neural structures. Patients with referred pain may not have a history of injury and have few signs suggesting local abnormalities. An increase in neural tension may suggest that referred pain is a contributing to thigh pain. The modified Thomas's test (Fig. 25.2h) is the most specific neural tension test for a patient with anterior thigh pain.

If the modified Thomas's test reproduces the patient's anterior thigh pain and altering the neural tension (e.g. passive knee flexion/extension) affects the pain, the lumbar spine and psoas muscle should be examined carefully. Any area(s) of abnormality should be treated and both the local signs (e.g. reproduction of pain with functional testing) and neural tension tests should be repeated to assess any changes. As with any soft tissue injury, local and referred factors may combine to produce the patient's symptoms. Commonly there is hypomobility of the upper lumbar intervertebral segments on the affected side associated with a tight psoas muscle. Mobilization of the hypomobile segments will often significantly reduce symptoms. Deep soft tissue treatment to the psoas muscle may also be effective (Fig. 25.10).

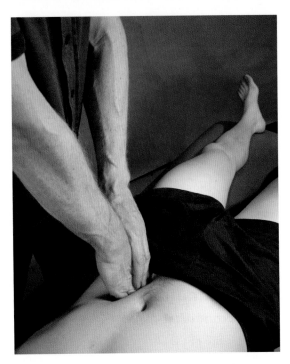

Figure 25.10 Deep soft tissue treatment to the psoas muscle

References

1. Gerrard DF. The use of padding in rugby union. An overview. *Sports Med* 1998; 25: 329–32.

2. Diaz JA, Fischer DA, Rettig AC, et al. Severe quadriceps muscle contusions in athletes—a report of three cases. *Am J Sports Med* 2003; 31(2): 289–93.

3. Robinson D, On E, Halperin N. Anterior compartment syndrome of the thigh in athletes—indications of conservative management. *J Trauma* 1992; 32: 183–6.

4. Tsuno MM, Shu GJ. Myositis ossificans. *J Manipulative Physiol Ther* 1990; 13: 340–2.

5. Danchilk JJ, Yochum TR, Aspergren DD. Myositis ossificans traumatica. *J Manipulative Physiol Ther* 1993; 16: 605–14.

6. Orchard JW. Intrinsic and extrinsic risk factors for muscle strains in Australian football. *Am J Sports Med* 2001; 29(3): 300–3.

7. Hughes C IV, Hasselman CT, Best TM, et al. Incomplete, intrasubstance strain injuries of the rectus femoris muscle. *Am J Sports Med* 1995; 23(4): 500–6.

8. Hasselman CT, Best TM, Hughes IV C, et al. An explanation for various rectus femoris strain injuries using previously undescribed muscle architecture. *Am J Sports Med* 1995; 23(4): 493–9.

9. Rask MR, Lattig GJ. Traumatic fibrosis of the rectus femoris muscle. *JAMA* 1972; 221: 268–9.

10. Temple HT, Kuklo TR, Sweet DE, et al. Rectus femoris muscle tear appearing as a pseudotumor. *Am J Sports Med* 1998; 26: 544–8.

11. Cross TM, Gibbs N, Houang MT, et al. Acute quadriceps muscle strains: magnetic resonance imaging features and prognosis. *Am J Sports Med* 2004; 32(3): 710–19.

12. Johnson AW, Weiss CB, Wheeler DL. Stress fractures of the femoral shaft in athletes—more common than expected. A new clinical test. *Am J Sports Med* 1994; 22: 248–56.

Posterior Thigh Pain

CHAPTER

26

WITH ANTHONY SCHACHE

Anatomy

The hamstring muscle group (Fig. 26.1) consists of three main muscles: biceps femoris, semimembranosus and semitendinosus. Biceps femoris has two heads, with the short head originating from the linea aspera and thus only acting on the knee joint.

Biceps femoris has a dual innervation, with the long head being innervated by the tibial portion of the sciatic nerve (L5, S1–3), whereas the short head

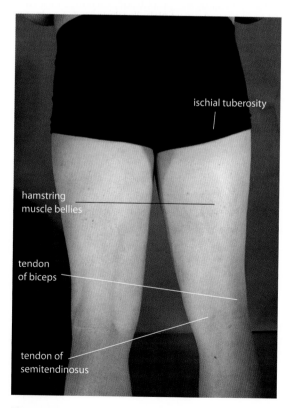

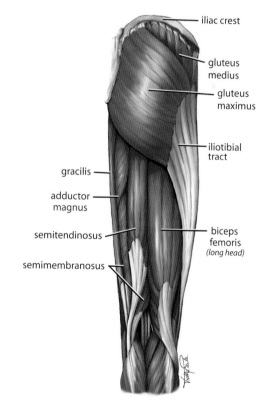

Figure 26.1 Anatomy of the posterior thigh

(a) Surface anatomy

(b) Muscles of the posterior thigh

is innervated by the common peroneal division (L5, S1–2).

The posterior portion of the adductor magnus is sometimes considered functionally as a hamstring due to its anatomical alignment. Adductor magnus is involved in hip extension and adduction and has innervation from the tibial portion of the sciatic nerve, like the majority of the hamstring group.

Clinical perspective

The effective management of posterior thigh pain is dependent upon correct diagnosis. Initially, the practitioner must determine whether the injury to the posterior thigh is a muscle strain or pain referred from elsewhere. This is not always a simple process. However, if not established, the athlete, practitioner and coach may be frustrated by a recurrent injury that hinders a successful return to sport.

In healthy individuals, a strain to a large muscle group such as the hamstrings is the result of a substantial force. The athlete should recall a particular point in time that the incident occurred and whether a significant force was applied to the muscle. Practitioners should be reticent to diagnose a muscle strain in the absence of these findings. Often this fundamental but common mistake will lead to inappropriate treatment. Tethering of neural structures or fascial strains in the posterior thigh can also occur as an incident, however, appropriate examination will reveal whether the injury has a fascial or neural component. The causes of posterior thigh pain are shown in Table 26.1.

 PRACTISE PEARL The challenge in patients with posterior thigh pain is to distinguish between a hamstring muscle strain and referred pain from the lumbar spine or gluteal muscle trigger points.

History

Posterior thigh pain that is not the result of a hamstring strain will require skilful clinical reasoning to determine the cause. This involves not only an intricate knowledge of the local anatomy and possible abnormalities but also an understanding of the structures that can refer pain into this region. Practitioners should be aware of the wide variety of assessment and treatment techniques used around the pelvis in order to make an accurate diagnosis. Systems of treatment often are associated with a specific diagnosis. Therefore, a common fault in manual medicine is to make the diagnosis based on what best fits with the treatment technique of choice.

The inability to utilize alternative techniques leads a practitioner to the inevitable conclusion that the presenting injury can only be a result of a diagnosis that fits in with the technique they are most competent in using. For example, a practitioner unskilled in sacroiliac management is unlikely to ever diagnose referred pain from the SIJ as a cause of hamstring pain.

History taking has the same goals and objectives as any other area in sports medicine. However, because there are so many causes of posterior thigh pain, the clinician, having taken the history, must be able to formulate a definite set of goals for the subsequent examination. Otherwise, time will limit the examination or there will be confusion with the vast amount of information collected.

Table 26.1 Causes of posterior thigh pain

Common	Less common	Not to be missed
Hamstring muscle strains	Referred pain	Tumors
Acute	Sacroiliac joint	Bone tumors
Recurrent	Tendinopathy	Vascular
Hamstring muscle	Bursitis	Iliac artery endofibrosis
contusion	Semimembranous	
Referred pain	Ischiogluteal	
Lumbar spine	Fibrous adhesions	
Neural structures	'Hamstring syndrome' (Chapter 22)	
Gluteal trigger points	Chronic compartment syndrome of the posterior thigh	
	Apophysitis/avulsion fracture of the ischial tuberosity (in adolescents)	
	Nerve entrapments	
	Posterior cutaneous thigh	
	Sciatic	
	Adductor magnus strains	
	Myositis ossificans, hamstring muscle	

The important points to consider in the history of the patient with posterior thigh pain are listed below. Note that this is a guide only and is not comprehensive.

1. Level of activity
   (a) Has a change in training caused injury?
   (b) Is there an adequate base of training?
2. Occupation/lifestyle
   (a) What factors outside of sport could be aggravating the condition (e.g. prolonged sitting at work, bending over with young children)?
3. Incident
   (a) Yes: consider strain, fascial/neural trauma.
   (b) No (not a strain!): consider overuse, referred pain, alternative abnormality.
4. Progress since injury
   (a) Slow: indicates a more severe injury.
   (b) Erratic: strain is being aggravated by activity or injury is not a strain.
5. Aggravating factors
   (a) Incident related: useful for specificity of rehabilitation (e.g. acceleration injuries require acceleration in the rehabilitation program).
   (b) Non-incident related: eradication or modification for recovery and prevention (e.g. sitting at a computer causing back/hamstring pain requires ergonomic modification).
6. Behavior with sport
   (a) Warms up with activity, worse after— inflammatory pathology.
   (b) Starts minimal or with no pain, builds up with activity but not as severe after— claudicant, either neurological or vascular.
   (c) Sudden onset: mechanical (e.g. strain).
7. Night pain
   (a) Sinister pathology.
   (b) Inflammatory condition.
8. Site of pain
   (a) Posterior thigh and lower back: lumbar referral or neuromotor/biomechanical mediator.
   (b) Buttock, SIJ without lower back symptoms: trigger points.
   (c) Ischial: tendinopathy/bursitis.
9. Presence of neurological symptoms
   (a) Nerve involvement.
10. Recurrent problem
    (a) Extensive examination and rehabilitation required.

Examination

All examinations should commence with observation and palpation. The remainder of the examination will depend on information gathered in the history. It is beneficial to have several quick tests to screen for various factors that commonly cause hamstring pain. However, once the most likely cause of pain has been identified, the most appropriate technique of assessment should be implemented to identify the exact nature of the problem. The initial examination should be thorough but not excessive. Contributing factors or alternative sources of pain in the hamstring group can be evaluated in subsequent examinations.

1. Observation
   (a) standing (Fig. 26.2a)
   (b) walking
   (c) lying prone
2. Active movements
   (a) lumbar movements
   (b) hip extension
   (c) knee flexion
   (d) knee extension
3. Passive movements
   (a) hamstring muscle stretch (Fig. 26.2b)
4. Resisted movements
   (a) knee flexion
   (b) hip extension
   (c) eccentric hamstring contraction (Fig. 26.2c)
5. Functional tests
   (a) kicking
   (b) running
   (c) sprint starts
6. Palpation
   (a) hamstring muscles (Fig. 26.2d)
   (b) ischial tuberosity
   (c) gluteal muscles (Fig. 26.2e)
7. Special tests
   (a) neural tension: slump test (Fig. 26.2f)
   (b) lumbar spine examination (Chapter 21)
   (c) sacroiliac joint (Chapter 22)
   (d) assessment of lumbopelvic stability (Chapter 11)
   (e) biomechanical analysis (video)

Investigations

Investigations of posterior thigh pain may be useful in defining the source of pain but practitioners must not take these findings in isolation from the rest of the examination. Both ultrasound and MRI can be used to confirm the presence of a muscle tear in cases where the diagnosis is in doubt clinically.

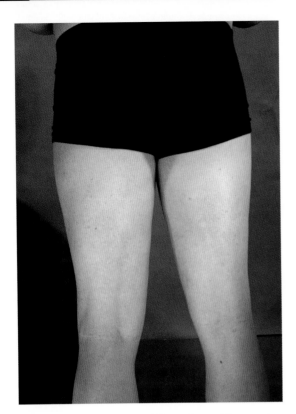

Figure 26.2 Examination of the patient with posterior thigh pain

(a) Observation. Look for wasting, bruising or swelling of the posterior thigh. Observation of gait is also important. Observation of the lumbar spine may show the presence of an excessive lordosis or relative asymmetry. A lateral view may demonstrate excessive lumbar lordosis or anterior pelvic tilt

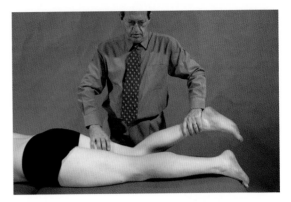

(c) Resisted movement—eccentric hamstring contraction. If pain is not produced by concentric contraction, an eccentric hamstring contraction should be performed as shown. This can be performed by rapid extension and catch or resistance against the force of the examiner's hand, which slowly extends the knee

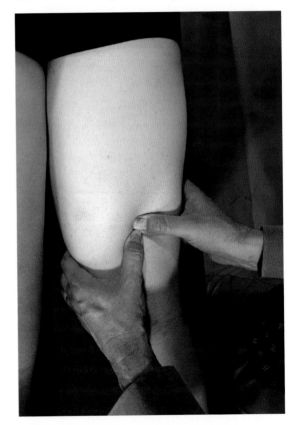

(d) Palpation. Commence with the belly of the hamstring muscle with the knee in partial flexion. Palpation should also be performed during muscle contraction and with the muscle on stretch. The hamstring origin should also be palpated

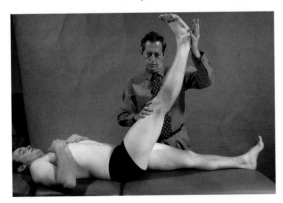

(b) Passive movement—hamstring muscle stretch. The leg is raised to the point where pain is first felt and then to the end of range, pain permitting. Movement should be compared to the uninjured side

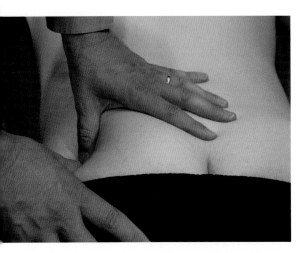

(e) Palpation—gluteal muscles. Palpate the gluteal muscles for trigger points that are taut bands, which are usually exquisitely tender locally and may refer pain into the hamstring muscle

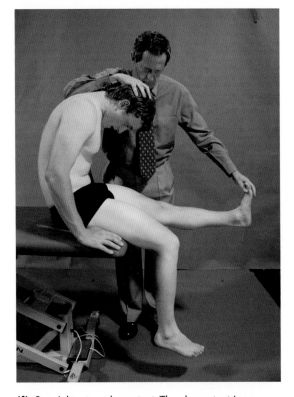

(f) Special tests—slump test. The slump test is an essential part of the examination of the patient with posterior thigh pain (Chapter 8). The slump test plays an important role in differentiating between hamstring muscle injuries and referred pain to the hamstring region from the lumbar spine

Hamstring muscle strains

Acute, moderate or severe hamstring strains are common injuries among sprinters, hurdlers and long jumpers. They also occur in other sports involving sprinting, especially football and field hockey. There is a tendency towards an increased incidence with increasing age. Hamstring injuries occur frequently despite the prevalence of stretching and strengthening programs.

Epidemiology

Hamstring muscle injuries are a common injury in sports that involve high-speed running and kicking. They are the most common and most prevalent injury in Australian football, constituting 15% of all injuries, with the average professional Australian Football League (AFL) club having six injuries per club (40 players) and 21 missed matches per club per season.[1] Similarly, in British soccer, hamstring injuries make up 12% of all injuries[2, 3] with an average of five per club per season, resulting in 15 matches and 90 days missed. The average injury caused the player to miss an average of 18 days and three matches.[4]

Hamstring muscle injuries have the highest recurrence rate of all injuries with a recurrence rate of 34% in AFL football[1] and 12% in British soccer.[4]

Biomechanics of hamstring injury

The majority of hamstring muscle injuries occur in the biceps femoris muscle, mainly at the muscle–tendon junction.[4–6] They are usually a non-contact injury and mostly occur during sprinting.

During maximal sprinting the hamstrings become highly active in the terminal swing phase as they work eccentrically to decelerate the swinging tibia and control extension of the knee. The hamstrings then remain active into the initial stance phase, whereby they work concentrically as an extensor of the hip joint.[4, 7–9] Recent studies have demonstrated that during unperturbed sprinting the point of failure is most likely to occur during the terminal swing phase just prior to foot strike.[10, 11] It is at this point that the hamstrings are maximally activated and are approaching peak length.[12]

Factors that predispose to hamstring strain

Predisposing factors are generally divided into intrinsic (person-related) and extrinsic (environment-related) factors.

Intrinsic predisposing factors

Age

Several studies have shown that increasing age is a risk factor for hamstring muscle injury,[4, 13–16] even when the confounding factor of previous injury is removed.[8] Community level Australian footballers over 23 years old were four times as likely to sustain a hamstring strain than those younger than 23.

This relationship may be related to decreased strength (see below). This may be due to an age-related reduction in muscle fiber size and number, leading to a loss of mass and strength. Thus age-related denervation of muscle fibers may lead to increased risk.[15] It has also been suggested that it may be due to age-related lumbar spinal degeneration, leading to L5 and S1 nerve impingement, thus resulting in hamstring and calf muscle fiber denervation, which then leads to decreased muscle strength.[16]

Previous injury

Previous hamstring injury is a major risk factor,[8, 14, 17, 18] but past history of injury is associated with reduced strength so this may be a confounder.[16] Previous calf muscle,[16] knee or groin injuries have also been associated with an increased likelihood of hamstring injury.[8]

Race

There is an increased incidence of hamstring injury in those of black[4] or Aboriginal[8] ethnic origin.

Flexibility

Prospective studies have shown either a significant association between pre-season hamstring muscle tightness and subsequent development of a hamstring muscle injury,[19] or a tendency towards a statistical relationship.[15, 20]

Retrospective studies are of less value as any associated muscle weakness may be the result, rather than the cause, of the muscle injury. The retrospective studies have shown mixed results.[21–23]

A survey of stretching practises among professional football teams in the United Kingdom found that more hamstring strains occurred in those teams that did not stretch regularly and/or hold their stretches for long periods.[24]

One study suggested that decreased quadriceps flexibility (<52° knee flexion) had an increased risk of hamstring injury.[15]

Strength

Low hamstring strength has been shown in most studies to be a significant predictor of hamstring muscle strain injury.[23, 25–28] However, this has been contradicted by other studies.[29, 30] Retrospective studies have shown that those with a history of hamstring injury have significantly weaker hamstrings.[21, 31, 32]

It may be that the actual length at which peak torque in the muscle is developed is most important rather than the magnitude of the peak torque itself. Footballers with a history of hamstring strain develop peak torque at angles representing shorter muscle length, which therefore makes them vulnerable to load in the muscle under lengthened situations.[33]

Neuromyofascial

A number of authors have suggested a relationship between increased neural tension and posterior thigh pain.[34, 35] The presence of myofascial trigger points in the gluteal and hamstring muscles appears to be associated with decreased flexibility and possible increased motor firing of the muscle.

Lumbopelvic stability

Neuromuscular control of the lumbopelvic region, including anterior and posterior pelvic tilt, may be needed to create optimal function of the hamstrings in sprinting and high-speed skilled movement. Changes in pelvic position could lead to changes in length–tension relationships or force–velocity relationships.[36] Improvements in lumbopelvic stability appear to assist in the rehabilitation program.[36]

Joint dysfunction

As mentioned above, age-related lumbar spinal degeneration leading to L5 and S1 nerve impingement may lead to hamstring and calf muscle fiber denervation, which then leads to decreased muscle strength.[16]

An increased incidence of lumbar lordosis was also noted in a group of players who had a history of hamstring strain in the previous 12 months when compared to an uninjured group.[22]

In those with hamstring strains the innominate bone at the sacroiliac joint ipsilateral to the hamstring strain was found to be tilted anteriorly.[37] A bilateral anterior pelvic tilt has been associated with weakness of the transversus abdominis, which may make the hamstrings functionally tighter.

Extrinsic predisposing factors

Warm-up

A physiological warm-up consisting of isometric contractions increases the amount of force and length of stretch that the muscle can absorb prior to tearing.[38] There appears to be clinical evidence that muscle strain injuries, in general, are more likely to occur without adequate warm-up.[39–41]

Fatigue

Fatigued muscles are able to absorb less energy.[42] Hamstring injuries are more common at the end of matches and training sessions in soccer,[4] have a higher incidence in the fourth quarter of Rugby union,[43] and occur infrequently during warm-up of the first quarter in Australian football.[44]

Fatigue may induce physiological changes within the muscle, as well as altered coordination, technique or concentration, predisposing the player to injury.[43] The dual innervation of biceps femoris could lead to asynchrony in the activation of separate parts of the muscle and result in inefficiencies. Abnormalities in running style may be the consequence of fatigue, increasing the workload of the stabilizing biarticular muscles around the pelvis.[45] When footballers become fatigued during sprinting there is an earlier activation of the biceps femoris and semitendinosus muscles.[46]

Fitness level

Inadequate pre-season training resulting in low fitness levels may contribute to an increased hamstring injury rate.[2, 47]

Training modalities

Too much emphasis on aerobic training instead of more high-intensity running/acceleration drills has been suggested as a causative factor.[48] Abrupt increases in training volume and intensity may also contribute to injury risk.[49]

Additional specific predisposing factors in recurrent hamstring injuries

- Inadequate rehabilitation: this may lead to deficits in strength and/or flexibility.
- Angle of peak torque: as mentioned above, footballers with a history of hamstring strain develop peak torque at angles representing shorter muscle length, which therefore makes them vulnerable to load in the muscle under lengthened situations.[33]
- Neural tension: injury may result in increases in neural tension.[34, 35]

Prevention of hamstring muscle injuries

Stretching

A warm-up stretching program was found to statistically reduce the number of hamstring injuries in a military population.[50]

Strengthening program

Correcting strength deficits can lower injury to the hamstrings.[27, 31] Pre-season hamstring muscle strengthening using an open chain weight machine reduced the number of minor hamstring injuries but not the number of significant injuries.[51] Specific eccentric training (see below) may be more important in view of the mechanism of injury.

Thermal pants

The use of thermal pants has been suggested to have a role in reducing the recurrence of hamstring injuries.[52]

Combined programs

A number of multifactorial programs appear to have been effective in reducing the number of hamstring injuries. The programs have included:

- increasing the amount of anaerobic interval rather than aerobic training, stretching while muscle is fatigued, sport-specific training drills, and closed chain rather than open chain leg weights[48]
- a program combining general interventions such as improved warm-up, regular cool down, and a series of exercises to improve stability of ankle and knee joints, flexibility and strength of the trunk, hip and leg muscles, as well as to improve coordination, reaction time and endurance—this was found to be effective in reducing injuries in soccer players, including thigh injuries[53]
- a pre-season conditioning program consisting of sport-specific cardiovascular conditioning, plyometric work, sport cord drills, strength training and flexibility exercises in a group of soccer players.[47]

Clinical features

The main aim of the clinical history, examination and investigations is to differentiate between the significant hamstring tear and neuromyofascial referred pain primarily from gluteal trigger points but also from lumbar spine and SIJ structures. The clinical features of the two are shown in Table 26.2.

Imaging

Ultrasound and MRI have both been found to be effective in depicting hamstring injuries (Fig. 26.3). Ultrasound may be the preferred imaging technique due to lower costs, however, MRI is more sensitive

Table 26.2 Clinical features of hamstring muscle tear and referred hamstring pain

Hamstring muscle tear	Referred hamstring pain
Sudden onset	May be sudden onset or gradual feeling of tightness
Moderately severe pain	Usually less severe, may be cramping or 'twinge'
Disabling—difficulty walking, unable to run	Often able to walk/jog pain-free
Markedly reduced stretch	Minimal reduction in stretch
Markedly reduced contraction against resistance	Full or near to full muscle strength against resistance
Local hematoma, bruising	No local signs
Marked focal tenderness	Variable tenderness, usually non-specific
Slump test negative	Slump test frequently positive
May have gluteal trigger points	Gluteal trigger points that reproduce hamstring pain on palpation or needling
May have abnormal lumbar spine/SIJ signs	Frequently have abnormal lumbar spine/SIJ signs
Abnormal ultrasound/MRI	Normal ultrasound/MRI

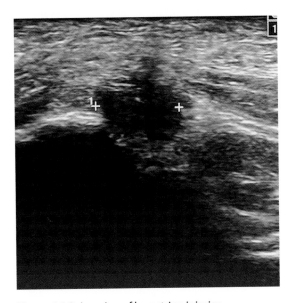

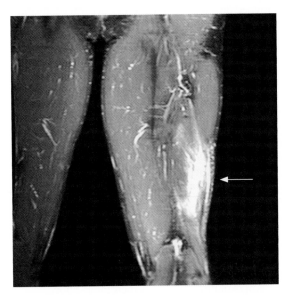

Figure 26.3 Imaging of hamstring injuries

(a) Ultrasound showing hypoechoic area (between electronic calipers, +)

(b) MRI demonstrating area of edema in hamstring consistent with muscle tear

for follow-up imaging of healing injuries. The longitudinal extent of the strain as measured on MRI is a strong predictor of the amount of time needed until an athlete can return to competition.[5]

Management of hamstring strain

There is very little scientific evidence on which to base one's management of hamstring injuries. Only one study has compared the efficacy of two treatment regimens,[36] so much of the regimen described below is on the basis of our clinical experience. Clearly, further research needs to be performed in this area.

The management of hamstring muscle injuries is summarized in Table 26.3.

Acute management

Acute injuries should always be assessed before any treatment, including ice, is administered.

Table 26.3 Management of hamstring injury

First 48 hours
RICE
Early mobilization
Pain-free, active knee extension while sitting
(Fig. 26.4) following 10–15 minutes of ice

Subsequent
Stretching
Hamstrings (Fig. 26.5)
Antagonist muscles
Quadriceps
Iliopsoas
Strengthening
Hamstrings
Concentric (Fig. 26.8a)
Eccentric (Fig. 26.8b)
Gluteals and adductor magnus (Fig. 26.9)
Soft tissue treatment
Hamstrings (Fig. 26.6a, b)
Gluteal trigger points (Fig. 26.6d)
Neural stretching (Fig. 26.7)
Spinal mobilization
Cross-training bike
Running program (below)
Stability program (Figs 26.10, 26.11; Chapter 11)

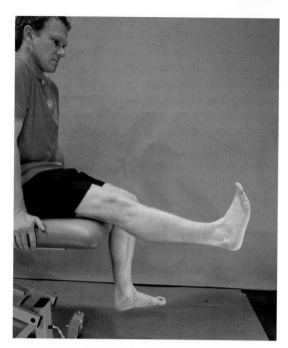

Figure 26.4 Active pain-free knee extension in the acute phase

The RICE program should be commenced. Pain-free, active knee extension may be performed while sitting following 10–15 minutes of ice (Fig. 26.4). This active stretching of the hamstring is conducted for 5 minutes and the whole process may be repeated every hour in the initial phase. The athlete may actually wake every few hours to use this technique in order to ensure inflammation settles as quickly as possible. This process normally takes place over two to three days or until inflammation has settled.

Medication

The role of NSAIDs in the treatment of acute muscle injuries such as the hamstring is controversial. The most common recommendation in the literature is short-term use (three to seven days) starting immediately after injury.[9, 17] The intended aim of using NSAIDs is to keep the inflammatory process under control and to provide analgesia.[54] However, the normal healing process could be blunted as a result and the repair response delayed.[55] There is a case to delay treatment with NSAIDs until two to four days after injury because the drugs interfere with chemotaxis of cells, which is necessary for the repair and remodeling of regenerating muscles.[9]

Only one study has examined the use of NSAIDs in hamstring injuries and found no additional benefit with NSAIDs over physiotherapy alone for the treatment of acute hamstring injuries.[56]

We do not believe there is sufficient evidence to justify the use of NSAIDs in hamstring injuries. It makes more sense to use simple analgesics (paracetamol [acetaminophen]) in the first 48 hours for pain relief. The only situation where we recommend that a short course of NSAIDs may be helpful is if there is an excessive inflammatory response in the muscle as a result of early mobilization and aggressive exercise therapy (see below).[57]

One study showed favorable results with intramuscular corticosteroid injection in American football players with acute hamstring injuries.[58] Previously, the use of corticosteroids in acute muscle strains had been clearly contraindicated because they were thought to lead to a delayed elimination of hematoma and necrotic tissue, as well as retardation of muscle regeneration.[57] There are concerns regarding the retrospective nature of the National Football League (NFL) study and lack of control group, so we caution against the use of corticosteroids in this situation until further clinical trials are conducted.

Stretching

In the acute phase, pain-free range of motion should be achieved as soon as possible. If there is long-term loss of range of motion, then specific stretching should be undertaken to focus on the affected area (Fig. 26.5).

Soft tissue therapy

At an appropriate time depending on the severity of the injury, soft tissue techniques can be used in the treatment of hamstring strains. The distal musculo-tendinous region is palpated and treated in knee flexion with the foot resting on the therapist's shoulder. Digital ischemic pressure and sustained myofascial tension (Figs 26.6b, c) are used. Abnormalities of the gluteal muscles may be associated with hamstring strains. These regions may be treated in a side-lying position using elbow ischemic pressure with the tissue on stretch and the muscle contracting (Fig. 26.6d).

Manual therapy

The presence of a degree of hypomobility in any segment of the lumbar spine, found on examination, should be treated (Chapter 21). If increased neural tension is found at examination, neural stretches should be included in the treatment regimen (Fig. 26.7).

Strengthening

Strengthening is an essential component of prevention and rehabilitation of hamstring injuries. Muscle strengthening should be specific for deficits in motor

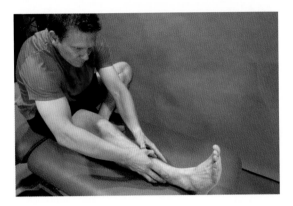

Figure 26.5 Hamstring stretches

(a) Hamstring stretch with contralateral knee flexion. The lower leg can be placed in different degrees of external and internal rotation to maximize the effectiveness of the stretch

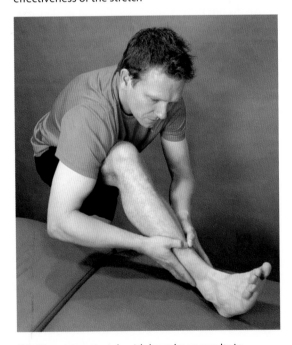

(b) Hamstring stretch with bent knee results in maximal stretch to the upper hamstrings

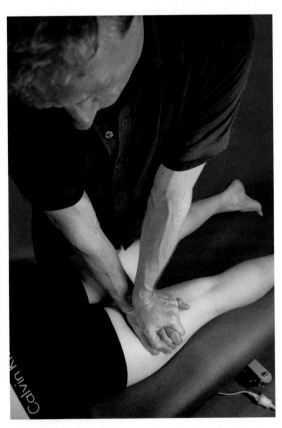

Figure 26.6 Soft tissue techniques in the treatment of hamstring injuries

(a) Sustained compression force to hamstring

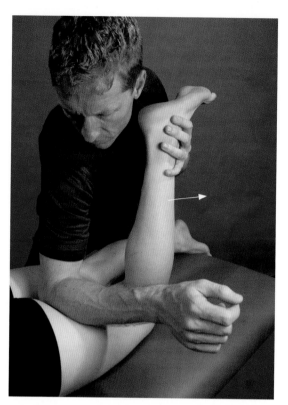

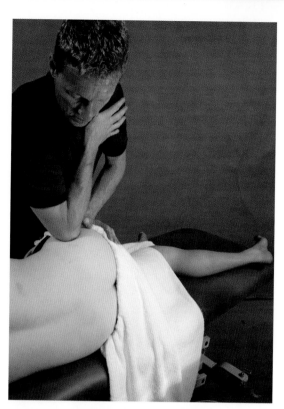

(b) Sustained myofascial tension combined with passive knee extension. The hand or the elbow (illustrated) is kept stationary and the release is performed by passively extending the knee (arrow)

(d) Treatment of the gluteal region in a side-lying position using elbow ischemic pressure with the muscle contracting

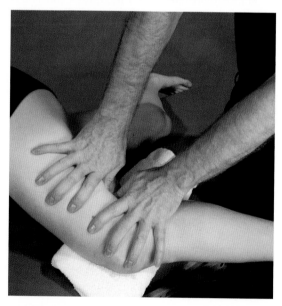

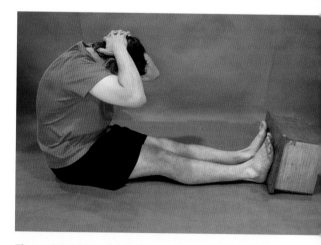

(c) Digital ischemic pressure to the distal biceps femoris tendon

Figure 26.7 Neural stretch. Stretching of neural structures should be performed as part of the treatment of hamstring pain if tightness has been detected on neural tension testing. These neural stretches may be performed with the aid of a therapist or by the patient as shown

unit recruitment, muscle bulk, type of contraction (e.g. eccentric/concentric) and ability to develop tension at speed.

In view of the probable mechanism of hamstring injury (see above), it is likely that eccentric strength is particularly important in recovery and prevention of recurrence of hamstring strains. Muscle strengthening is mode-specific, in other words concentric muscle exercises lead to increases in concentric strength, eccentric muscle exercises lead to increases in eccentric strength, with little or no crossover.[59, 60] Therefore, to increase eccentric hamstring muscle strength it is necessary to perform eccentric muscle training. The use of the Nordic eccentric exercise (Fig. 26.8b) has

been shown to be more effective than traditional concentric strengthening in developing eccentric hamstring strength.[60]

Taking into consideration the phase of the sprinting action where hamstring injuries occur, the ideal exercise would be eccentric to decelerate the very high angular knee velocity with maximum force production around 30° of knee flexion. No exercise exactly mimics that situation but, after some weeks of the Nordic hamstring training program, many athletes are able to stop the downward motion completely before touching the ground (i.e. at about 30° of knee flexion) using their hamstrings alone, even after being pushed by a partner at considerable speed. When an athlete can reach this stage, the characteristics of the Nordic hamstring exercise appear to resemble the typical injury situation: eccentric muscle action, high forces, near full knee extension.

Eccentric training has been shown to shift the point of peak torque development (see above) towards a more lengthened position,[61] which may make the muscle less vulnerable to repeated injury.

Eccentric muscle training results in muscle damage and delayed onset muscle soreness in those unaccustomed to it. Therefore, any eccentric strengthening program should allow adequate time for recovery, especially in the first few weeks. The protocol used for the Nordic strengthening program in Mjolsnes study is shown in Table 26.4.[60]

Strengthening exercises for the hamstring group should therefore consist of a mixture of concentric and eccentric exercises, as shown in Figure 26.8. Table 26.5 provides regimen guidelines for hamstring strengthening.

Muscles that assist the hamstrings

Not only should the hamstring itself be considered but also the muscles that assist the activity of the hamstring. Waters and colleagues found that at least 50% of the total hip moment is provided by the gluteal muscles in an isometric contraction of hip extension.[62] It seems reasonable to hypothesize that if gluteal strength is inadequate in a sprinting athlete, the hamstrings will be overloaded. The adductor magnus should also be considered as an important hip extensor. Therefore, strengthening of the hamstring group should always include specific work to ensure adequate gluteal and adductor magnus conditioning (Fig. 26.9).

Core stability

Neuromuscular control of the lumbopelvic region, including anterior and posterior pelvic tilt, may

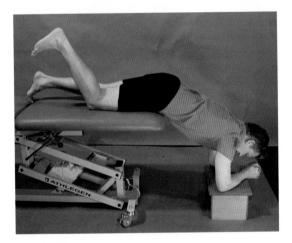

Figure 26.8 Strengthening exercises

(a) Concentric and eccentric exercises—prone. From a position of hip flexion, the knee is flexed (concentric) and/or extended and stopped just prior to full extension ('drop-and-catch') (eccentric). Weights can be added gradually and speed can be increased progressively

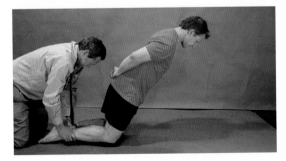

(b) Nordic eccentric hamstring exercise—patients allow themselves to fall forward and then resist the fall for as long as possible using their hamstrings

Table 26.4 Training protocol for Nordic hamstring exercises

Week	Sessions per week	Sets and repetitions	Load
1	1	2 × 5	Load is increased as subject can withstand the forward fall longer. When managing to withstand the whole ROM for 12 repetitions, increase load by adding speed to the starting phase of the motion. The partner can also increase loading further by pushing at the back of the shoulders.
2	2	2 × 6	
3	3	3 × 6–8	
4	3	3 × 8–10	
5–10	3	3 sets, 12, 10, 8 repetitions	

ROM = range of motion.

Table 26.5 Recommended regimen for hamstring strengthening

Weight	Load	Reps	Sets	Rest time	Speed	Regularity
Motor unit recruitment	60 RM	15	6	30 s	Concentric 2 s Eccentric 2 s	3 per day
Strength	6–8 RM	6–8	3–5	2 min	Concentric 1 s Eccentric 3 s	Once per 1–2 days
Hypertrophy	8–12 RM	8–12	6	2 min	Concentric 1 s Eccentric 3 s	Once per 1–2 days
Power	40 RM	15	3–4	3–4 min	Quick with control	Once per 2–3 days

RM = repetition maximum.

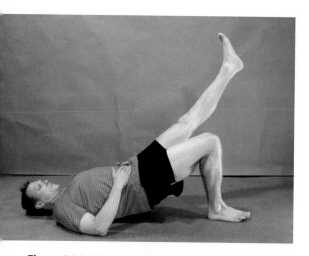

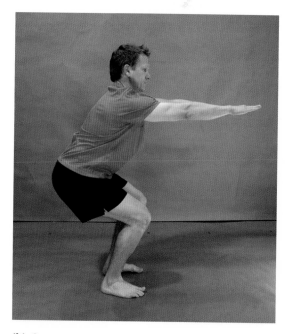

Figure 26.9 Hip strengthening exercises

(a) One-legged bridging

(b) Squat

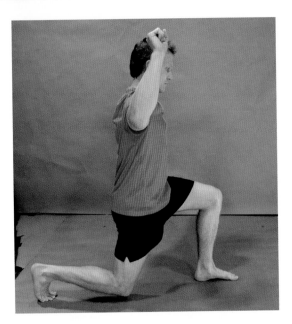

(c) Split squat

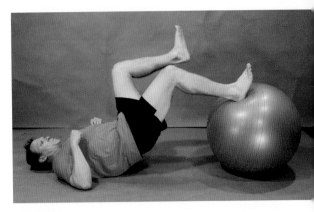

(b) Single-leg ball rollout

be needed to create optimal function of the hamstrings in sprinting and high-speed skilled movement. Changes in pelvic position could lead to changes in length–tension relationships or force–velocity relationships.[36]

A rehabilitation program consisting of progressive agility and stabilization exercises (Fig. 26.10) has been shown to be more effective in promoting return to sport and in preventing injury recurrence in athletes who have sustained an acute hamstring strain than

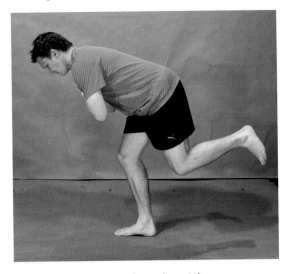

(c) Single-leg stance with trunk straight

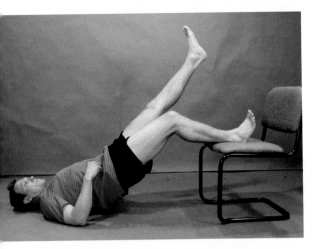

Figure 26.10 Agility and stablization exercises

(a) Bridge catch

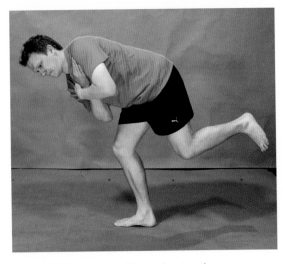

(d) Single-leg stance with trunk rotated

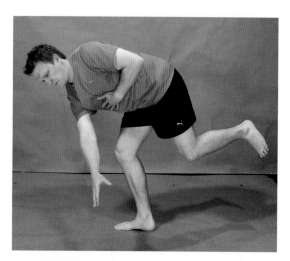

(e) Single leg stance with trunk rotated and with further stretch reaching out with arm

Table 26.6 Progressive hamstring running program

1. 2 km jog
2. 2 km varying pace up to 75% of maximum
3. Run throughs: accelerate 40 m, constant speed
   20 m (time 3.5 s), decelerate 40 m (×3)

35 m	20 m	35 m (×3)
30 m	20 m	30 m (×3)
25 m	20 m	25 m (×3)
20 m	20 m	20 m (×3)
15 m	20 m	15 m (×3)

4. Run throughs: accelerate 40 m, constant speed
   20 m (time 2.5 s), decelerate 40 m (×3)

35 m	20 m	35 m (×3)
25 m	20 m	25 m (×3)
20 m	20 m	20 m (×3)
15 m	20 m	15 m (×3)
10 m	20 m	10 m (×3)

5. Running out to catch ball—uncontested (×5)
6. Running out to catch ball—contested (×5)
7. Running and picking up ball—contested (×5)

has a more traditional stretching and strengthening exercise program.[36]

Progressive running program

PRACTISE PEARL Early commencement of a progressive running program is an important part of a rehabilitation following a hamstring muscle injury.

Scientific studies need to be performed to validate this program but physiotherapists with over 20 years experience of this program are convinced of its effectiveness. The basic principles are listed below with further detail in Table 26.6.

1. Running program starts 48 hours after injury.
2. 20 minute running sessions twice a day.
3. Preceded by 10 minutes of gentle hamstring stretching.
4. Commences with jogging with short stride (shuffle).
5. Patient encouraged to increase stride length and pace gradually over the session as the ache allows.
6. Interval running over 100 m (~110 yd) with acceleration, maintenance and deceleration phases.
7. If there is even the slightest increase in pulling sensation through the hamstring, then the session must immediately cease. The athlete should apply ice and the program can be attempted again as early as the next 12 hours.
8. Finish with 10 minutes of gentle hamstring stretching and then apply ice to the injured area for 10 minutes.

Criteria for return to sport

There is no standard time for return to sport after hamstring injury as every hamstring injury is different. No scientific studies have examined the outcomes of various return to play strategies.[63] It does not appear that the MRI appearance is a good indicator of readiness to return to play. Abnormalities on MRI tend to persist well after athletes are back to full sport.[5]

The length of time is proportional to the severity of the injury. Generally, an athlete with a mild hamstring strain may be able to return to sport in 12–18 days if optimally treated (Table 26.3).

Rather than a specific time frame it is preferable to have definite criteria for return to sport:

- Completion of progressive running program
- Full range of movement (equal to uninjured leg)
- Full strength (equal or almost equal to uninjured leg)
  - 90[17]–95%[31, 45] of eccentric strength of uninjured leg
- Pain-free maximal contraction
- Functional tests
  - Sprinting from a standing start
  - Abrupt changes of pace during run
  - Side stepping
  - Bending to catch ball at full speed (if appropriate for the sport)
- Successful completion of a full week of maximal training

It is important to continue the strengthening program for a few weeks after return to sport.

Referred pain to posterior thigh

The possibility of referred pain should always be considered in the athlete presenting with posterior thigh pain. Hamstring pain may be referred from the lumbar spine, the SIJ or from soft tissues, for example, the proximal fibers of the gluteus maximus and especially gluteus medius and the piriformis muscle (Fig. 26.11). Often, there is a history of previous or current low back pain.

The slump test (Fig. 26.2f) should be used to detect neural tightness. The test is positive when the patient's hamstring pain is reproduced and subsequently relieved with reduction of the neural tension by neck extension. Examination may reveal reduced range of movement of the lumbar spine, tenderness and/or stiffness of lumbar intervertebral joint(s) or tenderness over the area of the SIJ.

A positive slump test is strongly suggestive of a referred component to the patient's pain. However, a negative slump test does not exclude the possibility of referred pain and the lumbar spine should be carefully examined to detect any intervertebral segment hypomobility. Systematic soft tissue palpation of the hip extensors, abductors and rotators should also be performed.

Trigger points

Trigger points are common sources of referred pain to both the buttock (Chapter 22) and posterior thigh. The most common trigger points that refer pain to the mid hamstring are in the gluteus minimus, gluteus medius and piriformis muscles. The clinical syndrome associated with posterior thigh pain without evidence of hamstring muscle injury on MRI and reproduction of the patient's pain on palpation of gluteal trigger points is now well recognized and extremely common.[64]

The clinical features are described in Table 26.2. The patient will often complain of a feeling of tightness, cramping, 'twinge' or a feeling that the hamstring is 'about to tear'. On examination there may be some localized tenderness in the hamstring although it is usually not focal and there is restriction in hamstring and gluteal stretch. Firm palpation of the gluteal muscles will detect tight bands that contain active trigger points, which when firmly palpated are extremely tender, refer pain into the hamstring and elicit a 'twitch response'.

Treatment involves deactivating the trigger point either with ischemic pressure using the elbow (Fig. 26.12a) or dry needling (Fig. 26.12b). Following the

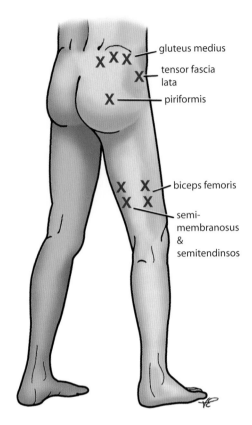

Figure 26.11 Pattern of referred pain to the hamstrings from trigger points

local treatment the tight muscle groups, the gluteals and hamstrings, should be stretched.

Lumbar spine

The lumbar spine is a source of pain referral to the posterior thigh. Unfortunately, it is difficult to distinguish between sources based on the behavior and distribution of the pain. Pain may be referred from the disk, zygoapophyseal joints, muscles, ligaments or any structure that can produce pain locally in the lumbar spine.[65]

Nerve root compression may also be a cause of hamstring pain. Diagnostic blocks and provocation injections have been advocated to isolate sources of pain in the lumbar spine. However, in the clinical setting, this is often not possible. It is important to examine the lumbar spine carefully (Chapter 21). This will assist in the identification of the lumbar spine as a source of hamstring pain. It is also important to remember that the lumbar spine may be a cause of lumbar pain indirectly. For example, the lumbar spine may cause a biomechanical block to extension of the lower limb, resulting in overload of the SIJ and referred pain to the hamstring group.

The slump technique (Fig. 26.2f) has been advocated as a method of treatment of hamstring pain in AFL footballers.[34] This is a quick test and it can be carried out rapidly to assess the relevance of neural structures as a cause of hamstring strain.

True nerve root compression is usually more definitive in its presentation. The patient may have associated neurological symptoms, such as numbness and loss of foot eversion. The management of these injuries usually involves an extended period of rest and, in certain cases, an epidural injection. In extreme cases, surgical decompression of the nerve root may be warranted.

Spondylolisthesis and spondylolysis have both been implicated as a source of hamstring pain and tightness.[66] Examination findings of positive lumbar quadrant tests or single leg standing lumbar extension are suggestive of either condition and can be confirmed with isotopic bone scan and CT. Stabilization programs are the treatment of choice as it has been shown that the deep abdominal muscles are deficient in people with back pain as a result of spondylolisthesis and spondylysis.[67] In severe cases, corticosteroid injection under X-ray control into the deficient pars interarticularis may be effective in reducing pain from spondylolysis.

Hamstring pain occurring in the sporting environment can often be due to loading of the lumbar spine outside of the training and competition environment. Pain in the hamstring may be the result of referred pain from the lumbar spine as a result of prolonged sitting or bending forward. Athletes in sedentary occupations should be aware that sitting posture is a cause of injury to the hamstring. Travel involving prolonged sitting prior to training and competition may cause injury. This includes car, bus or airplane travel, and care should be undertaken to limit prolonged sitting and to provide adequate lumbar support.

Lumbar referred hamstring pain may also be the result of repeated forward bending or squatting. This occurs in many manual occupations or in those with young children. Again, correct posture and lifting should be taught, along with strategies for limiting the frequency and load of bending.

Sacroiliac complex

The SIJ can refer pain into the hamstring or cause indirect pain in the hamstring similar to the lumbar spine. The SIJ is discussed in Chapter 22.

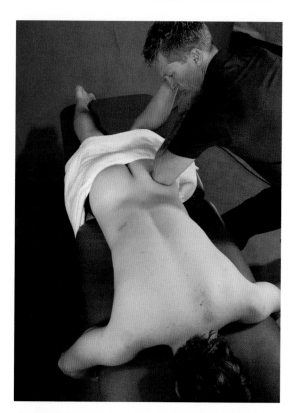

Figure 26.12 Treatment of gluteal trigger points

(a) Elbow pressure

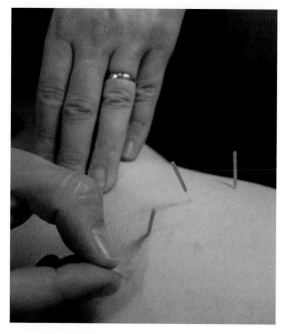

(b) Dry needling

Less common causes

Nerve entrapments

The hamstring group is supplied by the tibial branch of the sciatic nerve except for the short head of the biceps femoris, which is supplied by the peroneal branch of the sciatic nerve. These nerves arise from the lumbosacral plexus, specifically from the roots of L5, S1 and S2.

Nerve damage can occur at a variety of sites resulting in pain in the posterior thigh. Compression of the nerve roots of the sacral plexus will often result in pain into the hamstring group. Usually this is distinguished from other conditions by the identification of associated neurological symptoms such as alteration in sensation, loss of the Achilles reflex or weakness in muscles not in the hamstring group, such as the ankle evertors.

The sciatic nerve may be damaged at any point along its pathway as a result of direct impact or pelvic trauma. Compression of the nerve at the level of the piriformis has been described as an alternative cause of sciatica.[68] However, work by McCrory and Bell suggests that it is not only the piriformis but also the other hip external rotators that may cause compression of the sciatic nerve.[69]

The peripheral nerves of the body may also be a source of posterior thigh pain. The posterior cutaneous nerve of the thigh (PCNT) and the inferior cluneal nerve supply the skin over the posterior thigh. The PCNT has been described as the source of pain in piriformis syndrome as an alternative to the sciatic nerve.[69] If symptoms do not extend below the knee and there is no associated loss of neurological function in the structures supplied by the sciatic nerve, then the PCNT should be considered.

Upper hamstring tendinopathy

Tendinopathy of the hamstring may occur at the origin or the insertion of the hamstring muscle group. Both present with the typical inflammatory pattern of warming up with activity and an increase in pain post activity. Tenderness is easily elicited over the tendon with associated thickening.

Proximal hamstring tendinopathy is often associated with repetitive sprinting and instability of pelvic mechanics. There may be some difficulty differentiating it from ischial bursitis, which tends to be more a result of friction with sitting on hard surfaces or 'hamstring syndrome', which has more neurological symptoms. Upper hamstring tendinopathy may respond to transverse frictions in the short term and this will often allow an athlete to continue performing. However, the prognosis is usually protracted. A hamstring strengthening program should be commenced.

This condition is often resistant to treatment. We have had some success with extracorporeal shock wave treatment.

Ischial bursitis

It is often difficult to distinguish between hamstring tendinopathy and ischial bursitis. Both conditions have an inflammatory pain pattern at the origin of the hamstring muscle. An inflamed bursa is not readily palpated, however, athletes tend to complain of pain when sitting on hard surfaces where the ischium is under pressure. Ultrasound or MRI can confirm the presence of a fluid-filled bursa.

Anti-inflammatory medications combined with ice and rest are of limited benefit. Cortisone injections can be performed under X-ray control but the results are not always satisfactory.

Lower hamstring tendinopathy

Lower hamstring tendinopathy is often the result of large volumes of resisted flexion knee exercises. It also occurs in sprinters. The pain pattern is inflammatory and the pain is localized to the tendons of the hamstring group. Posterior capsular pain should be differentiated from tendinopathy. Pain associated with knee hyperextension, such as in kicking, is usually capsular. Management consists of anti-inflammatory agents, taping to reduce load and appropriate rehabilitation focusing on biomechanical defects.

Adductor magnus strains

Adductor magnus strains are rare but, when they do occur, behave similarly to a hamstring strain. The mechanism tends to be more of a rotatory action of eccentric internal rotation on one hip. Prognosis tends to be far better than hamstring strains; therefore, it is important to differentiate it from strains in the hamstring. The key to differentiating this condition is careful palpation to elicit the precise location of the tissue damage. Side-lying on the affected leg allows that hamstring group to fall laterally so that ready access can be made to the adductor magnus.

Compartment syndrome of the posterior thigh

While not as common as lower leg compartment syndromes, a compartment syndrome of the posterior thigh is occasionally seen. Patients present with dull pain, stiffness, cramps and weakness of the posterior thigh during and after training.[70] Two groups of patients with this syndrome are seen: endurance athletes without a history of trauma, and those with a history of hamstring injury.

Conservative management has not been successful and posterior fasciotomy of the thigh appears to be an effective treatment.[70]

Avulsion of the hamstring from the ischial tuberosity

Avulsion of the hamstring from the ischial tuberosity is seen in two groups of patients: adolescents who instead of sustaining a hamstring muscle tear, tear their hamstring from its bony attachment at the ischium, and older people, often with a history of chronic tendinopathy.

Young sportspeople in the 14–18 year age range are prone to avulsions of the ischial apophysis. Any young adult presenting with an incident of acute severe hamstring pain should be treated as if with an avulsion until proven otherwise. Plain X-ray or bone scan may be used to identify the avulsion. According to the literature, a separation of greater than 2 cm (1 in.) requires open reduction and internal fixation.[71] Separations of less than 2 cm (1 in.) are often managed conservatively, requiring eight to 12 weeks' rest. However, some caution should be exercised with conservative management as these athletes can be left with decreased power in their hamstrings, which limits future sporting performance. Occasionally, there is neurological involvement associated with this injury.[72]

In adults, complete rupture of the ischial origin of the hamstring muscles is relatively rare.[73, 74] The injury results from a sudden forceful flexion of the hip joint when the knee is fully extended and the hamstring muscles powerfully contracted. The most common activities associated with the rupture are waterskiing and power lifting. If treated with prompt surgery, the final functional results are good.

Vascular

Endofibrosis of the external iliac artery usually produces pain in the lateral and anterior thigh. However, in some cases, pain may be experienced in the posterior thigh. This condition is associated with cycling[75] and has been observed in triathletes. The pain is claudicant in nature. Pain may arise after 15–20 minutes of exercise but usually ceases immediately with the cessation of exercise.

On examination, a bruit is heard during the exercise that causes the pain. Diagnosis may be confirmed with echography or arteriography. If the condition is affecting performance, then treatment is either surgical or balloon dilation of the area where the artery is narrowed.

Recommended Reading

Croisier J-L. Factors associated with recurrent hamstring injuries. *Sports Med* 2004; 34(10): 681–95.

Drezner JA. Practical management: hamstring muscle injuries. *Clin J Sport Med* 2003; 13(1): 48–52.

Garrett WE Jr. Muscle strain injuries. *Am J Sports Med* 1996; 24(6): S2–S8.

Petersen J, Holmich P. Evidence based prevention of hamstring injuries in sport. *Br J Sports Med* 2005; 39(6): 319–23.

References

1. Orchard J, Seward H. Epidemiology of injuries in the Australian Football League, seasons 1997–2000. *Br J Sports Med* 2002; 36: 39–45.

2. Hawkins RD, Fuller CW. A prospective epidemiological study of injuries in four English professional football clubs. *Br J Sports Med* 1999; 33: 196–203.

3. Hawkins RD, Hulse MA, Wilkinson C, et al. The Association Football medical research programme: an audit of injuries in professional football. *Br J Sports Med* 2001; 35: 43–7.

4. Woods C, Hawkins RD, Maltby S, et al. The football association medical research programme: an audit of injuries in professional football—analysis of hamstring injuries. *Br J Sports Med* 2004; 38: 36–41.

5. Connell DA, Schneider-Kolsky ME, Hoving JL, et al. Longitudinal study comparing sonographic and MRI assessments of acute and healing hamstring injuries. *AJR Am J Roentgenol* 2004; 183: 975–84.

6. Koulouris G, Connell DA. Evaluation of the hamstring muscle complex following acute injury. *Skeletal Radiol* 2003; 32(10): 582–9.

7. Stanton P, Purdam C. Hamstring injuries in sprinting—the role of eccentric exercise. *J Orthop Sports Phys Ther* 1989; March: 343–9.

8. Verrall GM, Slavotinek JP, Barnes PG, et al. Clinical risk factors for hamstring muscle strain injury: a prospective study with correlation of injury by magnetic resonance imaging. *Br J Sports Med* 2001; 35: 435–40.

9. Petersen J, Holmich P. Evidence based prevention of hamstring injuries in sport. *Br J Sports Med* 2005; 39(6): 319–23.

10. Heiderscheit BC, Hoerth DM, Chumanov ES, et al. Identifying the time of occurrence of a hamstring strain injury during treadmill running: a case study. *Clin Biomech* 2005; 20(10): 1072–8.

11. Thelen DG, Chumanov ES, Hoerth DM, et al. Hamstring muscle kinematics during treadmill sprinting. *Med Sci Sports Exerc* 2005; 37(1): 108–14.

12. Wood GA. Biomechanical limitations to sprint running. In: Van Gheluwe B, Atha J, eds. *Current Research in Sports Biomechanics*. Basel: Karger, 1987: 58–71.

13. Arnason A, Tenga A, Engebretsen L, et al. A prospective video-based analysis of injury situations in elite male football: football incident analysis. *Am J Sports Med* 2004; 32(6): 1459–65.

14. Arnason A, Sigurdsson SB, Gudmundson A, et al. Risk factors for injuries in football. *Am J Sports Med* 2004; 32: S5–S16.

15. Gabbe BJ, Finch CF, Bennell KL, et al. Risk factors for hamstring injuries in community level Australian football. *Br J Sports Med* 2005; 39(2): 106–10.

16. Orchard JW. Intrinsic and extrinsic risk factors for muscle strains in Australian football. *Am J Sports Med* 2001; 29(3): 300–3.

17. Drezner JA. Practical management: hamstring muscle injuries. *Clin J Sport Med* 2003; 13(1): 48–52.

18. Garrett WE Jr. Muscle strain injuries. *Am J Sports Med* 1996; 24(6): S2–S8.

19. Witvrouw E, Danneels L, Asselman P, et al. Muscle flexibility as a risk factor for developing muscle injuries in male professional soccer players. a prospective study. *Am J Sports Med* 2003; 31(1): 41–6.

20. Rolls A, George K. The relationship between hamstring muscle injuries and hamstring muscle length in young elite footballers. *Phys Ther Sport* 2004; 5: 179–87.

21. Jonhagen S, Nemeth G, Eriksson E. Hamstring injuries in sprinters. The role of concentric and eccentric hamstring muscle strength and flexibility. *Am J Sports Med* 1994; 22(2): 262–6.

22. Hennessey L, Watson AW. Flexibility and posture assessment in relation to hamstring injury. *Br J Sports Med* 1993; 27: 243–6.

23. Orchard J, Marsden J, Lord S, et al. Preseason hamstring muscle weakness associated with hamstring muscle injury in Australian footballers. *Am J Sports Med* 1997; 25(1): 81–5.

24. Dadebo B, White J, George KP. A survey of flexibility training protocols and hamstring strains in professional football clubs in England. *Br J Sports Med* 2004; 38: 388–94.

25. Burkett LN. Investigation into hamstring strains: the case of the hybrid muscle. *J Sports Med* 1975; 3: 228–31.

26. Christensen C, Wiseman D. Strength, the common variable in hamstring strains. *J Athl Train* 1972; 7: 36–40.

27. Heiser T, Weber J, Sullivan G, et al. Prophylaxis and management of hamstring muscle injuries in intercollegiate football players. *Am J Sports Med* 1984; 12(5): 368–70.

28. Yamamato T. Relationship between hamstring strains and leg muscle strength. A follow up study of collegiate track and field athletes. *J Sports Med Phys Fitness* 1993; 33: 194–9.

29. Bennell K, Wajswelner H, Lew P, et al. Isokinetic strength testing does not predict hamstring injury in Australian rules footballers. *Br J Sports Med* 1998; 32: 309–14.

30. Dauty M, Potiron-Josse M, Rochcongar P. Consequences and prediction of hamstring muscle injury with concentric and eccentric isokinetic parameters in elite soccer players (Abstract). *Ann Readapt Med Phys* 2003; 46(9): 601–6.

31. Croisier J-L, Forthomme B, Namurois M-H, et al. Hamstring muscle strain recurrrence and strength performance disorders. *Am J Sports Med* 2002; 30(2): 199–203.

32. Worrell T, Perrin D, Gansneder B, et al. Comparison of isokinetic strength and flexibility measures between hamstring injured and noninjured athletes. *J Orthop Sports Phys Ther* 1991; 13: 118–25.

33. Brockett CL, Morgan DL, Proske U. Predicting hamstring strain injury in elite athletes. *Med Sci Sports Exerc* 2004; 36(3): 379–87.

34. Kornberg C, Lew P. The effect of stretching neural structures on grade one hamstring injuries. *J Orthop Sports Phys Ther* 1989; 10(12): 481–7.

35. Turl SE, George KP. Adverse neural tension: a factor in repetitive hamstring strain? *J Orthop Sports Phys Ther* 1998; 27(1): 16–21.

36. Sherry MA, Best TM. A comparison of 2 rehabilitation programs in the treatment of acute hamstring strains. *J Orthop Sports Phys Ther* 2004; 34: 116–25.

37. Cibulka MT, Rose SJ, Delitto A, et al. Hamstring muscle strain treated by mobilizing the sacroiliac joint. *Phys Ther* 1986; 66(8): 1220–3.

38. Safran MR, Seaber AV, Garrett WE Jr. Warm-up and muscular injury prevention: an update. *Sports Med* 1989; 8(4): 239–49.

39. Agre JC, Baxter TL. Musculoskeletal profile of male collegiate soccer players. *Arch Phys Med Rehabil* 1987; 68: 147–50.

40. Ekstrand J, Gillquist J, Moller M, et al. Incidence of soccer injuries and their relation to training and team success. *Am J Sports Med* 1983; 11: 63–7.

41. Dvorak J, Junge A, Chomiak J, et al. Risk factor analysis for injuries in football players: possibilities for a prevention program. *Am J Sports Med* 2000; 28(5): S69–S74.

42. Mair SD, Seaber AV, Glisson RR, et al. The role of fatigue in susceptibility to acute muscle strain injury. *Am J Sports Med* 1996; 24(2): 137–43.

43. Devlin L. Recurrent posterior thigh symptoms detrimental to performance in rugby union: predisposing factors. *Sports Med* 2000; 29(4): 273–87.

44. Verrall GM, Slavotinek JP, Barnes PG, et al. Diagnostic and prognostic value of clinical findings in 83 athletes with posterior thigh injury: comparison of clinical findings with magnetic resonance imaging documentation of hamstring muscle strain. *Am J Sports Med* 2003; 31(6): 969–73.

45. Croisier J-L. Factors associated with recurrent hamstring injuries. *Sports Med* 2004; 34(10): 681–95.

46. Pinniger GJ, Steele JR, Groeller H. Does fatigue induced by repeated dynamic efforts affect hamstring muscle function? *Med Sci Sports Exerc* 2000; 32: 647–53.

47. Heidt RS, Sweeterman LM, Carlonas RL, et al. Avoidance of soccer injuries with pre-season conditioning. *Am J Sports Med* 2000; 28(5): 659–62.

48. Verrall GM, Slavotinek JP, Barnes PG. The effect of sports specific training on reducing the incidence of hamstring injuries in professional Australian Rules football players. *Br J Sports Med* 2005; 39(6): 363–8.

49. Almeida SA, Williams KM, Shaffer RA, et al. Epidemiological patterns of musculoskeletal injuries and physical training. *Med Sci Sports Exerc* 1999; 31: 1176–82.

50. Hartig DE, Henderson JM. Increasing hamstring flexibility decreases lower extremity overuse injuries in military basic trainees. *Am J Sports Med* 1999; 27(2): 173–6.

51. Askling C, Karlson J, Thorstensson A. Hamstring injury occurrence in elite soccer players after pre-season strength training with eccentric overload. *Scand J Sci Med Sports* 2003; 13: 244–50.

52. Upton PAH, Noakes TD, Juritz JM. Thermal pants may reduce the risk of recurrent hamstring injuries in rugby players. *Br J Sports Med* 1996; 30: 57–60.

53. Junge A, Rosch D, Lars P, et al. Prevention of soccer injuries: a prospective intervention study in youth amateur players. *Am J Sports Med* 2002; 30(5): 652–9.

54. Obremsky WT, Seaber AV, Ribbeck BM, et al. Biomechanical and histologic assessment of a controlled muscle strain injury treated with piroxicam. *Am J Sports Med* 1994; 22(4): 558–62.

55. Saartok T. Muscle injuries associated with soccer. *Clin Sports Med* 1998; 17: 811–17.

56. Reynolds JF, Noakes TD, Schwellnus MP. Non-steroidal anti-inflammatory drugs fail to enhance healing of acute hamstring injuries treated with physiotherapy. *S Afr Med J* 1995; 85: 517–22.

57. Jarvinen TAH, Jarvinen TLN, Kaariainen M, et al. Muscle injuries: biology and treatment. *Am J Sports Med* 2005; 33(5): 745–64.

58. Levine WE, Bergfeld JA, Tessendorf W, et al. Intramuscular corticosteroid injection for hamstring injuries: a 13-year experience in the National Football League. *Am J Sports Med* 2000; 28(3): 297–300.

59. Kaminski TW, Wabbersen CV, Murphy RN. Concentric versus enhanced eccentric hamstring strength training: clinical implications. *J Athl Train* 1998; 33: 216–21.

60. Mjolsnes R, Arnason A, Osthagen T, et al. A 10-week randomized trial comparing eccentric vs. concentric hamstring strength training in well-trained soccer players. *Scand J Med Sci Sports* 2004; 14: 311–17.

61. Brockett CL, Morgan DL, Proske U. Human hamstring muscles adapt to eccentric exercise by changing optimum length. *Med Sci Sports Exerc* 2001; 33(5): 783–90.

62. Waters RL, Perry J, McDaniels JM, et al. The relative strength of the hamstrings during hip extension. *J Bone Joint Surg Am* 1973; 56A(8): 1592–7.

63. Orchard J, Best TM, Verrall GM. Return to play following muscle strains. *Clin J Sport Med* 2005; 15(6): 436–41.

64. Huguenin L, Brukner PD, McCrory P, et al. Effect of dry needling of gluteal muscles on straight leg raise: a randomised, placebo controlled, double blind trial. *Br J Sports Med* 2005; 39(2): 84–90.

65. Bogduk N. *Clinical Anatomy of the Lumbar Spine and Sacrum.* 4th edn. Edinburgh: Churchill Livingstone, 2004.

66. Barash HL, Galante JO, Lambert CN, Ray RD. Spondylolisthesis and tight hamstrings. *J Bone Joint Surg Am* 1970; 52A(7): 1319–28.

67. O'Sullivan PB, Twomey L, Allison GT. Dynamic stabilization of the lumbar spine. *Clin Rev Phys Rehab Med* 1997; 9(3 & 4): 315–30.

68. Puranen J, Orava S. The hamstring syndrome. A new diagnosis of gluteal sciatic pain. *Am J Sports Med* 1988; 16(5): 517–21.

69. McCrory P, Bell S, Bradshaw C. Nerve entrapment of the lower leg, ankle and foot in sport. *Sports Med* 2002; 32(6): 371–91.

70. Orava S, Rantanen J, Kujala UM. Fasciotomy of the posterior femoral muscle compartment in athletes. *Int J Sports Med* 1998; 19(1): 71–5.

71. Servant CTJ, Jones CB. Displaced avulsion of the ischial apophysis: a hamstring injury requiring internal fixation. *Br J Sports Med* 1998; 32: 255–7.

72. Street C, Burks R. Chronic complete hamstring avulsion causing foot drop: a case report. *Am J Sports Med* 2000; 28(4): 574–6.

73. Cross MJ, Vandersluis R, Wood D, et al. Surgical repair of chronic complete hamstring tendon rupture in the adult patient. *Am J Sports Med* 1998; 26(6): 785–8.

74. Klingele KE, Sallay PI. Surgical repair of complete proximal hamstring tendon rupture. *Am J Sports Med* 2002; 30(5): 742–7.

75. Abraham P, Saumet JL, Chevalier JM. External iliac artery endofibrosis in athletes. *Sports Med* 1997; 24(4): 221–6.

Acute Knee Injuries

WITH RANDALL COOPER, HAYDEN MORRIS AND LIZA ARENDT

CHAPTER

27

Acute injuries affecting the knee joint cause considerable disability and time off sport. They are common in all sports that require twisting movements and sudden changes of direction, especially the various football codes, basketball, netball and alpine skiing.

Functional anatomy

The knee contains two joints: the tibiofemoral joint with its associated collateral ligaments, cruciate ligaments and menisci; and the patellofemoral joint, which obtains stability from the medial retinaculum and the large patellar tendon passing anteriorly over

the patella. We refer to the tibiofemoral joint as the knee joint.

By understanding the role of the different ligaments and menisci in the knee joint, the clinician can better understand the mechanisms of injury, and also the likely consequences of injuries. The anatomy of the knee joint is shown in Figure 27.1.

The two cruciate ('cross') ligaments, anterior and posterior, are often referred to as the 'crucial' ligaments, such is their importance in sporting activity. They are named anterior and posterior in relation to their attachment to the tibia. The anterior cruciate ligament (ACL) runs posteriorly and superiorly from its attachment near the front of the tibial plateau to

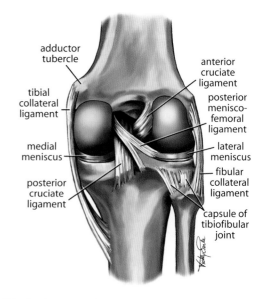

Figure 27.1 Anatomy of the knee joint

(a) The knee joint (anterior view)

(b) The knee joint (posterior view)

its femoral attachment at the posterolateral aspect of the intercondylar notch. The role of the ACL is to prevent forward movement of the tibia in relation to the femur, and to control rotational movement.

The posterior cruciate ligament (PCL) attaches on the posterior part of the tibial plateau and runs anterosuperiorly to its femoral attachment at the medial aspect of the intercondylar notch. The PCL prevents the femur from sliding forwards off the tibial plateau.

The ACL is essential for control in pivoting movements. Without an intact ACL, the tibia may rotate under the femur in an anterior–lateral direction. This is most common when an activity such as landing from a jump, pivoting or a sudden deceleration is attempted. The PCL serves to stabilize the body (femur) above the tibia. In its absence the femur wants to shift forward on the tibia. This shift forward is accentuated when one tries to run down an incline plane or down stairs.

The two collateral ligaments, the medial and lateral, provide medial and lateral stability to the knee joint. The superficial medial collateral ligament (MCL) originates from the medial epicondyle of the femur 3 cm (1.5 in.) above the joint line and passes downward as a thickened band to attach to the anteromedial aspect of the tibia about 8 cm (4 in.) from the joint line. This portion of the MCL is extra-capsular. The deep layer, or coronal ligaments, attaches to the joint margins and has an attachment from its deep layer to the medial meniscus. The MCL prevents excessive medial opening of the tibial–femoral joint.

The lateral collateral ligament (LCL) arises from the lateral epicondyle of the lateral border of the femur and passes downwards to attach to the head of the fibula. The LCL is a narrow strong cord with no attachment to the lateral meniscus. It serves to prevent lateral opening of the tibia on the femur during varus stress.

The two menisci, medial and lateral, are intra-articular and attach to the capsule layer at the level of the joint line. The menisci have an important role as a buffer absorbing some of the forces placed through the knee joint, thus protecting the otherwise exposed articular surfaces from damage. By increasing the concavity of the tibia, they play a role in stabilizing the knee. In addition, the menisci contribute to joint lubrication and nutrition. Thus, it is important to preserve as much of the menisci as possible after injury.

Clinical perspective

The acute knee injury of greatest concern to the athlete is the tear of the ACL. Meniscal injuries are common among sportspeople, either in isolation or combined with a ligament injury, for example, of the MCL or ACL. With the advent of arthroscopy and more sophisticated imaging techniques, it has become evident that the articular cartilage of the knee is often damaged in association with sports injuries including ligamentous or meniscal injuries. Cartilage damage, depending on the size and/or location, can have the most lasting negative consequence in regards to acute knee injuries. A list of acute knee injuries occurring in sport is shown in Table 27.1.

The main question the clinician needs to answer about the patient presenting with acute knee injury is, 'Does this patient have a significant knee injury?' A number of factors may help to provide the answer. These include:

- the mechanism of injury
- the amount of pain and disability at the time of injury
- the presence and timing of onset of swelling
- the degree of disability on presentation to the clinician.

Table 27.1 Causes of acute knee pain[a]

Common	Less common	Not to be missed
Medial meniscus tear	Patellar tendon rupture	Fracture of the tibial plateau
MCL sprain	Acute patellofemoral contusion	Avulsion fracture of tibial spine
ACL sprain (rupture)	LCL sprain	Osteochondritis dissecans (in adolescents)
Lateral meniscus tear	Bursal hematoma/bursitis	
Articular cartilage injury	Acute fat pad impingement	Complex regional pain syndrome type 1 (post injury)
PCL sprain	Avulsion of biceps femoris tendon	
Patellar dislocation	Dislocated superior tibiofibular joint	Quadriceps rupture

(a) All these conditions may occur in isolation or, commonly, in association with other conditions.

In the majority of cases, an acute knee injury can be diagnosed with an appropriate history and examination. The two main goals of assessment are:

1. to determine which structures have been damaged
2. to determine the extent of damage to each structure.

History

The first and most important step in taking the history is to invite the patient to tell his or her own story of the injury. Once the patient has had an unhurried opportunity to explain what happened, the practitioner may then wish to elicit additional aspects of the history.

Important components of the history include:

- a description of the precise mechanism of injury and the subsequent symptoms, for example, pain and giving way
- demonstration by the patient if possible, on the uninjured knee, of the stress applied at the time of injury
- the location of pain—pain associated with cruciate ligament injuries is often poorly localized (or emanates from the lateral tibial plateau); pain from injuries to the collateral ligaments is usually fairly well localized
- severity of pain—this does not always correlate with the severity of the injury, although most ACL injuries are usually painful immediately.

The degree and time of onset of swelling is an important diagnostic clue (Table 27.2). When a hemarthrosis is present, the swelling is usually considerable and develops within the first 1 or 2 hours following the injury. The causes of hemarthrosis are:

- major ligament rupture
  - ACL
  - PCL
- patellar dislocation
- osteochondral fracture
- peripheral tear of the meniscus, more common medially
- Hoffa's syndrome (acute fat pad impingement)
- bleeding diathesis (rare).

Note: Lipohemarthrosis (fat and blood in the knee) is caused by intra-articular fractures. Lipohemarthrosis will present in a similar manner to hemarthrosis.

An effusion that develops after a few hours or, more commonly, the following day is a feature of meniscal and chondral injuries. There is usually little effusion with collateral ligament injuries.

 PRACTISE PEARL If patients volunteer that they heard a 'pop', a 'snap' or a 'tear', the injury should be considered as an ACL tear until proven otherwise.

Patients presenting with a sensation of something having 'moved' or 'popped out' in the knee are usually thought to have a patellar dislocation. However, this symptom is more commonly associated with an ACL rupture. There may be associated 'clicking' or 'locking' and this is often seen with meniscal injuries. Locking is classically associated with a loose body or displaced meniscal tear. Locking does not mean locked in one knee position but is used when significant loss of passive range of motion is present, especially loss of full extension. It is helpful to ask the patient in what 'position' the knee locks. If the patient reports that the knee locks when it is straight, and does not bend, this usually is a manifestation of patellofemoral pain and injury—the kneecap is unable to engage in the groove secondary to pain.

The symptom of 'giving way' can occur with instability, such as in ACL deficiency. It may also occur with meniscal tears, articular cartilage damage, patellofemoral pain (Chapter 28) or severe knee pain. Patients with recurrent patellar dislocation and those with loose bodies in the knee can describe similar sensations. If a patient reports episodes of giving way on steps, this is most often a reflection of quadriceps weakness and/or pain, and rarely represents true kneecap instability.

The initial management of the injury and the degree of disability should be ascertained. A history of previous injury to either knee or any previous surgery should also be noted.

It is important to ascertain the patient's age, occupation, type of sport and leisure activities, and the level of sport played. All these factors may influence the type of treatment offered.

Table 27.2 Time relationship of swelling to diagnosis

Immediate (0–2 hours) (hemarthrosis)	Delayed (6–24) hours (effusion)	No swelling
ACL rupture Patellar dislocation	Meniscus	MCL sprain (superficial)

If the patient is a good historian, the diagnosis will be obvious in many cases. In the first two to three days following injury, examination can be difficult if the knee is painful and swollen.

Examination

The key feature of the knee examination is that each structure that may be injured must be examined. Clues to diagnosis are gleaned from the presence or absence of effusion, assessment of the state of the ligaments and menisci, and range of motion testing.

Examination includes:

A. Observation
  1. standing
  2. walking
  3. supine (Fig. 27.2a)
B. Active movements
  1. flexion
  2. extension
  3. straight leg raise
C. Passive movements
  1. flexion (Fig. 27.2b)
  2. extension (Fig. 27.2c)
D. Palpation
  1. patellofemoral joint (including patellar and quadriceps tendons)
  2. MCL
  3. LCL
  4. medial joint line (Fig. 27.2d)
  5. lateral joint line
  6. prone (e.g. hamstring tendons, Baker's cyst, gastrocnemius origins)
E. Special tests
  1. presence of effusion (Fig. 27.2e)
  2. stability tests
    (a) MCL (Fig. 27.2f)
    (b) LCL (Fig. 27.2g)
    (c) ACL
      (i) Lachman's test (Figs 27.2h–k)
      (ii) anterior drawer test (Fig. 27.2l)
      (iii) pivot shift test (Fig. 27.2m)
    (d) PCL
      (i) posterior sag (Fig. 27.2n)
      (ii) reverse Lachman's test
      (iii) posterior drawer test (Fig. 27.2o)
      (iv) external rotation test—active and passive
    (e) patella
      (i) medial and lateral patella translation (or mobility)
  3. flexion/rotation (McMurray's) test (Fig. 27.2p)

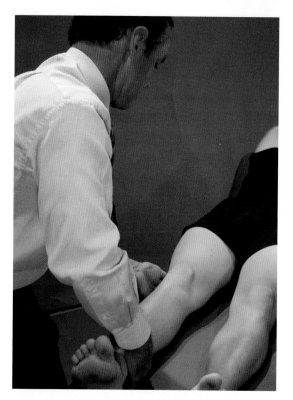

Figure 27.2 Examination of the patient with an acute knee injury

(a) Observation—supine. Look for swelling, deformity and bruising

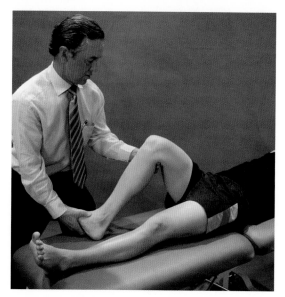

(b) Passive movement—flexion. Assess range of motion, end feel and presence of pain

4. patellar apprehension test (Fig. 27.2q)
5. patellofemoral joint (Chapter 28)
6. functional tests
    (a) squat test
    (b) hop test

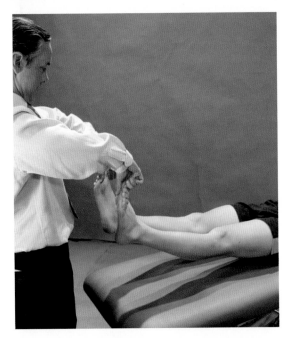

(c) Passive movement—extension. Hold both legs by the toes looking for fixed flexion deformity or hyperextension in the ACL, or PCL rupture. Overpressure may be applied to assess end range. This procedure may provoke pain in meniscal injuries

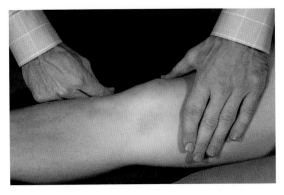

(e) Special tests—presence of effusion. Manually drain the medial subpatellar pouch by stroking the fluid in a superior direction. Then 'milk' the fluid back into the knee from above on the lateral side while observing the pouch for evidence that fluid is reaccumulating. This test is more sensitive than the 'patellar tap'. It is important to differentiate between an intra-articular effusion and an extra-articular hemorrhagic bursitis

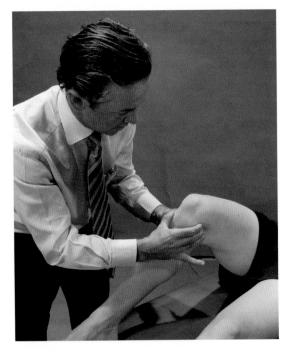

(d) Palpation—medial joint line. The knee should be palpated in 30° of flexion

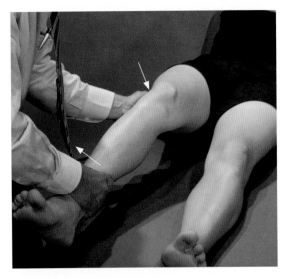

(f) Stability test—MCL. This is tested with the knee in full extension and also at 30° of flexion (illustrated). The examiner applies a valgus force, being careful to eliminate any femoral rotation. Assess for onset of any pain, extent of valgus movement and feel for end point. If the knee 'gaps' at full extension, there must be associated posterior cruciate injury

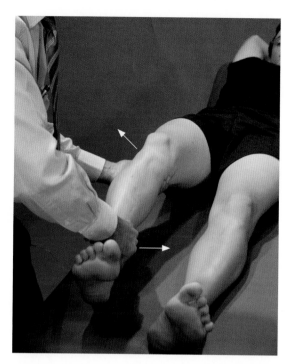

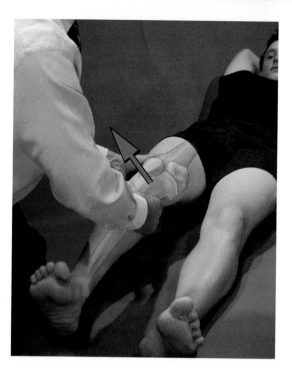

(g) Stability test—LCL. The LCL is tested in a similar manner to the MCL except with varus stress applied

(h) Stability test—Lachman's test. Lachman's test is performed with the knee in 15° of flexion, ensuring the hamstrings are relaxed. The examiner draws the tibia forward, feeling for laxity and assessing the quality of the end point. Compare with the uninjured side

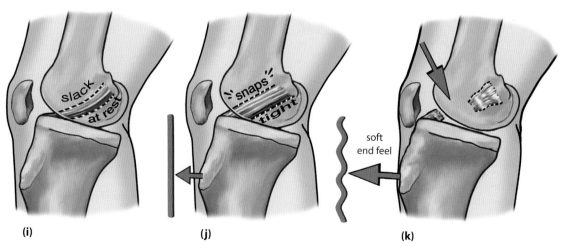

(i) **(j)** **(k)**

(i) The ACL is slightly slack in the start position
(j) When the ACL is intact, the ligament snaps tight and the examiner senses a 'firm'/'sudden' end feel
(k) When the ACL is ruptured, the Lachman's test results in a 'softer'/'gradual' end feel

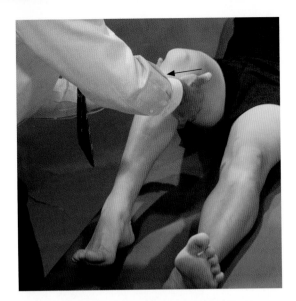

(l) Stability test—anterior drawer test. This is performed with the knee in 90° of flexion and the patient's foot kept stable. Ensure the hamstrings are relaxed with the index finger on the femoral condyles. The tibia is drawn anteriorly and assessed for degree of movement and quality of end point. The test can be performed with the tibia in internal and external rotation to assess anterolateral and anteromedial instability respectively

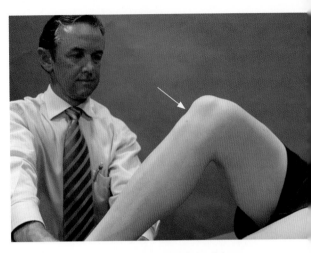

(n) Stability test—posterior sag. With both knees flexed at 90° and the patient relaxed, the position of the tibia relative to the femur is observed. This will be relatively posterior in the knee with PCL deficiency

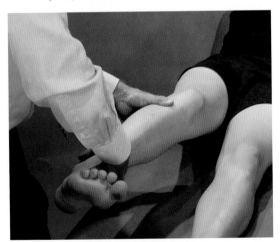

(m) Special test—pivot shift test. With the tibia internally rotated and the knee in full extension, a valgus force is applied to the knee. In a knee with ACL deficiency, the condyles will be subluxated. The knee is then flexed, looking for a 'clunk' of reduction, which renders the pivot shift test positive. Maintaining this position, the knee is extended, looking for a click into subluxation, which is called a positive jerk test

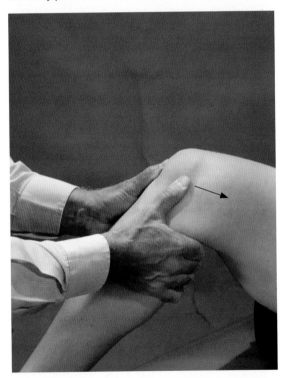

(o) Stability test—posterior drawer test. With the knee as for the anterior drawer test, the examiner grips the tibia firmly as shown and pushes it posteriorly. Feel for the extent of the posterior movement and quality of end point. The test can be repeated with the tibia in external rotation to assess posterolateral capsular integrity

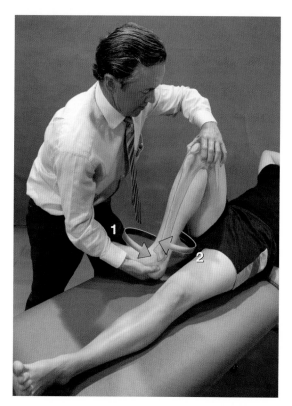

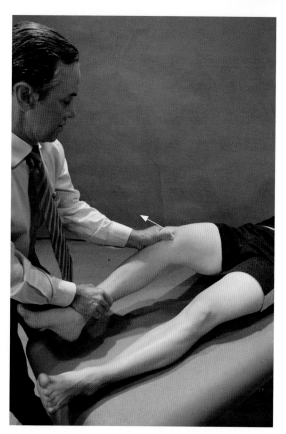

(p) Flexion/rotation (McMurray's) test. The knee is flexed and, at various stages of flexion, internal and external rotation of the tibia are performed. The presence of pain and a palpable 'clunk' is a positive McMurray's test and is consistent with meniscal injury. If there is no 'clunk' but the patient's pain is reproduced, then the meniscus may be damaged or there may be a patellofemoral joint abnormality

(q) Special tests—patellar apprehension test. The knee may be placed on a pillow to maintain 20–30° of flexion. Gently push the patella laterally. The test is positive if the patient develops apprehension with a sensation of impending dislocation

Investigations

X-ray

Clinicians often wonder whether or not to perform an X-ray in cases of an acute knee injury. More than 90% of radiographs ordered to evaluate knee injuries are normal. A set of decision criteria known as the Ottawa knee rule was developed in an adult emergency medicine setting in the mid 1990s (Table 27.3).[1]

Also, surgeons always wish to see preoperative films so there are no intraoperative surprises.

The main aim of performing an X-ray in cases of moderately severe acute knee injuries is to detect an avulsion fracture associated with an ACL injury or a tibial plateau fracture following a high-speed injury. An osteochondral fracture may be evident after patellar dislocation.

Table 27.3 Criteria for the Ottawa knee rule

A knee radiograph is indicated after trauma only when at least one of the following is present:

- patient age more than 55 or less than 18 years
- tenderness at the fibular head
- tenderness over the patella
- inability to flex the knee to 90° (this captures most hemarthrosis, fractures)
- inability to weight-bear for four steps at the time of the injury and when examined.

To these, we suggest a high index of suspicion for:

- high-speed injuries
- children or adolescents (who may avulse a bony fragment instead of tearing a cruciate ligament)
- if there is clinical suspicion of loose bodies.

MRI

MRI may be used as an adjunct to clinical assessment in cases of uncertain diagnosis, especially if a meniscal abnormality is suspected. MRI is also a useful investigation in determining the extent of ACL injury, articular cartilage damage and patellar tendon injury.[2-4] MRI should never be ordered in the absence of a thorough history and physical examination.

With the advent of MRI it was noted that significant knee injuries were associated with the presence of edema in the subchondral region. This phenomenon is known as a bone bruise. Clinically, a bone bruise is associated with pain, tenderness, swelling and delayed recovery. The presence of a bone bruise indicates substantial articular cartilage damage.[5]

Ultrasound examination

High-quality ultrasound examination of the patellar tendon is an excellent means of demonstrating partial tears of this tendon. A complete rupture should be obvious clinically.

Ultrasound examination can also detect the size and location of bursal swelling, and identify intra- versus extra-articular swelling if necessary.

Arthroscopy

Arthroscopy may be used as an investigation, a treatment or both. In most cases when the diagnosis is evident from the clinical assessment, it is used as a treatment method, while also confirming the clinical diagnosis. However, on occasions when the clinical picture is unclear and the patient has persistent pain not responding to treatment, diagnostic arthroscopy is performed.

Immediately before arthroscopy, the surgeon performs an examination under anesthesia (EUA). The combination of EUA and arthroscopy provides the clinician with both an assessment of the stability of the knee and a view of the affected structures. Depending on the findings, it is usually possible to treat the abnormality during the same procedure.

Meniscal injuries

Acute meniscal tears occur when the shear stress generated within the knee in flexion and compression combined with femoral rotation exceeds the meniscal collagen's ability to resist these forces.[6] The medial meniscal attachment to the medial joint capsule decreases its mobility, thereby increasing its risk for injury compared with the more mobile lateral meniscus.[7]

Degenerative meniscal tears occur in the older population frequently without an inciting event.

The different types of meniscal tear are shown in Figure 27.3.

Clinical features

The history can provide a mechanism and a sense of the severity of meniscal tears. The clinical features are listed below.

- The most common mechanism of meniscal injury is a twisting injury with the foot anchored on the ground, often by another player's body.
- The twisting component may be of comparatively slow speed. This type of injury is commonly seen in football and basketball players.
- The degree of pain associated with an acute meniscal injury varies considerably. Some patients may describe a tearing sensation at the time of injury.

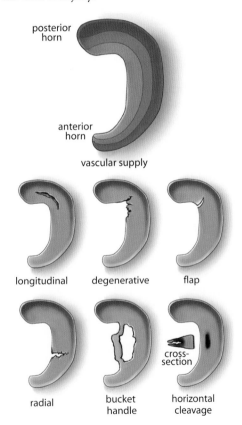

Figure 27.3 Meniscus tear orientation and zones of vascularity; these drawings are of a medial meniscal tear

- A small meniscal tear may cause no immediate symptoms; it may become painful and cause knee swelling over 24 hours.
- Small tears may also occur with minimal trauma in the older athlete as a result of degenerative change of the meniscus.
- Patients with more severe meniscal injuries, for example, a longitudinal ('bucket handle') tear, present with more severe symptoms. Pain and restriction of range of motion occur soon after injury. Intermittent locking may occur as a result of the torn flap, the 'bucket handle', impinging between the articular surfaces. This may unlock spontaneously with a clicking sensation. This often occurs in association with ACL tears. In these patients a history of locking may be due to either the ACL or the meniscal injury.

On examination, the signs of a meniscal tear include:

- joint line tenderness (palpated with the knee flexed at 45–90°)
- joint effusion—this is usually present, although absence of an effusion does not necessarily rule out meniscal damage
- pain—usually present on squatting, especially with posterior horn tears
- restricted range of motion of the knee joint—this may be due to the torn meniscal flap or the effusion.

The flexion/rotation (McMurray's) test (Fig. 27.2p) is positive when pain is produced by the test and a clunk is heard or felt that corresponds to the torn flap being impinged in the joint. However, it is not necessary to have a positive McMurray's test (i.e. a clunk) to make a diagnosis of a torn meniscus. The hyperflexion portion of the McMurray's test provokes pain in most meniscal injuries. Pain produced by

flexion and external rotation is often indicative of medial meniscal damage, whereas pain on internal rotation indicates lateral meniscal pain. Asking patients where they feel pain during hyperflexion maneuvers gives a suggestion of the location of the tear, medial or lateral.

MRI examination is the investigation of choice. This can aid management if the MRI shows either a complex tear or minimal damage or, more rarely, a peripheral meniscus tear. If meniscal tearing is minimal and stable without displacement, clinical progress remains the best measure of non-operative management. Peripheral meniscus tears, depending on the length of the tear, may be surgically addressed. Diagnostic arthroscopy for meniscus injury is rarely performed in centers where MRI is available.

Treatment

The management of meniscal tears varies depending on the severity of the condition. At one end of the spectrum, a small tear or a degenerative meniscus should initially be treated conservatively. On the other hand, a large painful 'bucket handle' tear, causing a locked knee, requires immediate arthroscopic surgery. The majority of meniscal injuries fall somewhere between these two extremes and the decision on whether to proceed immediately to arthroscopy must be made on the basis of the severity of the symptoms and signs, as well as the demands of the athlete. Experienced clinicians use the clinical features shown in Table 27.4 as a guide for choosing either conservative or surgical treatment.

The aim of surgery is to preserve as much of the meniscus as possible. Some meniscal lesions are suitable for repair by meniscal suture, which can be performed with an arthroscope. The decision as to whether or not to attempt meniscal repair is based on several factors, including acuity of the tear, age

Table 27.4 Clinical features of meniscal injuries that may affect prognosis

Factors that may indicate that conservative treatment is likely to be successful	Factors that may indicate that surgery will be required
Symptoms develop over 24–48 hours after injury	Severe twisting injury, athlete is unable to continue playing
Injury minimal or no recall of specific injury	Locked knee or severely restricted range of motion
Able to weight-bear	Positive McMurray's test (palpable clunk)
Minimal swelling	Pain on McMurray's test with minimal knee flexion
Full range of movement with pain only at end of range of motion	Presence of associated ACL tear
Pain on McMurray's test only in inner range of flexion	Little improvement of clinical features after 3 weeks of conservative treatment
Previous history of rapid recovery from similar injury	
Early degenerative changes on plain radiographs	

of the patient, stability of the knee, and tear location and orientation. The outer one-third of the meniscus rim has a blood supply, and tears in this region can heal. The tear with the best chance of a successful repair is an acute longitudinal tear in the peripheral one-third of the meniscus in a young patient with a concomitant ACL reconstruction.[8] Degenerative, flap, horizontal cleavages and complex meniscal tears are poor candidates for repair.[7] Young patients have a higher success rate. Peripheral meniscus tears in otherwise stable knees without concomitant ligament damage have a reduced success rate.[9]

Partial tears may require removal of the damaged flap of the meniscus. Patients with degenerative tears with no or minimal cartilage wear will be less symptomatic than those patients with concomitant cartilage damage.

Rehabilitation after meniscal surgery

Rehabilitation should commence prior to surgery. In this period it is important to:

- reduce pain and swelling with the use of electrotherapeutic modalities and gentle range of motion exercises
- maintain strength of the quadriceps, hamstrings, and hip abductor and extensor muscles
- protect against further damage to the joint (patient may use crutches if necessary)
- explain the surgical procedure and the post-operative rehabilitation program to the patient.

The precise nature of the rehabilitation process will depend on the extent of the injury and the surgery performed. Arthroscopic partial meniscectomy is usually a straightforward procedure followed by a fairly rapid return to activity. Some athletes with a small isolated medial meniscal tear are ready to return to sport after four weeks of rehabilitation. The rehabilitation process usually takes longer if there has been a more complicated tear of the meniscus, especially if the lateral meniscus is injured. The presence of associated abnormalities, such as articular cartilage damage or ligament (MCL, ACL) tears, will necessarily slow down the rehabilitation process.

If the athlete returns to play before the knee is properly rehabilitated, he or she may not experience difficulty during the first competition but may be prone to develop recurrent effusions and persistent pain. A successful return to sport after meniscal knee surgery should not be measured by the time to play the first match but rather the time to play the second!

Rehabilitation principles after arthroscopic partial meniscectomy are:

- to control pain and swelling
- to regain pain-free active range of motion
- graduated weight-bearing
- progressive strengthening within the available range of motion
- progressive balance, proprioceptive, and coordination exercises
- return to functional activities.

A typical rehabilitation program following arthroscopic partial meniscectomy is shown in Table 27.5. The suggested rehabilitation program may be varied depending on progress. It is important that this and other suggested rehabilitation programs contained in this chapter should only be considered as guidelines. Every patient is different and will differ in his or her response to injury, surgery and rehabilitation.

Close monitoring is essential during post-meniscectomy rehabilitation as the remaining meniscus and underlying articular cartilage slowly increase their tolerance to weight-bearing. Constant reassessment after progressively more difficult activities should be performed by the therapist monitoring the rehabilitation program. The development of increased pain or swelling should result in the program being slowed or revised accordingly.

Conservative management of meniscal injuries

Conservative management of relatively minor meniscal injuries will often be successful, particularly in the athlete whose sporting activity does not involve twisting activities. The principles of conservative management are the same as those following partial meniscectomy (Table 27.5), although the rate of progress may vary depending on the clinical features.

The criteria for return to sport following meniscal injury, treated surgically or conservatively, are shown below. If appropriate rehabilitation principles have been followed, then the criteria will usually all be satisfied:

- absence of effusion
- full range of movement
- normal quadriceps and hamstring function
- normal hip external rotator function
- good proprioception
- functional exercises performed without difficulty
- training performed without subsequent knee symptoms

Table 27.5 Rehabilitation program for conservative management of meniscal injury and following arthroscopic partial meniscectomy

Phase	Time post injury	Goal of phase	Physiotherapy	Exercise program	Functional/sport-related activity
Phase 1	0–1 week	Control swelling Maintain knee extension Knee flexion to 100°+ 4/5 quadriceps strength 4+/5 hamstring strength	Cryotherapy Electrotherapy Compression Manual therapy Gait re-education Patient education	Gentle ROM (extension and flexion) Quadriceps/VMO setting Supported (bilateral) calf raises Hip abduction and extension Hamstring pulleys/rubbers Gait re-education drills Light exercise bike	Progress to FWB and normal gait pattern
Phase 2	1–2 weeks	Eliminate swelling Full ROM 4+/5 quadriceps strength 5/5 hamstring strength	Cryotherapy Electrotherapy Compression Manual therapy Gait re-education Exercise modification and supervision	ROM drills Quadriceps/VMO setting Mini squats and lunges Leg press (double, then single leg) Step-ups Bridges (double, then single leg) Hip abduction and extension with rubber tubing Single-leg calf raises Gait re-education drills Balance and proprioceptive drills (single leg)	Swimming (light kick) Exercise bike Walking
Phase 3	2–3 weeks	Full ROM Full strength Full squat Dynamic proprioceptive training Return to running and restricted sport-specific drills	Manual therapy Exercise/activity modification and supervision	As above—increase difficulty, repetitions and weight where appropriate Jump and land drills Agility drills	Running Swimming Road bike Sport-specific exercises (progressively sequenced) e.g. running forwards, sideways, backwards, sprinting, jumping, hopping, changing direction, kicking
Phase 4	3–5 weeks	Full strength, ROM and endurance of affected limb Return to sport-specific drills and restricted training and match play	As above	High level sport-specific strengthening as required	Return to sport-specific drills, restricted training and match play

FWB = full weight-bearing. ROM = range of motion. VMO = vastus medialis obliquus.

- simulated match situations undertaken without subsequent knee symptoms.

Medial collateral ligament injury

Injury to the MCL usually occurs as a result of a valgus stress to the partially flexed knee. This can occur in a non-contact mechanism such as downhill skiing, or in contact sports when an opponent falls across the knee from lateral to medial. MCL tears are classified on the basis of their severity into grade I (mild, first degree), grade II (moderate, second degree) or grade III (complete, third degree).

In patients with a grade I MCL sprain, there is local tenderness over the MCL on the medial femoral condyle or medial tibial plateau but usually no swelling. When a valgus stress is applied at 30° of flexion, there is pain but no laxity. Ligament integrity is intact.

A grade II MCL sprain is produced by a more severe valgus stress. Examination shows marked tenderness, sometimes with localized swelling. A valgus stress applied at 30° of knee flexion causes pain. Some laxity (typically <5 mm [<0.05 in.]) is present but there is a distinct end point. Ligament integrity is compromised but intact throughout its length.

A grade III sprain of the MCL results from a severe valgus stress that causes a complete tear of the ligament fibers. The patient often complains of a feeling of instability and a 'wobbly knee.' The amount of pain is variable and frequently not as severe as one would expect given the nature of the injury. On examination, there is tenderness over the ligament and valgus stress applied at 30° of flexion reveals gross laxity without a distinct end point. This test may not provoke as much pain as incomplete tears of the ligament due to complete disruption of the nociceptive fibers of the ligament.

Grade III MCL injuries are frequently associated with a torn ACL, but rarely associated with medial meniscus injury. The presentation of medial joint line tenderness and lack of full extension is more a reflection of MCL injury. The lateral meniscus is more at risk because the mechanism of injury typically opens the medial side and compresses the lateral side.

While swelling is uncommon in grade 1 sprains, it may occasionally be seen with grade 2 injuries. In grade 3 sprains there is associated capsular tearing (deep fibers and superficial) and fluid escapes so some degree of swelling is common although a tense effusion is not present.

Distal MCL injuries have a tendency to recover more slowly.[10]

Treatment

The treatment of MCL injuries involves a conservative rehabilitation program. Patients with grade III MCL injuries that have been treated conservatively have been shown to return to sport as well as those treated surgically.[11] The rehabilitation program following MCL injury varies depending on the severity. A typical rehabilitation program for milder MCL injuries (grade I and mild grade II) is shown in Table 27.6.

A hinged knee brace (Fig. 27.4a) provides support and protection to the injured MCL during the rehabilitation process.

The more severe MCL injury (the severe grade II or grade III tear) requires a longer period of rehabilitation. An example of a rehabilitation program following a moderate-to-severe MCL injury is shown in Table 27.7.

Anterior cruciate ligament tears

Tears of the ACL are relatively common among sportspeople. Over 100 000 ACL reconstructions are performed annually in the United States.[12] They occur most frequently in those who play sports involving pivoting (e.g. football, basketball, netball, soccer, European team handball, gymnastics, downhill skiing). The incidence rate of ACL tears is between 2.4 and 9.7 times higher in female athletes competing in similar activities.[13–17]

ACL tears may occur in isolation or in combination with associated injuries, particularly meniscal and articular cartilage injury, or injury to the MCL.[18] They are the most common cause of prolonged absence from sport.

Clinical features

The majority of ACL tears occur in a non-contact situation, when the athlete is landing from a jump, pivoting or decelerating suddenly. The jumping mechanism is more likely to be associated with an accompanying meniscal injury.[19] The mechanism of non-contact injury has come under intense scrutiny in recent years. It is common for it to result from an action that the injured athlete has performed repeatedly in their career, often a simple maneuver. Video analysis has shown that at times a trivial contact with another body part, such as a touch to the shoulder or hand, can precede the injury.

The typical features of the history include the following:

Table 27.6 Rehabilitation of a mild MCL injury (see Figs 27.5 and 27.6)

Phase	Goal of phase	Time post injury	Physiotherapy treatment	Exercise program	Functional/sport-related activity
Phase 1	Control swelling Knee flexion to 100°+ Allow +20° extension 4/5 quadriceps strength 4+/5 hamstring strength	0–1 week	Cryotherapy Electrotherapy Compression Manual therapy Gait re-education Patient education	Gentle ROM (flexion mainly) Quadriceps/VMO setting Supported (bilateral) calf raises Hip abduction and extension Hamstring pulleys/rubbers Gait re-education drills	Progress to FWB and normal gait pattern
Phase 2	Eliminate swelling Full flexion ROM Allow +10° extension 4+/5 quadriceps strength 5/5 hamstring strength Return to light jogging	1–2 weeks	Cryotherapy Electrotherapy Compression Manual therapy Gait re-education Exercise modification and supervision	ROM drills Quadriceps/VMO setting Mini squats and lunges Leg press (double, then single leg) Step-ups Bridges (double, then single leg) Hip abduction and extension with rubber tubing Single-leg calf raises Gait re-education drills Balance and proprioceptive drills (single leg)	Straight line jogging Swimming (light kick) Road bike With hinged knee brace
Phase 3	Full ROM Full strength Full squat Dynamic proprioceptive training Return to running and restricted sport-specific drills	2–4 weeks	Manual therapy Exercise/activity modification and supervision	As above—increase difficulty, repetitions and weight where appropriate Jump and land drills Agility drills	Progressive running Swimming Road bike Sport-specific exercises (progressively sequenced) e.g. running forwards, sideways, backwards, sprinting, jumping, hopping, changing direction, kicking
Phase 4	Full strength, ROM and endurance of affected limb Return to sport-specific drills and restricted training and match play	3–6 weeks	As above	High level sport-specific strengthening as required	Return to sport-specific drills, restricted training and match play With hinged knee brace

FWB = full weight-bearing. ROM = range of motion. VMO = vastus medialis obliquus.

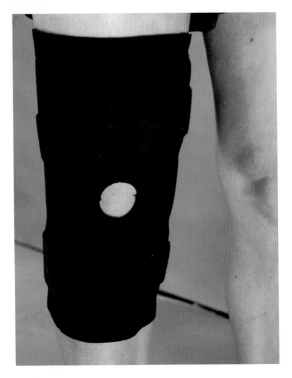

Figure 27.4 Splints

(a) Hinged knee brace

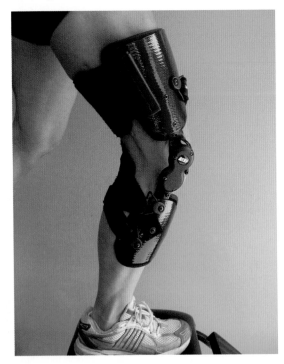

(b) Limited motion knee brace

- The patient often describes an audible 'pop', 'crack' or feeling of 'something going out and then going back'.
- Most complete tears of the ACL are extremely painful, especially in the first few minutes after injury.
- Athletes are initially unable to continue their activity. Occasionally pain will limit further activity and this is usually associated with a large tense effusion. This is the clinical feature of a hemarthrosis. Occasionally, swelling is minimal or delayed. At times the athlete tries to recommence the sporting activity and feels instability or a lack of confidence in the knee. Occasionally the athlete may resume playing and suffer an acute episode of instability.

Most athletes with an ACL tear present to a sports medicine practitioner between 24 and 48 hours following the injury. At this stage it may be difficult to examine the knee. The best time to examine a patient with this condition is in the first hour following the injury before the development of a tense hemarthrosis, which limits the examination. After a few days when the swelling has started to settle and the pain is less intense the examination becomes easier to perform in most cases.

After ACL rupture the examination findings are typical:

- athletes have restricted movement, especially loss of extension
- they may have widespread mild tenderness
- lateral joint tenderness is often present, as the knee stretches the lateral joint capsule while subluxating
- medial joint line tenderness may be present if there is an associated medial meniscus injury.

 The Lachman's test[20] (Figs 27.2h–k) is positive in ACL disruption and is the most useful test for this condition. Students should learn to master this test.

A positive pivot shift (or jerk) test (Fig. 27.2m) is diagnostic of ACL deficiency but it requires the patient to have an intact MCL and iliotibial band. In cases of acute injuries, especially with associated injury (e.g. meniscal tear), the pivot shift test is difficult to perform as the patient is unable to relax sufficiently. The anterior drawer test (Fig. 27.2l) is usually positive in cases of ACL tears but is the least specific test. It should always be compared with the other side as often there is a degree of laxity present prior to injury.

Table 27.7 Rehabilitation of a moderate-to-severe MCL injury (see Figs 27.5 and 27.6)

Phase	Time post injury	Goal of phase	Physiotherapy treatment	Exercise program	Functional/sport-related activity
Phase 1	0–4 weeks	Control swelling Knee flexion to 90°+ Allow +30° extension 4/5 quadriceps strength 4+/5 hamstring strength	Limited motion knee brace (limited 0–30°) Cryotherapy Electrotherapy Compression Manual therapy Gait re-education Patient education	Exercises done in brace Gentle flexion ROM Extension ROM to 30° only Quadriceps/VMO setting Supported (bilateral) calf raises Hip abduction and extension Hamstring pulleys/rubbers Gait drills	Initially NWB/PWB Progress to FWB Walking (normal gait pattern)
Phase 2	4–6 weeks	FWB Eliminate swelling Full ROM 4+/5 quadriceps strength 5/5 hamstring strength	Removal of brace 4–6 weeks Cryotherapy Electrotherapy Compression Manual therapy Gait re-education Exercise modification and supervision	ROM drills Quadriceps/VMO setting Mini squats and lunges Leg press (double, then single leg) Step-ups Bridges (double, then single leg) Hip abduction and extension with rubber tubing Single-leg calf raises Gait re-education drills Balance and proprioceptive drills (single leg)	Swimming (light kick) Road bike Walking
Phase 3	6–10 weeks	Full ROM Full strength Full squat Dynamic proprioceptive training Return to light jogging Return to running and restricted sport-specific drills	Manual therapy Exercise/activity modification and supervision	As above—increase difficulty, repetitions and weight where appropriate Jump and land drills Agility drills	Straight line jogging with hinged knee brace (no earlier than 6 weeks) Running Swimming Road bike Sport-specific exercises (progressively sequenced) e.g. running forwards, sideways, backwards, sprinting, jumping, hopping, changing direction, kicking
Phase 4	8–10/12 weeks	Full strength, ROM and endurance of affected limb Return to sport-specific drills and restricted training and match play	As above	High level of sport-specific strengthening as required	Return to sport-specific drills, restricted training and match play With hinged knee brace for first 2–4 weeks

FWB = full weight-bearing. NWB = non-weight-bearing. PWB = partial weight-bearing. ROM = range of motion. VMO = vastus medialis obliquus.

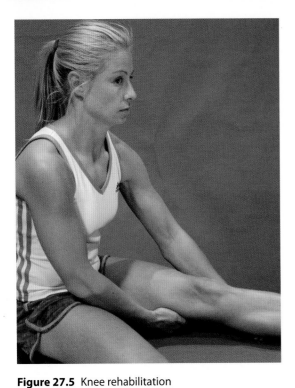

Figure 27.5 Knee rehabilitation

(a) Quadriceps drills—isometric contraction

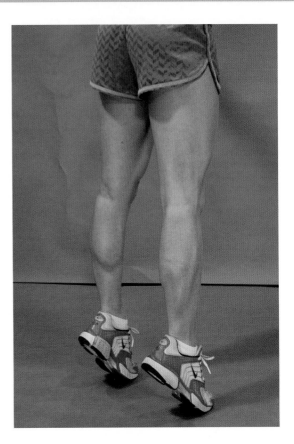

(c) Double-leg calf raise. Progression of the double-leg calf raise should incorporate an increase in range, sets and repetition, and speed of movement. The eccentric component should be emphasized

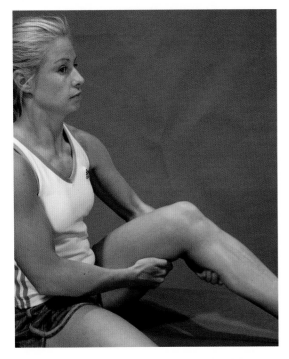

(b) Assisted knee flexion. Place hands behind the thigh and pull the knee into flexion

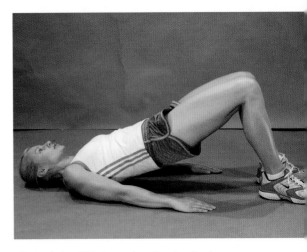

(d) Bridging. This is used to develop both core muscular strength and proprioception

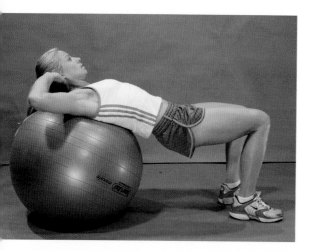

(e) Bridging with Swiss ball. A Swiss ball may be used to progress the exercise

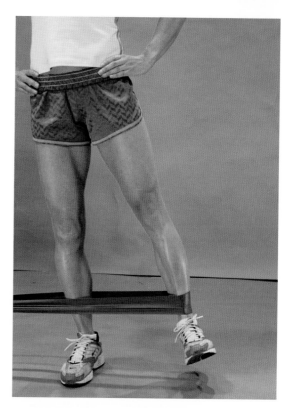

(g) Hip abduction with rubber tubing

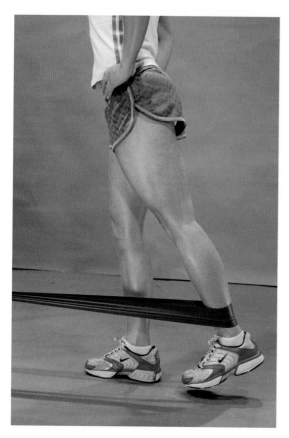

(f) Hip extension—with rubber tubing

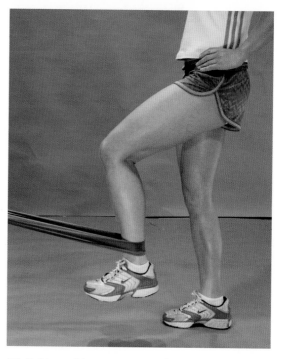

(h) Rubber tubing eccentric stride catch—standing

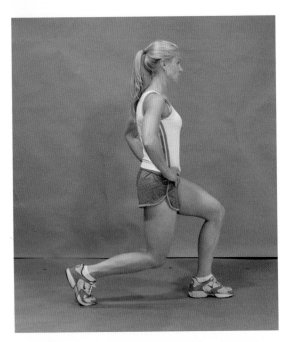

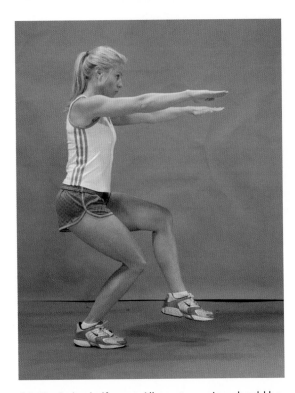

(i) Lunge—performed as shown. Progression involves a combination of increasing the number of sets and repetitions, increasing the depth of the lunge, and finally by holding additional weight

(k) Single-leg half squat. All squat exercises should be pain-free. The squat may be aided by the use of a Swiss ball. Particular attention must be given to technique, control of the pelvis, hip and knee. Progression of the squat is similar to that of progression of the leg press exercise

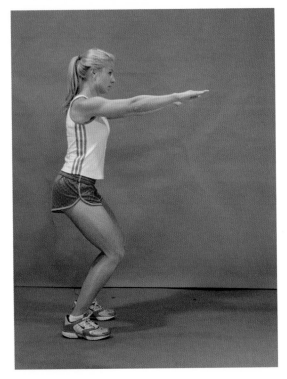

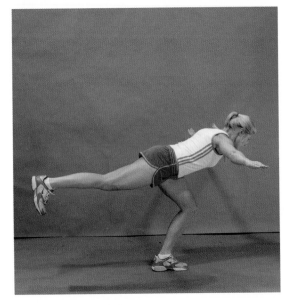

(j) Double quarter squat

(l) Arabesque single-leg squat

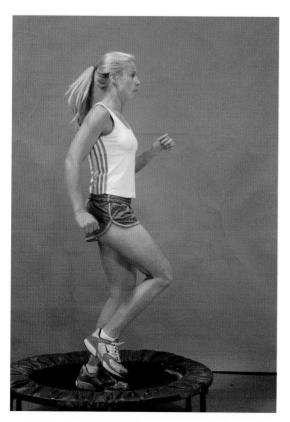

(m) Rebounder—jogging. Jogging and bounding are common rebounder exercises

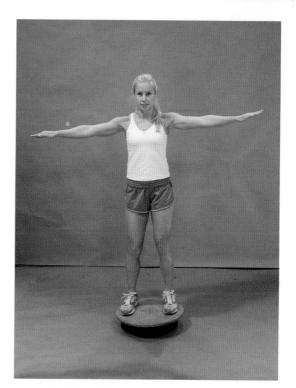

(o) Wobble board

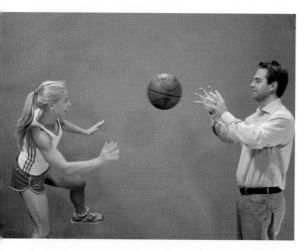

(n) Rebounder (not shown)—static proprioceptive hold/throwing ball. The rebounder can be used for a variety of proprioceptive and balance exercises. Ball throwing or 'eyes closed' exercises can provide an excellent functional challenge

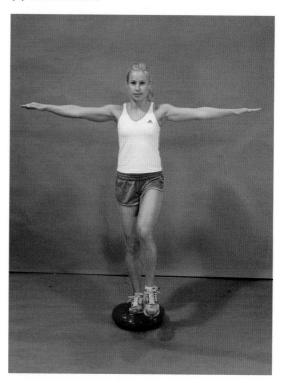

(p) Dura disk balance

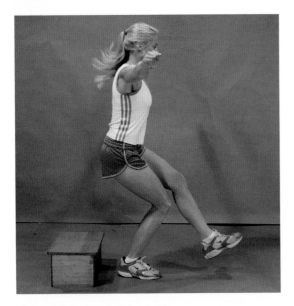

Figure 27.6 Functional activities

(a) Jump and land from block. This exercise may be used to reciprocate functional movements in many sports. Begin the exercise from a small height and jump without rotation. This exercise can be progressed by increasing the height of the jump and rotating 90° during the jump

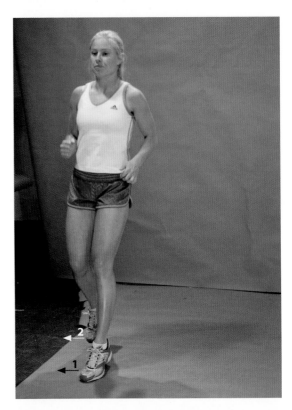

(c) Carioca exercises

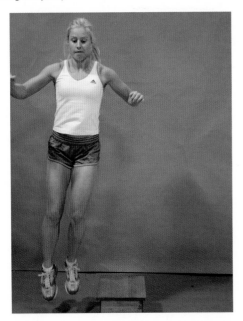

(b) Plyometric jumps over block—lateral. Plyometric exercises should only be included in the later stages of rehabilitation. Each plyometric exercise should be sport-specific

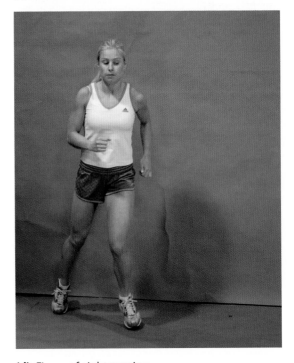

(d) Figure of eight running

X-ray of the knee should be performed when an ACL tear is suspected. It may reveal an avulsion of the ligament from the tibia or a 'Segond' fracture (anterior–lateral capsular avulsion)[21] at the lateral margin of the tibial plateau (Fig. 27.7); this is pathognomonic of an ACL rupture. MRI may be useful in demonstrating an ACL tear (Fig. 27.8) when the diagnosis is uncertain clinically.

A bone bruise is usually (>80%)[17] present in conjunction with an ACL injury. The most common site is over the lateral femoral condyle (Fig. 27.9). The bone bruise is most likely caused by impaction between the posterior aspect of the lateral tibial plateau and the lateral femoral condyle during displacement of the joint at the time of the injury. The presence of a bone bruise indicates impaction trauma to the articular cartilage.[5]

The degree to which bone bruises result in permanent injury to the cartilage continues to be investigated. At present it is not clear whether the presence of a bone bruise is significant in the long term. It may be that those patients with a bone bruise are

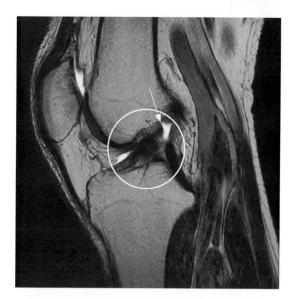

Figure 27.8 MRI of anterior cruciate ligament (circled) showing the precise location of the tear (arrow)

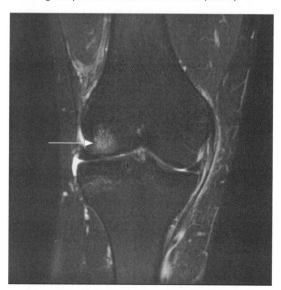

Figure 27.9 MRI showing a bone bruise of the lateral femoral condyle in association with an ACL tear

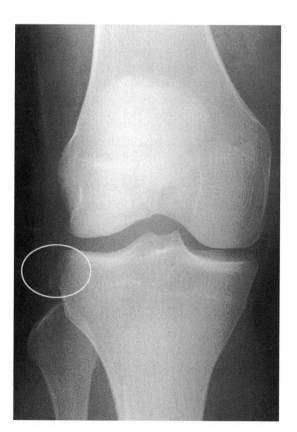

Figure 27.7 X-ray showing a Segond fracture

more prone to the development of osteoarthritis. It is also not clear at this time whether the presence of a bone bruise should result in a slower rehabilitation process with reduced loading of the knee in the first few months after injury. However, most clinicians would favor a conservative course of treatment in this regard, and limit pounding activities for three months post bone bruise.

Conservative or surgical treatment?

There are several areas of controversy regarding the management of ACL injuries. These include the relative merits of conservative versus surgical management; the use of braces to prevent ACL injury or control ACL deficiency; whether surgery should be performed immediately after the injury or should be delayed; the relative merits of the various surgical techniques; and the different rehabilitation programs followed after surgery.

Once the diagnosis is made, the decision on whether to opt for initial conservative or surgical management is dependent on a number of factors:

- the age of the patient
- the degree of instability
- associated abnormalities (e.g. MCL tear, meniscal tear)
- whether or not the patient performs pivoting sports
- the patient's occupation (e.g. firefighter, police)
- social factors, such as cost of treatment or time off work.

The degree of instability may be assessed by a number of parameters. Clinical examination of the knee is not always a reliable indication of functional stability. If the patient is undergoing arthroscopy, then EUA will provide an opportunity to assess knee stability. A pivot shift test, difficult to perform in the conscious patient with a recent injury, should be performed at this time. A positive pivot shift test is indicative of a significant degree of knee instability. In the patient with longer term ACL deficiency, symptoms such as recurrent episodes of giving way indicate instability. For those patients whose knee shows appropriate strength on functional testing and whose knee gives way with activities of daily living despite adequate strength, an ACL reconstruction is recommended. Many surgeons would advocate ACL reconstruction in patients with concomitant meniscal injuries.

The decision is also influenced by the demands placed on the knee. In a young athlete who plays a pivoting sport, such as football or basketball, the demands placed on the knee will be considerable. However, an athlete who is prepared to confine activity to those sports that do not involve a large amount of twisting, turning and pivoting may be able to function adequately without an intact ACL. The patient must be reminded that repeated episodes of giving way greatly increase the development of osteoarthritis. Despite this, there is no scientific evidence that reconstruction reduces the incidence of long-term osteoarthritis.

Another important factor to assess is the likelihood of the patient adhering to a comprehensive, time-consuming rehabilitation program after surgery. If the patient indicates a lack of willingness to undertake appropriate rehabilitation, surgery may not be successful. Other factors to consider are the cost of surgery and the amount of time off work.

Surgery should be recommended for those athletes wishing to participate in a high-speed sport with constant change of direction and pivoting. Other cases are assessed on their merit, taking into account the factors previously mentioned. As with other conditions, a trial of conservative management does not rule out the possibility of eventual surgery.

Surgical treatment

There are numerous surgical techniques used in the treatment of ACL injuries. As ACL tears are usually in-substance tears and therefore not suitable for primary repair, reconstruction of the ACL is the surgical treatment of choice. Numerous methods of ACL reconstruction have been described. ACL reconstructions were originally performed via an arthrotomy (opening the knee capsule with a surgical incision). With the advance of arthroscopic techniques, ACL reconstructions are now performed 'arthroscopically aided' through a small incision with arthroscope. This utilizes small incisions to help visualize and make the tunnels for placement of the ACL graft. Depending on the type of graft, incisions to harvest the graft and secure the tunnels will be made as well.

The aim of an ACL reconstruction is to replace the torn ACL with a graft that reproduces the normal kinetic functions of the ligament. In most cases, an autogenous graft, taken from around the knee joint, is used. The most common grafts used are the bone–patellar tendon–bone (BTB) autograft involving the central third of the patellar tendon, or the hamstring (semitendinosus +/− gracilis tendons) graft. The decision on whether to perform a patellar tendon or hamstring reconstruction is dependent on a number of factors.

Among orthopedic surgeons there is considerable debate on the patellar tendon versus hamstring tendon subject. A systematic review published in 2004 showed no difference in failure rate, range of motion, or isokinetic strength of arthrometer testing of knee laxity between the two techniques.[22] Our view is that each case should be considered on its merit, taking into account some of the differences in potential post-operative problems. For example, after patellar tendon reconstruction, pain with kneeling is common and approximately 50% of patients develop anterior knee pain. Patients who have a hamstring graft ACL reconstruction have decreased end range knee flexion power. The potential problems need to be addressed in the rehabilitation program and for that reason we advocate slightly different rehabilitation regimens for the two types of surgery.

Other graft options include allografts (the transplantation of cadaver tissue such as ligaments or tendons). Allografts have been used successfully for many years and are associated with decreased morbidity and patients' return to their daily activities more quickly. It has been suggested that allografts may also be associated with earlier return to sport, however, there is little evidence to support this theory.[17] The incorporation of allograft tissue appears to take at least as long as autograft tissue and arguably longer; therefore, many consider delaying the return to full sporting activities for eight to nine months.

Patient information about what happens during ACL reconstruction surgery is provided in the box. This is also available as a downloadable PDF file at <www.clinicalsportsmedicine.com>.

The timing of ACL reconstruction after an acute injury has come under review. Traditionally, ACL reconstructions were performed as soon as practical after the injury. However, there is evidence that delaying the surgery may decrease the post-operative risk of arthrofibrosis (see below).[23] Initial reports suggested three weeks as the appropriate delay in surgery. More important than a specific time is the condition of the knee at the time of surgery. The injured knee should have little or no swelling, have near full range of motion, and the patient should have a normal gait. This period until surgery is a time for active rehabilitation ('prehabilitation').

Combined injuries

Injuries of the ACL rarely occur in isolation. The presence and extent of other injuries may affect the way in which the ACL injury is managed.

Associated injury to the MCL (grades I–III) poses a particular problem due to the tendency to develop stiffness after this injury. Most orthopedic surgeons would initially treat the MCL injury in a limited motion knee brace for a period of six weeks, during which time the athlete would undertake a comprehensive rehabilitation program (see above). Only then would the ACL reconstruction be performed.

Rehabilitation after ACL reconstruction

Traditional methods of management after ACL reconstruction included a lengthy period of non-weight-bearing and knee immobilization. Early muscle activity around the knee joint was discouraged due to concerns regarding the integrity of the graft and its fixation. This program led to weakness and stiffness around the knee joint with impaired proprioception and poor function. A fixed flexion deformity was common due to the prolonged extension block, while there was usually prolonged loss of full flexion. Patellofemoral joint problems were also common during the rehabilitation process.

Management principles have changed dramatically in recent years, resulting in greatly accelerated rehabilitation after ACL reconstruction.[24] These management principles have changed as surgical techniques have changed. There is now a better understanding of the strengths of grafts and the strength of fixation techniques. There is no difference in joint laxity or clinical outcome between those who underwent accelerated rehabilitation compared to those with a non-accelerated program at two years post surgery.[25]

Without an open arthrotomy the extensor mechanism has been better preserved. The principle of complete immobilization has been replaced with protected mobilization, with a resultant dramatic decrease in stiffness and increase in range of motion of the knee joint. This has allowed earlier commencement of a strengthening program and rapid progression to functional exercises. The average time for rehabilitation after ACL reconstruction to return to sport has been reduced from around 12 months to six to nine months.

Rehabilitation must commence from the time of injury, not from the time of surgery, which may be days, weeks or months later.[26] Pre-operative management aims to reduce pain, swelling and inflammation, thus reducing the amount of intra-articular fibrosis and resultant loss of range of motion, strength and function. Immediately after injury, treatment should commence, including interferential stimulation, ultrasound and TENS, as well as strengthening exercises for the quadriceps, hamstring, hip extensor, hip abductor and calf muscles. Pain-free range of motion exercises should also be performed.

This period is also an opportunity for explanation of the hospital protocol and the progression and goals of the rehabilitation program. The therapist should set a realistic goal, taking into consideration the individual patient and the type of surgery performed. It is helpful to provide a written explanation as well. If

What happens during ACL reconstruction surgery?

The surgical reconstruction technique involves harvesting the tendon (patellar or hamstring, Fig. 27.10a) through a small incision and threading the tendon through tunnels drilled in the bones. The most crucial part of the operation is the points of entry of the tibial and femoral tunnels, and then the fixation of the graft.

The tibial attachment should be in the center of the previous anterior cruciate attachment (at the level of the inner margin of the anterior portion of the lateral meniscus). The femoral attachment is to the so-called isometric point. This is a position in the intercondylar notch on the femur at which the graft is at a fixed tension throughout the range of knee movement.

Once the graft attachment areas have been delineated and prepared, the graft is fixed by one of a variety of different methods. These methods include interference screw fixation (Fig. 27.10b), staples or the tying of sutures around fixation posts. The better the quality of graft fixation, the more comfortable one is in advancing rehabilitation in the first weeks after surgery. Improvement in the quality of graft fixation is a major reason for advancement of rehabilitation in the first weeks after ACL surgery, as it is the weakest link in the first six to eight weeks after ACL reconstruction surgery.

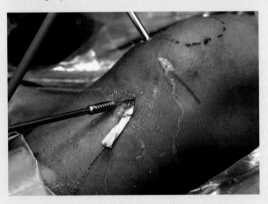

(b) Replacing the ruptured ACL with the graft tendon tissue; interference screw shown

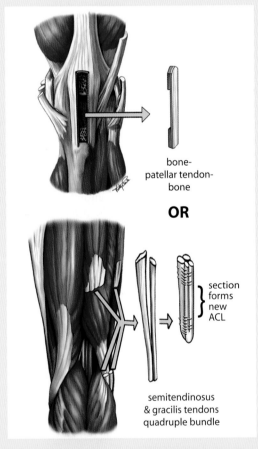

bone-
patellar tendon-
bone

OR

section
forms
new
ACL

semitendinosus
& gracilis tendons
quadruple bundle

Figure 27.10 The key steps in the process of ACL reconstruction

(a) Harvesting graft tissue for the patellar tendon (top panel) or semimembranosus/gracilis tendon ('hamstring graft') ACL reconstruction

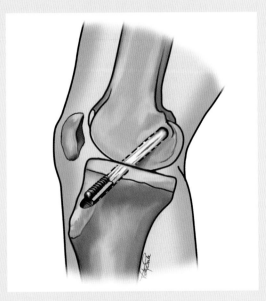

(c) After surgery—the knee with the new graft or 'neoligament' in place

necessary, the post-operative knee brace should be fitted and the use of crutches taught.

Immediately following surgery, weight-bearing status is largely determined by concomitant injuries (e.g. meniscal repair). Isolated ACL reconstructions are typically treated as weight-bearing as tolerated, using a brace and/or crutches until adequate quadriceps muscle strength is restored. Instructions should be given regarding the use of crutches as the patient will progress from limited weight-bearing to full weight-bearing for the first two weeks.

The rehabilitation programs for patellar tendon and hamstring tendon graft ACL reconstructions are slightly different due to the need to prevent the particular complications associated with each type of reconstruction. The main problem with the patellar tendon graft is anterior knee pain (see below). Therefore, attention must be paid to this area during the rehabilitation program with the use of soft tissue therapy to the patellar tendon, accompanied by a strengthening program for the tendon, and patellar taping (Chapter 28) to prevent patellofemoral and fat pad problems. The hamstring graft should be treated as though the patient has had a hamstring tear (Chapter 26), with an appropriate rehabilitation program to restore full range of motion and strength.

The major change in rehabilitation programs over the past few years is the incorporation of a core stability program along with increased emphasis on proprioceptive and balance exercises. These exercises have been used in successful ACL prevention programs (see below). Despite the widespread acceptance of these elements into rehabilitation programs, the two randomized trials have not shown convincing evidence of their efficacy.[27, 28]

The rehabilitation program is shown in Table 27.8. The time frames in the table are a guideline only and must be adjusted depending on the progress of the individual patient. It is essential to rehabilitate each patient individually, taking into consideration the extent of damage to the knee (e.g. articular cartilage damage), the patient's adherence to the exercise program, the amount of stiffness, which varies considerably between patients, and the eventual functional aims of the patient (e.g. daily activities, high level sport).

The patient must be taught to monitor the signs and symptoms around the knee following each work-out. Ice may need to be applied if pain, inflammation or swelling is present.

The timing of return to sport is dependent on several different factors, including the surgeon's assessment, the nature of the sport, the therapist's and coach's opinion and the confidence of the patient. Most surgeons support that ACL graft maturation takes up to six months, and advocate a six-month return to sport as an initial guideline. Beyond this temporal guideline, functional testing should be used to help assess readiness to return to sport.

Functional tests include agility tests, the standing vertical jump and the 'Heiden hop'. The patient performs the 'Heiden hop' by jumping as far as possible using the uninjured leg, landing on the injured leg. Athletes with good function are able to land solid with a single hop, to 'stick it'. Those with functional disability step further or take another small hop. Another way of testing function is by incorporating sport-specific drills. Isokinetic testing may be used to evaluate muscle strength. Quadriceps strength should be at least 90% of the uninjured leg and hamstring strength at least 100%. In the light of all these factors and the varying progress of different athletes and the sport to which they are returning, the time for return to sport after ACL reconstruction may vary from four to 12 months.

The use of a brace on return to sport is not necessary but may help the athlete's confidence. The use of a functional brace in the later stages of rehabilitation and on return to sport has not been shown to be helpful.[29, 30] There is some evidence that wearing a neoprene compression sleeve improves proprioception after ACL reconstruction.[31] Some sporting codes have restrictions on the type of brace and material used.

The research into the effectiveness of various rehabilitation techniques has generally been of poor quality and thus limited conclusions can be drawn. The research evidence is summarized in Table 27.9.

Problems encountered during ACL rehabilitation

Apart from surgical complications (e.g. infection, deep venous thrombosis), a number of secondary problems may occur during the rehabilitation process.

Patella problems

Patellofemoral pain may occur on the injured or the uninjured side. Patients may present with typical symptoms of patellofemoral pain (Chapter 28) but often will not comment on the presence of anterior knee pain as they assume that it is part of the normal process following surgery. The patient should always be asked about symptoms at the front of the knee and the patellofemoral joint should be examined at each visit.

Table 27.8 Rehabilitation following ACL reconstruction (see Figs 27.5 and 27.6)

Phase	Goal of phase	Time post surgery	Physiotherapy treatment	Exercise program	Functional/sport-related activity
Prehabilitation (preoperative rehabilitation)	No/minimal swelling Restore full ROM, particularly extension General 4+/5 lower limb strength or better Patient education—anatomy, surgical procedure, rehabilitation commitment, and goal setting	N/A	Cryotherapy Electrotherapy Compression Manual therapy Gait re-education Exercise modification and supervision	Dependent on ability of patient. In early stages, follow the exercise program from phase 1 and progress to phase 2. If patient has high level of function, start with exercise program from phase 2 and progress weights and repetitions as appropriate	Walking Bike riding Swimming (light kick and no breaststroke)
Phase 1	PWB–FWB Eliminate swelling 0–100° ROM 4+/5 quadriceps strength 5/5 hamstring strength	0–2 weeks	Cryotherapy Electrotherapy Compression Manual therapy Gait re-education Patient education	Gentle flexion ROM Extension ROM to 0° Quadriceps/VMO setting Supported (bilateral) calf raises Hip abduction and extension Hamstring pulleys/rubbers Gait drills	Nil
Phase 2	No swelling Full knee hyperextension Knee flexion to 130°+ Full squat Good balance and control Unrestricted walking	2–12 weeks	Cryotherapy Electrotherapy Compression Manual therapy Gait re-education Exercise modification	ROM drills Quadriceps/VMO setting Mini squats and lunges Leg press (double, then single leg) Step-ups Bridges (double, then single leg) Hip abduction and extension with rubber tubing Single-leg calf raises Gait re-education drills Balance and proprioceptive drills (single leg)	Walking Exercise bike

Table 27.8 Rehabilitation following ACL reconstruction (see Figs 27.5 and 27.6) *(continued)*

Phase	Goal of phase	Time post surgery	Physiotherapy treatment	Exercise program	Functional/sport-related activity
Phase 3	Full ROM Full strength and power Return to jogging, running, and agility Return to restricted sport-specific drills	3–6 months	Manual therapy Exercise/activity modification and supervision	As above—increase difficulty, repetitions and weight where appropriate Jump and land drills Agility drills	Straight line jogging Swimming (light kick) Road bike Straight line running at 3 months Progressing to sport-specific running and agility (progressively sequenced) e.g. running forwards, sideways, backwards, sprinting, jumping, hopping, changing directions, kicking
Phase 4	Return to sport	6–12 months	As above	High-level sport specific strengthening as required	Progressive return to sport, e.g. restricted training, unrestricted training, match play, competitive match play

FWB = full weight-bearing. PWB = partial weight-bearing. ROM = range of motion. VMO = vastus medialis obliquus.

Table 27.9 Rehabilitation techniques after anterior cruciate ligament reconstruction with evidence of effectiveness

- Immediate weight-bearing[32]
- Closed kinetic chain exercises selecting knee joint motions of less than 60°[33]
- Open kinetic chain exercises with knee angles greater than 40° of flexion[34, 35]
- High-intensity neuromuscular electrical stimulation (NMES) in addition to voluntary exercises for improving isometric quadriceps muscle strength[36]

A number of different factors may predispose to the development of patellofemoral pain. Commonly, the lateral structures around the patellofemoral joint, especially the lateral retinaculum and the iliotibial band, are tight. Weakness of the vastus medialis obliquus or proximal gluteal muscles may also be an important component, as may an altered gait pattern, typically associated with excessive subtalar pronation. An overemphasis on knee extension exercises and squats in the exercise program can cause patellofemoral problems. These patellofemoral problems occur not only with patellar tendon graft reconstructions but also with the hamstring tendon graft reconstructions.

The infrapatellar fat pad is frequently damaged by the arthroscope and may be the source of considerable discomfort after reconstruction. Taping techniques (Chapter 28) can be used to unload the fat pad.

Another complication seen after patellar tendon ACL reconstruction is inferior displacement of the patella (patella baja) due to traction on the patella by tight infrapatellar soft tissue structures. Patellar tendinopathy (Chapter 28) is also seen following ACL reconstruction, especially with patellar tendon grafts.

A common and as yet unexplained finding in cases of chronic ACL insufficiency and reconstruction is severe trochlea chondral damage.

Low back pain

Low back pain is not uncommon in the early stages of the rehabilitation program when it may be due to the use of crutches and to altered gait patterns. It usually occurs in patients who have a prior history of low back pain.

Lower limb stiffness

Stiffness in the foot and ankle commonly occurs as a result of a period of non-weight-bearing and the wearing of a brace. Tightness of the Achilles tendon is common. These problems typically present on return to running. Full range of motion of these joints should be maintained early in the rehabilitation program with mobilization and stretching in addition to active plantarflexion/dorsiflexion exercises.

Soft tissue stiffness (arthrofibrosis)

The rehabilitation program and its rate of progression will be influenced by the intrinsic tissue stiffness or laxity of the patient. This depends on the nature of the patient's collagen and appears to correlate with generalized ligamentous stiffness or laxity throughout the body. Patients with stiff soft tissues may develop a large bulky scar with adhesions after ACL reconstruction. These patients are usually slow to regain full flexion and extension, and the knee may require passive mobilization by the therapist. Patients tend to have tight lateral structures around a stiff patellofemoral joint. This is known as arthrofibrosis.[37]

Treatment involves encouraging active movement, early passive mobilization, massage and encouraging early activity. Efforts to control swelling are critical. It may be helpful to remove the brace earlier than usual in these patients. Severe cases may require arthroscopic scar resection as well as a vigorous rehabilitation program.

As mentioned previously, delaying the surgery until all signs of the hemarthrosis have disappeared and full range of motion has been regained appears to reduce the likelihood of arthrofibrosis developing.

Soft tissue laxity

The group of patients classified as having 'loose' soft tissue, are characterized by generalized increased ligamentous laxity. These patients tend to rapidly gain good range of motion in extension and flexion. They are treated by prolonging the time in the brace and restricting the range available. Range of motion exercises are discouraged, mobilization contraindicated and full extension work reduced to avoid stretching the graft. The rehabilitation program is slowed in these patients to allow time for the graft to develop as much scar tissue as possible.

Conservative management

When the clinical diagnosis of an ACL tear is made and the patient opts for initial conservative management, an arthroscopy should probably be performed. The aim of this arthroscopy is to assess stability of the knee under anesthesia, to wash out the hemarthrosis, and to assess and treat other injuries such as meniscal tears and articular cartilage damage. The presence of articular cartilage damage is indicative of a poor prognosis. These patients tend to have persistent problems with pain and swelling even after surgery. This is aggravated if a full or partial meniscectomy is required, as the stresses placed on the articular cartilage are increased.

Derotation knee braces may be used as part of the conservative management of ACL tears to provide additional stability when playing sport (e.g. downhill skiing). The effectiveness of these braces varies depending on the degree of instability and the type of brace.

The rehabilitation program for the conservatively managed ACL injury is similar to management after reconstruction (Table 27.8). The principles of initial reduction of swelling and pain, restoration of full range of motion, increase of muscle strength and power, functional rehabilitation and, finally, return to sport all apply. Depending on the degree of instability and other associated abnormalities (e.g. articular cartilage damage), the rate of progress may be slower or faster than after a reconstruction. The final stages of the rehabilitation program, the agility work and sport-specific drills, may not be possible in the patient with ACL deficiency. Conservative treatment of ACL injuries is most successful in sports that are not dependent on jumping and pivoting motions.

Outcomes after ACL treatment

While the general consensus among the surgical and sporting communities is that those sustaining an ACL injury make a full recovery after ACL reconstructive surgery, research findings suggest that is not always the case. Three main outcome measures are used to determine the success or otherwise of ACL treatment:

1. return to sport
2. reinjury rate
3. prevalence of osteoarthritis.

Return to sport

The majority of those who have an ACL reconstruction have good to excellent knee function and most (65–88%) are able to return to sport within the first year.[38–41] Thus, surgery is effective in allowing injured athletes to resume their sports career.[42]

Among patients treated non-operatively, the return rate ranges from 19% to 82%.[43, 44] Athletes who successfully return to sport after non-operative treatment probably represent a selected group with functionally stable knees and a strong motivation to continue pivoting sport despite their injury.[42]

While most athletes return to their previous sport after ACL reconstruction, there is some evidence that they may stop playing earlier than their non-injured counterparts.[43, 45, 46] In the only study in which the reduction in sport participation can be related to a control group, Roos et al.[44] found that 30% of those who had ACL injury were active after three years compared with 80% of controls, and that after seven years none of the elite injured players were active regardless of the type of treatment.

Although the initial return to sport rate is high, previously injured athletes retire at a higher rate than athletes without previous ACL injury.[42] The reason for this may be that many of the athletes who return to sport experience significant knee problems such as instability, reduced range of motion and/or pain.[43]

Reinjury rate

The incidence of graft failure is generally of the order of 3–6% in most studies.[47] There is some evidence from a meta-analysis that the failure rate may be lower in patellar tendon autografts,[48] although another systematic review failed to show a difference.[22] There also appears to be an increased risk of rupturing the contralateral ACL in patients who have already had an ACL injury. There may also be an increased risk of other knee injuries (e.g. meniscal, articular cartilage injury) after ACL injury, particularly in those managed non-operatively. Reinjury appears to be most likely in the first 12 months after surgery.[22]

Osteoarthritis

ACL rupture is associated with a significant risk of development of osteoarthritis (OA); it may be that the initial injury itself may influence the development of OA irrespective of what treatment is used or how the knee is loaded during subsequent years. Whereas previously it was thought that an isolated ACL injury was quite common, we now know that bone bruising (as seen on MRI) occurs in more than 80% of cases of ACL tears. Bone bruising is highly associated with articular cartilage damage. Meniscal injury is found in 75% of cases of ACL tears and this also predisposes to the development of OA. Long-term follow-up studies of patients who have undergone ACL reconstruction with more modern techniques have shown that nearly all patients develop radiological signs of OA after 15–20 years.[43] Many of these patients are, however, asymptomatic.

Although it was recognized that ACL injuries treated non-operatively were associated with an increased risk of OA, it had been hoped that ACL reconstruction, by restoration of knee anatomy and reduction of instability, would eliminate, or substantially reduce, the incidence of OA. At this time, however, there is no evidence that ligament reconstruction prevents the future development of OA.[43, 46, 49–51] It seems that the important predictor of future OA is the damage to other structures, such as the menisci and articular cartilage, at the time of the injury.

A related, important sports medicine question is, 'Does returning to active sport increase the likelihood of developing OA, or does it bring this event on more quickly?' No studies have evaluated this phenomenon but it is reasonable to assume that intense weight-bearing activity involving pivoting would accelerate the degenerative process compared to in someone who remained sedentary or took up a non-weight-bearing sport (e.g. cycling, swimming). We and others[42, 52] propose that athletes who have undergone an ACL reconstruction should receive advice about the likelihood of developing OA, and the possibility that returning to active sports participation will accelerate its development. Many professional and dedicated athletes may decide to continue their sport in spite of that advice, but it is the duty of health professionals to enable them to make an informed decision.

Gender difference

In light of the increased prevalence of ACL injuries in female athletes discussed previously, attention has been to possible differences in outcome after ACL reconstruction between males and females. The majority of studies show increased post-surgical laxity in females but no difference in graft failure, activity level, or subjective or functional assessment.[38, 53–57]

Prevention of ACL injury

As 60–80% of ACL injuries occur in non-contact situations, it seems likely that the appropriate prevention efforts are warranted. In ball sports two common mechanisms cause ACL tears:

1. a cutting maneuver[58–60]
2. one leg landing.

Cutting or sidestep maneuvers are associated with dramatic increases in the varus–valgus and internal rotation moments. The ACL is placed at greater risk with both varus and internal rotation moments. The typical ACL injury occurs with the knee externally rotated and in 10–30° of flexion when the knee is placed in a valgus position as the athlete takes off from the planted foot and internally rotates with the aim of suddenly changing direction (Fig. 27.11a).[61, 62] The ground reaction force falls medial to the knee

joint during a cutting maneuver and this added force may tax an already tensioned ACL and lead to failure. Similarly in the landing injuries, the knee is close to full extension.

High-speed activities such as cutting or landing maneuvers require eccentric muscle action of the quadriceps to resist further flexion. It may be hypothesized that vigorous eccentric quadriceps muscle action may play a role in disruption of the ACL. Although this normally may be insufficient to tear the ACL, it may be that the addition of a valgus knee position and/or rotation could trigger an ACL rupture.

One question that is often asked is why the ACL tears in situations and maneuvers that the athlete has performed many times in the past. Frequently,

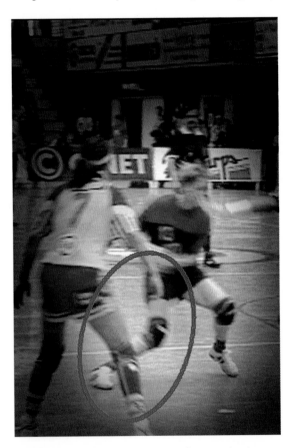

Figure 27.11 Abnormal positions that may lead to ACL injury

(a) The typical position during the cutting maneuver which leads to ACL injury

PHOTO COURTESY OF ODD-EGIL OLSEN, OSLO SPORTS TRAUMA RESEARCH CENTRE

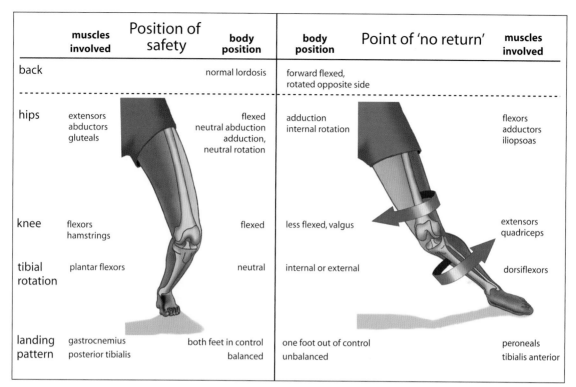

	muscles involved	Position of safety	body position	body position	Point of 'no return'	muscles involved
back			normal lordosis	forward flexed, rotated opposite side		
hips	extensors abductors gluteals		flexed neutral abduction adduction, neutral rotation	adduction internal rotation		flexors adductors iliopsoas
knee	flexors hamstrings		flexed	less flexed, valgus		extensors quadriceps
tibial rotation	plantar flexors		neutral	internal or external		dorsiflexors
landing pattern	gastrocnemius posterior tibialis		both feet in control balanced	one foot out of control unbalanced		peroneals tibialis anterior

(b) The positions of safety and of 'no return'

there is some external factor that renders the athlete susceptible. The athlete could be off balance, be pushed or held by an opponent, be trying to avoid collision with an opponent, or have adopted an unusually wide foot position. These perturbations may contribute to the injury by causing the athlete to plant the foot so as to promote unfavorable lower extremity alignment; this may be compounded by inadequate muscle protection and poor neuro-muscular control.[62] Fatigue and loss of concentration may also be a factor.

What has become recognized is that unfavorable body movements in landing and pivoting can occur, leading to what has become known as the 'functional valgus' or 'dynamic valgus' knee, a pattern of knee collapse where the knee falls medial to the hip and foot. This has been called by Ireland the 'position of no return', or perhaps it should be termed the 'injury prone position' since there is no proof that one cannot recover from this position (Fig. 27.11b).[63] Intervention programs aimed to reduce the risk of ACL injury are based on training safer neuromuscular patterns in simple maneuvers such as cutting and jump landing activities.

The mechanism of ACL injury in skiing is different from that in jumping, running and cutting sports such as football and basketball. In skiing, most ACL injuries result from internal rotation of the tibia with the knee flexed greater than 90°, a position that occurs when a skier who is falling backwards catches the inside edge of the tail of the ski.[64] Intervention programs in skiing are aimed at increasing the skier's awareness of patterns that are injurious to the knee, and giving alternative strategies in the hope of avoiding these patterns altogether.

Why do females tear their ACLs at three times the rate of males?

The rate of non-contact ACL injury among female athletes is considerably higher (×2–8) than that in males at comparable risk (exposure) and in comparable activities. At present, four main areas are being investigated to explain this discrepancy:

1. anatomical
2. hormonal
3. shoe surface interface
4. neuromuscular.

Anatomical differences

A number of anatomical differences between women and men have been proposed as contributing factors to the greater rupture rates of ACLs in females. These differents in females include:

- smaller size and different shape of the intercondylar notch[65, 66]
- wider pelvis and greater Q angle
- greater ligament laxity.[67]

Although anatomical differences may play a role in ACL injury risk, since there is little that one can change in one's anatomy, focus has turned to that which may be able to be changed.

Hormonal differences

Females have a unique hormonal cycle, and estrogen has long been implicated as a risk factor in the higher ACL injury rates in females. Estrogen receptors were detected in the human ACL[68] and more recently relaxin receptors were found on female but not male ACLs.[69] Research examining a possible relationship between phase of the menstrual cycle and ACL injury has shown conflicting results.[14, 70–74]

If estrogen level is a risk factor, it is not likely at the material level of ligament strength, as mechanical tests of ligament failure have not shown any difference in strength between ligaments in two studies of different animal models when levels of estrogen were modified.[75, 76]

If hormones have a role to play in ACL injury risk, most researchers believe they are mediated through the neuromuscular system and that a direct relationship is unlikely.[77]

Shoe–surface interface

The shoe–surface interface can be affected by a number of factors. In team handball a higher friction coefficient rate led to an increase in ACL tears.[78, 79] A higher rate of ACL injuries was found in footballers who wore cleats placed on the peripheral margin of the sole with a number of smaller pointed cleats positioned interiorly.[80] An uneven playing surface may also be a factor. A difference in rainfall or the type of grass may also contribute to alterations in the shoe–surface interface (Chapter 6).[81]

Neuromuscular factors

The balance of muscle power and recruitment pattern between the quadriceps and hamstring muscles is crucial to functional knee stability. Controlling the rotation of the limb under the pelvis in pivoting and landing is critical to controlling knee stability, and reducing or eliminating the functional valgus knee. Quadriceps contraction increases ACL strain between 10° and 30° of flexion. An eccentric quadriceps muscle contraction can produce forces beyond those required for ACL tensile failure.[82]

The hamstrings, in contrast, are ACL agonists, so any weakness, increased flexibility or delayed motor signal to the hamstrings may increase the susceptibility to ACL injury.[83] Female athletes rely more on their quadriceps muscles and respond to anterior tibial translation by activating their quadriceps first rather than their hamstrings.[84] Males, given a similar force, activate their hamstrings first to dynamically stabilize their knee, thus preventing displacement of the tibia on the femur.[85] This difference in the timing of muscle firing patterns has been thought to be related to the increased risk of injury in females. This study, along with Hewett et al.'s work,[86] which shows that females are more 'quadriceps dominant' than males, has led to the concept of a quadriceps dominant limb being a risk factor for serious knee injury, including injury to the ACL.

In addition to muscle strength and firing patterns, females land from a jump or pivot with less hip and knee flexion than do males.[86] This is what Hewett et al. refer to as 'ligament dominance'.[87] Training more flexion at the knee and hip in landing maneuvers has been shown to reduce valgus moments at the knee.

Risk equation

Uhorchak et al.[67] showed that a combination of female gender, decreased notch width, increased body mass index and generalized joint laxity were strong predictors of ACL injuries. This gives firm support to the notion of a 'risk equation', where no one factor predicts injury but, when combined, can increase injury risk with certain factors.

Prevention programs

Given the importance of neuromuscular factors in the etiology of ACL injuries, numerous programs have aimed to improve neuromuscular control during standing, cutting, jumping and landing.[86, 88–92] The components of the neuromuscular training programs are (Table 27.10):

1. balance training
2. landing with increased flexion at the knee and hip
3. controlling body motions, especially in deceleration and pivoting maneuvers

4. some form of feedback to the athlete during training of these activities.

A meta-analysis[93] of the six published prevention programs demonstrated an overall positive effect in reducing ACL injuries, with a total of 29 ACL injuries in the prevention group compared to 110 in the control group. Three of the six programs showed significant reduction, while two of the remaining three demonstrated positive trends and reduced odds ratios. The conclusion from this meta-analysis was that prevention programs may be effective provided that plyometrics, balance and strengthening exercises are incorporated into the training program, that the training be performed more than once a week, and that the program should continue for at least six weeks. The component of the programs which correlated best with ACL injury reduction was high-intensity plyometric movements that progressed beyond foot-work and agility.[93]

Although, as mentioned above, the mechanism of ACL injury in skiing is different, neuromuscular conditioning also successfully prevented ACL injury.[64] Ski injury prevention programs teach skiers to recognize and respond with appropriate strategies to dangerous situations and to avoid potentially compromising positions.[83]

Factors not yet fully explored include the role of individual athlete compliance, failure to comply with neuromuscular training (i.e. how quickly do we forget what we learn?), and what is the ideal age to teach these techniques (i.e. does age matter?). Do all athletes benefit from these intervention techniques or can we identify the 'at-risk' athlete and train that athlete differently? These are the questions on which interventionists will be focusing future direction and research.

ACL rupture among children with open physes

ACL injuries are common in children and adolescents.[94] Traditionally, surgical reconstruction of the ACL in children with open physes has not been recommended due to the risk of growth abnormalities resulting from surgical violation of the physes. There are, however, concerns that non-operative or delayed operative management risk meniscal and/or cartilage injuries, leading to premature degenerative disease.

There is increasing clinical evidence that the risk of damage to the physes is minimal, especially with various surgical techniques currently available to minimize physeal trauma. Most surgeons currently

Table 27.10 ACL prevention program[77]

Week	Exercises
Floor exercises	
1	Running and planting, partner running backwards and giving feedback on the quality of the movement, change position after 20 s
2	Jumping exercise: right leg, right leg over to left leg, left leg and finishing with a two-foot landing with flexion in both hips and knees
3	Running and planting (as in week 1), now doing a full plant-and-cut movement with the ball, focusing on knee position (Fig. 27.12a)
4	Two players together, two-leg jump forward and backwards, 180° turn and the same movement backwards; partner tries to push the player out of control but still focusing on landing technique
5	Expanding the movement from week 3 to a full plant and cut, then a jump shot with two-legged landing
Mat exercises	
1	Two players each standing on one leg on the mat, throwing to each other (Fig. 27.12b)
2	Jump shot from a box (30–40 cm [~1 ft] high) with a two-foot landing with flexion in hip and knees
3	'Step' down from box with one-leg landing with flexion in hip and knee
4	Two players both standing on balance mats trying to push partner out of balance, first on two legs, then on one leg
5	The players jump on a mat, catching the ball, then take a 180° turn on the mat
Wobble board exercises	
1	Two players standing two-legged on the board, throwing to each other
2	Squats on two legs, then on one leg
3	Two players throwing to each other, one foot each on the board
4	One foot on the board, bouncing the ball with eyes shut
5	Two players, both standing on balance boards trying to push partner out of balance, first on two legs, then on one leg (Fig. 27.12c)

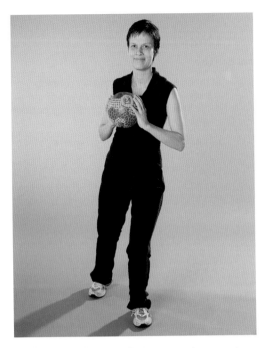

Figure 27.12 Examples of ACL prevention exercises

(a) Floor exercise

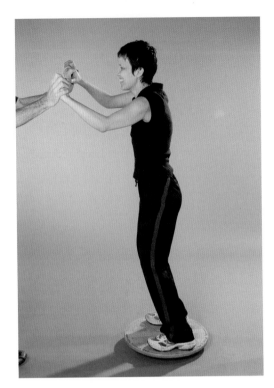

(c) Wobble board exercise

recommend ACL reconstruction in younger patients with open growth plates. In the adolescent patient approaching skeletal maturity, fixation of the ACL graft is performed in the same manner as in an adult, and graft choice is either the patella or hamstring tendons. In the younger patients, techniques are used to minimize the damage to the physes.[95] These include using only soft tissue for graft choice (such as hamstrings) to avoid a bone plug in the tunnel at the growth plate. Tunnels are made smaller in diameter and on the tibia they are slightly more vertical. On the femur one can avoid the growth plate altogether and use the 'over the top' technique of ACL graft placement. These techniques can be individualized to meet the needs of the surgeon and the patient, depending on the age and maturation of the patient.

Posterior cruciate ligament tear

The PCL is the primary restraint to posterior drawer, and secondary restraint to external rotation. Isolated

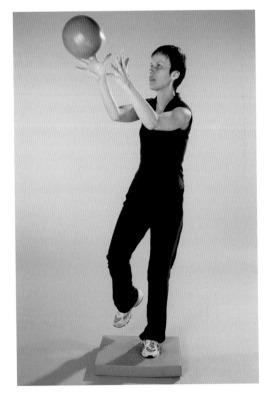

(b) Mat exercise

sectioning of the PCL results in an increased posterior translation of the knee under a posterior tibial load. This increase in laxity is relatively small at full extension and most pronounced at 90° of flexion. Only small rotatory or valgus/varus laxity results from isolated PCL injury.

Up to 60% of PCL injuries involve disruption of the posterolateral structures. The primary stabilizers are the lateral collateral ligament (LCL) and the popliteus complex. They provide varus and external rotatory stability to the knee respectively. When both the PCL and posterolateral structures are cut, posterior laxity is significantly increased.[96]

Tears of the PCL do not appear to be as common as of the ACL, due partly to the greater strength of the PCL. However, the condition is under-diagnosed.

PCL injuries are often associated with meniscal and chondral injury. The incidence of associated meniscal tears varies from 16% to 28%. Longitudinal tears of the anterior horn of the lateral meniscus are the most common location. There is also a high incidence of radial tears in the middle or posterior lateral meniscus.[97]

The incidence of significant chondral damage with isolated PCL injury was not thought to be as high as with ACL injury, but a recent study showed chondral damage in 52% of those with PCL tears, with lesions of grade III or more found in 16%.[97]

Clinical features

The mechanism of PCL injury is usually a direct blow to the anterior tibia with the knee in a flexed position. This can be from contact with an opponent, equipment or falling onto the hyperflexed knee. Hyperextension may also result in an injury to the PCL and posterior capsule.

The patient complains of poorly defined pain, mainly posterior, sometimes involving the calf. On examination, there is usually minimal swelling as the PCL is an extrasynovial structure. The posterior drawer test (Fig. 27.2o) is the most sensitive test for PCL deficiency. This is performed in neutral, internal and external rotation. A posterior sag of the tibia (Fig. 27.2n), and pain and laxity on a reverse Lachman's test may be present. PCL rupture is particularly disabling for downhill skiers, who rely on this ligament for stability in the tucked up position adopted in racing.

PCL tears are graded I, II and III on the position of the medial tibial plateau relative to the medial femoral condyle at 90° of knee flexion (the posterior drawer position). The tibia normally lies approximately 1 cm (0.4 in.) anterior to the femoral condyles in the resting position. In grade I injuries the tibia continues to lie anteriorly to the femoral condyles but is slightly diminished (0–5 mm [0–0.2 in.] laxity). In grade II injuries the tibia is flush with the condyles (5–10 mm [0.2–0.4 in.] laxity). When the tibia no longer has a medial step and can be pushed beyond the medial femoral condyle (>10 mm [>0.4 in.] laxity), it is classified as a grade III injury.[98]

It is important to distinguish between isolated PCL injury and a combined PCL and posterolateral corner injury. In isolated PCL tears, there is a decrease in tibial translation in internal rotation due primarily to the influence of the MCL.[99]

X-ray should be performed to exclude a bony avulsion from the tibial insertion of the PCL (best seen on lateral tibia radiographs). If a fracture is present, acute surgical repair is undertaken. Stress radiographs provide a non-invasive measure of sagittal translation compared to the uninjured knee. It is considered that more than 7–8 mm (>0.3 in.) of posterior translation is indicative of a PCL tear.

MRI has a high predictive accuracy in the diagnosis of the acute PCL injury,[100] but a lesser accuracy in chronic injuries. If an injury to the posterolateral corner is suspected, MRI can be helpful but to view this region properly usually requires a specific imaging protocol. When the MRI requisition states that injury to the posterolateral corner is suspected, the radiologist can optimize the imaging protocol.

Treatment

PCL rupture can generally be managed conservatively with a comprehensive rehabilitation program. A suggested program emphasizing intensive quadriceps exercises is shown in Table 27.11. More severe injuries (grade III) should be immobilized in extension for the first two weeks.

Results show that patients with isolated PCL tears have a good functional result despite ongoing laxity after an appropriate rehabilitation program. Regardless of the amount of laxity, half of the patients in one large study returned to sport at the same or higher level, one-third at a lower level and one-sixth did not return to the same sport.[101]

Surgical reconstruction is indicated when the PCL injury occurs in combination with other posterolateral structures or where significant rotatory instability is present.

Table 27.11 Rehabilitation of a PCL tear (see Figs 27.5 and 27.6)

Phase	Goal of phase	Time post injury	Physiotherapy treatment	Exercise program	Functional/sport-related activity
Phase 1	PWB–FWB Eliminate swelling 0–100° ROM 4+/5 quadriceps strength 5/5 hamstring strength	0–2 weeks	Cryotherapy Electrotherapy Compression Manual therapy Gait re-education Patient education	Gentle flexion ROM Extension ROM to 0° Quadriceps/VMO setting Supported (bilateral) calf raises Hip abduction and extension Hamstring pulleys/rubbers Gait drills	Nil
Phase 2	No swelling Full ROM 4+/5 quadriceps strength 5/5 hamstring strength	2–4 weeks	Cryotherapy Electrotherapy Compression Manual therapy Gait re-education Exercise modification	ROM drills Quadriceps/VMO setting Mini squats and lunges Leg press (double, then single leg) Step-ups Bridges (double, then single leg) Hip abduction and extension with rubber tubing Single-leg calf raises Gait re-education drills Balance and proprioceptive drills (single leg)	Walking Exercise bike
Phase 3	Full ROM Full strength and power Return to jogging, running, and agility Return to restricted sport-specific drills	4–6 weeks	Manual therapy Exercise/activity modification and supervision	As above—increase difficulty, repetitions and weight where appropriate Jump and land drills Agility drills	Straight line jogging Swimming (light kick) Road bike Straight line running Progressing to sport-specific running and agility (progressively sequenced) e.g. running forwards, sideways, backwards, sprinting, jumping, hopping, changing directions, kicking
Phase 4	Return to sport	6–10 weeks	As above	High-level sport-specific strengthening as required	Progressive return to sport, e.g. restricted training, unrestricted training, match play, competitive match play

FWB = full weight-bearing. PWB = partial weight-bearing. ROM = range of motion. VMO = vastus medialis obliquus.

Lateral collateral ligament tears

LCL tears are much less common than MCL tears. They are usually due to a severe, high-energy, direct varus stress on the knee and are graded in a similar fashion to MCL sprains. Differential diagnosis may be an avulsion of the biceps femoris tendon. Clinicians should be aware that local tenderness on the posterolateral corner of the knee may also occur with ACL tears.

Complete tears of the LCL are usually associated with other instabilities, such as PCL rupture, and may result in posterolateral rotatory instability of the knee. These tears are best treated by acute surgical repair in conjunction with repair of other damaged ligaments. Chronic reconstruction of the LCL is difficult and results are poor. A varus knee with lateral and/or posterolateral instability appears to be associated with worse results. An osteotomy is necessary for treatment of this ligament injury, with or without a reconstruction of the ligament itself.

Articular cartilage damage

Since the introduction of arthroscopy and MRI, considerable insight has been gained into the role of articular cartilage (chondral) damage as a cause of symptoms and signs in the knee joint. Articular cartilage damage may occur as an isolated condition in which chondral or subchondral damage is the primary pathology, or in association with other injuries, such as ligamentous instability resulting from MCL, ACL or PCL injuries. ACL tears are associated with a high incidence of damage to the medial femoral condyle, lateral femoral condyle and lateral tibial plateau. Articular cartilage damage may also be seen in association with meniscal injury and patellar dislocation. Chondral injury is graded according to the Outerbridge classification and more recently the International Cartilage Repair Society (ICRS) grading system (Tables 27.12, 27.13). Articular cartilage damage varies from gross, macroscopically evident defects in which the underlying bone is exposed (grade IV), to microscopic damage that appears normal on arthroscopy but is soft when probed (grade I).

Articular cartilage damage in the knee has both short-term and long-term effects. In the short term, it causes recurrent pain and swelling. In the longer term, it accelerates the development of osteoarthritis. Various methods have been used to encourage healing of articular cartilage defects. These include

Table 27.12 ICRS classification of chondral defects

1. Superficial lesions
   A. Soft indentation
   B. Superficial fissures or cracks
2. Lesions < 50% cartilage depth
3. A. Lesions >50 % depth
   B. Down to calcified layer
   C. Down to but not through subchondral bone
   D. Blisters
4. Very abnormal into subchondral bone

Table 27.13 Outerbridge classification of chondral defects

1. Softening
2. <1 cm (<0.4 in.) partial thickness lesion
3. >1 cm (>0.4 in.) defect, deeper
4. Subchondral bone exposed

microfracture (piercing the subchondral bone with an 'ice pick' to recruit pluripotential stem cells from the marrow), mosaic plasty (osteochondral plugs are taken from the trochlea margin and implanted within the injured area), and autologous chondrocyte implantation, where cultured chondrocytes (harvested from the patient and cultured in the laboratory) are reimplanted to the chondral defect. Gene therapy and bone morphogenetic proteins are currently in the experimental stage.

There is currently considerable debate as to the efficacy of the various treatments and as yet no consensus on optimal treatment has been reached. Although short-term reduction of symptoms has been shown with these treatments, long-term reduction of arthritic disability has not been shown. As yet, no method of treatment has been able to reproduce true hyaline cartilage with its complex layered structure.

An effective method of promoting scar tissue formation in damaged articular cartilage is by continuous passive motion. Continuous passive motion has been shown to stimulate formation of hyaline-like fibrocartilage in the chondral defect, especially in the immediate post-operative period. This should be supplemented by low load, non-weight-bearing exercise such as swimming and cycling. Following articular cartilage injury, the athlete may have to modify his or her training to reduce the amount of weight-bearing activity and substitute activities such as swimming and cycling.

When an injury (e.g. patellar dislocation, ACL or MCL tear) requires a lengthy period of partial or non-weight-bearing, particular attention must be paid to preserving the integrity of the articular cartilage. This is done with continuous passive motion, a hydrotherapy program, swimming or cycling.

Other methods of reducing stress on the damaged articular cartilage include correction of biomechanical abnormalities, attention to ensure symmetry of gait and the use of a brace to control any instability. Pool running may also be helpful and the minitrampoline is used in the early stages of running and agility work to reduce load bearing. Proprioceptive exercises and strength exercises are also important.

Acute patellar trauma

Acute trauma to the patella (e.g. from a hockey stick or from a fall onto the kneecap) can cause a range of injuries from fracture of the patella to osteochondral damage of the patellofemoral joint with persisting patellofemoral joint pain. In some athletes, the pain settles without any long-term sequelae.

If there is suspicion of fracture, X-ray should be obtained. It is important to be able to differentiate between a fracture of the patella and a bipartite patella. A skyline view of the patella should be performed in addition to normal views.

If there is no evidence of fracture, the patient can be assumed to be suffering acute patellofemoral inflammation. This can be a difficult condition to treat. Treatment consists of NSAIDs, local electrotherapy (e.g. interferential stimulation, TENS) and avoidance of aggravating activities such as squatting or walking down stairs. Taping of the patella may alter the mechanics of patellar tracking and therefore reduce the irritation and pain (Chapter 28).

Fracture of the patella

Patellar fractures can occur either by direct trauma, in which case the surrounding retinaculum can be intact, or by indirect injury from quadriceps contraction, in which case the retinaculum and the vastus muscles are usually torn.

Undisplaced fractures of the patella with normal continuity of the extensor mechanism can be managed conservatively, initially with an extension splint. Over the next weeks as the fracture unites, the range of flexion can be gradually increased and the quadriceps strengthened in the inner range.

Fractures with significant displacement, where the extensor mechanism is not intact, require surgical treatment. This involves reduction of the patella and fixation, usually with a tension band wire technique. The vastus muscle on both sides also needs to be repaired. The rehabilitation following this procedure is as for undisplaced fracture.

Patella dislocation

Patella dislocation occurs when the patella moves out of its groove laterally onto the lateral femoral condyle. Acute patella dislocation may be either traumatic with a good history of trauma and development of a hemarthrosis following injury, or atraumatic, which usually occurs in young girls with associated ligamentous laxity, does not have a good history of trauma, and is accompanied by mild-to-moderate swelling.

Clinical features

Patients with traumatic patella dislocation usually complain that, on twisting or jumping, the knee suddenly gave way with the development of severe pain. Often the patient will describe a feeling of something 'popping out'. Swelling develops almost immediately. The dislocation usually reduces spontaneously with knee extension; however, in some cases this may require some assistance or regional anesthesia (e.g. femoral nerve block).

A number of factors predispose to dislocation of the patella:

- femoral anteversion
- shallow femoral groove
- genu valgum
- loose medial retinaculum
- tight lateral retinaculum
- vastus medialis dysplasia
- increased Q angle
- patellar alta
- excessive subtalar pronation
- patellar dysplasia
- general hypermobility.

The main differential diagnosis of patella dislocation is an ACL rupture. Both conditions have similar histories of twisting, an audible 'pop', a feeling of something 'going out' and subsequent development of hemarthrosis.

On examination, there is usually a gross effusion, marked tenderness over the medial border of the patella and a positive lateral apprehension test when attempts are made to push the patella in a lateral direction. Any attempt to contract the quadriceps muscle aggravates the pain. X-rays, including anteroposterior, lateral, skyline and intercondylar views, should be performed to rule out osteochondral fracture or a loose body.

Treatment

Treatment of traumatic patella dislocation depends on presentation. Relatively atraumatic dislocations are treated conservatively. Traumatic first- or second-time dislocations (hemarthrosis present) are treated with arthroscopic washout and debridement. Recurrent dislocation is treated with surgical stabilization.

The most important aim of rehabilitation after patellofemoral dislocation is to reduce the chances of a recurrence of the injury. As a result, the rehabilitation program is lengthy and emphasizes core stability, pelvic positioning, vastus medialis obliquus strength and stretching of the lateral structures when tight. A suggested rehabilitation program is shown in Table 27.14.

The most helpful addition to patellofemoral rehabilitation in the recent past is increased emphasis on core stability. Similar to ACL intervention exercises, rotational control of the limb under the pelvis is critical to knee and kneecap stability.

Less common causes

Patellar tendon rupture

The patellar tendon occasionally ruptures spontaneously. This is usually in association with a sudden severe eccentric contraction of the quadriceps muscle, which may occur when an athlete stumbles. There may have been a history of previous corticosteroid injection into the tendon. A previous history of patellar tendinopathy is uncommon.

Patients complain of a sudden acute onset of pain over the patellar tendon accompanied by a tearing sensation and are unable to stand. On examination, there is a visible loss of fullness at the front of the knee as the patella is retracted proximally. The knee extensor mechanism is no longer intact and knee extension cannot be initiated.

Surgical repair of the tendon must be followed by intensive rehabilitation. Full recovery takes six to nine months and there is often some residual disability.

Bursal hematoma

Occasionally, an acute bursal hematoma or acute pre-patellar bursitis occurs as a result of a fall onto the knee. This causes bleeding into the pre-patellar bursa and subsequent inflammation.

This usually settles spontaneously with firm compression bandaging. If not, the hematoma should be aspirated and the bloodstained fluid removed. Anti-inflammatory medication may also

be appropriate. This injury is often associated with a skin wound (e.g. abrasion) and therefore may become infected. Adequate skin care is essential. If the bursa recurs, then aspiration followed by injection of a corticosteroid agent may be required. If conservative treatment fails, arthroscopic excision of the bursa is indicated.

Fat pad impingement

Acute fat pad impingement (often incorrectly referred to as 'Hoffa's syndrome') usually occurs as a result of a hyperextension injury. As the fat pad is the most sensitive part of the knee, this condition may be extremely painful.[102] There may be an inferiorly tilted lower pole of the patella predisposing to injury. On examination, tenderness is distal to the patella but beyond the margin of the patellar tendon. A hemarthrosis may be present.

This can be an extremely difficult condition to treat. The basic principles of treatment are a reduction of aggravating activities, electrotherapeutic modalities to settle inflammation and resumption of range of movement exercises as soon as possible. Taping of the patella may help in reducing the amount of tilt and impingement (Chapter 28). If conservative management is not successful, arthroscopic joint lavage and resection of the fat pad can be helpful.

Fracture of the tibial plateau

Tibial plateau fracture is seen in high-speed injuries such as falls while skiing, wave-jumping or horse-riding. This condition needs to be excluded when diagnosing collateral ligament damage with instability. The patient complains of severe pain and inability to weight-bear. Fractures are associated with a lipo-hemarthrosis, which can be detected on a horizontal lateral X-ray by the presence of a fat fluid level. CT scan is helpful in defining the fracture.

Minimally displaced fractures should be treated by six weeks of non-weight-bearing in a hinged knee brace (Fig. 27.4a). Displaced fractures (Fig. 27.13) or fractures with unstable fragment(s) require internal fixation. Displaced vertical split fractures may be fixed percutaneously during arthroscopy.

Tibial plateau fractures are commonly associated with meniscal or ACL injuries. In these cases arthroscopic assessment is required. Following recovery from a tibial plateau fracture, weight-bearing activity may need to be reduced as the irregular joint surface predisposes to the development of osteoarthritis.

Table 27.14 Rehabilitation program following patella dislocation (see Figs 27.5 and 27.6)

Phase	Time post injury	Goal of phase	Physiotherapy treatment	Exercise program	Functional/sport-related activity
Phase 1	0–2 weeks	Control swelling Maintain knee extension Isometric quadriceps strength	Extension splint (removal dependent on surgeon/physician) Cryotherapy Electrotherapy PFJ taping Manual therapy	Quadriceps drills (supine) Bilateral calf raises Foot and ankle Hip abduction	Progress to FWB
Phase 2	2–6 weeks	No swelling Full extension Flexion to 100° 4+/5 quadriceps strength 5/5 hamstring strength	Cryotherapy Electrotherapy Compression Manual therapy Gait re-education Exercise modification	ROM drills Quadriceps/VMO setting Mini squats and lunges Bridges (double, then single leg) Hip abduction and extension with rubber tubing Single-leg calf raises Gait re-education drills Balance and proprioceptive drills (single leg)	Walking Exercise bike
Phase 3	6–8 weeks	Full ROM Full strength and power Return to jogging, running, and agility Return to restricted sport-specific drills	Manual therapy Exercise/activity modification and supervision	As above—increase difficulty, repetitions and weight where appropriate Single-leg squats Single-leg press Jump and land drills Agility drills	Straight line jogging Swimming (light kick) Road bike Straight line running Progressing to sport-specific running and agility (progressively sequenced) e.g. running forwards, sideways, backwards, sprinting, jumping, hopping, changing directions, kicking
Phase 4	8–12 weeks	Return to sport	As above	High-level sport-specific strengthening as required	Progressive return to sport, e.g. restricted training, unrestricted training, match play, competitive match play

FWB = full weight-bearing. PFJ = patellofemoral joint. ROM = range of motion. VMO = vastus medialis obliquus.

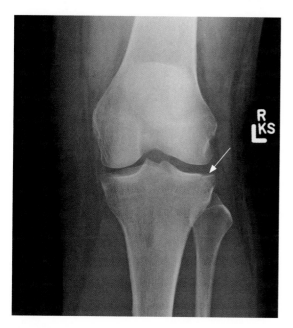

Figure 27.13 X-ray of a tibial plateau fracture

Superior tibiofibular joint injury

Acute dislocation of the superior tibiofibular joint occurs occasionally as a result of a direct blow. The patient complains of pain in the area of the joint and may be aware of obvious deformity. The lateral popliteal nerve may be damaged with this injury.

Sprain of the tibiofibular joint is more common. The patient complains of local pain aggravated by movement and, on examination, there is local tenderness and some anteroposterior instability. Treatment consists of rest and local electrotherapeutic modalities. Rarely, a chronic instability of the superior tibiofibular joint develops, which may need surgical stabilization.

Ruptured hamstring tendon

Spontaneous rupture of one of the distal hamstring tendons at the knee occurs occasionally during sprinting. Sudden onset of pain is localized to either the biceps femoris tendon or the semitendinosus tendon. Pain and weakness is present with resisted hamstring contraction. These injuries often require surgical exploration and repair, followed by protection in a limited motion brace.

Coronary ligament sprain

The coronary ligament is the name given to the deep portion of the fibrous joint capsule attached to the periphery of each meniscus and connected to the adjacent margin of the tibia.

A sprain of the coronary ligament may occur as a result of a twisting injury. These sprains may be difficult to differentiate from a meniscal injury. There is no joint effusion associated with this injury and usually minimal joint line swelling. There is, however, joint line tenderness and McMurray's test may be painful.

Arthroscopy may be required to differentiate coronary ligament sprains from meniscal tears. At arthroscopy, the only abnormality is occasional localized hemorrhage. Coronary ligament sprain is often associated with a grade I MCL sprain.

Recommended Reading

Aagaard H, Verdonk R. Function of the normal meniscus and consequences of meniscal resection. *Scand J Med Sci Sports* 1999; 9: 134–140.

Agel J, Bershadsky B, Arendt EA. Hormonal therapy: ACL and ankle injury. *Med Sci Sports Exerc* 2006; 38(1): 7–12.

Arnold T, Shelbourne KD. A perioperative rehabilitation program for anterior cruciate ligament surgery. *Physician Sportsmed* 2000; 28(1): 31–44.

Beynnon BD, Johnson R, Abate JA, et al. Treatment of anterior cruciate ligament injuries, Part 1. *Am J Sports Med* 2005; 33(10): 1579–602.

Beynnon BD, Johnson R, Abate JA, et al. Treatment of anterior cruciate ligament injuries, Part 2. *Am J Sports Med* 2005; 33(11): 1751–67.

Gillquist J, Messner K. Anterior cruciate ligament reconstruction and the long term incidence of gonarthrosis. *Sports Med* 1999; 27(3): 143–56.

Kvist J. Rehabilitation following anterior cruciate ligament reconstruction. *Sports Med* 2004; 34(4): 269–80.

Margheritini F, Rihn J, Musahl V, et al. Posterior cruciate ligament injuries in the athlete. An anatomical, biomechanical and clinical review. *Sports Med* 2002; 32(6): 393–408.

Myklebust G, Bahr R. Return to play guidelines after anterior cruciate ligament surgery. *Br J Sports Med* 2005; 39: 127–31.

Pyne SW. Current progress in meniscal repair and postoperative rehabilitation. *Curr Sports Med Rep* 2002; 1: 265–71.

Risberg MA, Lewek M, Snyder-Mackler. A systematic review of evidence for anterior cruciate ligament rehabilitation: how much and what type? *Phys Ther Sport* 2004; 5: 125–45.

Shaw T. Accelerated rehabilitation following anterior cruciate ligament reconstruction *Phys Ther Sport* 2002; 3: 19–26.

Shea KG, Apel PJ, Pfeiffer RP. Anterior cruciate ligament injury in paediatric and adolescent patients. *Sports Med* 2003; 33(6): 455–71.

Silvers HJ, Giza E, Mandelbaum BR. Anterior cruciate ligament tear prevention in the female athlete. *Curr Sports Med Rep* 2005; 4: 341–3.

Thomee P, Wahrborg P, Borjesson M, Thomee R, Eriksson B, Karlsson J. A new instrument for measuring self-efficacy in patients with an anterior cruciate ligament injury. *Scand J Med Sci Sports* 2005; 15: 1–7.

Wind WM, Bergfeld JA, Parker RD. Evaluation and treatment of posterior cruciate ligament injuries. Revisited. *Am J Sports Med* 2004; 32(7): 1765–75.

Woo SL-Y, Debski RE, Withrow JD, et al. Biomechanics of knee ligaments. *Am J Sports Med* 1999; 27: 533–43.

Recommended Websites

The website of the University of Minnesota Orthopaedics' Sports Medicine Institute has useful videos of all aspects of the acute knee examination. See: <http://www.sportsdoc.umn.edu>.

The important information websites for ACL prevention are:

- www.med.uio.no
- www.cincinnatichildrens.org/svc/prog/sports-med/human
- www.aclprevent.com/aclprevention.htm
- www.vermontskisafety.com
- www.ostrc.no

References

1. Stiell IG, Greenberg GH, Wells GA, et al. Prospective validation of a decision rule for the use of radiography in acute knee injuries. *JAMA* 1996; 275(8): 611–15.

2. McNally EG. Magnetic resonance imaging of the knee. *BMJ* 2002; 325: 115–16.

3. Prikett WD, Ward SI, Matava MJ. Magnetic resonance imaging of the knee. *Sports Med* 2001; 31(15): 997–1019.

4. Sanders TG, Miller MD. A systematic approach to magnetic resonance imaging interpretation of sports medicine injuries of the knee. *Am J Sports Med* 2005; 33(1): 131–48.

5. Johnson DL, Urban WP, Caborn DNM, et al. Articular cartilage changes seen with magnetic resonance imaging-detected bone bruises associated with acute anterior cruciate ligament rupture. *Am J Sports Med* 1998; 26(3): 409–14.

6. DeHaven KE, Bronstein RD. Arthroscopic medial meniscus repair in the athlete. *Clin Sports Med* 1997; 16: 69–86.

7. Pyne SW. Current progress in meniscal repair and postoperative rehabilitation. *Curr Sports Med Rep* 2002; 1: 265–71.

8. Rodeo SA. Instructional course lectures, the American Academy of Orthopaedic Surgeons—arthroscopic meniscal repair with use of the outside-in technique. *J Bone Joint Surg Am* 2000; 82A: 127–41.

9. Cannon WD, Vittori JM. The incidence of healing in arthroscopic meniscal repairs in ACL-reconstructed knees vs. stable knees. *Am J Sports Med* 1992; 20(2): 176–81.

10. Arendt E. *OKU Orthopaedic Knowledge Update: Sports Medicine 2.* 2nd edn. Rosemont, IL: American Academy of Orthopaedic Surgeons, 1999.

11. Indelicato PA. Isolated medial collateral injuries in the knee. *J Am Acad Orthop Surg* 1995; 3(1): 9–14.

12. Owings MF, Kozak LJ. Ambulatory and inpatient procedures in the United States 1996. *Vital Health Stat 13* 1998; 139: 1–119.

13. Arendt E, Dick R. Knee injuries patterns among men and women in collegiate basketball and soccer. NCAA data and review of literature. *Am J Sports Med* 1995; 23: 694–701.

14. Arendt EA, Agel J, Dick R. Anterior cruciate ligament injury patterns among collegiate men and women. *J Athl Train* 1999; 34: 86–92.

15. Garrick JG, Requa RK. Anterior cruciate ligament injuries in men and women: how common are they? In: Griffin LY, ed. *Prevention of Noncontact ACL Injuries.* Rosemont, IL: American Academy Orthopaedic Surgeons, 2001: 1–10.

16. Agel J, Arendt E, Bershadsky B. Anterior cruciate ligament injury in national collegiate athletic association basketball and soccer: a 13 year review. *Am J Sports Med* 2005; 33(4): 524–30.

17. Beynnon BD, Johnson RJ, Abate JA, et al. Treatment of anterior cruciate ligament injuries, Part 1. *Am J Sports Med* 2005; 33(10): 1579–602.

18. Barber FA. What is the terrible triad? *Arthroscopy* 1992; 8(1): 19–22.

19. Paul JJ, Spindler KP, Andrish JT, et al. Jumping versus nonjumping anterior cruciate ligament injuries: a comparison of pathology. *Clin J Sport Med* 2003; 13(1): 1–5.

20. Logan MC, Williams A, Lavelle J, et al. What really happens during the Lachman test? A dynamic MRI analysis of tibiofemoral motion. *Am J Sports Med* 2004; 32(2): 369–75.

21. Segond P. Recherches cliniques et expérimentales sur les épanchements sanguins du genou par entorse. *Prog Med* 1879; 7: 297–9, 319–21, 340–1.

22. Spindler KP, Kuhn JE, Freedman KB, et al. Anterior cruciate ligament reconstruction autograft choice: bone-tendon-bone versus hamstring: does it really matter? A systematic review. *Am J Sports Med* 2004; 32(8): 1986–95.

23. Shelbourne KD, Patel DV. Timing of surgery in anterior cruciate ligament-injured knees. *Knee Surg Sports Traumatol Arthrosc* 1995; 3: 148–56.

24. Shelbourne KD, Nitz P. Accelerated rehabilitation after anterior cruciate ligament reconstruction. *Am J Sports Med* 1990; 18(3): 292–9.

25. Beynnon BD, Uh BS, Johnson RJ, et al. Rehabilitation after anterior cruciate ligament reconstruction: a prospective, randomized, double-blind comparison of programs administered over 2 different time intervals. *Am J Sports Med* 2005; 33(3): 347–59.

26. Shelbourne KD, Klootwyk TE, DeCarlo MS. Rehabilitation program for anterior cruciate ligament reconstruction. *Sports Med Arthrosc Rev* 1997; 5: 77–82.

27. Liu-Ambrose T, Taunton JE, MacIntyre D, et al. The effects of proprioceptive or strength training on the neuromuscular function of the ACL reconstructed knee. *Scand J Med Sci Sports* 2003; 13: 115–23.

28. Cooper RL, Taylor NF, Feller JA. A randomised controlled trial of proprioceptive and balance training after surgical reconstruction of the anterior cruciate ligament. *Res Sports Med* 2005; 13: 217–30.

29. McDevitt ER, Taylor DC, Miller MD, et al. Functional bracing after anterior cruciate ligament reconstruction: a prospective, randomised, multi-center study. *Am J Sports Med* 2004; 32: 1887–92.

30. Risberg MA, Holm I, Steen H, et al. The effect of knee bracing after anterior cruciate reconstruction: a prospective, randomised study with two years' follow up. *Am J Sports Med* 1999; 27: 76–83.

31. Kuster MS, Grob K, Kuster M, et al. The benefits of wearing a compression sleeve after ACL reconstruction. *Med Sci Sports Exerc* 1999; 31(3): 368–71.

32. Tyler TF, McHugh MP, Gleim GW, et al. The effect of immediate weightbearing after anterior cruciate ligament reconstruction. *Clin Orthop* 1998; 357: 141–8.

33. Bynum EB, Barrack RL, Alexander AH. Open versus closed kinetic chain exercises after anterior cruciate ligament reconstruction: a prospective randomised study. *Am J Sports Med* 1995; 23: 401–6.

34. Beynonn BD, Fleming BC. Anterior cruciate ligament strain in-vivo: a review of previous work. *J Biomech* 1998; 31: 519–25.

35. Steinkamp LA, Dillingham MF, Markel MD, et al. Biomechanical considerations in patellofemoral joint rehabilitation. *Am J Sports Med* 1993; 21: 438–44.

36. Snyder-Mackler L, Delitto A, Bailey SL, et al. Strength of the quadriceps femoris muscle and functional recovery after reconstruction of the anterior cruciate ligament. A prospective randomized clinical trial of electrical stimulation. *J Bone Joint Surg Am* 1995; 77A: 1166–73.

37. Eakin CL. Knee arthrofibrosis: prevention and management of a potentially devastating condition. *Physician Sportsmed* 2001; 29(3): 31–42.

38. Corry IS, Webb JM, Clingeleffer AJ, et al. Arthroscopic reconstruction of the anterior cruciate ligament. A comparison of patellar tendon autograft and four-strand tendon autograft. *Am J Sports Med* 1999; 27: 444–54.

39. Feller JA, Webster KE. A randomised comparison of patellar tendon and hamstring tendon anterior cruciate ligament reconstruction. *Am J Sports Med* 2003; 31(4): 564–73.

40. Gobbi A, Ty B, Mahajan S, et al. Quadrupled bone-semitendinosus anterior cruciate ligament reconstruction: a clinical investigation in a group of athletes. *Arthroscopy* 2003; 19: 691–9.

41. Siegel MG, Barber-Westin SD. Arthroscopic-assisted outpatient anterior cruciate ligament reconstruction using the semitendinosus and gracilis tendons. *Arthroscopy* 1998; 14: 268–77.

42. Myklebust G, Bahr R. Return to play guidelines after anterior cruciate ligament surgery. *Br J Sports Med* 2005; 39(3): 127–31.

43. Myklebust G, Holm I, Maehlum S, et al. Clinical, functional, and radiologic outcome in team handball players 6 to 11 years after anterior cruciate ligament injury: a follow-up study. *Am J Sports Med* 2003; 31(6): 981–9.

44. Roos H, Ornell M, Gardsell P, et al. Soccer after anterior cruciate ligament injury: an incompatible combination? A national survey of incidence and risk factors and a 7 year follow up of 310 players. *Acta Orthop Scand* 1995; 66: 107–12.

45. Fink C, Hoser C, Hackl W, et al. Long term outcome of operative or non-operative treatment of anterior cruciate ligament rupture: is sports activity a determining variable? *Int J Sports Med* 2001; 22: 304–9.

46. von Porat A, Roos EM, Roos H. High prevalence of osteoarthritis 14 years after an anterior cruciate ligament tear in male soccer players: a study of radiographic and patient relevant outcomes. (a). *Am Rheum Dis* 2004; 63(3): 269–73.

47. Salmon L, Russell V, Musgrove T, et al. Incidence and risk factors for graft rupture and contralateral rupture after anterior cruciate ligament reconstruction. *Arthroscopy* 2005; 21(8): 948–57.

48. Freedman KB, D'Amato MJ, Nedeff DD, et al. Arthroscopic anterior cruciate ligament reconstruction: a meta-analysis comparing patellar tendon and hamstring tendon autografts. *Am J Sports Med* 2003; 31(1): 2–11.

49. Lohmander LS, Ostenberg A, Englund M, et al. High prevalence of knee osteoarthritis, pain, and functional limitations in female soccer players twelve years after anterior cruciate ligament injury. *Arthritis Rheum* 2004; 50: 3145–52.

50. Fithian DC, Paxton EW, Stone ML, et al. Prospective trial of a treatment algorithm for the management of the anterior cruciate ligament injured knee. *Am J Sports Med* 2005; 33(3): 335–46.

51. Feller J. Anterior cruciate ligament rupture: is osteoarthritis inevitable? *Br J Sports Med* 2004; 38(4): 383–4.

52. Brukner P. Return to play. A personal perspective. *Clin J Sport Med* 2005; 15(6): 459–60.

53. Barber-Westin SD, Noyes F, Andrews M. A rigorous comparison between sexes of results and complications after anterior cruciate reconstruction. *Am J Sports Med* 1997; 25: 514–25.

54. Noojin FK, Barret GR, Hartzog CW, et al. Clinical comparison of intra-articular anterior cruciate ligament reconstruction using autogenous semitendinosus and gracilis tendons in men versus women. *Am J Sports Med* 2000; 28: 783–9.

55. Ferrari JD, Bach BRJ, Bush-Joseph CA, et al. Anterior cruciate ligament reconstruction in men and women: an outcome analysis comparing gender. *Arthroscopy* 2001; 17: 588–96.

56. Gobbi A, Domzalski M, Pascual J. Comparison of anterior cruciate ligament reconstruction in male and female athletes using the patellar tendon and hamstring autografts. *Knee Surg Sports Traumatol Arthrosc* 2004; 12: 534–9.

57. Salmon LJ, Refshauge KM, Russell VJ, et al. Gender differences in outcome after anterior cruciate ligament reconstruction with hamstring tendon autograft. *Am J Sports Med* 2006; 34(4): in press.

58. McLean SG, Huang X, van den Bogert AJ. Association between lower extremity posture at contact and peak knee valgus moment during sidestepping: implications for ACL injury. *Clin Biomech* 2005; 20(8): 863–70.

59. McLean SG, Huang X, Su A, et al. Sagittal plane biomechanics cannot injure the ACL during sidestep cutting. *Clin Biomech* 2004; 19(8): 828–38.

60. McLean SG, Walker K, Ford KR, et al. Evaluation of a two dimensional analysis method as a screening and evaluation tool for anterior cruciate ligament injury. *Br J Sports Med* 2005; 39(6): 355–62.

61. Olsen OE, Myklebust G, Engebretsen L, et al. Injury mechanisms for anterior cruciate ligament injuries in team handball: a systematic video analysis. *Am J Sports Med* 2004; 32(4): 1002–12.

62. Teitz CC. Video analysis of ACL injuries. In: Griffin LY, ed. *Prevention of Noncontact ACL Injuries*. Rosemont, IL: American Academy Orthopaedic Surgeons, 2001.

63. Ireland ML. Anterior cruciate ligament injuries in young female athletes. *Your Patient & Fitness* 1996; 10(5): 26–30.

64. Ettlinger CF, Johnson RJ, Shealy JE. A method to help reduce the risk of serious knee sprains incurred in alpine skiing. *Am J Sports Med* 1995; 23: 531–7.

65. Souryal TO, Freeman TR. Intercondylar notch size

66. LaPrade RF, Burnett QM. Femoral intercondylar notch stenosis and correlation to anterior cruciate ligament injuries: a prospective study. *Am J Sports Med* 1994; 22: 198–203.

67. Uhorchak JM, Scoville CR, Williams GN, et al. Risk factors associated with noncontact injury of the anterior cruciate ligament: a prospective four year evaluation of 859 west point cadets. *Am J Sports Med* 2003; 31: 831–42.

68. Liu S, al-Shaikh R, Panossian V, et al. Primary immunolocalization of estrogen progesterone target cells in the human anterior cruciate ligament. *J Orthop Res* 1996; 14(4): 526–33.

69. Hame SL, Oakes DA, Markolf KL. Injury to the anterior cruciate ligament during alpine skiing: a biomechanical analysis of tibial torque and knee flexion angle. *Am J Sports Med* 2002; 30(4): 537–40.

70. Wojtys EM, Huston LJ, Boynton MD, et al. The effect of the menstrual cycle on anterior cruciate ligament injuries in women as determined by hormone levels. *Am J Sports Med* 2002; 30(2): 182–8.

71. Beynnon BD, Bernstein I, Belislea, et al. The effect of estradiol and progesterone on knee and ankle laxity. *Am J Sports Med* 2005: 33: 1298–304.

72. Moller-Nielsen J, Hammar M. Women's soccer injuries in relation to the menstrual cycle and oral contraceptive use. *Med Sci Sports Exerc* 1989; 21(2): 126–9.

73. Myklebust G, Maehlum S, Holm I, et al. A prospective cohort study of anterior cruciate ligament injuries in elite Norwegian team handball. *Scand J Med Sci Sports* 1998; 8(3): 149–53.

74. Slauterbeck JR, Fuzie SF, Smith MP, et al. The menstrual cycle, sex hormones and anterior cruciate ligament injury. *J Athl Train* 2002; 37(3): 275–8.

75. Seneviratne A, Attia E, Williams RJ, et al. The effect of estrogen on ovine anterior cruciate ligament fibroblasts: cell proliferation and collagen synthesis. *Am J Sports Med* 2004; 32(7): 1613–18.

76. Strickland SM, Belknap TW, Turner SA, et al. Lack of hormonal influences on mechanical properties of sheep knee ligaments. *Am J Sports Med* 2003; 31(2): 210–15.

77. Griffin LY, Albohm MJ, Arendt EA, et al. Update on ACL injury prevention: theoretical and practical considerations. *Am J Sports Med* 2006; in press.

78. Myklebust G, Engebretsen L, Braekken IH, et al. Prevention of anterior cruciate ligament injuries in female team handballers: a prospective study over three seasons. *Clin J Sports Med* 2003; 13: 71–8.

79. Olsen OE, Myklebust G, Engebretsen L, et al. Relationship between floor type and risk of ACL injury in team handball. *Scand J Med Sci Sports* 2003; 13(5): 299–304.

80. Lambson RB, Barnhill BS, Higgins RW. Football cleat design and its effect on anterior cruciate ligament injuries. *Am J Sports Med* 1996; 24(2): 155–9.

81. Orchard J, Seward H, McGivern J, et al. Intrinsic and extrinsic risk factors for anterior cruciate ligament injury in Australian footballers. *Am J Sports Med* 2001; 29(2): 196–200.

82. Woo SL-Y, Debski RE, Withrow JD, et al. Biomechanics of knee ligaments. *Am J Sports Med* 1999; 27(4): 533–43.

83. Boden BP, Griffin LY, Garrett WE Jr. Etiology and prevention of noncontact ACL injury. *Physician Sportsmed* 2000; 28(4): 53–60.

84. Huston LJ, Wojtys E. Neuromuscular performance characteristics in elite female athletes. *Am J Sports Med* 1996; 24: 427–36.

85. Griffin LY. Non contact ACL injuries: is prevention possible? Hormonal and neuromuscular factors may explain prevalence in women. *J Musculoskelet Med* 2001; 18: 507–16.

86. Hewett TE, Lindenfield TN, Riccobene JV, et al. The effect of neuromuscular training on the incidence of knee injury in female athletes. A prospective study. *Am J Sports Med* 1999; 27: 699–706.

87. Hewett TE, Myer TD, Ford KR. Reducing knee and anterior cruciate ligament injuries among female athletes: a systematic review of neuromuscular training interventions. *J Knee Surg* 2005; 18: 82–8.

88. Heidt RS, Sweeterman LM, Carlonas RL, et al. Avoidance of soccer injuries with pre-season conditioning. *Am J Sports Med* 2000; 28(5): 659–62.

89. Sodermann K, Werner S, Pietila T, et al. Balance board training: prevention of traumatic injuries of the lower extremities in female soccer players? A prospective randomised intervention study (a). *Knee Surg Sports Traumatol Arthosc* 2000; 8(6): 356–63.

90. Mandelbaum BR, Silvers HJ, Watanabe DS, et al. Effectiveness of a neuromuscular and proprioceptive training program in preventing anterior cruciate ligament injuries in female athletes: 2-year follow-up. *Am J Sports Med* 2005; 33(7): 1003–10.

91. Myklebust G, Engebretsen L, Braekken IH, et al. Prevention of anterior cruciate ligament injuries in female team handball players: a prospective intervention study over three seasons. *Clin J Sport Med* 2003; 13: 71–8.

92. Petersen W, Braun C, Bock W, et al. A controlled prospective case-control study of a prevention training program in female team handball players: the German experience. *Arch Orthop Trauma Surg* 2005; 125(9): 614–21.

93. Hewett TE, Ford KR, Myer GD. Anterior cruciate ligament injuries in female athletes. Part 2, a meta-analysis of neuromuscular interventions aimed at injury prevention. *Am J Sports Med* 2006; 34(3): 490–8.

94. Shea KG, Apel PJ, Pfieffer RP. Anterior cruciate ligament injury in paediatric and adolescent patients. *Sports Med* 2003; 33(6): 455–71.

95. Bales CP, Guettler JH, Moorman CT III. Anterior cruciate ligament injuries in children with open physes: evolving strategies of treatment. *Am J Sports Med* 2004; 32(8): 1978–85.

96. Harner CD, Hoher J. Evaluation and treatment of posterior cruciate ligament injuries. *Am J Sports Med* 1998; 26(3): 471–82.

97. Hamada M, Shino KM, Mitsuoka T, et al. Chondral injury associated with acute isolated posterior cruciate ligament injury. *Arthroscopy* 2000; 16: 59–63.

98. Wind WM Jr, Bergfeld JA, Parker RD. Evaluation and treatment of posterior cruciate ligament injuries: revisited. *Am J Sports Med* 2004; 32(7): 1765–75.

99. Bergfeld JA, McAllister DR, Parker RD, et al. The effects of tibial rotation on posterior translation in knees in which the posterior cruciate ligament has been cut. *J Bone Joint Surg Am* 2001; 83A: 1339–43.

100. Gross ML, Groiver JS, Bassett LW, et al. Magnetic resonance imaging of the posterior cruciate ligament: clinical use to improve diagnostic accuracy. *Am J Sports Med* 1992; 20: 732–7.

101. Shelbourne KD, Davis TJ, Patel DV. The natural history of acute, isolated, nonoperatively treated posterior cruciate ligament injuries. A prospective study. *Am J Sports Med* 1999; 27(3): 276–83.

102. Dye SF, Vaupel GL, Dye CS. Conscious neurosensory mapping of the internal structures of the human knee without intraarticular anesthesia. *Am J Sports Med* 1998; 26(6): 773–7.

Anterior Knee Pain

WITH KAY CROSSLEY, JILL COOK, SALLIE COWAN AND
JENNY McCONNELL

Anterior knee pain is the most common presenting symptom in many physiotherapy and sports
physician practises.[1] It contributes substantially to the
20–40% of family practise consultations that relate to
the musculoskeletal system.[2] Two common causes of
anterior knee pain in sportspeople are patellofemoral
pain and patellar tendinopathy. The anterior knee
anatomy is depicted in Figure 28.1.

In this chapter, we first outline a practical approach
to assessing the patient with anterior knee pain,
particularly with a view to distinguishing the common conditions; we then detail their management.
The chapter concludes with an outline of other causes
of anterior knee pain such as fat pad impingement,
which may mimic features of both patellofemoral
pain and patellar tendinopathy.

Clinical approach

Distinguishing between patellofemoral pain and
patellar tendinopathy as a cause of anterior knee pain
can be difficult as their clinical features can be similar.
Furthermore, on occasions, the two conditions may
both be present. The causes of anterior knee pain are
listed in Table 28.1.

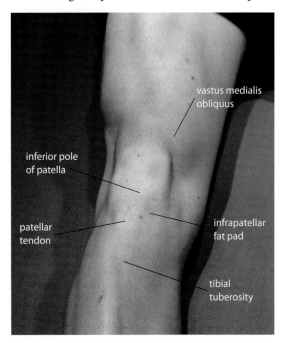

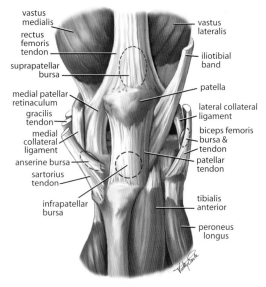

Figure 28.1 Anterior aspect of the knee

(a) Surface anatomy

(b) Anatomy

Table 28.1 Causes of anterior knee pain

Common	Less common	Occasionally seen/specific populations	Not to be missed
Patellofemoral pain Patellar tendinopathy	Synovial plica Pre-patellar bursitis Quadriceps tendinopathy Infrapatellar bursitis Patellofemoral instability Fat pad impingement	Sinding-Larsen–Johansson lesion Tenoperiostitis of upper tibia Stress fracture of the patella Osgood-Schlatter lesion	Referred pain from the hip Osteochondritis dissecans Slipped capital femoral epiphysis Perthes' disease Tumor (especially in the young)

History

There are a number of important factors to elicit from the history of a sportsperson with the general presentation of 'anterior knee pain'. These include the specific location of the pain, the nature of aggravating activities, the history of the onset and behavior of the pain, and any associated clicking, giving way or swelling.

Although it may be difficult for the patient with anterior knee pain to be specific, the area of pain often gives an important clue as to which structure is contributing to the pain. For example, retropatellar or peripatellar pain suggests that the patellofemoral joint (PFJ) is a likely culprit, lateral pain localized to the lateral femoral epicondyle indicates iliotibial band friction syndrome (Chapter 29), and inferior patellar pain implicates the patellar tendon or infrapatellar fat pad. The patient who presents with bilateral knee pain is more likely to have patellofemoral pain or tendinopathy than an internal derangement of both knees.

The type of activity that aggravates the anterior knee pain also aids diagnosis. Consider two contrasting scenarios that both describe pain at the infrapatellar region. In one case, precipitating activities, such as basketball, volleyball, high, long or triple jumps, involve repetitive loading of the patellar tendon. This suggests the diagnosis of patellar tendinopathy. On the other hand, if a swimmer presented reporting pain following tumble turning or vigorous kicking in the pool, where there had been no eccentric load on the tendon but a forceful extension of the knee, the practitioner should suspect an irritated fat pad. The mechanism of injury and the aggravating features are critical to accurate diagnosis.

The onset of typical patellofemoral pain is often insidious but it may present secondary to an acute traumatic episode (e.g. falling on the knee) or post other knee injury (e.g. meniscal, ligament) or knee surgery. The patient presents with a diffuse ache, which is usually exacerbated by loaded activities, such as stair ambulation or running. Sometimes patellofemoral pain is aggravated by prolonged sitting ('movie-goer's knee'), but sitting tends to aggravate pain of patellar tendinopathy so is not diagnostic of patellofemoral pain. Pain during running that gradually worsens is more likely to be of patellofemoral origin, whereas pain that occurs at the start of activity, settles after warm-up and returns after activity is more likely to be patellar tendinopathy. Table 28.2 is an aid to clinical differentiation of patellofemoral pain, patellar tendinopathy and fat pad impingement. As these conditions can coexist, accurate diagnosis can be challenging.

A history of recurrent crepitus may suggest patellofemoral pain. A feeling that the patella moves laterally at certain times suggests recurrent patellofemoral instability. An imminent feeling of giving way may be associated with patellar subluxation, patellofemoral pain or meniscal abnormality, although frank, dramatic giving way is usually associated with anterior cruciate ligament instability (Chapter 27). Nevertheless, giving way due to muscle inhibition, or due to pain, is not uncommon in anterior knee pain presentations.

A history of previous knee injury or surgery may be important, for example, patellofemoral pain is a well-recognized complication of posterior cruciate ligament injury (Chapter 27). An injury that is associated with an effusion may result in inhibition of the vasti (reduced magnitude and onset of timing on EMG). This inhibition appears to be more profound in the vastus medialis obliquus (VMO), especially at smaller knee effusion volumes.[3] Preferential inhibition of the VMO has the potential to set up an imbalance in the medial and lateral forces on the patella, predisposing to patellofemoral pain. Significant knee swelling is rare in primary anterior knee pain and generally suggests additional intra-articular abnormality. However, a small effusion may be present with patellofemoral pain.

Table 28.2 Comparison of the clinical features of three common causes of anterior knee pain. Note that these conditions may coexist

Signs	Patellofemoral pain	Patellar tendinopathy	Fat pad impingement
Onset	Running (especially downhill), steps/stairs, hills, any weight-bearing activities involving knee flexion (e.g. distance running)	Activities involving jumping and/or changing direction (e.g. basketball, volleyball, high jump, netball, bounding, ballet, climbing stairs)	Often, but not always, sudden onset with hyperextension injury
Pain	Non-specific or vague, may be medial, lateral or infrapatellar, aggravated by activities that load the PFJ	Usually around inferior pole of patella, aggravated by jumping and early to mid squat	Usually around inferior pole of patella, aggravated by prolonged standing, stairs, knee extension
Inspection	Generally normal or VMO wasting	Generally quadriceps wasting	Puffiness may be apparent around tendon, which may make pole of patella appear to be displaced posteriorly
Tenderness	Usually medial or lateral facets of patella but may be tender in infrapatellar region. May have no pain on palpation due to areas of patella being inaccessible	Most commonly inferior pole of patellar tendon attachment. Occasionally at distal attachment to tibial tuberosity, rarely in midtendon	Tender in fat pad region, inferior pole of patella and deep to tendon
Swelling	May have small effusion, swelling, suprapatellar or infrapatellar	Rare. Tendon may be increased in thickness	May have a 'puffy' appearance
Clicks/clunks	Occasional	No	No
Crepitus	Occasionally under patella	No	No
Giving way	Due to quadriceps inhibition (occasional) or subluxation	Occasionally due to quadriceps inhibition	No
Knee range of motion	May be decreased in severe cases but usually normal	Usually normal, no pain with overpressure	Active extension may be painful in acute fat pad impingement; passive overpressure into extension is generally painful
Quadriceps contraction in extension	Note quality of movement, not usually painful	Some cases more painful	Painful when acute
PFJ movement	May be restricted in any direction. Commonly restricted medial glide due to tight lateral structures	May have normal PFJ biomechanics. In combined problem will have PFJ signs	Normal or posteriorly displaced inferior pole of the patella
VMO	May have obvious wasting, weakness or more subtle deficits in tone and timing	May have generalized quadriceps weakness	May be normal or weak
Functional testing	Squats, stairs may aggravate. PFJ taping should decrease pain	Decline squats aggravate pain. PFJ taping has less effect	Aggravated by squats. PFJ taping should decrease pain if inferior pole of patella is tilted up

PFJ = patellofemoral joint. VMO = vastus medialis obliquus.

Previous treatment and the patient's response to that treatment should be noted. If treatment was unsuccessful, it is essential to determine whether the failure was due to incorrect diagnosis, inappropriate treatment or poor patient compliance.

Examination

Initially, the primary aim of the clinical assessment is to determine the most likely cause of the patient's pain. Since location of tenderness and aggravating factors are integral to the differential diagnosis, it is critical to reproduce the patient's anterior knee pain. This is usually done with either a double- or single-leg squat (Fig. 28.2c). A squat done on a decline[4] may make the test more specific to the anterior knee. The clinician should palpate the anterior knee carefully to determine the site of maximal tenderness.

Examination includes:

1. Observation
   (a) standing (Fig. 28.2a)
   (b) walking
   (c) supine (Fig. 28.2b)
2. Functional tests
   (a) squats
   (b) step-up/step-down
   (c) jump
   (d) lunge (Fig. 28.2c)
   (e) double- then single-leg decline squat
3. Palpation
   (a) patella (Fig. 28.2d) and inferior pole
   (b) medial/lateral retinaculum
   (c) patellar tendon
   (d) infrapatellar fat pad (Fig. 28.2e)
   (e) tibial tubercle
   (f) effusion
4. PFJ assessment
   (a) static assessment of patella position
       (i) superior
       (ii) inferior
       (iii) medial glide (Fig. 28.2f)
       (iv) lateral glide
   (b) dynamic assessment of patella position
   (c) assessment of vasti function
5. Flexibility
   (a) lateral soft tissue structures
       (i) quadriceps
       (ii) hamstring
       (iii) iliotibial band
       (iv) gastrocnemius
6. Special tests (to exclude other pathology)
   (a) examination of knee joint (Chapter 27)
   (b) examination of hip joint (Chapter 23)

(c) examination of lumbar spine (Chapter 21)
(d) neural tension tests (neural Thomas test, slump test)

Investigations

Imaging may be used to confirm a clinical impression obtained from the history and examination. Structural imaging includes conventional radiography, ultrasound, CT and MRI. Occasionally, radionuclide bone scan is indicated to evaluate the 'metabolic' status of the knee (e.g. after trauma, in suspected stress fracture).

The majority of patients with patellofemoral pain syndrome will require either no imaging, or plain radiography consisting of a standard AP view, a true lateral view with the knee in 30° of flexion, and an axial view through the knee in 30° of flexion. Plain radiography can detect bipartite patella and

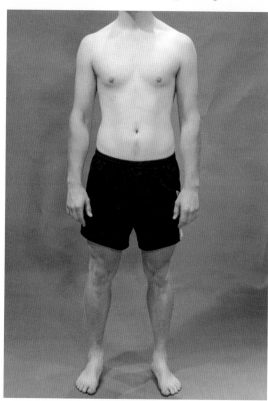

Figure 28.2 Examination of the patient with anterior knee pain

(a) Observation—standing. Observe the patient from the front looking at lower limb alignment, including femoral torsion, patella alignment or any signs of muscle wasting

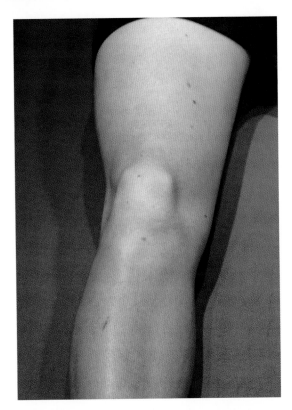

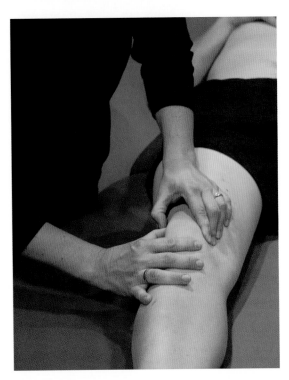

(d) Palpation—the patella and the medial and lateral facets are palpated for tenderness

(b) Observation—supine. Observe for lower limb alignment, effusion, position of the patella and any evidence of patella tilt or rotation

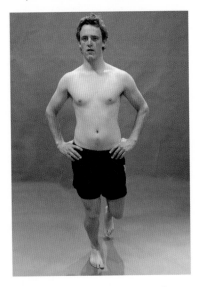

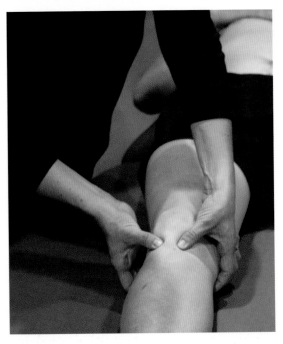

(c) Functional tests. If the patient's pain has not already been reproduced, functional tests such as squat, lunge (as illustrated), hop, step-up, step-down or eccentric drop squat should be performed

(e) Palpation—palpate the inferior pole of the patella, the patellar tendon attachment and the infrapatellar fat pad

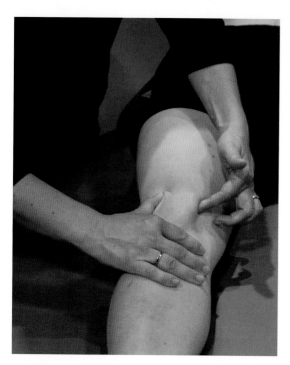

(f) Passive movement—patella glide. The patella is passively moved medially (shown), laterally, superiorly and inferiorly and the range and quality of movement is noted. Movement should be compared with the other side

osteoarthritis, provide evidence of an increased likelihood of Sinding-Larsen–Johansson lesion, as well as rule out potentially serious complications such as tumor or infection. Although CT and three-dimensional CT have been used to assess the PFJ, MRI is gaining increasing popularity as an investigation of patellofemoral pain, and the unstable patella, because of its capacity to image the patellar articular cartilage.[5]

MRI displays high signal abnormality in patellar tendinopathy. Ultrasound hypoechogenicity and excessive vascularity also indicate that patellar tendinopathy may be a diagnosis. However, in asymptomatic athletes or those with symptoms from another source in the anterior knee, the patellar tendon may reveal regions of 'abnormal' imaging.[6–8] Dynamic, loaded MRI may become a useful tool for the future but at present it is not utilized clinically.

Patellofemoral pain

After defining the condition and briefly reviewing the functional anatomy, we discuss predisposing factors and their clinical assessment in detail as this underpins the clinical strategies for prevention. We then provide a contemporary evidence-based, but clinically relevant, treatment program.

What is patellofemoral pain?

Patellofemoral pain is the preferred term used to describe pain in and around the patella. Synonyms include PFJ syndrome, anterior knee pain and chondromalacia patellae. Patellofemoral pain is an 'umbrella' term used to embrace all peripatellar or retropatellar pain in the absence of other pathologies. Since the cause of the pain may differ between patients, it is appropriate to review the potential sources of patellofemoral pain.[9] Numerous structures in the PFJ are susceptible to overload. A number of extra- and intra-articular components of the knee can generate neurosensory signals that ultimately result in of the patient feeling pain. Patellofemoral articular cartilage cannot directly be a source of pain, but a cartilage lesion may lead to chemical or mechanical synovial irritation or be associated with subchondral bone pain through edema or erosion.[10, 11] Peripatellar synovitis, in the absence of obvious cartilage damage, must be considered as one of the main causes of patellofemoral pain.[9] Soft tissues such as the lateral retinaculum have been implicated as a potent source of patellofemoral pain.[12–16] Another highly potent source of pain is the infrapatellar fat pad. It is highly innervated and is intimately related to the pain-sensitive synovium.[9, 17, 18]

Functional anatomy

At full extension, the patella sits lateral to the trochlea. During flexion, the patella moves medially and comes to lie within the intercondylar notch until 130° of flexion, when it starts to move laterally again.[19] The patella's mediolateral excursion is controlled by the quadriceps muscles, particularly the VMO and vastus lateralis components. With increasing knee flexion, a greater area of patellar articular surface comes into contact with the femur, thus offsetting the increased load that occurs with flexion. Loaded knee flexion activities subject the PFJ to loads many times the body weight, ranging from 0.5 times body weight for level walking to seven to eight times body weight for stair climbing.[20] Anatomically, the lateral structures of the PFJ are much stronger than the medial structures, so any imbalance in the forces will cause the patella to drift laterally.

Factors that may contribute to development of pain

Increased PFJ load instigates the development of patellofemoral pain. Factors that influence PFJ load can be considered in two categories: extrinsic and intrinsic. During physical activities the extrinsic load is created by the body's contact with the ground (ground reaction force) and is therefore moderated by body mass, speed of gait, surfaces and footwear. The number of loading cycles and frequency of loading are also important. During weight-bearing activities, any increase in the amount of knee flexion will increase the PFJ load. Therefore, when an individual experiences an increase in the magnitude of the PFJ load (e.g. higher training volume, increased speed of running, hill/stair running or bounding), this may overload the PFJ structures sufficiently to initiate a painful process.

Intrinsic factors can influence both the magnitude and the distribution of the PFJ load. Distribution of load is conceptualized as movement of the patella within the femoral trochlea: patella tracking. The factors that can influence patella tracking may be considered as 'remote' or 'local'. Considering the patient as a whole, 'remote' factors that affect patella tracking include femoral internal rotation, knee valgus, tibial rotation, subtalar pronation, and muscle flexibility.[21] Local factors that influence patella movement include patella position, soft tissue tension and neuromuscular control of the medial and lateral components of the vasti.

So how does an increase in PFJ load result in patellofemoral pain? Dye[22] described a concept whereby injury to the PFJ musculoskeletal tissues results from supraphysiological loads—either a single maximal load or lower magnitude repetitive load. Injury to these tissues initiates a cascade of events encompassing inflammation of the peripatellar synovium through to bone stress. Thus, any number of pain-sensitive structures can result in the conscious sensation of patellofemoral pain.[22]

Given this, when the initial subjective and objective examinations are completed and the diagnosis of patellofemoral pain is confirmed, the clinician should assess the contribution of various extrinsic and intrinsic factors to the development of patellofemoral pain. This assessment is crucial in the planning of an appropriate treatment regimen. The history will elucidate valuable information pertaining to extrinsic factors but clinical examination is usually required to evaluate most intrinsic contributing factors ('remote' and 'local').

'Remote' contributing factors

The following 'remote' factors may contribute to the development of patellofemoral pain:

- increased femoral internal rotation
- increased knee valgus
- increased tibial rotation
- increased subtalar pronation
- inadequate flexibility.

It is important to assess the patient in static postures as well as functional activities. Some factors may become more obvious during specific functional tasks, such as the step-down or single-leg squat, where the postural demands are high. Once a potential contributing factor has been identified, the clinician must investigate the mechanisms that will require intervention (Table 28.3).

Increased femoral internal rotation

Clinical observation of the patient in standing reveals internally rotated femurs, often manifesting as 'squinting patellae' where the patella are both facing medially. During gait (walking or running) further internal rotation of the thigh can often be observed and may be visualized as an apparent knee valgus. Similar observations are noted during the step-down or single-leg squat test.

Increased knee valgus

In standing, genu valgum is apparent with an increased Q angle. This is often exaggerated during gait, possibly associated with a midstance valgus thrust. The step-down and single-leg squats are associated with an increase in knee valgus position, which may manifest as an increased hip adduction or a lateral pelvic drop owing to weakness of the gluteus medius.

Increased tibial rotation

Increased structural or functional tibial rotations can affect PFJ loads directly, and also functionally through transferred rotations to the femur. Importantly, tibial rotations are coupled strongly with the motion of the subtalar joint. While limited information is available on the assessment or treatment of structural tibial rotation in isolation, functional rotation is often addressed in association with femoral or subtalar rotations.

Increased subtalar pronation

Subtalar pronation can be observed in standing and during gait. The assessment of the extent and significance of this motion is described in Chapter 35.

Table 28.3 'Remote' factors that can contribute to patellofemoral pain and their possible mechanisms

Factor	Possible mechanisms	Confirmatory assessments
Increased femoral internal rotation	Structural: • femoral anteversion Inadequate strength: • hip external rotators • hip abductors Altered neuromotor control: • hip external rotators • hip abductors Range of motion deficits: • hip	Radiographic—MRI, X-ray Clinical assessment Manual muscle test (Figs 28.3a, b) Clinical strength—hand-held dynamometer Biofeedback ROM tests: • clinical (Fig. 28.3c)/inclinometer • figure '4' test
Increased knee valgus	Structural: • genu varum • tibial varum • coxa varum Inadequate strength: • hip external rotators • hip abductors • quadriceps • hamstrings Altered neuromotor control: • hip external rotators • hip abductors • lumbopelvic muscles Range of motion deficits: • hip	Radiographic—long leg X-ray Clinical—goniometer/inclinometer Manual muscle test (Figs 28.3a, b) Clinical strength—hand-held dynamometer Active gluteal and TFL trigger points Biofeedback Active gluteal and TFL trigger points ROM tests: • clinical (Fig. 28.3c)/inclinometer • figure '4' test
Subtalar pronation		See Chapter 35
Muscle flexibility	Rectus femoris TFL/ iliotibial band Quadriceps Hamstrings Gastrocnemius	See Chapter 25 See Chapter 29 (Fig. 28.3d) See Chapter 25 See Chapter 26 See Chapter 31

ROM = range of motion. TFL = tensor fascia lata.

Inadequate flexibility

Inadequate flexibility or reduced compliance of the musculotendinous unit can be observed in all of the muscles that affect the knee. Aberrations in pelvis and hip motion may be influenced by muscles such as the tensor fascia lata (and its iliotibial band), rectus femoris and the hamstrings, whereas knee function may be affected by the quadriceps, hamstrings and gastrocnemius.

Local contributing factors

Local factors that can contribute to the development of patellofemoral pain are:

• patella position

• soft tissue contributions
• neuromuscular control of the vasti.

Patella position

Clinical examination provides valuable information on the structural and functional relationships of the PFJ (Table 28.4). The practitioner should carefully assess passive movement of the patella in all directions (medial [Fig. 28.2f], lateral, superior, inferior). Additionally, the position of the patella needs assessing in relation to the femur for tilt, rotation and glide. While the tests for patella position are not functional and may not be repeatable,[23, 24] clinical examination of the patella position remains a useful tool for clinical decision making.

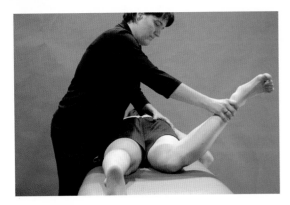

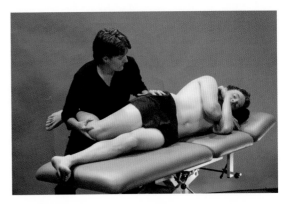

Figure 28.3 Assessment of 'remote' factors

(a) Hip external rotator strength may be assessed in prone, with the knees together and flexed to 90°. Strength can either be graded manually (illustrated) and compared with the other side, or measured with a hand-held dynamometer

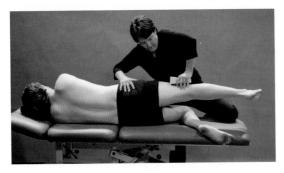

(b) Hip abductor strength may be assessed in supine or side-lying (illustrated). Strength can either be graded manually and compared with the other side, or measured with a hand-held dynamometer (illustrated)

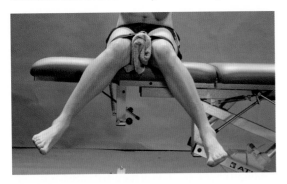

(c) Hip internal rotation range can be assessed in supine, prone or in sitting (illustrated). Range can either be estimated visually and compared with the other side (illustrated) or measured with a goniometer or inclinometer

(d) Flexibility of the iliotibial band/tensor fascia lata (ITB/TFL) complex can be assessed in supine with a modified Thomas test or in side-lying (shown). In either position, the hip is passively extended. Using the Thomas test position, the amount of hip abduction is either noted visually, or measured. Greater hip abduction is associated with tightness of the ITB/TFL complex. In the side-lying position, the ITB/TFL tightness is observed as an increased resistance to hip adduction

Soft tissue contributions

The contribution of the superficial and deep soft tissues to the PFJ mechanics can, in part, be obtained from the structural and functional assessments of patella position. Further information is available through palpation to gain an impression of the compliance of the lateral and medial soft tissues. Clinical assessment of the soft tissues is summarized in Table 28.4 and Figure 28.4.

Neuromuscular control of the vasti

Clinical examination of the vasti provides considerable insight into their function (Table 28.4, Fig. 28.5). Frank muscle wasting and weakness may be obvious, but apparently normal muscle bulk does not ensure normal function. It is important also to assess the timing of the VMO contractions to ensure they are synchronous with the rest of the quadriceps mechanism. The vasti should be assessed in a number of positions or activities, including those that are functionally relevant to the patient.

Treatment of patellofemoral pain

The management of a patient with patellofemoral pain requires an integrated approach that may include:

- reduction of pain and inflammation
- addressing extrinsic contributing factors

Table 28.4 Local factors that can contribute to patellofemoral pain

Factor	Clinical observation	
	Structural	Functional (with quadriceps contraction)
Patella position		
Lateral displacement	Patella displaced laterally, closer to the lateral than medial femoral condyle Restricted medial glide (Fig. 28.2f)	Patella moves laterally
Lateral tilt	Difficult to palpate lateral border, high medial border Lateral tilt increases with passive medial glide	Patella tilts laterally
Posterior tilt	Inferior patella pole displaced posteriorly, often difficult to palpate due to infrapatellar fat pad	Inferior pole moves further posteriorly. A 'dimple' may appear in the infrapatellar fat pad
Rotation	Long axis of the patella is not parallel with the long axis of the femur	Increase in rotation
Patella alta	High riding patella	NA
Soft tissue contributions		
Tight lateral structures	Lateral patella displacement or tilt Palpation of lateral structures (Fig. 28.4)	Lateral patella displacement or tilt (see above)
Compliant medial structures	Lateral patella displacement or tilt	Lateral patella displacement or tilt
Overall hypermobility	NA	Increased patella mobility in all directions
Vasti neuromuscular control		
Reduced activity of quadriceps (general)	Reduced muscle bulk of quadriceps	Reduced muscle strength
Delayed onset of VMO relative to VL	Reduced muscle bulk of VMO	Delayed onset of VMO relative to VL Assess in functional positions Biofeedback can assist (Fig. 28.5)
Reduced magnitude of VMO relative to VL	Reduced muscle bulk of VMO	Poor quantity/quality of VMO Assess in functional positions Biofeedback can assist
Altered reflex response	Reduced muscle bulk of VMO	Tendon tap

NA = not applicable. VL = vastus lateralis. VMO = vastus medialis obliquus.

- addressing intrinsic contributing factors:
  - 'remote' factors
  - local factors.

Immediate reduction of pain

The first priority of treatment is to reduce pain. This may require some or all of the following: rest from aggravating activities, ice, a short course of NSAIDs, electrotherapeutic modalities (e.g. ultrasound) and techniques such as mobilization (Fig. 28.6) or dry needling (Fig. 28.7) or acupuncture. Taping should have an immediate pain-relieving effect (Fig. 28.8).

Addressing extrinsic contributing factors

While initially it is vital to advise the patient to reduce the load on the PFJ, as rehabilitation progresses it is essential that any extrinsic factors that may have been placing excessive load on the PFJ (e.g. training, shoes, surfaces) are discussed and modified if necessary.

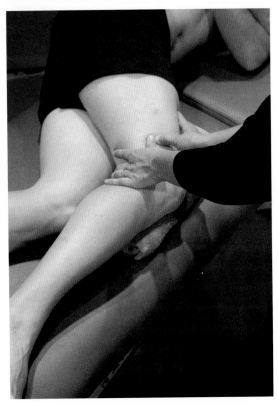

Figure 28.4 Clinical examination of lateral soft tissue contribution. The iliotibial band and lateral retinacular structures are palpated for any reduced compliance

Addressing intrinsic contributing factors

The clinician should have ascertained from the outset whether any intrinsic factors may have contributed to the development of the patient's pain. These potentially contributing factors should be addressed from the earliest treatment. The combination of treatment techniques should be based on the assessment and individualized for each person. 'Remote' intrinsic factors may be addressed through hip muscle retraining,[21, 25] improving musculotendinous compliance or foot orthoses. Local intrinsic factors may be addressed with techniques such as patella taping or bracing, improving lateral soft tissue compliance, generalized quadriceps strengthening or vasti retraining.

Patella taping

The aim of taping is to correct the abnormal position of the patella in relation to the femur. Patella taping reduces patellofemoral pain substantially and immediately.[26–31] However, the mechanism of the effect is still being investigated. In the short term, patella taping

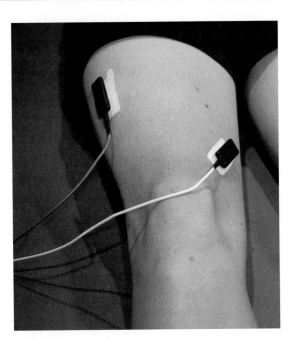

Figure 28.5 Clinical examination of neuromotor control of the vasti. The quality (amount and timing) of the vastus medialis obliquus and vastus lateralis components of the quadriceps can be assessed in a number of positions, including supine, sitting and standing. In these positions the patients is asked to contract the quadriceps. The clinician can either observe or palpate the quality of the contraction in these positions. A surface EMG biofeedback (illustrated) may be used to provide useful information to the clinician on the relative contribution of the vasti during quadriceps contractions across the various positions

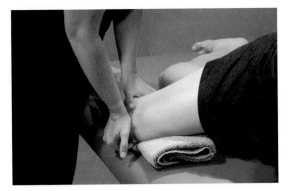

Figure 28.6 Mobilization of the patella is usually performed supine or side-lying (illustrated). The most commonly used mobilization techniques involve a medial glide component and may also include a medial tilt component

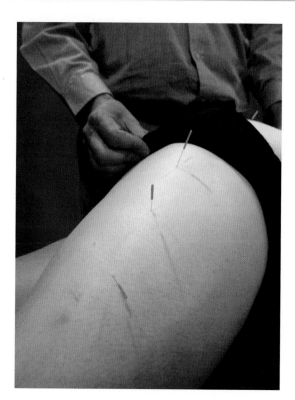

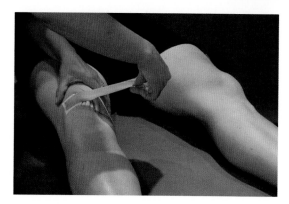

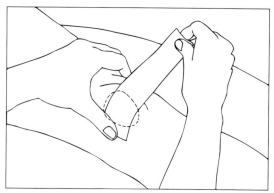

Figure 28.7 Dry needling of the vastus lateralis, tensor fascia lata and gluteals may provide immediate reduction in patellofemoral pain

Figure 28.8 Patella taping techniques

(a) Knee taped showing medial glide. Tape is applied to the lateral aspect of the patella. The patella is glided medially and the tape anchored to the skin over the medial aspect of the knee. When taping is completed, skin creases should be evident on the inside of the knee, indicating adequate tension on the patella

speeds the onset timing of the VMO relative to the vastus lateralis;[26, 32] its effect on vasti muscle activation is inconclusive.[27, 28, 33, 34] Further short-term effects of patella taping include improved knee function during gait.[28, 35] Taping is an effective interim measure to relieve patellofemoral pain while other contributing factors (e.g. VMO dysfunction, altered hip control) are being corrected.

A commonly used technique involves taping the patella with a medial glide (Fig. 28.8a). It may also require correction of abnormal lateral tilt (Fig. 28.8b), rotation (Fig. 28.8c) or inferior tilt (Fig. 28.8d). The taping is performed with rigid strapping tape. It is important that the clinician recognizes a posteriorly displaced inferior pole of the patella, as taping the patella too low will increase the patient's symptoms.

Patella taping effects should be assessed immediately using a pain-provoking activity such as a single- or double-leg squat. If the tape has been applied correctly, the post-taping squat will be less painful. If all or some pain persists, the tape should be altered, possibly including a component for tilt or rotation

or both. If patients are able to perform strengthening exercises pain-free without tape, then exercises alone will usually correct the abnormality. Most people, however, require tape to perform the exercises and, initially, to continue their sporting activities. Acute cases of patellofemoral pain may initially need tape applied 24 hours a day until the condition settles. The tape time is then gradually reduced.

Adverse skin reactions can occur beneath the rigid tape. Therefore, the area to be taped should be shaved and a protective barrier applied beneath the rigid strapping tape to reduce both the reaction to the zinc oxide in the tape adhesive and the reaction to shearing stresses on the skin. This can be achieved with adhesive gauze tape (Hypafix or Fixomull) applied to the area to be taped. A protective barrier or plastic skin can also be used in patients with extremely

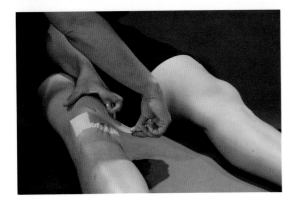

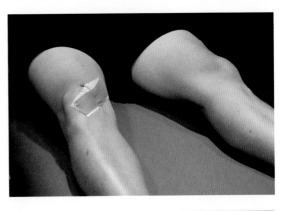

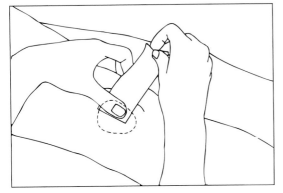

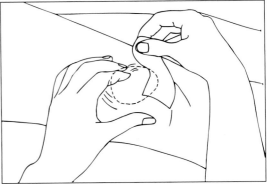

(b) Knee taped showing correction of lateral tilt. Tape is applied to the medial aspect of the patella and secured to the soft tissue on the inner aspect of the knee

(c) Knee taped showing correction of rotation. Tape is applied to the inferior pole of the patella and taken medially and superiorly to rotate the patella

sensitive skin. If skin irritation still occurs, the patient must be advised to remove the tape. Treatment with a hydrocortisone cream may be necessary. Patients with fair skin seem to have particularly sensitive skin and need to be monitored closely.

Braces

Some braces (Fig. 28.9) are commercially available to maintain medial glide. Recent studies have demonstrated that patellar braces are able to reduce patella displacement, increase patella contact area[36] and reduce the PFJ stress[37] in individuals with patellofemoral pain. However, a randomized controlled trial of such a brace did not find any benefit of the brace over a 'sham' knee sleeve or a general quadriceps strengthening program.[38] Braces are less specific than taping and do not specifically address tilt or rotation; but they may have a role in those patients who are unable to wear tape or who suffer recurrent patella subluxation or dislocation.

Improving lateral soft tissue compliance

Stretching of tight lateral structures such as the lateral retinaculum is beneficial. This is best done in a side-lying position with the knee flexed. The therapist glides the patella medially using the heel of the hand for a sustained stretch (Fig. 28.10). Other simple stretching techniques can be performed by the patient.

Vasti retraining

The first step in a VMO training program is for the patient to learn to contract the muscle. The patient should palpate the VMO while contracting their quadriceps in various degrees of knee flexion and/or in different activities to determine which position gives the best contraction. A dual channel biofeedback machine may also be used. The patient needs to have minimal patellofemoral pain before these exercises can become effective, otherwise muscle action may be inhibited. Therefore, taping may be required to relieve the pain and allow contractions to occur. The

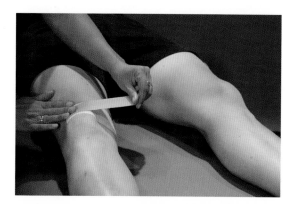

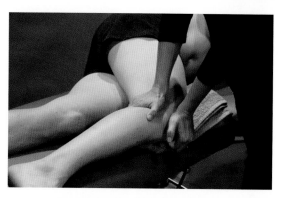

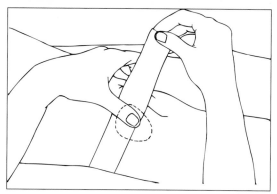

(d) Knee taped showing correction of inferior tilt. Tape is applied across the superior pole of the patella with sufficient firmness to elevate the inferior pole

Figure 28.10 Stretching of lateral structures. With the patient in a side-lying position, the patella is mobilized in a medial direction. This can be combined with soft tissue therapy (e.g. transverse gliding, friction) to the lateral structures

patient should attempt to recruit the VMO to contract before the rest of the quadriceps.

What types of exercises are most appropriate in training? Current evidence suggests that the VMO cannot be exercised in isolation and that no exercise appears to be preferential for activation of the VMO. Therefore, for each patient it is important to find and use the training position where the patient can attain a consistent VMO activation.

Initially, VMO exercises may commence in sitting with the knee at 90°, the foot on the floor and the patient palpating the VMO to facilitate muscle activation. A dual channel biofeedback machine or, in some cases, a muscle stimulator may assist the process. To ensure that the vasti are trained in positions that they are required to function, the patient should begin training in a weight-bearing position and perform functional exercises with steadily increasing load and difficulty as soon as possible. The final aim of training is to achieve a carryover from functional exercises to functional activities. The patient should perform small numbers of exercises frequently throughout the day. A series of graded VMO exercises is demonstrated in Figure 28.11.

Generalized strengthening exercises

Quadriceps strengthening exercises performed in the absence of other interventions (e.g. taping, bracing) may be effective in the management of patellofemoral pain. The available evidence does not support the effectiveness of one exercise regimen over another. Therefore, for many patients a generalized strengthening program may be sufficient to relieve their pain and reduce their disability.[38] However, clinically it

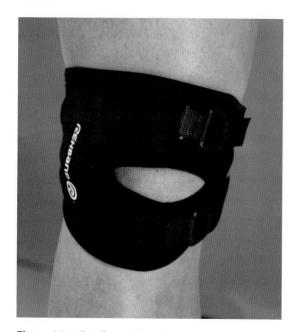

Figure 28.9 Patella stabilizing brace

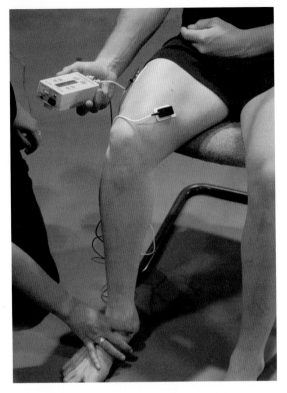

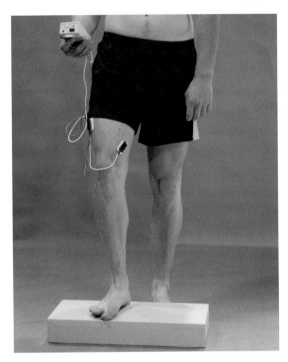

(c) Step-up with biofeedback machine in place

Figure 28.11 Vastus medialis obliquus training exercises

(a) Seated

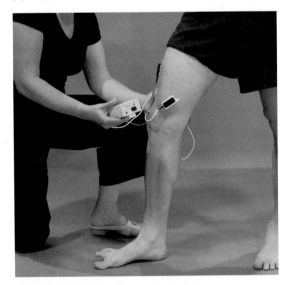

(b) VMO retraining could progress to small range flexion and extension movements in the walk stance position, with the VMO constantly active. This can then be progressed to a lunge

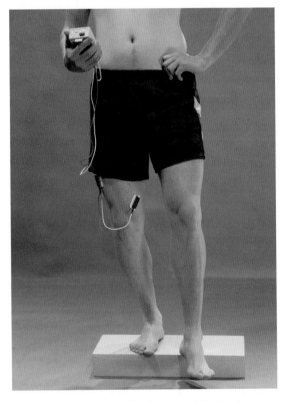

(d) Step-down with biofeedback machine in place

appears that a number of patients are unable to achieve restoration of pain-free function of their PFJ without specific retraining of the vasti.

Hip muscle strengthening

Retraining the hip abductors and external rotators helps to stabilize the lateral pelvis and to control internal hip rotation; this has been associated with pain reduction in patients with patellofemoral pain.[25] These exercises may be performed initially in non-weight-bearing positions and then progressed to weight-bearing positions (Fig. 28.12a). As soon as it is possible and practical, the patient must be taught to activate the hip abductors and external rotators, in combination with the VMO, during combined exercises (Fig. 28.12b). The emphasis of all retraining exercises will be on maintaining the activation of these muscles and correct alignment of the hip (i.e. neutral rotation) during weight-bearing flexion tasks (e.g. lunge, step-up and step-down, Fig. 28.12c).

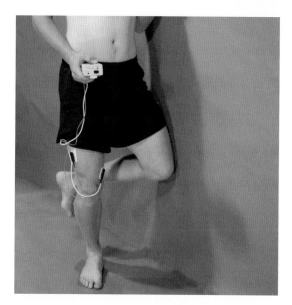

(b) Hip stability exercise. Training the hip external rotators and abductors in weight-bearing on one leg, with the contralateral leg against the wall. In this position the patient is asked to abduct the contralateral leg into the wall and at the same time externally rotate the weight-bearing leg. This should be combined with VMO contractions where required.

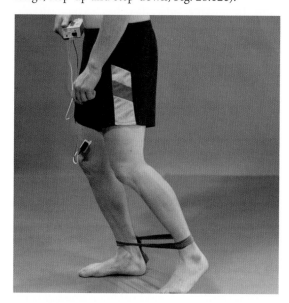

Figure 28.12 Hip muscle strengthening exercises

(a) Hip abduction and external rotation training in weight-bearing. Some patients should commence their hip retraining exercises in non-weight-bearing positions (prone, supine or side-lying). Once these have been mastered, the exercises should be progressed to weight-bearing, where combined hip external rotation, abduction and extension exercises can be performed. The use of resistance (illustrated) will increase the complexity of this exercise for both the weight-bearing and non-weight-bearing leg. These exercises should be combined with VMO activation.

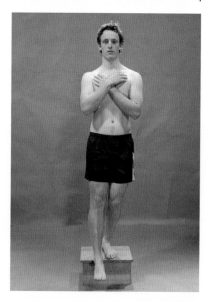

(c) Retraining hip muscles during a functional task. Functional retraining of the hip abductors and external rotators can be achieved by asking the patient to activate these muscles to maintain a neutral pelvis position during functional activities, such as lunges, step-ups and step-downs (shown).

Improving musculotendinous compliance

Attention must also be paid to improving the compliance of the hip flexors, quadriceps, hamstring and calf muscles as well as the iliotibial band through stretches, soft tissue techniques (Fig. 28.13) or dry needling (Fig. 28.7). Restoration of optimal muscle and fascial length is the goal. Transverse friction and transverse gliding should be applied to focal regions of thickening. Sustained myofascial tension (myofascial release) is the technique of choice to correct fascial thickening and shortening (Fig. 28.13).

In-shoe foot orthoses

If the assessment of the subtalar joint and tibial rotations indicates that an intervention is required, the clinician might consider either active retraining of the extrinsic muscles of the foot, taping, soft foot orthoses or rigid foot orthoses. These are outlined in Chapter 5. It is important to consider that in-shoe foot orthoses are effective in the management of patellofemoral pain. However, as with many other interventions, the mechanism of treatment effects is not known. It is possible that an orthosis may exert a positive effect through neuromuscular rather than mechanical mechanisms.

Evidence base for physical interventions

A number of controlled clinical trials have assessed the effectiveness or efficacy of physical interventions for patellofemoral pain (Table 28.5). Most trials have incorporated a number of techniques into their treatment program. While these reflect some aspects of clinical practise due to the inclusion of a variety of treatment techniques, mostly the interventions are not individualized to the patients' needs. A few studies have evaluated one aspect of intervention in isolation. These studies have enabled the assessment of a single treatment strategy, but the study results may not be generalized to the clinical scenarios. Treatment options that have gained popularity more recently have not been evaluated as thoroughly. Table 28.5 summarizes the level 1 (systematic reviews) and level 2 (controlled clinical trials) evidence of the evaluation of physical interventions for patellofemoral pain. While these studies represent the highest levels of evidence available, the quality of the various studies is varied.

Surgery—to be avoided

Experienced clinicians will have observed that the need for surgery in patellofemoral pain has been greatly reduced. This is likely due to the availability of evidence-based, exercise-based, physical interventions. To our knowledge, there has been no surgical randomized controlled trial showing the effectiveness of treatments such as chondroplasty or lateral release for patellofemoral pain. Thus, at a time when systematic reviews (level 1 evidence) argue for physical therapies for this condition, it would appear that such avenues should be tried repeatedly and with various expert therapists before being abandoned in favor of a hoped-for surgical miracle. We note that poor surgical outcomes have been reported and often patellofemoral pain is worsened after surgery.[64]

Patellofemoral instability

Patients with patellofemoral instability complain of a sensation of the patella slipping or moving laterally on certain movements. This may be followed by pain and swelling. The condition can arise by either or both of two distinct mechanisms. 'Primary' patellofemoral instability is more common among women than men.

Primary patellofemoral instability

This condition has the same predisposing factors as patellofemoral pain and the pattern of tenderness around the patella may be similar. Examination reveals patella hypermobility with apprehension and pain when the patella is pushed laterally by the examiner. Factors that predispose to this condition include generalized ligamentous laxity, patella alta (a patella that is located more superiorly than normal), trochlear dysplasia, and a lateralized tibial tuberosity.

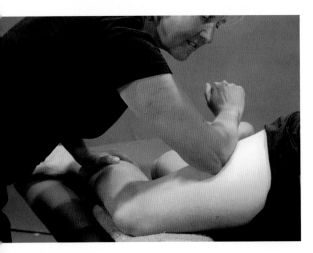

Figure 28.13 Soft tissue therapy—sustained myofascial tension of the iliotibial band

Table 28.5 Summary of level 1 (systematic reviews) and level 2 (controlled clinical trials) evidence investigating physical interventions for patellofemoral pain

Intervention	Effect of intervention	Level of evidence	Reference
Multimodal intervention	Positive	Level 1	Bolga & Malone 2005;[39] Bizzini et al. 2003[40] Crossley et al. 2001[41]
	Positive	Level 2	Whittingham et al. 2004;[42] Crossley et al. 2002;[43] Clark et al. 2000;[44] Harrison et al. 1999;[45] Eburne & Bannister 1996[46]
Taping	Positive	Level 1	Aminaka & Gribble 2005;[31] Crossley et al. 2001[41]
	Positive	Level 2	Whittingham et al. 2004[42]
	No effect	Level 2	Clark et al. 2000;[44] Kowall et al. 1996[47]
	Insufficient evidence	Level 1	Bizzini et al. 2003[40]
Bracing	Insufficient evidence	Level 1	D'Hondt et al. 2002;[48] Bizzini et al. 2003;[40] Crossley et al. 2001[41]
	Negative	Level 2	Finestone et al. 1993;[49] Miller et al. 1997[50]
Mobilization/ manipulation	Insufficient evidence	Level 1	Bizzini et al. 2003;[489] Crossley et al. 2001[41]
	No effect	Level 2	Rowlands & Brantingham 1999;[51] Taylor & Brantingham 2004[52]
Strengthening exercises	Positive	Level 1	Bizzini et al. 2003;[40] Heintjes et al. 2003[53]
	Positive	Level 2	Witvrouw et al. 2004;[54] Witvrouw et al. 2000;[55] Schneider et al. 2001;[56] Timm 1998;[57] Thomee 1997;[58] Stiene et al. 1996;[59] McMullen et al. 1980[60]
Stretching	NA	NA	NA
Hip muscle retraining	NA	NA	NA
Foot orthoses	Insufficient evidence	Level 1	D'Hondt et al. 2002;[48] Bizzini et al. 2003;[40] Crossley et al. 2001[41]
	Positive	Level 1	Arroll et al. 1997[61]
	Positive	Level 2	Eng & Pierrynowski 1993[62]
	No effect	Level 2	Wiener-Ogilvie & Jones 2004[63]

NA = none available.

Treatment of patellofemoral instability parallels that of patellofemoral pain. Acute management aims to reduce pain and swelling and a knee extension brace may provide temporary immobilization after an initial episode. The patient may use crutches for either partial or non-weight-bearing in that instance. Rehabilitation requires a VMO retraining program as outlined for patellofemoral pain (above). Surgery is indicated if a properly managed conservative program fails. Surgical approaches aim to correct the predisposing factors, and techniques used include arthroscopic

medial plication. Following surgery, an intensive rehabilitation program is vital.

Secondary patellofemoral instability

Secondary instability results from a primary dislocation episode (see Chapter 27 for acute management) that is likely to have arisen because of rupture of the medial patellofemoral ligament. This ligament is the main static restraint to lateral patella translation. It acts like a guy rope on a tent. Individuals with persistent patellofemoral instability after an acute dislocation may require additional investigations. Radiographs may reveal evidence of osteochondral damage to the articular surface of the patella and femur as well as predisposing anatomical abnormalities. Arthroscopy may be required to remove a loose osteochondral fragment, and, if appropriate, the medial patellofemoral ligament may need reconstruction.[65] As with surgery for primary instability, surgery for secondary instability also requires aggressive rehabilitation.

Fat pad irritation/ impingement

Fat pad syndrome was first described by Hoffa in 1903 to describe a condition where the infrapatellar fat pad was impinged between the patella and the femoral condyle due to a direct blow to the knee. More commonly, fat pad irritation occurs with repeated or uncontrolled hyperextension of the knee. The condition can be extremely painful and debilitating, as the fat pad is one of the most pain-sensitive structures in the knee.[9] Chronic fat pad irritation is relatively common and often goes unrecognized. The pain is often exacerbated by extension maneuvers, such as straight leg raises and prolonged standing, so it needs to be recognized early so that appropriate management can be implemented.

Clinical findings include localized tenderness and puffiness in the fat pad with the inferior pole of the patella being displaced posteriorly (Table 28.2). Patients often have hyperextension of the knees (genu recurvatum) associated with increased anterior pelvic tilt.

A popular clinical approach consists of treating the inferiorly tilted patella by taping across the superior surface of the patella to lever the inferior pole forward and relieve impingement of the fat pad (Fig. 28.8d). Unloading of the fat pad may be required to relieve the symptoms further. To unload the fat pad, a 'V' tape is placed below the fat pad, with the point of the 'V' at the tibial tubercle coming wide to the medial and lateral joint lines. As the tape is being pulled towards the joint line, the skin is lifted towards the patella, thus shortening the fat pad (Fig. 28.14). Muscle training and improving lower limb biomechanics is the basis of clinical management. Our clinical impression is that surgery should be avoided if possible. To date, there have been no randomized controlled trials of surgery for this condition.[66]

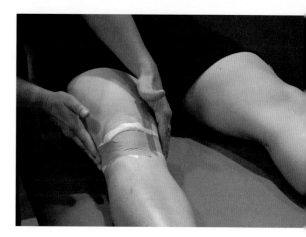

Figure 28.14 Fat pad unloading tape. Tape is applied in a 'V' from the tibial tuberosity to the joint lines. The fat pad region is pinched to unload the fat pad while applying the tape. This tape is often combined with taping the superior pole of the patella (Fig. 28.8d) in the treatment of fat pad impingement. This elevates the inferior pole of the patella

Patellar tendinopathy

There have been advances in understanding the histopathology, imaging and surgical outcomes in this condition in the past decade. Nevertheless, successful management of the jumping athlete with patellar tendinopathy remains a major challenge for the practitioner and patient.

Nomenclature

Patellar tendinopathy was first referred to as 'jumper's knee' due to its frequency in jumping sports (e.g. basketball, volleyball, high, long and triple jumps).[67] However, the condition also occurs in sportspeople who change direction and may occur in sportspeople who do not perform either jumping or change of direction. The term 'patellar tendinitis' is a misnomer as the pathology underlying this condition is degenerative tendinosis rather than inflammatory 'tendinitis' (see below).[68] Fortunately, the term patellar tendinitis is falling out of favor. On balance, patellar tendinopathy is probably the most appropriate general label for this condition (Chapter 2).[69]

Pathology and pathogenesis of patellar tendinopathy

Normal tendon is seen as white and glistening to the naked eye but the patellar tendon of patients undergoing surgery for patellar tendinopathy contains soft, yellow-brown tissue adjacent to the lower pole of the patella (Fig. 28.15). This macroscopic appearance is commonly labeled 'mucoid degeneration'. Under the light microscope, symptomatic patellar tendons do not consist of tight parallel collagen bundles but instead are separated by a large amount of mucoid ground substance that gives them a disorganized and discontinuous appearance. Clefts in collagen and occasional necrotic fibers suggest microtearing. There is also small vessel ingrowth. This histopathological picture, which is called 'tendinosis', is identical in tendons with both macroscopically evident partial tears and those without.[70] These regions of tendon degeneration correspond with areas of increased signal on MRI and hypoechoic regions on ultrasound.[68]

Pain and disuse associated with patellar tendinopathy may lead to poor VMO function and altered PFJ biomechanics. Regardless of the cause, the PFJ needs to be excluded as a source of pain in patients presenting with patellar tendinopathy.

Clinical features

The clinical features of patellar tendinopathy are outlined in Table 28.2. The patient complains of anterior knee pain aggravated by activities such as jumping, hopping and bounding. The most common site of tendinopathy is the deep attachment of the tendon to the inferior pole of the patella. Distal lesions are less common and midsubstance lesions have been reported.[71] The tendon is tender on palpation either at the inferior pole or in the body of the tendon. There is frequently associated thickening of the tendon. The most effective position for palpation is shown in Figure 28.16. Expert clinicians also assess possible precipitating factors, such as muscle tightness of the quadriceps and hamstring muscles, increased neural tension or abnormal biomechanics of the pelvis, PFJ or lower leg. Calf weakness is common in patients with patellar tendinopathy.

It is important to reproduce the patient's pain on examination. In less severe cases it may be necessary to perform a functional activity, such as a squat or hop, to reproduce the pain. As these activities also load the PFJ, taping to correct the PFJ followed by reassessment may help to differentiate between the two conditions or at least indicate if the PFJ should also be treated.

An alternative method of monitoring the clinical progress of patellar tendinopathy can be performed using the VISA questionnaire (Table 28.6) [72, 73] This simple questionnaire takes less than 5 minutes to

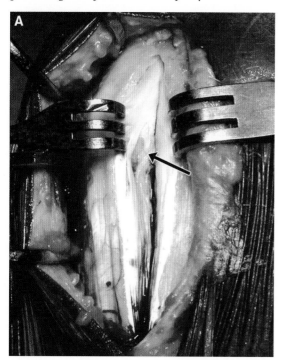

Figure 28.15 Intraoperative photograph showing the pathology that appears consistent with tendinosis. Note the darker region within the deep surface (arrow)—this is the markedly abnormal tissue

(SHELBOURNE KD, HENNE TD, GRAY T. RECALCITRANT PATELLAR TENDINOSIS IN ELITE ATHLETES. *AM J SPORTS MED*, 34(7) P. 1141–6 (2006), PUBLISHED BY SAGE PUBLICATIONS)

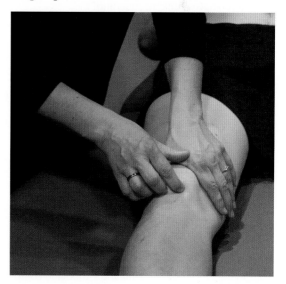

Figure 28.16 Position of palpation of the patellar tendon. Pressure on the superior pole of the patella tilts the inferior pole, allowing more precise palpation of the tendon origin

Table 28.6 Victorian Institute of Sport Assessment (VISA) questionnaire

1. For how many minutes can you sit pain free?

POINTS

0 min | | | | | | | | | | | 100 min

0 1 2 3 4 5 6 7 8 9 10

2. Do you have pain walking downstairs with a normal gait cycle?

POINTS

Strong severe pain | | | | | | | | | | | No pain

0 1 2 3 4 5 6 7 8 9 10

3. Do you have pain at the knee with full active non-weight-bearing knee extension?

POINTS

Strong severe pain | | | | | | | | | | | No pain

0 1 2 3 4 5 6 7 8 9 10

4. Do you have pain when doing a full weight-bearing lunge?

POINTS

Strong severe pain | | | | | | | | | | | No pain

0 1 2 3 4 5 6 7 8 9 10

5. Do you have problems squatting?

POINTS

Unable | | | | | | | | | | | No problem

0 1 2 3 4 5 6 7 8 9 10

6. Do you have pain during or immediately after doing 10 single leg hops?

POINTS

Strong severe pain/ unable | | | | | | | | | | | No pain

0 1 2 3 4 5 6 7 8 9 10

7. Are you currently undertaking sport or other physical activity?

POINTS

0 ☐ Not at all

4 ☐ Modified training ± modified competition

7 ☐ Full training ± competition but not at same level as when symptoms began

10 ☐ Competing at the same or higher level as when symptoms began

Table 28.6 Victorian Institute of Sport Assessment (VISA) questionnaire *(continued)*

8. Please complete EITHER A, B or C in this question.
   - If you have no pain while undertaking sport please complete Q8A only.
   - If you have pain while undertaking sport but it does not stop you from completing the activity, please complete Q8B only.
   - If you have pain that stops you from completing sporting activities, please complete Q8C only.

A. If you have no pain while undertaking sport, for how long can you train/practise?

POINTS

NIL	1–5 min	6–10 min	11–15 min	>15 min
☐	☐	☐	☐	☐
0	7	14	21	30

OR

B. If you have some pain while undertaking sport, but it does not stop you from completing your training/practise, for how long can you train/practise?

POINTS

NIL	1–5 min	6–10 min	11–15 min	>15 min
☐	☐	☐	☐	☐
0	4	10	14	20

OR

C. If you have pain that stops you from completing your training/practise, for how long can you train/practise?

POINTS

NIL	1–5 min	6–10 min	11–15 min	>15 min
☐	☐	☐	☐	☐
0	2	5	7	10

TOTAL SCORE ☐ 100

complete and once patients are familiar with it they will be able to complete most of it themselves.

Investigations

Ultrasound examination and MRI are the investigations of choice in patellar tendinopathy, although clinicians must appreciate that these imaging modalities do not have 100% sensitivity and specificity for the condition (Fig. 28.17). Ultrasound examination with Doppler will assess the vascularity present in the tendon. This is important as increased vascularity has been associated with pain.

Treatment

Treatment of patellar tendinopathy requires patience and a multifaceted approach, which is outlined in Table 28.7. It is essential that the practitioner and patient recognize that tendinopathy that has been present for

months may require a considerable period of treatment associated with rehabilitation before symptoms disappear (Chapter 2). Conservative management of patellar tendinopathy requires appropriate strengthening exercises, load reduction, correcting biomechanical errors, and soft tissue therapy. An innovation has been the use of sclerotherapy of neovessels with polidocanol. Surgery is indicated after a considered and lengthy conservative program has failed. This section outlines the physical therapy approach of correction of biomechanics that might be contributing to excessive load on the tendon, targeted exercise therapy and soft tissue treatment before outlining medical treatments including medication, sclerotherapy and surgery.

Relative load reduction: modified activity and biomechanical correction

There are numerous ways of reducing the load on the patellar tendon without resorting to complete

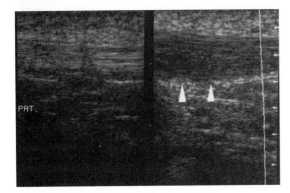

Figure 28.17 Imaging appearances in athletes with patellar tendinopathy

(a) Ultrasound images showing normal tendon on the left and the characteristic thickened tendon with regions of loss of echogenicity (arrowed) on the right. This appearance, although only mildly abnormal compared with some cases (e.g. Fig. 28.17b), already corresponds with the histopathology of tendon degeneration—tendinosis

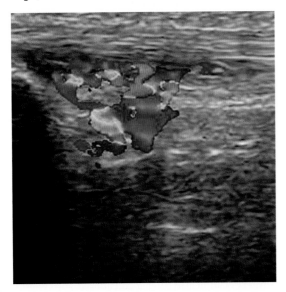

(b) Ultrasound appearance of a patellar tendon with greater morphological (structural) abnormality. There is a clearly demarcated region of hypoechogenicity and an abnormal amount of vascularity. This appearance may be asymptomatic[74] and is certainly not, per se, an indication for surgery

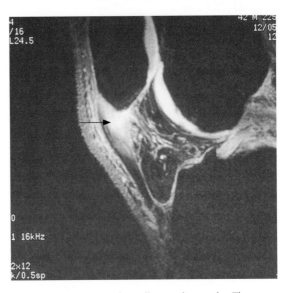

(c) MRI appearance of patellar tendinopathy. The key feature is the area of increased (bright) signal (arrowed). Symptoms do not correlate precisely with the severity of imaging appearances[8, 75]

Table 28.7 Overview of management of patellar tendinopathy

- A patient presenting with persistent painful patellar tendinopathy for the first time may require 3–6 months to recover. A patient with a longstanding history may require 6–12 months to return, pain-free, to competition without recurrence.
- Relative tendon unloading is critical for treatment success. This is achieved by activity modification and assisted by biomechanical correction.
- Progressive strengthening is the treatment of choice in patellar tendinopathy. Effective exercise prescription requires thorough assessment of the patient's functional capacity and a skilful approach to increasing demand on the tendon.
- It takes between 6 and 12 months to return to full competitive sport after successful patellar tendon surgery. Thus, the treating physician must be sure that an appropriate conservative treatment program has failed before suggesting a tendon needs surgery.

rest or immobilization. Relative rest means that the patient may be able to continue playing or training if it is possible to reduce the amount of jumping or sprinting, or the total weekly training hours.

Strengthening and correcting biomechanics improves the energy-absorbing capacity of the limb both at the affected musculotendinous unit and at the hip and ankle. The ankle and calf are critical in absorbing the initial landing load transmitted to the knee.[76] Biomechanical studies reveal that about

40% of landing energy is transmitted proximally.[77] Thus, the calf complex must function well to prevent more load than necessary transferring to the patellar tendon.

Better landing techniques can decrease patellar tendon load. Compared with flat-foot landing, forefoot landing generates lower ground reaction forces and, if this technique is combined with a large range of hip or knee flexion, vertical ground reaction forces can be reduced by a further 25%.[77]

Biomechanical correction requires assessment of both anatomical and functional shortcomings. Anatomical variants that may contribute to patellar tendinopathy include foot, ankle and hip deficiencies.

There are numerous functional biomechanical abnormalities. Inflexibility of the hamstrings, iliotibial band and calf muscles, as well as restricted ankle range of motion, are likely to increase the load on the patellar tendon. Hamstring tightness (decreased sit and reach test) is associated with an increased prevalence of patellar tendinopathy.[78] Weakness of the gluteal, quadriceps and calf muscles leads to fatigue and aberrant movement patterns that may alter forces acting on the knee during activity. Therefore, proximal and distal muscles also need assessment in patients with patellar tendinopathy.

Cryotherapy

Cryotherapy (e.g. ice) is a popular adjunct to treatment but if the patient finds no clinical benefit from this modality, there is no rationale for persisting.

Strengthening

At least six papers document the effectiveness of strengthening exercises on patellar tendinopathy. These can be divided into two groups: those studies that investigated exercises on a decline board and those using other exercises.

Three papers suggested that exercise-based interventions such as squatting, isokinetics and weights reduced the pain of patellar tendinopathy.[79-81] More recent studies have investigated the effectiveness of exercise on a 25° decline board—a method specifically loading the extensor mechanism of the knee.[82] Two randomized trials reported improvements in pain, function and return to sport with exercise, although time frames for improvement varied.[4, 83] Importantly, there was no improvement in pain or jump performance among the treatment group compared with those who undertook no exercise when the intervention occurred during competition period.[84]

An effective strength program embraces the principles outlined in Table 28.8. Commonly prescribed exercises are illustrated in Figure 28.18. When and how a strengthening program should begin is outlined in the box.

Table 28.8 Strengthening program for treatment of patellar tendinopathy

Timing	Type of overload	Activity
0–3 months	Strength and strength endurance	Hypertrophy and strengthen the affected muscles, focus attention on all anti-gravity muscles
3–6 months	Power and speed endurance	Weight-bearing speed-specific loads
6+ months	Combinations dependent on sport (e.g. load, speed)	Sport-specific rehabilitation

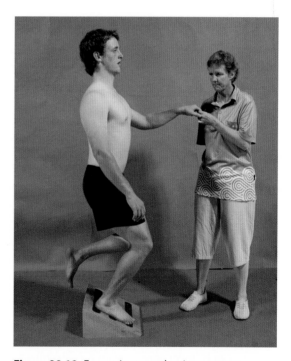

Figure 28.18 Eccentric strengthening program—patellar tendon

(a) Single-leg squat on decline board

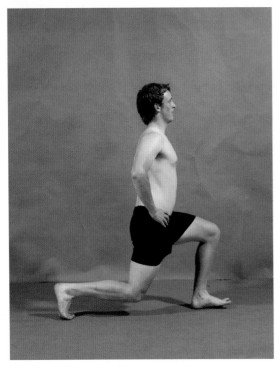

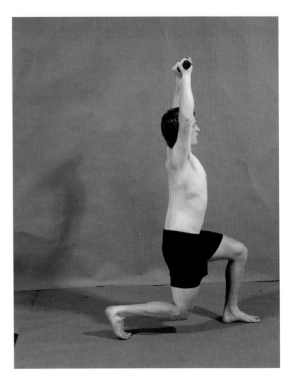

(b) Lunge

(c) Lunge with weights

When should patellar tendon strengthening begin?

Therapists often have concerns as to when and how they should begin a strengthening program. Even athletes with the most severe cases of patellar tendinopathy should be able to begin some weight-based strength and other exercises, such as calf strength and isometric quadriceps work, in standing. On the other hand, the athlete who has not lost a lot of knee strength and bulk can progress quickly to the speed part of the program.

Both pain and the ability of the musculotendinous unit to do the work should guide the amount of strengthening to be done. If pain is a limiting factor, then the program must be modified so that the majority of the work occurs without aggravating symptoms 24 hours after exercise. A subjective clinical rating system, such as the VISA questionnaire (Table 28.6), administered at about monthly intervals, will help both the therapist and the patient measure progress.

If pain is under control, then it is essential to monitor the ability of the limb to complete the exercises with control and quality. Exercises should

only be progressed if the previous work load is easily managed, pain is controlled and function is satisfactory.

Athletes with patellar tendinopathy tend to 'unload' the affected limb to avoid pain, so they commonly have not only weakness but also abnormal motor patterns that must be reversed. Strength training must graduate quickly to incorporate single-leg exercises (Fig. 28.18) as the athlete can continue to unload the affected tendon when exercising using both legs. Thus, exercises that target the quadriceps specifically, such as single-leg extensions, may have a place in the rehabilitation of patellar tendinopathy. Similarly, when the athlete is ready, increase the load on the quadriceps by having the patient stand on a 25° decline board to do squats. Compared with squatting on a flat surface, this reduces the calf contribution during the squat.

The therapist should progress the regimen by adding load and speed and then endurance to each of those levels of exercise. Combinations such as load and speed, or height and load, then follow. These end-stage exercises can provoke tendon pain and are only recommended after a prolonged rehabilitation period and when the sport demands intense loading. In several sports it may not be necessary to add potentially aggravating activities such as jump training to the rehabilitation program, whereas in volleyball, for example, it is vital.

Finally, the overall exercise program must correct aberrant motor patterns such as stiff landing mechanics (discussed above) and pelvic instability. For example, weight-bearing exercises must be in a functionally required range and the pelvis position must be monitored and controlled at all times. The common errors in rehabilitation strength programs are listed in Table 28.9.

Table 28.9 Common reasons why rehabilitation programs fail at various stages

Early failure	Late failure
Insufficient strength training	Failure to monitor the patient's symptoms
Progression of rehabilitation program is too quick	Rehabilitation and strength training ends on return to training, instead of continuing throughout the return to sport
Inappropriate loads during rehabilitation (too little, too much)	No speed rehabilitation Plyometrics training performed inappropriately, is not tolerated or unnecessary

Soft tissue therapy

Two studies compared soft tissue therapy/transverse friction to other treatments.[79, 85] In one, the main outcome measures did not differ between groups.[85] In the other, a three-arm trial of ultrasound, transverse friction and exercise provided a reduction in pain to 0%, 20% and 100% of participants, respectively.[79] Nevertheless, two studies are insufficient to suggest that soft tissue therapy may not be helpful in certain clinical settings, and it remains a popular treatment.

Digital ischemic pressure to trigger points in the calf muscles and transverse friction to the tendon are used in some centers (Fig. 28.19). If tightness in the quadriceps muscle is present, sustained myofascial tension can be performed on the quadriceps muscle with the knee flexed.

Pharmacotherapy

There have been three studies of pharmacotherapy in the treatment of patellar tendinopathy. Two studies investigated the effect of corticosteroid administered by iontophoresis, phonophoresis or injection,[86, 87] and one study investigated the effect of sclerosing injections.[88] Iontophoresis with corticosteroid improved outcome compared to phonophoresis as it may introduce corticosteroid into target tissue more effectively than phonophoresis.[86] Capasso et al.[87] reported that aprotinin offered a better outcome than either corticosteroid or placebo. The time from onset of patellar tendinopathy to recruitment into the study was not stated, hence some subjects may have had short-term

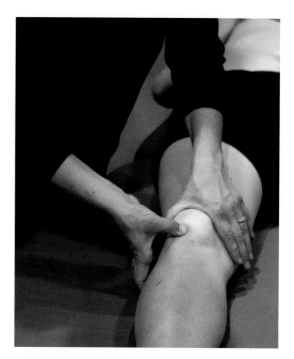

Figure 28.19 Massage therapy—transverse friction of the patellar tendon

symptoms that had responded to anti-inflammatory medication. Outcome measures in this study were based on the Kelly grading system[89] and the study used an unblinded clinical investigator.

Neovascularization is a cornerstone of tendon pathology and is the target of treatment by Alfredson and Ohberg.[88] This prospective trial investigated sclerosing injections on pain and function in the patellar tendon. Eighty per cent of subjects returned to their previous level of competition and pain reductions were also significant (visual analog scale reduced from 81 to 10). The authors suggest that the results of this treatment on those with long-term tendon pain (mean, 23 months) challenge the need for surgery for patellar tendinopathy.

In a high-quality randomized control trial of elite athletes with patellar tendinopathy, Norwegian investigators found that sclerosing injections with polidocanol resulted in a significant improvement in knee function and reduced pain in patients with patellar tendinopathy.[90]

Surgery

The first randomized trial that compared surgical treatment and conservative management of patellar tendinopathy was published in 2006.[90] There was no significant difference in outcome between groups; thus, surgical intervention provided no benefit over conservative management. Thus the clinical implication is that surgery is not a 'quick fix' for patellar tendinopathy.[90]

Three patellar tendon surgical studies reported a prospective design.[75, 91] In two of them, between 73% and 100% of the subjects reported good results. In the third, Testa et al.[92] investigated the efficacy of percutaneous tenotomy and reported that the technique was more effective for the treatment of midtendon pathology than it was for proximal tendon pathology. The diagnosis of a midtendon lesion was made on clinical grounds (palpation) and seven subjects had normal imaging results. Nearly 40% of participants in this study reported poor results and isokinetic testing revealed persistent strength deficits. Given that midtendon pathology is relatively rare, this study may have limited clinical utility.

There is no consensus as to the optimal surgical technique to use, with surgeons performing either a longitudinal or a transverse incision over the patellar tendon and generally excising abnormal tissue. Some surgeons excise the paratenon, while others suture it after having performed the longitudinal tenotomies and excision of the tendinopathic area. There has been some enthusiasm for possible arthroscopic debridement of the posterior portion of the patellar tendon and results published to date appear similar to those of patients undergoing open surgery.[93]

We recommend surgery only after a thorough, high-quality conservative program has failed. Surgeons must advise patients that while symptomatic benefit is very likely, return to sport at the previous level cannot be guaranteed (60–80% likelihood).[93, 94] Time to return to the previous level of sport, if achieved, is likely to take between six and 12 months.[93, 94]

Partial tendon tears: acute versus chronic

The term 'partial tear' is used to refer to either of two clinical entities. One use refers to the sudden significantly painful episode, which is associated with disability, and this corresponds to a substantial tear of an area of pathology of the patellar tendon. This 'acute' partial tear is not dissimilar to a complete 'rupture' of the tendon (Fig. 28.20a), except that some tendon remains intact. This is discussed in Chapter 27. If the partial tear is very large, causes major disability and shows no improvement in two to three weeks, early surgery may be justified to stimulate some healing response in the tendon.

A small partial tear of the patellar tendon (Fig. 28.20b) may also occur and this is often diagnosed at ultrasonography and is difficult to differentiate from an area of tendinosis. Alternatively, it may be an incidental finding on ultrasound examination. This type of partial tear is part of the continuum of tendinosis and can be managed as such. The indication for surgery of a small partial tear is failed conservative management.

Less common causes

Synovial plica

The importance of the synovial plica, a synovial fold found along the medial edge of the patella, has been a matter of considerable debate. An inflamed plica may cause variable sharp pain located anteriorly, medially or posteriorly. The patient may complain of sharp pain on squatting. On examination, the plica is sometimes palpable as a thickened band under the medial border of the patella. It should only be considered as the primary cause of the patient's symptoms when the patient fails to respond to appropriate management of patellofemoral pain. In this case, and in the presence of a tender thickened band, arthroscopy should be performed and the synovial plica removed.

Osgood-Schlatter lesion

Osgood-Schlatter lesion is an osteochondrosis (Chapter 40) that occurs at the tibial tuberosity. This is a common condition in girls of about

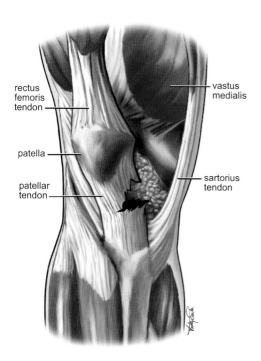

10–12 years and boys of about 13–15 years (but these ages vary) and results from excessive traction on the soft apophysis of the tibial tuberosity by the powerful patellar tendon. It occurs in association with high levels of activity during a period of rapid growth and is associated with a change in the tendon.

Treatment consists of reassurance that the condition is self-limiting. Whether or not to play sport depends on the severity of symptoms. Children with mild symptoms may wish to continue to play some or all sport; others may choose some modification of their programs. If the child prefers to cease sport because of pain, that decision should be supported. However, the amount of sport played does not seem to affect the time the condition takes to heal.

Sinding-Larsen–Johansson lesion

This uncommon lesion is one of the group of osteo-chondroses found in adolescents (Chapter 40). It is an important differential diagnosis in young patients with pain at the inferior pole of the patella. Treatment is outlined in Chapter 40.

Quadriceps tendinopathy

Pain arising at the quadriceps tendon at its attachment to the patella occurs occasionally, mainly in the older athlete and in weightlifters as the quadriceps tendon is loaded more in a deeper squat. It is characterized by tenderness along the superior margin of the patella and pain on resisted quadriceps contraction. Treatment follows the same principles as treatment of patellar tendinopathy. Differential diagnosis is suprapatellar pain of PFJ origin and bipartite patella.

Occasionally the condition responds well to self-applied transverse friction massage to the direct site of pain. Correction of focal thickening in the quadriceps muscle is also required and is achieved with sustained myofascial tension, transverse glides and stretching.

Bursitis

There are a number of bursae around the knee joint. These are shown in Figure 28.21. The most commonly affected bursa is the pre-patellar bursa. Pre-patellar bursitis ('housemaid's knee') presents as a superficial swelling on the anterior aspect of the knee. This must be differentiated from an effusion of the knee joint. Acute infective pre-patellar bursitis, common in those who kneel a lot, should be identified and treated quickly. Infrapatellar bursitis can also cause anterior knee pain that may mimic

Figure 28.20 Two types of partial tear of the patellar tendon

(a) A large partial tear is similar to an acute tendon rupture

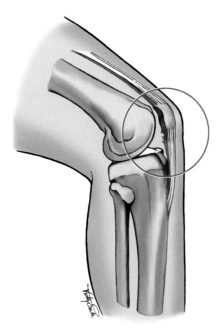

(b) A small partial tear that can result from overuse

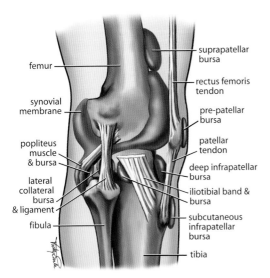

femur

synovial
membrane

popliteus
muscle
& bursa

lateral
collateral
bursa
& ligament

fibula

suprapatellar
bursa

rectus femoris
tendon

pre-patellar
bursa

patellar
tendon

deep infrapatellar
bursa

iliotibial band &
bursa

subcutaneous
infrapatellar
bursa

tibia

Figure 28.21 Bursae around the knee joint

patellar tendinopathy; this bursa forms part of an enthesis organ of the distal insertion and, thus, can be challenging to treat.

Treatment of mild cases of bursitis includes NSAIDs. More severe cases require aspiration and infiltration with a corticosteroid agent and local anesthesia, followed by firm compression bandaging and rest for 48 hours. If, despite these measures, there are several recurrences, surgical bursectomy may be required.

Recommended Reading

Cook JL, Khan KM. What is the most appropriate treatment for patellar tendinopathy? In: MacAuley D, Best T, eds. *Evidence-Based Sports Medicine*. London: BMJ Books, 2002: 422–41.

Crossley K, Bennell K, Green S, Cowan S, McConnell J. Physical therapy for patellofemoral pain: a randomized, double-blinded, placebo-controlled trial. *Am J Sports Med* 2002; 30(6): 857–65.

Crossley K, Bennell K, Green S, McConnell J. A systematic review of physical interventions for patellofemoral pain syndrome. *Clin J Sport Med* 2001; 11(2): 103–10.

Elias DA, White LM. Imaging of patellofemoral disorders. *Clin Radiol* 2004; 59(7): 543–57.

Hoksrud A, Öhberg L, Alfredson H, Bahr R. Ultrasound-guided sclerosis of neovessels in painful chronic patellar tendinopathy—a randomized controlled trial. *Am J Sports Med* 2006; in press.

McConnell J, Bennell K. Conservative management of anterior knee pain: the McConnell program. In Sanchis-Alfonso V, ed. *Anterior Knee Pain and Patellar Instability*. London: Springer-Verlag, 2006: 167–84.

Sanchis-Alfonso V, ed. *Anterior Knee Pain and Patellar Instability*. London: Springer-Verlag, 2006.

References

1. Baquie P, Brukner P. Injuries presenting to an Australian sports medicine centre: a 12-month study. *Clin J Sport Med* 1997; 7(1): 28–31.

2. Taunton JE, Ryan MB, Clement DB, McKenzie DC, Lloyd-Smith DR, Zumbo BD. A retrospective case-control analysis of 2002 running injuries. *Br J Sports Med* 2002; 36(2): 95–101.

3. Torry MR, Decker MJ, Viola RW, O'Connor DD, Steadman JR. Intra-articular knee joint effusion induces quadriceps avoidance gait patterns. *Clin Biomech* 2000; 15(3): 147–59.

4. Purdam CR, Jonsson P, Alfredson H, Lorentzon R, Cook JL, Khan KM. A pilot study of the eccentric decline squat in the management of painful chronic patellar tendinopathy. *Br J Sports Med* 2004; 38(4): 395–7.

5. Elias DA, White LM. Imaging of patellofemoral disorders. *Clin Radiol* 2004; 59(7): 543–57.

6. Cook JL, Khan KM, Kiss ZS, Purdam CR, Griffiths L. Reproducibility and clinical utility of tendon palpation to detect patellar tendinopathy in young basketball players. *Br J Sports Med* 2001; 35: 65–9.

7. Cook JL, Khan KM, Kiss ZS, et al. Asymptomatic hypoechoic regions on patellar tendon ultrasound: a 4-year clinical and ultrasound followup of 46 tendons. *Scand J Med Sci Sports* 2001; 11: 321–7.

8. Shalaby M, Almekinders LC. Patellar tendinitis: the significance of magnetic resonance imaging findings. *Am J Sports Med* 1999; 27: 345–9.

9. Dye SF, Vaupel GL, Dye CC. Conscious neurosensory mapping of the internal structures of the human knee without intraarticular anesthesia. *Am J Sports Med* 1998; 26(6): 773–7.

10. Insall J, Falvo KA, Wise DW. Chondromalacia patellae. A prospective study. *J Bone Joint Surg Am* 1976; 58A(1): 1–8.

11. Fulkerson JP. Diagnosis and treatment of patients with patellofemoral pain. *Am J Sports Med* 2002; 30(3): 447–56.

12. Fulkerson JP, Gossling HR. Anatomy of the knee joint lateral retinaculum. *Clin Orthop* 1980; 153: 183–8.

13. Fulkerson JP, Tennant R, Jaivin JS, Grunnet M. Histologic evidence of retinacular nerve injury associated with patellofemoral malalignment. *Clin Orthop* 1985; 197: 196–205.

14. Sanchis-Alfonso V, Rosello-Sastre E, Monteagudo-Castro C, Esquerdo J. Quantitative analysis of nerve changes in the lateral retinaculum in patients with isolated symptomatic patellofemoral malalignment. A preliminary study. *Am J Sports Med* 1998; 26(5): 703–9.

15. Sanchis-Alfonso V, Rosello-Sastre E. Immunohistochemical analysis for neural markers of the lateral retinaculum in patients with isolated symptomatic patellofemoral malalignment. A neuroanatomic basis for anterior knee pain in the active young patient. *Am J Sports Med* 2000; 28(5): 725–31.

16. Witonski D, Wagrowska-Danielewicz M. Distribution of substance-P nerve fibers in the knee joint in patients with anterior knee pain syndrome. A preliminary report. *Knee Surg Sports Traumatol Arthrosc* 1999; 7(3): 177–83.

17. Duri ZA, Aichroth PM, Dowd G. The fat pad. Clinical observations. *Am J Knee Surg* 1996; 9(2): 55–66.

18. Tsirbas A, Paterson RS, Keene GCR. Fat pad impingement: a missed cause of patellofemoral pain? *Aust J Sci Med Sport* 1991; 23: 24–6.

19. Fulkerson J. *Disorders of the Patellofemoral Joint*. 3rd edn. Baltimore: Williams & Wilkins, 1997.

20. Matthews L, Sonstegard D, Henke J. Load bearing characteristics of the patellofemoral joint. *Acta Orthop Scand* 1977; 48: 511–16.

21. Ireland ML, Willson JD, Ballantyne BT, Davis IM. Hip strength in females with and without patellofemoral pain. *J Orthop Sports Phys Ther* 2003; 33(11): 671–6.

22. Dye SF. The pathophysiology of patellofemoral pain: a tissue homeostasis perspective. *Clin Orthop* 2005; 436: 100–10.

23. Watson C, Propps M, Galt W, Redding A, Dobbs D. Reliability of measurements obtained using McConnell's classification of patellar orientation in symptomatic and asymptomatic subjects. *J Orthop Sports Phys Ther* 1999; 29: 378–85.

24. McConnell J. Invited commentary. *J Orthop Sports Phys Ther* 1999; 29: 388–90.

25. Tyler TF, Nicholas SJ, Mullaney MJ, McHugh MP. The role of hip muscle function in the treatment of patellofemoral pain syndrome. *Am J Sports Med* 2006; in press.

26. Cowan SM, Bennell KL, Hodges PW. Therapeutic patellar taping changes the timing of vasti muscle activation in people with patellofemoral pain syndrome. *Clin J Sport Med* 2002; 12(6): 339–47.

27. Ng GY, Cheng JM. The effects of patellar taping on pain and neuromuscular performance in subjects with patellofemoral pain syndrome. *Clin Rehabil* 2002; 16(8): 821–7.

28. Salsich GB, Brechter JH, Farwell D, Powers CM. The effects of patellar taping on knee kinetics, kinematics, and vastus lateralis muscle activity during stair ambulation in individuals with patellofemoral pain. *J Orthop Sports Phys Ther* 2002; 32(1): 3–10.

29. Wilson T, Carter N, Thomas G. A multicenter, single-masked study of medial, neutral, and lateral patellar taping in individuals with patellofemoral pain syndrome. *J Orthop Sports Phys Ther* 2003; 33(8): 437–43; discussion 444–8.

30. Christou EA. Patellar taping increases vastus medialis oblique activity in the presence of patellofemoral pain. *J Electromyogr Kinesiol* 2004; 14(4): 495–504.

31. Aminaka N, Gribble PA. A systematic review of the effects of therapeutic taping on patellofemoral pain syndrome. *J Athl Train* 2005; 40: 341–51.

32. Gilleard W, McConnell J, Parsons D. The effect of patellar taping on the onset of vastus medialis obliquus and vastus lateralis muscle activity in persons with patellofemoral pain. *Phys Ther* 1998; 78(1): 25–32.

33. Cowan SM, Hodges PW, Crossley KM, Bennell KL. Patellar taping does not change the amplitude of electromyographic activity of the vasti in a stair stepping task. *Br J Sports Med* 2006; 40(1): 30–4.

34. Cerny K. Vastus medialis oblique/vastus lateralis muscle activity ratios for selected exercises in persons with and without patellofemoral pain syndrome. *Phys Ther* 1995; 75(8): 672–83.

35. Powers CM, Landel R, Sosnick T, et al. The effect of patellar taping on stride characteristics and joint motion in subjects with patellofemoral pain. *J Orthop Phys Ther* 1997; 26(6): 286–91.

36. Powers CM, Ward SR, Chan LD, Chen YJ, Terk MR. The effect of bracing on patella alignment and patellofemoral joint contact area. *Med Sci Sports Exerc* 2004; 36(7): 1226–32.

37. Powers CM, Ward SR, Chen YJ, Chan LD, Terk MR. The effect of bracing on patellofemoral joint stress during free and fast walking. *Am J Sports Med* 2004; 32(1): 224–31.

38. Lun VM, Wiley JP, Meeuwisse WH, Yanagawa TL. Effectiveness of patellar bracing for treatment of patellofemoral pain syndrome. *Clin J Sport Med* 2005; 15(4): 235–40.

39. Bolga L, Malone T. Exercise prescription and patellofemoral pain: evidence for rehabilitation. *J Sports Rehabil* 2005; 14: 72–88.

40. Bizzini M, Childs JD, Piva SR, et al. Systematic review of the quality of randomized controlled trials for patellofemoral pain. *J Orthop Sports Phys Ther* 2003; 33: 4–20.

41. Crossley K, Bennell K, Green S, McConnell J. A systematic review of physical interventions for patellofemoral pain syndrome. *Clin J Sport Med* 2001; 11(2): 103–10.

42. Whittingham M, Palmer S, Macmillan F. Effects of taping on pain and function in patellofemoral pain syndrome: a randomized controlled trial. *J Orthop Sports Phys Ther* 2004; 34(9): 504–10.

43. Crossley K, Bennell K, Green S, Cowan S, McConnell J. Physical therapy for patellofemoral pain: a randomized,

double-blinded, placebo-controlled trial. *Am J Sports Med* 2002; 30(6): 857–65.

44. Clark DI, Downing N, Mitchell J, et al. Physiotherapy for anterior knee pain: a randomised controlled trial. *Ann Rheum Dis* 2000; 59(9): 700–4.

45. Harrison EL, Sheppard MS, McQuarrie AM. A randomized controlled trial of physical therapy treatment programs in patellofemoral pain syndrome. *Physio Can* 1999; Spring: 93–106.

46. Eburne J, Bannister G . The McConnell regimen versus isometric quadriceps exercises in the management of anterior knee pain. A randomised prospective controlled trial. *The Knee* 1996; 3: 151–3.

47. Kowall MG, Kolk G, Nuber GW, Cassisi JE, Stern SH. Patellar taping in the treatment of patellofemoral pain. A prospective randomized study. *Am J Sports Med* 1996; 24(1): 61–6.

48. D'Hondt N E, Struijs PA, Kerkhoffs GM, et al. Orthotic devices for treating patellofemoral pain syndrome. *Cochrane Database Syst Rev* 2002; 2: CD002267.

49. Finestone A, Radin EL, Lev B, Shlamkovitch N, Wiener M, Milgrom C. Treatment of overuse patellofemoral pain. Prospective randomized controlled clinical trial in a military setting. *Clin Orthop* 1993; 293: 208–10.

50. Miller MD, Huinkin DT, Wisnowski JW. The efficacy of orthotics for anterior knee pain in military trainees. *Am J Knee Surg* 1997; 10: 10–13.

51. Rowlands BW, Brantingham JW. The efficacy of patellar mobilization in patients suffering from patellofemoral pain syndrome. *J Neuromusc Sys* 1999; 7(4): 142–9.

52. Taylor KE, Brantingham JW. An investigation into the effect of exercise combined with patella mobilization/manipulation in the treatment of patellofemoral pain syndrome: a randomized, assessor-blinded, controlled clinical pilot trial. *Eur J Chiro* 2003; 51(1): 5–17.

53. Heintjes E, Berger MY, Bierma-Zeinstra SMA, et al. Exercise therapy for patellofemoral pain syndrome. *Cochrane Database System Rev* 2003; 4.

54. Witvrouw E, Danneels L, Van Tiggelen D, et al. Open versus closed kinetic chain exercises in patellofemoral pain: a 5-year prospective randomized study. *Am J Sports Med* 2004; 32: 1122–30.

55. Witvrouw E, Lysens R, Bellemans J, et al. Open versus closed kinetic chain exercises for patellofemoral pain syndrome. *Am J Sports Med* 2000; 28(5): 687–94.

56. Schneider F, Labs K , Wagner S. Chronic patellofemoral pain syndrome: alternatives for cases of therapy resistance. *Knee Surg Sports Traumatol Arthrosc* 2001; 9: 290–5.

57. Timm KE. Randomized controlled trial of protonics on patellar pain, position, and function. *Med Sci Sports Exerc* 1998; 30: 665–70.

58. Thomee R. A comprehensive treatment approach for patellofemoral pain syndrome in young women. *Phys Ther* 1997; 77(12): 1690–703.

59. Stiene HA, Brosky T, Reinking MF, et al. A comparison of closed kinetic chain and isokinetic joint isolation in patients with patellofemoral dysfunction. *J Orthop Sports Phys Ther* 1996; 24(3): 136–41.

60. McMullen W, Roncarati A, Koval P. Static and isokinetic treatments of chondromalacia patella: a comparative investigation. *J Orthop Sports Phys Ther* 1980; 12(6): 256–66.

61. Arroll B, Ellis-Pegler E, Edwards RA, et al. Patellofemoral pain syndrome: a critical review of the clinical trials on nonoperative therapy. *Am J Sports Med* 1997; 25(2): 207–12.

62. Eng JJ, Pierrynowski MR. Evaluation of soft foot orthotics in the treatment of patellofemoral pain syndrome. *Phys Ther* 1993; 73(2): 62–8; discussion 68–70.

63. Wiener-Ogilvie S, Jones RB. A randomised trial of exercise therapy and foot orthoses as treatment for knee pain in primary care. *Br J Podiatr* 2004; 7(2): 43–9.

64. Gecha SR, Torg JS. Clinical prognosticators for the efficacy of retinacular release surgery to treat patellofemoral pain. *Clin Orthop* 1990; 253: 203–8.

65. Schottle PB, Fucentese SF, Romero J. Clinical and radiological outcome of medial patellofemoral ligament reconstruction with a semitendinosus autograft for patella instability. *Knee Surg Sports Traumatol Arthrosc* 2005; 13(7): 516–21.

66. Saddik D, McNally EG, Richardson M. MRI of Hoffa's fat pad. *Skeletal Radiol* 2004; 33(8): 433–44.

67. Blazina ME, Kerlan RK, Jobe FW, Carter VS, Carlson GJ. Jumper's knee. *Orthop Clin North Am* 1973; 4: 665–78.

68. Khan KM, Bonar F, Desmond PM, et al. Patellar tendinosis (jumper's knee): findings at histopathologic examination, US and MR imaging. *Radiology* 1996; 200: 821–7.

69. Maffulli N, Khan KM, Puddu G. Overuse tendon conditions. Time to change a confusing terminology. *Arthroscopy* 1998; 14: 840–3.

70. Khan KM, Cook JL, Bonar F, Harcourt P, Astrom M. Histopathology of common overuse tendon conditions: update and implications for clinical management. *Sports Med* 1999; 27: 393–408.

71. Maffulli N, Binfield PM, Leach WJ, King JB. Surgical management of tendinopathy of the main body of the patellar tendon in athletes. *Clin J Sport Med* 1999; 9: 58–62.

72. Visentini PJ, Khan KM, Cook JL, et al. The VISA score: an index of the severity of jumper's knee (patellar tendinosis). *J Sci Med Sport* 1998; 1: 22–8.

73. Khan KM, Maffulli N, Coleman BD, Cook JL, Taunton JE. Patellar tendinopathy: some aspects of basic science and clinical management. *Br J Sports Med* 1998; 32: 346–55.

74. Cook JL, Khan KM, Harcourt PR, et al. Patellar tendon ultrasonography in asymptomatic active athletes reveals hypoechoic regions: a study of 320 tendons. *Clin J Sport Med* 1998; 8: 73–7.

75. Khan KM, Visentini PJ, Kiss ZS, et al. Correlation of US and MR imaging with clinical outcome after open patellar tenotomy: prospective and retrospective studies. *Clin J Sport Med* 1999; 9: 129–37.

76. Richards DP, Ajeman SV, Wiley JP, Zernicke RF. Knee joint dynamics predict patellar tendinitis in elite volleyball players. *Am J Sports Med* 1996; 24(5): 676–83.

77. Cook JL, Khan KM, Kiss ZS, Griffiths L. Patellar tendinopathy in junior basketball players: a controlled clinical and ultrasonographic study of 268 patellar tendons in players aged 14–18 years. *Scand J Med Sci Sports* 2000; 10(4): 216–20.

78. Cook JL, Khan KM, Kiss ZS, Purdam C, Griffiths L. Prospective imaging study of asymptomatic patellar tendinopathy in elite junior basketball players. *J Ultrasound Med* 2000; 19: 473–9.

79. Stasinopoulos D, Stasinopoulos I. Comparison of effects of exercise programme, pulsed ultrasound and transverse friction in the treatment of chronic patellar tendinopathy. *Clin Rehabil* 2004; 18(4): 347–52.

80. Jensen K, Di Fabio RP. Evaluation of eccentric exercise in treatment of patellar tendinitis. *Phys Ther* 1989; 69: 211–16.

81. Cannell LJ, Taunton JE, Clement DB, Smith C, Khan KM. A randomized clinical trial of the efficacy of drop squats or leg extension/leg curl exercises to treat clinically-diagnosed jumper's knee in athletes. *Br J Sports Med* 2001; 35: 60–4.

82. Purdam C, Cook JL, Hopper D, Khan KM. Discriminative ability of functional loading tests for adolescent jumper's knee. *Phys Ther Sport* 2003; 4(1): 3–9.

83. Young JC, Cook JL, Purdam C, Kiss ZS, Alfredson H. Eccentric decline squat protocol offers superior results at 12 months compared with traditional eccentric protocol for patellar tendinopathy in volleyball players. *Br J Sports Med* 2005; 39: 102–5.

84. Visnes H, Hoksrud A, Cook J, Bahr R. No effect of eccentric training on jumper's knee in volleyball players during the competitive season: a randomized clinical trial. *Clin J Sport Med* 2005; 15(4): 227–34.

85. Wilson J, Sevier T, Helfst R, Honong E, Thomann A. Comparison of rehabilitation methods in the treatment of patellar tendinitis. *J Sport Rehabil* 2000; 9: 304–14.

86. Pellechia G, Hamel H, Behnke P. Treatment of infrapatellar tendinitis: a combination of modalities and transverse friction massage versus iontophoresis. *J Sport Rehabil* 1994; 3: 1315–45.

87. Capasso G, Testa V, Maffulli N, Bifulco G. Aprotinin, corticosteroids and normosaline in the management of patellar tendinopathy in athletes: a prospective randomized study. *Sports Exerc Injury* 1997; 3: 111–15.

88. Alfredson H, Ohberg L. Neovascularisation in chronic painful patellar tendinosis—promising results after sclerosing neovessels outside the tendon challenge the need for surgery. *Knee Surg Sports Traumatol Arthrosc* 2005; 13(2): 74–80.

89. Kelly DW, Carter VS, Jobe FW, et al. Patellar and quadriceps ruptures—jumper's knee. *Am J Sports Med* 1984; 12: 375–80.

90. Hoksrud A, Öhberg L, Alfredson H, Bahr R. Ultrasound-guided sclerosis of neovessels in painful chronic patellar tendinopathy—a randomized controlled trial. *Am J Sports Med* 2006; in press.

91. Panni AS, Tartarone M, Maffulli N. Patellar tendinopathy in athletes. Outcome of nonoperative and operative management. *Am J Sports Med* 2000; 28(3): 392–7.

92. Testa V, Capasso G, Maffulli N, Bifulco G. Ultrasound guided percutaneous longitudinal tenotomy for the management of patellar tendinopathy. *Med Sci Sports Exerc* 1999; 31: 1509–15.

93. Coleman BD, Khan KM, Kiss ZS, Bartlett J, Young DA, Wark JD. Outcomes of open and arthroscopic patellar tenotomy for chronic patellar tendinopathy: a retrospective study. *Am J Sports Med* 2000; 28: 183–90.

94. Coleman BD, Khan KM, Maffulli N, Cook JL, Wark JD. Studies of surgical outcome after patellar tendinopathy: clinical significance of methodological deficiencies and guidelines for future studies. *Scand J Med Sci Sports* 2000; 10(1): 2–11.

Lateral, Medial and Posterior Knee Pain

Although acute knee injuries and anterior knee pain are very common presentations in sports medicine practice, patients presenting with lateral, medial or posterior knee pain can also provide challenges to the practitioner.

Lateral knee pain

Pain about the lateral knee (Fig. 29.1) is a frequent problem, especially among distance runners. The most common cause of lateral knee pain is iliotibial band friction syndrome (ITBFS). With repeated knee flexion/extension, the iliotibial band (ITB) rubs against the prominent lateral epicondyle of the femur. Training errors and biomechanical abnormalities can precipitate ITBFS. Patellofemoral syndrome (Chapter 28) may also present as lateral knee pain. In the older active person, degeneration of the lateral meniscus or lateral compartment osteoarthritis should be considered.

The biceps femoris tendon may become inflamed as it passes posterolaterally to the knee and inserts into the head of the fibula. This occurs in sprinters and footballers. Injuries of the superior tibiofibular

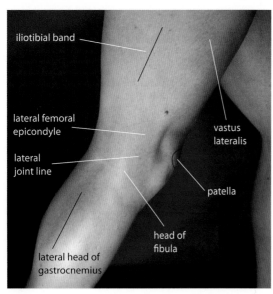

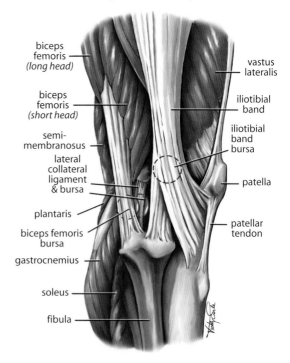

Figure 29.1 Lateral aspect of the knee

(a) Surface anatomy

(b) Anatomy of lateral aspect of the knee

joint may cause lateral knee pain. It is not uncommon for lateral knee pain to occur as a result of referred pain from the lumbar spine. The causes of lateral knee pain are shown in Table 29.1.

History

A history of overuse may be suggestive of ITBFS or biceps femoris tendinopathy. If there is a history of excessive downhill running or running on an uneven surface, ITBFS may be implicated. If the pain tends to occur with sprinting or kicking activities, biceps femoris tendinopathy is more likely. Lateral knee pain following knee or ankle injury may indicate the superior tibiofibular joint or lateral meniscus as the site of injury.

The pain of biceps femoris tendinopathy is maximal initially on activity and settles with warming up, returning following activity or the next day. With progression of the condition, pain may persist during exercise and be sufficient to cause the athlete to cease sporting activity. ITB pain usually does not lessen with activity. Pain on sudden twisting or a history of giving way or locking may be indicative of degenerative lateral meniscus problems. Pain associated with excessive lateral pressure syndrome increases with activity. As the population of active individuals who are over 50 years old increases, the diagnosis of lateral compartment osteoarthritis must be considered.

The presence of back pain may suggest referred pain from the lumbar spine. Associated neurological symptoms such as weakness and paresthesia in the lower leg may indicate common peroneal nerve entrapment.

Examination

Full assessment of the ligaments of the knee (Chapter 27) should be included in the examination. Biomechanical examination should also be performed.

1. Observation
   (a) standing
   (b) walking
   (c) supine
   (d) side-lying
2. Active movements
   (a) knee flexion
   (b) knee extension
   (c) repeated knee flexion (0–30°) (Fig. 29.2a)
   (d) tibial rotation
3. Passive movements
   (a) knee flexion/extension
   (b) tibial rotation (Fig. 29.2b)
   (c) superior tibiofibular joint
       (i) accessory glides (Fig. 29.2c)
   (d) muscle stretches
       (i) ITB (Ober's test) (Fig. 29.2d)
       (ii) quadriceps
       (iii) hamstring
4. Resisted movements
   (a) knee flexion (Fig. 29.2e)
   (b) tibial rotation
5. Functional movements
   (a) hopping
   (b) squat
   (c) jumping
6. Palpation
   (a) lateral femoral epicondyle (Fig. 29.2f)
   (b) lateral joint line
   (c) lateral retinaculum
   (d) lateral border of patella
   (e) superior tibiofibular joint
   (f) biceps femoris tendon
   (g) gluteus medius
7. Special tests
   (a) full knee examination (Chapter 27)
       (i) effusion (Fig. 29.2g)
       (ii) McMurray's test (Fig. 29.2h)

Table 29.1 Causes of lateral knee pain

Common	Less common	Not to be missed
Iliotibial band friction syndrome	Patellofemoral syndrome	Common peroneal nerve injury
Lateral meniscus abnormality	Osteoarthritis of the lateral	Slipped capital femoral epiphysis
Minor tear	compartment of the knee	Perthes' disease
Degenerative change	Excessive lateral pressure syndrome	
Cyst	Biceps femoris tendinopathy	
	Superior tibiofibular joint sprain	
	Synovitis of the knee joint	
	Referred pain	
	Lumbar spine	
	Neural	

(b) neural tension tests
  (i) prone knee bend
  (ii) slump (Fig. 29.2i)
(c) lumbar spine (Chapter 21)
(d) biomechanical assessment (Chapter 5)
  (Fig. 29.2j)

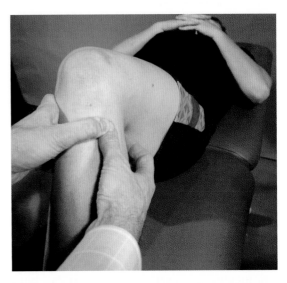

(c) Passive movements—accessory anteroposterior glide to superior tibiofibular joint

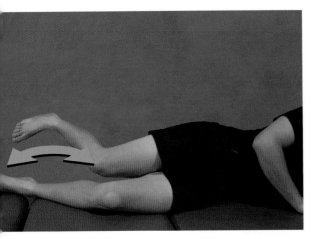

Figure 29.2 Examination of the patient with lateral knee pain

(a) Active movements—repeated flexion from 0° to 30°. This may reproduce the patient's pain if ITBFS is the cause. It can be performed in a side-lying position (illustrated), standing or as a squat

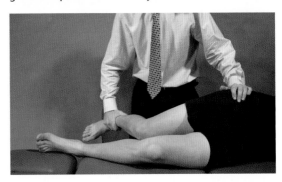

(d) Passive movement—ITB stretch. This is performed in a side-lying position with the hip in neutral rotation and knee flexion. The hip is extended and then adducted. If the ITB is tight, knee extension will occur with adduction (Ober's test)

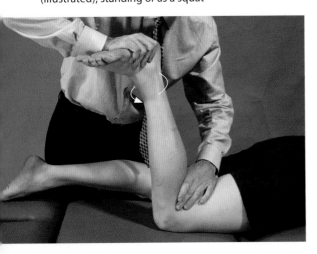

(b) Passive movements—tibial rotation. This is performed in knee flexion to assess superior tibiofibular joint movement

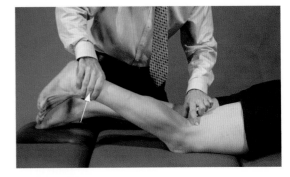

(e) Resisted movement—knee flexion. Concentric or eccentric contractions may reproduce the pain of biceps femoris tendinopathy

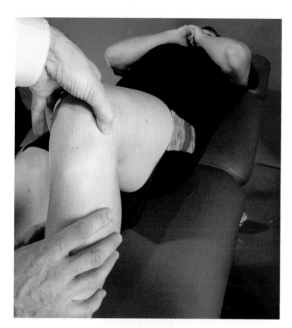

(f) Palpation—lateral femoral epicondyle

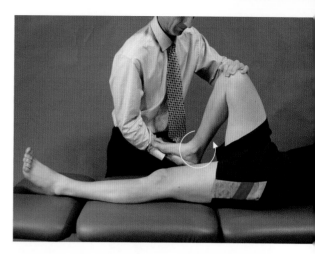

(h) Special tests—McMurray's test. The knee is flexed and, at various stages of flexion, internal and external rotation of the tibia are performed. The presence of pain and a palpable 'clunk' is a positive McMurray's test and is consistent with meniscal injury. If there is no 'clunk' but the patient's pain is reproduced, then the meniscus may be damaged or there may be patellofemoral joint abnormality

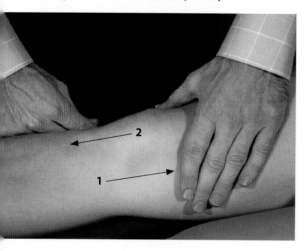

(g) Special test—knee effusion. Manually drain the medial subpatellar pouch by stroking the fluid in a superior direction. Then 'milk' the fluid back into the knee from above while observing the pouch for evidence that fluid is reaccumulating

Investigations

X-ray is useful in cases of persistent lateral knee pain in the older athlete to exclude lateral compartment osteoarthritis. A diagnostic local anesthetic injection can be used to differentiate local soft tissue pain (e.g. ITBFS) from any possible intra-articular or referred pain. Ultrasound or MRI may be useful to identify

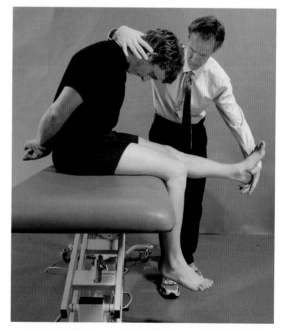

(i) Special tests—neural tension test. The slump test should be performed

the presence of a bursa under the ITB.[1] However, in the majority of patients with lateral knee pain, investigations are not required.

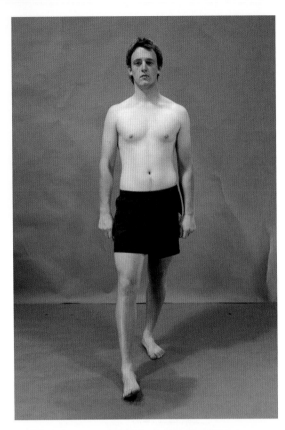

(j) Special tests—biomechanical assessment. Full lower limb biomechanical assessment should be performed while standing, walking and lying. Abnormal pelvic movements (e.g. excessive lateral tilt) should be noted

Iliotibial band friction syndrome

ITBFS occurs as a result of friction between the ITB and the underlying lateral epicondyle of the femur (Fig. 29.3a) Friction (or impingement) occurs near foot strike, predominantly in the foot contact phase, between the posterior edge of the iliotibial band and the underlying lateral femoral epicondyle. Runners have an average knee flexion angle of 21° at foot strike, with friction occurring at, or slightly below, 30° of flexion (Fig. 29.3b).[2] Substantial variation occurs in the width of the iliotibial bands between individuals, which may affect predisposition to ITBFS. Downhill running predisposes the runner to ITBFS because the knee flexion angle at foot strike is reduced. Sprinting and faster running on level ground are less likely to cause or aggravate ITBFS because, at foot strike, the knee is flexed beyond the angles at which friction occurs.

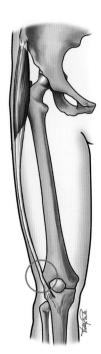

Figure 29.3 Site of ITB friction over the lateral epicondyle

(a) anterior view

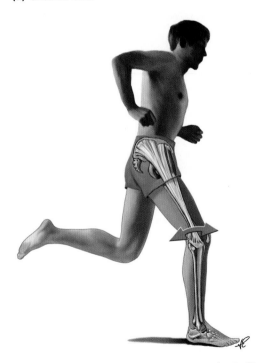

(b) lateral view—friction occurs at around 30° of knee flexion

Traditionally, it was thought that friction might lead to the development of ITB tendinopathy or inflammation of an anatomical bursa lying between the tendon and the lateral epicondyle. Recent clinical studies with MRI suggest the main abnormality is local fluid in an adventitious (secondary) bursa and that the ITB tendon itself generally remains intact.[1] This suggests the pathology is *not* a tendinopathy (Chapter 2).

Runners with ITBFS have been found to be weaker in knee flexion and knee extension, with decreased braking forces.[3] Studies have shown that runners with ITBFS have significant weakness of their hip abductors in the affected limb,[4] and have a decreased ability of the hip abductors to eccentrically control abduction.[5]

Clinical features

The athlete with ITBFS complains of an ache over the lateral aspect of the knee aggravated by running. If running a consistent course, pain seems to come on at about the same distance/time on each run. Longer runs or those down hill or on cambered courses are particularly aggravating.

On examination, tenderness is elicited over the lateral epicondyle of the femur 2–3 cm (~1 in.) above the lateral joint line. Crepitus may also be felt. Repeated flexion/extension of the knee may reproduce the patient's symptoms.

Ober's test (Fig. 29.2d) may reveal ITB tightness. This may be secondary either to tightness of the ITB fascia distally, shortening of the tensor fascia lata or gluteus maximus muscles proximally, or excessive development of the vastus lateralis, placing increased tensile load on the ITB.

The body of the ITB should be palpated for the presence of trigger points and focal areas of tightness. Tightness of the gluteal muscles and tensor fascia lata are commonly associated with ITBFS. The presence of trigger points in the tensor fascia lata, gluteus minimus and gluteus medius may contribute to ITBFS.

Hip abduction strength should also be assessed as weakness of hip abductors is associated with ITBFS.[4] Another study also found weakness in the hip flexors, but increased hip adductor strength, in addition to the abductor weakness.[6]

Two other common associations with ITBFS are inappropriate training and abnormal biomechanics, as both subject the ITB to extra load.

Excessive pronation may lead to increased internal rotation of the tibia. Increased varus alignment of the foot and lower limb may lead to varus strain on the knee. Excessive lateral tilting of the pelvis (Chapter 5) may place increased strain on the lateral thigh. A functional video analysis of the running action of patients with ITBFS may be required to detect bio-mechanical abnormality.

Imaging is not usually required to confirm the diagnosis of ITBFS. Both ultrasound and MRI will show thickening of the ITB over the lateral femoral condyle at the knee and often a fluid collection deep to the ITB at the same site.[7]

Treatment

Treatment of ITBFS includes:

- Activity modification. Avoid all pain-provoking activities such as downhill running.
- Symptomatic relief using ice, analgesics and electrotherapeutic modalities (e.g. TENS, interferential stimulation, ultrasound). Corticosteroid injection into the bursa between the ITB tendon and the lateral epicondyle reduces pain in acute cases (Fig. 29.4).[8]
- Soft tissue therapy aimed at correcting excessive tightness in the ITB and related structures (e.g. tensor fascia lata, quadriceps, hip abductors, rotators and extensors). Deep friction massage has not been found to be successful.[9] The most effective soft tissue techniques in the treatment of ITBFS are sustained myofascial release (Fig. 29.5a), ischemic pressure to the body of the ITB (Fig. 29.5b), and dry needling to ITB trigger points (Fig. 29.5c). Self massage can be performed with a foam roll (Fig. 29.5d) Gluteal trigger point (Fig. 22.9) dry needling (Fig. 29.5e) and ischemic pressure should also be performed.

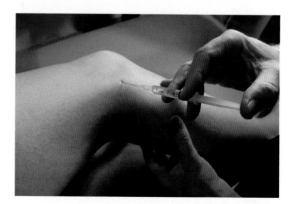

Figure 29.4 Corticosteroid injection into the bursa between the ITB tendon and the underlying lateral femoral condyle

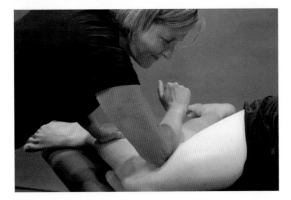

Figure 29.5 Treating tight myofascial structures

(a) Sustained myofascial tension to the proximal ITB

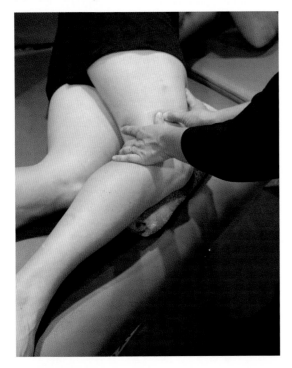

(b) Ischemic pressure to the body of the ITB

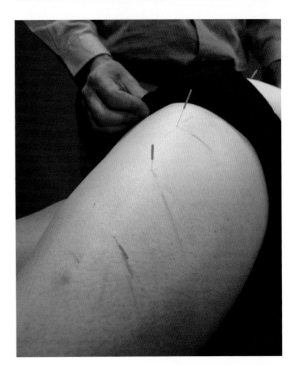

(c) Dry needling to ITB trigger points

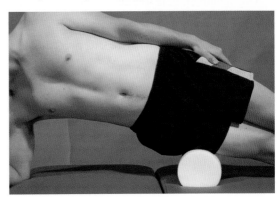

(d) Foam roll self massage to the ITB

- Frequent stretching of the ITB and other tight muscles with occasional sustained ITB stretches for 3 minutes to maintain fascial tissue length (Fig. 29.6). Adding an overhead arm extension to the normal ITB stretch increases the force generated in lengthening the ITB.[10]
- Strengthening of the lateral stabilizers of the hip/hip abductors (Fig. 29.7).

- Biomechanical abnormalities such as excessive subtalar pronation or excessive lateral tilting of the pelvis should be corrected.
- Surgery to release the ITB and excise the bursa may be indicated if conservative management fails. Methods used include excision of a triangular area of the ITB from the area overlying the lateral condyle when the knee is in a 30° position,[11] transection of the posterior half of the width of the ITB over the lateral condyle,[12] Z-lengthening of the iliotibial band,[13] or distal detachment and multiple puncture.[14]

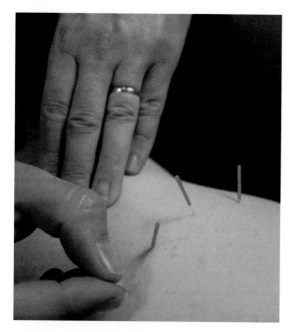

(e) Dry needling to gluteal trigger points

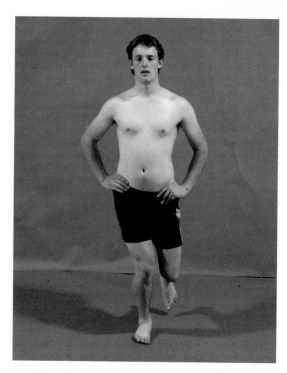

Figure 29.7 Strengthening exercises for the external hip rotators

(a) Exercise involves the patient standing on one leg and slowly performing a squat maintaining pelvic stability

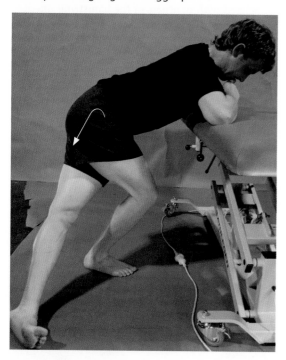

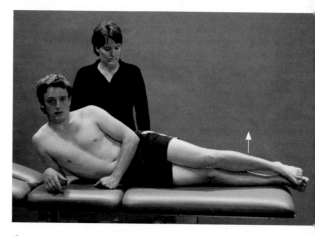

(b) Hip abduction in side-lying

Figure 29.6 ITB stretch—the ITB on the left side is being stretched. The symptomatic leg is extended and adducted across the uninvolved leg. The patient exhales and slowly flexes the trunk laterally to the opposite side until a stretch is felt on the side of the hip

- Resume running when there is no local tenderness and the strengthening exercises can be performed without pain. Initially run on alternate days and avoid downhill running.

Lateral meniscus abnormality

Meniscal abnormality and its typical acute clinical presentation are discussed in Chapter 27. However, degeneration of the lateral meniscus can also present as gradual-onset lateral knee pain. Thus, if a runner presents complaining of lateral knee pain that comes on after 20 minutes of running and is aggravated by running up hills, the practitioner should not automatically assume that the patient has ITBFS—the problem may relate to a degenerative meniscus. Careful physical examination should help distinguish the conditions. The meniscus is tender along the joint line, 2–3 cm below the site of tenderness in ITBFS. McMurray's test in full flexion (Fig. 29.2h) should also help to distinguish the conditions, as it should be positive when a meniscal injury is present and negative in cases of ITBFS.

Note that a degenerative meniscus can present as a painful or non-painful lump at the lateral joint line. This is sometimes misdiagnosed as an ITB bursa. If there is doubt as to the correct diagnosis, MRI is the investigation of choice.

Osteoarthritis of the lateral compartment of the knee

Lateral knee pain can also be caused by degeneration of the lateral tibial plateau and this is often found in conjunction with meniscal injury. Early in the disease, the patient often gives a history of increasing knee pain with activity and stiffness after resting.

As the disease progresses, the patient experiences pain at night that may disturb sleep associated with morning stiffness, usually for less than half an hour. In the early stages of the condition, examination may only reveal a small effusion.

A very useful investigation is weight-bearing plain X-ray. This has greater sensitivity than views taken with the patient supine. Initial treatment of osteoarthritis includes symptomatic relief with analgesia and NSAIDs if required, modification of activity and exercise prescription, together with weight loss if indicated. Intra-articular hyaluronic acid supplements (viscosupplements) have a similar efficacy to NSAIDs but the patient does not have to take tablets daily.[15, 16] Patients with severe clinical symptoms may require unicompartmental[17] or, eventually, total knee replacement.

Excessive lateral pressure syndrome

Excessive lateral pressure syndrome (lateral patellar compression syndrome) occurs when there is excessive pressure on the lateral patellofemoral joint resulting from a tight lateral retinaculum. This pressure may lead to increased bone strain on the lateral patella, inflammation of the lateral retinaculum and ITBFS.

The increased bone strain on the lateral patella may lead to development of a vertical stress fracture or even separation of the lateral patellar fragment. This must be differentiated radiologically from the congenital bipartite patella. The separated fragment is in the superolateral aspect of the patella. MRI has been used to image this condition.[18]

Initial treatment consists of patellofemoral mobilization and soft tissue therapy to the lateral retinaculum. Taping techniques rarely help. Surgical lateral retinacular release or even removal of the lateral patellar fragment is occasionally required.[19]

Biceps femoris tendinopathy

Biceps femoris tendinopathy occurs with excessive acceleration and deceleration activities. The pain can be produced with resisted flexion, especially with eccentric contractions (Fig. 29.2e). It is often associated with tightness of the hamstring muscles. Stiffness of the lumbar spine may contribute to hamstring tightness. Ultrasound examination may help confirm the diagnosis.

Treatment is based on the general principles of the treatment of tendinopathy: relative rest, soft tissue therapy (Fig. 29.8), stretching and strengthening, especially eccentric strengthening (Fig. 29.9).

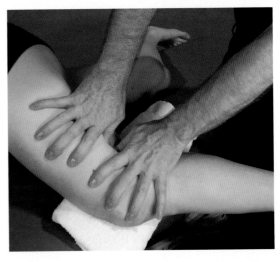

Figure 29.8 Soft tissue therapy in the treatment of biceps femoris tendinopathy. Ischemic pressure at the musculotendinous junction (shown) and muscle belly can be effective

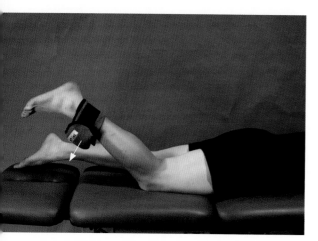

Figure 29.9 Eccentric strengthening exercises in the treatment of biceps femoris tendinopathy. Drop-and-catch is performed in prone positions (Chapter 26). This may be progressed to include hip flexion (i.e. patient lying over the end of the bed)

Superior tibiofibular joint injury

Superior tibiofibular joint injury may result from direct trauma or in association with rotational knee or ankle injuries. Pain occurs with activities demanding tibial rotation (e.g. pivoting, cutting). The patient may feel the pain distally in the shin and not localize the pain to the superior tibiofibular joint. On examination, the joint is tender and there may be either restricted or excessive movement on passive gliding of the superior tibiofibular joint (Fig. 29.2c).

Manual mobilization is an effective treatment for the stiff tibiofibular joint. Excessively mobile joints are more difficult to treat. Local electrotherapy may help relieve pain. Strengthening of the tibial rotators may help support the joint. Predisposing factors, such as excessive pronation, which place greater torsional forces through the joint, require correction. Occasionally in patients who fail to respond to conservative measures, a corticosteroid injection may be used. For patients with chronic pain or instability, surgical options include arthrodesis, fibular head resection, and proximal tibiofibular joint capsule reconstruction.[20]

Referred pain

Pain may refer from the lumbar spine to the lateral aspect of the knee. Referred pain is usually a dull ache and is poorly localized. The slump test may be positive. The lumbar spine should be examined in patients presenting with atypical lateral knee pain.

Medial knee pain

Pain about the medial knee (Fig. 29.10) is less common than anterior and lateral knee pain. The causes of medial knee pain are shown in Table 29.2.

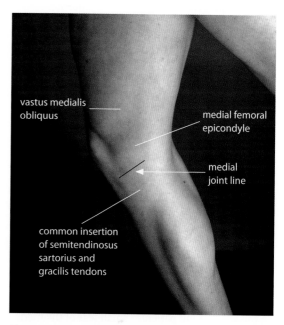

Figure 29.10 Medial aspect of the knee

(a) Surface anatomy

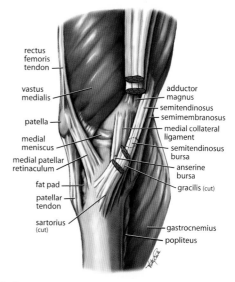

(b) Anatomy (ADAPTED FROM THE *CIBA COLLECTION OF MEDICAL ILLUSTRATIONS*, REPRODUCED BY COURTESY OF CIBA-GEIGY LIMITED, BASEL, SWITZERLAND. ALL RIGHTS RESERVED)

Table 29.2 Causes of medial knee pain

Common	Less common	Not to be missed
Patellofemoral syndrome	Synovial plica	Tumor (in the young)
Medial meniscus	Pes anserinus	Slipped capital femoral epiphysis
Minor tear	Tendinopathy	Referred pain from the hip
Degenerative change	Bursitis	Perthes' disease
Cyst	Medial collateral ligament	
	Grade I sprain/bursitis	
	Pellegrini-Stieda lesion	
	Osteoarthritis of the medial	
	compartment of the knee	
	Referred pain	
	Lumbar spine	
	Hip joint	
	Neural	

Patellofemoral syndrome

In most cases of medial knee pain, the pain is actually anteromedial and is most frequently due to patellofemoral syndrome. The patellofemoral joint commonly refers pain to the medial aspect of the knee. The patellofemoral syndrome has been discussed in Chapter 29.

Medial meniscus abnormality

In the young adult patient, a small tear of the medial meniscus may cause a synovial reaction and medial knee pain (Fig. 29.11). In the older patient, gradual degeneration of the medial meniscus can present as gradual-onset medial knee pain. The clinical scenario is similar to that described for a lateral meniscal abnormality above. The patient is generally aged over 35 years and complains of clicking and pain with certain twisting activities, such as getting out of a car or rolling over in bed. Examination reveals joint line tenderness and a positive McMurray's test (Fig. 29.2h). MRI is the investigation of choice. Treatment is as for an acute meniscal injury—conservative management is warranted but, if this fails, arthroscopic partial medial menisectomy is indicated.

Osteoarthritis of the medial compartment of the knee

The patient is generally in the age group that is prone to osteoarthritis (commonly >50 years). There may be a history of acute ligament injury in the past that makes him or her prone to osteoarthritis. In the early stages, it is very difficult to distinguish this condition clinically from medial meniscal injury. If weight-bearing X-rays are normal, MRI can distinguish the two conditions using specific articular cartilage sequences, including

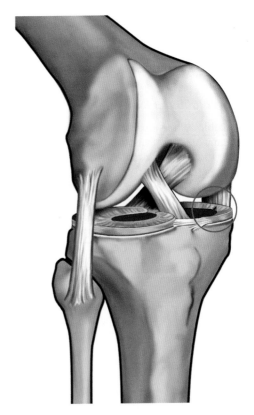

Figure 29.11 Medial meniscus tear—a common cause of medial knee pain

the technique of delayed gadolinium-enhanced MRI of cartilage (dGEMRIC), which estimates cartilage quality.[21] Management of osteoarthritis includes symptomatic relief with analgesia and NSAIDs, modification of activity and exercise prescription,[16] together with weight loss if indicated. Viscosupplementation is an effective treatment for osteoarthritis of the knee with beneficial effects on pain, function and patient global assessment, especially at the fifth to 13th week post-injection period.[15, 22]

A randomized clinical trial found that a custom-made, valgus-producing functional knee (unloader) brace provided significant benefit in this population of patients aged in their 60s.[23] Biomechanical studies have shown that these braces maintain condylar separation.[24] Whether similar results are found in younger, more active patients with significant medial joint osteoarthritis remains to be studied. If clinical symptoms are persistent and severe, referral to an orthopedic surgeon is warranted. Surgical intervention may include high tibial osteotomy and total knee replacement.

Pes anserinus tendinopathy/bursitis

The pes anserinus ('goose's foot') is the combined tendinous insertion of the sartorius, gracilis and semitendinosus tendons at their attachment to the tibia (Fig. 29.10b). The pes anserinus bursa lies between this insertion and the periosteum and may become inflamed as a result of overuse in swimmers (particularly breaststrokers), cyclists or runners.

Pes anserinus tendinopathy/bursitis is characterized by localized tenderness and swelling. Active contraction or stretching of the medial hamstring muscles reproduces pain. Treatment follows the general principles of tendinopathy/bursitis management. Excessive tightness will often be evident in the associated muscles. Clinical experience has found corticosteroid injection into the bursa to be extremely effective.

Pellegrini-Stieda syndrome

Pellegrini-Stieda syndrome is a disruption of the femoral origin of the medial collateral ligament with calcification at the site of injury. It can be a difficult lesion to assess before radiological changes become evident. It may follow direct trauma or, less frequently, a grade II or III sprain of the medial collateral ligament. Note that imaging abnormalities exist in asymptomatic individuals.[25]

Pellegrini-Stieda syndrome is an important cause of knee stiffness. The patient complains of difficulty straightening the leg and twisting. Examination reveals marked restriction in joint range of motion with a tender lump in the proximal portion of the medial collateral ligament. Treatment consists of active mobilization of the knee joint and infiltration of a corticosteroid agent to the tender medial collateral ligament attachment if pain persists.

Other causes of medial knee pain

A grade I medial collateral ligament sprain or bursitis may often present without a history of any major trauma. The medial collateral ligament may also become inflamed as a result of activities that put a constant valgus strain on the knee, such as swimming breaststroke. This condition is commonly referred to as 'breaststroker's knee' and is actually a first degree sprain of the medial collateral ligament or inflammation of the medial collateral ligament bursa due to excessive stress. A synovial plica may present as medial knee pain (Chapter 28).

Posterior knee pain

The diagnosis of pain about the posterior knee (Fig. 29.12) may be difficult. Posterior knee pain is a common site of referred pain from the lumbar spine and from the patellofemoral joint. Alternatively, local structures (e.g. popliteus, biceps femoris tendon) may cause posterior knee pain. A knee effusion is a common cause of pain and tightness of the back of the knee. The causes of posterior knee pain are shown in Table 29.3.

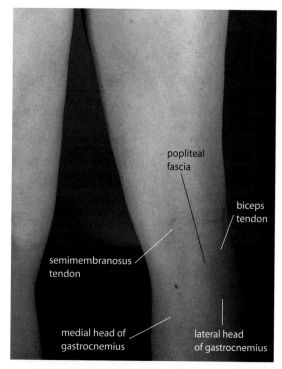

Figure 29.12 Posterior aspect of the knee

(a) Surface anatomy

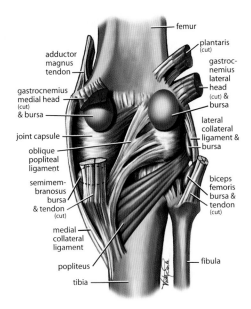

femur

plantaris (cut)

adductor magnus tendon

gastrocnemius lateral head (cut) & bursa

gastrocnemius medial head (cut) & bursa

lateral collateral ligament & bursa

joint capsule

oblique popliteal ligament

semimembranosus bursa & tendon (cut)

biceps femoris bursa & tendon (cut)

medial collateral ligament

popliteus

fibula

tibia

(b) Anatomy (ADAPTED FROM THE *CIBA COLLECTION OF MEDICAL ILLUSTRATIONS*, REPRODUCED BY COURTESY OF CIBA-GEIGY LIMITED, BASEL, SWITZERLAND. ALL RIGHTS RESERVED)

History

Posterior knee pain precipitated by acceleration or deceleration (e.g. downhill running, kicking, sprinting) is likely to be biceps femoris or popliteus tendinopathy. Pain described as a poorly localized dull ache not directly related to activity suggests referred pain. The presence of low back pain or patellofemoral symptoms provides a diagnostic clue. A previous acute knee injury may have caused an effusion with development of a Baker's cyst.

Examination

In the examination of the posterior aspect of the knee, it is important to differentiate between local and referred causes of pain. The slump test may indicate whether the pain is referred from the lumbar spine or neural structures. It is also important to detect the

presence of an effusion as this may be the cause of the posterior knee pain.

1. Observation
   (a) standing (Fig. 29.13a)
   (b) prone
2. Active movements
   (a) flexion
   (b) extension
   (c) tibial rotation
3. Passive movements
   (a) flexion
   (b) extension
   (c) tibial rotation
   (d) muscle stretch—hamstrings
4. Resisted movements
   (a) knee flexion
   (b) knee flexion in external tibial rotation (Fig. 29.13b)
   (c) external tibial rotation (Fig. 29.13c)
5. Palpation (Fig. 29.13d)
   (a) hamstring tendons
   (b) popliteus
   (c) joint line
   (d) gastrocnemius origin
6. Special tests
   (a) knee effusion
   (b) examination of knee joint (Chapter 27)
   (c) neural tension—slump test (Fig. 29.2i)
   (d) examination of lumbar spine (Chapter 21)
   (e) biomechanical examination (Chapter 5)

Investigations

Investigations are not appropriate in most cases of posterior knee pain. Ultrasound may confirm the presence of a Baker's cyst or identify a tendinopathy. MRI or arthroscopy are the investigations of choice if the diagnosis remains difficult.

Popliteus tendinopathy

The popliteus muscle arises from the posteromedial border of the proximal tibial metaphysis and travels

Table 29.3 Causes of posterior knee pain

Common	Less common	Not to be missed
Knee joint effusion	Popliteus tendinopathy	Deep venous thrombosis
Referred pain	Baker's cyst	Claudication
Lumbar spine	Gastrocnemius tendinopathy	Posterior cruciate ligament sprain
Patellofemoral joint		
Neural tension		
Biceps femoris tendinopathy		

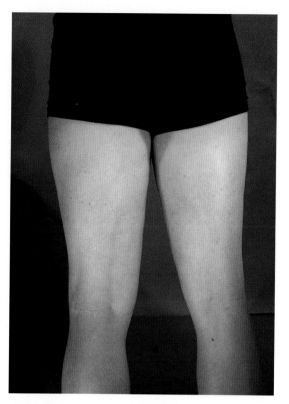

Figure 29.13 Examination of patient with posterior knee pain

(a) Observation—standing. Obvious swelling or fullness of the posterior aspect of the knee joint suggests a Baker's cyst. Inspection may reveal a biomechanical abnormality

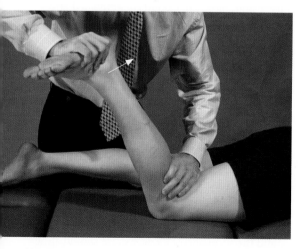

(b) Resisted movements—knee flexion in external tibial rotation. Resisted contraction of the popliteus tendon

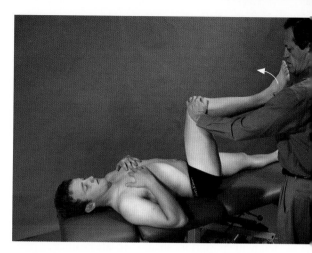

(c) Resisted movement—popliteus. With the patient supine, hips and knees flexed to 90° and the leg internally rotated, the patient is asked to 'hold it there' while the examiner applies an external rotation force

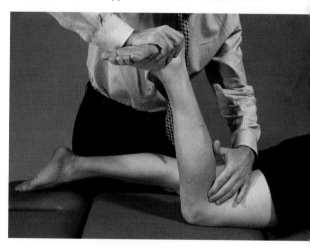

(d) Palpation. This should be performed with the knee in flexion. Tenderness can be elicited over the hamstring tendons (shown), gastrocnemius origin or popliteus. It is helpful for the patient to gently contract and relax individual muscles that are being palpated in order for the examiner to precisely pinpoint the site of pain

proximally beneath the lateral head of the gastrocnemius to insert on the lateral femoral condyle. It also has attachments to the fibula and the lateral meniscus. The popliteus has a number of actions:

• primary internal rotator of the tibia

- during initial flexion from an extended position it will unlock the knee
- acts with the quadriceps and posterior cruciate ligament to prevent forward displacement of the femur on the tibia during deceleration and downhill running
- provides varus and valgus stability
- allows retraction of the posterior horn of the lateral meniscus during knee flexion.

Popliteus region pain may arise from the popliteus muscle, its tendon or the popliteus–arcuate ligament complex. These structures lie close together and thus pain in this area is difficult to isolate. Pain is most commonly due to an increased range of tibial rotation following posterior capsule–arcuate ligament strain. The popliteus may then become injured as a result of a direct stretch or because it is used excessively to try to maintain posterolateral instability. Occasionally, it suffers overuse in acceleration/deceleration activities.

The main clinical finding is tenderness on palpation along the proximal aspect of the tendon (Fig. 29.13d). With the patient prone, palpate commencing near the posterolateral corner medial to the biceps tendon and palpate along the medial joint line. Resisted knee flexion in external tibial rotation will be painful in popliteus injuries (Fig. 29.13b). Garrick and Webb[26] describe a test for the popliteus with the patient supine, hips and knees flexed to 90° and the leg internally rotated. The patient is asked to 'hold it there' while the examiner applies an external rotation force (Fig. 29.13c). The clinician should assess active and passive tibial rotation. Excessive rotation may underlie repeated strain to the area. Restricted range of motion may also produce pain. Lower limb biomechanics should be assessed.

Treatment includes strengthening of the tibial rotators (Fig. 29.14) and hamstring muscles. Massage therapy and mobilization may help to correct any restriction of tibial rotation, knee flexion or rotation. Posterior knee structures, especially the hamstring muscles, should be stretched. NSAIDs, electrical stimulation and ultrasound may prove useful adjuncts to rehabilitation.

The popliteus works with the quadriceps to stabilize the knee, so any weakness or fatigue in the quadriceps puts excessive strain on the popliteus and should be corrected. An eccentric strengthening program for the quadriceps should be commenced.

Patients who fail to respond to the above regimen may respond to a corticosteroid injection posteriorly into the point of maximal tenderness.[27]

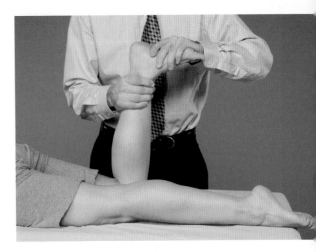

Figure 29.14 Strengthening of the tibial rotators. This may be performed against manual resistance (illustrated), with pulleys, rubber tubing resistance or with isokinetic machines

Gastrocnemius tendinopathy

With overuse, the origin of the medial gastrocnemius at the posterior femoral condyle occasionally becomes painful. This may result from excessive hill running or a rapid increase in mileage. Examination may reveal local tenderness. Pain may be reproduced on resisted knee flexion, calf raise with the knee in extension, jumping, hopping or, occasionally, with stretch of the gastrocnemius muscle. Treatment consists of ice, electrotherapy, soft tissue therapy to correct generalized or focal abnormalities of the gastrocnemius muscle and, most importantly, a graduated stretching/strengthening program (Chapter 32).

Biceps femoris tendinopathy

Biceps femoris tendinopathy has been described above under lateral knee pain (p. 546).

Baker's cyst

Baker's cyst is a chronic knee joint effusion (Fig. 29.15) that herniates between the two heads of the gastrocnemius. It occurs most commonly secondary to degenerative or meniscal abnormality. The amount of swelling may fluctuate. Examination findings are a swollen, tender mass over the posterolateral joint line. There may be other signs of intra-articular abnormality and the suspicion of a Baker's cyst should always lead to a full assessment of the knee joint. MRI will both confirm the presence of the cyst and may identify the underlying degenerative or meniscal cause.[28]

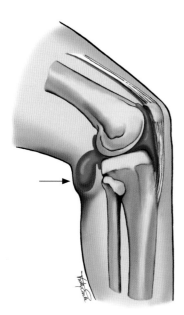

Figure 29.15 Baker's cyst (arrowed)—knee joint effusion herniating posteriorly; usually secondary to degenerative or meniscal pathology

Occasionally the cyst may rupture, leading to lower leg swelling simulating venous thrombosis. A ruptured cyst usually displays a 'crescent sign'—an ecchymotic ('bruised') area around the malleoli.

Treatment of the Baker's cyst involves treatment of the associated abnormality.

Deep venous thrombosis

Deep venous thrombosis usually presents as calf pain (Chapter 31) but may occasionally present as posterior knee pain. It usually occurs after surgery or following a period of immobilization.

Claudication

Claudication can occasionally present as posterior knee pain (Chapter 29). It can occur in young adults, not only in the older person. Popliteal artery entrapment syndrome usually presents as calf pain (Chapter 31).

Recommended Reading

Fredericson M, Guilet M, DeBenedictis L. Quick solutions for iliotibial band syndrome. *Physician Sportsmed* 2000; 28(2): 53–68.

Fredericson M, Wolf C. Iliotibial band syndrome in runners. Innovations in treatment. *Sports Med* 2005; 35: 451–9.

Muche JA, Lento PH. Posterior knee pain and its causes. *Physician Sportsmed* 2004; 32(3): 23–30.

Nyland J, Lachman N, Kocabey Y, et al. Anatomy, function, and rehabilitation of the popliteus musculotendinous complex. *J Orthop Sports Phys Ther* 2005; 35: 165–79.

Petsche TS, Selesnick FH. Popliteus tendonitis. Tips for diagnosis and management. *Physician Sportsmed* 2002; 30(8): 27–31.

References

1. Muhle C, Ahn JM, Yeh L, et al. Iliotibial band friction syndrome: MR findings in 16 patients and MR arthrographic studies of six cadaveric knees. *Radiology* 1999; 212: 103–10.
2. Orchard J, Fricker PA, Abud AT, et al. Biomechanics of iliotibial band friction syndrome in runners. *Am J Sports Med* 1996; 24(3): 375–9.
3. Messier SP, Edwards DG, Martin DF, et al. Etiology of iliotibial band friction syndrome in distance runners. *Med Sci Sports Exerc* 1995; 27(7): 951–60.
4. Fredericson M, Cookingham CL, Chaudhari AM, et al. Hip abductor weakness in distance runners with iliotibial band syndrome. *Clin J Sport Med* 2000; 10: 169–75.
5. Fredericson M, Wolf C. Iliotibial band syndrome in runners. *Sports Med* 2005; 35(5): 451–9.
6. Niemuth PE, Johnson RJ, Myers MJ, et al. Hip muscle weakness and overuse injuries in recreational runners. *Clin J Sport Med* 2005; 15(1): 14–21.
7. Nishimura G, Yamato M, Tamai K, et al. MR findings in iliotibial band syndrome. *Skeletal Radiol* 1997; 26(9): 533–7.
8. Gunter P, Schwellnus MP. Local corticosteroid injection in iliotibial band friction syndrome in runners: a randomised controlled trial. *Br J Sports Med* 2004; 38: 269–72.
9. Brosseau L, Casimiro L, Milne S, et al. Deep transverse friction massage for treating tendinitis. *Cochrane Database Syst Rev* 2002; 4: CD003529.
10. Fredericson M, White JJ, MacMahon JM, et al. Quantitative analysis of the relative effectiveness of 3 iliotibial band stretches. *Arch Phys Med Rehabil* 2002; 83(5): 589–92.
11. Martens M, Librecht P, Burssens A. Surgical treatment of the iliotibial band friction syndrome. *Am J Sports Med* 1989; 17(5): 651–4.
12. Drogset JO, Rossvoll I, Grontvedt T. Surgical treatment of iliotibial band friction syndrome. A retrospective study of 45 patients. *Scand J Med Sci Sports* 1999; 9: 296–8.

13. Richards DP, Alan Barber F, Troop RL. Iliotibial band z-lengthening. *Arthroscopy* 2003; 19(3): 326–9.

14. Zenz P, Huber M, Obenaus CH, et al. Lengthening of the iliotibial band by femoral detachment and multiple puncture. A cadaver study. *Arch Orthop Trauma Surg* 2002; 122(8): 429–31.

15. Altman RD, Moskowitz R. Intraarticular sodium hyaluronate (hyalgan) in the treatment of patients with osteoarthritis of the knee: a randomized clinical trial. *J Rheumatol* 1998; 25: 2203–12.

16. Petrella RJ, Bartha C. Home based exercise therapy for older patients with knee osteoarthritis: a randomized clinical trial. *J Rheumatol* 2000; 27(9): 2215–21.

17. Squire MW, Callaghan JJ, Goetz DD, et al. Unicompartmental knee replacement. A minimum 15 year follow-up study. *Clin Orthop* 1999; 367: 61–72.

18. Shellock FG, Stone KR, Crues JV. Development and clinical application of kinematic MRI of the patellofemoral joint using an extremity MR system. *Med Sci Sports Exerc* 1999; 31(5): 788–91.

19. Panni AS, Tartarone M, Patricola A, et al. Long-term results of lateral retinacular release. *Arthroscopy* 2005; 21(5): 526–31.

20. Sekiya JK, Kuhn JE. Instability of the proximal tibiofibular joint. *J Am Acad Orthop Surg* 2003; 11(2): 120–8.

21. Bashir A, Gray ML, Hartke J, et al. Nondestructive imaging of human cartilage glycosaminoglycan concentration by MRI. *Magn Reson Med* 1999; 41: 857–65.

22. Bellamy N, Campbell J, Robinson V, et al. Viscosupplementation for the treatment of osteoarthritis of the knee. *Cochrane Database Syst Rev* 2005; 18(2): CD005321.

23. Kirkley A, Webster-Bogaert S, Litchfield RB, et al. The effect of bracing on varus gonarthrosis. *J Bone Joint Surg Am* 1999; 81A: 539–48.

24. Komistek RD, Dennis DA, Northcut EJ, et al. An in vivo analysis of the effectiveness of the osteoarthritic knee brace during heel-strike of gait. *J Arthroplasty* 1999; 14: 738–42.

25. Niitsu M, Ikeda K, Ijima T, et al. MR imaging of Pellegrini-Stieda disease. *Radiat Med* 1999; 17: 405–9.

26. Garrick JG, Webb DR. *Sports Injuries: Diagnosis and Management*. Philadelphia: WB Saunders, 1990.

27. Petsche TS, Selesnick FH. Popliteus tendinitis. Tips for diagnosis and management. *Physician Sportsmed* 2002; 30(8): 27–31.

28. Muche JA, Lento PH. Posterior knee pain and its causes: a clinician's guide to expediting diagnosis. *Physician Sportsmed* 2004; 32(3): 23–30.

Shin Pain

WITH CHRIS BRADSHAW, MATT HISLOP AND MARK HUTCHINSON

Shin pain is a common complaint among athletes, particularly in distance runners. The term 'shin splints' is commonly used by runners as a non-descript reference regarding their leg pain. Historically, the term 'shin splints' has also been used by medical professionals to describe the pain along the medial border of the tibia commonly experienced by runners or to describe shin pain in general. Neither use of the term is pathologically precise. There are multiple unique causes with defined pathophysiologies that should lead the clinician to a more specific diagnosis of shin pain in athletes. The importance of a more accurate and specific diagnosis allows for more targeted treatment with improved outcomes and a higher rate of return to sport. Therefore, it is strongly recommended that the term 'shin splints' be abandoned by healthcare providers in favor of a more specific, anatomical and diagnostic terminology.

Clinical perspective

Shin pain in athletes generally involves one or more of several pathological, anatomically specific processes.

1. *Bone stress.* A continuum of increased bone damage exists from bone strain to stress reaction and stress fracture.
2. *Vascular insufficiency.* This includes a reduction in arterial inflow, such as with popliteal artery entrapment, or vascular outflow due to venous insufficiency, thrombotic disease or vascular collapse owing to elevated intracompartmental pressures.
3. *Inflammation.* Inflammation develops at the insertion of muscles, particularly the tibialis posterior and soleus, and fascia to the medial border of the tibia.
4. *Raised intracompartmental pressure.* The lower leg has a number of muscle compartments, each enveloped by a thick inelastic fascia. The muscle compartments of the lower leg are shown in Figure 30.1. As a result of overuse/inflammation, these muscle compartments may become swollen and painful, particularly if there is excessive fibrosis of the fascia.
5. *Nerve entrapment* (e.g. superficial peroneal nerve).

The differentiation between these processes and the narrowing of the differential diagnosis begins with historical clues, narrowed by clinical examination findings, and confirmed with specific targeted imaging or clinical tests (Table 30.1). It is important to remember that two or three of these conditions

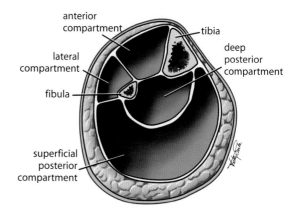

Figure 30.1 Cross-section of lower leg

(a) The various muscle compartments

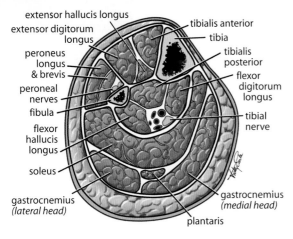

extensor hallucis longus
extensor digitorum longus
peroneus longus & brevis
peroneal nerves
fibula
flexor hallucis longus
soleus
gastrocnemius (lateral head)

tibialis anterior
tibia
tibialis posterior
flexor digitorum longus
tibial nerve
gastrocnemius (medial head)
plantaris

(b) The individual muscles, nerves and vessel

may exist simultaneously. For instance, it is not uncommon to have a stress fracture develop in a patient with chronic periostitis. Periostitis or stress fracture may lead to intracompartmental swelling and tip a patient on the edge of symptomatic exertional compartment syndrome over the edge. This interrelationship is demonstrated in Figure 30.2. These coexisting conditions are usually managed differently, and this explains why patients continue to have leg pain when only one condition has been addressed. The less common differential diagnoses for leg pain include tendinopathy, nerve entrapment, vascular claudication, neurogenic claudication, deep venous thrombosis, infection (osteomyelitis), metabolic bone disease, and tumors of bone and soft tissues, which may, in rare cases, effect prognosis and outcome of leg pain in athletes.

Role of biomechanics

Clinical experience suggests that abnormal biomechanics predisposes some individuals to pain on the anterior or medial border of the tibia (shin pain). Both extremes of foot type can contribute to the incidence of shin pain in athletes (Chapter 5). A rigid, cavus foot has limited shock absorption, thus increasing the impact pressure on the bone. In athletes with excessive pronation, the muscles of the superficial (soleus) and deep compartments (tibialis posterior, flexor hallucis longus, flexor digitorum longus) are placed at a relatively lengthened position and are required to contract eccentrically harder and longer to resist pronation after heel strike. On toe-off, these muscles must contract concentrically over a greater length to complete the transition to a supinated foot creating a rigid lever for push off. With fatigue, these muscles fail

to provide the normal degree of shock absorption. The chronic traction at the muscles' origins can, in turn, lead to chronic medial tibial periostitis (historically termed 'shin splints'). In chronic cases this mechanism can contribute to the presentation of stress fractures or deep compartment syndromes.

The athlete with excessive pronation may also develop lateral shin pain or stress injuries of the fibula. Pronation of the fixed foot creates an obligate internal tibial rotation. With repetitive excessive pronation, the tibia and fibula are exposed to repetitive rotational (torque) stresses. These stresses are transferred across the fibula, tibia, and proximal and distal tibiofibular articulations. Based on these biomechanical stresses, overuse can lead to stress reactions or stress fracture not only of the tibia but also of the fibula.

Motor imbalance can also lead to stress injuries in the lower extremity. Tight calf muscles, which commonly occur as a result of hard training, will restrict ankle dorsiflexion and increase the tendency for excessive pronation, leading to increased internal rotation of the tibia. Posterior tibial tendon weakness or deficiency can likewise contribute to foot pronation. Ankle instability secondary to chronic ankle sprains will obligate the athlete to overuse the peroneal tendons to compensate for ankle stability. This overuse can be just enough to send an athlete with borderline compartment syndrome over the brink to symptomatic complaints. To understand biomechanics clearly and have a foundation on which to create a differential diagnosis of leg pain, a complete knowledge of lower leg anatomy is essential (Figs 30.1, 30.3). When the presentation is atypical, one must expand the possibilities and consider a broad differential diagnosis for potential causes of leg pain in athletes (Table 30.2).

History

Taking a good history is essential for the correct diagnosis of athletes with leg pain. Asking the right questions should narrow the diagnosis. Clarifying the pain and assessing the mechanism is the key to the history. The history should be thorough and assess the presence of associated features with the pain such as paresthesias or muscle hernia.[1] A complete history should include a broad review of systems to discover other facets such as metabolic disturbances, prior surgical procedures, developmental problems, contributing medical issues, and social issues such as smoking. When the diagnosis does not classically fit the simple pain screen, a broader differential should be considered.

Table 30.1 The clinical characteristics and imaging features of common causes of shin pain in athletes

Site	Pain	Effect of exercise	Associated features	Tenderness	Investigations
Bone stress reaction or stress fracture	Localized Acute or sharp Subcutaneous medial tibial surface or fibula	Constant or increasing Worse with impact	Exacerbated by vibration (tuning fork) and ultrasound	Subcutaneous medial tibial surface or fibula	X-ray may be negative Use magnified views Look for callous or periosteal reaction MRI can stage severity and define prognosis but is non-specific
Medial tibial periostitis	Diffuse pain on posterior medial border of tibia; variable intensity	Decreases as athlete warms up and stretches	Worse in the morning and after exercise Pes planus	Posterior medial edge of tibia at muscular insertions	X-rays negative Bone scan shows diffuse uptake MRI shows diffuse edema and periosteal thickening
Chronic exertional compartment syndrome	No pain at rest; ache, tightness, gradually building with exertion	Specific onset variable between athletes, usually 10–15 minutes into exercise Decreases with rest	Occasional muscle weakness or dysfunction with exercise Paresthesia of nerve in affected compartment is possible	None at rest Antero and lateral more common with exertion Occasionally related to palpable muscle herniation (superficial peroneal nerve)	X-rays negative Bone scans negative Exertional compartment pressure testing is diagnostic Exertional MRI assessment may also be diagnostic
Popliteal artery entrapment	Pain in calf with exertion not anterolateral 'Atypical compartment syndrome'	Worse with exertion, especially active ankle plantarflexion	Pulses may be diminished with palpation or Doppler ultrasound with active plantarflexion	Rarely in proximal calf	X-rays negative MRI may reveal hypertrophic or abnormal insertion of medial gastrocnemius MRA (arteriography) with provocative maneuvers is diagnostic
Muscle–tendon injuries Strains Tendinopathy	Pain at pathological site with resisted stretch	Pre-exercise stretching usually helps	Good response to NSAIDs and ice	Pain can be at muscle belly, muscle–tendon junction, tendon, or tendon insertion	Rarely required X-rays usually negative MRI gives best view of soft tissue pathology

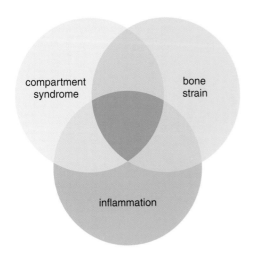

Figure 30.2 Possible interrelationship between the pathological sources of leg pain

The key questions and the responses that may give a clue to the diagnosis are listed in the box opposite.

Examination

In the examination of the patient with leg pain, it is important to palpate the site of maximal tenderness and assess the consistency of soft tissue. At rest, the physical examination for certain diagnoses (specifically chronic exertional compartment syndrome) is often unrewarding and the patient may be completely asymptomatic. The astute clinician will ask the athlete to reproduce their pain or symptoms via exertion or impact. This can be done on the athlete's playing surface, on a treadmill, or in and about the clinician's office by having the athlete run stairs or run around the block. A complete examination should be sequential, repeated the same way with each patient and include observation, analysis of muscle function and range of motion, anatomically directed palpation, functional testing and diagnosis-specific testing (Fig. 30.4).

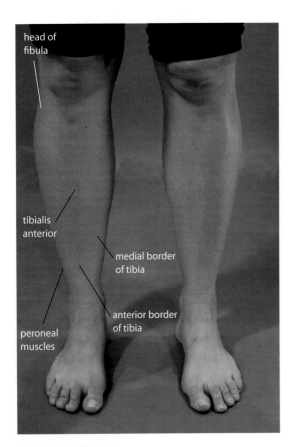

Figure 30.3 The leg

(a) Surface anatomy of the leg

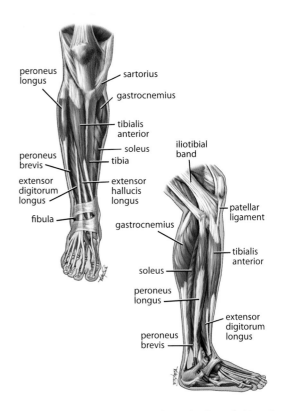

(b) Anatomy of the lower leg from the front (left) and lateral aspect (right) (ADAPTED FROM THE *CIBA COLLECTION OF MEDICAL ILLUSTRATIONS*, REPRODUCED BY COURTESY OF CIBA-GEIGY LIMITED, BASEL, SWITZERLAND. ALL RIGHTS RESERVED)

Question	Response
Was there an acute onset of pain?	Fractures and tendon ruptures are usually acute traumatic events. In athletes, the acute onset of pain may be preceded by low grade chronic pain of a stress fracture or tendinosis.
Is the pain chronic but stable?	Pain that is getting worse over time should raise concerns of a tumor.
Do you have a history of injury or prior leg pains?	Old fractures or injuries can lead to scar tissue, stiffness and pain.
Is the pain worse with impact?	Stress fractures are classically exacerbated with impact. Medial tibial periostitis and muscle strains may also be made worse with loading and resistance.
Is the pain worse with exertion?	Pain that is absent at rest but presents with exertion is classic for exertional compartment syndrome. However, popliteal artery entrapment can have a similar presentation, but with posterior rather than anterior/lateral pain.
Does the pain improve with warm-up and stretching?	Medial tibial periostitis and muscle strains will frequently improve with pre-exercise stretching, whereas stress fractures and exertional compartment syndrome will not.
Does the pain get worse with stretching or resistance?	Resistance given to the muscle tendon units, including their origins and insertions, should exacerbate the symptoms related to medial tibial periostitis and muscle tendon strains and tendinopathy.
Where is the pain? Is the pain focal? Is the pain diffuse?	The anatomical site of pain is the best physical clue to diagnosis. Focal pain over bone should raise suspicion of a stress fracture, focal pain over the muscle–tendon is likely to be a muscle strain or tendinopathy, diffuse pain over the posteromedial border of the tibia is likely to be medial tibial periostitis.
Do you have swelling with the pain? Is it diffuse? Is it focal?	Localized swelling is possible with a contusion, a stress fracture or muscle herniation. Diffuse swelling may indicate more significant injury, vascular problems such as deep venous thrombosis, or diffuse inflammatory problems such as medial tibial periostitis.
Do you feel electric shooting pain? Do you have weakness with the pain? Do you get numbness with the pain?	Electric shooting pain, dermatomal loss of sensation, and sclerotomal loss of motor power usually indicate nerve injury, entrapment or radiculopathy. Always check the lumbar spine.
Does the pain get better with ice or NSAIDs?	Pathologies associated with inflammation should improve with cryotherapy and anti-inflammatories. Osteoid osteomas (benign bone tumors) are known to have a significant response to aspirin (ASA).
Do you have pain at night?	Pain that wakes a patient up at night should raise concern about tumors.

1. Observation: Assesses lower limb alignment (varus/valgus, tibial torsion, pes planus), swelling, bruising, asymmetry.
   (a) standing (Fig. 30.4a)
   (b) walking—assess gait mechanics (forwards, backwards, on toes, on heels)
   (c) lying
2. Active movements: Assess motor function and range of motion.
   (a) plantarflexion/dorsiflexion—check pulses in full plantar or dorsiflexion; if diminished, consider popliteal artery entrapment
   (b) inversion/eversion
3. Passive movements: Assess true joint range of motion. May exacerbate pain in compartment syndromes.
   (a) plantarflexion (Fig. 30.4b)
   (b) dorsiflexion (Fig. 30.4c)
   (c) inversion/eversion
4. Resisted movements: Assess motor function. May exacerbate pain in muscle strains and tendinopathy.
   (a) plantarflexion/dorsiflexion
   (b) inversion/eversion
5. Functional tests
   (a) hopping—requires motor strength and

Table 30.2 Causes of shin pain

Common	Less common	Not to be missed
Muscle strains/ruptures	Referred pain from spine	Tumors
Abrasions and contusions	Chronic compartment syndrome	Osteosarcoma
Stress fracture	Superficial posterior	Osteoid osteoma
Acute fracture	Vascular insufficiency/claudication	Infection (osteomyelitis, cellulitis)
Medial tibial periostitis	Deep venous thrombosis (Chapter 31)	Acute compartment syndrome
Periosteal contusion	Popliteal artery entrapment	(Chapter 44)
Chronic compartment	Femoral endarteritis	Chronic transition to acute
syndrome	Atherosclerotic disease	compartment syndrome
Anterior	Superficial peroneal nerve entrapment	Chronic ankle injuries and
Lateral (peroneal)	Muscle herniations	Maisonneuve fracture
Deep posterior	Baker's cysts or ganglion cysts	*Rare and unusual*
	Osgood-Schlatter disease	
	Pes anserine bursitis	Syphilis
	Proximal tibiofibular subluxation	Sickle-cell anemia
	Achilles tendinopathy	Hyperparathyroidism
	Electrolyte and metabolic disturbances	Sarcoidosis
	Dehydration cramping	Rickets
		Paget's disease of bone
		Erythema nodosum

landing skills; rigid landing on heels exacerbates the pain of stress fracture
(b) jumping
(c) running—may bring on pain of exertional compartment syndrome; athletes should always reproduce complaints
(d) calf raises (Fig. 30.4d)
6. Palpation: Evaluate pain distribution, warmth, swelling, pitting edema, posterior cords or the presence of crepitus with motion.
(a) tibia (Fig. 30.4e)—focal pain indicates stress fracture, diffuse pain over posterior medial border of tibia indicates medial tibial periostitis
(b) fibula—the entire fibula should be palpated to identify focal pain related to a stress fracture; severe eversion/external rotation ankle sprains may injure the syndesmotic connection between the tibia and fibula and be associated with a proximal fibula fracture (Maisonneuve fracture)
(c) gastrocnemius, plantaris and soleus muscles (Fig. 30.4f)
(d) gastrocnemius–soleus aponeurosis (Fig. 30.4g)—assess for swelling and focal tenderness
(e) superficial and deep posterior compartment (Fig. 30.4h)
(f) anterior and lateral compartment—post-exertion palpation may reveal tenseness in exertional compartment syndrome or

a palpable localized mass due to muscle herniation
7. Special tests
(a) stress fracture test (Fig. 30.4i)—vibration may exacerbate pain associated with a stress fracture; applying a vibrating tuning fork along the subcutaneous border of the tibia is a convenient and inexpensive test easily applied in the training room or office
(b) biomechanical examination (Chapter 5)

Investigations

After taking the history and physical examination, an extended work-up should target the most likely diagnosis. Routine radiography is inexpensive and commonly performed but is rarely obviously positive in the diagnosis of leg pain. Careful inspection of the cortical borders with a hot lamp and magnification may increase the opportunity to visualize a subtle radiolucent line indicating a stress fracture. Repeating the study two to three weeks after the onset of pain may reveal periosteal reaction or a more obvious radiolucent line.

Historically, radioisotopic bone scan was the next test in line to confirm the presence of a stress fracture or medial tibial periostitis. Bone scans are sensitive but not particularly specific. For stress fractures, a discrete, focal area of increased uptake is seen on either the tibia or fibula (Fig. 30.5a). In chronic periostitis, the bone scan may show patchy areas of increased uptake

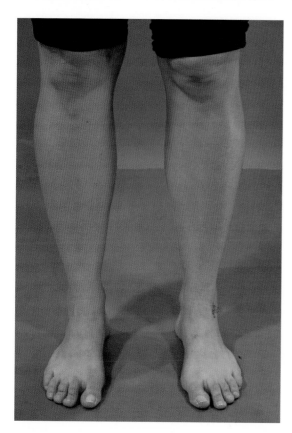

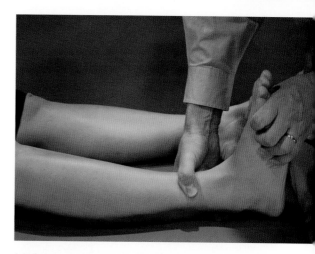

(c) Passive movement—dorsiflexion. Measure the degree of passive dorsiflexion compared with the other side

Figure 30.4 Examination of the patient with leg pain

(a) Observation—standing. Assess lower limb alignment, swelling, bruising and any evidence of subperiosteal hematoma

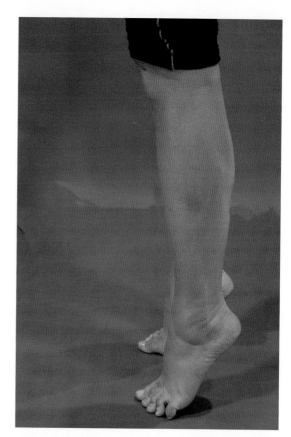

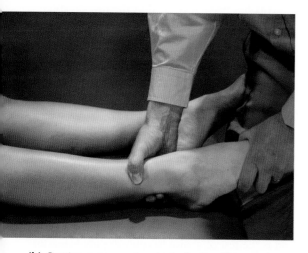

(b) Passive movement—plantarflexion. This may be restricted in anterior compartment syndrome

(d) Functional tests—calf raises. If pain has not been reproduced, ask the patient to perform repeated movements, such as hopping, running or calf raises (illustrated)

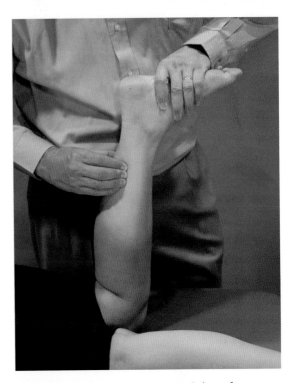

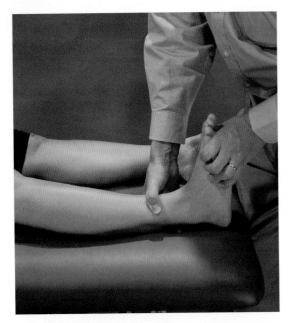

(e) Palpation—tibia. Palpate for the exact site of focal tenderness, feeling perpendicular to bone. Bony irregularity may occur along the medial tibial border with chronic periostitis

(g) Palpation—soleus aponeurosis. Palpate for sites of tenderness and associated taut bands that may be a precipitating factor in the development of inflammatory shin pain

along the medial border of the tibia (Fig. 30.5b). The absence of uptake does not preclude the diagnosis of periostitis. No identifiable changes on bone scan are associated with compartment syndrome.[2]

MRI has been advocated as the investigation of choice in patients with leg pain on the basis of its sensitivity to evaluate bony lesions, marrow changes, soft tissue injuries, and correlate these findings with clinical symptoms.[3] Typically, a stress fracture will appear on MRI as an area of periosteal edema (Fig. 30.5c). The severity of injury documented on MRI (bone edema only, unicortical radiolucent line or bicortical radiolucent line) has been directly correlated with healing time.[4, 5] Medial tibial periostitis will show a broader area of edema with thickening of the posterior medial periosteum. MRI may also confirm the diagnosis of a muscle strain or muscle herniation, as well as benign (lipoma, cysts, osteoid osteoma) and malignant tumors. MRA (magnetic resonance arteriography) with dynamic plantarflexion is the test of choice to confirm popliteal artery entrapment syndrome (Chapter 31). The role of MRI in the diagnosis of compartment syndromes is still

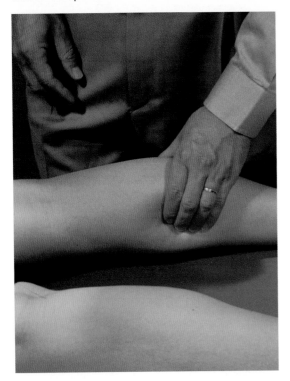

(f) Palpation—soleus muscle belly. A pincer grip is used

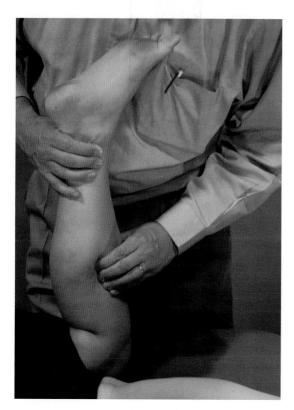

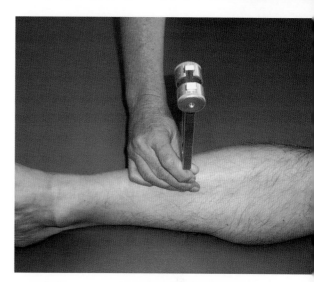

(i) Special test—stress fracture. Percussing, using a tuning fork or applying ultrasound over the site of tenderness can provoke pain in the presence of a stress fracture

(h) Palpation—deep posterior compartment. This is palpated through the relaxed overlying muscles. In compartment pressure syndrome, the entire compartment feels tight in contrast to the localized tissue tightness of chronic muscle strain. Muscle or fascial hernias are occasionally found. The superficial posterior compartment should also be palpated

unclear.[3, 4, 6–9] Pre- and post-exertion MRI scans may reveal intracompartmental edema, confirming the diagnosis of exertional compartment syndrome; however, this is an expensive way to confirm this diagnosis when more cost-efficient tests are available.

Intracompartmental pressure measurement (Chapter 9) is considered the gold standard in confirming the diagnosis of chronic exertional compartment syndrome in the athlete.[7] Pre- and immediate post-exertion measurements are essential to confirm the diagnosis. Devices used to measure the pressure have ranged from a wall blood pressure monitor with intravenous tubing and a three-way stopcock (Whiteside's technique), the transducer and pump used for an arterial line, laboratory systems, and hand-held devices. In each case, the fascia is punctured percutaneously with either a hollow bore needle or a needle with a side port, followed by measurements via that device

or by placement of a slit catheter. The latter two are more reproducible.

The anterior compartment is relatively easy to find. The deep posterior compartment or, if present, a tibialis posterior compartment, may be more difficult but are usually accessed posterior to the posteromedial edge of the tibia. Some authors recommend the use of ultrasound guidance to ensure correct catheter placement,[10] but we have not encountered any problems. The normal compartment pressure range is 0–10 mmHg. Positive pressures include at-rest or exertional pressures over 25 mmHg or elevation of at-rest pressures greater than 10 mmHg. Pressures from 10–20 mmHg or elevated pressures that decrease with exercise are considered inconclusive. Other authors have promoted the use of non-invasive methods such as near infra-red spectroscopy and results are promising but require further validation before general use.[9]

A summary of the recommended techniques and the appropriate exercises to produce pain is shown in Table 30.3.

Additional investigations for more atypical causes of leg pain include:

- EMG/nerve conduction studies:
  — peripheral nerve entrapments and metabolic neuropathy
- Ankle/brachial index:
  — vascular claudication

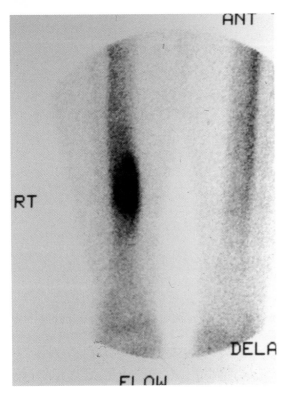

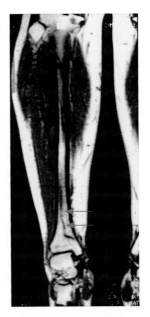

(c) MRI appearance of stress fracture of the tibia showing fracture line (faint) in the presence of marrow edema

- Venous Doppler ultrasound:
  — deep venous thrombosis
- Laboratory:
  — white blood cell count with differential—infection or osteomyelitis
  — ESR (erythrocyte sedimentation rate)—inflammation, rheumatological conditions
  — sickle-cell preparation—sickle-cell anemia
  — urine analysis with uromyoglobin—rhabdomyolyis
  — creatine phosphokinase, myoglobin—rhabdomyolysis, myopathy
  — prothrombin time (PT), activated partial thromboplastin time (APTT)—deep venous thrombosis
  — D-dimer—deep venous thrombosis
  — metabolic panel—hypokalemia, hypocalcemia, hypomagnesia, etc.
  — T_3 (triiodothyronine), T_4 (thyroxine), TSH (thyroid stimulating hormone)—thyroid myopathy

Stress fracture of the tibia

Stress fractures are more commonly a cause of shin pain in athletes in impact, running and jumping sports. Overall limb and foot alignment as well as limb length discrepancy may also play a role. The

Figure 30.5 Characteristic appearances on imaging

(a) Stress fracture

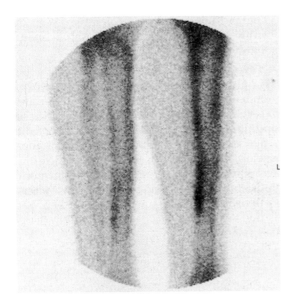

(b) Traction periostitis

Table 30.3 Compartment pressure testing

Compartment	Location of catheter	Exacerbating exercise	Compartment pressures (N = 10 mmHg, post exercise 5 min)
Deep posterior	Junction of lower and middle third of tibia Aim deep posteriorly just behind the posteromedial tibial border	Treadmill/running Stairs Run/jump Pulleys in PF/DF Repeated calf raises Isokinetic PF with IV/EV Sport-specific challenges	>25 mmHg post exercise
Superficial posterior	Aim more posteriorly from deep posterior entry into medial gastrocnemius or soleus	Treadmill Stairs Repeated calf raises	>30 mmHg
Anterior	Mid-belly of tibialis anterior Anterior to intermuscular septum (halfway between fibula and anterior border of tibia)	Repeated DF Treadmill/running Stairs Sport-specific challenges	>30 mmHg
Lateral (peroneal)	Mid-belly of peroneals Posterior to intermuscular septum	Repeated IV/EV Treadmill/running Stairs	>30 mmHg

Ankle movements: PF = plantarflexion, DF = dorsiflexion, IV = inversion, EV = eversion, N = normal.

incidence of stress fractures is increased by playing on more rigid, unforgiving surfaces. Approximately 90% of tibial stress fractures will affect the posteromedial aspect of the tibia, with the middle third and junction between the middle and distal thirds being most common. Proximal metaphyseal stress fractures may be related to more time loss from sports as they do not respond as well to functional bracing, which allows earlier return to play.

Stress fractures on the anterior edge of the tibia, the tension side of the bone, are more resistant to treatment and have a propensity to develop a non-union when compared to the risk of posteromedial stress fractures. A simple memory tool for the problematic anterior tibial stress fracture is 'anterior is awful'.

A classic case presentation for a routine posteromedial stress fracture is as follows:

- Gradual onset of leg pain aggravated by exercise.
- Pain may occur with walking, at rest or even at night.
- Examination—localized tenderness over the tibia.
- Biomechanical examination may show a rigid, cavus foot incapable of absorbing load, an excessively pronating foot causing excessive muscle fatigue or a leg length discrepancy.
- Tenderness to palpation along the medial border with obvious tenderness. (Note that,

occasionally, a stress fracture of the posterior cortex produces symptoms of calf pain (Chapter 31) rather than leg pain.)
- Bone scan and MRI appearances of a stress fracture of the tibia are shown in Figures 30.5a and 30.5c. MRI scan is of particular value as the extent of edema and cortical involvement has been directly correlated with the expected return to sport.[5]
- A CT scan may also demonstrate a stress fracture (Fig. 30.6).

Treatment

Prior to initiating treatment or during the treatment plan, it is important to identify which factors precipitated the stress fracture. The most common cause is an acute change in training habits, such as a significant increase in distance over a short period of time, beginning double practice days after laying off training for a season, or a change to a more rigid playing surface. Shoe wear, biomechanics and repetitive impact sports such as running and gymnastics have also been implicated. The athlete's coach can play a key role in modifying training patterns to reduce the risk of these injuries. In women, reduced bone density due to hypoestrogenemia secondary to athletic amenorrhea (the female athlete triad) may be a contributing factor. All female athletes with a

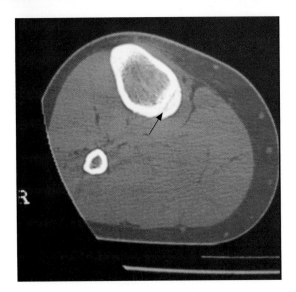

Figure 30.6 CT appearance of stress fracture of the tibia

first-time stress fracture should be screened for the female athlete triad (Chapter 41).

The classic treatment plan is as follows:

- Initial period of rest (sometimes requiring a period of non-weight-bearing on crutches for pain relief) until the pain settles.
- The use of a pneumatic brace has been described. Studies have shown a markedly reduced return to activity time with such use compared with average times in two of three studies[11,12] and compared with a 'traditional treatment' group in the third.[13] In this latter study the brace group returned to full, unrestricted activity in an average of 21 days compared with 77 days in the traditional group. The brace should extend to the knee as the mid-leg version may actually increase the stresses across a mid shaft stress fracture. Once a stress fracture is 'clinically healed', the athlete is advised to use the brace during practise and competition. Clinical healing implies minimal to no palpable pain at the fracture site and minimal to no pain with activities in the brace. Using this plan, there have been no reported cases of progression to complete catastrophic fracture of the tibia.
- If pain persists, continue to rest from sporting activity until the bony tenderness disappears (four to eight weeks).
- Once the patient is pain-free when walking and has no bony tenderness, gradually progress the

quality and quantity of the exercise over the following month. The athlete should be asked to continue to use a pneumatic brace to complete the current season until an appropriate period (four to eight weeks) of rest can occur.

- Cross-training with low-impact exercises, including swimming, cycling and deep-water running, maintains conditioning and reduces risk of recurrence.
- Pain associated with soft tissue thickening distal to the fracture site can be treated by soft tissue techniques.
- General principles of return to activity following overuse injury should be followed (Chapter 12).

Prevention of recurrence

To prevent recurrence, it is important to:

- determine whether excessive training and biomechanics precipitated the stress fracture
- ensure adequate calorie balance, as inadequate intake is a risk factor for stress fractures.

Alternative treatments, including electrical stimulation[14] and low-intensity pulsed ultrasound,[15] have shown some promise in case studies to have a beneficial effect on the speed of stress fracture healing in limited populations (professional and Olympic athletes) where a rapid return to sport is vital. A pilot study[16] suggests that intravenous use of the bisphosphonate pamidronate also shows promise in decreasing the time away from sport for tibial stress fractures. The quality of science of these studies is level 4 (case series only) and better designed case controlled studies are necessary to recommend their general application.

Stress fracture of the anterior cortex of the tibia

Stress fractures of the anterior cortex of the mid shaft of the tibia need to be considered separately as they are prone to delayed union, non-union and complete fracture.[17] Stress fracture of the anterior cortex of the medial third of the tibia presents with diffuse dull pain aggravated by physical activity. The bone is tender to palpation at the site of the fracture and periosteal thickening as evidenced by a palpable lump may be present if the symptoms have been experienced for some months. Isotopic bone scan (Fig. 30.7a) shows a discrete focal area of increased activity in the anterior cortex. The radiographic appearance at this stage shows a defect in the anterior cortex, which is termed 'the dreaded black line' (Fig. 30.7b). This

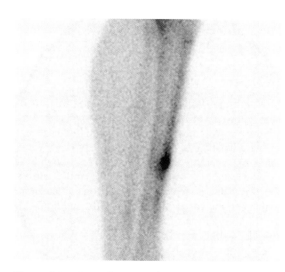

Figure 30.7 Stress fracture of the anterior cortex of the tibia

(a) Bone scan appearance

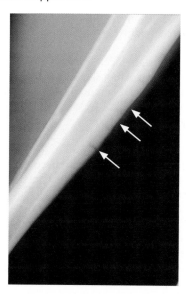

(b) Plain X-ray appearance of multiple 'dreaded black lines'

appearance is due to bony resorption and is indicative of non-union.

The mid-anterior cortex of the tibia is thought to be vulnerable to non-union for two reasons: the area has a relatively poor blood supply and is also an area under tension due to the morphological bowing of the tibia. Excessive anterior tibial bowing is often noted in association with this fracture. In general, the prognosis for these resistant stress injuries is guarded

with an elevated risk of delayed or non-union. One study presented some success with the use of pneumatic air braces in this population, thus avoiding the need for surgery.[18] However, the average return to unrestricted activities was 12 months with this form of treatment. Other options for treatment include pulsed electromagnetic stimulation,[19] surgical excision and bone grafting[20] and transverse drilling at the fracture site.[21] Chang and Harris described five cases treated with intramedullary tibial nailing.[22] They had two excellent results and three good results.

Our current treatment protocol is as follows:

- Immediate application of a pneumatic brace.
- Discontinue anti-inflammatory medications and smoking.
- Thorough screening for associated nutritional, metabolic and biomechanical risk factors.
- For all elite level athletes, application of electrical or ultrasonic bone stimulation.
- If no progress by four to six months, intramedullary rodding plus/minus bone grafting, debridement or drilling is recommended.

Medial tibial traction periostitis

As noted previously, there has been a tendency in the past to categorize all shin pain, especially that which is not a stress fracture, under the term 'shin splints'.[23, 24] Indeed, 'shin splints' is more of a vague symptom athletes describe for leg pain most commonly along the posterior medial border of the tibia. Some clinicians have labeled the process medial tibial stress syndrome (MTSS)[25] which, unfortunately, is also less than ideal as it does not accurately represent the pathophysiology of the process. With the advent of imaging techniques such as isotopic bone scan, CT and MRI, we are now able to make more precise anatomical and pathological diagnoses of patients with leg pain. The most descriptive term that accounts for the inflammatory, traction phenomenon on the medial aspect of the leg more common in runners is medial tibial periostitis or medial tibial traction periostitis.

The patient with medial tibial traction periostitis complains of diffuse pain along the medial border of the tibia (the junction of the lower third and upper two-thirds of the tibia), which usually decreases with warming up. More focal pain should alert the examiner to the possibility of a stress fracture. The athlete can often complete the training session but pain gradually recurs after exercise and is worse the following morning. Historically the tibialis posterior was thought to be the source of the pain, but more recently the soleus and flexor digitorum longus have been implicated.[26]

A number of factors may contribute to the increased stress and traction on the posterior medial aspect of the tibia. These include excessive pronation (flat feet),[27] training errors, shoe design, surface type, muscle dysfunction, fatigue and decreased flexibility. The biomechanics of medial tibial traction periostitis relate to the sequence of events that occurs with walking and running.[28] During midstance, foot pronation provides shock absorption and an accommodation to the varied terrain. The medial soleus is the strongest plantarflexor and invertor of the foot. The soleus muscle eccentrically contracts to resist pronation. Excessive pronation due to pes planus or overuse combined with repetitive impact loading leads to chronic traction over its insertion onto the periosteum on the posterior medial border of the tibia, leading directly to medial tibial traction periostitis.

Metabolic bone health may also contribute. Athletes with pain related to medial tibial traction periostitis were found to have lower bone mineral density at the affected region compared with control and athletic control subjects. Bone mineral density was also decreased on the unaffected side in subjects with unilateral symptoms.[29] These athletes regained normal bone mineral density after recovery from their symptoms.[30] Reduced bone density or bone conditioning to stress may contribute to the increased risk of medial tibial traction periostitis seen in female military recruits. A study examining possible risk factors for the development of medial shin pain in military recruits showed that females were three times as likely to develop the syndrome.[31] Beyond gender, no other risk factors of statistical significance were noted, but increased hip range of motion (both internal and external rotation) and lower lean calf girth were associated with medial shin pain in the male recruits.[31]

Radiographs are routinely negative with medial tibial traction periostitis; however, with careful inspection some periosteal reaction can be seen in some patients and localized swelling can be seen in others. Isotopic bone scan may show patchy, diffuse areas of increased uptake along the medial border of the tibia, as shown in Figure 30.5b. This is in contrast to stress fractures, which should show focal uptake. In early stages, however, the bone scan appearance may also be normal. MRI was found to have similar sensitivity and specificity to isotope bone scan.[8] Interestingly, there were a number of abnormal bone scan and MRI appearances in the asymptomatic control group in that study.[8]

Treatment

Most athletes will present with a long history of complaints, having tried a number of home remedies, stretches, medicines or cold treatment. It is of benefit to assess what has been attempted and what provided relief or exacerbated the problem. Even though heat or whirlpool may improve flexibility and warm up muscles, it also increases the circulation to the region, which can increase symptoms of inflammation.

The foundation of treatment is based on symptomatic relief, identification of risk factors and treating the underlying pathology. Symptomatic treatment begins with rest, ice and anti-inflammatory medications. Switching to pain-free cross-training activities such as swimming or cycling can keep the athlete active. In resistant cases, immobilization and protected weight-bearing may be necessary to rest the chronic tension placed on the soleus insertion with repeated weight-bearing. Taping techniques are only effective if they control foot pronation. Perhaps the most important facet of treatment is based on a careful assessment of foot alignment and gait mechanics. Permanent relief can occasionally be achieved through appropriate shoe wear and the application of cushioned orthoses (for shock absorption assistance) with a semi-rigid medial arch support (to support the pronated foot).

Alternative modalities can be effective in relieving pain and should be considered in patients with medial tibial traction periostitis. The entire calf muscle should be assessed for areas of tightness or focal thickening that can be treated with appropriate soft tissue techniques (Chapter 31). Digital ischemic pressure should be applied to the thickened muscle fibers of the soleus, flexor digitorum longus and tibialis posterior adjacent to their bony attachment, avoiding the site of periosteal attachment, which may prove too painful (Fig. 30.8a). The effect may be enhanced by adding passive dorsiflexion and plantarflexion while digital ischemic pressure is applied. Transverse frictions should be used on focal regions of muscle thickening in the soleus and flexor digitorum longus. Abnormalities of the tibialis posterior may be treated through the relaxed overlying muscles. Sustained myofascial tension can be applied parallel to the tibial border, releasing the flexor digitorum longus, and along the soleus aponeurosis in the direction of normal stress with combined active ankle dorsiflexion (Fig. 30.8b). Vacuum cupping techniques can be effective but it is important to remain clear of the tibial border to avoid causing capillary damage (Fig. 30.8c).

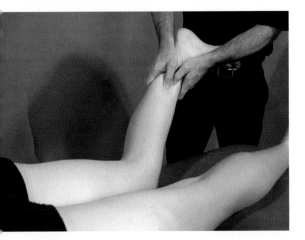

Figure 30.8 Soft tissue therapy in the treatment of inflammatory shin pain

(a) Digital ischemic pressure to the medial soleus aponeurosis and flexor digitorum longus. This can be performed with passive and active dorsiflexion

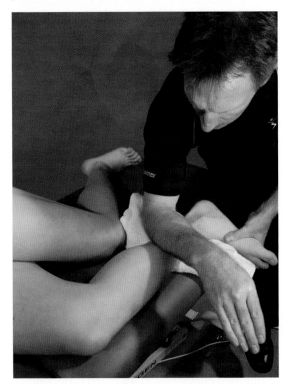

(b) Sustained myofascial tension along the soleus aponeurosis with passive ankle dorsiflexion

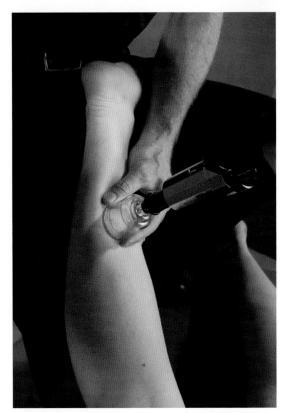

(c) Vacuum cupping

Physiotherapy programs have focused on motor strengthening and flexibility, especially proprioceptive neuromuscular facilitation (PNF) stretching. In addition, electrical stimulation, iontophoresis and ultrasound have been attempted with mixed results. Prolotherapy, injection with agents intended to accelerate the healing process, has also been performed but very little quality research is available to validate its efficacy. In resistant cases, surgical release (with or without periosteal tissue resection or ablation) of the superficial and posterior compartments off their conjoined insertion onto the posteromedial border of the tibia can be performed with a projected success rate of 70% improvement in high-performance elite athletes.[32, 33]

Chronic exertional compartment syndrome

Compartment syndrome is defined as increased pressure within a closed fibro-osseous space, causing reduced blood flow and reduced tissue perfusion, which subsequently leads to ischemic pain and possible permanent damage to the tissues of the compartment.[34] It may be acute, chronic (exertional), or convert from chronic to acute. Chronic exertional compartment syndrome with stress fractures and medial tibial traction periostitis are key components of the differential diagnosis of shin pain in athletes, especially in distance runners and those athletes in aerobic training. The syndrome is frequently bilateral.

Even though, classically, exertional compartment syndrome was thought to be an ischemic phenomenon like acute compartment syndrome, the exact etiology of chronic exertional compartment syndrome is still unclear. Repetitive overuse followed by associated inflammation may lead to fibrosis and therefore reduced elasticity of the fascia surrounding the muscle compartments. As a result, when the patient exercises, the muscles attempt to expand but are unable to do so. Biopsies have revealed abnormally thickened, non-compliant fascia.[35] A series of biopsies at the fascial–periosteal interface revealed varying degrees of fibrocytic activity, chronic inflammatory cells, vascular proliferation as well as a decrease in collagen irregularity, suggesting an attempt at remodeling was taking place.[36] Owing to this stiffened, abnormal fascial compartment, when the patient exercises, the muscle attempts to expand but is unable to do so. This results in increased pressure and, therefore, pain. As noted previously, ischemia is likely to play a role; however, this has not been substantiated well via scientific study. It is possible that within a tight fascial compartment the normal consequence of metabolic activity during exercise would lead to an increase in pressure sufficient to compromise tissue perfusion at the capillary level. Birtles et al.[37] induced similar symptoms to those of compartment syndrome by restricting venous flow during exercise. However, conflicting evidence via nuclear magnetic resonance spectroscopy studies[38] and MIBI imaging[39] has been unable to conclusively prove or disprove an ischemic role.

Typical clinical features of chronic exertional compartment syndrome are the absence of pain at rest with increasing achy pain and a sensation of tightness with exertion. Symptoms usually significantly dissipate within several minutes of rest but an ache may remain for up to 30 minutes. Rarely, athletes will develop paresthesia or motor weakness with exertion. At rest, physical examination is usually unremarkable. With exertion, palpable tenseness within the compartment may be appreciated and the presence of muscle bulges or herniations may be visualized. The most common compartment involved is the anterior compartment presenting with anterolateral pain with exertion. The other two common compartments are

the lateral compartment, which may present with paresthesia in the distribution of the superficial peroneal nerve to the dorsum of the foot, and the deep posterior compartment, usually associated with posteromedial tibial pain. Involvement of the superficial posterior compartment is quite rare.

Investigations and screening should always include an assessment of limb and foot alignment, evaluation of the biomechanical demands of the specific sport including court surface and shoe wear, a history of previous injuries or trauma, and a screen for overlapping pathology such as stress fractures, medial tibial traction periostitis, and metabolic and nutritional factors. Radiographs are frequently obtained as an inexpensive screening tool for associated bone pathology. The definitive diagnosis is made on the basis of intracompartmental pressure measurements (Table 30.3). Recently, the use of near infra-red spectroscopy has shown promise as a non-invasive alternative.[9]

Deep posterior compartment syndrome

Deep posterior compartment syndrome typically presents as an ache in the region of the medial border of the tibia or as chronic calf pain. Beware the multiple other causes of calf pain including popliteal artery entrapment syndrome (Chapter 31). The deep posterior compartment contains the flexor hallucis longus, flexor digitorum longus and tibialis posterior (Fig. 30.1). Occasionally, a separate fascial sheath surrounds the tibialis posterior muscle, forming an extra compartment that is particularly liable to provoke symptoms.[40]

Active, passive or resisted motion of these muscles may exacerbate pain. The patient describes a feeling of tightness or a bursting sensation. Pain increases with exercise. There may be associated distal symptoms (e.g. weakness, pins and needles on the plantar aspect of the foot), which may be indicative of tibial nerve compression. Small muscle hernias occasionally occur along the medial or anterior borders of the tibia after exercise.

On examination, there may be tenderness along the medial aspect of the tibia but this is often relatively mild. Due to the deep nature of the compartment, palpable fascial tightness is less obvious in comparison to anterior or lateral compartment syndromes. Nonetheless, the experienced clinician may be able to discern the difference between palpable tightness in the deep compartment and fascial thickening and induration found in association with traction periostitis.

Routinely all four compartments should be measured pre- and post-exertion in athletes in whom chronic exertional compartment syndrome is suspected. To measure deep posterior compartment pressures, the needle or catheter is inserted from the medial aspect through two layers of fascia aiming posterior to the tibia (Fig. 30.9). Exercises, including running or jumping, stair-climbing, use of pulleys in plantarflexion and dorsiflexion or repeated calf raises, or isokinetic resistance machines can be used to exacerbate complaints. Routinely, we ask patients to run 5 minutes into their pain to assure a valid test. It is important to reproduce the patient's pain, otherwise the test is not considered valid.

Post-exertional measurements must be obtained immediately after ceasing exercise and may be repeated again after 10 minutes. Normal compartment pressures are regarded as being between 0 and 10 mmHg.[41] For the diagnosis of chronic compartment syndrome, maximal pressure during exercise of greater than 35 mmHg, an elevation of pressures greater than 10 mmHg, or a resting post-exercise pressure greater than 25 mmHg is necessary (Table 30.3). If pressure takes more than 5 minutes to return to normal, this may also be significant.

Treatment of isolated deep posterior exertional compartment syndrome usually begins with a conservative regimen of reduced exercise and deep soft tissue therapy. Longitudinal release work with passive and active dorsiflexion is performed to reduce fascial thickening (Fig. 30.10). Transverse friction is used to treat chronic muscular thickening. Dry needling of the deep muscles or prolotherapy may also be helpful. Assessment and correction of any biomechanical abnormalities, especially excessive pronation, must be included.

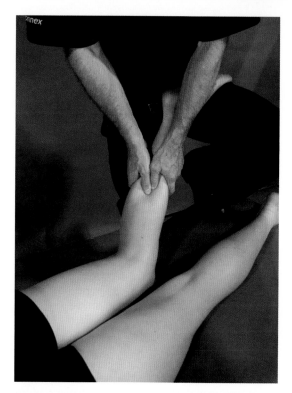

Figure 30.10 Soft tissue therapy in the treatment of deep posterior compartment syndrome—longitudinal release to reduce fascial thickening. Active or passive dorsiflexion improves the release

Isolated deep posterior exertional compartment syndrome is uncommon and may be confused with medial tibial traction periostitis, popliteal artery entrapment syndrome, vascular claudication and stress fractures. Indeed, it is not surprising that initial treatment is the same as that for medial tibial traction periostitis. However, if pressures are elevated and symptoms are refractory to treatment, surgical release may be necessary.

The surgical approach is along the posterior medial edge of the tibia and may be performed through a single or two small incisions. The saphenous vein lies directly along the path to the fascial insertion onto the posteromedial border of the tibia. Extreme care must be used to control all bleeding at the time of surgery as injury to one of the branches is common and increases the risk of post-operative hematoma or cellulitis.[42]

Some authors have suggested a benefit of fasciectomy (removal of a portion of fascial tissue) over fasciotomy (simple incision) due to concerns that the fascial insertion and sheath reforms.[10] They

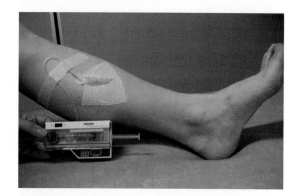

Figure 30.9 Compartment pressure testing—deep posterior compartment. The Stryker catheter is inserted into the deep posterior compartment

argue that this periosteal stripping serves an added role of treating any associated medial tibial traction periostitis as well as assuring release of any anatomical variations of tibialis posterior compartments. Due to the extensive nature of the procedure and increased risk of complications, in patients who have positive anterior/lateral compartment pressures but only borderline pressures in the deep compartment, recommendations to restrict releases and treatment to the affected compartment seem prudent.[42]

Anterior and lateral exertional compartment syndromes

The anterior compartment contains the tibialis anterior, extensor digitorum longus, extensor hallucis longus and peroneus tertius muscles as well as the deep peroneal nerve, and the lateral (peroneal) compartment contains the peroneus longus and brevis tendons as well as the superficial peroneal nerve. For anterior compartment pathology, pain during exertion is felt just lateral to the anterior border of the shin and paresthesia may present in the first web space. For lateral compartment pathology, pain is palpated just anterior to the fibula and paresthesia may occur to the dorsum of the foot. The intermuscular septum (raphe) between the two compartments can be visualized in thin individuals by looking for the indentation of skin when you squeeze the soft tissues between the anterior border of the tibia and fibula.

Examination will be normal or there may be palpable generalized tightness of the anterior or lateral compartment with focal regions of excessive muscle thickening. It is also important to assess the plantarflexors, especially the soleus and gastrocnemius. If these antagonists are tight, they may predispose to anterior compartment syndrome. Muscle herniation may be palpable with exertion approximately 5–7 cm (2–3 in.) proximally to the distal tip of the fibula where the superficial peroneal nerve penetrates through the lateral compartment fascia. Diagnosis of anterior and lateral exertional compartment syndromes is confirmed with pre- and post-exertional compartment testing (Table 30.3).

Treatment is based on the same principles as for the deep posterior compartment. Any and all contributing factors should be assessed and treated. Lowering the heel in the athlete's shoe or orthoses may reduce the load of the anterior muscles and alleviate pain. Sustained myofascial tension techniques combined with passive and active plantarflexion are effective in restoring fascial flexibility (Fig. 30.11a). Focal regions of muscular thickening should be treated

with transverse friction or dry needling. In addition, because the anterior and lateral compartments are superficial, vacuum cupping may be attempted (Fig. 30.11b). Accurate cup placement is required to avoid

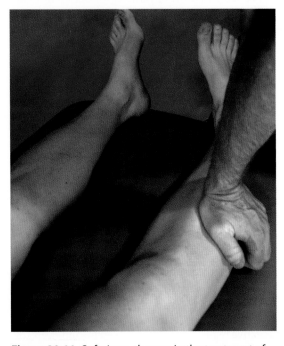

Figure 30.11 Soft tissue therapy in the treatment of anterior compartment syndrome

(a) Sustained myofascial tension with active or passive plantarflexion

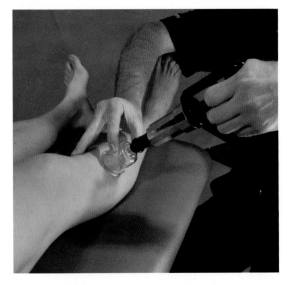

(b) Vacuum cupping

excessive capillary and periosteal damage. It is also helpful to treat tightness of the posterior compartment (antagonist muscles) with sustained myofascial tension (grade III) combined with passive and active dorsiflexion.

Unfortunately, when the diagnosis is pressure positive and classic, and no contributing or overlapping factors are identified, conservative treatment frequently fails and surgical release is necessitated. Fasciectomy is rarely necessary for anterior and lateral compartment releases, with minimal incision, percutaneous and endoscopically assisted releases approaching 90% success rate. Special care is essential to visualize the superficial peroneal nerve at the time of surgery to avoid iatrogenic injury.

Acute compartment syndromes are usually associated with trauma. Intracompartmental pressures are significantly elevated and do not settle with rest. Emergency surgical release is essential to avoid ischemic injury to the extremity. This emergency is covered more completely in Chapter 44; however, it is important to be knowledgable of a number of case reports in which acute anterior compartment syndromes were brought on by exercise and overuse.[43, 44] When pain does not settle in an appropriate time frame, conversion of an exertional compartment syndrome to an acute compartment syndrome should be considered.

Outcomes of surgical treatment of exertional compartment syndrome

Fasciotomy plus/minus fasciectomy is the standard surgical treatment for both anterior and deep posterior compartment syndromes. The majority (80–90%) of patients undergoing this procedure have a satisfactory result, with many being able to return to their previous level of sport.[45–47] However, a significant percentage of patients either fail to improve after surgery or after a period of improvement have a recurrence of symptoms. Some studies suggest that failure and recurrences are more common in the deep posterior compartment,[46–49] possibly due to failure to release the tibialis posterior,[10, 46] whereas another study showed a worse outcome in the anterior compartment.[50] Micheli et al. compared outcomes by gender and noted a slightly decreased rate of successful outcomes in female patients.[51]

In a study of 18 patients who underwent revision surgery,[52] increased pressure was found only in a localized area at the site of the scar in 60% of patients, whereas 40% had high pressures throughout the compartment. They found that the exuberant scar tissue was thicker, denser and more constricting than was the original fascia. Eight of the 18 patients had entrapment of the superficial peroneal nerve with numbness and paresthesiae over the dorsum of the foot with exertion, positive Tinel sign, and localized tenderness over the nerve, exacerbated by active dorsiflexion and eversion, as well as passive inversion and plantarflexion. All those with peroneal nerve entrapment had a good result from the revision surgery, whereas only 50% of those without nerve entrapment had a satisfactory outcome. Slimmon et al.[50] reported a 60% excellent or good outcome after a minimum of two years in 50 patients who underwent fasciectomy. Fifty-eight per cent were exercising at a lower level than before the injury and, of those, 36% cited the return of their compartment syndrome or the development of a different lower leg compartment syndrome as the reason for the reduction in exercise levels.

The foundation of a successful surgical result begins with a proper anatomical diagnosis. Care must be taken to confirm the diagnosis pre-operatively with intracompartmental pressure measurement as well as to treat any associated or contributing factors. Surgery should target the specific anatomical pathology. Avoiding release of all four compartments in every patient unless pre-operative testing provides definitive indication will reduce the risk of surgical complications. Meticulous control of intra-operative bleeding will reduce the risk of post-operative hematoma and cellulitis. Due to the extensive subcutaneous dissection, post-operative cellulitis or infection is more common than some other procedures. Perioperative antibiotics and post-operative cryotherapy can reduce this risk. If identified in the post-operative period, the surgeon should have a relatively low threshold to return to the operating room and perform early irrigation. The absolute indication for fasciectomy in contrast to fasciotomy is not clear as the former may increase the risk of bleeding and post-operative stiffness. Perhaps the most common complication is post-operative stiffness, which can be avoided by early and aggressive post-operative mobilization.

Rehabilitation following compartment syndrome surgery

The following protocol is recommended:[2]

- Perioperative antibiotics and cryotherapy to reduce complications of infection, hematoma and cellulitis.
- Range of motion exercises of the knee and ankle in the immediate post-operative period—full plantarflexion and dorsiflexion is encouraged.

- Three to five days of limited weight-bearing on crutches, then full weight-bearing as tolerated.
- Once the wounds have healed, a strengthening program including cycling and swimming should commence.
- Gradual return to light jogging at about four to six weeks after surgery.
- Full sports participation is anticipated at six to eight weeks if one compartment is released, and eight to 12 weeks if both legs and multiple compartments are released.
- The athlete should be pain-free with 90% strength regained prior to full sports participation.

Less common causes

Stress fracture of the fibula

Stress fractures of the fibula are not seen as frequently as stress fractures of the tibia. As the fibula plays a minimal role in weight-bearing, this stress fracture is usually due to muscle traction or torsional forces placed through the bone. In the athlete with excessive subtalar pronation, the peroneal muscles are forced to contract harder and longer during toe-off. Examination may reveal local tenderness and pain on springing the fibula proximal to the site of the stress fracture.

This injury is usually not as painful on weight-bearing as is stress fracture of the tibia. It is treated symptomatically with rest from activity until bony tenderness settles. Due to poorer rotational control, knee-high pneumatic braces may not be as effective as on the tibia. There should then be a gradual increase in the amount of activity. Soft tissue abnormalities should be corrected. This injury is often associated with a biomechanical abnormality such as excessive pronation or excessive supination.

Referred pain

Referred pain is not a common cause of shin pain in athletes but should be considered in cases with persistent and atypical pain. Pain may be referred from the lumbar spine, proximal nerve entrapment, the knee joint (Baker's cyst, meniscal cysts), the superior tibiofibular joint (instability or ganglion cyst) and, occasionally, the ankle joint (instability, Maisonneuve fracture).

Nerve entrapments

Within the leg itself, nerve entrapment of either the superficial peroneal nerve in the lateral compartment or the deep peroneal nerve in the anterior compartment can occur due to trauma[53] or a tight brace or cast. Fascial entrapment at the level of the fibular head is also seen occasionally.[54]

The tibial nerve in the deep posterior compartment is less commonly involved with entrapment but can be injured with trauma. Pain and sensory changes may occur. The diagnosis is suggested by the presence of motor or sensory changes and confirmed with nerve conduction studies performed pre- and post-exercise. Surgery may be required to alleviate these conditions.

Vascular entrapments

Popliteal artery entrapment syndrome usually presents with calf pain and is therefore more fully described in Chapter 31 but may rarely present as pain in the anterior compartment.[55, 56] It can be misdiagnosed as anterior compartment syndrome because they both present with claudicant-type pain. However, the pain from popliteal artery entrapment disappears immediately on cessation of exercise, whereas compartment syndrome pain often persists for approximately 30 minutes as an aching sensation. Even though deep venous thrombosis is most commonly posterior, chronic venous stasis changes can occur anteriorly and may be evidence of systemic disease.

Developmental issues

Juvenile tibia vara (Blount disease) usually presents owing to deformity rather than pain. Osgood-Schlatter disease is a traction apophysitis at the insertion of the patellar tendon onto the tibial tuberosity seen commonly among adolescent athletes. Patients usually present with pain and tenderness at the tibial tuberosity (Chapter 40). 'Growing pains' may affect the leg and are usually a diagnosis of exclusion. Intermittent achy pain exacerbated by periods of active growth with completely negative imaging and investigations are characteristic. The youngest reported patient treated with surgical release for pressure-positive chronic exertional compartment syndrome was 12 years old and it is unclear whether this patient would have grown out of the problem at maturity.

Acute bony injuries

Periosteal contusion

Periosteal contusion occurs as a result of a direct blow from a hard object such as a football boot. It can be extremely painful at the time of injury but the pain usually settles relatively quickly. Persistent pain may occur because of a hematoma having formed under the periosteum. There will be local tenderness and bony swelling. Treatment consists of rest and protection.

Fractured tibia and fibula

Combined fractures of the tibia and fibula are often due to indirect violence in landing from a jump on a twisted foot. The tibia or fibula may be injured individually by a direct blow. Weight-bearing will be impossible in cases of displaced fracture of the tibia. Fracture of the tibia is often compound and visible through damaged skin. An isolated fracture of the fibula may exhibit only local tenderness. An isolated fractured fibula (except where it involves the ankle joint) requires analgesia only. However, the ankle and knee joint must be carefully examined for associated injuries. The management of a combined fracture is that for fracture of the tibia. Patients with compound (open) fractures should be admitted to hospital.

Many closed tibial fractures can be treated conservatively as long as angulation is minimal. This involves an above-knee plaster with the knee slightly flexed and the ankle in 90° of dorsiflexion. The limb is elevated for three to seven days until swelling subsides. A check X-ray should be taken after casting. Patients should be reviewed at six to eight weeks, at which time they may be able to be placed in a hinged knee cast.

Bony union requires eight to 12 weeks; however, 16 to 20 weeks are required for consolidation. Physiotherapy after removal of the plaster is aimed at regaining full range of knee flexion and quadriceps muscle strength. Activities such as swimming can be resumed immediately after removal of the plaster but multidirectional running sports must wait until range of movement and muscle strength have returned to normal. There is a strong trend towards early surgical fixation of unstable tibial fractures with intramedullary nailing, which allows athletes earlier weight-bearing, conditioning activities, return to sport, and obviates the risk of potential malunion.

Recommended Reading

Batt ME. Shin splints: a review of terminology. *Clin J Sport Med* 1995; 5: 53–7.

Beck BR. Tibial stress injuries. An aetiological review for the purposes of guiding management. *Sports Med* 1998; 26(4): 265–79.

Blackman P. Exercise-related lower leg pain—compartment syndromes. *Med Sci Sports Exerc* 2000; 32(3 suppl.): S4–S10.

Bradshaw C. Exercise-related lower leg pain—vascular. *Med Sci Sports Exerc* 2000; 32(3 suppl.): S34–S36.

Brukner P. Exercise-related lower leg pain—an overview. *Med Sci Sports Exerc* 2000; 32(3 suppl.): S1–S3.

Detmer DE. Chronic shin splints. Classification and management of medial tibial stress syndrome. *Sports Med* 1986; 3: 436–46.

Edwards PH, Wright, ML. Hartman JF. A practical approach for the differential diagnosis of chronic leg pain in the athlete. *Am J Sports Med* 2005; 33(8): 1241–9.

McCrory P. Exercise-related lower leg pain—neural. *Med Sci Sports Exerc* 2000; 32(3 suppl.): S11–S14.

Pell RF, Khanuja HS, Cooley R. Leg pain in the running athlete. *J Am Acad Orthop Surg* 2004; 12(6): 396–404.

Styf J. Chronic exercise induced pain in the anterior aspect of the lower leg. An overview of the diagnosis. *Sports Med* 1989; 7(5): 331–9.

References

1. Pedowitz RA, Hargens AR. Acute and chronic compartment syndromes. In: Garrett WE, Speer KP, Kirkendall DT, eds. *Principles and Practice of Orthopaedic Sports Medicine*. Philadelphia: Lippincott, Williams & Wilkins; 2000; 87–97.

2. Blackman PG. A review of chronic exertional compartment syndrome in the lower leg. *Med Sci Sports Exerc* 2000; 32(3): S4–S10.

3. Fredericson M, Bergman G, Hoffman KL, et al. Tibial stress reaction in runners. Correlation of clinical symptoms and scintigraphy with a new magnetic resonance imaging grading system. *Am J Sports Med* 1995; 23(4): 472–81.

4. Yao L, Johnson C, Gentili A, et al. Stress injuries of bone—analysis of MR staging criteria. *Acad Radiol* 1998; 5(1): 34–40.

5. Arendt E, Agel J, Heikes C, et al. Stress injuries to bone in college athletes: a retrospective review of experience at a single institution. *Am J Sports Med* 2003; 31(6): 959–68.

6. Dunbar MJ, Stanish WD, Vincent NE. Chronic exertional compartment syndrome. In: Harries M, Williams C, Stanish WD, et al., eds. *Oxford Textbook of Sports Medicine*. Oxford: Oxford University Press, 1998; 669–78.

7. Amendola A, Rorebeck CH, Vellett D, et al. The use of magnetic resonance imaging in exertional compartment syndromes. *Am J Sports Med* 1990; 18(1): 29–34.

8. Batt ME, Ugalde V, Anderson MW, et al. A prospective controlled study of diagnostic imaging for acute shin splints. *Med Sci Sports Exerc* 1998; 30(11): 1564–71.

9. van den Brand JGH, Nelson T, Verleisdonk EJMM, et al. The diagnostic value of intracompartmental pressure measurement, magnetic resonance imaging, and near-infrared spectroscopy in chronic exertional compartment syndrome: a prospective study in 50 patients. *Am J Sports Med* 2005; 33(5): 699–704.

10. Hislop M, Tierney P, Murray P, et al. Chronic exertional compartment syndrome: the controversial 'fifth' compartment of the leg. *Am J Sports Med* 2003; 31(5): 770–6.

11. Dickson TB, Kichline PD. Functional management of stress fractures in female athletes using a pneumatic leg brace. *Am J Sports Med* 1987; 15: 86–9.

12. Whitelaw GP, Wetzler MJ, Levy AS, et al. A pneumatic leg brace for the treatment of tibial stress fractures. *Clin Orthop* 1991; 270: 302–5.

13. Swenson EJ, DeHaven KE, Sebastianelli WJ, et al. The effect of pneumatic leg brace on return to play in athletes with tibial stress fractures. *Am J Sports Med* 1997; 25(3): 322–8.

14. Benazzo F, Mosconi M, Baeccarisi G, et al. Use of capacitive coupled electric fields in stress fractures in athletes. *Clin Orthop* 1995; 310: 145–9.

15. Warden SJ. A new direction for ultrasound therapy in sports medicine. *Sports Med* 2003; 33(2): 95–107.

16. Stewart GW, Brunet ME, Manning MR, et al. Treatment of stress fractures in athletes with intravenous pamidronate. *Clin J Sport Med* 2005; 15(2): 92–4.

17. Brukner PD, Bennell KL, Matheson GO. *Stress Fractures.* Melbourne: Blackwell Scientific, 1999.

18. Batt ME, Kemp S, Kerslake R. Delayed union stress fractures of the anterior tibia: conservative management. *Br J Sports Med* 2001; 35: 74–7.

19. Rettig AC, Shelbourne KD, McCarroll JR, et al. The natural history and treatment of delayed union and non-union stress fractures of the anterior cortex of the tibia. *Am J Sports Med* 1988; 16: 250–5.

20. Green NE, Rogers RA, Lipscomb AB. Nonunions of stress fractures of the tibia. *Am J Sports Med* 1985; 13(3): 171–6.

21. Orava S, Karpakka J, Hulkko A, et al. Diagnosis and treatment of stress fractures located at the mid-tibial shaft in athletes. *Int J Sports Med* 1991; 12: 419–22.

22. Chang PS, Harris RM. Intramedullary nailing for chronic tibial stress fractures. A review of five cases. *Am J Sports Med* 1996; 24(5): 688–92.

23. Bates P. Shin splints—a literature review. *Br J Sports Med* 1985; 19(3): 132–7.

24. Detmer DE. Chronic shin splints. Classification and management of medial tibial stress syndrome. *Sports Med* 1986; 3: 436–46.

25. Mubarak SJ, Gould RN, Fon Lee Y, et al. The medial tibial stress syndrome: a cause of shin splints. *Am J Sports Med* 1982; 10: 201–5.

26. Beck BR, Osternig LR. Medial tibial stress syndrome. The location of muscles in the leg in relation to symptoms. *J Bone Joint Surg Am* 1994; 76A(7): 1057–61.

27. Bennett JE, Reinking MF, Pluemer B, et al. Factors contributing to the development of medial tibial stress syndrome in high school runners. *J Orthop Sports Phys Ther* 2001; 31(9): 504–10.

28. Pell RF, Khanuja HS, Cooley R. Leg pain in running. *J Am Acad Orthop Surg* 2004; 12(6): 396–404.

29. Magnusson HK, Westlin NE, Nykvist F, et al. Abnormally decreased regional bone density in athletes with medial tibial stress syndrome. *Am J Sports Med* 2001; 29(6): 712–15.

30. Magnusson HI, Ahlborg HG, Karlsson C, et al. Low regional tibial bone density in athletes with medial tibial stress syndrome normalizes after recovery from symptoms. *Am J Sports Med* 2003; 31(4): 596–600.

31. Burne SG, Khan KM, Boudville PB, et al. Risk factors associated with exertional medial tibial pain: a 12 month prospective clinical study. *Br J Sports Med* 2004; 38(4): 441–5.

32. Detmer DE. Chronic shin splints: classification and management of medial tibial stress syndrome. *Sports Med* 1986; 3: 436–46.

33. Holen KJ, Engebretsen L, Grontvedt T, et al. Surgical treatment of medial tibial stress syndrome (shin splint) by fasciotomy of the superficial posterior compartment of the leg. *Scand J Med Sci Sports* 1995; 8: 40–5.

34. Fraimont MJ, Adamson GJ. Chronic exertional compartment syndrome. *J Am Acad Orthop Surg* 2003; 11(4): 268–76.

35. Hurschler CR, Vanderby D, Martinez DA, et al. Mechanical and biochemical analysis of tibial compartment fascia in chronic compartment syndrome. *Ann Biomed Eng* 1994; 22: 430–5.

36. Barbour TDA, Briggs CA, Bell SN, et al. Histology of the fascial-periosteal interface in lower limb chronic deep posterior compartment syndrome. *Br J Sports Med* 2004; 38: 709–17.

37. Birtles DB, Rayson MP, Casey A, et al. Venous obstruction in healthy limbs: a model for chronic compartment syndrome? *Med Sci Sports Exerc* 2003; 35(10): 1638–44.

38. Balduini FC, Shenton DW, O'Connor KH, et al. Chronic exertional compartment syndrome: correlation of compartment pressure and muscle ischaemia utilising 31p-NMR spectroscopy. *Clin Sports Med* 1993; 12(1): 151–65.

39. Owens S, Edwards P, Miles K, et al. Chronic compartment syndrome affecting the lower limb: MIBI perfusion imaging as an alternative to pressure monitoring: two case reports. *Br J Sports Med* 1999; 33: 49–53.

40. Davey JR, Rorebeck CH, Fowler PJ. The tibialis posterior muscle compartment. An unrecognised cause of exertional

compartment syndrome. *Am J Sports Med* 1984; 12(5): 391–7.

41. Pedowitz RA, Hargens AR, Mubarak SJ, et al. Modified criteria for the objective diagnosis of chronic compartment syndrome of the leg. *Am J Sports Med* 1990; 18(1): 35–40.

42. Hutchinson MR, Bederka B, Kopplin M. Anatomic structures at risk during minimal-incision endoscopically assisted fascial compartment releases in the leg. *Am J Sports Med* 2003; 31(5): 764–9.

43. Esmail AN, Flynn JM, Ganley TJ, et al. Acute exercise-induced compartment syndrome in the anterior leg: a case report. *Am J Sports Med* 2001; 29(4): 509–12.

44. McKee MD, Jupiter JB. Acute-exercise-induced bilateral anterolateral leg compartment syndrome in a healthy young man. *Am J Orthop* 1995; 24: 862–4.

45. Fronek J, Mubarak SJ, Hargens AR, et al. Management of chronic exertional anterior compartment syndrome of the lower extremity. *Clin Orthop* 1986; 207: 253–62.

46. Howard JL, Mohtadi NGH, Wiley JP. Evaluation of outcomes in patients following surgical treatment of chronic exertional compartment syndrome in the leg. *Clin J Sport Med* 2000; 10: 176–84.

47. Rorabeck CH, Fowler PJ, Nott L. The results of fasciotomy management of chronic exertional compartment syndrome. *Am J Sports Med* 1988; 16: 224–7.

48. Schepsis AA, Gill SS, Foster TA. Fasciotomy for exertional anterior compartment syndrome: is lateral compartment release necessary? *Am J Sports Med* 1999; 27(4): 430–5.

49. Wallensten R. Results of fasciotomy in patients with medial tibial syndrome or chronic anterior-compartment syndrome. *J Bone Joint Surg Am* 1983; 65A: 1252–5.

50. Slimmon D, Bennell K, Brukner P, et al. Long-term outcome of fasciotomy with partial fasciectomy for chronic exertional compartment syndrome of the lower leg. *Am J Sports Med* 2002; 30(4): 581–7.

51. Micheli L, Solomon R, Solomon J, et al. Outcomes of fasciotomy for chronic exertional compartment syndrome. *Am J Sports Med* 1999; 27: 197–201.

52. Schepsis AA, Fitzgerald M, Nicoletta R. Revision surgery for exertional anterior compartment syndrome of the lower leg: technique, findings, and results. *Am J Sports Med* 2005; 33(7): 1040–7.

53. Jackson DL. Superficial peroneal nerve palsy in a football player. *Physician Sportsmed* 1990; 18(5): 67–74.

54. Leach RE, Purnell MB, Saito A. Peroneal nerve entrapment in runners. *Am J Sports Med* 1989; 17(2): 287–91.

55. Bradshaw C. Exercise-related lower leg pain—vascular. *Med Sci Sports Exerc* 2000; 32(3): S34–S36.

56. Stager A, Clement D. Popliteal artery entrapment syndrome. *Sports Med* 1999; 28(1): 61–70.

Calf Pain

WITH CHRIS BRADSHAW AND MATT HISLOP

Calf pain is a common presenting complaint and if not managed appropriately it can persist for months or recur and cause frustration for both patient and practitioner. Both acute and chronic calf pain often stem from injury to the calf muscle. The term 'calf muscle' refers to the gastrocnemius and soleus muscles. The more superficial muscle, the gastrocnemius, has medial and lateral heads that arise from the femoral condyles, while the deeper soleus arises from the upper fibula and the medial tibial border. These muscles have a joint tendon, the Achilles, which inserts onto the calcaneus. As a biarthrodial muscle extending over the knee and the ankle, the gastrocnemius is thought to be more susceptible to injury than a uniarthrodial muscle. The anatomy of the calf is shown in Figure 31.1.

Clinical perspective

Injuries to the musculotendinous complex are by far the most common causes of calf pain. Muscle strains occur most commonly in the medial head of the gastrocnemius or near the musculotendinous junction. A sudden burst of acceleration, such as stretching to play a ball in squash or tennis, may precipitate injury. The calf region is also a common site of contusion caused through contact with playing equipment or another player. Muscle strains and contusions are acute injuries that present with typical histories that are usually easily distinguishable.

Some patients present with intermittent episodes of cramping pain in the calf that may be due to recurrent minor calf muscle strain, which is a result of inadequately rehabilitated scar tissue. However, the possibility of referred pain from the lumbar spine, neural or myofascial structures should always be considered.

The calf is the most common site in the body of muscle cramps. Cramps may occur at rest or during or after exercise taken in any environmental conditions—they are not specific to exercise or exercise in heat. They tend to occur in the more acclimatized

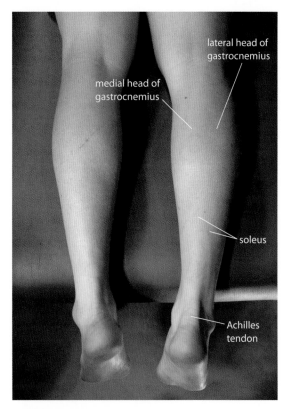

Figure 31.1 Anatomy of the calf

(a) Surface anatomy

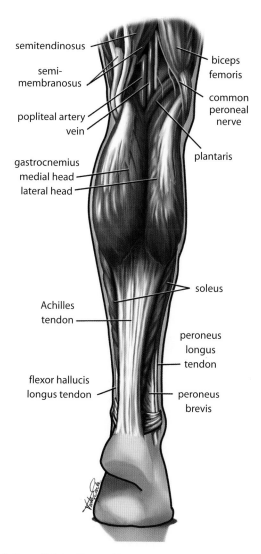

(b) Superficial calf muscles

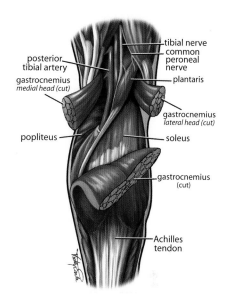

(c) Removal of the gastrocnemius showing the underlying soleus muscle

and conditioned athlete and probably result from alterations in spinal neural reflex activity activated by fatigue in susceptible individuals.

The calf is also a common site of the phenomenon known as delayed onset muscle soreness (Chapter 2). This may occur after the first training session following a lay-off or when excessive eccentric muscle contractions are performed, for example, plyometrics. Lateral calf pain may be due to a direct blow, referred pain from the superior tibiofibular joint, peroneal muscle strain or fibular stress fracture. The causes of calf pain are listed in Table 31.1.

Biomechanical factors may predispose to calf pain. Excessive subtalar pronation may overload the

soleus and gastrocnemius muscles as they supinate and plantarflex the foot for propulsion. This can cause muscle tightness and soreness and may predispose to muscle strain or tendinopathy. Muscle overload can promote muscular hypertrophy, which can predispose to the development of a compartment syndrome (Chapter 30).

History

The most important aspect of the history is the description of the onset of pain. A sudden onset of a tearing sensation in the calf is diagnostic of calf muscle strains. The patient is usually able to localize the site of the tear. The degree of disability, both immediately after the injury and subsequently, is a guide to the severity of the tear.

In patients with chronic mild calf pain, a history of a previous acute injury may be significant. The practitioner should ask about the treatment and quality of rehabilitation of the previous injury. A history of low back pain may be a clue to referred pain. The practitioner should also be alert to the possibility of referred pain if the calf pain is variable rather than constant. If there is no obvious precipitating cause of calf pain, the possibility of deep venous thrombosis after long car or airplane trips, or recent surgery, needs to be explored. Claudicant pain that comes on with exertion and then disappears may indicate proximal vascular occlusion by atheroma or entrapment (e.g. femoral or iliac artery stenosis, Fig. 4.6) or exertional compartment syndrome.

Table 31.1 Causes of calf pain

Common	Less common	Not to be missed

Muscle strains
  Gastrocnemius
  Soleus
Muscle contusion
  Gastrocnemius
Muscle cramp
Referred pain
  Lumbar spine
  Myofascial structures
Delayed onset muscle
  soreness
	Superficial posterior compartment syndrome
	Deep posterior compartment syndrome (Chapter 30)
	Referred pain
	  Superior tibiofibular joint
	  Knee (Baker's cyst, posterior cruciate ligament, posterior
	    capsular sprain)
	Entrapment
	  Popliteal artery
	  Endofibrosis of external iliac artery
	Stress fracture of the fibula
	Stress fracture of the posterior cortex of the tibia
	(Chapter 30)
	Varicose veins
		Deep venous thrombosis
		Arterial insufficiency

 Acute calf muscle strains are common among middle-aged athletes, particularly in racquet sports.

Examination

The aims of examination in the patient with acute calf strain are to determine the site and the severity of the injury as well as detecting any predisposing factors such as chronic calf muscle tightness. Examination of a patient with chronic or intermittent calf pain requires not only palpation of muscles but also assessment of neural tension (slump test, Chapter 8) and examination of the lumbar spine. It is important to palpate the entire length of the muscle bellies and their associated aponeuroses for areas of muscle and fascial tightness and thickenings that may predispose to injury.

1. Observation
   (a) standing
   (b) walking
   (c) prone
2. Active ankle movements
   (a) plantarflexion/dorsiflexion (standing) (Fig. 31.2a)
   (b) plantarflexion/dorsiflexion (prone)
3. Passive ankle movements
   (a) dorsiflexion (knee flexion) (Fig. 31.2b)
   (b) dorsiflexion (knee extension) (Fig. 31.2c)
   (c) muscle stretch
       (i) gastrocnemius (Fig. 31.2d)
       (ii) soleus (Fig. 31.2e)
4. Resisted movements
   (a) dorsiflexion
5. Functional tests
   (a) hop
   (b) jump
   (c) run
6. Palpation
   (a) gastrocnemius (Fig. 31.2f)

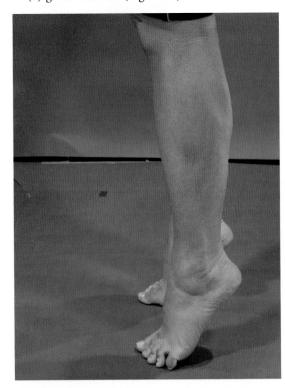

Figure 31.2 Examination of the patient with calf pain

(a) Active movement—plantarflexion/dorsiflexion (standing). The functional competence can be assessed during a bilateral or unilateral heel raise-and-drop until pain is reproduced

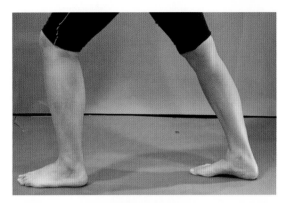

(**d**) Stretch—gastrocnemius. Examine with the knee in full extension and heel on the ground

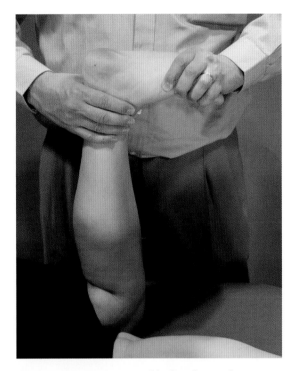

(**b**) Passive movement—ankle dorsiflexion (knee flexion). Examine with the knee flexed and add overpressure

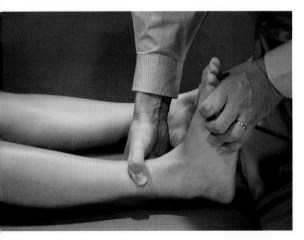

(**c**) Passive movement—ankle dorsiflexion (knee extension). Examine with the knee extended and add overpressure (Homan's sign)

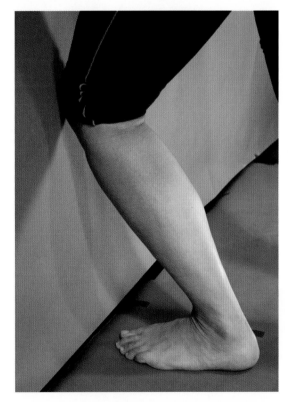

(**e**) Stretch—soleus (lunge test). The patient should flex the knee so that it passes vertically over the third toe to prevent excessive pronation. Record the range of motion and compare both sides

   (b) soleus
   (c) posterior knee
   (d) superior tibiofibular joint
7. Special tests
   (a) Thomson's test (Fig. 31.2g)

   (b) Homan's sign (Fig. 31.2c)
   (c) neural tension test—slump test (Fig. 31.2h)
   (d) gluteal trigger points
   (e) lumbar spine (Chapter 21)
   (f) biomechanical examination (Chapter 5)

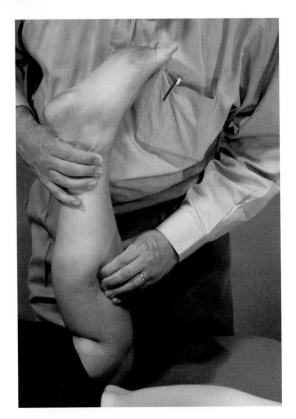

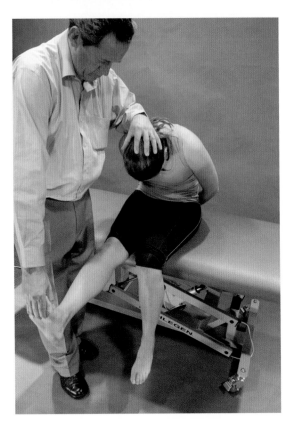

(f) Palpation. The patient should actively contract and relax the muscles and the ankle should be moved passively through dorsiflexion and plantarflexion during palpation. The gastrocnemius may be palpated in the relaxed position by placing the knee in flexion and the ankle in plantarflexion. Feel for swelling and defects in muscle or tendon tissue

(h) Special test—neural tension test (slump test)

Investigations

Although investigations are generally not required in an athlete with calf pain, ultrasound or MRI may occasionally be useful in evaluating an injury that is not following the normal healing pattern. These imaging modalities can differentiate between a muscle strain and a contusion if not clinically evident. If deep venous thrombosis is suspected, a Doppler scan may be required.

Gastrocnemius muscle strains

Acute strain

Acute strain of the gastrocnemius muscle occurs typically when the athlete attempts to accelerate from a stationary position with the ankle in dorsiflexion, or when lunging forward, such as while playing tennis or squash. Sudden eccentric overstretch, such as when an athlete runs onto a kerb and the ankle drops suddenly into dorsiflexion, is another common mechanism.

The exact moment of injury was caught on video in the case of a famous Australian batsman whose

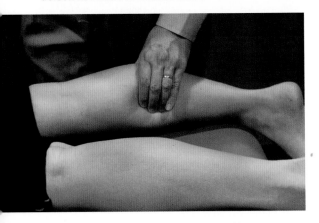

(g) Special test—Thomson's test. The calf is squeezed. If no ankle plantarflexion occurs, there has been a complete tear of the Achilles tendon or musculotendinous junction

gastrocnemius strain occurred when his entire body weight was over his foot on the injured side with the center of mass well in front of the leg. The gastrocnemius muscle–tendon complex was at close to maximal length, and the muscle–tendon length was also constant at the time. Therefore, the injury probably occurred just as the muscle–tendon complex was moving from an eccentric to an isometric phase.[1]

The patient complains of an acute, stabbing or tearing sensation usually either in the medial belly of the gastrocnemius or at the musculotendinous junction.

Examination reveals tenderness at the site of muscle strain. Stretching the gastrocnemius reproduces pain (Fig. 31.2d), as does resisted plantarflexion with the knee extended. In grade III muscle tears, there may be a palpable defect.

Assess functional competence of the injured muscle by asking the patient to perform a bilateral heel raise. If necessary, a unilateral heel raise, a heel drop or hop may be used to reproduce the pain. This places the muscle under progressively greater load concentrically and eccentrically. Calf muscle strain can be graded as shown in Table 31.2.

The tightness of the muscle itself should be assessed as overuse may often lead to palpable rope-like bands or local tissue thickening, which may predispose to further injury.

Treatment

Initial treatment aims to reduce pain and swelling with the use of ice and electrotherapeutic modalities (e.g. TENS, magnetic field therapy, interferential stimulation). Crutches may be necessary if the patient is unable to bear weight. A heel raise should be used on both the injured and uninjured side.

Gentle stretching of the gastrocnemius to the level of a feeling of tightness (Fig. 31.3) can begin soon after injury. Muscle strengthening should start after 24 hours. This involves a progression of exercises,

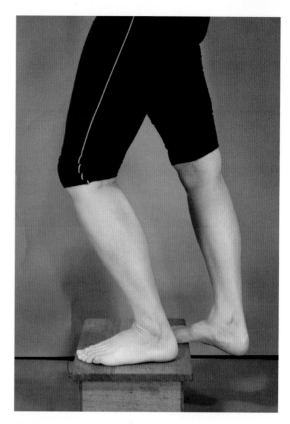

Figure 31.3 Stretching exercise for the right gastrocnemius muscle with the knee in full extension. This can be performed over a step or with the foot placed against a wall to increase the stretch

commencing with concentric bilateral calf raise, followed by unilateral calf raise with the gradual addition of weights and, finally, eccentric calf lowering over a step gradually increasing speed, then adding weights (Fig. 31.4). Low-impact cross-training such as stationary cycling or swimming can be commenced as soon as pain allows.

Table 31.2 Grading of calf strains

Grade	Symptoms	Signs	Average time to return to sport
I	Sharp pain at time of (or after) activity, may be able to continue	Pain on unilateral calf raise or hop	10–12 days
II	Unable to continue activity	Active plantarflexion pain Significant loss of dorsiflexion Bilateral calf raise pain	16–21 days
III	Immediate severe pain at musculotendinous junction	Thomson's test positive Defect palpable	6 months after surgery

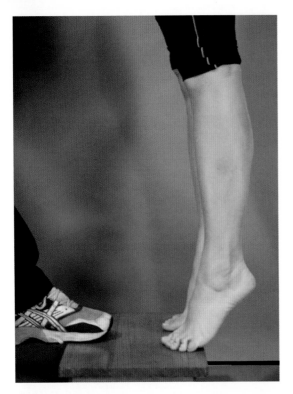

Figure 31.4 Strengthening exercises for the gastrocnemius muscle

(a) Bilateral calf raise

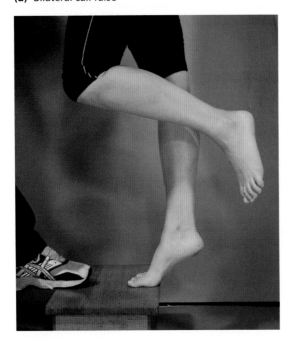

(b) Unilateral calf raise

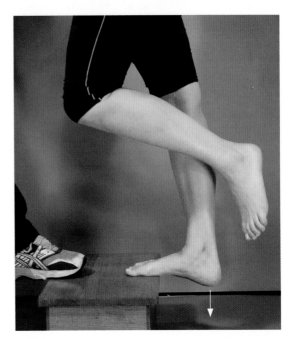

(c) Eccentric lowering

When active weight-bearing muscle contraction is pain-free, sustained myofascial tension should be performed on the muscle belly (Fig. 31.5) with digital ischemic pressure to focal areas of increased tone and/or tenderness. Endeavor to correct possible predisposing factors, such as calf muscle tightness, that may arise from poor biomechanics. Athletes should undergo a graduated return to weight-bearing, progressing through walking, easy jogs and, as eccentric strength returns, include sprint and change of direction drills.

'Tennis leg'

The term 'tennis leg' refers to an acute muscle tear in the older athlete characterized by sudden onset of severe calf pain and significant disability. The injury is invariably associated with extensive bruising and swelling, and can be mistaken for a deep venous thrombosis. The most common site is the medial head of gastrocnemius, but occasionally the plantaris muscle is involved.

Chronic strain

Chronic gastrocnemius muscle strain may occur as an overuse injury or following inadequate rehabilitation of an acute injury. Inadequate rehabilitation results in disorganized, weak scar tissue that is susceptible to further injury.

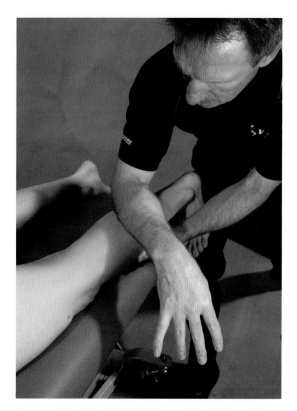

Figure 31.5 Soft tissue therapy—sustained myofascial tension to the muscle belly of the gastrocnemius

Treatment consists of transverse friction and longitudinal gliding soft tissue therapy at the site of excessive scar tissue and along the entire musculo-tendinous unit. Stretching serves to restore normal muscle length and stretches should be held for at least 15 seconds.[2] The practitioner must ensure that the patient is prescribed sufficient concentric and eccentric strengthening. Alfredson et al. have described a progressive eccentric strengthening program that required patients to perform three sets of 15 heel drops (with a straight knee, Fig. 31.4c, and also with a bent knee) twice a day, seven days a week.[3] The intensity of the exercise was increased by adding hand weights.

Soleus muscle strains

Strains of the soleus muscle are a relatively common sports injury. Although patients with soleus strains can present with sudden onset pain, they commonly report a history of increasing calf tightness over a period of days or weeks. Often walking and jogging are more painful than sprinting. The medial third

of the fibers of the soleus and its aponeurosis are prone to become hard and inflexible, particularly in athletes with excessive subtalar pronation. This tissue is susceptible to strain, especially at its junction with adjacent 'normal' tissue.

Examination reveals tenderness deep to the gastrocnemius, usually in the lateral aspect of the soleus muscle. Both the soleus stretch (Fig. 31.2e) and resisted soleus contraction provoke pain. This can be differentiated from the stretch and contraction that provoke pain in gastrocnemius strains (Fig. 31.2d).

Treatment of soleus muscle strains involves the use of heel raise and stretching (lunge). Soft tissue therapy is directed at the site of the lesion as well as tissue proximally and distally (Fig. 31.6). Strengthening exercises (Fig. 31.7) are prescribed for the soleus muscle. Orthoses may be required to control excessive pronation.

Accessory soleus

The soleus accessory muscle is a relatively rare (0.7–5.5%) anatomical variant and is found to be bilateral in 10% of cases. It usually appears as a soft

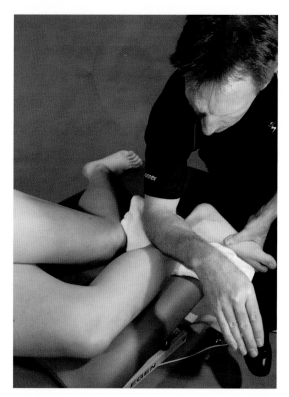

Figure 31.6 Soft tissue therapy—sustained myofascial tension to the soleus muscle

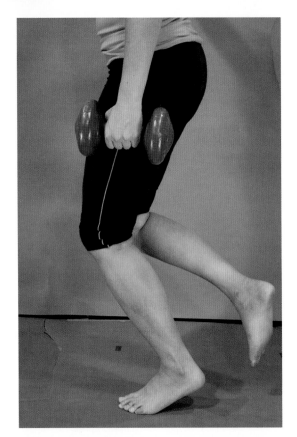

Figure 31.7 Strengthening exercises for the soleus muscle—calf raise with bent knee. This can be made more difficult by adding weights or having the patient drop down over the end of a step

tissue mass bulging medially between the distal part of the tibia and the Achilles tendon and may be mistaken for a tumor or an inflammatory lesion.[4] Athletes may be noted to have a fullness on inspection of their Achilles region from behind.

It may be asymptomatic (25%) or associated with chronic exertional compartment syndrome or posterior tibial nerve compression (tarsal tunnel syndrome). Presentation is usually during adolescence due to muscle hypertrophy.

X-ray generally shows soft tissue swelling between the deep compartment and the Achilles tendon, which obscures or obliterates Kager's triangle on the lateral radiograph of the ankle. The appearance of normal muscle on MRI allows the clinician to distinguish it from both abnormal muscle and soft tissue tumors.[5]

Asymptomatic cases require no treatment. If pain or discomfort is present, either fasciotomy alone or with excision of the accessory muscle is recommended.[4]

Claudicant-type calf pain

A common presentation to a sports physician is the patient who complains of a claudicant-type calf pain with exercise. The differential diagnosis in this patient is a vascular cause (popliteal artery entrapment, atherosclerotic disease, endofibrosis), neuromyofascial causes (referred pain or nerve entrapment) or compartment syndrome (deep posterior or superficial).

Vascular causes

Vascular causes of exercise-induced lower limb pain are uncommon and difficult to diagnose. The pain of vascular entrapment is difficult to differentiate from that caused by compartment syndrome and nerve entrapment, although there are subtle differences in the relationship of the pain to the bout of exercise. Post-exercise examination of the peripheral pulses and arterial bruits is vital and the diagnosis can be confirmed by Doppler ultrasound, ankle–brachial ratios and angiography. It may also be important to perform compartment pressure tests and nerve conduction studies to rule out coexisting conditions.

Popliteal artery entrapment

Popliteal artery entrapment syndrome is often not recognized and misdiagnosed as a compartment syndrome but can cause exercise-induced calf pain.[6] The syndrome was first described as a cause of exercise-induced leg pain in 1879. There are two types of popliteal artery entrapment syndrome: anatomical and functional.

The classically described anatomical abnormality is a variation in the anatomical relationship between the popliteal artery as it exits the popliteal fossa and the medial head of the gastrocnemius muscle. Five such variations have been described, the commonest being an abnormal medial head of the gastrocnemius muscle, the accessory part of which is observed to pass behind the popliteal artery. Other observed abnormalities include a tendinous slip arising from the medial head of the muscle, an abnormal plantaris muscle and multiple muscle abnormalities involving the lateral and medial heads of the gastrocnemius and the plantaris. Rarer anatomical variations of popliteal artery entrapment syndrome include entrapment of the artery at the level of the adductor hiatus and an isolated entrapment of the anterior tibial artery as it passes through the interosseous membrane.

The term 'functional' popliteal artery entrapment syndrome was first described by Rignault et al. in 1985[7] and describes a situation where no anatomical abnormality is visible at surgical exploration. It is hypothesized that muscle contraction (active plantarflexion of the ankle) compresses the artery between muscle and the underlying bone. This may explain why the syndrome is commonly seen in healthy young athletes with hypertrophied gastrocnemius muscles.[6]

The pain of popliteal artery entrapment syndrome is claudicant pain felt in the calf or anterior aspect of the leg. The pain is brought on by exercise and the severity of the symptoms is related to the intensity of exercise. Cessation of exercise tends to bring about rapid relief from the pain. This compares with the classic pain pattern of compartment syndrome, which is related to the volume of exercise and tends to settle over a period of around half an hour after exercise. If exercise is attempted on consecutive days, the pain from a compartment syndrome is often more severe on the second day. The pain from popliteal artery entrapment syndrome is unaffected by exercise on the previous day. The pain can be paradoxically more severe on walking than on running. This is believed to be due to the more prolonged contraction of the gastrocnemius muscle while walking.

Roughly 10% of patients with popliteal artery entrapment syndrome present with signs and symptoms of either acute or chronic limb ischemia with paresthesia, discoloration of the foot and toes, temperature change, rest pain and tissue necrosis.[8]

Examination at rest can sometimes identify a popliteal artery bruit with forceful, active ankle plantarflexion or passive dorsiflexion, but examining the patient immediately post-exercise is important in making the diagnosis. Immediately post-exercise a popliteal artery bruit may be heard and the peripheral pulses will be either weak or absent.

Non-invasive investigations include post-exercise ankle–brachial pressures and Doppler ultrasound. The definitive diagnosis is made on angiography but it is important for the radiologist to image the arterial tree with the patient actively plantarflexing and actively and passively dorsiflexing the ankle. In our experience, unfortunately, there appears to be a significantly high rate of false positive tests using this method. Correlation between the investigation results and clinical suspicion is therefore vital.

Treatment involves open surgical exploration of the popliteal fossa and division of the offending fascial band. There is some suggestion that the presence of chronic entrapment of the popliteal artery can lead to endothelial damage, which may lead to accelerated atherosclerotic disease in later life. Early treatment is recommended to prevent the development of popliteal artery damage and the need for grafting.[9]

Atherosclerotic vessel disease

Atherosclerotic vessel disease classically affects middle-aged sedentary patients. However, some athletes, particularly in the veteran or masters class, fall into the category of middle-aged or elderly and possess risk factors that predispose them to atherosclerosis. Pain may be felt in the thigh or the calf and is typically claudicant. With progression of the disease, the intensity of exercise needed to produce symptoms decreases. At rest, the peripheral pulses may be difficult to palpate or absent. An arterial bruit may also be heard at rest. The presence of such bruits may be enhanced by examining the patient post-exercise. The gold standard diagnostic test is Doppler ultrasound, although pre- and post-exercise ankle–brachial ratios can be used as a non-invasive screening test. Angiography can confirm the diagnosis. Surgical treatments include angiographic balloon catheter dilatation or stenting, open endarterectomy or bypass surgery. Bypass surgery is the most commonly used surgical technique for atherosclerotic vessel disease and its success depends on the extent of the disease and on the viability of the smaller distal vessels.

Endofibrosis

Endofibrotic disease can cause exercise-related calf pain, although more commonly the pain is felt in the thigh. Typically the lesion occurs in the proximal external iliac artery—but may extend distally towards the origin of the femoral artery beneath the inguinal ligament. It is bilateral in 15% of cases.

External iliac artery endofibrosis has been described in professional cyclists and causes exercise-related thigh or calf pain that is related to the intensity of cycling. The pain is therefore most commonly felt while racing, climbing a hill or riding into a strong wind. The pain is typically relieved rapidly by a drop in the intensity of exercise. It is postulated that the cycling position may cause folding of the artery and result in micro-traumatic lesions, and psoas hypertrophy has also been postulated to be involved.

Examination at rest may reveal a positional bruit heard over the femoral artery with the hip held in flexion. The diagnosis is made clinically by examining the patient immediately post-exercise, detecting a bruit over the femoral artery and weak or absent distal pulses. Pre- and post-exercise ankle–brachial ratios screen for the diagnosis, which is anatomically confirmed with angiography. Arterial ultrasound or echography can also be useful in visualizing the endofibrotic lesion.

Non-surgical techniques for the treatment of external iliac artery endofibrosis include angioplastic balloon catheter dilatation and stenting, which can be planned for and performed at the time of angiography. Surgical techniques include bypass surgery and open endarterectomy. Use of these techniques has made a return to top level cycling and triathlon possible in patients. However, long-term follow-up of such patients has not been carried out.

The natural history of this pathology is not certain. However, Abraham et al. suggest that it is non-progressive once high level sport is ceased. They advise that an athlete who is reducing his/her sporting level, and who is asymptomatic with activities of daily living and submaximal, be managed conservatively but followed up regularly.[10]

Neuromyofascial causes

The neural component of calf pain can be assessed with the use of the slump test (Fig. 31.2h). This may reproduce the patient's calf pain. If pain is relieved by cervical extension, neural structures may be contributing to the patient's pain.

The most common source of referred pain is myofascial trigger points in the gluteal muscles. Myofascial pain may present as an episode of sudden sharp pain and mimic a calf strain, as pain of more gradual onset accompanied by tightness, or as muscle cramps. Treatment consists of ischemic pressure or dry needling to the trigger points followed by muscle and neural stretching.

The joints of the lumbar spine may occasionally refer pain to the calf. This should be suspected clinically if the pain is somewhat variable in location or if there is a history of recurrent 'calf strains'.

The knee joint may also refer pain to the calf (Chapter 29). This may be due to a Baker's cyst, a posterior cruciate ligament injury in which bleeding may track down into the calf, from a strain of the posterior capsule of the knee joint or a popliteus muscle injury.

Nerve entrapments

Nerve entrapments around the calf include tibial nerve entrapment (rare) secondary to a Baker's cyst; popliteal artery aneurysm or ganglion resulting in ankle inverter and toe flexor weakness and paresthesia to the sole of the foot; and sural nerve entrapment, which may result from compression (ski boots, casts),

mass lesions, trauma or thrombophlebitis causing pain and paresthesia in the lateral heel and foot.

The sural nerve may be compressed in a fibrous arch that thickens the superficial sural aponeurosis around the opening through which the nerve passes. Intense physical training may lead to an increase in the sural muscle mass, which in turn compromises the sural nerve in its trajectory through the unyielding and inextensible superficial sural aponeurosis. The nerve may also become trapped in scar tissue.[11]

Investigations can include nerve conduction studies plus/minus looking for a space-occupying lesion. Management includes conservative measures such as neural stretches, fascial massage or cortisone injections, and failing this consideration of surgical exploration and/or neurolysis.

Superficial compartment syndrome

Patients with superficial posterior compartment syndrome, the least common of the lower leg compartment syndromes, present with calf pain. The superficial compartment contains the gastrocnemius and soleus muscles, which are enclosed in a fascial sheath. Symptoms are similar to those of the other compartment syndromes with pain aggravated by activity and relieved by rest. An elevated compartment pressure confirms the diagnosis during and after exercise (Table 29.3). Treatment consists of soft tissue therapy or, if this is unsuccessful, surgery.

Patients with either deep posterior compartment syndrome or stress fracture involving the posterior cortex of the tibia may present with calf pain instead of, or as well as, shin pain (Chapter 30).

Conditions not to be missed

Deep venous thrombosis occurs occasionally in association with calf injuries. The post-injury combination of lack of movement, disuse of the muscle pump and the compressive effect of swelling may all lead to venous dilatation, pooling and a decrease in the velocity of blood flow. Certainly athletes who sustain a calf muscle injury should avoid long airplane flights in the days after injury.

Deep venous thrombosis is seen rarely after arthroscopy.[12] After uncomplicated ACL knee reconstruction, deep venous thrombosis and pulmonary embolus proved fatal in an otherwise healthy 30-year-old. The diagnosis should be suspected when the patient has constant calf pain, tenderness, increased temperature and swelling. Homan's sign (passive dorsiflexion) is positive (Fig. 31.2c). The presence of deep venous thrombosis may be confirmed by Doppler scan and venography.

Recommended Reading

Abraham P, Bouye P, Quere I, et al. Past, present and future of arterial endofibrosis in athletes. *Sports Med* 2004; 34(7): 419–25.

Best TM. Soft-tissue injuries and muscle tears. *Clin Sports Med* 1997; 16: 419–34.

Stager A, Clement D. Popliteal artery entrapment syndrome. *Sports Med* 1999; 28(1): 61–70.

References

1. Orchard J, Alcott E, James T, et al. Exact moment of a gastrocnemius muscle strain captured on video. *Br J Sports Med* 2002; 36: 222–3.

2. Roberts JM, Wilson K. Effects of stretching duration on active and passive range of motion in the lower extremity. *Br J Sports Med* 1999; 33: 259–63.

3. Alfredson H, Pietila T, Jonsson P, et al. Heavy-load eccentric calf muscle training for the treatment of chronic Achilles tendinosis. *Am J Sports Med* 1998; 26(3): 360–6.

4. Christodoulou A, Terzidis I, Natsis K, et al. Soleus accessorius, an anomalous muscle in a young athlete: case report and analysis of the literature. *Br J Sports Med* 2004; 38: e38.

5. Buschmann WR, Cheung Y, Jahss MH. Magnetic resonance imaging of anomalous leg muscles: accessory soleus, peroneus quartus and the flexor digitorum longus accessorius. *Foot Ankle* 1991; 12: 109–16.

6. Stager A, Clement D. Popliteal artery entrapment syndrome. *Sports Med* 1999; 28(1): 61–70.

7. Rignault DP, Pailler JL, Lunerl F. The 'functional' popliteal entrapment syndrome. *Int Angiol* 1985; 4: 341–8.

8. Barbaras AP. Popliteal artery entrapment syndrome. *Br J Hosp Med* 1985; 34(5): 304.

9. Baltopoulos P, Fillipou DK, Sigala F. Popliteal artery entrapment syndrome. Anatomic or functional syndrome? *Clin J Sport Med* 2004; 14: 8–12.

10. Abraham P, Bouye P, Quere I, et al. Past, present and future of arterial endofibrosis in athletes. *Sports Med* 2004; 34(7): 419–25.

11. Fabre T, Montero C, Gaujard E, et al. Chronic calf pain in athletes due to sural nerve entrapment. *Am J Sports Med* 2000; 28(5): 679–82.

12. Jaureguito JW, Greenwald AE, Wilcox JF, et al. The incidence of deep venous thrombosis after arthroscopic knee surgery. *Am J Sports Med* 1999; 27: 707–10.

Pain in the Achilles Region

WITH HÅKAN ALFREDSON AND JILL COOK

Although Achilles—the legendary warrior and hero of Homer's *The Iliad*—died as a result of an arrow that pierced the midportion of his tendon, today's patient with a painful presentation in this region usually has a good long-term prognosis.[1] Nevertheless, runners have a 15 times greater risk of Achilles tendon rupture, and 30 times greater risk of tendinopathy than do sedentary controls.[2] This chapter highlights clinically useful evidence-based treatments for pain in the Achilles region.[3, 4]

Functional anatomy

The key structures that contribute to pain in the Achilles region (posterior heel and proximal towards the calf) are illustrated in Figure 32.1. The Achilles tendon, the thickest and strongest tendon in the human body,[5] is the combined tendon of the gastrocnemius and soleus muscles. The tendon has no synovial sheath but is surrounded by a paratenon (also known as peritendon), which is continuous with the perimysium of the muscle and the periosteum of the calcaneus. Pain in the main body of the tendon (2–3 cm [1–1.5 in.] above the insertion, which we refer to as the 'midportion') appears to respond much better to treatment than pain at the insertion itself. The bursae are important potential sources of pain, as is the superolateral tubercle of the calcaneum, which, when excessively large, is called a 'Haglund's deformity'. A large and rather square-shaped calcaneum appears to predispose to bursitis. The posterior process of the talus approximates the Achilles insertion and, thus, can contribute to pain in this region. Blood vessels enter the Achilles tendon from the deep surface (Fig. 32.1c); this is where abnormal vessels are ablated using sclerotherapy (see p. 603).

Clinical perspective

Acute tendon rupture is most common among men aged 30–50 years (mean age, 40 years); it causes sudden severe disability. Most textbooks suggest that rupture limits active plantarflexion of the affected leg—but beware, the patient can often plantarflex using an intact plantaris and the long toe flexors.

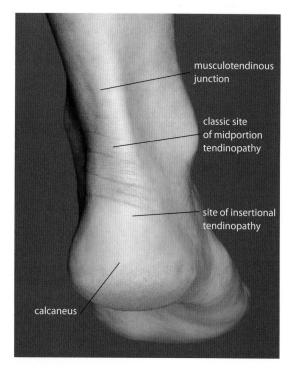

Figure 32.1 The Achilles region

(a) Surface anatomy

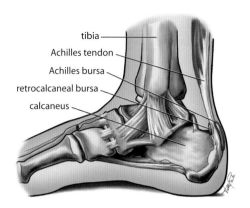

(b) Anatomy

normal

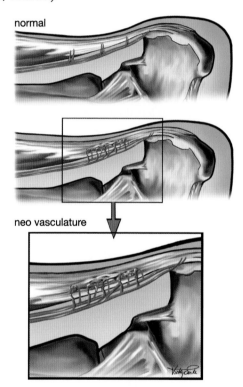

neo vasculature

(c) Stylized and magnified depiction to illustrate abnormal vasculature in Achilles tendinosis

 The key diagnostic test is the 'calf squeeze test' (also called Simmond's or Thomson's test) (see Fig. 32.2h).

Overuse Achilles tendon injuries—tendinopathy—may arise with increased training volume or intensity but may also arise insidiously. Because the prognosis for midportion Achilles tendinopathy is much better than for insertional tendinopathy, these conditions

should be distinguished clinically. The condition that was previously called 'Achilles tendinitis' is not truly an inflammatory condition and, thus, should be referred to as 'Achilles tendinopathy'.[6] Chapter 2 details the pathology that underlies the common tendinopathies.

The main differential diagnoses of gradual onset pain in the Achilles region arise from the neighboring anatomy (Table 32.1). There are two bursae in this region: the retrocalcaneal bursa, which lies between the posterior aspect of the calcaneus and the insertion of the Achilles tendon, and the Achilles bursa, which lies between the insertion of the Achilles tendon and the skin (Fig. 32.1b). The posterior process of the talus or a discrete anatomical variant, the os trigonum, can each be involved in posterior impingement syndrome (Chapter 34). This is most commonly seen in ballet dancers but occurs occasionally in sprinters and in football players. Other, much less common differential diagnoses include dislocation of the peroneal tendons, an accessory soleus muscle, irritation or neuroma of the sural nerve, and systemic inflammatory disease. These pathologies cause pain in and also *around* the Achilles tendon; true tendon pain is almost always confined to the tendon itself.

In adolescents, it is important to consider the diagnosis of Sever's lesion, a traction apophysitis at the insertion of the Achilles tendon into the calcaneus (Chapter 40). Referred pain is a very rare cause of pain in the Achilles region.

History

The athlete with overuse tendinopathy notices a gradual development of symptoms and typically complains of pain and morning stiffness after increasing activity level. Pain diminishes with walking about or applying heat (e.g. a hot shower). In most cases, pain diminishes during training, only to recur several hours afterwards.

The onset of pain is usually more sudden in a partial tear of the Achilles tendon. In this uncommon condition, pain may be more disabling in the short term. As the histological abnormality in a partial tear and in overuse tendinopathy are identical (see below), we do not emphasize the distinction other than to suggest that time to recovery may be longer in cases of partial tear. A history of a sudden, severe pain in the Achilles region with marked disability suggests a complete rupture. The patient often reports hearing a 'shot'.

Examination

Palpate the painful area for tenderness, thickening and crepitus (a 'crackling' feeling that arises because

Table 32.1 Causes of pain in the Achilles region

Common	Less common	Not to be missed

Midportion Achilles tendinopathy (this includes tendinosis, paratendinitis and partial tears)
Posterior impingement syndrome
Insertional Achilles tendinopathy including retrocalcaneal bursitis and Haglund's disease
Sever's lesion (adolescents)
	Achilles bursitis
	Accessory soleus muscle
	Referred pain
	  Neural structures
	  Lumbar spine
		Achilles tendon rupture
		Achilles tendinopathy due to the inflammatory arthropathies (Chapter 50)

of the hydrophilic [water-attracting] excess matrix proteins found in the peritendon). Also, seek possible predisposing factors, such as unilateral calf tightness, joint stiffness at the ankle or subtalar joints, and abnormal lower limb biomechanics. If the Achilles tendon seems to be the cause of pain, and the examiner is confident that the tendon is intact, the examination should aim to provoke tendon pain during tendon-loading activity. In most patients, simple single-leg heel-raises will be sufficient to cause pain. In more active individuals, however, it may be necessary to ask the patient to hop on the spot, or hop forward, to further load the tendon and reproduce pain. In some athletes repeated loading (i.e. multiple hops, jumps) tests may be necessary to evaluate the tendon fully. These functional tests provide a baseline against which treatment response can be compared. Another method of monitoring the clinical progress of Achilles tendinopathy is to use the VISA questionnaire[7] (Table 32.2, this is also available as a downloadable PDF file at <www.clinicalsportsmedicine.com>). This simple questionnaire takes less than 5 minutes to complete

Table 32.2 Victorian Institute of Sport Assessment (VISA-A) questionnaire

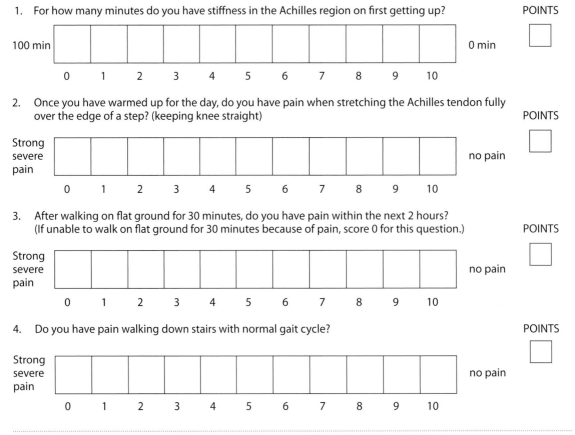

1. For how many minutes do you have stiffness in the Achilles region on first getting up?   POINTS

100 min   0 min

    0 1 2 3 4 5 6 7 8 9 10

2. Once you have warmed up for the day, do you have pain when stretching the Achilles tendon fully over the edge of a step? (keeping knee straight)   POINTS

Strong severe pain   no pain

    0 1 2 3 4 5 6 7 8 9 10

3. After walking on flat ground for 30 minutes, do you have pain within the next 2 hours? (If unable to walk on flat ground for 30 minutes because of pain, score 0 for this question.)   POINTS

Strong severe pain   no pain

    0 1 2 3 4 5 6 7 8 9 10

4. Do you have pain walking down stairs with normal gait cycle?   POINTS

Strong severe pain   no pain

    0 1 2 3 4 5 6 7 8 9 10

Table 32.2 Victorian Institute of Sport Assessment (VISA-A) questionnaire *(continued)*

5.   Do you have pain during or immediately after doing 10 (single leg) heel raises from a flat surface?   POINTS

Strong
severe   no pain
pain

      0   1   2   3   4   5   6   7   8   9   10

6.   How many single-leg hops can you do without pain?   POINTS

0   10

      0   1   2   3   4   5   6   7   8   9   10

7.   Are you currently undertaking sport or other physical activity?   POINTS

   0 ☐ Not at all

   4 ☐ Modified training ± modified competition

   7 ☐ Full training ± competition but not at same level as when symptoms began

  10 ☐ Competing at the same or higher level as when symptoms began

8.   Please complete *either* A, B or C in this question.
   •   If you have no pain while undertaking Achilles tendon loading sports, please complete Q8A only.
   •   If you have pain while undertaking Achilles tendon loading sports but it does not stop you from completing the activity, please complete Q8B only.
   •   If you have pain that stops you from completing Achilles tendon loading sports, please complete Q8C only.

A.   If you have no pain while undertaking Achilles tendon loading sports, for how long can you train/practise?

                                                  POINTS

    NIL   1–10 min   11–20 min   21–30 min   >30 min

     0   7   14   21   30

B.   If you have some pain while undertaking Achilles tendon loading sports but it does not stop you from completing your training/practise, for how long can you train/practise?

                                                  POINTS

    NIL   1–10 min   11–20 min   21–30 min   >30 min

     0   4   10   14   20

C.   If you have pain that stops you from completing your training/practise in the Achilles tendon loading sports, for how long can you train/practise?

                                                  POINTS

    NIL   1–10 min   11–20 min   21–30 min   >30 min

     0   2   5   7   10

TOTAL SCORE (/100)   ☐ %

and once patients are familiar with it they can complete most of it themselves.

Examination involves:

1. Observation
   (a) standing
   (b) walking
   (c) prone (Fig. 32.2a)
2. Active movements
   (a) plantarflexion
   (b) dorsiflexion
3. Passive movements
   (a) plantarflexion
   (b) plantarflexion with overpressure (Fig. 32.2b)
   (c) dorsiflexion
   (d) subtalar joint (Fig. 32.2c)
   (e) muscle stretch
       (i) gastrocnemius (Fig. 32.2d)
       (ii) soleus (Fig. 32.2e)
4. Resisted movements
   (a) plantarflexion—calf raises
5. Functional tests
   (a) single-leg calf raises
   (b) hop (Fig. 32.2f)
   (c) eccentric drop
6. Palpation
   (a) Achilles tendon (Fig. 32.2g)
   (b) retrocalcaneal bursa
   (c) posterior talus
   (d) calf muscle
7. Special test
   (a) Prone inspection for tendon rupture
   (b) Simmond's calf squeeze test[8] (Fig. 32.2h)
   (c) biomechanical assessment (Chapter 5)

Investigations

Plain radiographs are of limited value but, if symptoms are longstanding, they may reveal a Haglund's deformity, a prominent superior projection of the calcaneus (Fig. 32.3a), or spurs projecting into the tendon. This is associated with insertional tendinopathy and may also precipitate retrocalcaneal bursitis. Posterior impingement can be shown radiographically using functional views (see Fig. 32.14). X-ray may reveal calcification in the tendon itself but, unless severe (Fig. 32.3b), this can be asymptomatic.

In symptomatic patients, both ultrasound and MRI (Figs 32.3c–f) often reveal an abnormal signal in the Achilles tendon that generally corresponds with the histopathology of tendinosis described below (pp. 597–606). Ultrasound and MRI can help distinguish different causes of pain in the Achilles region (e.g. highlight whether the Achilles bursa or the

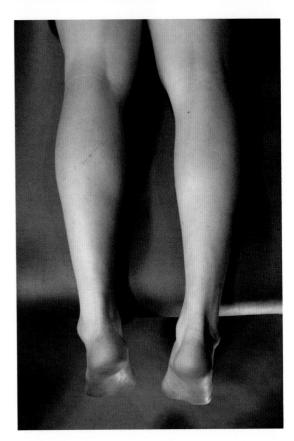

Figure 32.2 Examination of the patient with pain in the Achilles region

(a) Observation—prone. Look for swelling of the tendon and wasting of the calf muscle

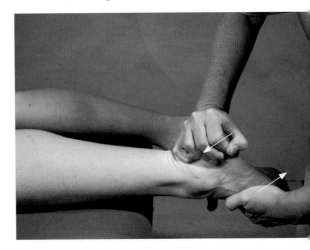

(b) Passive movement—plantarflexion. This will be painful if posterior impingement is present. Overpressure can be applied

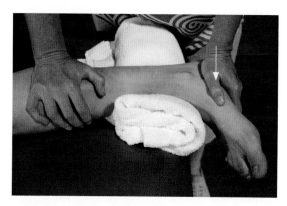

(c) Passive movement—subtalar joint. Restricted subtalar joint movement is a potential cause of Achilles region pain and a contributory factor to abnormal biomechanics

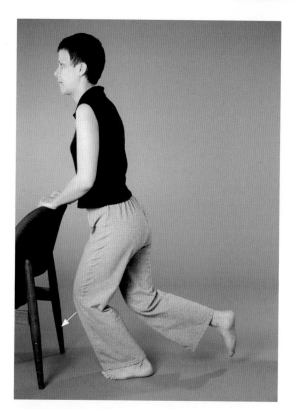

(e) Passive movement—muscle stretch (soleus). The patient stands upright and keeps the knee flexed. The foot should remain in a neutral position

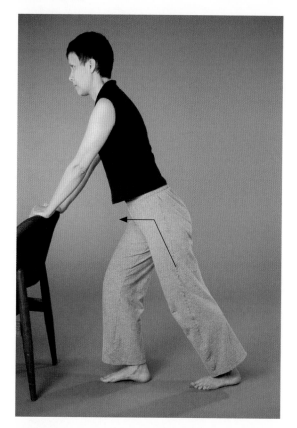

(d) Passive movement—muscle stretch (gastrocnemius). The patient stands so that body weight causes overpressure. The knee must remain extended and the heel remains in contact with the floor. The foot remains in neutral by keeping the patella in line with the third metatarsal. Compare the stretch on both sides

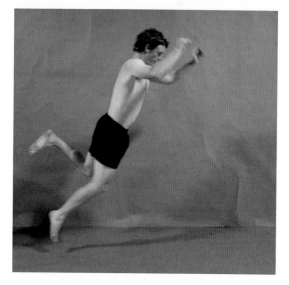

(f) Functional tests. These can be used to reproduce pain, if necessary, or to test strength. Tests include double-leg and single-leg calf raises, hops forward (illustrated), eccentric drops and lunge

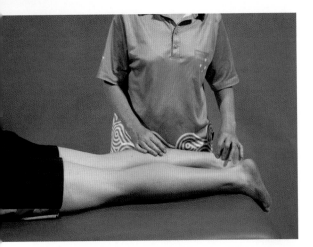

(g) Palpation—prone. Palpate the site of pain. Palpate the tendon and paratenon while the tendon moves to determine which structure is involved. Palpate the gastrocnemius, soleus and retrocalcaneal bursa(e)

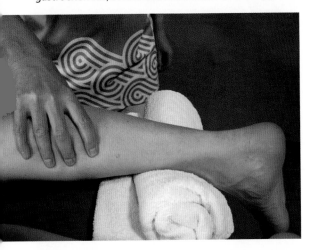

(h) Special test—Simmond's (Thomson's) calf squeeze test for Achilles tendon rupture. The practitioner squeezes the fleshy part of the calf. The test is positive if the foot fails to plantarflex

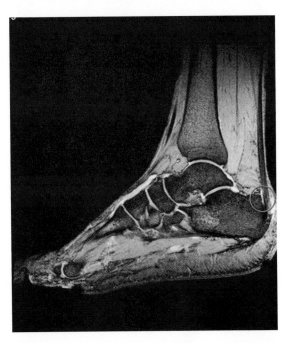

Figure 32.3 Imaging findings in patients presenting with Achilles pain

(a) MRI showing the prominent calcaneum of Haglund's deformity and associated tendon and bursal pathology

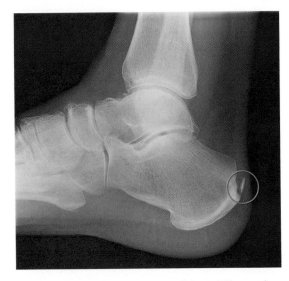

(b) Calcification in the insertion of the Achilles tendon. Patients can be managed according to the symptoms of tendinopathy (see p. 597)

Achilles tendon insertion is abnormal in patients with pain at the distal tendon). Color Doppler ultrasound is being used increasingly in tendinopathies; it provides information about the extent of the characteristic abnormal vascularity. It may also provide a target for treatment (see sclerotherapy p. 603). Because of the variability in imaging and its inconsistent clinical correlation,[9, 10] the results of imaging should not dominate

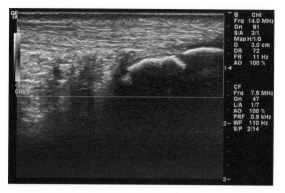

(c) Gray-scale ultrasound appearance of a normal Achilles tendon

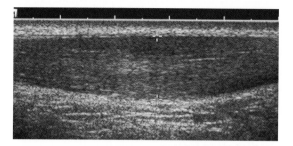

(d) Gray-scale ultrasound appearance of an Achilles tendon with mild morphological abnormality

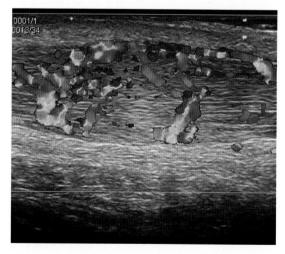

(e) Color Doppler ultrasound appearance showing abnormal vessels in symptomatic tendinopathy

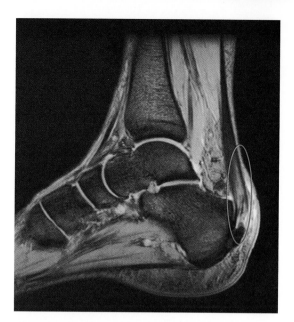

(f) MRI appearance showing mild morphological abnormality

Midportion Achilles tendinopathy

It is important to distinguish between midportion and insertional Achilles tendinopathy as they differ in their prognosis and response to treatment. We briefly review the pathology of Achilles tendinopathy, list expert opinion of the factors that predispose to injury, and summarize the clinical features of the condition. The subsequent section details the treatment of midportion tendinopathy.

Histopathology and basic molecular biology

When operating on patients with chronic Achilles tendinopathy, the surgeon generally finds a degenerative lesion characterized by an intratendinous, poorly demarcated, dull-grayish discoloration of the tissue with a focal loss of normal fiber structure (Fig. 32.4a).[13] A partial tear or rupture, defined as a macroscopic discontinuity involving a small proportion of the tendon cross-section, is seen in approximately 20% of cases. These tears always occur in a region of pre-existing pathology and do not occur in normal tendon tissue.[14] The paratendinous structures are either normal or contain edema or scarring. Importantly, when the symptomatic parts of such Achilles tendon tissue are examined under the light microscope, there is collagen fiber disarray (Fig. 32.4b). This applies equally

clinical decision making; variation in symptoms such as morning stiffness and load pain should direct treatment modification. Studies in many tendons have indicated that clinical outcomes are independent of imaging and change in imaging.[11, 12]

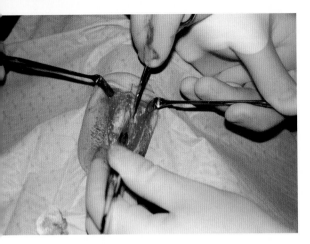

Figure 32.4 **(a)** Intraoperative photograph showing the appearance of tendinosis.

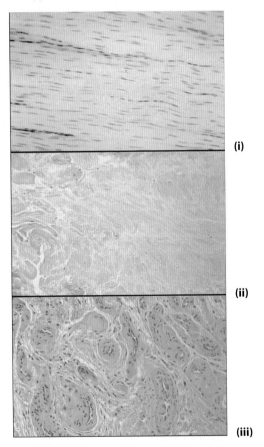

(i)

(ii)

(iii)

(b) Light microscopic appearance of this tissue: **(i)** appearance of normal tendon; **(ii)** collagen fiber disarray, loss of the characteristic parallel bundles, fewer cell nuclei; **(iii)** areas of abnormal vascularity and increasingly prominent cells (see also Figs 32.1c, 32.3e)

to areas of partial tear, which show hypervascularity without signs of tissue repair.[13] This histopathological picture is called 'tendinosis' and is identical in tendons with macroscopically evident partial tears and those without.[13] These regions of tendon disarray correspond with areas of increased signal on MRI and hypoechoic regions on ultrasound.[15]

It is noteworthy that inflammatory cells are absent in tendinosis. Also, intratendinous microdialysis[16, 17] and contemporary molecular biology techniques (cDNA arrays, real-time quantitative polymerase chain reaction) of appropriately prepared biopsy tissue[18] all failed to show evidence of prostaglandin-mediated inflammation. There are, however, signs of what Hart et al. have termed 'neurogenic inflammation'.[19] This is characterized by neuropeptides, such as substance P and calcitonin gene-related peptide (CGRP). It appears that peptidergic group IV nerve fibers release peptides from their terminals, starting various pathophysiological, and presumably painful, processes. While this field awaits further research advances, clinicians can endeavor to limit the onset of pathology by attending to the likely risk factors for Achilles tendinopathy.

Predisposing factors

Injury to the Achilles tendon occurs when the load applied to the tendon, either in a single episode or, more often, over a period of time, exceeds the ability of the tendon to withstand that load. Factors that may predispose to Achilles tendinopathy include:

- years of running
- increase in activity (distance, speed, gradient)
- decrease in recovery time between training sessions
- change of surface
- change of footwear (e.g. lower heeled spike, shoe with heel tab)
- excessive pronation[20] (increased load on gastrocnemius–soleus complex to resupinate the foot for toe-off) (Fig. 32.5)
- calf weakness
- poor muscle flexibility (e.g. tight gastrocnemius)
- joint range of motion (restricted dorsiflexion)
- poor footwear (e.g. inadequate heel counter, increased lateral flaring, decreased forefoot flexibility) (Chapter 6)
- genetic predisposition.[21]

Clinical features

The presentations of Achilles tendinopathy can vary as listed in Table 32.3.

Table 32.3 Clinical features associated with presentation of overuse Achilles tendinopathy (i.e. not a complete rupture)

Clinical feature or imaging finding	Variability in presentation with overuse Achilles tendinopathy
History	
Onset of pain	May be sudden, gradual but noticeable, or insidious
Severity of pain	May range from a minor inconvenience to profound pain with activity
Duration	May range from days to years
Disability	May be minimal, moderate or severe
Examination	
Extent of swelling/crepitus	Can range from being a major feature of the presentation to being absent
Extent of tenderness	May range from being pinpoint to extending throughout several centimeters of the tendon
Presence of a nodule	May or may not be present, and when present may vary in size

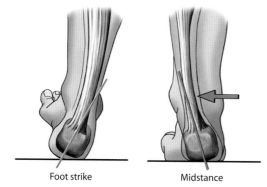

Foot strike   Midstance

Figure 32.5 Whipping action of the Achilles tendon produced by overpronation, a risk factor for midportion Achilles tendinopathy

Practise tips relating to imaging Achilles tendinopathy

There are various appearances of Achilles tendinopathy with imaging (Table 32.4). Thus, we recommend that the history and physical examination remain the keys to diagnosis. Until patients become familiar with the concept of tendinosis, imaging may help illustrate that the abnormality is one of collagen disarray and abnormal vasculature; this will help the patient understand the lengthy time course of healing.

Treatment of midportion Achilles tendinopathy

Level 2 evidence-based treatments for Achilles tendinopathy include heel-drop exercises, nitric oxide

Table 32.4 Variations in imaging findings in patients with overuse Achilles tendinopathy (i.e. not a complete rupture)

Investigation	Variations seen in clinical practise
Ultrasound—extent of swelling	Tendon swelling can be associated with tendon fiber damage (see below) or it can occur without discontinuity and swelling (e.g. fusiform swelling). It is possible to have a normal ultrasound scan with symptoms and signs of Achilles tendinopathy but differential diagnoses must be fully evaluated and excluded.
Ultrasound—discontinuity of tendon fibers	Tendon fibers may appear intact or extensively damaged on ultrasonography ('hypoechogenicity'). This is usually associated with tendon swelling.
MRI appearance	The MRI appearance can vary from essentially normal to a marked increase in abnormal signal, best seen on T2-weighted sequences. Another feature of tendinopathy is increased tendon diameter without signal.

donor therapy (glyceryl trinitrate [GTN] patches), sclerosing injections and microcurrent therapy (see below). In addition, experienced clinicians begin conservative treatment by identifying and correcting possible etiological factors. This may include relative rest, orthotic treatment (heel lift, change of shoes, corrections of malalignment) and stretching of tight muscles. Whether these 'commonsense' interventions contribute to outcome is unlikely to be tested.

Figure 32.6 illustrates a commonly used progression of treatment. The sequence of management options may need to vary in special cases such as the elite athlete, the person with acute tendon pain unable to fully bear weight, or the elderly patient who may be unable to complete the heel-drops. As always, the clinician should respond to individual patient needs and modify the sequence appropriately.

Alfredson's painful heel-drop protocol

In 1984, Curwin and Stanish[23] pioneered what they termed 'eccentric training' as therapy for tendon injuries. From this base, Alfredson and colleagues made three critical modifications.[24, 25] Firstly, they considered worsening pain as part of the normal recovery process; thus, they advised patients to continue with the full exercise program even as pain worsened on starting the program. Along those lines, if the patient experienced no pain doing the program, he or she was advised to increase the load until the exercises provoked pain (Fig. 32.7, Table 32.5). The second innovation was to incorporate two types of heel-drops into the program (see below); traditionally, only one type of heel-drop had been prescribed. Finally, they prescribed 180 heel-drops per day—a far larger number than had been recommended previously. Alfredson's 12-week program cured approximately 90% of those with midtendon pain and pathology.[25–27] In addition to the good clinical results, ultrasound and MRI follow-up demonstrated that patients' tendons returned towards normal appearance and thickness.[28]

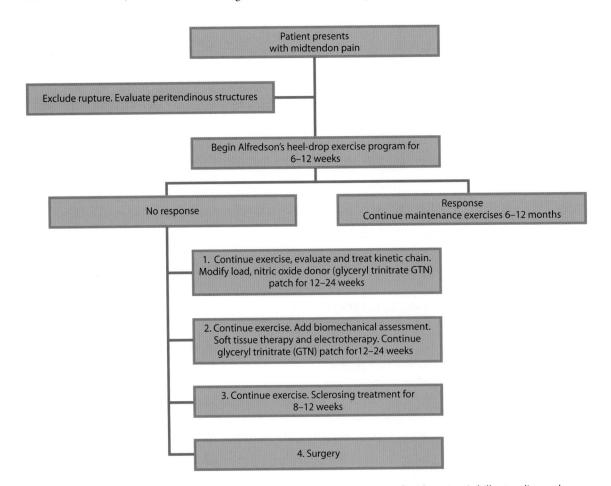

Figure 32.6 Flow chart showing one approach to the clinical management of midportion Achilles tendinopathy (modified from Alfredson et al.[22])

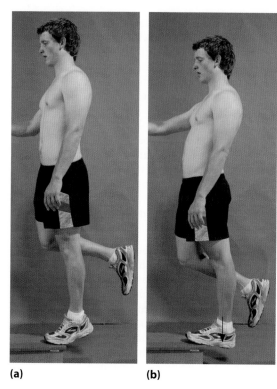
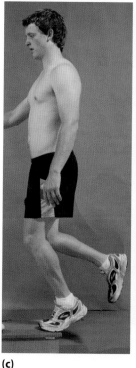
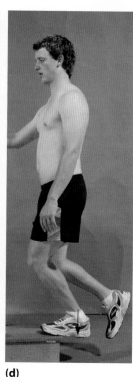

(a)   **(b)**   **(c)**   **(d)**

Figure 32.7 Alfredson's painful heel-drop protocol for Achilles tendinopathy. The heel-drop protocol consists of two key exercises: the 'gastrocnemius drop' and the 'soleus drop'.

(a) For the gastrocnemius drop, the patient begins in a demipointe position, with the heel raised and the knee fully extended.

(b) From the starting position, the patient lowers the heel so that the foot is parallel with the ground.

Variations on the heel-drop program may also be effective[29] but have not been as rigorously evaluated as have those used in patients in Alfredson's program.

 There is evidence to suggest that heel-drops promote superior clinical recovery than do heel-raises.[30]

(c) For the soleus drop, the patient again adopts the demipointe position with the heel raised, but for this exercise the knee should be flexed to 45° so that the soleus is engaged.

(d) The patient lowers the heel so that the foot is parallel with the ground.

In a study that compared these two types of exercises, 82% of patients who did the heel-drops were back to their previous activity level at the completion of treatment, whereas only 36% of those doing heel-raises achieved that outcome.[31]

Nitric oxide donor therapy

There is level 2 evidence to support nitric oxide donor therapy (glyceryl trinitrate [GTN] patches

Table 32.5 Alfredson's painful heel-drop protocol (180 drops/day)

Number of exercises	Exercise specifics	Exercise progression
3 × 15 repetitions 2 times daily 7 days/week for 12 weeks	Do exercise both with knee straight (fully extended) (Fig. 32.7a) and knee bent (flexed 45°) (Fig. 32.7b) over edge of a step Lower only (heel-drop) from standing on toes (i.e. raise back onto toes using unaffected leg or arms)	Do exercises until they become pain-free Add load until exercises are again painful Progressively add load up to 60 kg

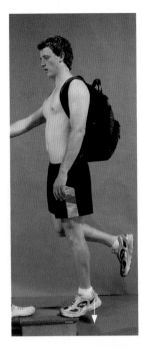

(e) To increase the load, additional weight can be added using a backpack or, where necessary, a weight machine

applied locally 1.25 mg/day).[32] Compared with the control group, the glyceryl trinitrate group showed reduced pain with activity by 12 weeks. In this group, 28 (78%) of 36 patients' tendons were asymptomatic with activities of daily living at six months, compared with 20 (49%) of 41 patients' tendons in the control group (Fig. 32.9b).

Glyceryl trinitrate (GTN) patches come in varying doses. A 0.5 mg patch should be cut in quarters and applied to the site of maximum pain for 24 hours at a time and then replaced (Fig. 32.9a). A 0.2 mg patch would best be cut in half and applied similarly.

Corticosteroid injection around and into tendon

The Cochrane database of systematic reviews concludes that peritendinous injection of corticosteroids in Achilles tendinopathy has short-term pain-relieving effects but no effect or detrimental effects in the longer term.[33, 34] Although intratendinous injection is generally contraindicated,[34] Danish researchers[35] injected corticosteroid intratendinously in six tendons with promising results. This, however, requires further research before being recommended.

How do heel-drops reduce pain in tendinopathy?

There are several possible explanations for the effectiveness of heel-drops but none have yet been proven. Heel-drops have an immediate and long-term influence on tendon. In the short-term, a single bout of exercise increases tendon volume and signal on MRI.[28] Heel-drops affect type 1 collagen production and, in the absence of ongoing insult, may increase tendon volume over the longer term.[36] Thus, heel-drops may increase tensile strength in the tendon over time. Repetitive loading and a lengthening of the muscle–tendon unit may therefore improve the capacity of the musculotendinous unit to affectively absorb load (Fig. 32.8).

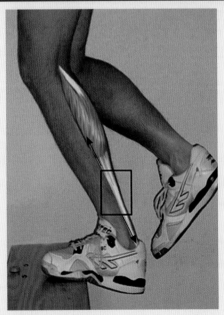

Figure 32.8 How heel-drops might work to improve Achilles tendon metabolism

Sclerosing injections

This treatment consists of using ultrasound guidance (Fig. 32.10a) while injecting a vascular sclerosant (polidocanol, an aliphatic, non-ionized, nitrogen-free substance with a sclerosing and anesthetic effect) in the area of neovascularization anterior to the tendon (Figs 32.10 b, c). Short-term (six month) evaluation of

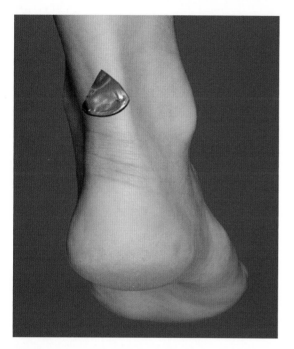

Figure 32.9 Nitric oxide donor therapy.

(a) A glyceryl trinitrate (GTN) patch is worn over the most painful site 24 hours a day for six months.

this treatment showed that eight of 10 tendons were pain-free after a mean of two treatments.[37] Tendons that were pain-free had no neovascularization outside or inside the tendon (Fig. 32.10d), but in the two unsuccessfully treated patients, vessels remained. Two-year follow-up of these patients showed that the same eight patients remained pain-free with no vessels in the tendon (unpublished data). Ultrasonographically, tendon thickness had decreased and the structure looked more normal.

In a small double-blind randomized controlled study[38] comparing the effects of injections of a sclerosing and a non-sclerosing substance (lignocaine [lidocaine] plus adrenalin [epinephrine]), two doses of the sclerosing substance led to five of 10 participants being satisfied with treatment; a further open-label treatment (injection) led to all remaining patients being satisfied. The placebo group, on the other hand, saw no patients satisfied after two placebo injections, and nine of 10 participants satisfied after open-label cross-over to the active agent.

Rehabilitation after sclerosing injection includes one to three days of rest, then gradually increased tendon-loading activity while being careful to avoid jumping, fast runs and heavy strength training during the first two weeks. After two weeks, such activities that load the tendon maximally are permitted.

After treating 500 patients with Achilles tendinopathy, the pioneers of this treatment (Alfredson et al.) reported three complications. Two patients have sustained total ruptures (one at the end of an 800-m track race eight weeks after treatment) and another patient who was treated in the midportion sustained a partial rupture in an area in which he previously

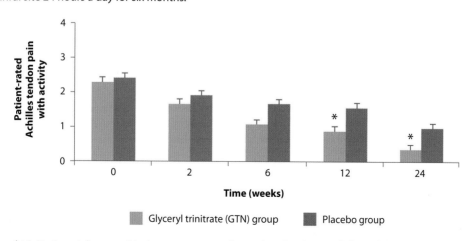

(b) Glyceryl trinitrate patches provided outcomes superior to the placebo patch for Achilles tendinopathy[4]
* = statistically significant difference ($P < 0.05$)

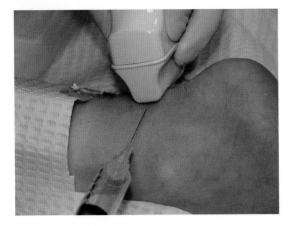

Figure 32.10 Sclerotherapy

(a) Ultrasound-guided sclerotherapy

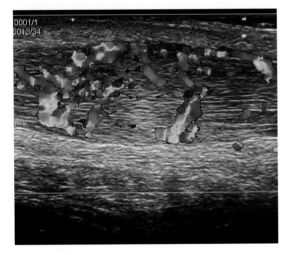

(b) Abnormal vessels—neovessels—before sclerotherapy

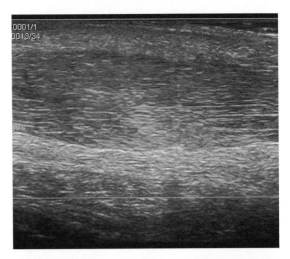

(c) Vessels absent immediately after sclerotherapy

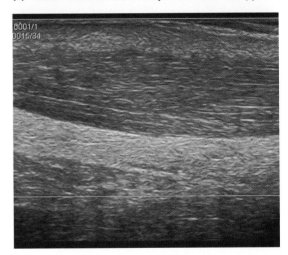

(d) Vessels are still absent 12 months after treatment in a pain-free patient

had four intratendinous corticosteroid injections. In summary, sclerosing therapy may have a role in patients who fail to respond to heel-drops and nitric oxide donor therapy. As with all innovative therapies, further research is needed to determine the long-term safety of this procedure. If the technique proves successful when used in other centers and at other tendon sites, it would strengthen the argument for more routine use.[39]

Electrophysical agents

There is little quality evidence supporting the use of electrophysical agents, including extracorporeal shock wave therapy,[40] in treating tendinopathy. Therapeutic ultrasound increases protein synthesis in tendons,[41] but there is an oversupply of poor quality protein in tendon suffering from overuse, so it may not improve the clinical outcome to further increase this substance.

A randomized trial[42] showed a superior outcome after treatment and one month later in patients who had undergone hyperthermia with low-frequency microwave compared with those treated with traditional ultrasound. Microcurrent applied for two weeks decreased pain at 12 months compared with conventional treatment.[43]

Adjunct conservative treatments

Biomechanical evaluation of the foot and leg is a clinically important part of Achilles tendon management. Although there is little empirical evidence to support the association between static foot posture and Achilles tendinopathy,[44] modification of foot posture in some patients can reduce pain and increase the capacity to load the tendon.[20]

Similarly, soft tissue therapy of the calf complex can assist rehabilitation (Fig. 32.11), as can tendon mobilization.[45] Frictions have been shown to increase the protein output of tendon cells;[46] however, similar to the effect seen with ultrasound, greater amounts of collagen and ground substance may not improve pain or pathology.

Surgical treatment

Surgical treatment procedures range from simple percutaneous tenotomy[47] to removal of tendon pathology via an open procedure. Percutaneous tenotomy resulted in 75% of patients reporting good or excellent results after 18 months.[48] The outcome of open surgery for Achilles tendinopathy was superior among patients whose tendons had diffuse disease, compared with those whose tendons had a focal area of tendinopathy.[49] At seven months post-surgery, 88% of those with diffuse disease had returned to physical activity, as had 50% of those with a focal lesion.

All Achilles tendon surgery requires early post-operative rehabilitation and this needs to continue for six to 12 months as final clinical results rely on the return of strength and functional capacity. Wise patients will continue with a maintenance program of physiotherapist-prescribed rehabilitation exercises even after having returned to training and competition.

Insertional Achilles tendinopathy, retrocalcaneal bursitis and Haglund's disease

These three 'diagnoses' are discussed together as they are intimately related in pathogenesis and clinical presentation.[50–53]

Relevant anatomy and pathogenesis

The Achilles tendon insertion, the fibrocartilaginous walls of the retrocalcaneal bursa that extend into the tendon (Fig. 32.1b) and the adjacent calcaneum form an 'enthesis organ' (Fig. 32.12).[54] The key concept is that at this site the tendon insertion, the bursa and the bone are so intimately related that a prominence of the calcaneum will greatly predispose to mechanical irritation of the bursa and the tendon. Also, there is significant strain on the tendon insertion on the posterior aspect of the tendon with dorsiflexion.[53] This then leads to a change in the nature of those tissues, consistent with the biological process of mechanotransduction (physical response to a mechanical load, Chapter 2).

We distinguish between the term 'Haglund's deformity', a descriptive label for prominence of the posterolateral calcaneum, and 'Haglund's disease', a clinical label for the clinical syndrome of a prominent, painful lateral portion of the retrocalcaneal bursa

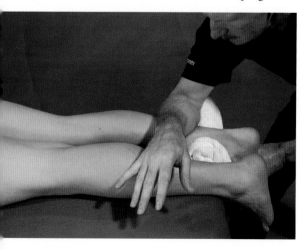

Figure 32.11 Soft tissue therapy to the belly of the calf muscles

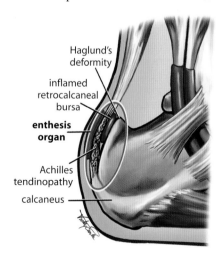

Haglund's deformity

inflamed retrocalcaneal bursa

enthesis organ

Achilles tendinopathy

calcaneus

Figure 32.12 The 'enthesis organ' illustrates why insertional Achilles tendinopathy is often associated with retrocalcaneal bursitis and calcaneal prominence

associated with a prominent superolateral superior calcaneus (the Haglund's deformity).[5] Thus, an asymptomatic patient may be found to have a Haglund's deformity on radiographs taken for another reason. This is important as the deformity, per se, is not an indication for treatment.

Insertional Achilles tendinopathy is not as common, or as well-researched, as midportion tendinopathy. The pathology is tendinosis, not inflammation,[55] and there is some local revascularization inside and outside the distal tendon.

Clinical assessment

Good clinical practise includes evaluation of the tendon, bursa and calcaneum by careful history, inspection of the region for bony prominence and local swelling as well as palpation of the area of maximal tenderness. Biomechanical abnormalities, joint stiffness and proximal soft tissue tightening can exacerbate an anatomical predisposition to retrocalcaneal bursitis; they warrant correction if present. Ultrasound and MRI can help to assess the extent of pathology in the tendon and the bursa. Radiography can complement clinical assessment of the calcaneum and will reveal tendon calcification, if present. If the pathology is truly in the tendon insertion, it is important to alert the patient that this is more challenging to treat than midportion tendinopathy. We iterate that symptoms of insertional Achilles tendinopathy, as with any enthesopathy, should raise suspicion about the possibility of the diagnosis of rheumatoid arthritis or spondyloarthopathy (Chapter 50).

Treatment

Treatment must consider the enthesis organ as a unit. Isolated treatment of insertional tendinopathy is generally unsuccessful. For example, Alfredson's painful heel-drop protocol (very effective in midportion tendinopathy) only achieved good clinical results in approximately 30% of cases of insertional tendinopathy.[56] However, in a pilot study of 11 patients with more than two years of chronic insertional tendinopathy, sclerosing of local neovessels with polidocanol cured eight patients at eight-month follow-up. Pain during tendon-loading activity, recorded on a visual analog scale, decreased from 82 mm (3.2 in.) before treatment to 14 mm (0.6 in.) after treatment. This success rate was encouraging as nine patients had multiple pathology as is usually the case (thickened retrocalcaneal bursae, calcification, loose fragment). A heel lift worn inside both shoes (0.5–1.0 cm [0.25–0.5 in.]) is a good practical way of unloading the region.

Sometimes symptoms appear to arise mainly from the retrocalcaneal bursa itself. In these cases the symptoms may respond to NSAIDs or intrabursal corticosteroid injection (0.5 mL of corticosteroid and 0.2 mL of local anesthetic agent). Abolition of pain after local anesthesia helps confirm the diagnosis. Following injection, the patient should rest for 48 hours and then slowly resume activity, building up to full activity over a period of two to three weeks.

If conservative management fails in cases of Haglund's disease where a deformity is present, surgery is indicated. Thus, surgery may be indicated in a larger proportion of patients with insertional Achilles tendinopathy and retrocalcaneal bursitis compared with in those with midportion Achilles tendinopathy.

In summary, insertional Achilles tendinopathy is commonly associated with retrocalcaneal bursitis and Haglund's disease—it is a condition of the 'enthesis organ'. This challenging condition should be distinguished from 'non-insertional' tendinopathy, which we call 'midportion' tendinopathy for simplicity. Accurate diagnosis is a key to identifying underlying conditions that may need to be treated (e.g. biomechanical abnormality, Haglund's deformity). The heel-drop program is not particularly effective in this enthesopathy. Surgical treatment and novel therapies, such as the sclerosant polidocanol, may be warranted in this condition. Spondyloarthropathy needs to be considered as a differential diagnosis.

Achilles tendon rupture (complete)

WITH JON KARLSSON

Complete rupture of the Achilles tendon classically occurs in athletes in their 30s or 40s. The typical patient is a 40-year-old male, and the male:female ratio is 10:1. The location of rupture is not associated with a 'watershed' area of poor blood supply.[57]

The patient describes feeling 'as if I was hit or kicked in the back of the leg'; pain is not always the strongest sensation. This is immediately followed by grossly diminished function. A snap or tear may be audible.

The patient will usually have an obvious limp but may have surprisingly good function through the use of compensatory muscles. That is, the patient may be able to walk, but not on the toes with any strength.

 Four clinical tests can greatly simplify examination of complete Achilles tendon rupture:

1. On careful inspection with the patient prone and both ankles fully relaxed, the foot on the side with the ruptured tendon hangs straight down (because of the absence of tendon tone); the foot on the non-ruptured side maintains a little plantarflexion.
2. Acutely, there may be a palpable gap in the tendon, approximately 3–6 cm (1.5–3 in.) proximal to the insertion into the calcaneus.
3. The strength of plantarflexion is markedly reduced.
4. Simmond's (also known as Thomson's) calf squeeze test is positive (Fig. 32.2h).[8]

Treatment of the acutely ruptured Achilles tendon may be either surgical (Fig. 32.13) or conservative.

Surgical management

Open surgical treatment of Achilles tendon rupture is associated with a 27% lower risk of rerupture compared with non-surgical treatment.[58] However, open operative treatment is associated with an 11% risk of complications, including infection, adhesions and disturbed skin sensitivity.[59] Another approach to reduce these complications is to perform surgery 'percutaneously' but this does not eliminate the risk of complications. Early post-operative mobilization with a functional brace reduced the complication rate compared with in those who had been managed with post-operative cast immobilization for eight weeks. Post-operative management depends on the type of surgery and the surgeon's post-operative protocols. Because range of movement and strength can be difficult to regain after rupture repair, earliest possible mobilization and rehabilitation is

recommended. A protocol consisting of open surgical end-to-end repair, a brief period of post-operative cast immobilization (one to two weeks), followed by controlled range of motion training until the eighth post-operative week provided excellent outcomes.[60]

Non-surgical management

Non-surgical management of an Achilles tendon rupture may be indicated in older patients, or patients with a low level of activity.[58] This involves cast immobilization, initially in a position of maximal plantarflexion to protect the tendon for four weeks, then after four weeks gradually reducing the amount of plantarflexion. The total immobilization time is eight weeks. Some, but not all, studies of this treatment method have reported residual lengthening of the Achilles tendon as well as the higher rerupture rate mentioned above. A recent meta-analysis of Achilles tendon rupture treatments concluded that there were insufficient data to draw conclusions about different non-operative treatment regimens.[58] It should, however, be borne in mind that non-surgical treatment leads to a high success rate provided that no rerupture occurs; thus, the main drawback of a non-surgical treatment protocol is the increased risk of rerupture. Recent studies have also discussed the possibility of treating the ruptured Achilles tendon with early range of motion without any surgical intervention. We look forward to those results with interest.

Posterior impingement syndrome

Posterior impingement syndrome of the ankle refers to impingement of the posterior talus by the adjacent aspect of the posterior aspect of the tibia in extremes of plantarflexion. An enlarged posterior tubercle of the talus (Fig. 32.14a) or an os trigonum (Fig. 32.14b) may be present. This condition is commonly found in ballet dancers, gymnasts and footballers, all of whom maximally plantarflex their ankles. It is also seen secondary to ankle plantarflexion/inversion injuries.

The os trigonum represents an unfused ossific center in the posterior process of the talus. This is a normal anatomical variant present in approximately 10% of the population. The pain arises because of the space-occupying nature of the bone; it does not depend on whether the bone is fused or not.

The diagnosis of posterior impingement syndrome is suggested by pain and tenderness at the posterior aspect of the ankle and confirmed by a positive posterior impingement test.

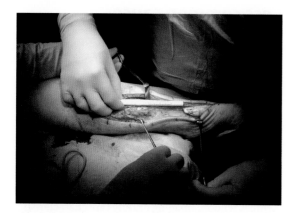

Figure 32.13 Intraoperative photograph showing the ruptured Achilles tendon. The surgeon is showing that the gap between the torn tendon ends exceeds 5 cm

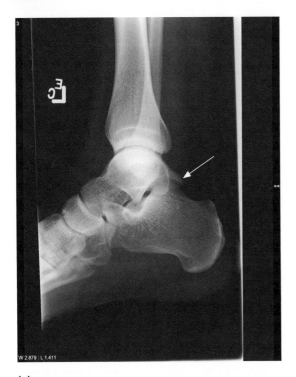

(a)

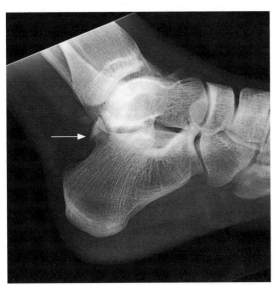

(b)

Figure 32.14 Posterior impingement. **(a)** Prominent posterior process of the talus (arrow) and **(b)** the os trigonum (arrow), both of which can be associated with posterior impingement

 PRACTISE PEARL Pain is reproduced on passive plantarflexion of the ankle (Fig. 32.2b).

If further confirmation is required, a small amount of a local anesthetic agent can be injected around the posterior talus and the impingement test performed without pain. Ideally, this test would be done under radiographic guidance so that there is certainty about the location of the injection. In practice, this is not always feasible and the test relies on the clinical accuracy of the practitioner.

Treatments that expert clinicians have used for posterior impingement syndrome include relative rest, manual mobilization of the subtalar, talocrural and midfoot joints, NSAIDs and electrotherapeutic modalities. In ballet dancers, forcing turnout and/or 'sickling' the foot can predispose to this condition, so technique assessment is essential. If the condition persists, a corticosteroid injection around the area of maximal tenderness may reduce pain. This is best done from the lateral side, as the medial aspect of the ankle contains the neurovascular bundle. Frequently, this condition does not respond to conservative management and requires surgical removal of the posterior process or the os trigonum. This can be done arthroscopically.

Sever's lesion

Sever's lesion or calcaneal apophysitis is a common insertional enthesopathy among adolescents (Chapter 40). It can be considered the Achilles tendon equivalent of Osgood-Schlatter lesion at the patellar tendon insertion.

Less common causes

Accessory soleus

Although considered a 'rare' cause of Achilles region pain, anatomical studies suggest that an accessory soleus is present in about 6% of people. This was mirrored in an Italian study of 650 athletes; 18 (2.7%) had an accessory soleus.[61] The condition is more common among men than women and the average age of presentation is 20 years. The primary presenting patterns are pain in the Achilles region during exercise (a 'compartment' type pain) with swelling, or painless swelling. When pain is present it arises in the Achilles tendon. Imaging findings are characteristic; plain radiographs show a soft tissue shadow posterior to the tibia obscuring the pre-Achilles fat pad. Ultrasound, CT and MRI can each confirm a mass with the same texture as muscle. In cases that are symptomatic, observation is an appropriate treatment but, if symptoms warrant, surgical removal of the accessory soleus is probably the best treatment.[62]

Other causes of pain in the Achilles region

Achilles bursitis (Fig. 32.1b) is generally caused by excessive friction, such as by heel tabs, or by wearing shoes that are too tight or too large. Various types of rather stiff boots (e.g. in skating, cricket bowling) can cause such friction, and the pressure can often be relieved by using a punch to widen the heel of the boot and providing 'donut' protection to the area of bursitis as it resolves.

Referred pain to this region from the lumbar spine or associated neural structures is unusual and always warrants consideration in challenging cases (Chapters 3, 35).

Recommended Reading

Alfredson H, Ohberg L. Sclerosing injections to areas of neo-vascularisation reduce pain in chronic Achilles tendinopathy: a double-blind randomised controlled trial. *Knee Surg Sports Traumatol Arthrosc* 2005; 13(4): 338–44.

Astrom M, Westlin N. No effect of piroxicam on Achilles tendinopathy. A randomized study of 70 patients. *Acta Orthop Scand* 1992; 63: 631–4.

Although over 15 years old, this study remains very relevant as it is one of the few trials that assessed NSAIDs for clinical outcome, and the graphs of outcome for placebo and NSAIDs are virtually superimposed.

Nilsson-Helander K, Thomeé R, Grävare-Silbernagel K, et al. The Achilles Tendon Total Rupture Score (ATRS). Development and validation. *Am J Sports Med* 2007 (in press).

O'Brien M. The anatomy of the Achilles tendon. *Foot Ankle Clin* 2005; 10(2): 225–38.

Paoloni JA, Appleyard RC, Nelson J, Murrell GA. Topical glyceryl trinitrate treatment of chronic noninsertional Achilles tendinopathy. A randomized, double-blind, placebo-controlled trial. *J Bone Joint Surg Am* 2004; 86A(5): 916–22.

Roos EM, Engstrom M, Lagerquist A, Soderberg B. Clinical improvement after 6 weeks of eccentric exercise in patients with mid-portion Achilles tendinopathy—a randomized trial with 1-year follow-up. *Scand J Med Sci Sports* 2004; 14(5): 286–95.

References

1. Paavola M, Kannus P, Paakkala T, Pasanen M, Jarvinen M. Long-term prognosis of patients with Achilles tendinopathy. An observational 8-year follow-up study. *Am J Sports Med* 2000; 28(5): 634–42.

2. Kujala UM, Sarna S, Kaprio J. Cumulative incidence of Achilles tendon rupture and tendinopathy in male former elite athletes. *Clin J Sport Med* 2005; 15(3): 133–5.

3. Alfredson H. Conservative management of Achilles tendinopathy: new ideas. *Foot Ankle Clin* 2005; 10(2): 321–9.

4. Paoloni JA, Appleyard RC, Nelson J, Murrell GA. Topical glyceryl trinitrate application in the treatment of chronic supraspinatus tendinopathy: a randomized, double-blinded, placebo-controlled clinical trial. *Am J Sports Med* 2005; 33(6): 806–13.

5. O'Brien M. The anatomy of the Achilles tendon. *Foot Ankle Clin* 2005; 10(2): 225–38.

6. Alfredson H. Chronic midportion Achilles tendinopathy: an update on research and treatment. *Clin Sports Med* 2003; 22(4): 727–41.

7. Robinson J, Cook JL, Purdam C, et al. The VISA-A questionnaire: a valid and reliable index of the clinical severity of Achilles tendinopathy. *Br J Sports Med* 2001; 35: 335–41.

8. Simmonds FA. The diagnosis of the ruptured Achilles tendon. *Practitioner* 1957; 179: 56–8.

9. Zanetti M, Metzdorf A, Kundert HP, et al. Achilles tendons: clinical relevance of neovascularization diagnosed with power Doppler US. *Radiology* 2003; 227(2): 556–60.

10. Khan KM, Forster BB, Robinson J, et al. Are ultrasound and magnetic resonance imaging of value in assessment of Achilles tendon disorders? A two year prospective study. *Br J Sports Med* 2003; 37(2): 149–53.

11. Cook JL, Khan KM, Kiss ZS, et al. Asymptomatic hypoechoic regions on patellar tendon ultrasound: a 4-year clinical and ultrasound follow-up of 46 tendons. *Scand J Med Sci Sports* 2001; 11: 321–7.

12. Khan KM, Visentini PJ, Kiss ZS, et al. Correlation of US and MR imaging with clinical outcome after open patellar tenotomy: prospective and retrospective studies. *Clin J Sport Med* 1999; 9: 129–37.

13. Astrom M, Rausing A. Chronic Achilles tendinopathy. A survey of surgical and histopathologic findings. *Clin Orthop* 1995; 316: 151–64.

14. Kannus P, Jozsa L. Histopathological changes preceding spontaneous rupture of a tendon. *J Bone Joint Surg Am* 1991; 73A: 1507–25.

15. Astrom M, Gentz CF, Nilsson P, Rausing A, Sjoberg S, Westlin N. Imaging in chronic Achilles tendinopathy:

a comparison of ultrasonography, magnetic resonance imaging and surgical findings in 27 histologically verified cases. *Skeletal Radiol* 1996; 25(7): 615–20.

16. Alfredson H, Forsgren S, Thorsen K, Fahlstrom M, Johansson H, Lorentzon R. Glutamate NMDAR1 receptors localised to nerves in human Achilles tendons. Implications for treatment? *Knee Surg Sports Traumatol Arthrosc* 2001; 9(2): 123–6.

17. Alfredson H, Thorsen K, Lorentzon R. In situ microdialysis in tendon tissue: high levels of glutamate, but not prostaglandin E2 in chronic Achilles tendon pain. *Knee Surg Sports Traumatol Arthrosc* 1999; 7(6): 378–81.

18. Alfredson H, Lorentzon M, Backman S, Backman A, Lerner UH. cDNA-arrays and real-time quantitative PCR techniques in the investigation of chronic Achilles tendinosis. *J Orthop Res* 2003; 21(6): 970–5.

19. Hart DA, Frank CB, Bray RC. Inflammatory processes in repetitive motion and overuse syndromes: potential role of neurogenic mechanisms in tendons and ligaments. In: Gordon SL, Blair SJ, Fine LJ, eds. *Repetitive Motion Disorders of the Upper Extremity*. Rosemont, IL: American Academy of Orthopaedic Surgeons, 1995: 247–62.

20. McCrory JL, Martin DF, Lowery RP, et al. Etiologic factors associated with Achilles tendinitis in runners. *Med Sci Sports Exerc* 1999; 31: 1374–81.

21. Mokone GG, Gajjar M, September AV, et al. The guanine-thymine dinucleotide repeat polymorphism within the tenascin-C gene is associated with Achilles tendon injuries. *Am J Sports Med* 2005; 33(7): 1016–21.

22. Alfredson H, Khan K, Cook J. An algorithm for managing Achilles tendinopathy: a primary care emphasis on treatment. *Br J Sports Med* 2007; in press.

23. Curwin S. The aetiology and treatment of tendinitis. In: Harries M, Williams C, Stanish WD, Micheli LJ, eds. *Oxford Textbook of Sports Medicine*. Oxford: Oxford University Press, 1994.

24. Alfredson H, Lorentzon R. Chronic Achilles tendinosis: recommendations for treatment and prevention. *Sports Med* 2000; 29(2): 135–46.

25. Alfredson H, Pietila T, Jonsson P, Lorentzon R. Heavy-load eccentric calf muscle training for the treatment of chronic Achilles tendinosis. *Am J Sports Med* 1998; 26: 360–6.

26. Fahlstrom M, Jonsson P, Lorentzon R, Alfredson H. Chronic Achilles tendon pain treated with eccentric calf-muscle training. *Knee Surg Sports Traumatol Arthrosc* 2003; 11(5): 327–33.

27. Roos EM, Engstrom M, Lagerquist A, Soderberg B. Clinical improvement after 6 weeks of eccentric exercise in patients with mid-portion Achilles tendinopathy—a randomized trial with 1-year follow-up. *Scand J Med Sci Sports* 2004; 14(5): 286–95.

28. Shalabi A, Kristoffersen-Wilberg M, Svensson L, Aspelin P, Movin T. Eccentric training of the gastrocnemius-soleus complex in chronic Achilles tendinopathy results in decreased tendon volume and intratendinous signal as evaluated by MRI. *Am J Sports Med* 2004; 32(5): 1286–96.

29. Silbernagel KG, Thomee R, Thomee P, Karlsson J. Eccentric overload training for patients with chronic Achilles tendon pain—a randomised controlled study with reliability testing of the evaluation methods. *Scand J Med Sci Sports* 2001; 11(4): 197–206.

30. Niesen-Vertommen SL, Taunton JE, Clement DB, Mosher RE. The effect of eccentric versus concentric exercise in the management of Achilles tendonitis. *Clin J Sport Med* 1992; 2: 109–13.

31. Mafi N, Lorentzon R, Alfredson H. Superior short-term results with eccentric calf muscle training compared to concentric training in a randomized prospective multicenter study on patients with chronic Achilles tendinosis. *Knee Surg Sports Traumatol Arthrosc* 2001; 9: 42–7.

32. Paoloni JA, Appleyard RC, Nelson J, Murrell GA. Topical glyceryl trinitrate treatment of chronic noninsertional Achilles tendinopathy. A randomized, double-blind, placebo-controlled trial. *J Bone Joint Surg Am* 2004; 86A(5): 916–22.

33. McLauchlan GJ, Handoll HH. Interventions for treating acute and chronic Achilles tendinitis. *Cochrane Database Syst Rev* 2001; 2: CD000232.

34. Shrier I, Matheson GO, Kohl HW. Achilles tendonitis: are corticosteroid injections useful or harmful. *Clin J Sport Med* 1996; 6: 245–50.

35. Koenig MJ, Torp-Pedersen S, Qvistgaard E, Terslev L, Bliddal H. Preliminary results of colour Doppler-guided intratendinous glucocorticoid injection for Achilles tendonitis in five patients. *Scand J Med Sci Sports* 2004; 14(2): 100–6.

36. Kjaer M, Langberg H, Miller BF, et al. Metabolic activity and collagen turnover in human tendon in response to physical activity. *J Musculoskelet Neuronal Interact* 2005; 5(1): 41–52.

37. Ohberg L, Alfredson H. Ultrasound guided sclerosis of neovessels in painful chronic Achilles tendinosis: pilot study of a new treatment. *Br J Sports Med* 2002; 36(3): 173–5; discussion 176–7.

38. Alfredson H, Ohberg L. Sclerosing injections to areas of neo-vascularisation reduce pain in chronic Achilles tendinopathy: a double-blind randomised controlled trial. *Knee Surg Sports Traumatol Arthrosc* 2005; 13(4): 338–44.

39. Hoksrud A, Öhberg L, Alfredson H, Bahr R. Ultrasound-guided sclerosis of neovessels in painful chronic patellar tendinopathy—a randomized controlled trial. *Am J Sports Med* 2006; in press.

40. Costa ML, Shepstone L, Donell ST, Thomas TL. Shock wave therapy for chronic Achilles tendon pain: a

randomized placebo-controlled trial. *Clin Orthop* 2005; 440: 199–204.

41. Parvizi J, Wu CC, Lewallen DG, Greenleaf JF, Bolander ME. Low-intensity ultrasound stimulates proteoglycan synthesis in rat chondrocytes by increasing aggrecan gene expression. *J Orthop Res* 1999; 17(4): 488–94.

42. Giombini A, Di Cesare A, Casciello G, Sorrenti D, Dragoni S, Gabriele P. Hyperthermia at 434 MHz in the treatment of overuse sport tendinopathies: a randomised controlled clinical trial. *Int J Sports Med* 2002; 23(3): 207–11.

43. Chapman-Jones D, Hill D. Novel microcurrent treatment is more effective than conventional therapy for chronic Achilles tendinopathy. *Physiotherapy* 2002; 88(8): 471–9.

44. Astrom M, Arvidson T. Alignment and joint motion in the normal foot. *J Orthop Sports Phys Ther* 1995; 22: 216–22.

45. Hunter G. The conservative management of Achilles tendinopathy. *Phys Ther Sport* 2000; 1: 6–14.

46. Davidson C, Ganion LR, Gehlsen G, et al. Rat tendon morphological and functional changes resulting from soft tissue mobilization. *Med Sci Sports Exerc* 1997; 29: 313–19.

47. Testa V, Capasso G, Maffulli N, Bifulco G. Ultrasound guided percutaneous longitudinal tenotomy for the management of patellar tendinopathy. *Med Sci Sports Exerc* 1999; 31: 1509–15.

48. Testa V, Capasso G, Benazzo F, Maffulli N. Management of Achilles tendinopathy by ultrasound-guided percutaneous tenotomy. *Med Sci Sports Exerc* 2002; 34(4): 573–80.

49. Paavola M, Kannus P, Orava S, Pasanen M, Jarvinen M. Surgical treatment for chronic Achilles tendinopathy: a prospective seven month follow up study. *Br J Sports Med* 2002; 36(3): 178–82.

50. Benjamin M, Moriggl B, Brenner E, Emery P, McGonagle D, Redman S. The "enthesis organ" concept: why enthesopathies may not present as focal insertional disorders. *Arthritis Rheum* 2004; 50(10): 3306–13.

51. de Palma L, Marinelli M, Meme L, Pavan M.

Immunohistochemistry of the enthesis organ of the human Achilles tendon. *Foot Ankle Int* 2004; 25(6): 414–18.

52. Canoso JJ. The premiere enthesis. *J Rheumatol* 1998; 25(7): 1254–6.

53. Lyman J, Weinhold PS, Almekinders LC. Strain behavior of the distal Achilles tendon: implications for insertional Achilles tendinopathy. *Am J Sports Med* 2004; 32(2): 457–61.

54. Rufai A, Ralphs JR, Benjamin M. Structure and histopathology of the insertional region of the human Achilles tendon. *J Orthop Res* 1995; 13(4): 585–93.

55. McGarvey WC, Palumbo RC, Baxter DE, Leibman BD. Insertional Achilles tendinosis: surgical treatment through a central tendon splitting approach. *Foot Ankle Int* 2002; 23(1): 19–25.

56. Ohberg L, Alfredson H. Sclerosing therapy in chronic Achilles tendon insertional pain—results of a pilot study. *Knee Surg Sports Traumatol Arthrosc* 2003; 11(5): 339–43.

57. Theobald P, Benjamin M, Nokes L, Pugh N. Review of the vascularisation of the human Achilles tendon. *Injury* 2005; 36(11): 1267–72.

58. Khan RJ, Fick D, Keogh A, Crawford J, Brammar T, Parker M. Treatment of acute Achilles tendon ruptures. A meta-analysis of randomized, controlled trials. *J Bone Joint Surg Am* 2005; 87(10): 2202–10.

59. Paavola M, Orava S, Leppilahti J, Kannus P, Jarvinen M. Chronic Achilles tendon overuse injury: complications after surgical treatment. An analysis of 432 consecutive patients. *Am J Sports Med* 2000; 28(1): 77–82.

60. Moller M, Lind K, Movin T, Karlsson J. Calf muscle function after Achilles tendon rupture. A prospective, randomised study comparing surgical and non-surgical treatment. *Scand J Med Sci Sports* 2002; 12(1): 9–16.

61. Rossi F, Dragoni S. Symptomatic accessory soleus muscle. Report of 18 cases in athletes. *J Sports Med Phys Fitness* 2005; 45(1): 93–7.

62. Leswick DA, Chow V, Stoneham GW. Resident's corner. Answer to case of the month #94. Accessory soleus muscle. *Can Assoc Radiol J* 2003; 54(5): 313–15.

Acute Ankle Injuries

WITH JON KARLSSON

Epidemiological data suggested that there were over 300 000 annual emergency department presentations with ankle sprains in the United Kingdom[1] and that 42 000 of these were 'severe'. The highest rates were in girls aged 10–14 years. Extrapolated to the populations of Australia and the United States, these UK data would equate to an ankle-injury related burden of 100 000 emergency department presentations annually in Australia, and 1.5 million annually in the United States.

Although the term 'sprained ankle' is sometimes thought to be synonymous with 'lateral ligament injury' and, thus, imply a rather benign injury, this is not always the case. If the ankle injury is indeed a lateral ligament sprain, inadequate rehabilitation can lead to prolonged symptoms, decreased sporting performance and high risk of recurrence. Thus, the first half of this chapter focuses on anatomy, clinical assessment and management of lateral ligament injuries after ankle sprain and two less common sequelae of ankle sprain—medial ligament injury and Pott's fracture.

The seemingly benign presentation of 'sprained ankle' can also mask damage to other structures in addition to the ankle ligaments, such as subtle fractures around the ankle joint, osteochondral fractures of the dome of the talus and dislocation or rupture of the peroneal tendons, in most cases the peroneus brevis tendon. Such injuries are frequently not diagnosed and thus cause ankle pain that persists much longer than would be expected with a straightforward ankle sprain. This is often referred to as 'the problem ankle' and this presentation is discussed in the second half of this chapter.

Functional anatomy

The ankle contains three joints (Fig. 33.1):

1. talocrural (ankle) joint
2. inferior tibiofibular joint
3. subtalar joint.

The talocrural or ankle joint (Fig. 33.1a) is a hinge joint formed between the inferior surface of the tibia and the superior surface of the talus. The medial and lateral malleoli provide additional articulations and stability to the ankle joint. The movements at the

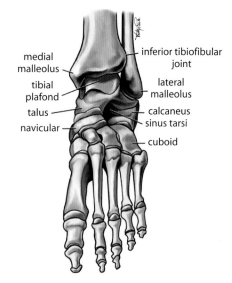

Figure 33.1 Anatomy of the ankle

(a) Talocrural (ankle) joint

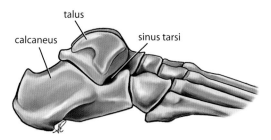

(b) Subtalar joint

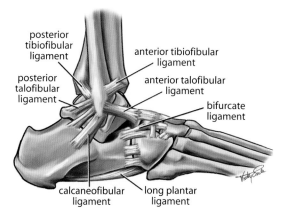

(c) Ligaments of the ankle joint—lateral view

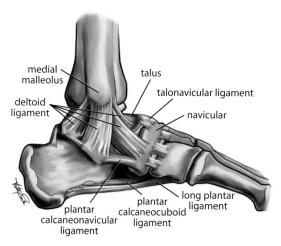

(d) Ligaments of the ankle joint—medial view

ankle joint are plantarflexion and dorsiflexion; the joint is least stable in plantarflexion. This leads to an increased number of injuries with the foot in the position of plantarflexion.

The inferior tibiofibular joint is the articulation of the distal parts of the fibula and tibia. The inferior tibiofibular joint is supported by the inferior tibiofibular ligament or syndesmosis. A small amount of movement is present at this joint and the rotational movement, even though minimal, is extremely important, for instance, for barefoot walking and running.

The subtalar joint (Fig. 33.1b), between the talus and calcaneus, is divided into an anterior and posterior articulation separated by the sinus tarsi. The main roles of the subtalar joint are to provide shock absorption, to permit the foot to adjust to uneven ground and to allow the foot to remain flat on the ground when the leg is at an angle to the surface. Inversion and eversion occur at the subtalar joint.

The ligaments of the ankle joint are shown in Figures 33.1c, d. The lateral ligament consists of three parts: the anterior talofibular ligament (ATFL), which passes as a flat and rather thin band from the tip of the fibula anteriorly to the lateral talar neck, the calcaneofibular ligament (CFL), which is a cord-like structure directed inferiorly and posteriorly, and the short posterior talofibular ligament (PTFL), which runs posteriorly from the fibula to the talus. The medial or deltoid ligament of the ankle is a strong, fan-shaped ligament extending from the medial malleolus anteriorly to the navicular and talus, inferiorly to the calcaneus and posteriorly to the talus. This ligament is strong and composed of two layers, one deep and the other more superficial. Accordingly, the deltoid ligament is infrequently injured.

Clinical perspective

Inversion injuries are far more common than eversion injuries due to the relative instability of the lateral joint and weakness of the lateral ligaments compared with the medial ligament. Eversion injuries are seen only occasionally. As the strong medial ligament requires a greater force to be injured, these sprains almost always take longer to rehabilitate. The differential diagnoses that must be considered after an ankle injury are listed in Table 33.1. The aim of the initial clinical assessment is to rule out an ankle fracture, if possible, and to diagnose the site of abnormality as accurately as possible.

History

The mechanism of injury is an important clue to diagnosis after ankle sprain. An inversion injury suggests lateral ligament damage, an eversion injury suggests medial ligament damage. If the injury has involved compressive forces on the ankle mortise, consider the possibility of osteochondral injury.

The onset of pain is very important. A history of being able to weight-bear immediately after an injury

Table 33.1 Acute ankle injuries

Common	Less common	Not to be missed
Ligament sprain	Osteochondral lesion of the talus	Complex regional pain syndrome type I (post-injury)
Lateral ligaments (Fig. 33.1c)	Ligament sprain/rupture Medial ligament injury	Greenstick fractures (children)
ATFL	AITFL injury	Sprained syndesmosis
CFL	Fractures	Tarsal coalition (may come to light as a result of an ankle sprain)
PTFL	Lateral/medial/posterior malleolus (Pott's)	
	Tibial plafond	
	Base of the fifth metatarsal	
	Anterior process of the calcaneus	
	Lateral process of the talus	
	Posterior process of the talus	
	Os trigonum	
	Dislocated ankle (fracture/dislocation)	
	Tendon rupture/dislocation	
	Tibialis posterior tendon	
	Peroneal tendons (longitudinal rupture)	

ATFL = anterior tibiofibular ligament. AITFL = anteroinferior tibiofibular ligament. CFL = calcaneofibular ligament. PTFL = posterior tibiofibular ligament.

with a subsequent increase in pain and swelling as the patient continues to play sport or walk about suggests a sprain (ligament injury) rather than a fracture. The location of pain and concomitant swelling and bruising generally gives an indication as to the ligaments injured. The most common site is over the anterolateral aspect of the ankle involving the ATFL. Occasionally in severe injuries, both medial and lateral ligaments are damaged. The degree of swelling and bruising is usually, but not always, an indication of severity.

The degree of disability, both immediately following the injury and subsequently, is an important indicator of the severity of the injury. The initial management, the use of the RICE regimen and the duration of restricted weight-bearing after the injury are important.

The practitioner should ask about a previous history of ankle injury and assess whether post-injury rehabilitation was adequate. Did the athlete use protective tape or braces after previous injury?

Examination

One aim of ankle examination is to assess the degree of instability present and thus the grade of the ligamentous injury. Another is to detect functional deficits, such as loss of range of motion, reduced strength and reduced proprioception. The practitioner should be alert for associated injuries and examine for them. For example, avulsion fracture of the base of the

fifth metatarsal is commonly overlooked but is easily detected by palpation.

Examination involves:

1. Observation
   (a) standing
   (b) supine
2. Active movements
   (a) plantarflexion/dorsiflexion (Fig. 33.2a)
   (b) inversion/eversion
3. Passive movements
   (a) plantarflexion/dorsiflexion
   (b) inversion/eversion (Fig. 33.2b)
4. Resisted movements
   (a) eversion (Fig. 33.2c)
5. Functional tests
   (a) lunge test (Fig. 33.2d)
   (b) hopping
6. Palpation
   (a) distal fibula
   (b) lateral malleolus
   (c) lateral ligaments (Fig. 33.2e)
   (d) talus
   (e) peroneal tendon(s)
   (f) base of fifth metatarsal
   (g) anterior joint line
   (h) dome of talus
   (i) medial ligament
   (j) sustentaculum tali
   (k) sinus tarsi
   (l) anteroinferior tibiofibular ligament (AITFL)

7. Special tests (comparison with other side necessary)
   (a) anterior drawer (Fig. 33.2f)
   (b) lateral talar tilt (increased inversion) (Fig. 33.2g)
   (c) proprioception (Fig. 33.2h)

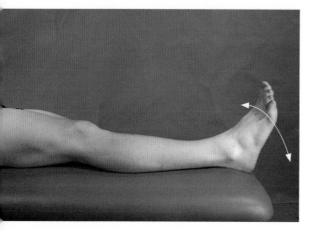

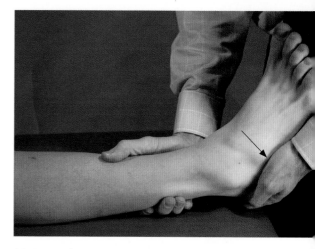

(c) Resisted movement—eversion. In acute, painful ankle injuries, resisted movements may not be possible. In cases of persistent pain following ankle injury, weakness of the ankle evertors (peroneal muscles) should be assessed

Figure 33.2 Examination of the patient with an acute ankle injury

(a) Active movement—plantarflexion/dorsiflexion. Assessment of dorsiflexion is important as restriction results in a functional deficit. Range of motion can be compared with the uninjured side. Tight calf muscles may restrict dorsiflexion. This can be eliminated by placing the knee in slight flexion

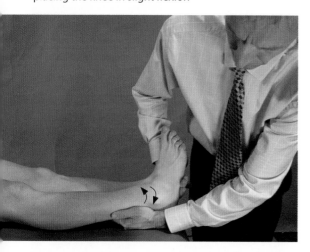

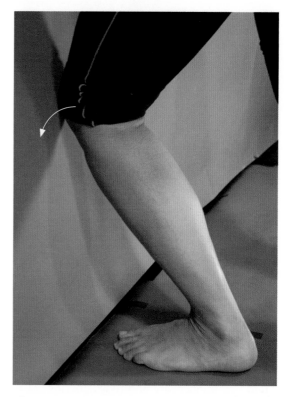

(b) Passive movement—inversion/eversion. Inversion is frequently painful and restricted in lateral ligament injury, while eversion is painful following injuries to the medial ligament. Increased pain on combined plantarflexion and inversion suggests ATFL injury

(d) Functional test—lunge test. Assess ankle dorsiflexion compared with the uninjured side. Note any pain. Other functional tests may be performed to reproduce the patient's pain if appropriate (e.g. single-leg standing, hopping)

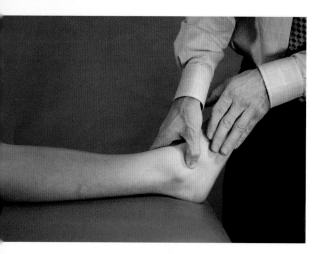

(e) Palpation—lateral ligament

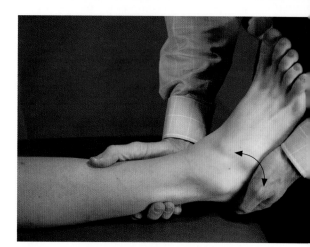

(g) Ligament testing—talar tilt. This tests integrity of the anterior talofibular and calcaneofibular ligaments laterally and the deltoid ligament medially. The ankle is grasped as shown and the medial and lateral movement of the talus and calcaneus are assessed in relation to the tibia and fibula. Pain on this test must also be noted

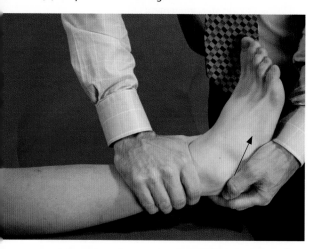

(f) Ligament testing—anterior drawer test. The ankle is placed in slight plantarflexion and grasped as shown. Pressure is exerted upwards and the degree of excursion (anterior drawer) is noted and compared with the uninjured side. This test assesses the integrity of the ATFL and CFL. Pain on this test should also be noted; if painful it may indeed mask injury to the ligament. Then the test should be repeated within five days. The most optimal time to test the integrity of the lateral ligaments is on the fifth post-injury day

Investigations

Many practitioners are unsure whether or not to X-ray a moderately severely sprained ankle where the patient has difficulty weight-bearing. For experienced sports medicine practitioners, palpation should reveal whether or not tenderness is greatest on bone (lateral or medial malleolus) or on ligament tissue itself. For

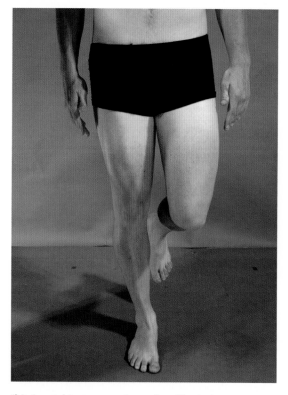

(h) Special test—proprioception. Single-leg standing with eyes closed may demonstrate impaired proprioception compared with the uninjured side

practitioners not as confident in physical examination, the Ottawa ankle rules provide very useful guidance (Fig. 33.3).[2] We recommend that X-rays of the ankle joint include the base of the fifth metatarsal to exclude avulsion fracture. If damage to the lower tibiofibular syndesmosis (AITFL) is suspected, special ankle mortise or syndesmosis views are required.

An osteochondral lesion of the talus may not be apparent on initial X-ray. If significant pain and disability persist despite appropriate treatment four to six weeks after an apparent 'routine' ankle sprain, a radioisotopic bone scan, CT or MRI is indicated to exclude an osteochondral lesion (see p. 624). If MRI is not available and the bone scan gives a positive result, a CT scan should be ordered to image the site of abnormality. Although MRI is very popular because it also images soft tissues, CT often provides superior images of bony damage.

Lateral ligament injuries

Lateral ligament injuries occur in activities requiring rapid changes in direction, especially if these take place on uneven surfaces (e.g. grass fields). They are also seen when a player, having jumped, lands on another competitor's feet. They are one of the most common injuries seen in basketball, volleyball, netball and most football codes.

The usual mechanism of lateral ligament injury is inversion and plantarflexion, and this injury usually damages the ATFL before the CFL. This occurs because the ATFL is taut in plantarflexion and the

CFL is relatively loose (Fig. 33.4). Also, the ATFL can only tolerate half the strain of the CFL before tearing. Complete tear of the ATFL, CFL and PTFL results in a dislocation of the ankle joint and is frequently associated with a fracture. Such an injury is rather infrequent, however. Isolated ligament ruptures of the CFL and especially the PTFL are rare.

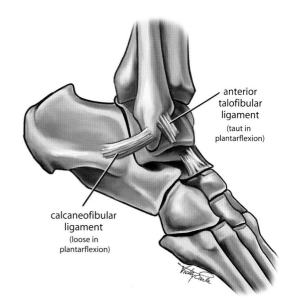

Figure 33.4 A plantarflexion injury can lead to injury of the anterior talofibular ligament before the calcaneofibular ligament

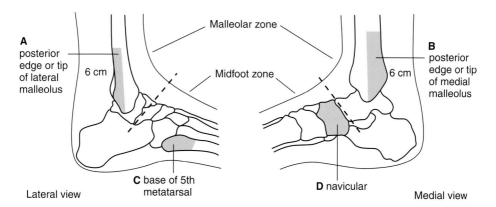

Figure 33.3 Ankle X-ray: recommendation 1. Ankle X-rays are only required if there is any pain in the malleolar zone and any one of these findings: bone tenderness at **A**; or bone tenderness at **B**; or inability to bear weight both immediately and at the clinical assessment (four steps). Foot X-ray: recommendation 2. Foot X-rays are only required if there is any pain in the midfoot zone, and any one of these findings: bone tenderness at **C**; or bone tenderness at **D**; or inability to bear weight both immediately and at the clinical assessment (four steps)

Ankle sprain may be accompanied by an audible snap, crack or tear, which, although often of great concern to the athlete and onlookers, has no particular diagnostic significance (unlike the case in knee ligament injuries where it has profound implications, Chapter 27). Depending on the severity of the injury, the athlete may continue to play or may rest immediately. Swelling usually appears rapidly, although occasionally it may be delayed some hours.

To assess lateral ligament injuries, examine all three components of the ligament and determine the degree of ankle instability. In a grade I tear there is no abnormal ligament laxity. It is important to compare both sides (assuming the other side has not been injured) as there is a large inter-individual variation in normal ankle laxity. Grade II injuries reveal some degree of laxity but have a firm end point. Grade III injuries show gross laxity without a discernible end point. All three grades are associated with pain and tenderness, although grade III tears may be least painful after the initial episode has settled. Grading of these injuries guides prognosis and helps determine the rate of rehabilitation.

Treatment and rehabilitation of lateral ligament injuries

The management of lateral ligament injuries of all three grades follows the same principles. After minimizing initial hemorrhage and reducing pain, the aims are to restore range of motion, muscle strength and proprioception, and then prescribe a progressive, sport-specific exercise program.

Initial management

Lateral ligament injuries require RICE treatment (Chapter 10). This essential treatment limits the hemorrhage and subsequent edema that would otherwise cause an irritating synovial reaction and restrict joint range of motion. The injured athlete must avoid factors that will promote blood flow and swelling, such as hot showers, heat rubs, alcohol or excessive weight-bearing. Gradually increased weight-bearing will, however, help reduce the swelling and increase the ankle motion, and enhances the rehabilitation.

Reduction of pain and swelling

Analgesics may be required. After 48 hours, gentle soft tissue therapy and mobilization may reduce pain. By reducing pain and swelling, muscle inhibition around the joint is minimized, permitting the patient to begin range of motion exercises.

The indications for the use of NSAIDs in ankle injuries are unclear. The majority of practitioners tend to prescribe these drugs after lateral ligament sprains although their efficacy has not been proven (Chapter 10). The rationale for commencing NSAIDs two to three days after injury is to reduce the risk of joint synovitis with early return to weight-bearing.

Restoration of full range of motion

If necessary, the patient may be non-weight-bearing on crutches for the first 24 hours but then should commence partial weight-bearing in normal heel–toe gait. This can be achieved while still using crutches or, in less severe cases, by protecting the damaged joint with strapping or bracing. Thus, partial and, ultimately, full weight-bearing can take place without aggravating the injury. Lunge stretches and accessory and physiological mobilization of the ankle (Fig. 33.5a), subtalar (Fig. 33.5b) and midtarsal joints should begin early in rehabilitation. As soon as pain allows, the practitioner should prescribe active range of motion exercises (e.g. stationary cycling).

Muscle conditioning

Active strengthening exercises, including plantarflexion, dorsiflexion, inversion and eversion (Fig. 33.6), should begin as soon as pain allows. They should be progressed by increasing resistance (a common method is to use rubber tubing). Strengthening eversion with the ankle fully plantarflexed is particularly important in the prevention of future lateral ligament injuries. Weight-bearing exercises (e.g. shuttle [Fig. 33.6b], wobble board exercises) are encouraged as soon as pain permits, preferably the first or second day after injury.

Proprioception

Proprioception is invariably impaired after ankle ligament injuries. The assessment of proprioception is shown in Figure 33.2h. The practitioner should begin proprioceptive retraining (Chapter 12) early in rehabilitation and these exercises should gradually progress in difficulty. An example of a common progression is balancing on one leg, then using the rocker board (Fig. 33.7a) or minitrampoline, and ultimately performing functional activities while balancing (Fig. 33.7b).

Functional exercises

Functional exercises (e.g. jumping, hopping, twisting, figure-of-eight running) can be prescribed when the athlete is pain-free, has full range of motion and adequate muscle strength and proprioception. Specific

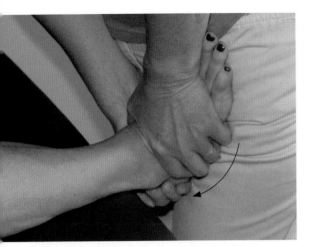

Figure 33.5 Mobilization of the ankle joint

(a) Ankle dorsiflexion. The calcaneus and foot are grasped to passively dorsiflex the ankle

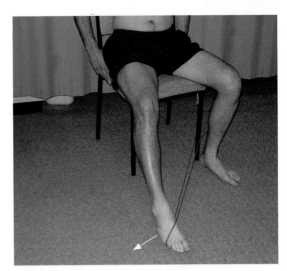

Figure 33.6 Strengthening exercises—eversion

(a) Using a rubber tube as resistance

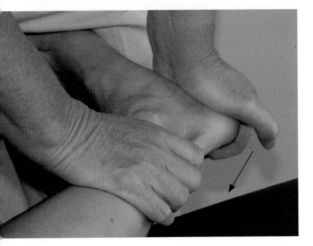

(b) Eversion mobilization techniques to restore subtalar joint movement after ankle sprain

technical training not only accelerates a player's return to sport but can also substantially reduce the risk of reinjury.[3-5] It should be borne in mind that approximately 75% of those who sustain an ankle ligament injury have had a previous injury, in many cases not fully rehabilitated.

Return to sport

Return to sport is permitted when functional exercises can be performed without pain during or after activity. While performing rehabilitation activities and upon return to sport, added ankle protection should be provided with either taping or bracing.

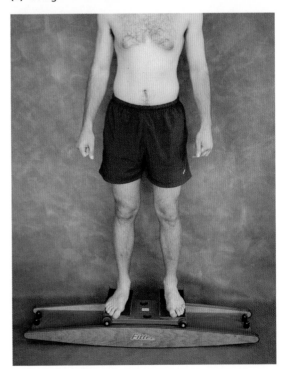

(b) Shuttle exercises

The relative advantages of taping and bracing have been discussed in Chapter 6. As both seem equally effective, the choice of taping or bracing depends on patient preference, cost, availability and expertise in applying tape.

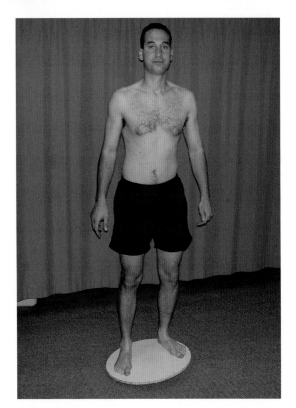

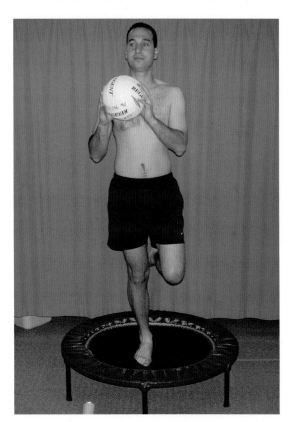

Figure 33.7 Proprioceptive retraining following acute ankle injury

(a) Rocker board

(b) Functional activity while balancing

Any athlete who has had a significant lateral ligament injury should use protective taping or bracing while playing sport for a minimum of six to 12 months post-injury.[4, 5] There are a number of methods to protect against inversion injuries. The three main methods of tape application are stirrups (Fig. 33.8a), heel lock (Fig. 33.8b) and the figure of six (Fig. 33.8c). Usually at least two of these methods are used simultaneously.

Braces have the advantage of ease of fitting and adjustment, lack of skin irritation and reduced cost compared with taping for a lengthy period. There are a number of different ankle braces available. The lace-up brace (Fig. 33.9) is popular and effective.

Treatment of grade III injuries

A 2002 Cochrane systematic review concluded that there was insufficient information from randomized trials to recommend surgery over conservative treatment of grade III ankle sprains.[6] They found that functional recovery (as measured by return to work) was quicker in those treated with rehabilitation, subsequent rate of ankle sprains was no different between groups, and there was more ankle stiffness in those treated surgically.[6] Finnish researchers compared surgical treatment (primary repair plus early controlled mobilization) with early controlled mobilization alone in a prospective study of 60 patients with grade III lateral ankle ligament injuries.[7] Of the patients treated with rehabilitation alone, 87% had excellent or good outcomes compared with 60% of patients treated surgically. Thus, early mobilization alone provided a better outcome than surgery plus mobilization in patients with complete tears of the lateral ankle ligaments. Dutch investigators have reported better long-term outcomes after surgery for lateral ligament rupture compared with rehabilitation but this conclusion was controversial.[8] Differences in 'rehabilitation' protocols can explain such contradictory study results.

In clinical practice, it is widely agreed that all grade III ankle injuries warrant a trial of initial conservative management over at least a six-week period, irrespective of the caliber of the athlete. If, despite appropriate

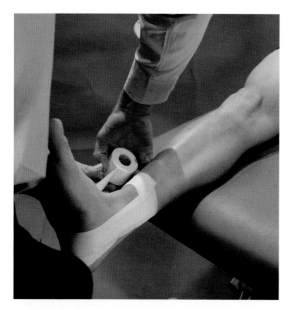

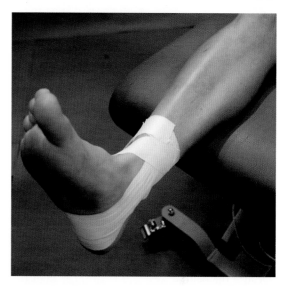

(c) Figure of six. This is applied over stirrups. Tape runs longitudinally along the lateral ankle, under the heel and is pulled up to loop back around the medial ankle as shown

Figure 33.8 Application of ankle tape

(a) Stirrups. After preparation of the skin, anchors are applied circumferentially. The ankle should be in the neutral position. Stirrups are applied from medial to lateral, and repeated several times until functional stability is achieved

rehabilitation and protection, the patient complains of recurrent episodes of instability or persistent pain, then surgical reconstruction of the lateral ligament is indicated. The preferred surgical method is anatomical reconstruction using the damaged ligaments; this method has been shown to produce good functional results in several studies. The ligaments are shortened

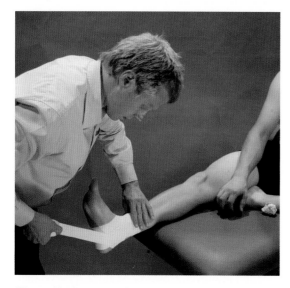

(b) Heel lock. One method used to limit inversion is taping commenced at the front of the ankle and then angled inferiorly across the medial longitudinal arch, then diagonally and posteriorly across the lateral aspect of the heel, and then continued medially over the back of the Achilles tendon to loop back anteriorly. Tape direction is thereafter reversed to restrict eversion

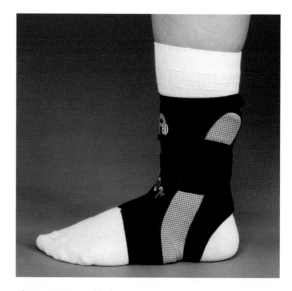

Figure 33.9 Ankle braces—a long lace-up brace is effective and comfortable

and reinserted to bone, and only if the ligament tissue is extremely damaged or even absent, may other methods such as tenodesis, in most cases using the peroneus brevis tendon, be considered. Following surgery, it is extremely important to undertake a comprehensive rehabilitation program to restore full joint range of motion, strength and proprioception. The principles of rehabilitation outlined on page 618 are appropriate. The anatomical reconstruction will produce good clinical results in more than 90% of patients. There is, however, increased risk of inferior results in cases of very longstanding ligament insufficiency and generalized joint laxity.

Less common causes

Medial (deltoid) ligament injuries

Because the deltoid ligament is stronger than the lateral ligament, and probably because eversion is a less common mechanism of ankle sprain, medial ankle ligament injuries are less common than lateral ligament injuries. Occasionally, medial and lateral ligament injuries occur in the same ankle sprain. Medial ligament injuries may occur together with fractures (e.g. medial malleolus, talar dome, articular surfaces). Medial ligament sprains should be treated in the same manner as lateral ligament sprains, although return to activity takes about twice as long (or more) as would be predicted were the injury on the lateral side.

Pott's fracture

A fracture affecting one or more of the malleoli (lateral, medial, posterior) is known as a Pott's fracture. It can be difficult to distinguish a fracture from a moderate-to-severe ligament sprain as both conditions may result from similar mechanisms of injury and cause severe pain and inability to weight-bear. Careful and gentle palpation can generally localize the greatest site of tenderness to either the malleoli (fracture) or just distal to the ligament attachment (sprain). X-ray is often required; the Ottawa rules (Fig. 33.3) are useful in these cases.

The management of Pott's fractures requires restoration of the normal anatomy between the superior surface of the talus and the ankle mortise (inferior margins of the tibia and fibula). If this relationship has been disrupted, internal fixation is almost always required.

Isolated undisplaced spiral fractures of the lateral malleolus (without medial ligament instability) and posterior malleolar fractures involving less than 25% of the articular surface are usually stable. These fractures can be treated symptomatically with early mobilization using crutches only in the early stages for pain relief.

Lateral malleolar fractures associated with medial instability, hairline medial malleolar fractures or larger undisplaced posterior malleolar fractures are potentially unstable but may be treated conservatively with six weeks of immobilization using a below-knee cast with extension to include the metatarsal heads. In cases of undisplaced or minimally displaced fractures, the immobilization time may be shortened considerably, using an ankle brace and early range of motion training. A walking heel may be applied after swelling has subsided (three to five days).

Displaced medial malleolar, large posterior malleolar, bimalleolar or trimalleolar fractures, or any displaced fracture that involves the ankle mortise, require orthopedic referral for open reduction and internal fixation. A comprehensive rehabilitation program should be undertaken following surgical fixation or removal of the cast. The aims of the rehabilitation program are to restore full range of motion, strengthen the surrounding muscles and improve proprioception. Guidelines for ankle rehabilitation are provided on page 618.

Maisonneuve fracture

This injury is found more commonly in patients presenting to emergency departments than in the sports setting, but occasionally high-impact sports injuries can cause this variant of the syndesmosis sprain. The injury involves complete rupture of the medial ligament, the AITFL (see below) and interosseous membrane, as well as a proximal fibular fracture. Surprisingly, non-weight-bearing X-rays may not demonstrate the fracture, and the unstable ankle can reduce spontaneously. Urgent referral to an orthopedic surgeon is necessary.[9]

Persistent pain after ankle sprain—'the problem ankle'

Most cases of ankle ligament sprain resolve satisfactorily with treatment—pain and swelling settle and function improves. However, as ankle sprain is such a common condition, there remains a substantial number of patients who do not progress well and complain of pain, recurrent instability, swelling and impaired function three to six weeks after injury. This is a very common presentation in a sports medicine practice and the key to successful management is accurate diagnosis. The ankle may continue to cause problems because of an undiagnosed fracture or other bony abnormality (Table 33.2). Alternatively, there may be ligament, tendon, synovial or neurological dysfunction (Table 33.3). In the remainder of this chapter, we discuss a clinical approach to managing patients with this presentation before detailing management of specific conditions.

Clinical approach to the problem ankle

The clinician should take a detailed history that clarifies whether the problem has arisen following an ankle sprain (the true 'problem ankle') or whether the patient has longstanding ankle pain that arose without a history of injury (see Chapter 34). The patient who has had inadequate rehabilitation will usually complain of persistent pain and limitation of function with increasing activity. Determine whether the rehabilitation was adequate by asking the patient to show you the exercises he or she performed in rehabilitation. Did therapy include range of motion exercises (particularly dorsiflexion), strengthening exercises (with the foot fully plantarflexed to engage the peroneal muscles) and proprioceptive retraining?

Examination of the inadequately rehabilitated ankle reveals decreased range of motion in the ankle joint (especially dorsiflexion), weak peroneal muscles and impaired proprioception. These findings can be reversed with active and passive mobilization of the ankle joint (Fig. 33.5), peroneal muscle strengthening (Fig. 33.6) and training of proprioception (Fig. 33.7). Other abnormalities can also cause this constellation of examination findings—remember that the ankle may be inadequately rehabilitated because of the pain of an osteochondral lesion of the talus.

If rehabilitation has been appropriate and symptoms persist, it is necessary to consider the presence of other abnormalities. Was it a high-energy injury that may have caused a fracture? Symptoms of intra-articular abnormalities include clicking, locking and joint swelling. The practitioner should palpate all the sites of potential fracture very carefully to exclude that condition.

Soft tissue injuries that can cause persistent ankle pain after sprain include chronic ligament instability, complex regional pain syndrome type 1 (formerly known as reflex sympathetic dystrophy, RSD) and, rarely, tendon dislocation or subluxation, or even

Table 33.2 Fractures and impingements that may cause the 'problem ankle'—persistent ankle pain after ankle injury

Fractures	Bony impingements[a]
Anterior process calcaneus	Anterior impingement
Lateral process talus	Posterior impingement
Posterior process talus (also os trigonum fracture)	Anterolateral impingement
Osteochondral lesion	
Tibial plafond chondral lesion	
Fracture of base of fifth metatarsal	

(a) Although impingements are included here in the bony causes, pain commonly arises from soft tissue impingement between bony prominences.

Table 33.3 Ligamentous, tendon and neurological causes of the 'problem ankle'—persistent ankle pain after ankle injury

Atypical sprains	Tendon injuries	Other soft tissue and neural abnormalities
Chronic ligamentous instability	Chronic peroneal tendon weakness	Inadequate rehabilitation
Medial ligament sprain	Peroneal tendon subluxation/ rupture	Chronic synovitis
Syndesmosis sprain (AITFL sprain)	Tibialis posterior tendon subluxation/rupture	Sinus tarsi syndrome
Subtalar joint sprain		Complex regional pain syndrome type 1

tendon rupture. Inflammation of the sinus tarsi (sinus tarsi syndrome) can be a cause of persistent ankle pain in its own right, but this syndrome can also occur secondary to associated fractures. Thus, even if the patient has features of the sinus tarsi syndrome, the clinician should still seek other injuries too.

Appropriate investigation is a key part of management of patients with the problem ankle. Both radioisotopic bone scan or MRI are able to distinguish soft tissue damage from bony injury; MRI is preferred in most cases. In soft tissue injuries, isotope activity in the bone phase is normal. If bony damage is present, isotope activity in the bone phase is increased. MRI can detect bony and soft tissue abnormalities but the clinician must remember that a subluxing tendon can appear normal on MRI. The conditions that are associated with the various findings on MRI and bone scan are listed in Figure 33.10.

Osteochondral lesions of the talar dome

It is not uncommon for osteochondral fractures of the talar dome to occur in association with ankle sprains, particularly when there is a compressive component to the inversion injury, such as when landing from a jump. The talar dome is compressed by the tibial plafond, causing damage to the osteochondral surface. The lesions occur most commonly in the superomedial corner of the talar dome, less commonly on the superolateral part.

Large fractures may be recognized at the time of injury. The fracture site will be tender and may be evident on X-ray (Fig. 33.11a). Usually, the lesion is not detected initially and the patient presents some time later with unremitting ankle aching, despite appropriate treatment for an ankle sprain. The patient often gives a history of progressing well following a sprain but then developing symptoms of increasing pain and swelling, stiffness and perhaps catching or locking as activity is increased. Reduced range of motion is often a prominent symptom.

Examination with the patient's foot plantarflexed at 45° to rotate the talus out of the ankle mortise may reveal tenderness of the dome of the talus. If this diagnosis is suspected, the practitioner should image the ankle with MRI (Fig. 33.11d) or isotopic bone scan (Fig. 33.11b). A positive bone scan should be supplemented with a CT scan (Fig. 33.11c) to determine the exact degree of injury. MRI alone provides anatomical and pathological data, and is as the investigation of choice. The grading of osteochondral fractures of the talar dome is shown in Table 33.4.

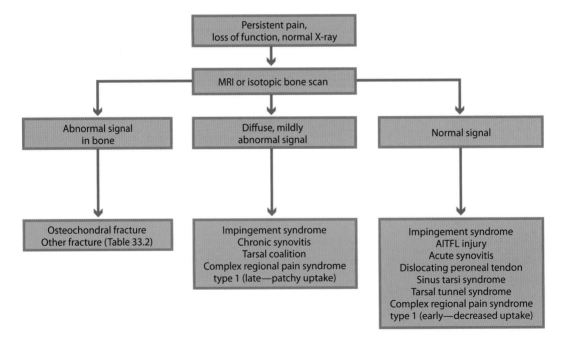

Figure 33.10 Investigation pathway in the patient with persistent ankle pain following an acute injury. When MRI is readily available it serves as an ideal first-line investigation for persistent ankle pain

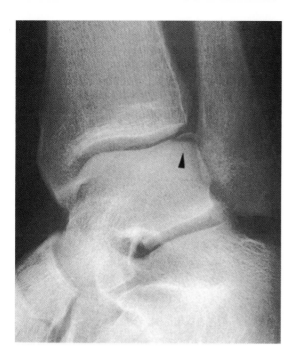

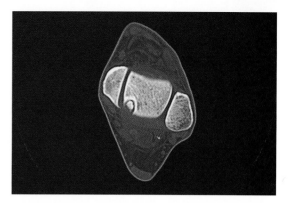

(c) CT scan (grade IV)

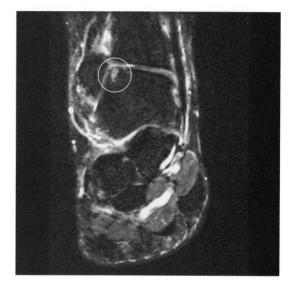

Figure 33.11 Osteochondral lesion of the talar dome

(a) X-ray

(d) MRI (grade I)

Chronic grade I and II lesions should be treated conservatively. The patient should avoid activities that cause pain and be encouraged to pedal an exercise bicycle with low resistance. Formerly, cast immobilization was advocated for these injuries, but joint motion without significant loading is now encouraged to promote articular cartilage healing. If there is pain, or symptoms of clicking, locking or giving persist beyond two to three months of this conservative management, ankle arthroscopy is indicated. A grade IIa, III or IV lesion also requires arthroscopic removal of the separated fragment or cyst and curetting and drilling of the fracture bed down to bleeding bone. After treatment of osteochondral lesions, a comprehensive rehabilitation program is required. Tibial plafond chondral lesions (see below) are managed identically.

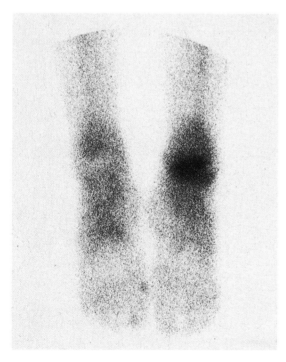

(b) Radioisotopic bone scan

Table 33.4 Grading of osteochondral fracture of the talar dome

Grade	Description	Investigation	Appearance
I	Subchondral fracture	MRI	
II	Chondral fracture	CT/MRI	
IIa	Subchondral cyst	CT/MRI	
III	Chondral fracture with separated but not displaced fragments	CT/MRI	
IV	Chondral fracture with separated and displaced fragment(s)	X-ray/CT/MRI	

Avulsion fracture of the base of the fifth metatarsal

Inversion injury may result in an avulsion fracture of the base of the fifth metatarsal either in isolation or, more commonly, in association with a lateral ligament sprain. This fracture results from avulsion of the peroneus brevis tendon from its attachment to the base of the fifth metatarsal.

X-rays should be examined closely. Avulsion fracture is characterized by its involvement of the joint surface of the base of the fifth metatarsal (Fig. 33.12). A potentially confusing fracture is the fracture of the proximal diaphysis of the fifth metatarsal that does not involve any joint surfaces. This fracture is known as the Jones' fracture and may often require internal fixation (Chapter 35). Although the mechanism can appear to be one of 'acute' injury, in most cases the Jones' fracture is a result of repetitive overuse (i.e. a stress fracture) of the proximal diaphysis of the fifth metatarsal. Fracture of the base of the fifth metatarsal may be treated conservatively with immobilization for pain relief followed after one to two weeks by protected mobilization and rehabilitation.

Other fractures

A number of other fractures may occasionally be seen as a result of acute ankle injuries (Fig. 33.13), alone or in association with ligamentous injury. They may appear quite subtle on plain X-ray.

Fractured lateral talar process

The lateral talar process is a prominence of the lateral talar body with an articular surface dorsolaterally for the fibula and inferomedially for the anterior portion of the posterior calcaneal facet (Fig. 33.13). Patients with a fracture of this process may present with ankle pain, swelling and inability to weight-bear for long periods. Examination reveals swelling and bruising

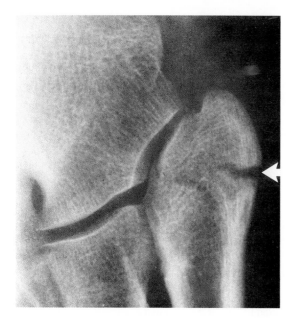

Figure 33.12 Avulsion fracture of the base of the fifth metatarsal

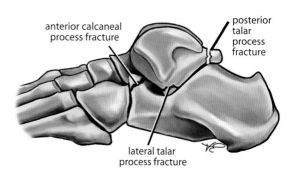

Figure 33.13 Fractures around the talus and calcaneus

over the lateral aspect of the ankle and tenderness over the lateral process, immediately anterior and inferior to the tip of the lateral malleolus. The fracture is best seen on the mortise view X-ray of the ankle. Undisplaced fractures may be treated in a short leg cast. Fractures displaced more than 2 mm (0.1 in.) require either primary excision or reduction and internal fixation. Comminuted fractures may require primary excision.

Fractured anterior calcaneal process

Fractures of the anterior calcaneal process may cause persistent pain after an ankle sprain. Palpation of the anterior calcaneal process, just anterior to the opening of the sinus tarsi (Fig. 33.13), is painless in patients with a tear of the ATFL but will cause considerable pain in those with a fracture of the anterior process. If plain X-rays (including oblique foot views) fail to show a fracture that is suspected clinically, isotopic bone scan or MRI/CT is indicated. If the fracture is small, symptomatic treatment may suffice. If large, it requires four weeks of non-weight-bearing cast immobilization or surgical excision of the fragment.

Tibial plafond chondral lesions

Tibial plafond (the inferior tibial articular surface, Fig. 33.1a) injuries may occur with vertical compression forces, such as a fall from a height. However, they can also complicate otherwise straightforward ankle sprains. The patient complains of difficulty weight-bearing, and examination reveals swelling and restricted dorsiflexion. As with talar dome lesions, X-ray is generally normal, so MRI/CT or isotopic bone scan are necessary to demonstrate the lesion. If imaging and clinical features are consistent with bony damage, arthroscopic debridement is indicated but ankle pain can persist for months to a year, even after treatment.

Fractured posterior process of the talus

Acute fractures of the posterior process of the talus (Fig. 33.13) occasionally occur and may require six weeks of cast immobilization or excision (see also Chapter 34). Acute os trigonum fractures may require surgical excision. This is often the result of an acute plantarflexion injury in kicking and has been seen in fencing.

Impingement syndromes

The impingement syndromes of the ankle are usually the result of overuse but are occasionally present as persistent pain following an acute ankle injury. For example, ballet dancers often suffer posterior impingement following lateral ankle sprain. Posterior impingement syndrome was discussed in Chapter 32. Anterior and anterolateral impingement syndromes are discussed in Chapter 34.

Tendon dislocation or rupture

Dislocation or rupture of the peroneal tendon can cause lateral ankle symptoms of the 'problem ankle' and tibialis posterior injury can cause similar symptoms medially.

Dislocation of peroneal tendons

The peroneal tendons are situated behind the lateral malleolus and fixed by the peroneal retinaculum. They are occasionally dislocated as a result of forceful passive dorsiflexion. This may occur when a skier catches a tip and falls forward over the ski. The peroneal retinaculum is then ripped off the posterior edge of the lateral malleolus and one or both of the tendons slip out of their groove. This dislocated tendon(s) may remain in its dislocated position or spontaneously relocate and subsequently become prone to recurrent subluxation. Examination reveals tender peroneal tendons that can be dislocated by the examiner, especially with ankle plantarflexion.

Treatment of dislocation of peroneal tendons is surgical replacement of the tendons in the peroneal groove and repair of the retinaculum, using bone anchors or drill holes. If the peroneal groove is shallow, in a few cases retinacular repair should be accompanied by deepening of the groove or rotation of the malleolus to better secure the tendons. Soft tissue repair, however, produces a good result in most cases.

Dislocation of the tibialis posterior tendon

Dislocation of the tibialis posterior tendon is extremely rare in sport. However, it occurs with ankle dorsiflexion and inversion so that strong contraction of the tibialis posterior muscle pulls the tendon out of its retinaculum using the malleolus as a fulcrum. The patient may complain of moderate, not exquisite, medial ankle pain and inability to weight-bear. Examination reveals swelling and bruising of the medial ankle above and about the medial malleolus with tenderness along the path of the tibialis posterior tendon. The tendon can be subluxed anteriorly and subsequently relocated posteriorly with the foot in the fully plantarflexed position. The diagnosis is clinical but ultrasonography or MRI (Fig. 33.14) may reveal fluid around the tendon.

Immediate surgical treatment is indicated to minimize the time that the tendon is dislocated while permitting primary repair of the flexor retinaculum and reattachment of the tibialis posterior sheath.[10] Post-operatively the ankle is immobilized in a below-knee plaster cast with a total of six weeks non-weight-bearing on the affected ankle. After the cast is removed, an ankle brace can be used to immobilize the ankle but active ankle motion is permitted three times daily while taking care to avoid resisted inversion. Weight-bearing can recommence at six weeks under physiotherapy/physical therapy supervision followed

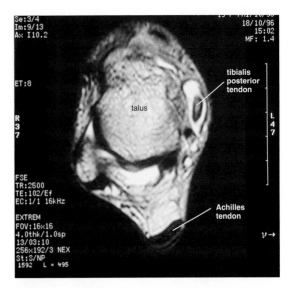

Figure 33.14 MRI appearance (T2-weighted) shortly after tibialis posterior tendon dislocation shows the tibialis posterior tendon (dark) in cross-section surrounded by abnormal fluid (high signal intensity). The tendon is in its normal position during this examination. If imaging had been delayed sufficiently, fluid would have been absent and the MRI appearance may have been normal

by strengthening and functional rehabilitation. In an elite ballet dancer, return to full performance occurred at five months post-surgery[11] and at eight years follow-up the dancer was still performing in a major professional company without recurrence.

Rupture of the tibialis posterior tendon

An athlete with a ruptured tibialis posterior tendon presents with pain in the region of the tubercle of the navicular extending to the posterosuperior border of the medial malleolus and along the posteromedial tibial border. Examination reveals thickening or absence (less frequent) of the tibialis posterior tendon and inability to raise the heel. A flattened medial arch is a classic sign but this may not be evident immediately. MRI is the investigation of choice in this condition, although ultrasound may also be helpful. Surgical repair is indicated as the tibialis posterior tendon is essential to maintain the normal medial arch of the foot.

Other causes of the problem ankle

Anteroinferior tibiofibular ligament injury

The AITFL is one component of the ankle syndesmosis. It may be damaged in more severe ankle injuries (Fig. 33.15) and it is occasionally associated with fractures (e.g. Maisonneuve fracture, see p. 622). This injury causes considerably more impairment than does a lateral ankle sprain. Palpation reveals maximal tenderness over the AITFL (Fig. 33.1c). Combined rotation of the foot and dorsiflexion of the ankle joint may reproduce the pain. Weight-bearing views are needed to improve the sensitivity of plain X-ray to detect this injury. Complete interruption to the syndesmosis may occur with very severe injuries. Widening of the ankle mortise is the diagnostic feature on X-ray. Orthopedic surgical referral is essential.

Post-traumatic synovitis

Some degree of synovitis will occur with any ankle injury due to the presence of blood within the joint. This usually resolves in a few days but may persist if there is excessive early weight-bearing, typically in athletes eager to return to training soon after their ankle sprain, or due to insufficient rehabilitation. These athletes will often develop persistent ankle pain aggravated by activity and associated with swelling. Synovitis of the ankle joint is also seen in athletes who have chronic mild instability because of excessive accessory movement of the ankle joint during activity.

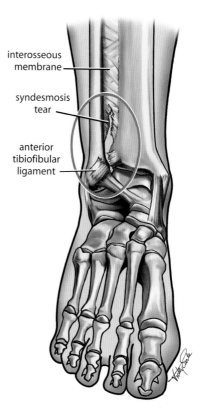

Figure 33.15 Anatomy of a syndesmosis sprain. This injury may be associated with medial malleolar fracture (not illustrated)

Treatment of synovitis includes NSAIDs, rest from aggravating activity and local electrotherapy. A corticosteroid injection into the ankle joint (Fig. 33.16) may be required. Injection should be followed by 48 hours of limited weight-bearing and gradual resumption of activity. Sometimes arthroscopy may be indicated.

When synovitis is associated with a degree of chronic instability, treatment involves taping or bracing. Such a patient can gain significant relief by wearing a brace for activities of daily living as well as sport. These patients may also benefit from ankle reconstructive surgery.

Sinus tarsi syndrome

The sinus tarsi syndrome may occur as an overuse injury secondary to excessive subtalar pronation (Chapter 34) or as a sequel to an ankle sprain. Pain occurs at the lateral opening of the sinus tarsi (Fig. 33.1b). The pain is often more severe in the morning and improves as the patient warms up.

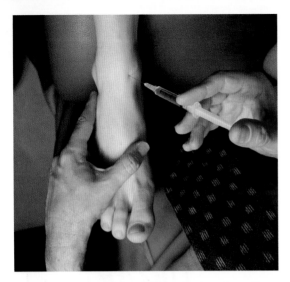

Figure 33.16 Corticosteroid injection into the ankle joint in the treatment of post-traumatic synovitis. The needle is inserted medial to the tibialis anterior tendon and directed posterolaterally

Forced passive inversion and eversion may both be painful. The most appropriate aid to diagnosis is to monitor the effect of injection of a local anesthetic agent into the sinus tarsi (Fig. 33.17).

Treatment consists of relative rest, NSAIDs, electrotherapeutic modalities, subtalar joint mobilization and taping to correct excessive pronation if present. If conservative management is unsuccessful, injection of corticosteroid and local anesthetic agents may help resolve the inflammation.

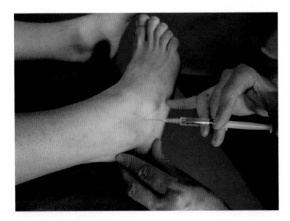

Figure 33.17 Injection into the sinus tarsi. The lateral opening of the sinus is maintained when the foot is inverted. The needle is directed towards the tip of the medial malleolus

Complex regional pain syndrome type 1

Complex regional pain syndrome (CRPS) type 1, formerly known as RSD (Chapters 3, 4), may occasionally complicate ankle injury. Initially, it appears that the patient with a 'sprained ankle' is improving but then symptoms begin to relapse. The patient complains of increased pain, swelling recurs and the skin may become hot or, more frequently, very cold. There may also be localized sweating, discoloration and hypersensitivity.

As early treatment substantially improves the prognosis in CRPS type 1, early diagnosis is imperative. Initial X-rays are normal. Later, patchy demineralization occurs and this can be seen as regions of decreased opacity on X-ray and areas of increased uptake on bone scan—the investigation of choice.[12] Tests of sympathetic function (Chapter 9) may confirm the diagnosis.[13]

It is most important that the peculiar nature of the condition be explained to the patient as it may be a particularly painful condition, even at rest. It remains very difficult to treat and there have been few controlled treatment trials for established CRPS type 1.[14] Physiotherapy may play a role[15] and ultrasound and hydrotherapy may facilitate range of movement exercises. Gabapentin, an anticonvulsant with a proven analgesic effect in various neuropathic pain syndromes, has shown mild efficacy as treatment for pain in patients with CRPS type 1.[16] Because CRPS type 1 is associated with regional osteoclastic overactivity (excessive bone turnover, as shown by increased uptake on radionuclide bone scan), a bisphosphonate medication (alendronate) was trialed in 39 patients.[17] In contrast to placebo-treated patients, all of the alendronate-treated patients had substantially reduced pain and improved joint mobility as early as the fourth week of treatment.

If the pain does not settle, chemical or surgical blockade is indicated. However, a Cochrane systematic review failed to support this therapy for relieving pain.[18] CRPS type 1 remains a very difficult condition to treat.

Recommended Reading

Bachmann LM, Kolb E, Koller MT, Steurer J, ter Riet G. Accuracy of Ottawa ankle rules to exclude fractures of the ankle and mid-foot: systematic review. *BMJ* 2003; 326(7386): 417.
A nice summary of the status of the Ottawa ankle rules 10 years after the original paper by Stiell et al. (see below).

Chan KM, Karlsson J. *ISAKOS-FIMS World Consensus Conference on Ankle Instability*. Stockholm: International Society of Arthroscopy, Knee Surgery and Orthopaedic Sports Medicine, 2005.

Kannus P, Renstrom P. Treatment for acute tears of the lateral ligament of the ankle. *J Bone Joint Surg Am* 1991; 73A: 305–12.

Remains a classic paper showing that these 'fathers of sports medicine' provided answers to many important questions nearly 20 years ago.

Osborne MD, Rizzo TD Jr. Prevention and treatment of ankle sprain in athletes. *Sports Med* 2003; 33(15): 1145–50.

Quisel A, Gill JM, Witherell P. Complex regional pain syndrome underdiagnosed. *J Fam Pract* 2005; 54(6): 524–32. Available online: <http://www.jfponline.com/Pages.asp?AID=1947>.

Stiell IG, Greenberg GH, McKnight RD, et al. Decision rules for the use of radiography in acute ankle injuries. *JAMA* 1993; 269: 1127–32.

Retained even in this third edition as a classic paper.

References

1. Bridgman SA, Clement D, Downing A, Walley G, Phair I, Maffulli N. Population based epidemiology of ankle sprains attending accident and emergency units in the West Midlands of England, and a survey of UK practice for severe ankle sprains. *Emerg Med J* 2003; 20(6): 508–10.

2. Bachmann LM, Kolb E, Koller MT, Steurer J, ter Riet G. Accuracy of Ottawa ankle rules to exclude fractures of the ankle and mid-foot: systematic review. *BMJ* 2003; 326(7386): 417.

3. Holme E, Magnusson SP, Becher K, Bieler T, Aagaard P, Kjaer M. The effect of supervised rehabilitation on strength, postural sway, position sense and re-injury risk after acute ankle ligament sprain. *Scand J Med Sci Sports* 1999; 9(2): 104–9.

4. Verhagen E, van der Beek A, Twisk J, Bouter L, Bahr R, van Mechelen W. The effect of a proprioceptive balance board training program for the prevention of ankle sprains: a prospective controlled trial. *Am J Sports Med* 2004; 32(6): 1385–93.

5. Verhagen EA, van Tulder M, van der Beek AJ, Bouter LM, van Mechelen W. An economic evaluation of a proprioceptive balance board training programme for the prevention of ankle sprains in volleyball. *Br J Sports Med* 2005; 39(2): 111–15.

6. Kerkhoffs GM, Handoll HH, de Bie R, Rowe BH, Struijs PA. Surgical versus conservative treatment for acute injuries of the lateral ligament complex of the ankle in adults. *Cochrane Database Syst Rev* 2002; 3: CD000380.

7. Kaikkonen A, Kannus P, Jarvinen M. Surgery versus functional treatment in ankle ligament tears. A prospective study. *Clin Orthop* 1996; 326: 194–202.

8. Pijnenburg AC, Bogaard K, Krips R, Marti RK, Bossuyt PM, van Dijk CN. Operative and functional treatment of rupture of the lateral ligament of the ankle. A randomised, prospective trial. *J Bone Joint Surg Br* 2003; 85B(4): 525–30.

9. Babis GC, Papagelopoulos PJ, Tsarouchas J, Zoubos AB, Korres DS, Nikiforidis P. Operative treatment for Maisonneuve fracture of the proximal fibula. *Orthopedics* 2000; 23(7): 687–90.

10. Rolf C, Guntner P, Ekenman I, Turan I. Dislocation of the tibialis posterior tendon: diagnosis and treatment. *J Foot Ankle Surg* 1997; 36(1): 63–5.

11. Khan KM, Gelber N, Slater K, Wark JD. Dislocated tibialis posterior tendon in a classical ballet dancer: a case report. *J Dance Med Sci* 1997; 1: 160–2.

12. Shehab D, Elgazzar A, Collier BD, et al. Impact of three-phase bone scintigraphy on the diagnosis and treatment of complex regional pain syndrome type I or reflex sympathetic dystrophy. *Med Princ Pract* 2006; 15(1): 46–51.

13. Perez RS, Keijzer C, Bezemer PD, Zuurmond WW, de Lange JJ. Predictive value of symptom level measurements for complex regional pain syndrome type I. *Eur J Pain* 2005; 9(1): 49–56.

14. Forouzanfar T, Koke AJ, van Kleef M, Weber WE. Treatment of complex regional pain syndrome type I. *Eur J Pain* 2002; 6(2): 105–22.

15. Oerlemans HM, Oostendorp RA, de Boo T, van der Laan L, Severens JL, Goris JA. Adjuvant physical therapy versus occupational therapy in patients with reflex sympathetic dystrophy/complex regional pain syndrome type I. *Arch Phys Med Rehabil* 2000; 81(1): 49–56.

16. van de Vusse AC, Stomp-van den Berg SG, Kessels AH, Weber WE. Randomised controlled trial of gabapentin in complex regional pain syndrome type 1 [ISRCTN84121379]. *BMC Neurol* 2004; 4: 13.

17. Manicourt DH, Brasseur JP, Boutsen Y, Depreseux G, Devogelaer JP. Role of alendronate in therapy for posttraumatic complex regional pain syndrome type I of the lower extremity. *Arthritis Rheum* 2004; 50(11): 3690–7.

18. Cepeda M, Carr D, Lau J. Local anesthetic sympathetic blockade for complex regional pain syndrome. *Cochrane Database Syst Rev* 2005; 4: CD004598.

Ankle Pain

WITH KAREN HOLZER

Sportspeople, particularly ballet dancers, footballers and high jumpers, may complain of ankle pain that is not related to an acute ankle injury (Chapter 33). Clinical management is simplified if the presentations are further divided into:

- medial ankle pain
- lateral ankle pain
- anterior ankle pain.

Note that the region that might be considered 'posterior ankle' pain is defined as the 'Achilles region' in this book (Chapter 32).

Medial ankle pain

Clinical experience suggests that the most common cause of medial ankle pain is tibialis posterior tendinopathy. Posterior impingement syndrome of the ankle (Chapter 32) may occasionally present as medial ankle pain. Flexor hallucis longus tendinopathy is not uncommon and may occur together with posterior impingement syndrome. Tarsal tunnel syndrome, in which the posterior tibial nerve is compressed behind the medial malleolus, may present as medial ankle pain with sensory symptoms distally. Causes of medial ankle pain are listed in Table 34.1. The anatomy of the region is illustrated in Figure 34.1.

History

In patients with medial ankle pain there is usually a history of overuse, especially running or excessive walking (tibialis posterior tendinopathy), toe flexion in ballet dancers and high jumpers (flexor hallucis longus tendinopathy) or plantarflexion in dancers and footballers (posterior impingement syndrome). Pain may radiate along the line of the tibialis posterior tendon to its insertion on the navicular tubercle or into the arch of the foot with tarsal tunnel syndrome. Sensory symptoms such as pins and needles or numbness may suggest tarsal tunnel syndrome.

Examination

Careful palpation and testing of resisted movements is the key to examination of this region.

Table 34.1 Causes of medial ankle pain

Common	Less common	Not to be missed
Tibialis posterior tendinopathy	Medial calcaneal nerve entrapment	Navicular stress fracture (Chapter 35)
Flexor hallucis longus tendinopathy	Calcaneal stress fracture	Complications of acute ankle injuries (Chapter 33)
	Tarsal tunnel syndrome	Complex regional pain syndrome type 1 (following knee or ankle injury)
	Talar stress fracture	
	Medial malleolar stress fracture	
	Posterior impingement syndrome (Chapter 32)	
	Referred pain from lumbar spine	

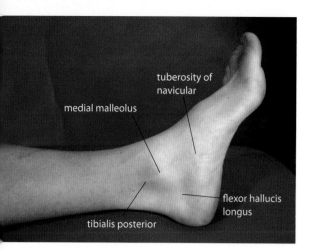

Figure 34.1 Medial aspect of the ankle

(a) Surface anatomy

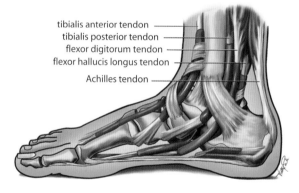

(b) Anatomy of the medial ankle

1. Observation
   (a) standing
   (b) walking
   (c) supine
2. Active movements
   (a) ankle plantarflexion/dorsiflexion
   (b) ankle inversion/eversion
   (c) flexion of the first metatarsophalangeal joint
3. Passive movements
   (a) as for active
   (b) subtalar joint
   (c) midtarsal joint
   (d) muscle stretches
       (i) gastrocnemius
       (ii) soleus
4. Resisted movement
   (a) inversion (Fig. 34.2a)
   (b) first toe flexion (Fig. 34.2b)

5. Functional tests
   (a) hop
   (b) jump
6. Palpation
   (a) tibialis posterior tendon (Fig. 34.2c)
   (b) flexor hallucis longus
   (c) navicular tubercle
   (d) ankle joint
   (e) midtarsal joint
7. Special tests
   (a) Tinel's test (Fig. 34.2d)
   (b) sensory examination (Fig. 34.2e)
   (c) biomechanical examination (Chapter 5)
   (d) lumbar spine examination (Chapter 21)

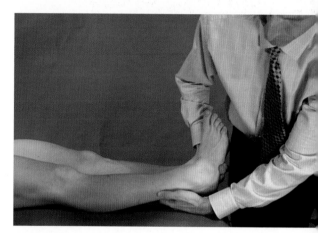

Figure 34.2 Examination of the patient with medial ankle pain

(a) Resisted movement—inversion (tibialis posterior)

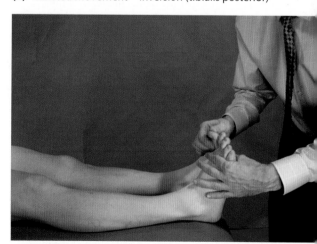

(b) Resisted movement—toe flexion (flexor hallucis longus)

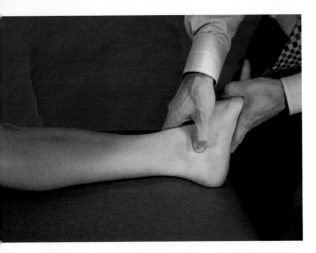

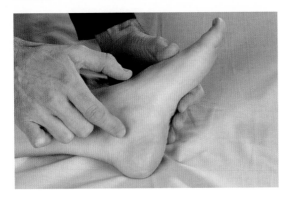

(c) Palpation—tibialis posterior tendon. The tibialis posterior tendon is palpated from posteromedial to the medial malleolus to its insertion at the navicular tubercle

(d) Special tests—Tinel's test. Tapping over the posterior tibial nerve in the tarsal tunnel may reproduce symptoms

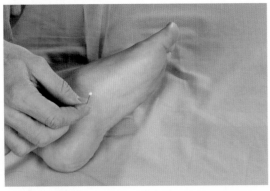

(e) Special tests—sensory examination of the medial aspect of the foot. Sensory deficits may occur with tarsal tunnel syndrome

Investigations

Plain X-ray should be performed when posterior impingement is suspected to confirm the presence of either a large posterior process of the talus or an os trigonum. A lateral view with the foot in a maximally plantarflexed position (posterior impingement view) can be useful to determine if bony impingement is occurring. A radioisotopic bone scan may show an area of mildly increased uptake at the posterior aspect of the talus in cases of chronic posterior impingement. In suspected cases of tendinopathy, ultrasonography or MRI may be indicated if pain has been longstanding or if there is doubt about the diagnosis. Nerve conduction studies should be obtained if tarsal tunnel syndrome is the likely diagnosis.

Tibialis posterior tendinopathy

The tibialis posterior tendon functions to invert the subtalar joint and is the main dynamic stabilizer of the hind foot against valgus (eversion) forces, in addition to providing stability to the plantar arch. It is the most anterior structure that passes behind the medial malleolus, then divides and sends attachments to the navicular tuberosity, the cuboid, cuneiforms, bases of the second to fourth metatarsals and the spring ligament.

Causes

The etiology of tibialis posterior tendinopathy is usually related to an overuse injury rather than an acute traumatic injury.

1. Overuse—often related to:
   (a) excessive walking, running or jumping
   (b) excessive subtalar pronation—this increases eccentric tendon loading during supination for toe-off
2. Acute
   (a) direct trauma—laceration
   (b) indirect trauma—eversion ankle sprain, ankle fracture
   (c) acute avulsion fracture
3. Inflammatory conditions
   (a) tenosynovitis secondary to rheumatoid arthritis, seronegative arthropathies

Chronic tendinopathy is characterized by collagen disarray and interstitial tears, and may eventually lead to tendon rupture.

Clinical features

- Medial ankle pain behind the medial malleolus and extending towards the insertion of the tendon.

- Swelling is very unusual—if present, it suggests substantial tendon injury or an underlying seronegative arthropathy.
- Tenderness along the tendon prominent posterior and inferior to the medial malleolus.
- Crepitus is occasionally present.
- Resisted inversion (Fig. 34.2a) will elicit pain and relative weakness compared with the contralateral side.
- A single heel raise test also viewed from behind will reveal lack of inversion of the hind foot, and if severe the patient may have difficulty performing a heel raise.

Investigations

MRI or ultrasound may confirm the diagnosis and reveal the extent of tendinosis. MRI is the most useful method of imaging tendons around the ankle. It is highly sensitive and specific for the detection of a rupture.[1,2] When compared with MRI, ultrasonography had a sensitivity and specificity of 80% and 90%, respectively.[3] In cases of suspected inflammatory tenosynovitis, blood tests for serological and inflammatory markers should be performed.

Treatment

Conservative care consists of controlling pain where needed with ice and prescribing concentric and eccentric tendon loading exercises (Fig. 34.3). Experienced clinicians often administer soft tissue therapy to the tibialis posterior muscle and tendon and prescribe a rigid orthosis to control excessive pronation. In severe

cases, a period of immobilization in an air cast has been prescribed to provide short-term symptom relief but this would be an extreme measure.

If an inflammatory arthropathy is present, antiinflammatory medications are indicated.

If there is tendon rupture (Chapter 33), or if conservative management fails to settle the condition, surgery is recommended. In the case of tenosynovitis a synovectomy may be performed, while in cases of severe tendinopathy or tendon rupture a reconstruction may be required.

Flexor hallucis longus tendinopathy

The flexor hallucis longus tendon flexes the big toe and assists in plantarflexion of the ankle. It passes posterior to the medial malleolus, and runs between the two sesamoid bones to insert into the base of the distal phalanx of the big toe.

Causes

Flexor hallucis longus tendinopathy may occur secondary to overuse, a stenosing tenosynovitis, pseudocyst or tendon tear. A common cause is overuse in a ballet dancer, as dancers repetitively go from flat foot stance to the *en pointe* position, when extreme plantarflexion is required. Wearing shoes that are too big and require the athlete to 'toe-grip' may also result in flexor hallucis longus tendinopathy.

This condition is often associated with posterior impingement syndrome (Chapter 32) as the flexor hallucis tendon lies in a fibro-osseous tunnel between the lateral and medial tubercles of the posterior process of the talus. Enlargement or medial displacement of the os trigonum puts pressure on the flexor hallucis longus at the point where the tendon changes direction from a vertical course dorsal to the talus to a horizontal course beneath the talus (Fig. 34. 4). This can cause tendon thickening and may result in 'triggering' of the tendon, when partial tearing and subsequent healing of the tendon produce excessive scar tissue.

Clinical features

- Pain on toe-off or forefoot weight-bearing (e.g. rising in ballet), maximal over the posteromedial aspect of the calcaneus around the sustentaculum tali.
- Pain may be aggravated by resisted flexion of the first toe or stretch into full dorsiflexion of the hallux.
- In more severe cases, there may be 'triggering' of the first toe, both with rising onto the balls

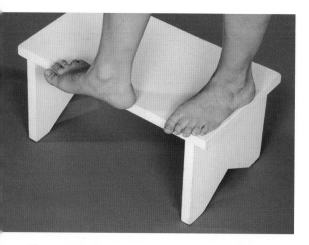

Figure 34.3 Eccentric exercises—tibialis posterior. Patient stands on the edge of a step and drops down into eversion, eccentrically contracting the tibialis posterior muscle

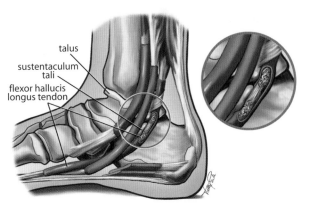

Figure 34.4 Flexor hallucis longus tendinopathy showing the tendon irritated near the medial malleolus.

of the foot (e.g. in ballet) and in lowering from this position. Triggering occurs when the foot is placed in plantarflexion and the athlete, unable to flex the hallux, but then with forcible active contraction of the flexor hallucis longus, is able to extend the interphalangeal or metatarsophalangeal joints of the toe. A snap or pop occurs in the posteromedial aspect of the ankle when this happens. Subsequent passive flexion or extension of the interphalangeal joint produces a painless snap posterior to the medial malleolus.

Investigations

MRI or ultrasound may both reveal pathology. The characteristic MRI sign is abrupt fluid cut-off in the tendon sheath; excessive fluid is found loculated around a normal-appearing tendon proximal to the fibro-osseous canal.[4]

Treatment

In the acute phase, treatment may include:

- ice
- avoidance of activities that stress the flexor hallucis longus tendon (e.g. dancer working at the barre but not rising *en pointe*)
- flexor hallucis longus strength and stretching exercises
- soft tissue therapy proximally in the muscle belly
- correction of subtalar joint hypomobility with manual mobilization
- control of excessive pronation during toe-off with tape or orthoses—this may be helpful but is difficult to achieve in dancers.

Prevention of recurrences should focus on a reduction in the amount of hip turnout, thus ensuring that the weight is directly over the hip, avoidance of hard floors, and using firm, well-fitting pointe shoes, so that the foot is well supported and no additional strain is placed on the tendon. Technique correction is important in ballet dancers with this condition as it is thought to arise not only from excessive ankle eversion or inversion with pointe work but also from proximal weakness, such as poor trunk control.[5]

Surgical treatment should be considered when persistent synovitis or triggering prevents dancing *en pointe*. Surgery involves exploration of the tendon and release of the tendon sheath.

Tarsal tunnel syndrome

Tarsal tunnel syndrome occurs as a result of entrapment of the posterior tibial nerve in the tarsal tunnel where the nerve winds around the medial malleolus. It may also involve only one of its terminal branches distal to the tarsal tunnel.

Causes

In approximately 50% of cases the cause of tarsal tunnel syndrome is idiopathic. It may also occur as a result of trauma (e.g. inversion injury to the ankle) or overuse associated with excessive pronation. Other less common causes include:

- ganglion
- talonavicular coalition
- varicose veins
- synovial cyst
- lipoma
- accessory muscle—flexor digitorum accessorius longus
- tenosynovitis
- fracture of the distal tibia or calcaneus.

Clinical features

- Poorly defined burning, tingling or numb sensation on the plantar aspect of the foot, often radiating into the toes.
- Pain is usually aggravated by activity and relieved by rest.
- In some patients the symptoms are worse in bed at night and relieved by getting up and moving or massaging the foot.
- Swellings, varicosities or thickenings may be found on examination around the medial ankle or heel.
- A ganglion or cyst may be palpable in the tendon sheaths around the medial ankle.

- Tenderness in the region of the tarsal tunnel is common.
- Tapping over the posterior tibial nerve (Tinel's sign) may elicit the patient's pain and occasionally cause fasciculations but this 'classic' sign is not commonly seen.
- There may be altered sensation along the arch of the foot.
- The distribution of the sensory changes in the foot needs to be differentiated from the typical dermatomal distribution of S1 nerve root compression.

Investigations

Nerve conduction studies should be performed.[6, 7] These not only help to confirm the diagnosis but they can also guide the surgeon as to the location of the nerve compression. Ultrasound or MRI may be required to assess for a space-occupying lesion as a cause of the syndrome. An X-ray and, if required, a CT scan should be performed in the case of excessive pronation or if a tarsal coalition is suspected.

Differential diagnosis

Differential diagnosis includes entrapment of the medial and/or lateral plantar nerves, or both, plantar fasciitis, intervertebral disk degeneration and other causes of nerve inflammation or degeneration.

Treatment

Conservative treatment should be attempted in those with either an idiopathic or biomechanical cause. Treatment with NSAID and, if required an injection of a corticosteroid agent into the tarsal tunnel may be helpful. If excessive pronation is present, an orthosis should be utilized.

Surgical treatment is required if there is mechanical pressure on the nerve. A decompression of the posterior tibial nerve and its branches should be performed, but only after both the diagnosis and site of nerve entrapment have been confirmed. Results of surgery have not been encouraging,[8] with a high perioperative complication rate.[9]

Stress fracture of the medial malleolus

Stress fracture of the medial malleolus is an unusual injury but should be considered in the runner presenting with persistent medial ankle pain aggravated by activity.[10, 11] Although the fracture line is frequently vertical from the junction of the tibial plafond and the medial malleolus, it may arch obliquely from the junction to the distal tibial metaphysis.

Clinical features

Athletes classically present with medial ankle pain that progressively increases with running and jumping activities. Often they experience an acute episode, which leads to their seeking medical attention. Examination reveals tenderness overlying the medial malleolus frequently in conjunction with an ankle effusion.

Investigations

In the early stages, X-rays may be normal, but with time a linear area of hyperlucency may be apparent, progressing to a lytic area and fracture line. If the X-ray is normal, a radioisotopic bone scan, CT (Fig. 34.5) or MRI will be required to demonstrate the fracture.

Treatment

If no fracture or an undisplaced fracture is evident on X-ray, treatment requires weight-bearing rest with an air-cast brace until local tenderness resolves, a period of approximately six weeks. If, however, a displaced fracture or a fracture that has progressed to non-union is present, surgery with internal fixation is required. Following fracture healing, the practitioner should assess biomechanics and footwear. A graduated return to activity is required.

Medial calcaneal nerve entrapment

The medial calcaneal nerve is a branch of the posterior tibial nerve arising at the level of the medial malleolus

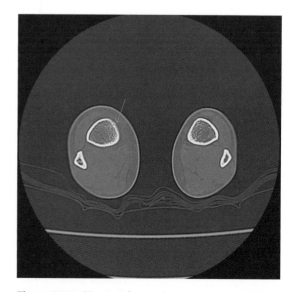

Figure 34.5 CT scan of stress fracture of the medial malleolus

or below and passing superficially to innervate the skin of the heel. Occasionally it may arise from the lateral plantar nerve, a branch of the posterior tibial nerve. It has been theorized that a valgus hind foot may predispose joggers to compression of this nerve branch.

Clinical features

Entrapment or irritation causes burning pain over the inferomedial aspect of the calcaneus, which often radiates into the arch of the foot, and is aggravated by running. Examination reveals tenderness over the medial calcaneus and a positive Tinel's sign. There is often associated excessive pronation.

Investigations

Nerve conduction studies can help confirm the diagnosis. Injection of local anesthetic at the point of maximal tenderness with a resultant disappearance of pain will confirm the diagnosis.

Treatment

Treatment involves minimizing the trauma to the nerve with a change of footwear or the use of a pad over the area to protect the nerve. Use of local electrotherapeutic modalities and transverse friction to the painful site may help to settle the pain. If this is not successful, injection of corticosteroid and local anesthetic agents into the area of point tenderness may be helpful. Surgery may be required to decompress the nerve.

Other causes

Two conditions that generally cause foot pain but may present as medial ankle pain are stress fractures of the calcaneus and the navicular (Chapter 35). Referred pain from neural structures may occasionally present as medial ankle pain. Entrapment of the medial plantar nerve generally causes midfoot pain but may present as medial ankle pain.

Lateral ankle pain

Lateral ankle pain is generally associated with a biomechanical abnormality. The two most common causes are peroneal tendinopathy and sinus tarsi syndrome. The causes of lateral ankle pain are listed in Table 34.2. The anatomy of the region is illustrated in Figure 34.6.

Examination

Examination is as for the patient with acute ankle injury (Chapter 33) with particular attention to testing resisted eversion of the peroneal tendons (Fig. 34.7a) and careful palpation for tenderness and crepitus (Fig. 34.7b).

Peroneal tendinopathy

The most common overuse injury causing lateral ankle pain is peroneal tendinopathy. The peroneus longus and peroneus brevis tendons cross the ankle joint within a fibro-osseous tunnel, posterior to the lateral malleolus. The peroneus brevis tendon inserts into the tuberosity on the lateral aspect of the base of the fifth metatarsal. The peroneus longus tendon passes under the plantar surface of the foot to insert into the lateral side of the base of the first metatarsal and medial cuneiform. The peroneal tendons share a common tendon sheath proximal to the distal tip of the fibula, after which they have their own tendon sheaths. The peroneal muscles serve as ankle dorsiflexors in addition to being the primary evertors of the ankle.

Table 34.2 Causes of lateral ankle pain

Common	Less common	Not to be missed
Peroneal tendinopathy	Impingement syndrome	Stress fracture of the distal fibula
Sinus tarsi syndrome	Anterolateral	Cuboid syndrome
	Posterior	Complex regional pain syndrome
	Recurrent dislocation of peroneal tendons	type 1 (following knee or ankle
	Stress fracture of the talus	trauma)
	Referred pain	
	Lumbar spine	
	Peroneal nerve	
	Superior tibiofibular joint	

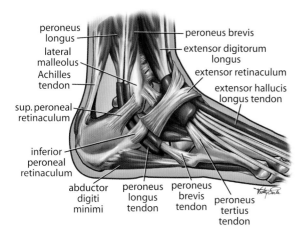

Figure 34.6 Lateral aspect of the ankle

(a) Anatomy of the lateral ankle

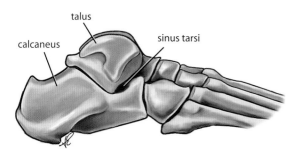

(b) Sinus tarsi

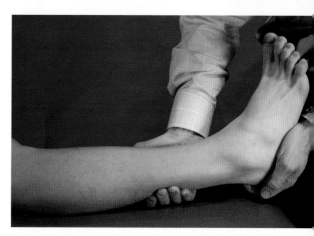

Figure 34.7 Examination of the patient with lateral ankle pain

(a) Resisted movement—eversion (peroneal muscles)

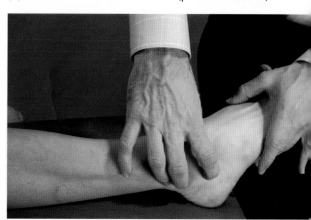

(b) Palpation—the peroneal tendons are palpated for tenderness and crepitus

Causes

Peroneal tendinopathy may occur either as a result of an acute ankle inversion injury or secondary to an overuse injury. Soft footwear may predispose to the development of peroneal tendinopathy.

Common causes of an overuse injury include:

1. excessive eversion of the foot, such as occurs when running on slopes or cambered surfaces[12]
2. excessive pronation of the foot
3. secondary to tight ankle plantarflexors (most commonly soleus) resulting in excessive load on the lateral muscles
4. excessive action of the peroneals (e.g. dancing, basketball, volleyball).

An inflammatory arthropathy may also result in the development of a peroneal tenosynovitis and subsequent peroneal tendinopathy.

It has been suggested that peroneal tendinopathy may be due to the excessive pulley action of, and abrupt change in direction of, the peroneal tendons at the lateral malleolus.

There are three main sites of peroneal tendinopathy:

1. posterior to the lateral malleolus
2. at the peroneal trochlea
3. at the plantar surface of the cuboid.

Clinical features

The athlete commonly presents with:

- lateral ankle or heel pain and swelling which is aggravated by activity and relieved by rest

- local tenderness over the peroneal tendons on examination, sometimes associated with swelling and crepitus (a true paratenonitis)
- painful passive inversion and resisted eversion, although in some cases eccentric contraction may be required to reproduce the pain
- a possible associated calf muscle tightness
- excessive subtalar pronation or stiffness of the subtalar or midtarsal joints that is demonstrated on biomechanical examination.

Investigations

MRI is the recommended investigation and shows characteristic features of tendinopathy—increased signal and tendon thickening.[13] If MRI is unavailable, an ultrasound may be performed. If an underlying inflammatory arthropathy is suspected, obtain blood tests to assess for rheumatological and inflammatory markers.

Treatment

Treatment initially involves settling the pain with rest from aggravating activities, analgesic medication if needed and soft tissue therapy. Stretching in conjunction with mobilization of the subtalar and midtarsal joints may be helpful. Footwear should be assessed and the use of lateral heel wedges or orthoses may be required to correct biomechanical abnormalities. Strengthening exercises should include resisted eversion (e.g. rubber tubing, rotagym), especially in plantarflexion as this position maximally engages the peroneal muscles.

In severe cases, surgery may be required, which may involve a synovectomy, tendon debridement or repair.

Sinus tarsi syndrome

The sinus tarsi (Fig. 34.6b) is a small osseous canal running from an opening anterior and inferior to the lateral malleolus in a posteromedial direction to a point posterior to the medial malleolus. The interosseus ligament occupies the sinus tarsi and divides it into an anterior portion, which is part of the talocalcaneonavicular joint, and a posterior part, which represents the subtalar joint. It is lined by a synovial membrane and in addition to ligament it contains small blood vessels, fat and connective tissue.

Causes

Although injury to the sinus tarsi may result from chronic overuse secondary to poor biomechanics (especially excessive pronation), approximately 70%

of all patients with sinus tarsi syndrome have had a single or repeated inversion injury to the ankle. It may also occur after repeated forced eversion to the ankle, such as high jump take off.

The sinus tarsi contains abundant synovial tissue that is prone to synovitis and inflammation when injured. An influx of inflammatory cells may result in the development of a low-grade inflammatory synovitis.

Other causes of sinus tarsi syndrome may include chronic inflammation in conditions such as gout, inflammatory arthropathies and osteoarthritis.

Clinical features

The symptoms of sinus tarsi syndrome include:

- pain which may be poorly localized but is most often centered just anterior to the lateral malleolus
- pain that is often more severe in the morning and may diminish with exercise
- pain that may be exacerbated by running on a curve in the direction of the affected ankle—the patient may also complain of ankle and foot stiffness, a feeling of instability of the hind foot and occasionally of weakness
- difficulty walking on uneven ground
- full range of pain-free ankle movement on examination but the subtalar joint may be stiff
- pain on forced passive eversion of the subtalar joint; forced passive inversion may also be painful due to damage to the subtalar ligaments
- tenderness of the lateral aspect of the ankle at the opening of the sinus tarsi and occasionally also over the anterior talofibular ligament; there may be minor localized swelling.

Diagnosis

The most appropriate diagnostic test is injection of 1 mL of a short-acting local anesthetic agent (e.g. 1% lignocaine [lidocaine]) into the sinus tarsi (Fig. 34.8). In sinus tarsi syndrome, this injection will relieve pain so that functional tests, such as hopping on the affected leg, can be performed comfortably (for diagnosis). An ankle X-ray may be performed to exclude degenerative changes of the subtalar joint. MRI may show an increased signal and fluid in the sinus tarsi.

Treatment

Conservative management includes relative rest, ice, NSAID and electrotherapeutic modalities. Mobilization of the subtalar joint is essential (Fig. 34.9). Rehabilitation involves proprioception and strength

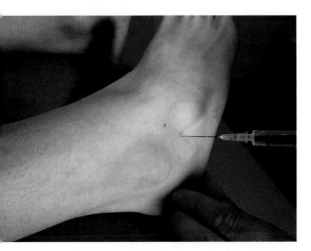

Figure 34.8 Local anesthetic injection. The needle is introduced into the lateral opening of the sinus tarsi with the foot in passive inversion. The needle should be directed medially and slightly posteriorly

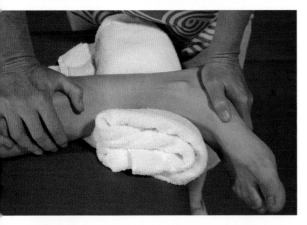

Figure 34.9 Mobilization of the subtalar joint is performed by medial-to-lateral transverse glide of the calcaneus on the talus with the patient side-lying and the ankle dorsiflexed

training. Biomechanical correction may be indicated. Direct infiltration of the sinus tarsi with corticosteroid and local anesthetic agents may prove therapeutic but it is important that all underlying abnormalities are also corrected.

Anterolateral impingement

Causes

Repeated minor ankle sprains or a major sprain involving the anterolateral aspect of the ankle may cause anterolateral impingement. An inversion sprain

to the anterior talofibular ligament may promote synovial thickening and exudation. Usually this is subsequently resorbed, but sometimes this is incomplete and the residual tissue becomes hyalinized and molded by pressure from the articular surfaces of the talus and fibula, where it may be trapped during ankle movements. A meniscoid lesion thus develops in the anterolateral gutter. It has also been suggested that meniscoid lesions may result from tears of the anterior talofibular ligament in which the torn fragment becomes interposed between the lateral malleolus and the lateral aspect of the talus. Another postulated cause of anterolateral ankle impingement is chondromalacia of the lateral wall of the talus with an associated synovial reaction.

Clinical features

The classic presentation is pain at the anterior aspect of the lateral malleolus and an intermittent catching sensation in the ankle in an athlete with a previous history of an ankle inversion injury. Examination may reveal tenderness in the region of the anteroinferior border of the fibula and anterolateral surface of the talus. The pain is relieved by tightening the tibialis posterior tendon and releasing the peroneal tendons. Proprioception may be poor.[14]

Investigations

Clinical assessment has been shown to be more reliable than MRI to diagnose this lesion.[15] An arthroscopic examination confirms the diagnosis. Corticosteroid injection may be helpful initially but, frequently, arthroscopic removal of the fibrotic, meniscoid lesion is required.

Posterior impingement syndrome

Posterior impingement syndrome sometimes presents as lateral ankle pain but more commonly as pain in the posterior ankle (Chapter 32).

Stress fracture of the talus

Stress fractures of the posterolateral aspect of the talus have been described in track and field athletes and football players.[16]

Cause

These stress fractures may develop secondary to excessive subtalar pronation and plantarflexion, resulting in impingement of the lateral process of the calcaneus on the posterolateral corner of the talus.[16] In pole vaulters, this injury is attributed to 'planting' the pole too late.

Clinical features

The main symptom is that of lateral ankle pain of gradual onset, made worse by running and weight-bearing. Clinical examination reveals marked tenderness and occasionally swelling in the region of the sinus tarsi.

Diagnosis

Typical isotopic bone scan and CT scan appearances are shown in Figure 34.10. MRI will also reveal the fracture, with the STIR sequence being most helpful.

Treatment

Treatment requires six weeks' cast immobilization and then a supervised graduated rehabilitation. In elite athletes, when a rapid recovery is required, or in the case of failure of conservative management, surgical removal of the lateral process has been shown to produce good results. As this injury is invariably associated with excessive pronation, biomechanical correction with orthoses is required before activity is resumed.

Referred pain

A variation of the slump test (Chapter 8) with the ankle in plantarflexion and inversion can be performed to detect increased neural tension in the peroneal nerve. If the test is positive, this position can be used as a stretch in addition to soft tissue therapy to possible areas of restriction (e.g. around the head of the fibula).

Anterior ankle pain

Pain over the anterior aspect of the ankle joint without a history of acute injury is usually due to either tibialis anterior tendinopathy or anterior impingement of the ankle. The surface anatomy of the anterior ankle is shown in Figure 34.11.

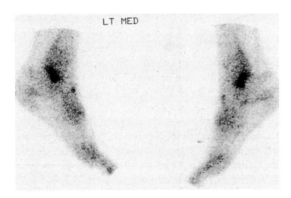

Figure 34.10 Stress fracture of the talus

(a) Isotopic bone scan

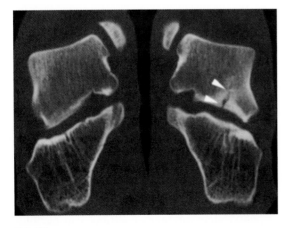

(b) CT scan

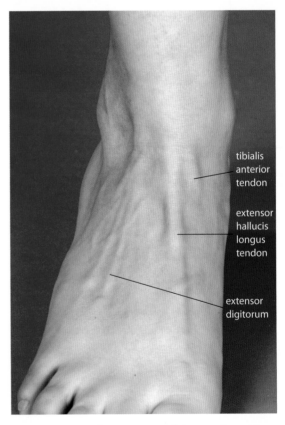

tibialis anterior tendon

extensor hallucis longus tendon

extensor digitorum

Figure 34.11 Surface anatomy of the anterior ankle showing tendons

Anterior impingement of the ankle

Anterior impingement of the ankle joint (anterior tibiotalar impingement) is a condition in which additional soft or bony tissue is trapped between the tibia and talus during dorsiflexion and may be the cause of chronic ankle pain or may result in pain and disability persisting after an ankle sprain. Although this syndrome has been called 'footballer's ankle', it is also seen commonly in ballet dancers.

Causes

Anterior impingement occurs secondary to the development of exostoses on the anterior rim of the tibia and on the upper anterior surface of the neck of talus (Fig. 34.12). The exostoses were initially described in ballet dancers and thought to be secondary to a traction injury of the joint capsule of the ankle that occurs whenever the foot was repeatedly forced into extreme plantarflexion. Subsequently the development of the exostoses has been attributed to direct osseous impingement during extremes of dorsiflexion, as occurs with kicking in football and the *plié* (lunge) in ballet. As these exostoses become larger, they impinge on overlying soft tissue and cause pain.

Ligamentous injuries following inversion injuries to the ankle may also result in anterior ankle impingement; it has been shown that the distal fascicle of the anterior inferior tibiofibular ligament may impinge on the anterolateral aspect of the talus.

Clinical features

The patient complains of:

- anterior ankle pain, which initially starts as a vague discomfort
- pain ultimately becoming sharper and more localized to the anterior aspect of the ankle and foot
- pain that is worse with activity, particularly with running, descending *plié* (lunge) in classical ballet, kicking in football or other activities involving dorsiflexion.

As the impingement develops, the patient complains of ankle stiffness and a loss of take-off speed.

Examination reveals tenderness along the anterior margin of the talocrural joint and, if the exostoses are large, they may be palpable. Dorsiflexion of the ankle is restricted and painful. The anterior impingement test (Fig. 34.13a), where the patient lunges forward maximally with the heel remaining on the floor, reproduces the pain.

Investigations

Lateral X-rays in flexion and extension show both exostoses and abnormal tibiotalar contact. Ideally performed weight-bearing in the lunge position, showing bone-on-bone impingement, confirms the diagnosis (Fig. 34.13b).

Treatment

In milder cases, conservative treatment consists of a heel lift, rest, modification of activities to limit dorsiflexion, NSAID and physiotherapy, including

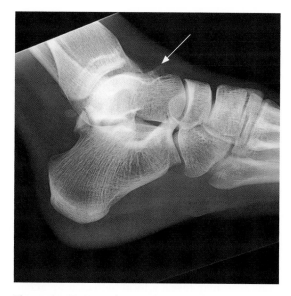

Figure 34.12 X-ray showing bony exostosis on the anterior talus

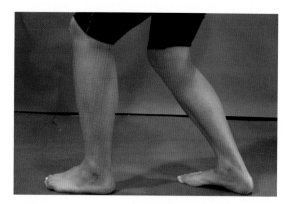

Figure 34.13 The anterior impingement test

(a) The patient lunges forward maximally and, if this reproduces his or her pain, the test is positive and suggests the diagnosis of anterior impingement

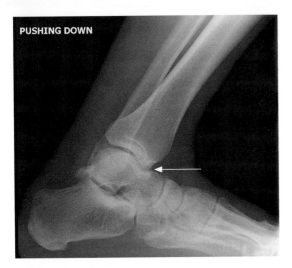

(b) The same position is used to take a lateral X-ray. A positive test reveals bone-on-bone impingement (arrowed) when the patient adopts the lunge position that reproduces pain

accessory anteroposterior glides of the talocrural joint at the end of range of dorsiflexion. Taping or orthoses may help control the pain if they restrict ankle dorsiflexion or improve joint instability, which has been shown to contribute to the development of anterior impingement.

More prominent exostoses may require surgical removal arthroscopically or as an open procedure.

Tibialis anterior tendinopathy

The tibialis anterior tendon is the primary dorsiflexor of the foot, in addition to adducting and supinating (inverting) the foot. It passes medially over the anterior ankle joint and runs to insert into the medial and plantar aspects of the medial cuneiform bone and the adjacent base of the first metatarsal.

Causes

Tendinopathy of the tibialis anterior may result from overuse of the ankle dorsiflexors secondary to restriction in joint range of motion, as may occur with a stiff ankle. It may also be due to downhill running, playing racquet sports involving constant change of direction, or with excessive tightness of strapping or shoelaces over the tibialis anterior tendon.

Clinical features

The main symptoms are pain, swelling and stiffness in the anterior ankle, which are aggravated by activity, especially running, and walking up hills or stairs. On examination, there is localized tenderness, swelling and occasionally crepitus along the tibialis anterior tendon. There is pain on resisted dorsiflexion and eccentric inversion.

Investigations

Ultrasound or MRI may be used to confirm the diagnosis and exclude tears of the tendon.

Treatment

Eccentric strengthening, soft tissue therapy and mobilization of the ankle joint are common treatments. Correction of biomechanics with orthoses may be helpful.

Inferior tibiofibular joint injury

The tibiofibular syndesmosis, consisting of the anterior and posterior inferior tibiofibular ligaments and interosseous membrane, maintains the joint between the distal tibia and fibula. It plays a dynamic role in ankle function.

Causes

Diastasis (separation) occurs with partial or complete rupture of the syndesmosis ligament. Ruptures of the syndesmosis are rarely isolated injuries but generally occur in association with deltoid ligament injuries or, more frequently, with fractures of either the fibula or the posterior and medial malleoli.

Clinical features

The classic presentation includes:

- anterior ankle pain following a moderate-to-severe ankle injury
- tenderness on examination located at the anterior aspect of the syndesmosis and interosseus membrane
- painful active external rotation of the foot. If there is severe disruption of the syndesmosis, the squeeze test is positive (i.e. proximal compression produces distal pain in the region of the interosseous membrane).

Investigations

Plain X-rays are recommended to exclude fractures and osseous avulsions. Mortise views may reveal widening of the syndesmosis. Stress X-rays in external rotation may demonstrate the diastasis. CT or MRI are required to exclude osteochondral lesions. Isotope bone scan may reveal a focal increased uptake in the region of the anterior tibiofibular ligament and interosseous membrane.

Treatment

Provided there is no widening of the distal tibiofibular joint, conservative management with rest, NSAIDs and physiotherapy is required. As the pain settles, strengthening, range of motion and proprioceptive exercises are introduced.

In more severe cases, when there is widening of the distal tibiofibular joint, surgery and insertion of a temporary syndesmosis screw is required.

Recommended Reading

Lau JT, Daniels TR. Tarsal tunnel syndrome: a review of the literature. *Foot Ankle Int* 1999; 20: 201–9.

Liu SH, Nguyen TM. Ankle sprains and other soft tissue injuries. *Curr Opin Rheumatol* 1999; 11: 132–7.

Mizel MS, Hecht PJ, Marymont JV, et al. Evaluation and treatment of chronic ankle pain. *J Bone Joint Surg Am* 2004; 86A: 622–31.

References

1. Hutchinson BL, O'Rourke EM. Tibialis posterior tendon dysfunction and peroneal tendon subluxation. *Clin Podiatr Med Surg* 1995; 12: 703–23.
2. Landorf K. Tibialis posterior tendon dysfunction. Early identification is the key to success. *Aust Podiatr* 1995; 29: 9–14.
3. Premkumar A, Perry MB, Dwyer AJ, et al. Sonography and MR imaging of posterior tibial tendinopathy. *AJR Am J Roentgenol* 2002; 178: 223–32.
4. Lo LD, Schweitzer ME, Fan JK, et al. MR imaging findings of entrapment of the flexor hallucis longus tendon. *AJR Am J Roentgenol* 2001; 176(5): 1145–8.
5. Khan K, Brown J, Way S, et al. Overuse injuries in classical ballet. *Sports Med* 1995; 19: 341–57.
6. Patel AT, Gaines K, Malamut R, et al. Usefulness of electrodiagnostic techniques in the evaluation of suspected tarsal tunnel syndrome: an evidence-based review. *Muscle Nerve* 2005; 32(2): 236–40.
7. Oh SJ, Meyer RD. Entrapment neuropathies of the tibial (posterior tibial) nerve. *Neurol Clin* 1999; 17: 593–615, vii.
8. Scalley TC, Schon LC, Hinton RY, et al. Clinical results following revision tibial nerve release. *Foot Ankle Int* 1994; 15: 360–7.
9. Pfeiffer WH, Cracchioto A 3rd. Clinical results after tarsal tunnel decompression. *J Bone Joint Surg Am* 1994; 76A: 1222–30.
10. Brukner P, Bennell K, Matheson G. *Stress Fractures*. Melbourne: Blackwell Scientific, 1999.
11. Kor A, Saltzman AT, Wempe PD. Medial malleolar stress fractures. Literature review, diagnosis and treatment. *J Am Podiatr Med Assoc* 2003; 93: 292–7.
12. Clarke HD, Kitaoka HB, Ehman RL. Peroneal tendon injuries. *Foot Ankle Int* 1998; 19: 280–8.
13. Tjin ATER, Schweitzer ME, Karasick D. MR imaging of peroneal tendon disorders. *AJR Am J Roentgenol* 1997; 168: 135–40.
14. Highet RM. Diagnosis of anterolateral ankle impingement: comparison between magnetic resonance imaging and clinical examination (letter). *Am J Sports Med* 1998; 26: 152–3.
15. Liu SH, Nuccion SL, Finerman G. Diagnosis of anterolateral ankle impingement. Comparison between magnetic resonance imaging and clinical examination [see comments]. *Am J Sports Med* 1997; 25: 389–93.
16. Bradshaw C, Khan K, Brukner P. Stress fracture of the body of the talus in athletes demonstrated with computer tomography. *Clin J Sport Med* 1996; 6: 48–51.

Foot Pain

WITH JASON AGOSTA AND KAREN HOLZER

Many practitioners consider the foot a difficult region to treat, largely because the anatomy seems rather complex (Figs 35.1, 35.2). If the foot is considered in its three distinct regions (Fig. 35.1)—the rear foot (calcaneus and talus), the midfoot (the cuneiforms and navicular medially, the cuboid laterally) and the forefoot (the metatarsals and phalanges)—the bony anatomy is greatly simplified. Soft tissue anatomy can be superimposed on the regional division of the foot (Figs 35.2c–e).

In keeping with this anatomical division of the foot, clinical assessment of foot pain is most conveniently considered in three anatomical regions (Fig. 35.1):

- heel pain (arising from the rear foot)
- midfoot pain
- forefoot pain.

Rear foot pain

The most common cause of rear foot (inferior heel) pain is plantar fasciitis. A lay term for this condition is 'heel spur(s)'. This condition occurs mainly in runners and the older adult, and is often associated with a biomechanical abnormality, such as excessive pronation or supination. Another common cause of heel pain is the fat pad syndrome or fat pad contusion. This is also known as a 'bruised heel' or a 'stone bruise'.

Less common causes of heel pain are stress fracture of the calcaneus and conditions that refer pain to this area such as tarsal tunnel syndrome (Chapter 34) or medial calcaneal nerve entrapment (Chapter 34). Causes of rear foot pain are listed in Table 35.1.

History

The pain of plantar fasciitis is usually of insidious onset, whereas fat pad damage may occur either as a result of a single traumatic episode (e.g. jumping from a height onto the heel) or from repeated heel strike (e.g. on hard surfaces with inadequate heel support). Plantar fasciitis pain is typically worse in the morning, improves with exercise at first and is aggravated by standing.

Examination

Examination of the patient with inferior heel pain is shown in Figure 35.3. Biomechanical assessment is an important component of the examination and must include ankle, subtalar and midtarsal joint

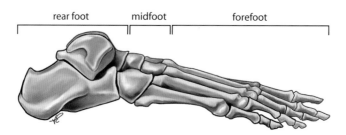

Figure 35.1 The regions of the foot—rear foot, midfoot and forefoot

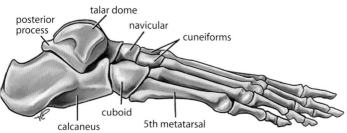

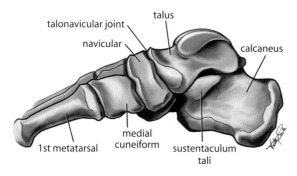

Figure 35.2 Anatomy of the foot

(a) Lateral view of the bones of the foot

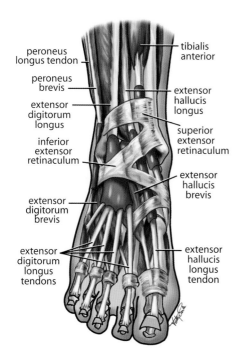

(b) Medial view of the bones of the foot

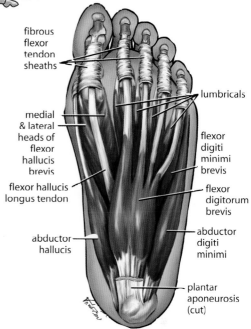

(d) Plantar view of the soft tissues of the foot—first layer

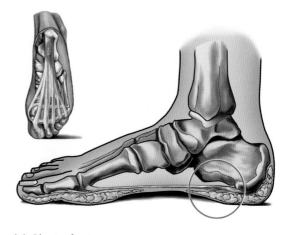

(c) Dorsal view of the soft tissues of the foot

(e) Plantar fascia

Table 35.1 Causes of rear foot and inferior heel pain

Common	Less common	Not to be missed
Plantar fasciitis	Calcaneal fractures	Spondyloarthropathies
Fat pad contusion	Traumatic	Osteoid osteoma
	Stress fracture	Regional complex pain syndrome
	Medial calcaneal nerve entrapment (Chapter 34)	type 1 (after knee or ankle
	Lateral plantar nerve entrapment	injury)
	Tarsal tunnel syndrome (Chapter 34)	
	Talar stress fracture (Chapter 34)	
	Retrocalcaneal bursitis (Chapter 32)	

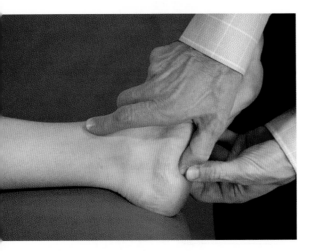

Figure 35.3 Examination of the rear foot

(a) Palpation—medial process of calcaneal tuberosity. Palpate plantar fascia attachment

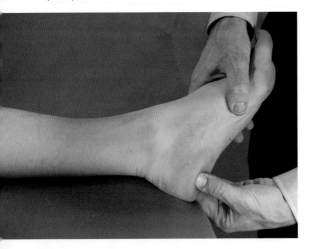

(b) Palpation—heel fat pad

range of motion. Inspection of running shoes is also important.

Investigations

X-ray only contributes to the clinical work-up of rearfoot pain in a small proportion of cases. It may reveal a calcaneal spur but, as this may or may not be symptomatic, it does not add clinical utility. Plain X-ray is generally normal in stress fractures of the calcaneus but if the injury has been present for many weeks, there may be a line of sclerosis (increased opacity). This appearance is characteristic of stress fracture in trabecular bone. Isotopic bone scan or MRI are the investigations of choice for stress fracture. MRI and ultrasound can each be used to confirm the presence and severity of plantar fasciitis. MRI reveals increased signal intensity and thickening at the attachment of the plantar fascia to the calcaneus at the medial calcaneal tuberosity, often with edema in the adjacent bone. Ultrasound reveals a characteristic region of hypoechogenicity. In plantar fasciitis, bone scan may demonstrate an increased uptake at the attachment of the plantar fascia at the medial calcaneal tuberosity as an incidental finding; it is not usually done for that purpose.

Plantar fasciitis

The plantar aponeurosis is composed of three segments, all arising from the calcaneus. The central, and clinically most important, segment arises from the plantar aspect of the posteromedial calcaneal tuberosity and inserts into the toes to form the longitudinal arch of the foot. The aponeurosis provides static support for the longitudinal arch and dynamic shock absorption. Plantar fasciitis, an overuse condition of the plantar fascia at its attachment to the calcaneus, is due to collagen disarray in the absence of inflammatory cells. Thus, the pathology resembles that of tendinosis (Chapter 2) and the condition should be more correctly referred to as plantar fasciosis[1] or fasciopathy. However, as neither of these terms is in common usage, we continue to use the traditional term, 'plantar fasciitis', in this book.

Causes

Individuals with pes planus (low arches or flat feet) or pes cavus (high arches) are at increased risk of developing plantar fasciitis. The flat foot deformity will place an increased strain on the origin of the plantar fascia at the calcaneus as the plantar fascia attempts to maintain a stable arch during the propulsive phase of the gait. In the cavus foot, there may be excessive strain on the heel area because the foot lacks the ability to evert in order to absorb the shock and adapt itself to the ground.

Plantar fasciitis commonly results from activities that require maximal plantarflexion of the ankle and simultaneous dorsiflexion of the metatarsophalangeal joints (e.g. running, dancing). In the older patient it may be related to excessive walking in inappropriate or non-supportive footwear.[2] In a matched case-control study, reduced ankle dorsiflexion was the most important risk factor.[2] Obesity and work-related weight-bearing are also independent risk factors.

Plantar fasciitis is commonly associated with tightness in the proximal myofascial structures, especially the calf, hamstring and gluteal regions. Presumably this is because the fascia is continuous throughout the lower limb.

Clinical features

The pain is usually of gradual onset and felt classically on the medial aspect of the heel. Initially, it is worse in the morning and decreases with activity, often to ache post-activity. Periods of inactivity during the day are generally followed by an increase in pain as activity is recommenced. As the condition becomes more severe, the pain may be present when weight-bearing and worsen with activity. There may be a history of other leg or foot problems in patients with abnormal biomechanics.

Examination reveals acute tenderness along the medial tuberosity of the calcaneus, and may extend some centimeters along the medial border of the plantar fascia. The plantar fascia is generally tight and stretching the plantar fascia may reproduce pain.

Assessment of the patient's gait may reveal either supination or pronation. Both an abducted gait and calf tightness may reduce the athlete's ability to supinate, increasing the strain on the plantar fascia.

Investigations

Ultrasound is the gold standard diagnostic investigation for plantar fasciitis, with swelling of the plantar fascia the typical feature. The thickness of the fascia may also be measured.

X-rays are often performed but are not essential for the diagnosis. X-ray may show a calcaneal spur (Fig. 35.4) but Lu and colleagues have confirmed that the spurs are not causally related to pain.[3] In their study, X-ray appearances were unrelated to pain and often worsened even when symptoms had completely resolved.[3]

Treatment

Treatment includes:

- avoidance of aggravating activity
- cryotherapy after activity
- NSAIDs, which are effective in some patients[4] but should be limited to seven to 10 days
- stretching of the plantar fascia (Fig. 35.5a),[5] gastrocnemius and soleus
- self massage with a frozen bottle or golf ball (Fig. 35.5b)
- strengthening exercises[6]—strengthening exercises for the intrinsic muscles of the foot are designed to improve longitudinal arch support and decrease stress on the plantar fascia;[7] a simple technique is to raise the toes and press them each individually to the floor
- taping (Fig. 35.5c)

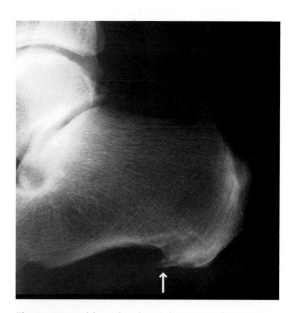

Figure 35.4 Although calcaneal spurs can be rather large, they are not causally associated with plantar fasciitis. They are also found in asymptomatic individuals, as in this case, on both feet when only one is symptomatic, and they can enlarge even after symptoms have resolved

- silicone gel heel pad (Fig. 35.5d)
- footwear with well-supported arches and midsoles[6]
- biomechanical correction with orthoses[8, 9]
- night splints[10–12] or Strasbourg sock (Fig. 35.5e)
- soft tissue therapy, both to the plantar fascia and proximal myofascial regions including calf, hamstrings and gluteals (Fig. 35.5f)
- corticosteroid injection[13] (Fig. 35.5g)—this may be useful in the short term but must be combined with other treatments such as stretching and biomechanical correction to prevent recurrence; there is some concern that injection is associated with an increased risk of rupture[14, 15] and fat pad atrophy
- iontophoresis[16]
- extracorporeal shock wave therapy—this has been used recently but research evidence of its efficacy has been conflicting[17, 18]
- surgery—this is sometimes required in patients who remain symptomatic despite appropriate treatment, and we have found this to be needed more in patients with a rigid, cavus foot whose plantar fascia tends to be shortened and thickened rather than in those with a pes planus foot type; we reiterate that the finding of a calcaneal spur on X-ray is not an indication for surgery
- plantar fasciectomy—in an uncontrolled case series of plantar fasciectomy with neurolysis of the nerve to the abductor digiti quinti muscle, 92% of patients had a 'satisfactory functional outcome'; time from surgery to return to work averaged nine weeks[19]

- minimally invasive endoscopic plantar fascia release—this is a promising procedure that is gaining acceptance among foot surgeons.[20, 21]

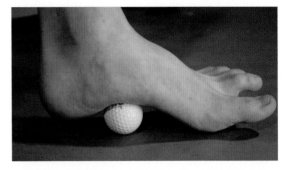

(b) Self massage with a golf ball

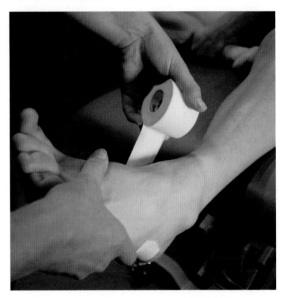

(c) Plantar fascia taping. The foot is placed into inversion by taping from the lateral aspect of the dorsum of the foot and across the plantar aspect before anchoring the tape to the skin over the medial arch

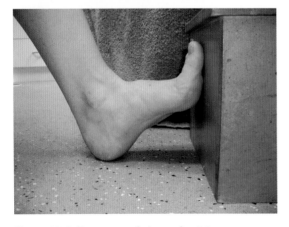

Figure 35.5 Treatment of plantar fasciitis

(a) Stretching the plantar fascia

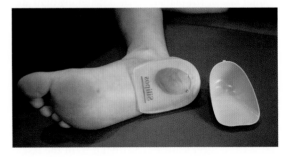

(d) A silicone gel heel pad and heel cup

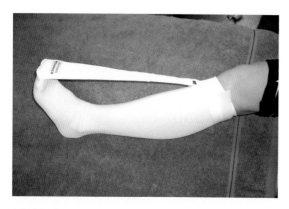

(e) Strasbourg sock

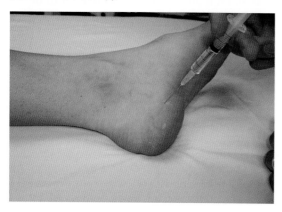

(f) Soft tissue therapy

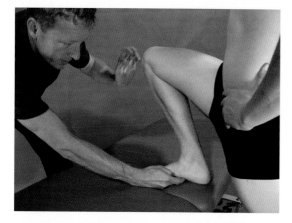

(g) Corticosteroid injection

Fat pad contusion

The fat pad, which is composed of an elastic fibrous tissue septa separating closely packed fat cells, acts as a shock absorber, protecting the calcaneus at heel strike.

Causes

Fat pad contusion or fat pad syndrome may develop either acutely after a fall onto the heels from a height or chronically because of excessive heel strike with poor heel cushioning or repetitive stops, starts and changes in direction.

Clinical features

The patient often complains of marked heel pain, particularly during weight-bearing activities. The pain is often felt laterally in the heel due to the pattern of heel strike. Examination reveals tenderness, often in the posterolateral heel region. There may be an area of redness.

Investigations

MRI often demonstrates edematous changes in the fat pad, with ill-defined areas of decreased signal intensity on T1-weighted images that increase in signal intensity on T2-weighted images.

Treatment

Treatment consists primarily of avoidance of aggravating activities, in particular, excessive weight-bearing, RICE and NSAIDs. As the pain settles, the use of a silicone gel heel pad (Fig. 35.5d) and good footwear are important as the athlete resumes activity. Heel lock taping (see Fig. 33.8b) will often provide symptomatic relief.

Calcaneal stress fractures

Calcaneal stress fractures[22] are the second most common tarsal stress fracture. They occur most commonly at two main sites: the upper posterior margin of the os calcis or adjacent to the medial tuberosity, at the point where calcaneal spurs occur.

Causes

Calcaneal stress fractures were first described among the military and are related to marching; they also occur in runners, ballet dancers and jumpers.

Clinical features

Patients give a history of insidious onset of heel pain that is aggravated by weight-bearing activities, especially running. Examination reveals localized tenderness over the medial or lateral aspects of the posterior calcaneus and pain that is produced by squeezing the posterior aspect of the calcaneus from both sides simultaneously.

Investigations

Plain X-ray may show a typical sclerotic appearance on the lateral X-ray, parallel to the posterior margin of the calcaneus (Fig. 35.6). Isotopic bone scan reveals a focal area of increased uptake or MRI reveals an area of high signal on a T2-weighted image.

Treatment

Treatment involves a reduction in activity and for those with marked pain a short period of non-weight-bearing may be required. Once pain-free, a program of gradually increased weight-bearing can occur. Stretching of the calf muscles and plantar fascia, and joint mobilization are important for long-term recovery. Soft heel pads, in conjunction with orthoses if required, are recommended.

Lateral plantar nerve entrapment

An entrapment of the first branch of the lateral plantar nerve (one of the terminal branches of the posterior tibial nerve after it passes through the tarsal tunnel) occurs between the deep fascia of the abductor hallucis longus and the medial caudal margin of the quadratus planus muscle.[23] Pain radiates to the medial inferior aspect of the heel and proximally into the medial ankle region. Patients do not normally complain of numbness in the heel or foot. A diagnostic injection with local anesthetic will confirm the diagnosis.

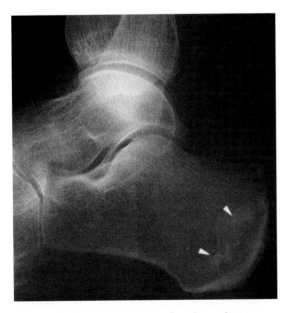

Figure 35.6 X-ray appearance of a calcaneal stress fracture

Treatment consists of rest, NSAIDs and iontophoresis.[23] Arch support using tape or an orthosis is helpful in athletes with excessive pronation. A corticosteroid injection may be required and occasionally surgical release may be necessary.

Midfoot pain

The midfoot is comprised of the three cuneiform bones, the cuboid and the navicular bones as well as the surrounding soft tissues (Figs 35.1, 35.2). The most common cause of midfoot pain is midtarsal joint sprain after ankle injury but the most important cause of midfoot pain is a stress fracture of the navicular bone. Tendinopathy of the extensor tendons is another common cause of midfoot pain. The causes of midfoot pain are listed in Table 35.2.

History

Acute onset of midfoot pain occurs with a sprain of the midtarsal joint or plantar fascia. Gradual pain is a sign of overuse injury, such as extensor tendinopathy, tibialis posterior tendinopathy or navicular stress fracture. In most conditions, pain is well localized to the site of the injury but in navicular stress fracture pain is poorly localized.

Examination

Examination involves palpation of the area of tenderness and a biomechanical examination to detect factors that predispose to injury. Examination of the midfoot is shown in Figure 35.7.

Investigations

If there is a clinical suspicion of a stress fracture of the navicular or the cuneiform, an X-ray should be performed. This rarely reveals a fracture, even if one is present, but it is useful to rule out tarsal coalition (p. 660), to show bony abnormalities such as talar beaking (osteophytes at the talonavicular joint) and accessory ossicles, and to exclude bony tumors. An isotopic bone scan (with CT scan if positive) or MRI should be performed if X-ray fails to reveal a stress fracture.

Stress fracture of the navicular

Stress fractures of the navicular are among the most common stress fractures seen in the athlete, especially in sports that involve sprinting, jumping or hurdling.[24] The stress fracture commonly occurs in the middle third of the navicular bone, a relatively avascular

Table 35.2 Causes of midfoot pain

Common	Less common	Not to be missed
Navicular stress fracture	Cuneiform stress fracture	Lisfranc's joint injury (fracture or
Midtarsal joint sprain	Cuboid stress fracture	dislocation)
Extensor tendinopathy	Stress fracture base 2nd metatarsal	Osteoid osteoma
Tibialis posterior tendinopathy	Peroneal tendinopathy	Complex regional pain syndrome
Plantar fascia strain	Abductor hallucis strain	type 1 (after knee or ankle
	Cuboid syndrome	injury)
	Tarsal coalition (in adolescents)	
	Köhler's disease (in young children)	
	Accessory navicular bone	

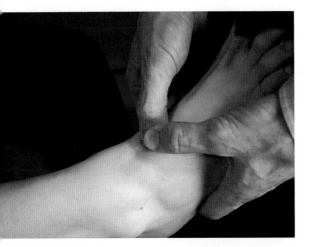

Figure 35.7 Examination of the midfoot

(a) Palpation—'N spot'. The proximal dorsal surface of the navicular is tender when a stress fracture is present

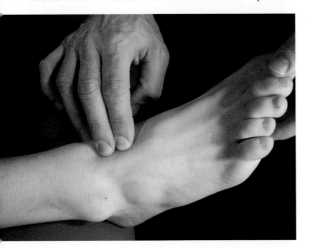

(b) Palpation—extensor tendons. These may be tender as they pass under the extensor retinaculum. The midtarsal joint and bones should be palpated

region of the bone. Stress fractures in this region are thus susceptible to delayed union.

Cause

A combination of overuse and training errors plays a significant role in the development of navicular stress fractures. Although the exact cause of a navicular stress fracture is not known, it is believed that impingement of the navicular bone occurs between the proximal and distal tarsal bones when the muscles exert compressing and bending forces.

Clinical features

The onset of symptoms is usually insidious, consisting of a poorly localized midfoot ache associated with activity. The pain typically radiates along the medial aspect of the longitudinal arch or the dorsum of the foot. The symptoms abate rapidly with rest.

Examination reveals localized tenderness at the 'N-spot', located at the proximal dorsal portion of the navicular. If palpation confirms tenderness over the 'N spot' (Fig. 35.7a), the athlete should be considered to have a navicular stress fracture until proven otherwise.

Investigations

Sensitivity of X-ray in navicular stress fracture is poor.[25] Thus, either isotopic bone scan (Fig. 35.8a) (with CT scan if positive, Figs 35.8b, c) or MRI (Fig. 35.8d) is required if clinical features suggest stress fracture. Poor positioning and scanning technique can lead to a navicular stress fracture being missed on CT scan.[26] Appropriate views require correct angling of the CT gantry and thin (2 mm [0.1 in.]) slices extending from the distal talus to the distal navicular.

Treatment

The treatment of a navicular stress *reaction* (no cortical breach) is weight-bearing rest, often in an air cast,

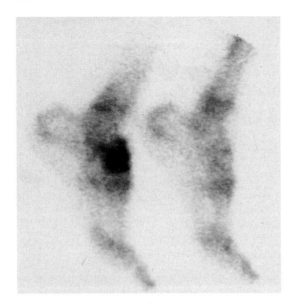

Figure 35.8 Navicular stress fracture

(a) Isotopic bone scan

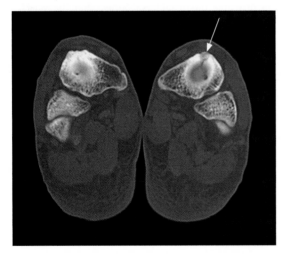

(b) CT scan showing undisplaced fracture (arrow)

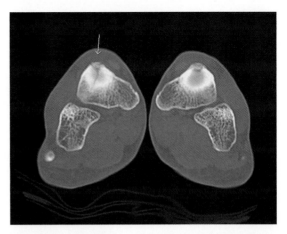

(c) CT scan showing more extensive Y-shaped fracture

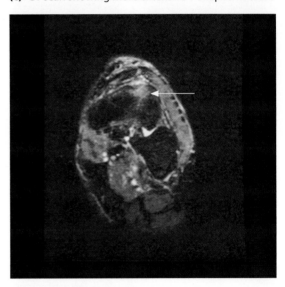

(d) T2-weighted MRI showing bone marrow edema

until symptoms and signs have resolved, followed by a graduated return to activity.

Treatment of navicular stress fracture is *strict* non-weight-bearing immobilization in a cast for six to eight weeks.[25] At the end of this period the cast should be removed and the 'N spot' palpated for tenderness. Generally, the 'N spot' will be non-tender but, if tenderness is present, the patient should have the cast reapplied for a further two weeks of non-weight-bearing immobilization. Management must be based on the clinical assessment as there is poor CT and MRI correlation with clinical union of the stress fracture (Fig. 35.9).[25, 27]

Often, patients with these fractures will present after a long period of pain or after a period of weight-bearing rest. All patients, even if they have been unsuccessfully treated with prolonged weight-bearing rest or short-term cast immobilization, should undergo cast immobilization for a six week period. This method of treatment produces excellent results and may be successful even in longstanding cases.

Some clinicians advocate surgical treatment with the insertion of a screw in cases where there is significant separation of the fracture (Fig. 35.8c). In cases of delayed or non-union, surgical internal fixation with or without bone grafting is required.

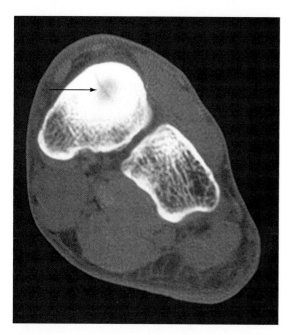

Figure 35.9 Imaging of navicular stress fracture does not necessarily mirror clinical recovery. This CT scan of a 26-year-old runner shows that the fracture line is still evident (arrow) but the patient had returned pain-free to all competition and had no further recurrences of stress fracture

Post-cast rehabilitation and prevention of recurrence

Following removal of the cast, it is essential to mobilize the stiff ankle, subtalar and midtarsal joints. The calf muscles require soft tissue therapy and exercise to regain strength. These must be done before resuming running. Activity must be begun gradually, slowly building up to full training over a period of six weeks. Predisposing factors to navicular stress fractures may include tarsal coalition, excessive pronation and restricted dorsiflexion of the ankle. These factors need to be corrected before resuming activity.

Extensor tendinopathy

The extensor (dorsiflexor) muscles of the foot comprise the tibialis anterior, extensor hallucis longus and brevis, and extensor digitorum longus and brevis. The insertions in the foot and actions of the extensor muscles are shown in Table 35.3.

Tibialis anterior tendinopathy is the most common tendinopathy occurring in the extensor muscles of the foot. Tendinopathies of the extensor hallucis longus and brevis and extensor digitorum longus and brevis muscles are rare.

Causes

The tibialis anterior tendon resists plantarflexion of the foot at heel strike and is, therefore, susceptible to overuse injury. Tendinopathy may be related to extensor muscle weakness or, alternatively, it may occur secondary to a recent increase in the training load or compression by excessively tight shoelaces. Stiffness of the first metatarsophalangeal joint and midfoot may contribute.

Clinical features

Generally after a period of overuse, the patient with extensor tendinopathy complains of an aching dorsal aspect of the midfoot. Examination may reveal tenderness, often with mild swelling, at the insertion of the tibialis anterior tendon at the base of the first metatarsal and the cuneiform. Resisted dorsiflexion and eccentric inversion may elicit pain.

Table 35.3 Extensor muscles, their insertions at the foot and their actions

Muscle	Insertion in foot	Action
Tibialis anterior	Medial cuneiform and base of 1st metatarsal	Dorsiflexes foot at ankle Inverts foot at subtalar and transverse tarsal joints Maintains medial longitudinal arch
Extensor digitorum longus	Extensor expansion of lateral four toes	Extends toes and dorsiflexes foot
Extensor hallucis longus	Base of distal phalanx of big toe	Extends big toe Dorsiflexes foot Inverts foot at subtalar and transverse tarsal joints
Extensor digitorum brevis	Long extensor tendons to 2nd–4th toes	Extends toes
Extensor hallucis brevis	Proximal phalanx of big toe	Extends big toe

Investigations

Both ultrasound and MRI may reveal swelling of the tendon at its insertion and exclude the presence of a degenerative tear.

Treatment

Popular clinical treatment involves relative rest, electrotherapeutic techniques and soft tissue therapy to the extensor muscles. Extensor muscle strengthening is advocated as is the case with other tendinopathies. The underlying precipitating cause needs to be addressed. This may include mobilization of the first ray, tarsometatarsal and midtarsal joints if the first metatarsophalangeal joint and midfoot is stiff; a change of lacing pattern or placing adhesive foam to the underside of the tongue of the shoe will help if compression by the shoelaces is the cause. Rarely, footwear will need to be replaced.

Midtarsal joint sprains

The midtarsal joint (Chopart's joint) consists of the talonavicular and calcaneocuboid joints. Other joints in the midtarsal area are the naviculocuneiform, cuboid cuneiform and intercuneiform joints.

Individual ligamentous sprains to the midtarsal joints are uncommon and if they occur usually affect the dorsal calcaneocuboid or bifurcate ligament, comprising the calcaneonavicular and calcaneocuboid ligament.

Injuries to the midtarsal joints are most commonly seen in gymnasts, jumpers and footballers.

Dorsal calcaneocuboid ligament injury

Patient presents with pain in the lateral midfoot following an inversion injury. Examination reveals localized tenderness and swelling at the dorsolateral aspect of the calcaneocuboid joint. Stress inversion of the foot elicits pain.

X-ray is required to exclude fracture. MRI may confirm the diagnosis. Electrotherapeutic modalities may be helpful and taping may provide additional support. Orthoses may be required. Following a joint sprain, joint inflammation occasionally develops. This generally responds well to NSAIDs but if it persists the patient may benefit from a corticosteroid injection into one of the midtarsal joints.

Bifurcate ligament injuries

Injuries to the bifurcate ligament may be associated with fractures to the anterior process of the calcaneus and may occur secondary to violent dorsiflexion, forceful plantarflexion and inversion injuries.

Patients present with lateral midfoot pain and swelling, usually following an ankle sprain or injury. Examination reveals local tenderness and occasionally swelling overlying the ligament, with pain elicited at the site with simultaneous forefoot supination and plantarflexion.

X-rays are required to assess for a fracture of the anterior process of the calcaneus. If present, a CT scan may be required for further assessment. An MRI scan can be used to confirm the joint/ligament sprain.

Treatment is similar to the dorsal calcaneocuboid sprain mentioned above. If a non-displaced or mildly displaced fracture of the anterior process of the calcaneum is present, four weeks' immobilization is required. If the fracture is displaced, surgery is required.

Lisfranc's joint injuries

The eponym Lisfranc's joint refers to the tarsometatarsal joints—the bases of the five metatarsals with their corresponding three cuneiforms and cuboid (Fig. 35.10). Injuries to these joints are given this eponym after Jacques Lisfranc, a surgeon in Napoleon's army who described an operation for amputation through the tarsometatarsal joint.

The spectrum of injuries of the Lisfranc's joint complex ranges from partial sprains with no displacement to complete tears with separation (diastasis) of the first and second metatarsal bones and, depending on the severity, different patterns of tarsal and metatarsal displacement (Fig. 35.11). Although Lisfranc's joint injuries ('midfoot sprains') are not common in the

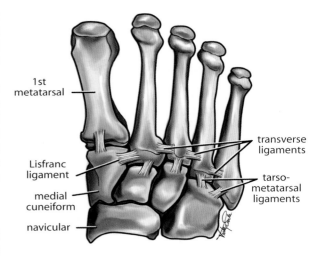

1st metatarsal

transverse ligaments

Lisfranc ligament

tarso-metatarsal ligaments

medial cuneiform

navicular

Figure 35.10 Ligamentous attachments of the Lisfranc's joint articulation

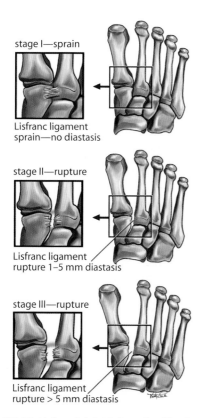

stage I—sprain

Lisfranc ligament
sprain—no diastasis

stage II—rupture

Lisfranc ligament
rupture 1–5 mm diastasis

stage III—rupture

Lisfranc ligament
rupture > 5 mm diastasis

Figure 35.11 Lisfranc's joint injury classification system

general population, they are the second most common foot injury in athletes. In athletes, they generally occur as a consequence of a low-velocity indirect force, in contrast to the general population, where they occur as a consequence of a high-velocity force.

Lisfranc's joint fracture–dislocation

Lisfranc's joint fracture–dislocation is rare in sport but because of its disastrous consequences if untreated, the diagnosis must be considered in all cases of 'midfoot sprain' in the athlete.

Causes

There are two main mechanisms of injury:

1. *Direct*: The direct injury is more uncommon and occurs as a simple crush injury to the tarsometatarsal joint region. There is no specific pattern of damage or distinctive appearance with a direct injury.
2. *Indirect*: The indirect mechanism is more common and generally occurs secondary to a longitudinal force sustained while the foot is

plantarflexed and slightly rotated. There are three common injury situations: longitudinal compression, a backward fall with the foot entrapped, and a fall on the point of the toes. The extent of the damage depends on the severity of the injury: in milder injuries the weak dorsal tarsometatarsal ligaments are ruptured, while with more severe injuries, there may also be fractures of the plantar aspect of the metatarsal base, or the plantar capsule may rupture and the metatarsal may displace dorsally. Thus, a fracture at the plantar base of a metatarsal can be a clue to a subtle Lisfranc's joint injury.

Clinical features

A patient with this injury may complain of midfoot pain and difficulty weight-bearing, following an acute injury by the mechanisms described above. Pain is classically aggravated by forefoot weight-bearing—the patient is unable to run on her or his toes and will feel pain on the push-off phase of running and sometimes during walking and on calf raises.

Often the presentation may be delayed, and the patient presents with ongoing midfoot pain and swelling, aggravated by running.

 Midfoot pain that persists for more than five days post-injury should raise suspicion of a Lisfranc's joint injury.

Examination reveals:

- tenderness with or without swelling on the dorsal midfoot, often with associated bruising in this region
- pain with combined eversion and abduction of the forefoot while the calcaneus is held still.

Neurovascular examination is mandatory as the dorsalis pedis artery can be compromised in the initial injury or by subsequent swelling of the foot.

Investigations

Plain X-rays while weight-bearing are recommended. Diastasis between the first and second metatarsal bases of greater than 2 mm (0.1 in.) (Fig. 35.12a) suggests a Lisfranc's joint injury, although in patients with a metatarsus adductus a 3 mm (0.15 in.) separation may be normal. In such cases, it is essential to take comparative weight-bearing X-rays of the non-injured side, as a difference in diastasis of greater than 1 mm (0.05 in.) between the two sides is considered diagnostic. Other radiological signs that may indicate an injury to the Lisfranc's joint include a 'fleck sign', which appears as a fleck fracture near the base of the second metatarsal or medial cuneiform or, in the lateral view, either dorsal displacement of the metatarsal bases relative to the tarsus or flattening of the medial longitudinal arch. However, often a dislocation may spontaneously reduce, and the foot on plain X-rays may appear normal despite the presence of severe soft tissue disruption.

MRI scans have been shown to be sensitive in detecting tears of the Lisfranc's ligament when plain X-rays appear normal, and should be performed if there is a possible midfoot injury. Isotopic bone scan in conjunction with weight-bearing plain X-rays and/or CT scans (Fig. 35.12b) have also been shown to be sensitive in the detection of Lisfranc's joint injuries.

Treatment

The treatment of a Lisfranc's joint injury depends on the degree of instability present.[28] In grade 1 injuries, where there is no instability (diastasis), conservative management is recommended with a non-weight-bearing in a cast or air cast for a six week period. Following removal of the cast, mobilization of the ankle and a calf strengthening program are required. Orthoses may be needed to correct the intrinsic alignment of the foot and to support the second metatarsal base. A graded return to activity is required.

If there is evidence of instability present, as in grade 2 and 3 injuries, surgical reduction and fixation is required. This may be performed either percutaneously or, in more difficult cases, an open operation may be needed. In the situation of a delay in diagnosis, similar treatment protocols are required.

This is a significant injury that has a much better prognosis if managed correctly initially rather than being salvaged once there is prolonged joint malalignment and non-union. A delay in diagnosis has been associated with a poor outcome, a prolonged absence from sport, and chronic disability due to ligamentous instability of the tarsometatarsal joint.

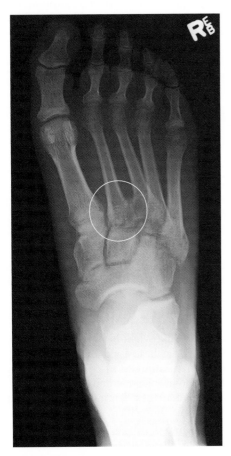

Figure 35.12 Lisfranc's fracture–dislocation

(a) Plain X-ray

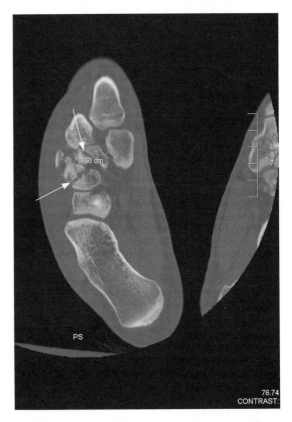

(b) CT scan showing fractures of medial and middle cuneiforms (arrows) with 0.30 cm of diastasis in the Lisfranc joint

Less common causes

First tarsometatarsal joint pain

In the excessively pronating foot, retrograde forces on the first ray result in the build-up of exostoses at the first metatarsal–cuneiform joint. These bone spurs may cause joint impingement and midfoot pain. The resultant limitation of dorsiflexion of the first ray subjects the second ray to an increased load that can damage the second metatarsal–cuneiform joint.

Treatment consists of correction of the abnormal foot mechanics with the use of orthoses and mobilization of restricted joint range of movement. Occasionally, surgery may be required to remove the bony exostoses.

Tibialis posterior tendinopathy

Tibialis posterior tendinopathy may present with medial foot pain when there is partial avulsion (tendinosis) at the insertion of the tendon into the navicular tuberosity. As with other overuse tendon injuries (Chapter 2), this condition has recently been shown to be a degenerative tendinosis rather than an inflammatory 'tendinitis'. This presentation can be more difficult to treat than the more common presentation of medial ankle pain arising from irritation of the tendon as it passes behind the medial malleolus (Chapter 34). Treatment principles for both presentations are outlined in Chapter 35. In younger patients, the accessory ossicle, the os navicularis (Fig. 35.13), may be avulsed. This requires orthoses and gradual

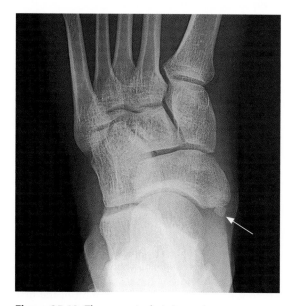

Figure 35.13 The os navicularis (arrow)

return to activity. Occasionally, surgery is indicated for failure of conservative management.

Peroneal tendinopathy

Peroneal tendinopathy is an overuse injury commonly associated with excessive pronation during the toe-off phase of gait. The peroneal tendon may become inflamed at the lateral aspect of the fibula (Chapter 34) or in the peroneal groove of the cuboid. Resisted eversion and hopping reproduce pain. Popular clinical treatment includes electrotherapeutic modalities, soft tissue therapy and correction of excessive pronation with orthoses. Resistance exercises are prescribed as for other tendinopathies. Remember that soft tissue massage proximal to the site of pain—in the muscle bellies in the mid-calf—can be very helpful in releasing the entire muscle–tendon complex.

Cuboid syndrome

Peroneal tendinopathy is often associated with the development of the cuboid syndrome.[29] Due to excessive traction of the peroneus longus, the cuboid becomes subluxated. Pain is experienced with lateral weight-bearing. There may also be a history of an inversion sprain. Most patients with this syndrome have excessively pronated feet but it is also seen in patients with lateral instability.

The peroneus longus subluxates the cuboid bone so that the lateral aspect is rotated dorsally and medially. There may be a visible depression over the dorsal aspect of the cuboid. Treatment involves a single manipulation to reverse the subluxation.[29] The cuboid should be pushed upward and laterally from the medial plantar aspect of the cuboid, as shown in Figure 35.14.

Plantar fascia strains

Acute strains of the plantar fascia in the midfoot region are relatively common and respond more quickly to treatment than does plantar fasciitis at the calcaneal attachment. There may be a history of one significant injury or repeated trauma.

Examination reveals well-localized tenderness over the plantar fascia that is aggravated by extension of the metatarsophalangeal joints. A palpable nodule may indicate a partial rupture of the plantar fascia. A short period of non-weight-bearing, a cast boot, local electrotherapeutic modalities, soft tissue therapy and taping (Fig. 35.5c) are all beneficial and the condition generally resolves in two to six weeks depending on the severity.

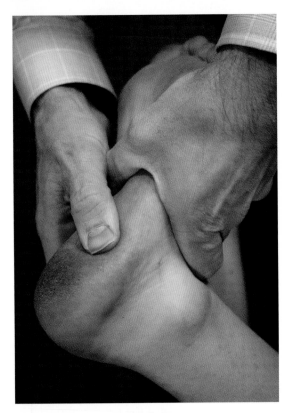

Figure 35.14 Manipulation of the cuboid in a superior and lateral direction in cuboid syndrome

Abductor hallucis strains

Abductor hallucis strains result in pain along the medial longitudinal arch and are often associated with excessive pronation. The abductor hallucis tendon is tender to palpate. Initial treatment consists of local electrotherapeutic modalities and taping.

Stress fracture of the cuboid

Stress fractures of the cuboid are not common and are thought to occur secondary to compression of the cuboid between the calcaneus and the fourth and fifth metatarsal bones when exaggerated plantarflexion is undertaken with or without inversion.[30] Treatment, in the absence of displacement, is non-weight-bearing for four to six weeks, followed by a graduated return to activity. If displacement is present, surgical reduction and fixation with or without a bone graft may be required.

Stress fracture of the cuneiforms

Stress fractures of the cuneiform bones are rare and have been described in military recruits and athletes.[31]

They are thought to occur secondary to repetitive loading of the bone. Management depends on the cuneiform bone involved: limited weight-bearing rest has been shown to effectively result in healing of medial cuneiform stress fractures; however, stress fractures of the intermediate cuneiform bone have been shown to require surgical reduction and fixation for adequate healing.[32]

Köhler's disease

Köhler's disease, or osteochondritis of the navicular, is found in children aged 2–8 years (Chapter 40).

Tarsal coalition

Congenital fusions of the foot bones usually present as midfoot pain. Tarsal coalitions[33] may be osseous, cartilaginous (synchondrosis), fibrous (syndesmosis) or a combination. A fibrous coalition is relatively mobile and therefore may not cause any pain on limited motion. As fibrous or cartilaginous coalitions ossify during adolescence, rear foot or midfoot joint range of motion decreases, placing additional stress on the talocrural (ankle) joint. The two most common tarsal coalitions occur at the calcaneonavicular joint or the talocalcaneal joint; 50–60% occur bilaterally.

Common presentations include an adolescent beginning sports participation or the person in their 20s complaining of pain after vigorous physical activity. They can also be brought to light after an ankle sprain as pain does not settle (Chapter 33). Because tarsal coalition alters foot biomechanics, it can present in adults with painful bony spurs at sites distant from the coalition (Fig. 35.15).

Examination often reveals reduced range of subtalar and midtarsal joint movement that may be painful at the end of range. Plain X-rays are the most useful diagnostic tool for osseous coalitions. MRI may be required to visualize a fibrous coalition.

Forefoot pain

Forefoot problems range from corns, calluses and nail problems to bone and joint abnormalities. Forefoot pain is especially common in athletes participating in kicking sports and among ballet dancers. The causes of forefoot pain are listed in Table 35.4.

History

Most causes of forefoot pain result from overuse and thus have an insidious onset. Occasionally, acute forefoot pain may result from a sprain of the first metatarsophalangeal joint ('turf toe'). The type of

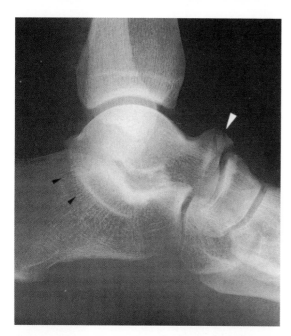

Figure 35.15 X-ray showing talocalcaneal coalition (black arrows) with a continuous cortical line joining the talus and sustentaculum tali, and talar beaking (white arrow) that results from abnormal subtalar movement

activity performed provides a clue to the cause of the patient's forefoot pain. The presence of sensory symptoms may indicate that a neuroma is present.

Examination

The key to examination of the patient with forefoot pain is careful palpation to determine the site of maximal tenderness. Biomechanical examination is necessary.

1. Observation (Fig. 35.16a)
2. Palpation
   (a) metatarsals (Fig. 35.16b)
   (b) first metatarsophalangeal joint (Fig. 35.16c)
   (c) sesamoid bone of the foot (Fig. 35.16d)
   (d) space between third and fourth metatarsal (Fig. 35.16e)

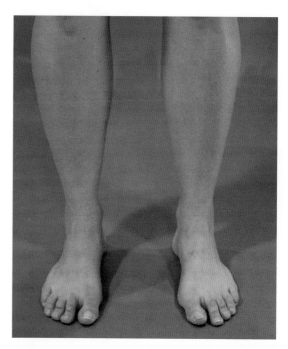

Figure 35.16 Examination of the patient with forefoot pain

(a) Observation for the presence of obvious abnormalities (e.g. hallux abducto-valgus, claw toes, Morton's foot, plantar warts, onychocryptosis, corns, callus)

Table 35.4 Causes of forefoot pain

Common	Less common	Not to be missed
Corns, calluses	Freiberg's osteochondritis	Complex regional pain syndrome type 1 (after ankle or knee injury)
Onychocryptosis	Joplin's neuritis	
Synovitis of the MTP joints	Stress fracture of the sesamoid	
First MTP joint sprain	Toe clawing	
Subungual hematoma	Plantar wart	
Hallux abducto-valgus	Subungual exostosis	
Hallux limitus	Stress fracture of the base of the 2nd metatarsal	
Morton's neuroma	Synovitis of the metatarsal–cuneiform joint	
Sesamoid pathology		
Stress fracture of the metatarsal		
Fracture of the 5th metatarsal		

MTP = metatarsophalangeal.

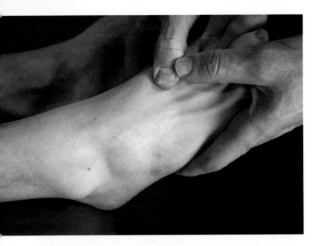

(b) Palpation—metatarsals

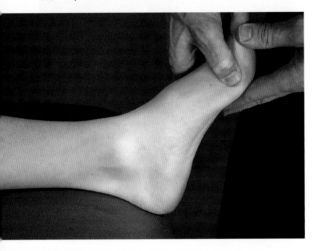

(c) Palpation—first metatarsophalangeal joint

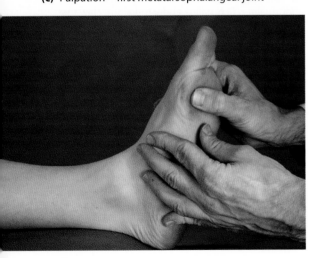

(d) Palpation—sesamoid

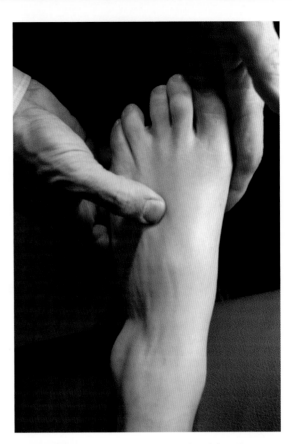

(e) Palpation—space between third and fourth metatarsal

Investigations

X-ray may show evidence of a healing stress fracture or acute fracture, the presence of hallux abducto-valgus, hallux limitus or a subungual exostosis. Isotopic bone scan or MRI may confirm the diagnosis of a stress fracture. An MRI or ultrasound can be used to determine the presence of a neuroma.

Stress fractures of the metatarsals

Stress fractures of the metatarsals in most series[22] have been shown to be the second most common stress fracture, second to the tibia. The most common metatarsal stress fracture is at the neck of the second metatarsal. This occurs in the pronating foot, when the first ray is dorsiflexed, resulting in the second metatarsal being subjected to greater load. The second metatarsal is also susceptible to stress fracture in the case of a Morton's foot, where the first ray is shorter than the second (Fig. 35.17). The base of the second metatarsal is firmly fixed in position next to the

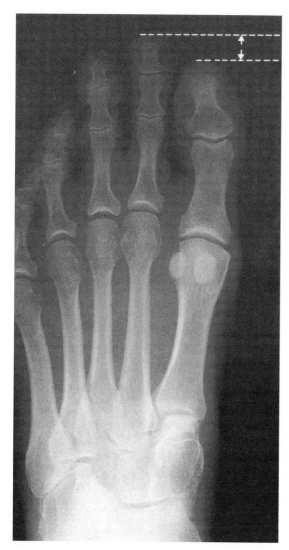

Figure 35.17 Morton's foot with the first ray shorter than the second

cuneiform bones, further increasing the likelihood of fracture. Stress fracture of the second metatarsal is common in ballet dancers. Stress fractures of the other metatarsals also occur, particularly in the third metatarsal if it is longer than the second.

Clinical features

The patient with a metatarsal stress fracture complains of forefoot pain aggravated by activity such as running or dancing. The pain is not severe initially but gradually worsens with activity. Examination reveals the presence of focal tenderness overlying the metatarsal.

Investigation

X-rays may reveal a radiolucent line or periosteal thickening if the fracture has been present for a few weeks (Fig. 35.18a). If the X-ray is negative, an isotopic bone scan (Fig. 35.18b) or MRI may confirm the diagnosis.

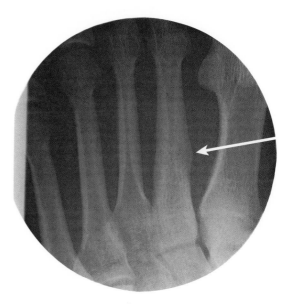

Figure 35.18 Stress fracture of the second metatarsal

(a) X-ray appearance—note the generalized cortical hypertrophy, as seen in ballet dancers

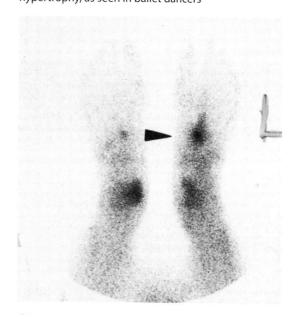

(b) Isotopic bone scan appearance

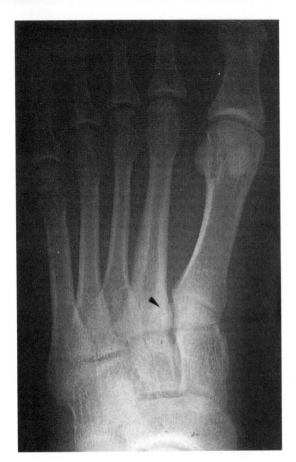

(c) Involving the second tarsometatarsal joint

Treatment

The management of most stress fractures is straight-forward, involving rest from weight-bearing aggra-vating activities for approximately four weeks. If the patient is required to be on his or her feet excessively, the use of an air cast may be required for one to two weeks until pain settles. The athlete should be allowed to recommence activity when he or she does not experience pain when walking and there is no local tenderness at the fracture site. A graduated exercise program should be instituted to return the athlete to full training and competition. Orthoses may be required to control abnormal foot mechanics. Any instability during forefoot weight-bearing may predispose to the development of a stress fracture.

Two stress fractures require special treatment: fractures of the base of the second metatarsal and fractures of the fifth metatarsal.

Fractures of the second metatarsal

An unusual fracture of the base of the second meta-tarsal involving the joint is seen in ballet dancers[22, 34–36] (Fig. 35.18c). This fracture should be treated by having the dancer remain non-weight-bearing on crutches until tenderness settles, usually at least four weeks. The differential diagnosis of second metatarsal stress fracture is chronic joint synovitis. Assessment of the early stage by an isotopic bone scan or MRI will assist diagnosis.

Fractures of the fifth metatarsal

Three different fractures affect the fifth metatarsal.[22, 37] The fracture of the tuberosity at the base of the fifth metatarsal (Fig. 33.12) has been described in Chapter 33 and is usually an avulsion injury that results from an acute ankle sprain. This uncomplicated fracture heals well with a short period of immobilization for pain relief.

A serious fracture of the fifth metatarsal is the fracture of the diaphysis known as a Jones' fracture (Fig. 35.19a). This may be the result of an inversion plantarflexion injury or, more commonly, as a result of overuse. A Jones' fracture requires six to eight weeks of non-weight-bearing cast immobilization[38] or, in situations when rapid return to activity is required, immediate surgical fixation with the percutaneous insertion of a screw. Non-union may be treated by bone grafting or screw fixation. More recently there has been a tendency to favor early screw fixation due to concerns regarding the high incidence of failure of cast treatment. In one study, early screw fixation resulted in quicker times to union and return to sport compared to cast treatment.[39] The average time to return to sport after this procedure appears to be approximately eight weeks, although early return to sport may predispose the athlete to re-fracture[40] and it may be wise to wait for full radiographic healing before return to sport.[41]

An acute spiral fracture of the distal third of the fifth metatarsal is seen, especially in dancers who suffer this fracture when they lose their balance while on demi pointe and roll over the outer border of the foot—'fouette fracture' (Fig. 35.19b). Undisplaced fractures of this type may be treated with weight-bearing rest, while displaced fractures may require four to six weeks of cast immobilization.

Metatarsophalangeal joint synovitis

Metatarsophalangeal joint synovitis (commonly referred to as 'metatarsalgia') is a common inflam-matory condition occurring most frequently in the

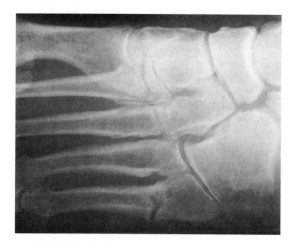

Figure 35.19 Fractures of the fifth metatarsal

(a) Diaphysis or Jones' fracture with slight separation. Sclerosis of the fracture margins suggests delayed union

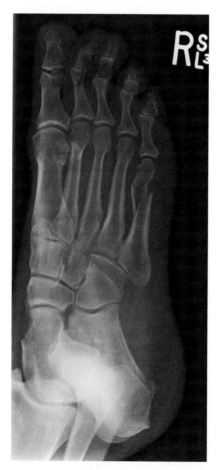

(b) Spiral fracture of the distal fifth metatarsal

second, third and/or fourth metatarsophalangeal joints, or isolated in the first metatarsophalangeal joints.

Causes

The metatarsophalangeal joints become inflamed, usually due to excessive pressure over a prolonged period. It is often related to:

- pes cavus or high arched foot
- excessive pronation of the foot
- clawing or hammer toes
- tight extensor tendons of the toes
- prominent metatarsal heads
- Morton's foot—there is a shortened first metatarsal, which results in an abnormal subtalar joint, and increased weight going through the second metatarsophalangeal joint.

Clinical features

The patient complains of pain aggravated by forefoot weight-bearing, particularly in the midstance and propulsion phases of walking. The pain is usually gradual in onset.

Examination reveals local tenderness on palpation. Pain is aggravated by passive forced flexion of the toe. It most commonly affects the second metatarsophalangeal joint, occasionally the first or third. There may be an associated skin lesion (e.g. a callus) over the plantar surface of the affected joint due to the excessive load. This injury may be caused by uneven distribution of load, especially with excessive pronation.

Investigations

X-rays should be performed to assess the degree of degeneration of the joint.

Treatment

Treatment requires appropriate padding to redistribute weight from the painful areas together with footwear that has adequate midsole cushioning. NSAIDs may be helpful and occasionally corticosteroid injection is required. The joint is injected via the dorsal surface, while longitudinal traction is placed on the toe to open the joint space.

First metatarsophalangeal joint sprain ('turf toe')

A sprain to the first metatarsophalangeal joint, otherwise known as a 'turf toe', is a common injury occurring in athletes in which the plantar capsule and ligament of the first metatarsophalangeal joint is damaged.

Cause

The classic mechanism of injury is usually that of a forced hyperextension to the first metatarsophalangeal joint, although occasionally a plantarflexion injury to the joint may result in this injury.

Predisposing risk factors include:

- competing or training on artificial turf
- pes planus or excessive pronation
- decreased preinjury ankle range of motion
- decreased preinjury metatarsophalangeal range of motion
- soft flexible footwear.

Clinical features

The athlete usually complains of localized pain, swelling and occasional redness at the first metatarsophalangeal joint following a 'bending' injury to the joint. The pain is classically aggravated by weight-bearing or movement of the big toe.

Examination reveals localized swelling and tenderness at the first metatarsophalangeal joint. In mild injuries plantar or plantar medial tenderness is present; in more severe injuries dorsal tenderness occurs. Passive plantarflexion and dorsiflexion of the first metatarsophalangeal joint are generally painful, and there may be a reduction in the range of movement in both directions.

Investigations

Plain X-rays are generally unremarkable, although occasionally small periarticular flecks of bone are noted, most likely indicating avulsion of the metatarsophalangeal capsule or ligamentous complex. Isotopic bone scans, although not generally performed, may demonstrate increased uptake in spite of normal X-rays.

Treatment

Treatment consists of ice, NSAIDs, electrotherapeutic modalities and decreased weight-bearing for at least 72 hours. Additional treatment may include taping (Fig. 35.20) and the use of stiff-soled shoes to protect the first metatarsophalangeal joint from further injury. Recovery generally takes three to four weeks.

A possible long-term sequel to this injury is the development of hallux limitus.

Hallux limitus

Hallux limitus is defined as a restriction in dorsiflexion of the hallux at the first metatarsophalangeal joint secondary to exostoses or osteoarthritis of the joint.

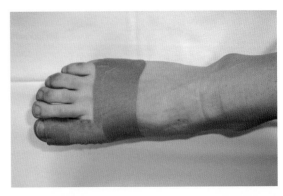

Figure 35.20 Taping to protect an injured first metatarsophalangeal joint

Often the term 'hallux rigidus' is used to describe the final progression of hallux limitus as ankylosis of the joint occurs.

The primary role of the hallux is to enable dorsiflexion of the first metatarsal during the propulsive phase of gait. It has been shown that approximately 60° of dorsiflexion is required for normal gait. Limitation of this range of motion results in problems with gait.

Causes

- Trauma—secondary to chondral damage
- Excessive pronation of the foot may increase the stresses on the joint and promote development of exostoses
- Repetitive weight-bearing dorsiflexion of the first metatarsophalangeal joint
- Autoimmune arthropathy (e.g. rheumatoid arthritis)
- Aberration of the first metatarsal or proximal phalanx
- Hypermobile first ray
- Muscle imbalance

Clinical features

The main presenting symptom is usually that of pain around the first metatarsophalangeal joint. The pain is often described as a deep aching sensation that is aggravated by walking, especially in high heels, or activities involving forefoot weight-bearing. Dorsal joint hypertrophy can be a source of irritation from footwear and may lead to pain secondary to skin or soft tissue irritation.

In patients with longstanding hallux limitus, a distinct shoe wear pattern is seen: the sole demonstrates wear beneath the second metatarsophalangeal joint and the first interphalangeal joint.

Examination reveals tenderness of the first metatarsophalanageal joint, especially over the dorsal aspect, often with palpable dorsal exostoses. There is a painful limitation of joint motion, the degree of limitation reflecting the severity of the arthrosis.

Investigations

Plain X-rays display the classic characteristics of degenerative osteoarthritis and the degree of degeneration observed will reflect the duration and severity of the condition. Features include joint space narrowing, sclerosis of the subchondral bone plate, osteophytic proliferation, flattening of the joint, sesamoid displacement and free bony fragments.

Treatment

Conservative management consists of an initial reduction in activity, NSAIDs, a cortisone injection if required, physiotherapy, and correction of biomechanical factors with orthoses and/or footwear. Conservative treatment often fails when hallux dorsiflexion is less than 50°. In extreme cases, cheilectomy (resection of all bony prominences of the metatarsal head and base of the proximal phalanx) is required. Occasionally, arthroplasty of the first metatarsophalangeal joint is indicated.

Hallux valgus

Hallux valgus is defined as a static subluxation of the first metatarsophalangeal joint. It is characterized by valgus (lateral) deviation of the great toe and varus (medial) deviation of the first metatarsal (Fig. 35.21).

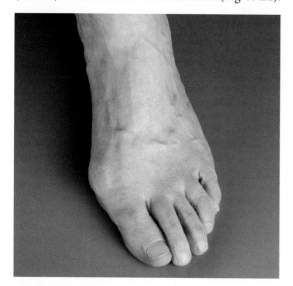

Figure 35.21 Hallux valgus

Bony exostoses develop around the first metatarsophalangeal joint, often with an overlying bursitis. In severe cases, exostoses limit first metatarsophalangeal joint range of motion and cause pain with the pressure of footwear.

Causes

The development of hallux valgus appears to occur secondary to a combination of intrinsic and extrinsic causes. Recognized causative factors include:

- constricting footwear (e.g. high heels)
- excessive pronation—increased pressure on the medial border of the hallux, resulting in deformation of the medial capsular structures
- others—cystic degeneration of the medial capsule, Achilles tendon contracture, neuromuscular disorders, collagen deficient diseases.

Clinical features

In the early phases hallux valgus is often asymptomatic, however, as the deformity develops, pain over the medial eminence occurs. The pain is typically relieved by removing the shoes or by wearing soft, flexible, wide-toed shoes. Blistering of the skin or development of an inflamed bursa over the medial eminence may occur. In severe deformity, lateral metatarsalgia may occur due to the diminished weight-bearing capacity of the first ray.

Examination reveals the hallux valgus deformity often with a tender swelling overlying the medial eminence.

Investigation

Plain X-rays should be performed to assess both the severity of the deformity and the degree of first metatarsophalangeal joint degeneration.

Treatment

Initial treatment involves appropriate padding and footwear to reduce friction over the medial eminence. Correction of foot function with orthoses is essential. In more severe cases surgery may be required to reconstruct the first metatarsophalangeal joint and remove the bony exostoses. Orthoses are often required after surgery.

Sesamoid injuries

The first metatarsophalangeal joint is characterized by the two sesamoid bones which play a significant part in the function of the great toe. Embedded within the two tendons of the flexor hallucis brevis, they function to:

- protect the tendon of flexor hallucis longus
- absorb most of the weight-bearing on the medial aspect of the forefoot
- increase the mechanical advantage of the intrinsic musculature of the hallux.

In approximately 30% of individuals, a bipartite medial or lateral sesamoid is present.

Causes

The sesamoid bones may be injured by traumatic fracture, stress fracture, sprain of a bipartite sesamoid and sprain of the sesamoid–metatarsal articulation. Sesamoid abnormality involves inflammatory changes and osteonecrosis around the sesamoid. The medial sesamoid is usually affected. Inflammation may be caused by landing after a jump, increased forefoot weight-bearing activities (e.g. sprinting and dancing) or after traumatic dorsiflexion of the hallux.

Pronation may cause lateral displacement or subluxation of the sesamoids within the plantar grooves of the first metatarsal. This subluxation of the sesamoids may lead to erosion of the plantar aspect of the first metatarsal, resulting in pain underneath the first metatarsal head, arthritic changes and ultimately decreased dorsiflexion.

Clinical features

The patient complains of pain with forefoot weight-bearing and will often walk with weight laterally to compensate. Examination reveals marked local tenderness and swelling overlying the medial or lateral sesamoid. Movement of the first metatarsophalangeal joint is usually painful and often restricted. Resisted plantarflexion of the great toe elicits both pain and weakness.

Investigations

Plain X-rays including an axial sesamoid view should be performed to assess for a sesamoid fracture. Isotopic bone scan or MRI scan is often required to detect early stress fractures and differentiate between a bipartite sesamoid sprain or inflammation and a fracture.

Treatment

Treatment of sesamoid inflammation is with ice, NSAIDs and electrotherapeutic modalities to reduce inflammation. Padding can distribute weight away from the sesamoid bones (Fig. 35.22) and technique correction is mandatory in activities such as dance. In ballet, this injury arises because of excessive rolling in of the foot, which is commonly due to 'forcing turnout'. Corticosteroid injection into the joint space between the sesamoid and metatarsal may prove effective if underlying abnormalities have been corrected. Orthoses are required if foot mechanics are abnormal. Treatment of sesamoid stress fractures, which occur particularly in basketballers, tennis players and dancers,[22] involves up to six weeks of non-weight-bearing in an air cast or short leg cast. These stress fractures are prone to non-union and, in the elite athlete or in those who have non-union, percutaneous fixation with a screw may be successfully performed. The surgical removal of a sesamoid bone should be avoided if possible as removal causes significant muscle imbalances and may contribute to a hallux abducto-valgus deformity. However, excision is required in cases of significant osteonecrosis. Partial sesamoidectomy has been used without success and there are now reports of an arthroscopic approach to this joint.[42]

Stress fracture of the great toe

Stress fractures of the proximal phalanx of the great toe have been reported in adolescent athletes.[22, 43] There appears to be an association with hallux valgus.

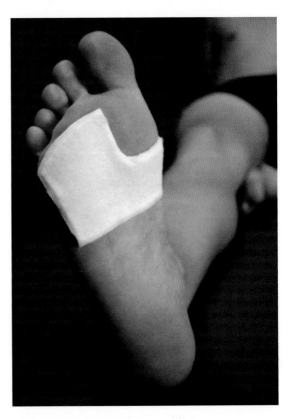

Figure 35.22 Sesamoiditis—padding

Treatment involves a period of non-weight-bearing rest of four to six weeks followed by graduated return to activity.

Freiberg's osteochondritis

Freiberg's disease or osteochondritis of the metatarsal head affects adolescents between the ages of 14 and 18 years (Chapter 40). The metatarsal head appears fragmented on X-ray. Offloading of the metatarsal heads using padding and orthoses is essential to prevent permanent metatarsal head flattening that may predispose to adult osteoarthritis.

Joplin's neuritis

Joplin's neuritis involves compression and irritation of the dorsal medial cutaneous nerve over the first metatarsal and first metatarsophalangeal joint. It usually occurs because of irritation from footwear and is common in patients with hallux abducto-valgus or exostoses around the first metatarsophalangeal joint.

The patient complains of pain radiating along the first ray into the hallux. Wearing appropriate footwear and using foam and felt to redistribute the load from the affected area generally provides relief. Orthoses may be required to prevent excessive pronation.

Morton's interdigital neuroma

So-called Morton's neuroma is not a true neuroma but a swelling of nerve and scar tissue arising from compression of the interdigital nerve, usually between the third and fourth metatarsals (Fig. 35.23a). The patient complains of pain radiating into the toes, often associated with pins and needles and numbness. Pain is increased by forefoot weight-bearing activities and with narrow-fitting footwear.

Examination reveals localized tenderness and, in cases of extensive chronic proliferation, there may be a palpable click on compression of the metatarsal heads. Excessive pronation contributes to metatarsal hypermobility and impingement of the interdigital nerve.

Treatment consists initially of ice to alleviate acute tenderness. Plantar metatarsal padding is used to spread the load over the metatarsals (Fig. 35.23b). Intrinsic foot muscle strengthening exercises are indicated to maintain or improve the transverse arch. However, in chronic cases, little improvement is seen with padding. Injection of corticosteroid and local anesthetic agents in conjunction with the padding may provide lasting relief. The use of orthoses

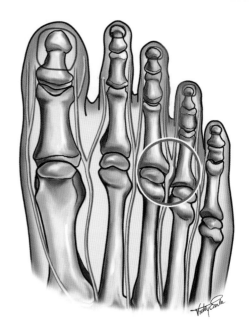

Figure 35.23 Morton's neuroma

(a) Location of nerve entrapment in Morton's neuroma

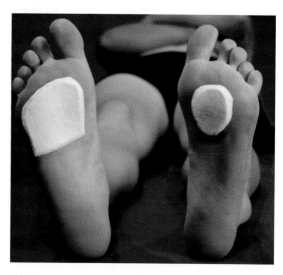

(b) Plantar metatarsal padding

is essential if excessive pronation is present. If the patient obtains no relief, surgical excision of the damaged nerve is indicated.

Toe clawing

Toe clawing occurs secondary to short, tight long flexor tendons (Fig. 35.24). During the propulsive

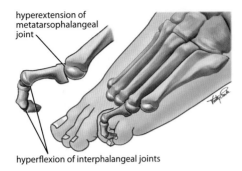

hyperextension of metatarsophalangeal joint

hyperflexion of interphalangeal joints

Figure 35.24 Toe clawing

phase of gait, the long flexors contract to stabilize the toes. In the unstable foot, the long flexors contract excessively during the propulsive phase and the toes claw the surface in an attempt to maintain stability.

Clawing of toes does not result in pain itself but excessive pressure on the prominent joints and ends of toes often causes painful skin lesions.

Corns and calluses

Excessive pressure on the skin may cause hypertrophy of the squamous cell layer of the epidermis, which manifests as corns and calluses. In the feet, corns and calluses result from uneven weight distribution and thus indicate abnormal foot biomechanics or poorly fitting footwear.

Treatment involves the removal of circumscribed corns and diffuse areas of callus with a scalpel, the wearing of well-fitting footwear and, if abnormal foot mechanics are present, orthoses. Petroleum jelly over the corn or callus and on the outside of the sock can also help.

Plantar warts

The papovavirus causes plantar warts when it enters the skin. The warts can be particularly painful on weight-bearing. They should be differentiated from corns. Applying lateral pressure or pinching will be painful in warts, whereas corns are more painful with direct pressure. Gentle paring with a scalpel will also reveal the characteristic appearance of a plantar wart with fine black dots within a defined margin of white or brown tissue.

Plantar warts are best treated with chemical solutions containing salicylic acid. The overlying hyperkeratosis should be removed weekly to allow the chemicals to penetrate the wart. Blistering and abscess formation occur and require debridement with a scalpel and the application of a dressing.

Subungual hematoma

Subungual hematoma occurs when direct trauma or repetitive pressure from footwear leads to bleeding under the toenails. Pain arises from increased pressure under the nail and, in cases of repetitive trauma, the nails appear black. The nail may eventually loosen from the nail bed.

Treatment of an acute subungual hematoma involves using a heated needle or paper clip to perforate the nail and release the collection of blood. Cover with a small dressing.

Subungual exostosis

A subungual exostosis develops because of direct trauma. The patient presents with pain on direct pressure to the nail. The nail plate may be displaced from the nail bed due to elevation from the exostosis. Treatment requires the wearing of loose-fitting footwear, appropriate cutting of the nail and padding. Surgery may be required to remove the bony exostosis.

Onychocryptosis

Onychocryptosis (ingrown toenail) arises from abnormal nail growth or poor nail cutting. Patients often present in acute pain with tenderness on gentle palpation. Nails are often infected. Treatment with local and oral antibiotic therapy is required. Conservative treatment involves elevating the offending corner of the nail plate from the soft tissue, cutting a small 'V' into the middle of the nail distally (to take pressure off the edges) and stretching the soft tissue away from the nail with a cotton bud.

Surgical management consists of resection of the outer aspect of the nail to prevent the nail border injuring the soft tissue. Resection involves anesthetizing the toe and removing the nail border with appropriate nail splitters and forceps. All abnormal tissue is removed and the nail matrix treated with phenol to prevent regrowth.

Recommended Reading

Dyck DD, Boyajian-O'Neill LA. Plantar fasciitis. *Clin J Sport Med* 2004, 14: 305–9.

Glazer JL, Brukner P. Plantar fasciitis. Current concepts to expedite healing. *Physician Sportsmed* 2004; 32(11): 24–8.

Hockenbury RT. Forefoot problems in athletes. *Med Sci Sports Exerc* 1999; 31(7 suppl.): S448–58.

Jaivin JS. Foot injuries and arthroscopy in sport. *Sports Med* 2000; 29: 65–72.

Khan K, Brown J, Way S, et al. Overuse injuries in classical ballet. *Sports Med* 1995; 19: 341–57.

May TJ, Judy TA, Conti M, et al. Current treatment of plantar fasciitis. *Curr Sports Med Rep* 2002; 1: 278–84.

Neely FG. Biomechanical risk factors for exercise-related lower limb injuries. *Sports Med* 1998; 26: 395–413.

Nigg BM. The role of impact forces and foot pronation: a new paradigm. *Clin J Sport Med* 2001; 11: 2–9.

Sherman KP. The foot in sport. *Br J Sports Med* 1999; 33: 6–13.

Simons SM. Foot injuries of the recreational athlete. *Physician Sportsmed* 1999; 27(1): 57–70.

Taunton JE, Ryan MB, Clement DB, et al. Plantar fasciitis: a retrospective analysis of 267 cases. *Phys Ther Sport* 2002; 3: 57–65.

References

1. Lemont H, Ammirati KM, Ulsen N. Plantar fasciitis: a degenerative process (fasciosis) without inflammation. *J Am Podiatr Med Assoc* 2003; 93(3): 234–7.

2. Riddle DL, Pulisic M, Pidcoe P, et al. Risk factors for plantar fasciitis: a matched case-control study. *J Bone Joint Surg Br* 2003; 85B(5): 872–7.

3. Lu H, Gu G, Zhu S. [Heel pain and calcaneal spurs]. *Chung Hua Wai Ko Tsa Chih* 1996; 34: 294–6.

4. Wolgin M, Cook C, Graham CM, et al. Conservative treatment of plantar heel pain: long term follow up. *Foot Ankle Int* 1994; 15: 97–102.

5. DiGiovanni BF, Nawoczenski DA, Lintal ME, et al. Tissue-specific plantar fascia-stretching exercise enhances outcomes in patients with chronic heel pain. A prospective randomized study. *J Bone Joint Surg Br* 2003; 85B(7): 1270–7.

6. Martin RL, Irrgang JJ, Cionti SF. Outcome study of subjects with insertional plantar fasciitis. *Foot Ankle Int* 1998; 19: 803–11.

7. Dyck DD, Boyajian-O'Neill LA. Plantar fasciitis. *Clin J Sport Med* 2004; 14: 305–9.

8. Pfeffer G, Bacchetti P, Deland J, et al. Comparison of custom and prefabricated orthoses in the initial treatment of proximal plantar fasciitis. *Foot Ankle Int* 1999; 20(4): 214–21.

9. Gross MT, Byers JM, Krafft JL, et al. The impact of custom semirigid foot orthotics on pain and disability for individuals with plantar fasciitis. *J Orthop Sports Phys Ther* 2002; 32: 149–57.

10. Batt ME, Tanji JL, Skattum N. Plantar fasciitis: a prospective randomized clinical trial of the tension night splint. *Clin J Sport Med* 1996; 6: 158–62.

11. Powell M, Post WR, Keener J, et al. Effective treatment of chronic plantar fasciitis with dorsiflexion night splints: a crossover prospective randomised outcome study. *Foot Ankle Int* 1998; 19(1): 10–18.

12. Probe RA, Baca M, Adams R, et al. Night splint treatment for plantar fasciitis. A prospective randomized study. *Clin Orthop* 1999; 368: 190–5.

13. Crawford E, Atkins D, Young P, et al. Steroid injection for heel pain: evidence of short term effectiveness: a randomized controlled trial. *Rheumatology* 1999; 38(10): 974–7.

14. Sellman JR. Plantar fascia rupture associated with corticosteroid injection. *Foot Ankle Int* 1994; 15(7): 376–81.

15. Acevedo JI, Beskin JL. Complications of plantar fascia rupture associated with corticosteroid injection. *Foot Ankle Int* 1998; 19: 91–7.

16. Gudeman SD, Eisele SA, Heidt RS Jr, et al. Treatment of plantar fasciitis by iontophoresis of 0.4% dexamethasone. *Am J Sports Med* 1997; 25(3): 312–16.

17. Crawford F, Thomas C. Interventions for treating plantar heel pain. *Cochrane Database Syst Rev* 2003; 3: CD000416.

18. Buchbinder R, Ptasznik R, Gordon J, et al. Ultrasound-guided extracorporeal shock wave therapy for plantar fasciitis: a randomized controlled trial. *JAMA* 2002; 288(11): 1364–72.

19. Sammarco GJ, Helfrey RB. Surgical treatment of recalcitrant plantar fasciitis. *Foot Ankle Int* 1996; 17: 520–6.

20. Jerosch J, Schunck J, Liebsch D, et al. Indication, surgical technique and results of endoscopic fascial release in plantar fasciitis (EFRPF). *Knee Surg Sports Traumatol Arthrosc* 2004; 12: 471–7.

21. O'Malley MJ, Page A, Cook R. Endoscopic plantar fasciotomy for chronic heel pain. *Foot Ankle Int* 2000; 21: 505–10.

22. Brukner PD, Bennell KL, Matheson GO. *Stress Fractures*. Melbourne: Blackwell Scientific, 1999.

23. Baxter D, Pfeffer G. Treatment of chronic heel pain by surgical release of the first branch of the lateral plantar nerve. *Clin Orthop* 1992; 279: 229–36.

24. Khan KM, Brukner PD, Kearney C, et al. Tarsal navicular stress fracture in athletes. *Sports Med* 1994; 17: 65–76.

25. Khan KM, Fuller PJ, Brukner PD, et al. Outcome of conservative and surgical management of navicular stress fracture in athletes. Eighty-six cases proven with computerized tomography. *Am J Sports Med* 1992; 20(6): 657–66.

26. Kiss ZA, Khan KM, Fuller PJ. Stress fractures of the tarsal navicular bone: CT findings in 55 cases. *AJR Am J Roentgenol* 1993; 160: 111–15.

27. Burne SG, Mahoney CM, Forster BB, et al. Tarsal navicular stress injury: long term outcome and clinico-radiological correlation using both computed tomography and magnetic resonance imaging. *Am J Sports Med* 2005; 33: 1875–81.

28. Nunley JA, Vertullo CJ. Classification, investigation, and management of midfoot sprains. Lisfranc injuries in the athlete. *Am J Sports Med* 2002; 30(6): 871–8.

29. Marshall P, Hamilton WG. Cuboid subluxation in ballet dancers. *Am J Sports Med* 1992; 20(2): 169–75.

30. Hermel MB, Gershon-Cohen J. The nutcracker fracture of the cuboid by indirect violence. *Radiology* 1953; 60: 850–4.

31. Khan KM, Brukner PD, Bradshaw C. Stress fracture of the medial cuneiform bone in a runner. *Clin J Sport Med* 1993; 3(4): 262–4.

32. Creighton R, Sonogar A, Gordon G. Stress fracture of the tarsal middle cuneiform bone. A case report. *J Am Podiatr Med Assoc* 1990; 80: 489–95.

33. Sakellariou A, Claridge RJ. Tarsal coalition. *Orthopedics* 1999; 22: 1066–73.

34. Harrington T, Crichton KJ, Anderson IF. Overuse ballet injury of the base of the second metatarsal. *Am J Sports Med* 1993; 21: 591–8.

35. Micheli LJ, Sohn RS, Soloman R. Stress fractures of the second metatarsal involving Lisfranc's joint in ballet dancers: a new overuse of the foot. *J Bone Joint Surg Am* 1985; 67A: 1372–5.

36. O'Malley MJ, Hamilton WG, Munyak J, et al. Stress fractures at the base of the second metatarsal in ballet dancers. *Foot Ankle Int* 1996; 17(2): 89–94.

37. Yu WD, Shapiro MS. Fractures of the fifth metatarsal. Careful identification for optimum treatment. *Physician Sportsmed* 1998; 26(2): 47–64.

38. DeLee JC, Evans JP, Julian J. Stress fracture of the fifth metatarsal. *Am J Sports Med* 1983; 11: 349–53.

39. Mologne TS, Lundeen JM, Clapper MF, et al. Early screw fixation versus casting in the treatment of acute Jones fractures. *Am J Sports Med* 2005; 33(7): 970–5.

40. Wright R, Fischer D, Shively R, et al. Refracture of proximal fifth metatarsal (Jones) fracture after intramedullary screw fixation in athletes. *Am J Sports Med* 2000; 28(5): 732–6.

41. Larson CM, Almekinders LC, Taft TN, et al. Intramedullary screw fixation of Jones fractures—analysis of failure. *Am J Sports Med* 2002; 30(1): 55–60.

42. Perez Carro L, Echevarria Llata JI, Martinez Argueros JA. Arthroscopic medial bipartite sesamoidectomy of the great toe. *Arthroscopy* 1999; 15: 321–3.

43. Pitsis GC, Best JP, Sullivan MR. Unusual stress fractures of the proximal phalanx of the great toe: a report of two cases. *Br J Sports Med* 2004; 38: e31.

The Patient with Longstanding Symptoms

A regular presentation in sports medicine is that of a patient who has already consulted a number of practitioners for diagnosis and treatment about what appears to be a musculoskeletal problem but whose symptoms remain unresolved.

Presentations of patients with longstanding symptoms may include:

- chronic low back pain or neck pain
- persistent tendinopathies
- multiple painful sites
- a persistent joint problem
- a non-healing fracture
- persistent foot pain.

Longstanding symptoms may be due to the conditions that masquerade as sports injuries (Chapter 4) but they may also be true musculoskeletal problems. Note that a condition that masquerades as a sports medicine condition may not produce longstanding symptoms as it may produce significant symptoms in the short term if not diagnosed (e.g. deep venous thrombosis and pulmonary embolism masquerading as a calf injury). We also suggest that the reader reviews Chapter 3, which discusses the multifactorial nature of chronic musculoskeletal pain with contributions from joints, muscles and neural structures. Unless all these contributors are recognized and eliminated, the result will be unsatisfactory.

The purpose of this chapter is to provide a clinical approach to the 'difficult' presentation. We do not suggest we have the answers for all, or even most, such presentations. Nevertheless, a systematic approach to this presentation can lead to successes. We use case histories to illustrate our suggestions. In our experience, the presentation of unresolved pain generally presents as a diagnostic challenge, or

a therapeutic challenge, so the chapter is structured to reflect this.

What is the diagnosis?

When you are referred a patient known to have a long history of problems, you may wish to schedule extra time when making the appointment to permit a thorough evaluation. If there is no forewarning that the patient has longstanding symptoms, we suggest explaining to the patient the need to revisit the entire history, examination and investigations thoroughly and that an additional appointment time will be needed to do this. In this way, the initial, perhaps 10–20 minute, consultation can be used to emphasize the importance of the problem and the rationale for treating it differently from a straightforward presentation.

Going back to square one

By definition, the problem began a long time earlier so it is crucial to obtain details of the earliest symptoms in the patient's own words rather than from a referral letter or discharge summary. For example, what has been evaluated as chronic knee pain for the past few years may have begun with a childhood knee injury that had been overlooked. After a thorough assessment of the presenting complaint, its time course and response to therapy, remember to ask about the past medical history and the past family history. Associated musculoskeletal symptoms that provide a clue to an alternative diagnosis may only arise by specific questioning.

For example, a 33-year-old woman who presented with chronic wrist pain unresponsive to physical therapies eventually recalled several episodes of joint swelling and pain in childhood that were attributed to playing sport. The history provided a vital clue to her final diagnosis of rheumatoid arthritis. A stockbroker with longstanding shoulder pain was surprised to be asked about previous neck pain. She had fallen from her horse two years earlier but an X-ray of her neck was normal and, as her neck pain settled, she no longer gave it any consideration. Failed therapy to her shoulder, including several corticosteroid injections, led to a review, and the history of neck injury, together with C3–4 tenderness on careful palpation, led to the eventual diagnosis of a significant facet joint hypomobility.

It is important for the practitioner to ask about the demands of work, as active individuals often attribute symptoms to sport when this may not always be the case. An executive attributed his shoulder pain to weight training, particularly to resting the squat bar on his shoulders, but careful history taking revealed that he always jammed the telephone into the crook of his shoulder for upwards of five hours per day. Examination revealed loss of triceps jerk and weakness in the C5–6 distribution. CT scan confirmed a lateral disk bulge that impinged the nerve root at its foraminal exit. Treatment consisted of a headset for the telephone and therapy to the neck, rather than avoidance of squats with weight on the neck.

A history of non-musculoskeletal symptoms may provide evidence of a systemic condition manifesting as long-term pain. A 42-year-old basketball coach was surprised to learn that his years of recalcitrant, but intermittent, midfoot pain could be linked to his psoriasis. These two aspects of his history had not been linked previously as he had provided the information about each in isolation when he saw different doctors and therapists about these problems.

Thorough examination

In cases of longstanding symptoms, the physical examination must be thorough (in scope) and meticulous (in attention to subtle details). The practitioner must always examine the spine, as referred pain commonly goes undiagnosed. A 44-year-old policeman who finally presented to the sports medicine clinic because of persistent chest pain had undergone a lot of cardiac and gastrointestinal investigations. Clearly, these conditions are important to rule out. Examination was able to reproduce his chest pain precisely by palpation of the mid-thoracic zygapophyseal joints. Careful observation and monitoring of his response to treatment confirmed this source of pain.

Continue to examine the patient thoroughly even if one abnormality has been found as there may be a combination of factors contributing to the current problem. A 65-year-old retired executive had an obvious clinical case of rupture of the proximal head of biceps. He functioned well but complained of persisting shoulder pain while sleeping. Examination revealed wasting of the infraspinatus and weakness of shoulder external rotation. Ultrasound confirmed a torn rotator cuff that may, or may not, have predated his biceps rupture. A strengthening program focused on the rotator cuff relieved his shoulder pain. This illustrates that although Occam's razor (to minimize the assumptions, i.e. aim to link symptoms to one diagnosis rather than multiple) is generally valid, and an extremely valuable medical principle, there can be exceptions.

The routine physical examination is not a very sensitive test for pain in athletic individuals, particularly elite performers. This is particularly true in ballet dancers and gymnasts. The diagnosis of a large central lumbar disk herniation was overlooked for months in a principal dancer with calf pain as he had 'full' flexion and 'normal' straight leg raise on examination. However, he was unable to lift his partners and, on closer examination, his straight leg raise was significantly reduced for him, although still greater than that for most patients. Thus, functional testing is an essential part of the examination, particularly if it is not possible to reproduce the patient's pain otherwise. If a patient has exercise-associated leg pain that only comes on after running, or riding, he or she should be encouraged to come to the consultation prepared to reproduce the pain by undertaking the activity.

Reassess the results of investigations

If an investigation provides a false negative result or is not interpreted correctly, it may lead to prolonged misdiagnosis.[1] Thus, practitioners must be prepared to re-examine investigation results, or repeat tests, where clinical suspicion demands. A 25-year-old woman with a classic longstanding history of traumatic rupture of her rotator cuff had undergone an ultrasound scan by very skilled ultrasound technicians that was reported correctly by the radiologist as being normal. Upon presentation as a patient with longstanding symptoms, MRI was performed, which revealed a full thickness tear of the cuff. Furthermore, it is possible for radiologists to miss subtle diagnoses, particularly if the clinical notes are brief or inaccurate. Remember that the radiologist may have over 60 images to examine for each MRI of the knee, or over 20 slices of a spine. If the clinical picture suggests that imaging should reveal an abnormality, the films should be reviewed, and there are countless examples where this has provided the solution for a patient with significant symptoms.

Consider appropriate tests that have not yet been performed. A 40-year-old retired ballet dancer had had years of shooting medial ankle pain that had been attributed to ankle osteoarthritis and investigated with X-ray and bone scan, both of which were consistent with early osteoarthritis. However, these appearances are not uncommon in former dancers. Careful clinical evaluation suggested the possibility of tarsal tunnel syndrome and nerve conduction tests confirmed the diagnosis.

Because of the wonderful advances that MRI has brought, there is a danger of accepting the myth that a normal MRI scan rules out an abnormality of any kind. The practitioner must remember that MRI will not detect most nerve-related abnormalities, such as referred pain or nerve entrapments. For example, MRI of the groin will be normal if the pain comes from obturator neuropathy.[2] Tendon dislocations and joint subluxations will appear normal if the MRI is performed when the tissue is enlocated. There are also technical aspects of MRI windowing and sequence selection that can cause abnormalities to escape detection. On balance, MRI provides much very useful diagnostic information but, as with all imaging, the clinician and the radiologist should collaborate to optimize the outcome for the patient.

Treatment

In some cases of longstanding symptoms, the diagnosis appears straightforward but the patient does not benefit from treatment. In these cases, the experienced practitioner will:

- ensure that the diagnosis is correct (and not combined with another abnormality)
- review details of the past treatment
- attempt to elicit the underlying cause of the problem
- consider a broad range of treatment options
- resist the temptation to resort to surgical intervention unless the indications for surgery are met.

Be sure the diagnosis is correct

Some conditions that can be easily misdiagnosed are listed in Table 36.1. On some occasions, patients are presumed to have a straightforward case of the condition listed as an 'obvious' diagnosis when they

Table 36.1 Some conditions that are not what they appear at first

'Obvious' diagnosis	True diagnosis
Migraine headache	Upper cervical zygapophyseal joint hypomobility
Rotator cuff tendinopathy	Glenohumeral joint instability (in the younger athlete) Acromioclavicular joint osteoarthritis (in the older athlete)
Tennis elbow	Cervical disk abnormality
Wrist 'tendinitis'	Cervical abnormality
Hip osteoarthritis	Upper lumbar spine disk degeneration
Persistent hamstring strain	Abnormal neural tension
Patellofemoral pain/knee osteoarthritis	Referred pain from hip
Bucket handle tear of the meniscus	Referred pain from a ruptured L4–5 disk
Patellar dislocation	Anterior cruciate ligament rupture
Osgood-Schlatter lesion (Chapter 40)	Osteoid osteoma tibial tuberosity
'Shin splints' (periostitis, tendinopathy)	Chronic compartment syndrome or stress fracture
Achilles tendinopathy	Posterior impingement Retrocalcaneal bursitis
Plantar fasciitis	Medial plantar nerve entrapment
Morton's neuroma	Referred pain from an L5–S1 disk prolapse

actually are suffering from the condition listed in the second column of the table.

Is there a persisting cause?

Assuming the diagnosis is correct, the practitioner must ask why the condition occurred. Persistent biomechanical problems are often culprits (Chapter 5). Examples of biomechanical errors that prevent treatment from being successful are given in Table 36.2.

Obtain details of treatment

The practitioner must discover the specific details of treatment. Even though Achilles tendinopathy may

Table 36.2 Common biomechanical causes of persistent symptoms

Symptom	Biomechanical fault that may be present
Shoulder pain in a volleyball player	Poor scapular stability
Shoulder pain in a swimmer	Limited trunk rotation
Elbow pain in a throwing athlete	Letting the elbow 'hang' because of trunk and lower limb weakness
Back pain in a tennis player	Failing to control lumbar hyperextension when serving
Anterior knee pain in a runner	Vastus medialis wasting and poor gluteal control of the pelvis (this might be best seen on a video of the athlete running)
Shin pain in ballet dancer	'Forcing turnout'—excessive tibial external rotation in an attempt to improve lower leg alignment
Achilles tendinopathy in a runner	Excessive rear foot varus that needs to be corrected with orthoses

have been treated many times, this does not guarantee that the appropriate eccentric strength training has been prescribed. We have seen many patients with tendinopathies whose treatment regimens have included ultrasound therapy, laser, shortwave diathermy, interferential stimulation, ice, heat and rest but whose strength training was limited to 10 concentric exercises once daily.

For example, a 30-year-old patient presented 18 months after having undergone a patellar lateral release procedure and chondroplasty (shaving the articular cartilage of the patella) for anterior knee pain. Her pain was similar to her preoperative pain but more intense. The indication for surgery had been 'failed conservative management', which had included patellar taping and an exercise program. Close questioning revealed that her pain had never been relieved by taping and that she had been unable to comply with the strengthening program because of persistent pain. A different therapist re-evaluated the patient and trialed various combinations of taping (Chapter 28) until the patient could perform a few single-leg step-downs without pain. The patient then undertook the knee and proximal core strengthening program and was totally pain-free at two months. At two-year follow-up she remained pain-free in daily life and had returned to her favorite sport—aerobics. The key to success was the time the therapist spent to experiment with various tape patterns until one proved successful. This case report demonstrates that the details of past therapy must be known so that appropriate treatments can be prescribed.

Similarly, many patients have had their backs 'treated' but never received targeted manual mobilization of hypomobile joints combined with an adequate lumbar stabilization program. This is particularly the

case in those countries where high-quality manual therapy is not readily available.

Make the multidisciplinary team available

A therapy that is commonly overlooked is that of soft tissue massage. The acceptance of and evidence base for massage is, fortunately, growing, and many patients with chronic musculoskeletal pain have benefited from deep, focused soft tissue therapy combined with an appropriate rehabilitation program. Treatment modalities such as trigger point therapy and prolotherapy may be indicated for specific patients. Rehabilitation may need to include exercise programs such as the Pilates' method, Feldenkrais, the Alexander method and forms of yoga or Tai Chi.

Appropriate referral

The sports medicine clinician can make a valuable contribution by referring to specific professionals who may have particular areas of expertise. If surgery is indicated, referral to a surgeon particularly experienced in that problem is preferable to referral to a generalist. Sports clinicians need to be familiar with a range of experts, including: pain management practitioners; someone who is very familiar with complex regional pain syndrome type 1; a rheumatologist who understands sports medicine; and a physiotherapist who is particularly adroit with the elderly or with the young athlete.

Summary

This chapter deals with a difficult presentation that is frustrating for patient and clinician. We believe that taking the time to acknowledge the genuine nature of the patient's problem, obtaining a thorough history and performing a detailed physical examination all contribute to patients realizing that they are being cared for. If the clinician reviews all the material at hand, he or she may discover a flaw in the assumption that has underpinned diagnosis or treatment to date.

Critical review of the investigations may suggest formal review of previous images or further investigations. To discover why treatment has been unsuccessful may require critical biomechanical assessment and a detailed analysis of what has already taken place. Broad consultation with multidisciplinary colleagues may provide novel insights and modern-day technologies mean that national and international experts can be readily consulted.

Recommended Reading

Kasper DL, Braunwald E, Fauci AS, et al., eds. The practice of medicine. In: *Harrison's Principles of Internal Medicine*. 16th edn. New York: McGraw-Hill, 2005: 1–5.

References

1. Khan KM, Tress BW, Hare WSC, et al. 'Treat the patient, not the X-ray': advances in diagnostic imaging do not replace the need for clinical interpretation. *Clin J Sport Med* 1998; 8: 1–4.
2. Bradshaw C, McCrory P, Bell S, et al. Obturator nerve entrapment. A cause of groin pain in athletes. *Am J Sports Med* 1997; 25: 402–8.

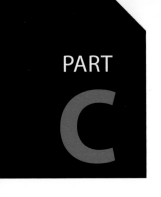

PART

C

Enhancing Sport Performance

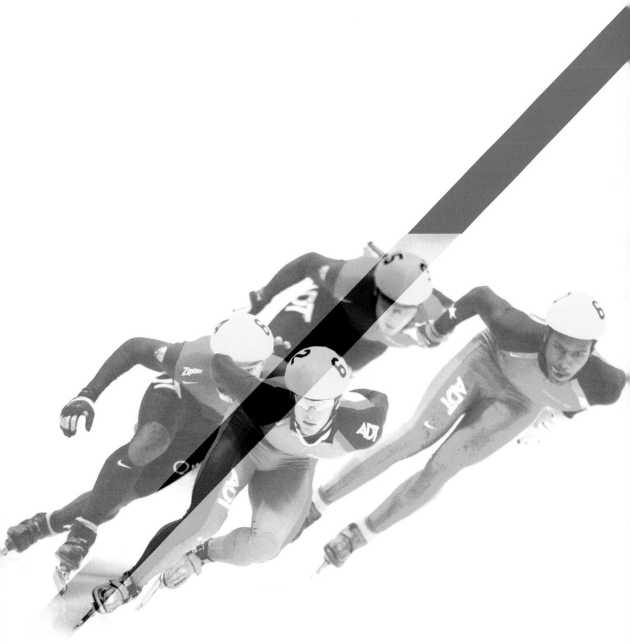

Maximizing Sporting Performance: Nutrition

WITH KAREN INGE AND LISA SUTHERLAND

> I wasn't feeling well in the first half. I felt down, man. I had three slices of pizza before the game and the food took me down.
>
> *Leroy Loggins, professional basketball player*

Nutrition is an important component of good health and of sporting performance. Optimum nutrition may help maximize athletic performance by:

- maximizing energy stores
- achieving ideal weight for performance
- ensuring sufficient intake of vitamins and minerals
- maintaining adequate hydration
- optimizing pre-competition and competition food intake.

Nutrition also plays a crucial role in aiding recovery from intense training and this was discussed in Chapter 6.

Maximizing energy stores

In this section we discuss carbohydrates and fats—the major fuels. Protein is discussed in the next section.

Carbohydrates and fats

Carbohydrate and fat are the two main sources of energy used in athletic activity.[1] Protein makes a relatively small contribution, which becomes more significant with the depletion of carbohydrate stores and inadequate energy intake.

Carbohydrate is stored in the liver and skeletal muscle in the form of glycogen. When required for energy, glycogen is released and broken down to provide the glucose necessary for energy. Glycogen stores are limited and need to be replenished daily.[2] The average amount of energy available from stored carbohydrate is only 8.4 MJ (2000 kcal), which would provide fuel for a run of approximately 40 km (25 miles). Endurance training increases the capacity of the muscles to store glycogen.[3] Untrained individuals have muscle glycogen stores of 80–90 mmol/kg, whereas trained individuals may have muscle stores as high as 130–135 mmol/kg.

Fat provides the body's largest store of potential energy. The energy storage capacity of fat is more than twice the equivalent quantity of carbohydrate or protein. Body fat content varies considerably from athlete to athlete. However, even the leanest athlete, who may have only 7 kg of body fat, would have enough energy stored as fat to run 1200 km (750 miles).

The fuel the body uses depends on the intensity and the duration of the exercise as well as the fitness and nutritional status of the individual.

Fuel for short duration/high-intensity exercise

In high-intensity exercise of short duration (1–2 minutes), almost all energy is supplied from glycogen stored in skeletal muscle.[4, 5] Carbohydrate is the only nutrient that provides energy when the muscles have insufficient oxygen for their needs. This type of exercise is called anaerobic exercise (Chapter 6) and produces lactic acid. Lactic acid impedes the mobilization of fat from adipose tissue, further increasing the reliance of muscles on glycogen as their supply of fuel.

Fat does not provide a significant fuel source during periods of high-intensity exercise; its breakdown is too slow to meet the athlete's needs.

Fuel for long duration/moderate-intensity exercise

Fat supplies a much higher proportion of energy in exercise of low-to-moderate intensity. During moderate exercise, increases in serum adrenalin (epinephrine) and growth hormone and decreases in insulin promote the release of free fatty acids from adipose tissue into the bloodstream. The longer the time spent exercising, the greater the contribution of fat as a fuel.

Fat may supply as much as 70% of the energy needs for exercise of moderate intensity lasting 4–6 hours. Endurance training increases the capacity of the aerobic pathway in the mitochondria to break down fat for energy and preserve glycogen. This delays the depletion of glycogen.

An important role of the athlete's diet is to supply sufficient carbohydrate to fill the glycogen storage sites in muscle.

 The ideal training diet for athletes, especially endurance athletes, requires 60–70% of energy to be taken in as carbohydrate and less than 30% as fat. This intake has considerably more carbohydrate and less fat than the average Western diet. To ensure an adequate carbohydrate intake, the estimated requirement should be based on grams per kilogram of body weight per day. For endurance athletes or athletes undertaking strenuous training sessions exceeding 90 minutes, a daily carbohydrate intake of between 8 and 10 g/kg of body weight is required for repletion of glycogen stores.

To replenish glycogen stores on a daily basis, following depletion by strenuous exercise, athletes should eat 1–1.2 g/kg per hour of carbohydrate for up to 4 hours after exercise depending on the level of depletion. In the short term, the sooner the carbohydrate is ingested after exercise, the more effective is the replenishment of glycogen stores. Unless there is adequate daily replenishment, glycogen stores eventually deplete. This glycogen depletion may present clinically as excessive fatigue, a feeling of sluggishness, heavy legs, staleness or an inability to maintain normal training intensity (Chapter 52). An 80 kg endurance athlete with a carbohydrate requirement of 8 g/kg of body weight per day requires 640 g of carbohydrate per day. This requires a high-carbohydrate diet. The carbohydrate content of common foods is given in Table 37.1 (this is also available as a downloadable PDF file at <www.clinicalsportsmedicine.com>). Some athletes can find it difficult to eat enough carbohydrate to replenish their stores and may benefit from consuming carbohydrates in liquid form (Table 37.2).

Glycemic index—a way of differentiating carbohydrates

In the past, carbohydrate-rich foods were categorized as simple (refined) carbohydrate, such as sugars, or complex (unrefined) carbohydrate, such as starches. However, these categories do not indicate how food is broken down and absorbed by the body. A more informative way to differentiate carbohydrates is by their glycemic index (GI). This is a ranking of the effect of carbohydrate-containing foods on blood sugar levels. Foods with a high GI (Table 37.3, this is also available as a downloadable PDF file at <www.clinicalsportsmedicine.com>) are quickly digested and absorbed into the bloodstream, resulting in a rapid and high rise in blood sugar levels. High GI carbohydrates are often recommended as a quickly digested and absorbed carbohydrate to be consumed during exercise and for immediate recovery post-exercise. Low GI foods are more slowly digested and result in a slower but continuous release of glucose into the blood. Low GI carbohydrates may be preferable for more sustained energy release and satiety effects, however, research is inconclusive and the total amount of carbohydrate consumed may be the most important factor for prolonged endurance exercise performance.

Protein—a fuel

The major role of protein for athletes is to repair and build muscle tissue. Protein can also be used as a fuel, although the contribution to energy production is generally small, contributing between 5% and 10% of total energy needs. Energy is obtained from the breakdown of dietary and tissue protein to amino acids, which are then converted to glucose. The contribution of protein to total energy increases with the duration of exercise and with depletion of carbohydrate stores.[6, 7]

The protein requirements of the endurance athlete, therefore, are considerably higher than those for the sedentary individual. The recommended daily intake (RDI) of protein for a sedentary person is 0.8 g/kg per day. The protein requirements for an endurance athlete are approximately 1.2–1.7 g/kg per day, with the higher levels required by athletes undertaking strenuous training.[8, 9] A 60 kg endurance athlete in heavy training would, therefore, require about 96 g of protein per day. The protein content of common foods is shown in Table 37.4 (this is also available as a downloadable PDF file at <www.clinicalsportsmedicine.com>).

Table 37.1 Carbohydrate content of foods

Food	Amount	Weight (g)	Energy (g)	Energy (kJ/kcal)	Carbohydrate (g)	Fiber (g)
Bread, wholemeal (whole-wheat)	1 slice	30	280	280 (67)	12	2
Bread roll, wholemeal	½ slice	30	300	301 (72)	13	2
Bread, pita	30 g	30	340	330 (80)	16	1
Muffin, English	1 half	40	330	330 (80)	15	1
Crumpet	1 average	50	390	389 (93)	20	2
Biscuit, plain	2 biscuits	20	270	272 (65)	13	1
Biscuit, plain, sweet	2 biscuits	17	320	318 (76)	12	0
Rice cakes	1½ cakes	19	290	288 (69)	15	1
Oats, rolled, cooked	¾ cup	195	410	414 (99)	17	3
Processed bran	½ cup	35	410	401 (96)	14	11
Weet-Bix	1½ biscuits	26	340	339 (81)	16	3
Vita Brits	1½ biscuits	26	340	339 (81)	16	3
Weeties	½ cup	25	350	351 (84)	17	3
Muesli, flakes	½ cup	22	350	351 (84)	15	1
Rice, brown, boiled	⅓ cup	60	370	368 (88)	19	1
Pasta, white, boiled	½ cup	75	370	372 (89)	18	1
Barley, pearl, boiled	½ cup	90	400	401 (96)	19	3
Potato, pale skin, baked	1 medium	100	310	305 (73)	15	1
Sweet potato, peeled, boiled	⅓ cup	71	220	217 (52)	12	1
Sweet corn, frozen, on cob	⅓ cup	48	190	188 (45)	8	2
Pea, green, boiled	1 cup	165	340	330 (80)	11	11
Parsnip, peeled, boiled	1 cup	150	310	314 (75)	15	4
Beetroot, peeled, boiled	6 slices	180	310	309 (74)	15	5
Turnip, white, peeled, boiled	1½ cup	360	320	322 (77)	14	11
Lentil, boiled	½ cup	105	310	309 (74)	10	4
Bean, kidney, fresh, boiled	½ cup	83	400	397 (95)	12	9
Bean, haricot/cannellini, boiled	½ cup	86	220	330 (80)	11	8
Salad bean, commercial	⅓ cup	63	380	376 (90)	15	3
Soup, bean, lentil, homemade	150 g	150	530	527 (126)	15	3
Potato and leek soup	300 g	300	370	364 (87)	14	2
Soup, medium, canned/ homemade	1 cup	264	420	418 (100)	17	1
Soup, light vegetable, canned	2 cups	528	520	523 (125)	18	3
Minestrone soup	300 g	300	280	280 (67)	13	4
Apple, golden delicious	1 average	123	220	221 (53)	13	2
Apricot, fresh, raw	3 medium	180	280	280 (67)	13	4
Banana, raw, peeled	½ average	50	200	200 (48)	12	1

continues

Table 37.1 Carbohydrate content of foods *continued*

Food	Amount	Weight (g)	Energy (g)	Energy (kJ/kcal)	Carbohydrate (g)	Fiber (g)
Cherry, raw	25 medium	100	210	209 (50)	11	2
Custard apple, raw, peeled	¼ medium	120	360	360 (86)	19	3
Fig, raw	4 pieces	160	270	267 (64)	13	4
Fig, dried	2 pieces	30	290	288 (69)	16	4
Grape, green sultana, raw	30 average	90	220	217 (52)	13	1
Kiwifruit, raw, peeled	2 medium	160	320	318 (76)	15	5
Melon, honeydew, raw	1 whole	240	320	318 (76)	16	2
Mango, raw, peeled	1 small	100	240	234 (56)	13	2
Mandarin, raw, peeled	3 whole	183	300	297 (71)	15	4
Nectarine, raw	3 medium	220	350	347 (83)	17	5
Orange, Valencia, raw	1 whole	160	240	242 (58)	12	3
Juice, orange, unsweetened	1 glass	204	290	288 (69)	16	1
Pear, Williams, raw, unpeeled	1 average	130	260	255 (61)	15	3
Peach, raw, unpeeled	2 medium	174	230	230 (55)	11	2
Peach, canned, in pear juice	⅔ cup	170	290	288 (69)	16	2
Tangerine, raw, peeled	2 large	200	200	200 (48)	10	4
Watermelon, raw, peeled	1½ cup	293	280	280 (67)	15	2
Milk, skim	1½ glasses	300	430	427 (102)	15	0
Milk, whole	1½ glasses	300	520	816 (195)	14	0
Yoghurt, low-fat, natural	1 tub	200	440	439 (105)	12	0
Ice-cream, vanilla	1½ scoops	67	570	569 (136)	14	0

Source: Nutlab 95. Canberra: Australian Government Publishing Service, 1995.

Table 37.2 Liquid carbohydrate supplements

Source	Amount	Carbohydrate (g)
Orange juice, 100% unsweetened	200 mL	15
Soft drink (pop)	200 mL	24
Low-fat milk	200 mL	11
Glucose powder	2 tspn	11
Polycose	1 tbsp	15
Ensure Plus	264 mL	47
Sustagen Sport	1 tbsp	13
Sustagen Gold	250 mL	35
Gatorade	200 mL	12

Source: Nutlab 95. Canberra: Australian Government Publishing Service, 1995.

Table 37.3 A guide to the glycemic index (GI)[a] of foods

Food group	Low GI	Intermediate GI	High GI
Breakfast cereals	All Bran Muesli Oats Porridge Special K Guardian	Mini Wheat Nutrigrain Sustain Vita Brits Weet-Bix	Coco Pops Corn Flakes Puffed Wheat Rice Bubbles Sultana Bran
Breads	Fruit loaf Grain Pumpernickel	Croissant Crumpet Pita Wholemeal (whole wheat)	Bagel Rye White
Crackers	Jatz	Ryvita Sao	Kavli Puffed crispbread Water crackers
Grains	Buckwheat Bulgur	Taco shells	
Rice	Doongara	Basmati	Calrose Brown Long grain
Pasta	Instant noodles Egg fettucine Ravioli Spaghetti Vermicelli		
Sweet biscuits	Oatmeal	Arrowroot Shredded Wheat Shortbread	Morning Coffee
Cakes	Apple muffin Banana cake Sponge cake		Waffles
Snack foods	Peanuts Potato crisps Chocolate	Popcorn Mars Bar Muesli bar	Corn chips Jelly beans Life Savers
Vegetables	Carrots Peas Sweet corn Sweet potato Yam	Beetroot New potato Pontiac potato	Parsnip Baked potato French fries Pumpkin Swede
Legumes	Baked beans Butter beans Chick peas Haricot beans Kidney beans Lentils Soya beans		Broad beans

continues

Table 37.3 A guide to the glycemic index (GI)[a] of foods *continued*

Food group	Low GI	Intermediate GI	High GI
Fruit	Apple Apricot (dried) Cherries Grapefruit Grapes Kiwifruit Orange Peach Pear Plum	Banana Mango Pawpaw Pineapple Raisins Rockmelon (cantaloupe) Sultanas	Watermelon
Dairy foods	Milk Flavored milk Ice-cream Yoghurt		
Drinks	Apple juice Orange juice	Cordial, soft drink (pop)	Lucozade

(a) GI ratio ranges: low GI foods, below 55; intermediate GI foods, 55–70; high GI foods, more than 70.

Table 37.4 Protein content of foods

Food	Amount	Weight (g)	Energy (kJ)	Energy (kcal)	Protein (g)
Milk, skim	1 cup	259	380	90	9
Milk, reduced fat	1 cup	260	540	129	10
Milk, whole	1 cup	258	700	167	9
Yoghurt, low-fat, natural	1 tub	200	450	108	12
Yoghurt, low-fat, flavored	1 tub	200	630	151	10
Yoghurt, flavored/fruit	1 tub	200	810	193	10
Cheese, cheddar	1 slice	20	340	81	5
Cheese, ricotta	20 g	20	120	29	2
Cheese, cottage, low-fat	20 g	20	75	18	4
Cheese, camembert	20 g	20	260	62	4
Cheese, cream	1 tbsp	20	280	67	2
Ice-cream, vanilla	600 g	600	480	114	3
Beef, fillet steak, lean	120 g	120	990	235	36
Chicken, boneless, baked, lean	120 g	120	940	224	34
Turkey, breast, baked, lean	120 g	120	780	186	35
Pork, boneless, cooked, lean	120 g	120	850	204	37
Ham, non-canned, lean and fat	1 slice	25	150	36	4
Lamb, boneless, cooked, lean	120 g	120	940	225	37
Fish, steamed	150 g	150	780	187	36
Oysters, raw	1 dozen	60	180	44	7

continues

Table 37.4 Protein content of foods *continued*

Food	Amount	Weight (g)	Energy (kJ)	Energy (kcal)	Protein (g)
Prawns, king, cooked	100 g	100	440	104	24
Egg, whole, hard-boiled	1 medium	47	300	71	6
Muesli flakes	1 cup	43	690	164	4
Weet-Bix	2 biscuits	30	400	95	3
Corn Flakes	1 cup	30	470	113	2
Bread, wholemeal (whole wheat)	1 slice	30	280	67	3
Rice cakes	1 serve	13	190	46	1
Crispbread, rye	1 biscuit	8	100	24	1
Biscuit, plain, dry	10 g	10	140	33	1
Potato, baked flesh	1 medium	100	310	73	3
Rice, brown, boiled	½ cup	90	570	135	3
Pasta, white, boiled	½ cup	75	370	89	3
Sweet corn, frozen, on cob	½ cup	80	440	106	2
Pea, green, boiled	½ cup	83	170	40	4
Broccoli, boiled	1 cup	152	150	37	7
Bean, green, boiled	1 cup	140	100	23	2
Apple, raw, unpeeled	1 medium	120	250	59	0
Pear, yellow-green, raw, unpeeled	1 medium	150	320	76	0
Orange, raw, peeled	1 medium	120	190	45	1
Banana, raw, peeled	1 average	140	420	100	2
Rockmelon (cantaloupe), raw, peeled	½ whole	120	110	26	1
Grape, green sultana	30 average	90	230	55	1
Brazil nut	20 g	20	560	133	3
Cashew nut	20 g	20	480	115	3
Almonds, unsalted	20 g	20	470	112	3
Peanuts, roasted, salted	20 g	20	520	124	5
Baked beans, canned in sauce	1 cup	272	775	185	13
Lentils, boiled	1 cup	211	620	148	14
Beans, kidney, fresh, boiled	200 g	200	960	229	26

Source: Nutlab 95. Canberra: Australian Government Publishing Service, 1995.

The combination of appropriate resistance training and adequate protein intake is essential to achieve muscle hypertrophy. The protein requirement of strength-training athletes is about 1.2–1.7 g/kg per day.[10, 11] An 80 kg strength-training athlete would, therefore, require about 96–136 g of protein per day.

The average Western diet contains a level of protein greater than 1 g/kg per day. The protein requirements of most athletes are usually met if 12–15% of total energy needs are provided by protein.

 It is important that the athlete also has an adequate carbohydrate and overall energy intake.

Some groups of athletes may be at risk of an inadequate protein intake. These include children and adolescents, lactating and pregnant women, and vegetarians. Vegetarians eating a narrow range of incomplete protein foods may be particularly at risk. Athletes on low-energy diets, those with multiple daily training sessions and those on very-high-carbohydrate diets may also be at risk of inadequate protein intake.

Achieving ideal body weight for performance

Many athletes attempt to alter their body composition, either by trying to put on weight (usually in the form of muscle) or by losing weight (usually in the form of fat). Certain sports require athletes to have large amounts of muscle mass. These include power events such as sprinting, throwing, weightlifting, power lifting and various football codes (soccer, Australian Rules, Rugby, American, Canadian). Some groups of athletes are required to be a particular weight to compete, such as lightweight rowers, boxers, martial arts exponents and jockeys. Other sports require extremely low body fat levels, such as gymnastics, distance running and ballet.

Therefore, accurate assessment of body composition is necessary in certain athletes. We note, however, that some coaches associate a certain percentage body fat level with improved performance, and that is not necessarily the case once the athlete has a healthy body composition for the sport. Each athlete needs to be aware of his or her own ideal body composition for performance.

Assessment of body composition

To assess body composition, the structural components of the body—muscle, bone and fat—are measured. Height and weight indices such as body mass index (BMI) are considered reasonable tools for predicting obesity in the general population; however, they are of little use for athletes as they do not provide reliable information about the relative composition of an individual's body.

Underwater or hydrostatic weighing has been used extensively in the assessment of body composition but has been shown to be inaccurate for certain groups in the community, in particular, young athletes. This method is susceptible to error due to variations in bone density.

In the clinical setting, the most practical method of obtaining information regarding body fat levels in athletes is skin-fold measurements. However, to minimize error, this should be used as the sum of skin folds from various standardized sites, rather than any

attempt made to predict percentage body fat from the skin-fold measurements.

The seven standard sites are shown in Figure 37.1. An example of average and range of skin-fold measurements for different sports is shown in Table 37.5. The sum of skin folds provides a reasonable estimation of body fat percentage and allows monitoring of changes. More sophisticated methods of measuring body composition, including MRI and dual-energy X-ray absorptiometry (DEXA), are available as research tools.

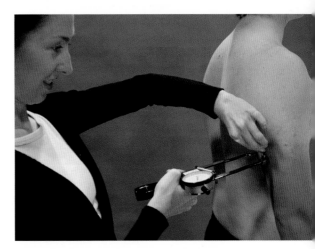

Figure 37.1 Examples of sites of skin-fold measurements

(a) Triceps—a vertical fold is raised on the midline of the posterior surface of the right arm

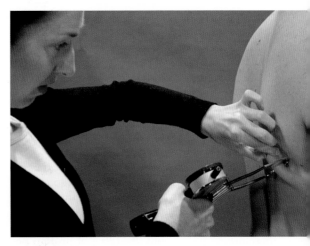

(b) Subscapular—the skin fold is raised just below and to the right of the inferior angle of the right scapula in the natural fold that runs obliquely downwards

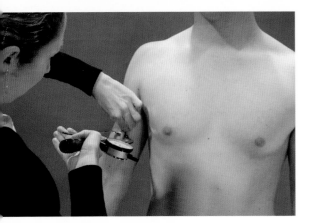

(c) Biceps—the fold is raised at the midline of the anterior surface of the right arm

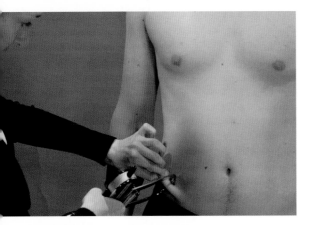

(d) Supraspinale—the site is located level with the undersurface of the tip of the anterior superior iliac spine. The natural fold is raised obliquely

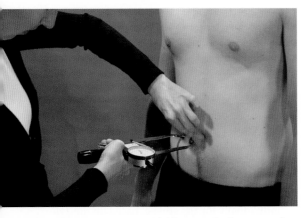

(e) Abdomen—a vertical fold is raised adjacent to the right of the umbilicus so that all the subcutaneous fat is raised parallel to the fold

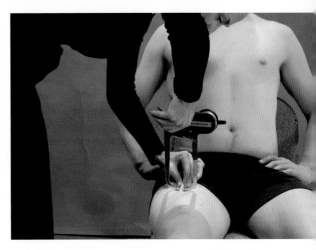

(f) Anterior thigh—the site is located halfway between the crease at the top of the thigh and the top of the kneecaps. The athlete is usually seated. The skin fold is grasped parallel to the long axis of the femur

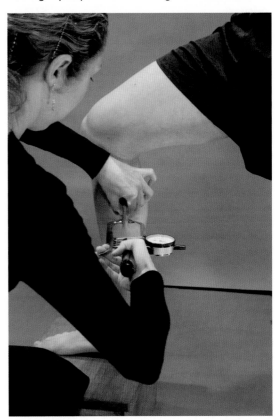

(g) Medial calf—the fold is grasped on the inner side of the calf where the muscle bulk is greatest. The athlete places the foot on a box or chair so that the knee is flexed at right angles

Table 37.5 Approximate mean (and range) of skin-fold measurements in elite athletes of various sports[a]

Sport	Men (mm)[a]	Women (mm)[a]
Basketball (guard/forward)	67 (45–100)	77 (41–132)
Cycling	54 (26–85)	62 (34–90)
Gymnastics	42 (28–60)	38 (27–58)
Hockey (field)	59 (38–108)	88 (48–140)
Rowing		
Lightweight	45 (36–65)	73 (55–105)
Heavyweight	67 (46–111)	88 (61–119)
Skiing		
Alpine	51 (31–82)	59 (31–87)
Nordic	46 (27–77)	74 (57–108)
Swimming	54 (34–108)	80 (45–155)
Track and field		
Sprint	56 (54–58)	60 (45–84)
Middle distance	39 (26–68)	59 (37–111)
Triathlon	40 (28–60)	56 (34–89)
Volleyball	57 (37–80)	91 (36–148)
Weightlifting	75 (34–190)	Not available
Water polo	70 (36–120)	96 (46–161)

(a) Sum of seven skin folds = triceps, subscapular, biceps, supraspinale, abdominal, anterior thigh, medial calf.
Adapted from Kerr D, Ackland T. Kinanthropometry: physique assessment of the athlete. In: Burke LM, Deakin V, eds. *Clinical Sports Nutrition*. 3rd edn. Sydney: McGraw-Hill, 2006: 53–72.

Skin-fold measurements are used particularly to monitor an individual's body fat status. For example, a trained anthropometrist can measures skin folds if there is concern regarding body composition, such as during attempted body fat reduction or while injured with reduced activity levels.

Dietary regimens for weight loss

Athletes may adhere to weight-reduction dietary regimens both for immediate weight loss prior to competition and for maintenance over a competitive season. Weight loss programs may incorporate diet only, or a combination of diet, weight loss aids and exercise. Many popular programs have the potential to compromise nutritional status, performance and overall health.

High-protein/low-carbohydrate diets such as the Zone diet and 'Dr Atkins' diet have been popular in recent years. These diets were formulated on the hypothesis that carbohydrate-rich foods rather than protein contribute most to increased body fat levels. Such diets, however, do not serve athletes well for several reasons. When protein intake is increased and carbohydrate intake decreased, the body responds by breaking down glycogen stores and by losing water. In addition, a loss of lean muscle tissue reduces metabolic rate and performance. This causes weight loss but not necessarily fat loss. Loss of glycogen and fluid from the body results in the athlete feeling tired, with subsequent delayed recovery from training and poor performance.[12]

Athletes in weight-dependent sports will often resort to strict dieting or complete fasting in an attempt to lose weight rapidly before 'weigh-in'. This usually causes weight loss but fluid, glycogen and lean muscle are also sacrificed in the process. The athlete is left tired and unable to perform optimally. In the long term the athlete who fasts may find it increasingly difficult to achieve and maintain a low body weight due to a reduction in basal metabolic rate.

Guidelines to help distinguish a sensible weight reduction program from a 'fad diet' include:

1. A safe weight loss program should be planned individually for the athlete, based on lifestyle and medical history.
2. A sensible program should meet dietary requirements from a wide variety of foods

from all the food groups rather than relying on vitamin and mineral supplementation.

3. A realistic goal for weight loss (approximately 0.5–1.0 kg per week) should be aimed for. Greater weight losses indicate a loss of fluid and lean muscle tissue in addition to body fat.

4. Information on outcomes from the program should be presented in a factual and specific manner rather than via anecdotes and testimonials.

5. Permanent weight loss is achieved through gradual but lifelong changes. Avoid programs that promise dramatic results or guarantee fast success.

6. Check that the program has been developed or recommended by a person qualified in the area of sports nutrition (e.g. sports dietitian).

Other methods of weight control

Appetite suppressants

These are the most common of the 'slimming pills' available and act to reduce hunger or give a feeling of being full with the aim of stopping the user from eating. Many of these pills have side-effects ranging from dry mouth, anxiety, insomnia and gastro-intestinal disturbances to headaches, drowsiness and nausea. These effects impair performance. The aim of these pills is to reduce the volume of food eaten and hence decrease kilojoule intake. In many cases, this means a reduction in nutrients such as carbohydrate and vitamins essential for maintaining energy levels. Appetite generally returns when the athlete stops using the pills, with a resultant increase in weight and body fat. Many of these pills are banned by the International Olympic Committee (Chapter 61).

Diuretics

Diuretics promote the excretion of water and salts by the kidneys. Thus, athletes use these drugs as a means of rapid weight loss for upcoming competition. The dehydration and electrolyte loss that follows increases the risks of cardiac arrhythmia. Because fat-free mass contains approximately 70% water, weight loss by dehydration occurs at the expense of intracellular and extracellular fluid. As a result, muscle endurance and work capacity are decreased. Even moderate dehydration will adversely affect muscular endurance. Diuretics are also on the International Olympic Committee's list of banned substances (Chapter 61).

Saunas

As with the use of diuretics, the result of sitting in a sauna is a loss of fluid rather than a reduction in body fat levels. Athletes and coaches should be strongly discouraged from employing methods of weight reduction involving dehydration.

The safe way to lose body fat

There are a number of considerations when planning a weight loss program—including whether or not the athlete has fat weight to lose! Let us illustrate our approach with a case history.

A 25-year-old professional footballer wants to lose body fat before the competitive season begins. His sum of seven skin-fold measurements is 90 mm, height is 185 cm and weight is 98 kg. In addition to football, he works part-time as a sales representative. He shares a house with two friends; however, they all do their own cooking and shopping. A brief dietary history revealed a typical daily intake, shown below.

Suboptimal diet

Breakfast

1 cup of coffee with milk

Mid morning

1 toasted cheese and ham sandwich

Lunch

1 white salad roll with ham and cheese, or
    1 hamburger
1 piece of fruit

Mid afternoon

1 medium chocolate bar

After training

'lots of water'

Dinner

2–3 glasses of beer
Steak or chops fried in pan, large serve
Boiled vegetables
Two scoops of ice-cream
or
Fast-food/telephone orders
    fish and chips
    1 medium pizza
    spaghetti carbonara

After dinner

Often potato crisps and/or chocolate bar
1 can soft drink (pop)

Analysis of this athlete's diet revealed a number of problems.

High fat intake

Many of the foods consumed are high in fat. The diet included obvious fats, such as margarine on sandwiches or toast and oil or butter used in cooking, but also 'hidden fats', such as those found in fatty meats, chocolate, potato crisps and deep-fried foods. By eliminating much of this fat, the athlete could increase the quantities of food he is consuming and still lose weight as his total energy intake will have been reduced.

Carbohydrate intake

The diet contains limited sources of low GI carbohydrates, with most carbohydrates coming from refined flour products and sugar. The athlete needs education regarding the GI of different foods and needs to be encouraged to space intake of low GI carbohydrates over the day. His energy levels were quite low; therefore smart carbohydrate choices will ensure that his training and recovery improves.

Lack of dietary fiber

Many of the athlete's food choices are foods that are low in dietary fiber. A high fiber diet (more than 30 g per day) is recommended and is particularly important for those attempting to reduce body fat levels. Fiber not only helps protect against diseases of the gastrointestinal tract but also promotes a feeling of satiety, as high-fiber foods often have a low GI. High-fiber foods are often lower in kilojoules and fat, and contain carbohydrate, vitamins and minerals.

Timing of meals

A regular intake of food over the day is the best way of maintaining a high metabolic rate and, hence, effectively controlling body fat levels. The athlete's tendency is to eat little during the day and large quantities of food in the evening when he relaxes. He also found he is still hungry later in the evening and is likely to eat high-fat snacks at this time.

Many athletes find difficulty distributing food intake evenly over the day. Time constraints in the morning and during the day mean that only small quantities of food are consumed at these times. Afternoon snacks are commonly missed if the athlete is training after work or school. All these factors can contribute to overeating at the evening meal. This athlete needs to spread out his food intake evenly, incorporating a high-carbohydrate snack several hours prior to training.

Lack of cooking/food preparation skills

A lack of time and knowledge often results in athletes being ill-equipped to prepare healthy meals at home. One of this athlete's major problems is his limited cooking skills, making food preparation a difficult task. He needs practical education, such as cooking classes, shopping tours and easy recipes. He needs advice on using pre-prepared foods, canned and frozen products and information on healthy choices when eating out or when ordering home-delivered meals.

Fluids

The athlete has two problems with his fluid intake. One is his tendency to dehydrate over the day and during training. The other problem is his choice of fluids. Soft drinks (pop) and alcohol are both significant sources of kilojoules in the diet but neither provides other useful nutrients. Flavored milk contains other vitamins and minerals such as calcium, riboflavin and protein. The athlete should be encouraged to select a low-fat flavored milk or mineral water, iced water, low joule soft drinks and low alcohol beverages.

New plan

A new program was devised for the athlete providing approximately 7500 kJ (1800 kcal), with 60% of energy from carbohydrate, 25% from fats (50 g), 15% from protein (67 g) and 38 g of fiber (see box). He was encouraged to drink plenty of water throughout the day.

Healthy nutritional plan

Breakfast

1 cup wholegrain cereal with ¾ cup of low-fat milk
1 piece fresh fruit (e.g. banana)
1 slice wholegrain or wholemeal (whole wheat) toast spread with 2 tspn jam or honey
1 glass 100% fruit juice

Snack

1 piece fresh fruit

Lunch

2 wholegrain sandwiches/rolls/pita bread each filled with lean meat/low-fat cheese/skinless chicken/turkey/tuna/salmon with plenty of salad
1 serve fresh fruit salad or 1 piece fresh fruit
water, low joule soft drink or plain mineral water

Pre-training snack

1 slice raisin bread, or English muffin
or 1 tub low-fat fruit yogurt
water

Post training

1 banana
water

Dinner

180 g lean meat or skinless poultry or 200 g fish
(cooked without added fats or oils)
1 cup steamed brown rice, or 1 large potato,
or 1½ cups pasta, plenty of vegetables,
including green leafy vegetables (e.g.
broccoli, silverbeet)
water

Guidelines for safe weight loss

1. Aim for a realistic weight loss of 0.5–1.0 kg
   per week. To achieve this requires a daily
   energy intake of 2.1–4.2 MJ below energy
   output.
2. The diet must be nutritionally adequate.
   Deficiencies of essential nutrients will
   compromise performance.
3. Increase complex carbohydrates. At least
   60–65% of total energy intake must come
   from mostly medium and low GI foods
   (Table 37.3) to ensure maximum glycogen
   stores.
4. Fat intake should be reduced.
5. Decrease alcohol intake. Alcohol is high in
   kilojoules, has little nutritional value and
   contributes to dehydration.
6. Regulate food intake. Meals should be spread
   evenly over the day. Skipping meals can lead
   to subsequent overeating and snacking on
   high-fat foods.

Bulking up

Many athletes wish to gain weight. An increase in muscle mass may increase power-to-weight ratio. This may be of advantage to athletes participating in a range of sports such as rowing, sprinting, throwing events, weightlifting, boxing and football.

Methods commonly used by athletes to gain weight

Athletes use a variety of methods in attempts to gain weight.[13]

High protein intake

The RDI of protein for the average person is 0.8 g/kg per day but athletes wishing to bulk up are advised to have a protein intake of 1.2–1.7 g/kg per day. However, a high protein intake will only result in gains in muscle mass if combined with an appropriate strength-training program, appropriate rest/recovery, and adequate carbohydrate consumption.[14, 15]

Protein powders have long been regarded by athletes involved in bodybuilding or strength training as a vital component of the training diet. The composition of protein powders may vary considerably. Many are simply based on skim milk powder with additional vitamins, minerals and certain amino acids. Most athletes can achieve adequate protein intake with a balanced food intake, however, protein powders are often considered a convenient form of protein, and consuming protein in liquid form can be useful for athletes with very high energy requirements or low appetite.

Many athletes wishing to bulk up have protein intakes considerably in excess of the recommended values.[13] There is no evidence that protein intakes two or three times higher than the RDI for athletes have any additional effect on increasing muscle bulk. Many athletes are also unaware that additional protein consumed above energy requirements will be stored as fat, rather than contributing to muscle stores. A high-protein diet may, in fact, indirectly result in inadequate carbohydrate intake, necessitating increased use of protein as a fuel. Excessive protein intake is associated with an increased risk of dehydration, gout and loss of calcium.

Amino acid supplements

Amino acid supplements are used by some athletes in the hope that their use will stimulate protein synthesis and muscle mass through an increase in production of human growth hormone by the pituitary gland.[16] The production of human growth hormone is affected by many factors, including the early phase of sleep, a protein meal, lowering of blood sugar and exercise. There is no evidence that ingestion of amino acids increases production of human growth hormone. If ingesting amino acid supplements did increase human growth hormone levels, there is still no evidence that this would augment muscle strength.

Dietary requirements for the athlete wishing to bulk up

A suitable weight gain diet should include the following:

1. High energy intake. An additional 2900–4200 kJ (700–1000 kcal) per day may be required for gains in lean body mass of 0.5–1 kg per week.
2. For strength athletes, up to 1.6–1.7 g/kg per day of protein is required.
3. 25–30% of energy as fat. In some cases this may need to be higher to enable the athlete to meet energy needs without having to consume huge quantities of food.
4. 60–65% of energy as carbohydrate (7–10 g/kg per day). Adequate glycogen stores are essential to supply fuel for muscles undergoing intense weight training. Regular intense strength training depletes glycogen stores, which must be replenished.

Other methods

Human growth hormone and anabolic steroids have also been used to increase muscle bulk. Both these substances are banned by the International Olympic Committee (Chapter 61).

Ensuring sufficient intake of vitamins and minerals

Vitamins and minerals are essential for certain metabolic processes and deficiencies are known to affect sporting performances.

Two questions often asked by athletes are:

1. Does exercise increase vitamin and/or mineral requirements?
2. Does vitamin and/or mineral supplementation improve sporting performance?

This chapter addresses question 1. Question 2 falls within the domain of Chapter 38.

The importance of an adequate supply of vitamins and minerals as a necessary part of normal body processes is well recognized. The role they play in enhancing sporting performance is less clear. Tables 37.6 and 37.7 (also available as downloadable PDF files at <www.clinicalsportsmedicine.com>) summarize the food sources, necessary part of functions, and possible

Table 37.6 Vitamins: food sources, major functions and possible importance in exercise

Vitamin	Food sources	Major functions	Possible importance in exercise
Water soluble			
Vitamin C (ascorbic acid)	Green leafy vegetables, parsley, capsicum, citrus fruits, currants, berry fruits, tropical fruits, tomatoes	Maintenance of connective tissue, cartilage, tendons and bone Facilitates absorption of iron Role in wound healing and muscle repair Protects against oxidants	Antioxidant Increased iron absorption Formation of adrenalin (epinephrine) Promotion of aerobic energy production
Vitamin B_1 (thiamine)	Meat (especially pork), yeast, wholegrains, nuts, all vegetables	Energy production through carbohydrate metabolism Nerve and heart function	Energy production from carbohydrate Hemoglobin formation
Vitamin B_2 (riboflavin)	Milk and milk products, yeast, organ meats, eggs, wholegrains, green leafy vegetables	Energy production through fat and protein metabolism Necessary for growth and development	Cofactor for energy release

continues

Table 37.6 Vitamins: food sources, major functions and possible importance in exercise *continued*

Vitamin	Food sources	Major functions	Possible importance in exercise
Niacin/nicotinic acid	Meat, liver, fish, eggs, yeast, some green leafy vegetables, peanuts, wholegrain products	A vital component of coenzymes concerned with energy processes	Energy release from carbohydrate and fat
Vitamin B_6 (pyridoxine)	Mainly high-protein products, wholegrains, yeast, cereals, vegetables, peanuts, bananas	Role in protein metabolism Role in glucose metabolism	Energy production from carbohydrate Formation of hemoglobin and oxidative enzymes
Vitamin B_{12} (cyanocobalamin)	Liver, meat, dairy products, oysters, sardines (not generally found in plant foods)	Formation of genetic materials Development of red blood cells	Red blood cell production
Folic acid	Liver, meat, fish, green leafy vegetables, orange juice	Formation of genetic materials Maintenance of normal red cell production Coenzyme in amino acid production	Red blood cell production
Pantothenic acid	Meat, poultry, fish, grains, cereals, legumes, yeast and egg yolk	Central role in carbohydrate metabolism, fats and proteins Role in nerve cell growth and function	Carbohydrate and fat synthesis
Biotin	Meat, egg yolk, fish, nuts, vegetables (also formed in intestines by bacteria)	Synthesis of carbohydrates, fats and proteins Role in nerve cell growth and function	Carbohydrate and fat synthesis
Fat soluble			
Vitamin A (retinol)	Liver, dairy foods, green leafy vegetables, fruits	Essential for normal growth and development Essential to prevent night blindness Maintenance of surface cells such as skin and lining of the gut	Antioxidant Prevention of red cell damage
Vitamin D (calciferol)	Eggs, butter, liver, fish oil, fortified margarine (also manufactured in the body by the action of sunlight on the skin)	Growth and mineralization of bones Aids in absorption of calcium and phosphorus from the diet	Calcium transport in muscles
Vitamin E (alpha-tocopherol)	Wheat germ, vegetable oils/margarine, nuts, seeds, wholegrain products, green leafy vegetables	Red blood cell production An antioxidant, may protect cell membranes	Antioxidant Prevention of red blood cell damage Promotion of aerobic energy production

continues

Table 37.6 Vitamins: food sources, major functions and possible importance in exercise *continued*

Vitamin	Food sources	Major functions	Possible importance in exercise
Vitamin K	Liver, meat, green leafy vegetables, soya beans, cauliflower, cabbage	Important in the blood clotting mechanism Facilitates action of some bone and kidney proteins	Nil known

Table 37.7 Minerals: food sources, functions and possible importance in exercise

Mineral	Some food sources	Some major functions	Possible importance
Macronutrients			
Calcium	Milk, cheese, yoghurt, green leafy vegetables, canned fish, sesame seeds	Bone structure Blood clotting Transmission of nerve impulses Muscle contraction	Muscle contraction Glycogen breakdown
Chlorine	Common table salt	Maintenance of electrolyte and fluid balance	
Magnesium	Most foods, especially wholegrain products, green leafy vegetables, fruits and other vegetables	Involved in regulation of protein synthesis, muscle contraction and body temperature regulation Essential cofactor in most energy production pathways	Muscle contraction Glucose metabolism
Phosphorus	Milk, poultry, fish and meat	Formation of bones and teeth (with calcium) Essential to normal functioning of B group vitamins Important role in the final delivery of energy to all cells, including muscle, in the form of ATP	Formation of ATP and creatine phosphokinase Release of oxygen from red blood cells
Potassium	Abundant in most foods, especially meat, fish, poultry, cereals, oranges, bananas, fresh vegetables and milk	Muscle function Nerve transmission Carbohydrate and protein metabolism Maintenance of body fluids and acid–base balance of blood	Nerve transmission Muscle contraction Glycogen storage
Sodium	Table salt, soy sauce, seafoods, dairy products, yeast spread	Important co-role with potassium to carry out functions mentioned above	Nerve impulse transmission Water balance
Micronutrients			
Chromium	Traces in meat and vegetables	Functions with insulin to help control glucose metabolism	Glucose metabolism

continues

Table 37.7 Minerals: food sources, functions and possible importance in exercise *continued*

Mineral	Some food sources	Some major functions	Possible importance
Cobalt	Meat, liver, milk, green leafy vegetables	Component of vitamin B_{12} May help prevent anemia and nervous system disorders	
Copper	Meat, vegetables, fish, oysters, drinking water from copper pipes	Component of many enzymes Role in hemoglobin formation	Oxygen transportation and utilization Linked with iron
Fluoride	Water supplies, tea and some small fish	Prevention of tooth decay Possible role in prevention of osteoporosis	
Iodine	Iodized salt, seafood	Component of thyroid hormones that regulate metabolic rate	
Iron	Liver, heart, lean red meat, dried apricots, kidney beans and green leafy vegetables	Formation of compounds essential to the transport and utilization of oxygen	Oxygen transport by red blood cells Muscle metabolism
Manganese	Wholegrain cereals, green leafy vegetables, wheat germ, nuts, bananas	Involvement in bone structure and nervous system activity Cofactor in carbohydrate metabolism	Energy metabolism
Molybdenum	Liver, legumes, wholegrains	Component of certain enzymes	
Selenium	Mainly high-protein foods, wholegrain products	Component of antioxidant enzyme helping to protect cells from oxidation by free radicals of oxygen	
Zinc	Meat, eggs, liver, oysters, wholegrain products, legumes	Component of many enzymes Aids in wound healing Growth Cofactor in protein and carbohydrate metabolism	Energy production in muscle cells
Cadmium, nickel, silicon, tin, vanadium	In most animal and plant foods	Uncertain	Uncertain

importance in exercise of the different vitamins and minerals, respectively.

The B complex vitamins

The B complex vitamins—thiamin (B_1), riboflavin (B_2), niacin, pyridoxine (B_6), cyanocobalamin (B_{12}), pantothenic acid, folate and biotin—combine to ensure proper digestion, muscle contraction and energy release. Because of the key role of these vitamins in energy metabolism, many athletes will supplement their diets with these vitamins.

Although requirements for some of the B complex vitamins may be increased during exercise, there is limited evidence to support any benefits of supplementation of these vitamins. In most cases, it appears that requirements may be met through the increased food intake of athletes in heavy training. More research is needed in this area.

Vitamin C

Although studies on the effect of vitamin C supplementation on performance have been contradictory, supplementation with vitamin C is extremely popular with both athletes and non-athletes. Vitamin C deficiency will affect the work capacity of athletes. Strenuous exercise may cause increased need for this vitamin, and there is an interest in the role of vitamin C as an antioxidant. An adequate intake of foods rich in vitamin C such as fresh fruit and vegetables is recommended.

Fat-soluble vitamins (A, D, E and K)

There have been very few studies of the relationship between the fat-soluble vitamins A and D and physical performance. To date, there appears to be no biological rationale to supplement vitamin A or D in athletes. Vitamins A and E are believed to act as antioxidants, although more research is required in this area. Vitamin E supplementation may play a potential role in helping to maintain red blood cells intact during exercise and may also assist muscle recovery following strenuous exercise.

Iron

Iron deficiency is a common problem among athletes, particularly female endurance athletes. True iron deficiency should not be confused with the dilutional pseudo-anemia associated with exercise and referred to as 'sports anemia'.[17] A number of factors may contribute to the development of iron deficiency.

Inadequate intake

The RDIs of iron for different population groups are shown in Table 37.8. The RDI of iron for menstruating females is considerably higher than for males. There are no specific RDIs for athletes, however, it is generally considered that regular activity may increase daily iron requirements significantly. Females with low energy intakes, commonly those concerned about weight gain, are susceptible to inadequate dietary intakes of iron. The average Western diet supplies

Table 37.8 Recommended daily intakes of iron

Age group (years)	Iron (mg)
Children	
4–11	6–8
Adolescents	
12–18	10–13
Men	
19–64	7
> 64	7
Women	
19–menopause	12–16
Postmenopausal	5–7
Pregnancy	+10–20

approximately 6–7 mg of iron per 4.2 MJ (1000 kcal). Energy intakes of 8.4 MJ (2000 kcal) or less may result in inadequate iron intake unless special measures are taken.[18]

Increased loss

Increased iron loss may occur at a number of sites in athletes. Blood loss from the gastrointestinal tract is common in athletes. Usually this is present in small amounts and not noticeable in the feces; however, accumulated losses may be considerable. It is uncertain whether this gastrointestinal blood loss is due to jarring of the colon associated with running or ischemic damage resulting from diversion of blood from the gut to the exercising muscles (Chapter 47).

Blood is also lost through the urine of athletes, especially distance runners. The bleeding usually occurs in the wall of the bladder, either due to a jarring effect from running or the stress of exercise.

Direct trauma to the muscles of the foot while running may also lead to destruction of red blood cells and subsequent iron loss. Minute amounts of iron (0.1–0.2 mg/L) are also lost in sweat. It is unlikely that this loss would make a significant contribution to iron deficiency.

Decreased absorption

Inadequate absorption of iron may also contribute to iron deficiency. The two forms of iron—heme and non-heme—have considerably different rates of absorption. Heme iron is found in all meat, poultry and fish, as well as liver and kidney. Up to 20% of heme iron is absorbed. Non-heme iron is found in nuts, legumes, cereals, leafy green vegetables and dried fruit and is less well absorbed. Vegetarians and other athletes who have low intakes of heme iron are susceptible to iron deficiency because of inadequate absorption. Ingested iron may combine with other substances to form complexes that are virtually insoluble and therefore poorly absorbed. Examples of these substances are phytic acid (found in cereal fiber) and tannins (found in tea).

A physiological response to insufficient iron intake is enhanced iron absorption. Iron-deficient endurance athletes, however, have decreased absorption rates compared with sedentary, iron-deficient control subjects. This suggests that exercise may impair absorption, perhaps due to reduced gut blood flow.

Stages of iron deficiency

The initial stage of iron deficiency is characterized by depletion of body iron stores. A sensitive indicator of iron deficiency in adults that is unaffected by a range of infectious and inflammatory conditions is soluble transferrin receptor (sTfR) levels. The normal range for soluble transferrin receptor is 3–9 mg/L and this level can rise three- to fourfold in iron deficiency. The traditional measure of iron stores, serum ferritin, is affected by physical activity and inflammation, so the soluble transferrin receptor test may prove to be the more sensitive and clinically useful test over time.

The development of iron-deficiency anemia is characterized by hemoglobin levels of less than 130 g/L (8 mmol/L) in males and less than 110 g/L (6.8 mmol/L) in females. Anemia is much less common in athletes than iron depletion.

Effect of iron deficiency on performance

Iron-deficiency anemia has a marked effect on athletic performance because reduced hemoglobin levels decrease the transport of oxygen to exercising muscles. In these circumstances, the athlete is likely to complain of tiredness, lethargy and poor performance and may appear pale.

While the effect of iron-deficiency anemia on performance is clear-cut, the effect of the depletion of body iron stores as indicated by lowered serum ferritin levels is less well understood. Studies have shown that tiredness is reduced and performance appears to be enhanced when serum ferritin levels return to normal after increased iron ingestion.

A possible explanation of the detrimental effect on athletic performance lies in the role of iron in energy metabolism. Iron deficiency results in decreased concentrations of the iron-containing enzyme, alpha-glycerophosphate oxidase, an enzyme involved in energy metabolism. Iron is also involved in energy metabolism through the cytochromes and the enzymes catalase, peroxidase, pyruvate-malate oxidase and xanthine oxidase.

Low serum ferritin levels are common in sportspeople. Female endurance athletes appear to be particularly susceptible, especially if they do not eat red meat.

Guidelines to ensure adequate iron intake

The iron content of common foods is shown in Table 37.9 (also available as a downloadable PDF at <www.clinicalsportsmedicine.com>). Ingestion of non-heme iron in conjunction with foods rich in vitamin C (e.g. citrus and tropical fruits, tomatoes, capsicums, parsley as well as fruit and vegetables juices) increases the absorption of iron (see box).[19] Eating meat at the same time as non-heme forms of iron increases the absorption of the non-heme iron.

Guidelines to increase body iron stores[19]

1. Eat (even small amounts of) lean red meat regularly (three to four times per week).
2. Eat liver and kidney.
3. Eat skinless poultry (particularly with dark flesh) and fish.
4. Include foods or drinks rich in vitamin C with each meal.
5. Increase consumption of wholegrain breads and iron-enriched breakfast cereal.
6. Vegetarian athletes need to pay particular attention to including plenty of iron-dense foods along with foods rich in vitamin C.
7. Avoid drinking tea with meals.
8. Do not take iron supplements unless instructed to do so by your medical practitioner or dietitian.

Occasionally, iron supplementation will be required in those athletes who continue to be symptomatic and are unable to elevate their serum ferritin levels to normal. This can be achieved orally or occasionally via intramuscular injection (clinicians should remain alert to possible anaphylaxis). Those susceptible to low iron levels should have their serum ferritin levels monitored as frequently as semi-annually.

Calcium

Calcium is essential for healthy bones, blood clotting, nerve transmission, muscle contraction and enzyme activation. The skeleton contain 99% of the body's calcium and the remaining 1% is distributed in membrane structures, soft tissues and body fluids.

Along with heredity, physical activity and hormones, calcium plays an important role in bone metabolism. The most important period for calcium intake is childhood and adolescence.[20] The RDIs of calcium are shown in Table 37.10.

Adequate calcium intake is essential to maintain bone mass. As calcium is a 'threshold nutrient' (i.e. a certain level is needed and beyond that no further benefit is obtained) many women with a normal diet have adequate intakes.[21] However, with aging, gastrointestinal absorption is reduced and, particularly in women 10 or more years postmenopausal, calcium supplementation has been shown to improve bone health.[22] Ammenorheic athletes may also benefit from supplementation although it must be remembered that the fundamental clinical limitation among

Table 37.9 Iron, magnesium and zinc content of common foods

Food	Amount	Magnesium (mg)	Iron (mg)	Zinc (mg)
Beef, fillet steak, grilled, lean	100 g	22	4.1	4.5
Lamb, chump chop, grilled, lean	100 g	29	3.5	4.8
Chicken, breast, baked, lean	100 g	23	0.9	1.7
Pork, boneless, cooked, lean	100 g	22	1.4	3.1
Veal, boneless, cooked, lean	100 g	23	2.1	3.8
Beef, liver, simmered	100 g	24	6.5	5.3
Pate, liver	30 g	5	2.8	1.1
Fish, steamed	100 g	31	0.4	0.7
Oyster, raw	½ dozen	30	2.3	38.7
Scallop, raw	6 average	17	0.6	2.1
Crab, boiled	100 g	27	1.0	9.1
Sardine, canned in oil, drained	6 whole	54	2.4	1.6
Tuna, canned in brine, drained	100 g	27	1.3	1.2
Salmon, canned in brine	100 g	25	1.7	2.1
Egg, whole, hard-boiled	1 medium	5	0.9	0.4
Broccoli, boiled	1 cup	32	1.5	1.0
Zucchini, green skin, boiled	1 cup	22	0.9	0.5
Spinach, English, boiled	1 cup	94	4.4	0.9
Silverbeet, boiled	1 cup	28	2.5	0.6
Pea, green, boiled	1 cup	35	1.8	1.3
Bean, green, boiled	1 cup	24	1.5	1.1
Lettuce, common, raw	2 leaves	8	0.6	0.2
Muesli flakes	1 cup	33	6.9	0.5
All Bran	1 cup	184	5.6	3.5
Weeties	1 cup	110	3.2	1.2
Bread, wholemeal	1 slice	18	0.7	0.4
Crispbread, rye	2 biscuits	13	0.5	0.3
Rice cakes	1 serve	44	0.4	0.8
Baked beans, canned in sauce	1 cup	68	4.4	1.4
Lentils, boiled	1 cup	53	4.2	1.9
Cashew nuts, roasted	30 g	75	1.4	0.6
Peanuts, raw	30 g	48	0.7	0.9
Sesame seeds	15 g	51	0.8	0.8
Rice, brown, boiled	1 cup	88	0.9	1.6
Pasta, wholemeal, boiled	200 g	78	3.6	1.2

Source: Nutlab 95. Canberra: Australian Government Publishing Service, 1995.

Table 37.10 Recommended daily intakes for calcium

Age group (years)	Calcium (mg)
Children	
4–7	800
Boys	
8–11	800
12–15	1200
16–18	1000
Girls	
8–11	900
12–15	1000
16–18	800
Men	
19–64	800
>64	800
Women	
19–54	800
>54	1000
Pregnancy	+300
Lactation	+400
Amenorrheic athletes	1200–1500

those athletes is total energy nutrition, not lack of calcium per se.

The richest sources of calcium in the Western diet are dairy products. The calcium content of common foods is shown in Table 37.11. Certain factors such as fiber, excessive salt or protein, caffeine or phosphorus tend to impair calcium absorption.

Some athletes avoid dairy products because of the perceived high fat content. However, most dairy products are now available in a low-fat form. In those athletes who are unwilling or unable to meet the RDI of calcium through food, calcium supplementation may be necessary. Salt and caffeine intake should be decreased to increase calcium retention.

Magnesium

Magnesium is present in the body in relatively large amounts. It may have a role at the cellular level affecting glucose metabolism in muscle and muscle contraction characteristics. During prolonged exercise, the serum magnesium concentration may decrease. There has been some concern that low serum magnesium levels during exercise could be due to excessive loss through sweating.

There is limited evidence that additional magnesium is of benefit to sporting performance. The magnesium content of common foods is shown in Table 37.9.

Zinc

Zinc has several important functions that may be associated with sporting performance. It is involved in all phases of growth and development, as well as in nutrient metabolism and energy production in the muscle cell.

Maintaining adequate zinc stores is important as losses may be increased in strenuous exercise. High-carbohydrate diets also tend to be lower in

Table 37.11 Some foods that contain over 200 mg of calcium per usual serve

Food	Amount	Energy (kJ)	Energy (kcal)	Calcium (mg)
Milk, whole	250 mL	700	170	294
Milk, skim	250 mL	380	90	319
Milk, low-fat	250 mL	540	129	356
Yoghurt, low-fat, natural	200 g	450	107	420
Yoghurt, natural	200 g	610	145	340
Yoghurt, flavored/fruit	200 g	810	193	360
Cheese, cheddar	35 g	590	140	270
Cheese, low-fat	35 g	480	115	280
Cheese, parmesan	35 g	650	160	400
Salmon, pink, canned in brine	100 g	720	170	310
Soy beverage, fortified	250 mL	650	155	290

Source: Nutlab 95. Canberra: Australian Government Publishing Service, 1995.

zinc. The zinc content of common foods is shown in Table 37.9.

While zinc deficiency impairs sporting performance, there is no evidence that supplementation will benefit the athlete. Side-effects of prolonged zinc supplementation include reduced high-density lipoprotein cholesterol levels (and increased risk of coronary heart disease) and interference with iron absorption, possibly leading to anemia.

Selenium

Selenium is a trace mineral that functions with vitamin E as an antioxidant. It is thought to play a role in muscle performance. Due to its possible toxicity, supplementation is not recommended.

Chromium

Chromium is an important factor in blood glucose homeostasis. Insulin resistance and hyperinsulinemia have been associated with low chromium status. Chromium supplementation is frequently used by individuals in an attempt to control blood glucose levels and for weight loss, however, research has yet to indicate any true benefits. Chromium picolinate has been promoted as an ergogenic aid for muscle development; however, these claims are, to date, unfounded.

Vitamin and mineral supplements

This topic is discussed in Chapter 38.

Maintaining adequate hydration

Water constitutes approximately 60% of the human body. It is an integral part of cells—required for lubrication, elimination of body waste and for the transportation of nutrients and gases throughout the body. Adequate hydration is essential for optimal athletic performance. The role of water is to:

1. Maintain blood volume. Inadequate fluid intake may result in a reduced blood volume and therefore a lower stroke volume.
2. Regulate body temperature. Exercise produces large amounts of heat, which must be eliminated from the body in order to maintain an appropriate body temperature. The body controls its own core temperature by transferring heat from muscle to the circulating blood. As the body core temperature increases, blood flow to the skin also increases. In moderate temperatures, this allows heat to be transferred to the environment by convection, radiation and, especially, evaporation through sweat (Chapter 53).

In warm-to-hot environmental conditions, the body must also dissipate heat absorbed externally in addition to that produced internally. In the absence of convection and radiation, the body must rely solely on the evaporation of sweat to regulate body core temperature. Adequate fluid intake is, therefore, vital to compensate for fluid lost through evaporation of sweat to prevent dehydration.

Clinical perspective

As water losses increase to 3–4% of body weight, athletic performance is impaired, urinary output is reduced and symptoms include dry mouth, flushed skin, nausea and lethargy. Fluid losses of 5–6% of body weight increase pulse rate and respiratory rate and affect concentration. Dizziness, weakness and mental confusion are associated with a fluid loss of approximately 8% of body weight. Prolonged physical activity in hot conditions may result in up to 3 L of fluid being lost per hour through sweat.

The most practical method of ensuring adequate fluid replacement, during and after exercise, is through regular assessment of body weight, especially early in the training program and in hot weather (Chapter 53). Monitoring urine color and volume is another useful method of assessing hydration, however, results must be interpreted with caution as a range of factors may influence these parameters. With increasing dehydration, urine becomes scant, more concentrated and appears darker.

Sports drinks

How quickly an individual rehydrates is determined by a number of factors, including the composition, volume and possibly temperature of the replacement fluid.[23] For any sports drink to be effective, it must leave the stomach quickly and be absorbed rapidly.

Many sports drinks contain carbohydrates in the form of glucose, fructose or a glucose polymer. Glucose solutions of less than 10% concentration appear to empty from the stomach quickly, while concentrations greater than 10% may inhibit gastric emptying. Glucose polymers (long chains of simple sugars linked together) may empty from the stomach at a faster rate than simple glucose and allow a greater amount of carbohydrate to be consumed. The ideal carbohydrate concentration is 4–8%.

Fructose appears to empty from the stomach relatively quickly; however, it is not absorbed from the small intestine as quickly as glucose. Large amounts may cause gastrointestinal distress and osmotic diarrhea.

In addition to carbohydrate, many sports drinks contain minerals, such as sodium, potassium, chloride and magnesium. The addition of sodium may be of benefit as it enhances fluid absorption in the small intestine. Sodium is also believed to enhance rehydration by reducing diuresis to promote maintenance of plasma osmolality and maintaining thirst. The level of sodium normally found in sports drinks ranges from 10 to 30 mmol/L. Low serum sodium levels (hyponatremia) have been reported in athletes involved in ultraendurance events who consumed large volumes of plain water or drinks with low sodium chloride content in conjunction with sodium losses through sweat. Losses of other electrolytes in sweat are relatively small and may be easily replaced by a balanced diet.

Drinking before exercise

The ideal fluid to consume prior to exercise depends on the time remaining before exercise and the likely duration of the exercise. Water may be consumed at any time prior to exercise. The ingestion of carbohydrate-containing beverages in the hours prior to exercise may provide an additional energy source. The volume tolerated is specific to individuals and specific needs, however, a large drink (300–500 mL) in the 10–15 minutes before activity may help to stimulate gastric emptying.

Drinking during exercise

Drinking carbohydrate–electrolyte replacement fluid during training and competition enhances performance in endurance activities that last more than 60 minutes. Where possible, athletes should aim to replace at least 80% of fluid loss: 150–200 mL of cold fluid should be consumed every 10–15 minutes. For the athletes with high fluid losses it may be difficult to replace fluid at a rate that matches losses and a certain level of dehydration may be unavoidable. Cooler fluids are generally more palatable and help to lower body core temperature. Warmer fluids may be used when exercise is carried out in cool environments. It is important to remember that thirst is not an accurate guide to hydration status.

Carbohydrate–electrolyte fluids may be particularly useful for day-long, multiple-event competitions in which there is inadequate time between events to replenish carbohydrate stores by eating solid foods. In this case, athletes should consume a dilute (4–8%) carbohydrate fluid at regular intervals, starting at most 30 minutes into the exercise. During short events, cool water is adequate.

Rehydration after exercise

For athletes undertaking moderate exercise in moderate temperature, cool water is an excellent post-exercise drink. Sweetened beverages may stimulate thirst and increase the amount of fluid consumed. The need for fluid replacement after exercise can be estimated by monitoring weight loss during the activity.

Athletes training each day at high intensities or at high temperatures may suffer from a prolonged state of dehydration. Drinking beverages containing sodium may help rehydrate these athletes. Sodium increases thirst and reduces fluid excretion. Carbohydrate–electrolyte beverages such as sports drinks generally contain sufficient sodium for this purpose. Oral rehydration solutions with a sodium content of more than 50 mmol/L may be useful for athletes with large fluid deficits, particularly if the next exercise session is not far away.

In addition to sodium, athletes in hard training should aim to ingest carbohydrate after the cessation of exercise. A practical, easily absorbed source of carbohydrate is a high-carbohydrate drink (e.g. sports drink or soft drink [pop]).

Caffeine

As well as the sports drinks currently available, athletes commonly drink beverages containing caffeine. These include coffee, tea, cocoa, cola and energy drinks. It has been suggested that the use of caffeinated drinks by endurance athletes increases the utilization of free fatty acids during prolonged exercise, thus sparing muscle glycogen. This effect is likely to be minimal for elite endurance athletes as training has conditioned their bodies to use fatty acids maximally. In addition, the large doses of carbohydrate recommended for athletes prior to competition may counteract the effects of caffeine by increasing insulin levels, thus inhibiting fatty acid release.

The potential ergogenic effect of caffeine may be related to the central nervous system through an increase in alertness and tolerance to fatigue.

The adverse effects of caffeine on performance must also be considered. Anxiety, nervousness, increased basal metabolic rate and heat production are detrimental side-effects of large doses of caffeine. Caffeine may also have a mild diuretic effect, however, the body retains much of the fluid in caffeinated fluids. Individuals vary in their response to caffeine.

Alcohol

Even small amounts of alcohol impair athletic performance. When advising athletes about the effects of alcohol, it is important to make them understand that drinking alcohol does not supply energy for exercise. Although a concentrated source of kilojoules, alcohol does not contribute to glycogen stores and, thus, does not fuel muscles. Drinking excessive alcohol increases body fat. The diuretic effect of alcohol also impairs athletic performance as it promotes dehydration. After competition, it is particularly important that athletes rehydrate adequately before consuming alcohol and that they consume some food to enhance recovery.

Guidelines that team clinicians have found useful in guiding sportspeople on the use of alcohol in sport include:

- avoid binge drinking
- avoid alcohol in the 24 hours prior to competition
- avoid alcohol if injured
- be aware of the dehydrating effect of alcohol
- be aware of the effect of alcohol on vasodilation/temperature regulation
- be aware of the energy value of alcohol
- if drinking alcohol, first rehydrate and then drink alcohol together with a nutritious meal.

Fluid intake in children and older adults

As children have a larger body surface-area-to-weight ratio than adults, they are more at risk of heat injury than adults. Children also have a lower sweating capacity and a lower cardiac output, which may further reduce their ability to transfer internal heat to the environment. Children may also produce more heat during activity and take longer to acclimatize to warmer temperatures (see also Chapter 40). Although previous guidelines recommend children ingest 300–400 mL of fluid prior to exercise and 100 mL of fluid every 20 minutes while active, there is a contemporary recognition that overdrinking is not to be encouraged and could cause harm. Thus, children, like adults, should drink 'ad libitum' (as they feel thirsty).

As the ability to cope with heat stress is reduced with age, older adults have diminished thermoregulatory function. They tend to respond less to thirst than younger athletes and subsequently drink less than they need to. They may also have reduced sweat volumes.

The effect of 'making weight' on fluid status

Some sports, particularly those with weight limits, require special consideration. In sports such as wrestling, boxing, lightweight rowing and martial arts, fluid deprivation is frequently used to achieve a lower than normal body weight. In addition to withholding fluids in the days prior to the event, athletes often also take diuretic tablets, wear sweat suits during training and take saunas to further deplete body fluid levels.

These practises may reduce muscle strength, impair body temperature regulation, decrease blood flow to the kidneys and, thus, decrease work performance. The few hours from weigh-in to competition may be insufficient time to re-establish fluid and electrolyte balance. To prevent the need to reduce body weight rapidly prior to competition, athletes should be encouraged to practice safe methods of reducing body fat levels in the weeks leading up to the event. Reducing weight by minimizing body fat stores will be more advantageous than reducing weight by dehydration. Athletes in weight-limited sports require regular dietary monitoring to ensure they optimize their energy levels while remaining under the weight limit.

Optimizing the pre-competition meal

A number of dietary techniques can aid performance. These techniques vary depending on the duration of the competition and subsequent fuel requirements.

Endurance sport

Inadequate glycogen may limit performance in endurance events lasting more than 1–1.5 hours but appropriate training and dietary manipulation can double the capacity of muscle to store glycogen. Training also increases reliance on fat as an exercise fuel, thus sparing glycogen stores.

Carbohydrate loading

Carbohydrate loading is widely used in various forms. Sports dietitians recommend that early in the week prior to competition athletes maintain a normal moderate-to-high carbohydrate diet as training gradually tapers. This will maintain steady levels of muscle glycogen. In the three to four days prior to competition, training is reduced even further and traditionally the carbohydrate content of the diet has been recommended to increase to 70–80% of the total intake simultaneously. Recent research indicates that it may be possible to achieve adequate muscle glycogen with increased carbohydrate intake for only 24 hours prior to competition. Carbohydrate loading appears to be most effective in trained athletes competing in events lasting longer than 60–90 minutes or in multiple-event competitions.

Short duration events

In shorter duration events of up to 1 hour it is unlikely that the body's glycogen stores will be exhausted. Nevertheless, it is important to maximize glycogen stores prior to competition. Training will already have built up the athlete's capacity to store glycogen. In the 24–36 hours before the event, training should be reduced while maintaining a normal training diet with emphasis on high carbohydrate intake.

Carbohydrate loading is not indicated for short duration events and may be a disadvantage for short, high-speed, explosive events in which excessive weight is a penalty. As much as 1.5 kg may be gained because of the water associated with glycogen storage during carbohydrate loading.

Bicarbonate loading

Bicarbonate loading is a nutritional technique used by some athletes performing high-intensity anaerobic activity such as an 800 m run or a 200 m swim.

The bicarbonate buffer system controls blood pH tightly during exercise. Intense exercise produces lactic acid, which causes fatigue and impairs performance. Sodium bicarbonate, an alkaline salt found in the blood, buffers lactic acid. Thus, athletes have used alkaline salts such as sodium bicarbonate (baking soda) in an attempt to improve performance in anaerobic type events. Alkaline loading does not appear to affect Vo_{2max}, heart rate or strength but has been shown to improve maximal performance during repeated short-term anaerobic tasks during training.

This positive effect has been noted with athletes consuming between 200 and 300 mg/kg of body weight of sodium bicarbonate. Side-effects are commonly associated with these dosages. These include nausea, vomiting, flatulence, diarrhea and muscle cramps.

Bicarbonate loading should not be attempted for the first time in an important competition. The effect of bicarbonate loading varies considerably between individuals and should be tested out in a training situation prior to use in competition.

Competition diet between events

Some sports require an athlete to compete several times a day (e.g. track and field, swimming). In these situations, the main nutritional priority is to replace fluids and replenish glycogen stores between events. If there is a time span of 2–3 hours between events, it will be possible to eat as well as drink. The advantage of eating solid foods is not only to restore glycogen but also to combat hunger. If the time between events is too short to consume solids, carbohydrate-containing fluids should be the priority. Liquid meals may also be useful in these situations, particularly if the athlete experiences pre-competition nerves.

The pre-event meal

There is no magic food or meal, which, if ingested prior to competition, will ensure success. Energy utilized during training or competition comes predominantly from foods consumed in the days prior to the event. However, in long duration, continuous activity, the pre-event meal makes an important contribution to energy stores. The pre-event meal will contribute little to muscle glycogen stores; nevertheless, it needs to be composed largely of carbohydrates to ensure adequate liver glycogen and blood glucose levels. For pre-event meals to be easily digested and quickly cleared from the gastrointestinal tract, the fat and fiber content should be kept low.

The timing of the pre-event meal is important. It is recommended that food be consumed at least 2–3 hours prior to competition to allow gastric emptying. Although the pre-event meal should be light and easily digested, it should be satisfying to prevent the onset of hunger and weakness during the event. A solid or liquid meal providing 1–4 g/kg of carbohydrate is recommended. Choices from within the 'athletes menu' section below are all appropriate as elements of a pre-game meal.

There is conflicting evidence regarding the effect of the GI of the pre-exercise meal on sustained energy levels and performance. The most important aspect is the total amount of carbohydrate consumed before and during exercise.

One of the most important considerations of the pre-event meal is the psychological aspect. The meal should be familiar, enjoyable and well tolerated. The pre-event meal is not an appropriate time to experiment with new foods. Athletes should experiment with different meal sizes and types during training to determine which type of meal is most appropriate.

The athlete's menu

Variety and taste are important factors influencing an athlete's ability to adhere to a high-carbohydrate, low-fat diet. Some tasty meal suggestions consistent with the guidelines discussed in this chapter are listed in the box below.

> #### Breakfast
> - Wholegrain cereal with low-fat milk and sliced bananas
> - Wholemeal (whole wheat) toast spread with fresh ricotta and fruit spread
> - Toasted wholegrain muffin topped with baked beans
> - Low-fat yogurt and fresh fruit with a sprinkle of rice bran
> - Pancakes topped with 'Fromage frais' and fresh strawberries
>
> #### Lunch
> - Wholemeal roll filled with chicken and salad
> - Pita bread pocket stuffed with tuna, tomato and spring onions
> - Baked jacket potato topped with salmon and low-fat cheese
> - Bowl of minestrone soup with fresh bread rolls
> - Stir-fried rice with vegetables
>
> #### Dinner
> - Lean grilled meat with jacket potatoes and steamed vegetables
> - Taco shells filled with lean mince and red kidney beans served with brown rice and salad
> - Vegetable lasagna made with low-fat cheese
> - Stir-fried chicken and Chinese vegetables served with brown rice
> - Spinach fettuccine with lentil and vegetable sauce
>
> #### Snacks
> - Low-fat yoghurt with fruit
> - Fresh, canned, stewed or dried fruit
> - Raisin bread, crumpets or muffins topped with jam, honey or syrup
> - Wholegrain breakfast cereal with low-fat milk
> - Rice cakes topped with sliced banana and honey

Conclusion

Nutrition plays an important role in maximizing athletic performance. Especially in elite competition, the differences between success and failure are usually very small. Maximizing performance with the use of these nutritional techniques can give an athlete the edge over his or her rivals.

Recommended Reading

Borsheim E, Tipton KD, Wolf SE, Wolfe RR. Essential amino acids and muscle protein recovery from resistance exercise. *Am J Physiol Endocrinol Metab* 2002; 283(4): E648–57.

Burke LM, Deakin V, eds. *Clinical Sports Nutrition*. 3rd edn. Sydney: McGraw-Hill, 2006.

Tipton KD, Wolfe RR. Exercise, protein metabolism, and muscle growth. *Int J Sport Nutr Exerc Metab* 2001; 11(1): 109–32.

Tipton KD, Wolfe RR. Protein and amino acids for athletes. *J Sports Sci* 2004; 22(1): 65–79.

Tipton KD, Borsheim E, Wolf SE, Sanford AP, Wolfe RR. Acute response of net muscle protein balance reflects 24-h balance after exercise and amino acid ingestion. *Am J Physiol Endocrinol Metab* 2003; 284(1): E76–89.

References

1. Burke LM, Hawley JA. Carbohydrate and exercise. *Curr Opin Clin Nutr Metab Care* 1999; 2(6): 515–20.
2. MacLaren D. The 'rise' of sports nutrition. *J Sports Sci* 1999; 17(12): 933–5.
3. Martin WH, Klein S. The use of endogenous carbohydrates and fat as fuels during exercise. *Proc Nutr Soc* 1998; 57(1): 49–54.
4. Borsheim E, Cree MG, Tipton KD, Elliott TA, Aarsland A, Wolfe RR. Effect of carbohydrate intake on net muscle protein synthesis during recovery from resistance exercise. *J Appl Physiol* 2004; 96(2): 674–8.
5. Miller SL, Tipton KD, Chinkes DL, Wolf SE, Wolfe RR. Independent and combined effects of amino acids and glucose after resistance exercise. *Med Sci Sports Exerc* 2003; 35(3): 449–55.
6. Tipton KD, Wolfe RR. Protein and amino acids for athletes. *J Sports Sci* 2004; 22(1): 65–79.
7. Phillips SM, Parise G, Roy BD, Tipton KD, Wolfe RR, Tamopolsky MA. Resistance-training-induced adaptations in skeletal muscle protein turnover in the fed state. *Can J Physiol Pharmacol* 2002; 80(11): 1045–53.
8. Bolster DR, Pikosky MA, Gaine PC, et al. Dietary protein intake impacts human skeletal muscle protein fractional synthetic rates after endurance exercise. *Am J Physiol Endocrinol Metab* 2005; 289(4): E678–83.
9. Tipton KD, Elliott TA, Cree MG, Wolf SE, Sanford AP, Wolfe RR. Ingestion of casein and whey proteins result in

muscle anabolism after resistance exercise. *Med Sci Sports Exerc* 2004; 36(12): 2073–81.

10. Durham WJ, Miller SL, Yeckel CW, et al. Leg glucose and protein metabolism during an acute bout of resistance exercise in humans. *J Appl Physiol* 2004; 97(4): 1379–86.

11. Phillips SM. Protein requirements and supplementation in strength sports. *Nutrition* 2004; 20(7–8): 689–95.

12. Cheuvront SN. The zone diet and athletic performance. *Sports Med* 1999; 27(4): 213–28.

13. Kreider RB. Dietary supplements and the promotion of muscle growth with resistance exercise. *Sports Med* 1999; 27(2): 97–110.

14. Rankin JW. Role of protein in exercise. *Clin Sports Med* 1999; 18(3): 499–511, vi.

15. Grandjean A. Nutritional requirements to increase lean mass. *Clin Sports Med* 1999; 18(3): 623–32.

16. Johnson WA, Landry GL. Nutritional supplements: fact vs. fiction. *Adolesc Med Clin* 1998; 9(3): 501–13, vi.

17. Fields KB. The athlete with anemia. In: Fields KB, Fricker PA, eds. *Medical Problems in Athletes*. Malden, MA: Blackwell Scientific, 1997: 258–65.

18. Ronsen O, Sundgot-Borgen J, Maehlum S. Supplement use and nutritional habits in Norwegian elite athletes. *Scand J Med Sci Sports* 1999; 9(1): 28–35.

19. Chatard JC, Mujika I, Guy C, Lacour JR. Anaemia and iron deficiency in athletes. Practical recommendations for treatment. *Sports Med* 1999; 27(4): 229–40.

20. Bailey DA, Martin AD, McKay HA, Whiting SJ, Mirwald R. Calcium accretion in girls and boys during puberty: a longitudinal analysis. *J Bone Miner Res* 2000; 15: 2245–50.

21. Kanis JA, Passmore R. Calcium supplementation of the diet. *BMJ* 1989; 298: 137–40, 205–8, 673–4.

22. Dawson-Hughes B, Harris SS, Krall EA, Dallal GE. Effect of calcium and vitamin D supplementation on bone density in men and women 65 years of age or older. *N Engl J Med* 1997; 337: 670–6.

23. Maughan RJ. The sports drink as a functional food: formulations for successful performance. *Proc Nutr Soc* 1998; 57(1): 15–23.

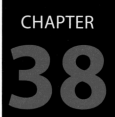

Maximizing Sporting Performance: To Use or Not to Use Supplements?

WITH JASON E. TANG AND STUART M. PHILLIPS

Clinicians are increasingly faced with requests by athletes and recreational sportspeople about the potential performance-enhancing benefits of supplements. Many sportspeople take supplements without discussing this with a clinician. As the array of supplements available is large, it is difficult for clinicians to remain up to date with the latest trends in this field.

This chapter aims to highlight the extent of supplement use and, thus, provide clinicians with practical background information that will aid in counseling athletes regarding categories of supplements in vogue in 2006/2007. We also provide website links that are likely to provide regular updates and we will update this time-sensitive chapter on our website <www.clinicalsportsmedicine.com>. Because dietary supplements are often cited as causes of 'inadvertent' positive drug tests, the chapter closes by discussing contamination of supplements—a category of compounds that does not undergo the same level of quality control that is applied to pharmaceuticals. This chapter complements material in Chapters 37 and 61.

Extent of use of supplements among sportspeople

Although it is impossible for clinicians to keep abreast of the latest and newest supplements available, sportspeople continually seek advice about supplement use. This tension is heightened by the fact that a large proportion of athletes use supplements. Among Canadian athletes who competed at the 1996 and 2000 Olympic Summer Games in Atlanta and Sydney, 69% and 74%, respectively, reported using some type of supplement ranging from vitamins to minerals and from creatine to amino acids.[1] The authors concluded that, 'Widespread use of supplements, combined with an absence of evidence of their efficacy and a concern for the possibility of "inadvertent" doping, underscore the need for appropriately focused educational initiatives in this area'. Surveys of recreational exercisers and college-aged athletes have reported rates close to 85% for supplement use, with use of supplemental protein, creatine and thermogenic enhancers (ephedra, caffeine) being higher in younger (<30 years) exercisers who were more concerned with muscle mass gain.[2] In addition, a sex-based dichotomy exists where females most often cite health as the number one reason for taking a supplement, whereas males cite the ability of a supplement to enhance speed and agility, strength and power, or muscle gain.[3]

While it may seem trite, one of the easiest questions to answer regarding supplement use for athletes is perhaps the most salient: 'Does this stuff work?'. By 'work' most athletes are asking whether it enhances either health, performance or, in some cases, immune function. Insofar as performance is concerned, however, athletes seem to overlook the fact that any supplement that has the potential to be ergogenic will be, or perhaps has already been, banned by sports regulatory agencies. Despite this and the evidence for their efficacy being, at best, questionable, certain supplements remain relatively popular due to the promise of enhancing performance.

As sportspeople have not been trained to appreciate 'levels of evidence', personal testimonies of 'stars' carry great weight; thus, advice from other athletes on the latest and greatest supplement can strongly influence athletes' decisions. The Internet and coaches' opinions are also important sources

CHAPTER 38 MAXIMIZING SPORTING PERFORMANCE: TO USE OR NOT TO USE SUPPLEMENTS?

38

of information on supplement use. The axiom that a certain supplement 'works for me!' is also an oft-heard statement from athletes. Sadly, the supplement user fails to consider the answer to the question of whether an athlete has had success because of, or in spite of, taking a supplement.

Some evidence exists to support the thesis that the nutritional habits of many supplement users are often suboptimal. This suggests room for improved performance via appropriate nutrition as outlined in Chapter 37 and by attention to appropriate recovery (Chapter 7). In addition, athletes quite often report that they take supplements (particularly those of vitamins and minerals and sometimes amino acids/protein) to 'ensure that they are getting enough'.[2, 3] Athletes are woefully under-informed about supplements; thus, if clinicians have a sound foundational knowledge about key categories of supplements and are able to stay current with popular supplements they will gain trust from the athletes who seek their expertise. From this position of trust there may be the opportunity to counsel the athlete on ways to improve performance through appropriate nutrition, training (Chapter 6) and recovery (Chapter 7).

Supplements for strength and power sports

Supplement use by strength and power sport athletes typically occurs in conjunction with the performance of resistance exercise, the primary goal being to maximize gains in muscle mass. Three commonly used categories of supplements among those engaged in strength and power sports are proteins and amino acids, beta-hydroxy-beta-methylbutyrate (HMB), and various forms of male steroid hormone precursors. This chapter focuses on the first two categories as the latter is covered in Chapter 61.

Proteins and amino acids

Proteins and amino acids are perhaps the most widely used supplements by strength and power sport athletes. The rationale for their use seems reasonable; strength and power are a function of muscle mass and amino acids are the building blocks of this tissue. Most athletes feel that very high protein intakes (2–3 g/kg per day) are required to build and maintain muscle mass. Although it is known that insufficient protein intake will limit muscle growth and repair, there is little evidence to support recommending protein and/or amino acid supplements to athletes already eating a well-balanced diet.

The current recommended daily allowance (RDA) for protein is 0.8 g/kg per day; however, the RDA does not take physical activity into account. Studies examining nitrogen balance in athletes (used as an index of protein requirements) have suggested that individuals engaged in strength training may require slightly higher protein intakes (1.2–1.7 g/kg per day) than sedentary individuals.[4] While it is likely to be true that novices require slightly higher protein intakes than the RDA, considerable evidence exists to suggest that dietary protein requirements may be reduced following resistance training.[5] Indeed, it appears that with training individuals become more efficient in their protein utilization. Thus, most athletes who train regularly are probably already consuming sufficient protein in their diet to meet any increased protein requirement that may exist as a consequence of their activity.[6]

Athletes are likely to ask clinicians about the benefits of supplementing with specific individual amino acids such as glutamine, leucine, lysine, arginine and ornithine. Glutamine is an amino acid that is purported to support immune function and also increase muscle growth. Evidence to support either effect is completely lacking, however. A very thorough review of glutamine's potential efficacy in supporting enhanced immune function with exercise found that the balance of evidence showed no effect of the amino acid on any aspect of immune function.[7] Glutamine's other touted role as a 'cell volumizer' or an 'anticatabolic' agent to enhance muscle mass gains with resistance exercise is also without good evidence, at least in healthy persons.[7]

The branched-chain amino acids (BCAA: leucine, isoleucine, valine) are often used by power sport athletes as anabolic agents and by many classes of athletes as agents to combat central fatigue and 'improve focus'. There is no good evidence to suggest that supplemental BCAAs (leucine as an individual branched chain has been the most commonly studied) serve as potential anabolic growth promoters, at least not in a chronic sense of promotion of muscle hypertrophy.[8] However, there are observations in humans and animals that BCAAs and leucine in particular are acutely anticatabolic and have potential anabolic properties.[9] While it is highly debatable whether BCAA administration can combat central fatigue, defined as a loss of central drive from the motor cortex resulting in muscle fatigue, most recent reviews of this mechanism failed to support the existence of such an effect.[8–10]

Growth-hormone promoting amino acids such as arginine and aspartate are also ineffective. In perhaps the longest supplement trial to date, male athletes received a daily oral dose of arginine (5.7 g) and aspartate (8.7 g) for a total of four weeks. No effects were observed of the supplementation regimen on either maximal aerobic capacity or hormone levels (in particular growth hormone and testosterone) versus a lower supplement dose or a control group.[11] Further, it is debatable whether growth hormone even has any muscle-specific anabolic properties in healthy humans, particularly athletes.[12]

While protein and amino acid supplements may not be necessary with respect to achieving daily protein requirements, these types of supplements may be useful to some athletes for other reasons. For example, consuming a protein shake or energy bar is very convenient. In addition, diets consisting of higher protein contents (normally meat) can be associated with higher intakes of fat; athletes trying to attain a certain body composition may find supplements beneficial in this regard.

Two recent studies highlight another potential benefit of protein intakes higher than the RDA for athletes. Layman and colleagues[13] studied overweight women who consumed an energy-restricted diet (7100 kJ [1.7 kcal] per day) designed to promote weight loss via 'higher' protein intake (1.5 g/kg per day) compared with a group of women consuming a similar energy intake but protein at the RDA level (0.8 g/kg per day). Ten weeks after beginning the diet, all the women had lost similar amounts of weight but the composition of weight loss in those consuming the higher protein diet was significantly shifted towards fat rather than lean mass loss (6.3 g fat lost/g lean tissue lost versus only 3.8 g fat lost/g lean tissue lost in those consuming the higher protein). Extending these findings, a subsequent study showed that the addition of exercise to a higher protein diet resulted in the greatest retention of lean tissue and loss of fat mass compared to groups that performed similar exercise with lower protein intake or no exercise but dietary changes alone.[14] A very salient point here is that the diets contained protein from high-quality sources (meat and dairy) but it was not supplemental in nature. These two studies[13, 14] highlight that a higher protein diet (1.5 g/kg per day) would appear to be beneficial for athletes who are seeking weight loss since the result is greater fat loss than lean mass loss. Of course, most athletes consume this level of protein on a habitual basis.[6] This underscores the importance of involving a sports dietitian with athletes whenever possible (Chapters 1, 37). Appropriate nutrition can then meet the athlete's protein need (Chapter 37) without the athlete using supplements for which

there is no evidence of benefit. It is also noteworthy that many power sport athletes spend more money on ineffective (and possibly counterproductive) supplements each month than it would cost to benefit from advice from an expert sports dietitian.

Beta-hydroxy-beta-methylbutyrate (HMB)

HMB, a metabolite of the amino acid leucine, is a relatively new supplement with purported ergogenic effects. HMB is thought to directly attenuate protein breakdown[15] and contribute to cell membrane integrity by acting as a substrate for cholesterol synthesis.[16] A recent meta-analysis of nine studies examining HMB supplementation with resistance training reported 1.1% and 5.6% per month increases in lean body mass and strength, respectively, when compared to unsupplemented training.[16] However, the ergogenic potential of HMB appears to be restricted to untrained individuals as similar increases in lean body mass and strength have not been observed in trained and elite athletes.[17] Further research into the potential benefits of HMB supplementation is warranted. At this time, however, it appears that HMB may augment muscle mass and strength gains in novices, with no major risks associated with its use.[18, 19] A recent review serves as a good resource for clinicians on the subject of HMB.[20]

Supplements for weight-restricted sports

Unlike strength and power athletes who strive to increase body mass, participants in sports such as distance running, martial arts, boxing, gymnastics, rowing and ballet generally seek to minimize body mass (especially fat mass) as this may benefit performance. Supplements that promise to improve fat oxidation can, therefore, be quite attractive to these athletes.

Carnitine

Carnitine is a protein involved in the transfer of fatty acids from the cell into the mitochondria where they are oxidized. Supplementation with carnitine improves fat oxidation in individuals with carnitine deficiency, however, most healthy individuals and athletes are not deficient in carnitine. Moreover, carnitine is readily available from the diet through the consumption of red meat and dairy products; in addition, both the liver and kidney can synthesize this protein. Nonetheless, supplementation with carnitine has been hypothesized to increase fat oxidation by

CHAPTER 38 MAXIMIZING SPORTING PERFORMANCE: TO USE OR NOT TO USE SUPPLEMENTS?

38

increasing the ability of the cell to shuttle fatty acids into the mitochondria.

Evidence supporting the efficacy of carnitine supplementation is equivocal at best. Only a few studies have found beneficial effects of carnitine supplementation in healthy individuals.[21] However, it is unclear whether the acute changes in fat oxidation reported by such studies would translate into significant weight/fat loss in the long term. In addition, several investigations have reported no ergogenic effect of carnitine supplementation.[22, 23] Short-term supplementation with carnitine (4–6 g per day for 1–2 weeks) has had no effect on muscle carnitine concentrations, whereas long-term administration (2 g per day for 12 weeks) has also failed to increase muscle carnitine concentration.[24] It is possible that oral consumption of this protein simply results in its digestion and therefore the supplement never actually reaches its target tissue intact.

Supplements for high-intensity exercise

Although there are a plethora of products that are claimed to increase energy supply, few are supported by evidence. Creatine, alkaline loading and anti-oxidants are popular supplements that are discussed here. Caffeine is a stimulant that can cause a positive doping test result; it is discussed in Chapter 61.

Creatine

Creatine is a tripeptide synthesized from the amino acids arginine, glycine and methionine, primarily in the liver. Muscle does not synthesize creatine but instead absorbs it from the circulation. Creatine can also be obtained through the diet as it is abundant in both fish and meat. In the muscle, creatine is involved in the phosphagen energy system where phosphocreatine (PCr) is used to provide a rapid, but transient, source of energy during brief high-intensity bouts of exercise. Creatine also plays a critical role in the resynthesis of ATP, the energy currency of the cell.

Creatine supplementation increases both PCr and total creatine (TCr) in muscle tissue.[25] The loading regimen is usually three or four doses of 4–5 g daily for the first five days, followed by a maintenance dose of 2–3 g daily thereafter. One can also achieve the same relative muscle creatine content by supplementing with a dose of 3–4 g per day for 30 days.[26] With respect to resistance exercise, the increase in PCr should theoretically enhance the ability to perform work (e.g. weightlifting repetitions), which over

the course of training should translate into greater strength and muscle mass gains. Some, but not all, studies found an increase in strength and muscle mass when resistance training was accompanied by creatine supplementation. However, the initial mass gains associated with creatine supplementation have been largely attributed to water retention.[27]

The increase in PCr associated with creatine supplementation enhances short-term, high-intensity exercise such as sprinting, most likely through improved ATP resynthesis.[28] Creatine, however, does not affect endurance performance as PCr stores are quickly depleted within the first few seconds of exercise. Moreover, the increased body weight caused by fluid retention may actually be detrimental to the performance of endurance athletes. Several recent reviews on the efficacy of creatine on performance, using a wide variety of laboratory as well as field-based tests, have been published.[16, 29] Nissen and Sharp[16] concluded that creatine could positively affect body mass gain when the supplement and resistance training were combined. They reported that creatine supplementation increased lean mass and strength by quite minor amounts in novice weightlifters, more than the changes observed with resistance training alone.[16] Moreover, these effects are likely to be much larger for the uninitiated insofar as weightlifting is concerned because of the potential for much greater lean mass gain in this population compared to a well-trained athlete.

Similarly, Branch[29] found that body composition showed a shift towards greater lean mass gain with creatine supplementation while also improving repeated sprint performance and upper-body strength exercises. Despite these findings, Branch[29] observed that laboratory tests always showed a far greater effect than did field-based tests, which may highlight the fact that the effect of creatine may be somewhat diminished when athletes move from the laboratory to the field. Nonetheless, creatine does appear to hold some promise in enhancing sprint performance, particularly if the task is repetitive in nature. At the same time, creatine is not recommended for athletes where the added body weight associated with creatine supplementation may be likely to hinder performance.[16, 29]

As with all medications and supplements, some individuals experience adverse effects with creatine supplementation. These can include gastrointestinal discomfort, nausea, vomiting and diarrhea. Thus, athletes who have not taken creatine prior to competition should not hastily begin a regimen in the hope of some sudden ergogenic benefit. A story in the newspaper *USA Today* attributed the deaths of three American collegiate wrestlers in December 1999 to creatine use as all had creatine in their possession at the time of death. This implication, however, was not substantiated at the formal inquiries.

Renal dysfunction is a potentially significant side-effect of creatine supplementation, particularly in individuals with pre-existing renal disease.[26] Thus, individuals with pre-existing renal dysfunction or those at high risk of renal disease (i.e. diabetes, family history of kidney disease) should be monitored medically if considering creatine supplementation. A review of creatine's efficacy and safety can be found as a discussion paper from the American College of Sports Medicine.[26]

Alkaline loading

Performance of high-intensity exercise, for example, an 800 m run, a 200–400 m swim, or a track sprint cycling event, leads to a marked lowering of blood and muscle pH in athletes. The increased hydrogen ion (H^+) load has been theorized to result in reduced cross-bridge interaction during contraction and to even lower the force per active cross-bridge during contraction, both of which would manifest as fatigue. Regardless of the mechanism(s), buffering intramuscular H^+ by ingesting sodium bicarbonate or sodium citrate has been variably shown to increase performance over short distances (i.e. 800–1500 m; see Maughan et al.[17] for review). The mechanism for this effect is the induction of metabolic alkalosis, which raises the initial pH of the muscle such that subsequent decreases in intramuscular pH with sprinting are much lower.

Highly trained but non-elite (best 800 m time about 2:05 s) middle-distance runners performed a simulated 800 m race. When metabolic alkalosis was induced by sodium salt ingestion, they were able to run almost 3 seconds faster than in the placebo or control trials.[30] A more recent report indicated similar improvements (3–4 s) over a distance of 1500 m in runners who completed simulated races in about 4:15 seconds.[31] Reviewing evidence[17] concluded that the performance improvements seen in sub-elite athletes over distances of 800–1500 m, if translated to elite athletes, would result in highly significant performance enhancements (i.e. result in new world records in the 800 m and 1500 m events).[30, 31]

Doses at which sodium bicarbonate and/or sodium citrate are thought to be effective are in the order of 150–300 mg/kg of body weight.[17, 30, 31] Such a dose does, however, often result in complaints such as diarrhea, bloating, vomiting and other gastrointestinal distress. Maughan et al.[17] reported that anecdotally athletes have been unable to compete as a result of the severity of the symptoms associated with alkaline salt ingestion; hence, as an overall recommendation we suggest that athletes do not partake in loading of these supplements without undue caution and the knowledge that the adverse side-effects may prevent them from competing.

Antioxidants

Skeletal muscles produce free radicals both at rest and during contractile activity. Most free radicals generated in skeletal muscle are oxygen based. This is the result of the fact that skeletal muscle contains mitochondria, which have oxygen as their ultimate electron acceptor. Not all transfers of electrons to oxygen to form water (the terminal reaction catalyzed in the oxidative electron transport chain) occur perfectly, however, and reactive oxygen species can be produced. These reactive oxygen species have an unpaired electron, which results in a chemically unstable and highly reactive condition. Due to this unpaired electron these molecules will react with almost any cellular compound that they are in close proximity to, including cellular proteins, lipids and DNA. The result of this free-radical mediated chemical reaction is an increase in oxidative stress and impaired cellular function. Thus, compounds that might slow or completely quench the chain of free radical damage and oxidative stress would theoretically prevent undesirable cellular damage. Human cells have evolved an elaborate defense system to combat oxidative stress. Even though both enzymatic and non-enzymatic systems exist, only non-enzymatic defenses will be dealt with here.

The most common compounds taken by athletes that function as non-enzymatic antioxidants are vitamins, particularly vitamins E and C. Vitamin E is the only true antioxidant but vitamin C is required to regenerate vitamin E if it has become a vitamin E radical as a result of interaction with a cellular reactive oxygen species. A variety of evidence (reviewed in Powers et al.[32]) suggests that supplementation with antioxidants may support muscle function. However, in contrast to animal studies, investigations in humans have generally not demonstrated enhanced exercise performance after antioxidant supplementation. Powers et al.'s[32] review of at least six well-conducted studies concluded that supplementation with vitamin E, even when combined with high doses of vitamin C, showed no performance improvement.

CHAPTER 38 MAXIMIZING SPORTING PERFORMANCE: TO USE OR NOT TO USE SUPPLEMENTS?

38

Whether athletes are subject to greater oxidative stress, due to performing regular exercise, than their sedentary counterparts remains unclear. From a theoretical standpoint the increased oxygen flux through the mitochondrial respiratory chain during exercise could result in greater generation of reactive oxygen species and, thus, require antioxidant supplements. Again, evidence to support such a supposition is lacking. In fact, if exercise were to be associated with increased oxidative stress, one would theorize that the increased cellular damage would have adverse consequences and athletes might suffer a greater rate of cellular dysfunction, resulting in more adverse health consequences, than sedentary persons, which is not the case.[33]

At present there is little evidence to suggest that athletes would have a greater requirement for antioxidant vitamins, or gain a performance benefit. While supplemental vitamin use is not likely to harm the sportsperson, megadoses of vitamins are not recommended and may actually cause harm. Upper limits for daily intakes of vitamin E (1000 mg) and C (2000 mg) have been established within the current dietary reference intakes.

Other nutrients

Phytochemicals and zoochemicals are defined as nonessential nutrients found in plants and animal food, respectively, that may have health benefits associated with their ingestion. Examples of phytochemical compounds include lycopene (a carotenoid), genistein (an isoflavone) and quercetin (a flavanoid). Zoochemicals include such compounds as conjugated linoleic acids (CLA), a naturally occurring fat found in milk and beef, and omega-3 fatty acids such as eicosapentanoic acid (EPA) or docosahexanoic acid (DHA), fats found in high abundance in certain fish. The benefits ascribed to these compounds are many, ranging from fat loss (CLA), to cancer prevention (lycopene), a reduction in symptoms of menopause (genistein), and a reduction in heart disease risk (EPA and DHA). Even though purified supplements of lycopene, CLA, EPA, DHA and genistein are available, there is evidence to suggest that these chemicals are most beneficial in exerting health benefits when they are consumed in whole foods.[34] At this stage it is impossible to make hard recommendations on the intakes of such compounds. The most important impact that these compounds might have would be to improve athletes' health and/or immune function; however, at present the consumption of whole foods (Chapter 37) appears to be a far more beneficial, practical, and far less costly means of obtaining effective doses of phytochemicals and zoochemicals.

Supplement contamination

A number of athletes have failed doping controls and claimed that the positive result was due to inadvertent consumption of contaminated supplements. A recently published article contains some of the first data on a multinational survey of non-hormonal (i.e. no prohormone-based supplements) supplements sold over the counter from various countries around the world.[35] This report found that almost 15% of supplements contained androgenic steroids not listed on the label. These 'positive' supplements came from the United Kingdom, Italy, Germany, the United States and the Netherlands. Supplements contained androgenic steroid levels that varied, but when nandrolone prohormones were ingested to a total uptake of more than 1 μg, a level attained in only one or two of the manufacturer's recommended dose in some supplements, the subsequent positive doping results for norandrosterone persisted for several hours.[35] The source of contaminants in this study came from the following products: amino acids and protein powders, creatine, carnitine, ribose, guarana, zinc, pyruvate, HMB, *Tribulus terrestris*, vitamins and minerals, and herbal extracts.

Maughan[36] has recently commented on this phenomenon and makes the following very salient comment: 'Some of the doping cases involving nandrolone may be the result of inadvertent ingestion by athletes of nandrolone or one of its metabolic precursors. Even guilty athletes, however, protest their innocence, and the principle of strict liability, which means that the offence lies not in the intention to cheat but rather in the presence of a prohibited substance in the urine, means that such protestations have little effect on those responsible for enforcing the doping regulations.' Clearly available evidence suggests that supplements may be contaminated, albeit likely inadvertently. However, while the athlete may be unaware of what is contained in a supplement, it is still ultimately a case of caveat emptor and it will be the athlete who pays the price for ingesting these supplements if he or she tests positive for a banned substance.

Conclusion

A variety of supplements exist, which athletes are known to take in an attempt to enhance their overall health, immunity or performance, either for training or competition purposes. The decision as to whether an athlete would choose to take a certain supplement is likely to be due to a combination of factors, including efficacy (either directly or psychologically), cost, side-effects and contamination risk. One could argue that, in reality, supplements are unlikely to have an impact anywhere near the magnitude of good overall nutrition, reliable and consistent training, and appropriate rest/recovery. In fact, the point made at the outset of this chapter was that if a supplement is truly shown to be performance enhancing, it is more than likely that it will be banned. Athletes will continue to take supplements, however, and probably with increasing frequency. Three rather rudimentary questions need to addressed when an athlete asks for advice on supplement use:

1. Is the supplement safe?
2. Is the supplement legal?
3. Is the supplement effective?

With the risk of contamination being very real, the answer to question 2 is not always easy to discern. We conclude that many supplements, particularly dietary supplements, may be less beneficial than an appropriately planned diet.

Recommended Reading

Kim PL, Staron RS, Phillips SM. Fasted-state skeletal muscle protein synthesis after resistance exercise is altered with training. *J Physiol* 2005; 568(Pt 1): 283–90.

Maughan RJ. Contamination of dietary supplements and positive drug tests in sport. *J Sports Sci* 2005; 23(9): 883–9.

Maughan RJ, King DS, Lea T. Dietary supplements. *J Sports Sci* 2004; 22(1): 95–113.

Palisin T, Stacy JJ. Beta-hydroxy-beta-methylbutyrate and its use in athletics. *Curr Sports Med Rep* 2005; 4(4): 220–3.

References

1. Huang SH, Johnson K, Pipe AL. The use of dietary supplements and medications by Canadian athletes at the Atlanta and Sydney Olympic Games. *Clin J Sport Med* 2006; 16(1): 27–33.

2. Morrison LJ, Gizis F, Shorter B. Prevalent use of dietary supplements among people who exercise at a commercial gym. *Int J Sport Nutr Exerc Metab* 2004; 14(4): 481–92.

3. Froiland K, Koszewski W, Hingst J, Kopecky L. Nutritional supplement use among college athletes and their sources of information. *Int J Sport Nutr Exerc Metab* 2004; 14(1): 104–20.

4. Lemon PW. Effect of exercise on protein requirements. *J Sports Sci* 1991; 9: 53–70.

5. Tipton KD, Wolfe RR. Protein and amino acids for athletes. *J Sports Sci* 2004; 22(1): 65–79.

6. Phillips SM. Protein requirements and supplementation in strength sports. *Nutrition* 2004; 20(7–8): 689–95.

7. Castell L. Glutamine supplementation in vitro and in vivo, in exercise and in immunodepression. *Sports Med* 2003; 33(5): 323–45.

8. Gleeson M. Interrelationship between physical activity and branched-chain amino acids. *J Nutr* 2005; 135(6 suppl.): 1591S–1595S.

9. Matthews DE. Observations of branched-chain amino acid administration in humans. *J Nutr* 2005; 135(6 suppl.): 1580S–1584S.

10. Newsholme EA, Blomstrand E. Branched-chain amino acids and central fatigue. *J Nutr* 2006; 136(1 suppl): 274S–276S.

11. Abel T, Knechtle B, Perret C, Eser P, von Arx P, Knecht H. Influence of chronic supplementation of arginine aspartate in endurance athletes on performance and substrate metabolism—a randomized, double-blind, placebo-controlled study. *Int J Sports Med* 2005; 26(5): 344–9.

12. Rennie MJ. Claims for the anabolic effects of growth hormone: a case of the emperor's new clothes? *Br J Sports Med* 2003; 37(2): 100–5.

13. Layman DK, Boileau RA, Erickson DJ, et al. A reduced ratio of dietary carbohydrate to protein improves body composition and blood lipid profiles during weight loss in adult women. *J Nutr* 2003; 133(2): 411–17.

14. Layman DK, Evans E, Baum JI, Seyler J, Erickson DJ, Boileau RA. Dietary protein and exercise have additive effects on body composition during weight loss in adult women. *J Nutr* 2005; 135(8): 1903–10.

15. Smith HJ, Wyke SM, Tisdale MJ. Mechanism of the attenuation of proteolysis-inducing factor stimulated protein degradation in muscle by beta-hydroxy-beta-methylbutyrate. *Cancer Res* 2004; 64(23): 8731–5.

16. Nissen SL, Sharp RL. Effect of dietary supplements on lean mass and strength gains with resistance exercise: a meta-analysis. *J Appl Physiol* 2003; 94(2): 651–9.

17. Maughan RJ, King DS, Lea T. Dietary supplements. *J Sports Sci* 2004; 22(1): 95–113.

18. Gallagher PM, Carruthers JA, Godard MP, Schulze KE, Trappe SW. Beta-hydroxy-beta-methylbutyrate ingestion, part II: effects on hematology, hepatic and renal function. *Med Sci Sports Exerc* 2000; 32(12): 2116–19.

19. Nissen S, Sharp RL, Panton L, Vukovich M, Trappe S, Fuller JC Jr. Beta-hydroxy-beta-methylbutyrate (HMB) supplementation in humans is safe and may decrease cardiovascular risk factors. *J Nutr* 2000; 130(8): 1937–45.

20. Palisin T, Stacy JJ. Beta-hydroxy-beta-methylbutyrate and its use in athletics. *Curr Sports Med Rep* 2005; 4(4): 220–3.

21. Muller DM, Seim H, Kiess W, Loster H, Richter T. Effects of oral L-carnitine supplementation on in vivo long-chain

fatty acid oxidation in healthy adults. *Metabolism* 2002; 51(11): 1389–91.

22. Brass EP. Supplemental carnitine and exercise. *Am J Clin Nutr* 2000; 72(2 suppl.): 618S–623S.

23. Vukovich MD, Costill DL, Fink WJ. Carnitine supplementation: effect on muscle carnitine and glycogen content during exercise. *Med Sci Sports Exerc* 1994; 26(9): 1122–9.

24. Wachter S, Vogt M, Kreis R, et al. Long-term administration of L-carnitine to humans: effect on skeletal muscle carnitine content and physical performance. *Clin Chim Acta* 2002; 318(1–2): 51–61.

25. Kreider RB. Effects of creatine supplementation on performance and training adaptations. *Mol Cell Biochem* 2003; 244(1–2): 89–94.

26. Terjung RL, Clarkson P, Eichner ER, et al. American College of Sports Medicine roundtable. The physiological and health effects of oral creatine supplementation. *Med Sci Sports Exerc* 2000; 32(3): 706–17.

27. Tarnopolsky MA, Parise G, Yardley NJ, Ballantyne CS, Olatinji S, Phillips SM. Creatine-dextrose and protein-dextrose induce similar strength gains during training. *Med Sci Sports Exerc* 2001; 33(12): 2044–52.

28. Casey A, Greenhaff PL. Does dietary creatine supplementation play a role in skeletal muscle metabolism and performance? *Am J Clin Nutr* 2000; 72(2 suppl.): 607S–617S.

29. Branch JD. Effect of creatine supplementation on body composition and performance: a meta-analysis. *Int J Sport Nutr Exerc Metab* 2003; 13(2): 198–226.

30. Wilkes D, Gledhill N, Smyth R. Effect of acute induced metabolic alkalosis on 800-m racing time. *Med Sci Sports Exerc* 1983; 15(4): 277–80.

31. Bird SR, Wiles J, Robbins J. The effect of sodium bicarbonate ingestion on 1500-m racing time. *J Sports Sci* 1995; 13(5): 399–403.

32. Powers SK, DeRuisseau KC, Quindry J, Hamilton KL. Dietary antioxidants and exercise. *J Sports Sci* 2004; 22(1): 81–94.

33. Blair SN, Cheng Y, Holder JS. Is physical activity or physical fitness more important in defining health benefits? *Med Sci Sports Exerc* 2001; 33(6 suppl.): S379–S399; discussion S419–S420.

34. Liu J, Knappenberger KS, Kack H, et al. A homogeneous in vitro functional assay for estrogen receptors: coactivator recruitment. *Mol Endocrinol* 2003; 17(3): 346–55.

35. Geyer H, Parr MK, Mareck U, Reinhart U, Schrader Y, Schanzer W. Analysis of non-hormonal nutritional supplements for anabolic-androgenic steroids—results of an international study. *Int J Sports Med* 2004; 25(2): 124–9.

36. Maughan RJ. Contamination of dietary supplements and positive drug tests in sport. *J Sports Sci* 2005; 23(9): 883–9.

Maximizing Sporting Performance: Psychology Principles for Clinicians

WITH NOEL BLUNDELL

It is very common to hear a sporting champion acknowledging the contribution of his or her sports psychologist when making an acceptance speech at a major competition. On the other hand, often the players who most need psychological assistance do not realize it. Instead, they are likely to blame other factors (e.g. technique, fitness) for their poor performance. Barriers to athletes using sports psychology counseling include negative perceptions of psychology and its value, lack of sports psychology knowledge, and the challenges of psychologists integrating with players and coaching staff.[1] The clinician who sees the athlete for a 'medical' problem or 'injury' must be aware that psychological factors may contribute to each of the problems listed below:

- inconsistency in performance
- 'choking' under pressure
- personality clashes with players or officials
- poor performance when traveling
- diminishing performance as a season or tournament progresses
- failure to master a particular sport skill
- failure to meet team goals
- excess tiredness, recurrent illness/injury
- substance abuse
- domestic problems.

Advanced sports psychology for athlete performance is outside the scope of this book. The purpose of the chapter is to provide some background information for clinicians who work with teams and sportspeople regarding:

- fundamental psychological skills that can improve sports performance
- relaxation techniques

- how psychological skills can aid physical preparation for sport
- the role of a sports psychologist working with a sporting team.

Further references relating to the psychology of sport and rehabilitation are listed in the Recommended Reading (p. 724). Psychological aspects of the rehabilitation process[2] are discussed in Chapter 12.

Fundamental psychological skills

An athlete's psychological skill level determines whether tasks performed effortlessly at training can be reproduced in front of thousands of fans or under the scrutiny of a coach finalizing an Olympic squad. Even without training, successful athletes possess high levels of psychological skills. However, just as technique training can enhance motor skills, appropriate psychological training can often improve the consistency of an athlete's on-field performance.[3]

Control of arousal level for optimal performance

Performance—the execution of skills in a competitive environment before an audience or judges—is facilitated by the athlete being in the optimum psychological state (Fig. 39.1). Athletes often describe the feeling of being in their optimum arousal zone as 'feeling in sync' or 'being in the flow'.

Variations from optimal arousal impair performance.[4, 5] Under-arousal leads to inappropriate recognition of, and response to, on-field cues. More often, an athlete's arousal level becomes excessive, leading to an increase in muscular tension and subsequent

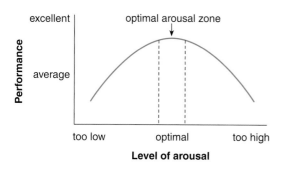

Figure 39.1 The inverted U: this demonstrates that performance is affected if an athlete is outside the optimal psychological state; the position of the curve varies between individuals and varies according to the complexity of the task

impairment of concentration, rhythm, coordination, timing and energy levels. A negative cycle develops, as shown in Figure 39.2.

Japanese elite athletes reported the optimal psychological state as one in which they felt relaxed, self-confident, highly motivated and completely focused. These appear to be primary elements for an optimal experience.[4]

Athletes seeking to achieve this state need to:

- understand that the performance arousal relationship follows an inverted U curve

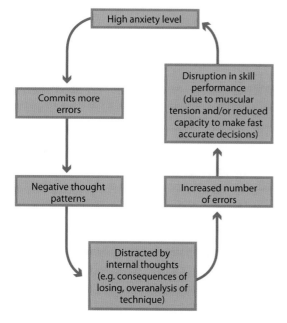

Figure 39.2 The negative cycle of decreasing performance and anxiety

- identify their peak performance state
- develop a competition day routine
- monitor their arousal level
- master techniques that allow adjustment of arousal level in either direction (e.g. mental imagery, progressive muscular relaxation, centering and positive self-talk)
- recognize situations that disturb their arousal level during performance.

Mental imagery

Mental imagery, also called mental rehearsal, is an experience that resembles sporting experience but occurs without the activity being performed. It is a mental skill that is useful in various situations. It may be used to modify arousal level, to enhance skill acquisition, to aid development of pre-competition and competition routines[6] and as a method of rehearsing other skills (i.e. motor skills, behavior modification). Thus, it is a widely used technique for improving sporting performance.

Downhill skiers provide a good example of the use of mental imagery. They can be seen—eyes closed, head moving from side to side—as they await clearance to begin their 'run' down the mountain. What they are doing is mentally rehearsing the act of skiing down the slope, shifting their body weight, changing direction smoothly, feeling the wind against their faces and flashing over the finish line.

As well as being used to enhance performance of 'closed skills' (when there are no variables other than the player and the ball, e.g. gymnastics, golf, serving at tennis), mental imagery can be used for 'open skills' where opponents influence the situation (e.g. track events, receiving serve).

Mental imagery can be used to develop coping strategies for sporting situations through a process known as 'stress inoculation'. Consider the tennis player who becomes so angry when he or she double-faults at a crucial time of a match that the next two games are lost as well. The player, through mental imagery, may recreate these circumstances but mentally practice remaining in control of the situation by using a coping strategy such as centering (see below). There are, however, potential dangers with this technique, which should only be introduced and controlled by a competent sports psychologist.

The danger lies in that the player may continue to mentally rehearse the double-fault and inadvertently become pre-programmed to serve the double-fault in the given set of circumstances. The sports psychologist must be sure that the athlete is competent at mental imagery, that the athlete knows how to use the coping strategy expertly and that the athlete focuses on 'successfully coping' and not on the anger in response to a double-fault.

Like all skills, mental imagery requires specific practise. Each motor skill must be completed entirely and at competition speed. It must be positive and successful—the athlete must be aware of negative images and feelings but should never rehearse failure.

The effectiveness of mental imagery is enhanced by deep relaxation. Successful mental imagers use as many senses as possible, such as hearing, feeling and smell, and not just sight. It would seem that mental imagery is more effective if the athlete is 'looking out' from within, as he or she would when performing, rather than being a spectator from the outside (as if watching him or herself on television), although the latter is still beneficial.

When should athletes use mental imagery?

Mental imagery should be used before practise sessions and, depending on the sport, before and during competition. Mental imagery should be undertaken three to four times a week for about 10 minutes per day (two 5-minute sessions) progressing to six to seven times per week during the last two weeks before the major competition. If the athlete performs mental imagery spontaneously, that is, in the course of daily activities, without a conscious attempt to do so, this should be encouraged. It is not advisable to perform mental imagery while trying to fall asleep the night before competition as imagery provokes an emotional state similar to that experienced in the competitive environment.

Progressive muscle relaxation

There are numerous techniques to obtain muscle relaxation. One simple, effective method is called progressive muscle relaxation. This involves contracting and relaxing specific muscle groups in turn. It teaches awareness of the feeling of relaxation to make the athlete more body-aware. It increases the ability to switch concentration from one anatomical region to another. This prepares the mind for the task of switching to appropriate cues, as necessary during sport. When first learning progressive muscle relaxation, many different muscle groups need to be contracted. Once the skill has been acquired, the pattern of muscle contraction depends on the athlete's preference and the sport being played (e.g. shoulders, neck and arms in a tennis player).

Centering

Progressive muscular relaxation requires several minutes to perform but the psychologically skilled athlete can produce a similar effect with a technique called centering that only requires a few seconds to perform. Thus, centering can be useful during competition.

An athlete who has mastered centering can change his or her arousal level with one breath, but this requires practise. At first, the procedure may appear stilted and the instructions listed in the box opposite excessively formal. However, with experience, the athlete develops a feel for centering and can incorporate it into the sporting routine, such as while leaning on a golf buggy waiting for an opponent to tee-off, or sitting in the chair between sets of tennis.

The breathing exercise, if undertaken successfully, will induce an enhanced level of relaxation and change the focus of attention. By focusing attention, monitoring the movement of the abdominal muscles and subsequently transferring attention to a point in the environment (e.g. the ball in tennis), the negative cycle is broken.

One method to learn centering is for athletes to practice for 3 minutes at a time for a total of 30 minutes a day and begin by completing sets of three long deep breaths. At first athletes may experience difficulty totally focusing their attention on monitoring abdominal movement. This, however, is critical and develops with practise. After a short time an athlete should be able to induce the desired effects by just taking one breath.

As athletes become more skilled at adjusting their arousal levels, they can use the technique less often. This is a sign of progress. By having a method whereby he or she can control anxiety, the athlete automatically tends to reduce anxiety.

Routine

Routine prepares the athlete mentally and physically for training or performance. Adopting specific pre-event routines improves consistency of performance. Routines are also useful in performing specific skills.

Routines for preparing for competition

Routines provide an overall structure for the athlete in the lead-up to competition and they can help put the player in the optimum arousal zone. The athlete must have the flexibility to modify the routine by adding to, or subtracting from, as competition schedules demand. Competition routine might begin two nights

Procedure for centering

1. Sit in a comfortable chair.
2. To release muscular tension in the face, smile slightly so that the lips are apart.
3. Flick the arms and then roll the head slightly, attempting to consciously relax the arm and neck muscles.
4. Close the eyes and drop the chin towards the chest.
5. (a) Take a long deep breath using the diaphragm, as shown in Figure 39.3. There should be minimal chest movement and absolutely no hunching or raising of the shoulders. Breathe in through the nose and out through the mouth. Do not take a deep breath expanding the lungs and chest as this further increases the muscular tension that is already present in the shoulder region because of anxiety.
   (b) While inhaling and exhaling, it is imperative that thoughts are focused on the movement of the abdominal muscles. Aim to monitor this movement to the exclusion of all else.
   (c) As you exhale, 'let yourself go', that is, allow the muscles to relax. You will know if you have been successful in this phase if you feel a release of muscular tension.
6. Repeat the technique three times. (If thoughts flash through your mind while taking a breath, it should not be regarded as a successful breath and must be repeated.)
7. After completion of the breathing exercise, it is important to immediately focus your attention on the most critical aspect of the environment, for example, the ball or the target.

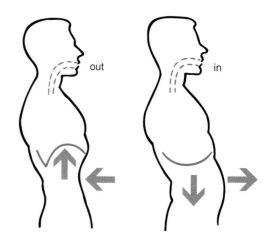

Figure 39.3 Diaphragmatic breathing in centering. The athlete should notice the stomach go out as he or she breathes in, and in as he or she breathes out. There should not be any use of the chest muscles

pitcher does not return to the key starting point in the routine, it is likely that the next pitch will not be productive. One practical and highly successful way of providing such athletes with feedback and reinforcing the need to re-start their routine is with the use of transceivers between the coach and athlete (see below).

Positive self-talk

Positive self-talk can assist an athlete to focus and obtain an optimum arousal level. Training for positive self-talk involves eradication of inappropriate thoughts, such as 'I can't get this shot', 'I never play well against Lauren', and replacing these with positive thoughts and words that reflect an appropriate focus on cues. In using positive self-talk, the player draws on past positive experiences, such as 'I've been here before, I know I can do it, focus on the job at hand'.

One way of teaching self-talk is with the aid of modern transceiver technology. By providing the athlete with a wireless ear piece, the sports psychologist can provide feedback to the athlete via the transceiver unit without compromising the integrity of the competitive environment. Without this device, the coach must interrupt practise to teach the athlete and this reduces psychological pressure and limits the integrity of the environment.

Although some devices allow the athlete and psychologist to communicate via transceivers, we believe that one-way messages from the sports psychologist are generally the most helpful way of using this new technology.

before competition and continue for several hours after the event.

An example of a routine for a swimmer who needs to compete on consecutive days is shown in the box on page 720.

Routines for performing skills

Routines can also be used to enhance the performance of closed skills. An example of a routine used by an international basketballer to shoot foul shots is given in the box on page 721.

A pitcher in baseball or softball (or a bowler in cricket) may have his or her routine disrupted. If the

Routine for preparation for competition for a swimmer competing on consecutive days

Afternoon—two days prior to first competition

5.00 p.m.	Light training
6.30 p.m.	Evening meal—high carbohydrate, plenty of fluid
9.00 p.m.	Sleep

Day before competition

7.00 a.m.	Wake up
8.00 a.m.	Light training—consisting only of the warm-up routine
9.30 a.m.	Breakfast
10.30 a.m.	Massage
12.30 p.m.	Lunch. Relax by watching TV, short walk, chatting with friends. Sleep
4.30 p.m.	Mental imagery routine
5.00 p.m.	Light training—consisting only of the warm-up routine
6.30 p.m.	Evening meal
8.00 p.m.	Stretching routine
9.00 p.m.	Sleep

Competition day (heats in morning, finals at night)

6.00 a.m.	Early rise (always rise at least 3 hours before racing), shower and stretch
6.30 a.m.	Breakfast: pre-event meal (Chapter 37)
7.00 a.m.	Travel to venue to arrive at least 1½ hours prior to race, listening to music on iPod on the way
7.30 a.m.	Get changed, stretch, pre-event massage
8.10 a.m.	Warm-up in pool
8.30 a.m.	Report to marshal area—mental imagery during this time
8.55 a.m.	Introductions
9.00 a.m.	Race
9.10 a.m.	Warm-down in diving pool
9.30 a.m.	Carbohydrate replacement—supplement
10.00 a.m.	Post-event massage
10.30 a.m.	Return to hotel/home/village
11.00 a.m.	Relax, sleep
2.00 p.m.	Late lunch (pre-race meal). Relax, may sleep (maximum 90 minutes)
4.30 p.m.	Travel to venue to arrive at least 1½ hours prior to race, listening to music on iPod on the way
5.30 p.m.	Get changed, stretch, pre-event massage
6.10 p.m.	Warm-up in pool
6.30 p.m.	Report to marshal area—mental imagery during this time
6.55 p.m.	Introductions
7.00 p.m.	Race
7.10 p.m.	Warm-down in diving pool
7.30 p.m.	Carbohydrate replacement—supplement
8.00 p.m.	Post-event massage
9.00 p.m.	Sleep

When an athlete uses the transceiver, the sports psychologist can provide feedback regarding the quality of concentration intensity, use of centering techniques, between point (pitch) routines, variations in emotional level, rhythm of the context and so on. This is done in the natural breaks in the practise (i.e. between points in a tennis match; between pitches in baseball/softball).

In clinical practise, excellent results occur when positive self-talk is enhanced with consistent feedback

Routine for shooting foul shots
• Whistle goes to signal foul.
• Walks to the foul line.
• Focuses on a spot on the ring (the same spot each time).
• Rehearses the movement without the ball.
• Receives the ball, bounces it four times while bent forward.
• Stands up straight, breathes in, relaxes the shoulders.
• Breathes out, shoots the ball, follows through.

to the player at appropriate times, particularly if the player is not inclined to provide such reinforcement. After a relatively short period players begin to look for the reinforcement and soon after start to positively reinforce themselves.

Goal-setting

Athletes often have conflicting goals that must be prioritized. Because of time constraints, they need to list specifically what is being attempted and plan long-, medium- and short-term goals. There may be some outcome-oriented goals (e.g. to make the Olympic team) but these goals are usually supported by specific, shorter term, task-oriented goals (e.g. to be able to press 150 kg by July, to run sub 10.2 seconds 100 m by August). These specific tasks are activities over which the athlete feels he or she has direct control. If short-term, task-oriented goals are met, then longer term goals should fall into place. Each different aspect of training (e.g. nutrition, strength, skill, psychological) needs goals, as do off-field factors such as schooling, career or family.

Modification of harmful psychological characteristics

Athletes have psychological characteristics that may be either beneficial or harmful to their sporting endeavors in different situations. By being made aware of their attributes, athletes can begin to understand why they react as they do in certain situations and learn to modify those behaviors that are harmful to their performance.

An example of harmful psychological characteristics can be described as the syndrome of the 'overmotivated underachiever' (Table 39.1).

This leads to a high anxiety level that manifests as poor decision making, lower concentration and disruption of skill production. The source of these problems is that the athlete is 'trying too hard' to be successful and hindering progress.[7] For example, athletes who had suffered tibial stress fractures scored higher on a type A behavior pattern inventory and exercise dependency compared with non-injured but otherwise matched runners.[8] A member of the sports medicine team may recognize these characteristics in a hard-training athlete who presents with symptoms such as those mentioned on page 716. In this situation, a sports psychologist can intervene. The sports psychologist can provide the athlete with insight into the problem and teach the techniques to alter the psychological characteristics that create the problem.

Psychological attributes also play an important role in how an athlete performs in team sports. Demonstration of physical courage, reaction to stressful situations such as being behind during competition or receiving an unfavorable refereeing decision, and ability to maintain focus and communication with other players are all determined by psychological attributes. Individuals can learn to control any attributes that are harmful to performance.

An entire team may aim to modify a single psychological attribute. A national women's field hockey team felt itself to be deficient in assertiveness, which manifested in some hesitancy on the pitch and some off-field compromises with nutrition and training schedules. The team psychologist provided assertiveness training, which was implemented both on and off the field in the 12 months leading up to the Olympic Games. Coaches and players felt that the ensuing behavioral change was a contributory factor to the eventual gold-medal-winning performance.

Mental skills' training and relaxation

Water flotation tanks

Some elite athletes use flotation tanks as part of their active recovery program. The flotation tank is a

Table 39.1 Features of the 'overmotivated underachiever'

- The athlete is generally highly motivated, usually intelligent and analytical.
- He or she tends to be obsessed with achieving inappropriate and unrealistic goals.
- The athlete tends to train hard and thus be extremely coachable but to suffer niggling injuries or persistent tiredness (Chapter 52).

bathtub-like enclave, half-filled with heavily salinated water so that the individual floats comfortably on the surface. Possible benefits of flotation include an increase in favorable mood states, improved capacity for sleep, the capacity for lower systolic and diastolic blood pressures and decreased plasma cortisol levels.[9, 10] The float tank can be used for relaxation therapy, mental imagery and watching tapes of selected performances.

Music

Music is widely used by athletes as part of their routine in preparation for sporting competition. Music can improve simple visual tasks in the laboratory and improve muscle contraction in the short term.[11, 12] One potential problem for those athletes unfamiliar with psychological training is that they may be listening to music that is having an inappropriate effect on their arousal level. The psychologically sophisticated athlete will use several different types of music depending on his or her arousal level. Nevertheless, it is unwise to change a well-established, successful formula.

Massage

Massage can be used not only to reduce tension but also to provide feedback to the athlete about muscle tension. This helps the athlete learn to monitor muscle tone. The therapeutic aspect of massage, removing abnormally tight tissue, also facilitates deep relaxation. It is highly advantageous to complement progressive relaxation techniques with deep therapeutic massage as the two techniques reinforce each other.

Mental skills' training aiding physical preparation for sport

Mental skills' training techniques can enhance several components of physical performance—physical attributes, sports skills and rehabilitation.

Facilitating physical training

Psychological training can help an athlete improve physical factors, such as speed and strength, but this is often overlooked. Centering improves the athlete's awareness of muscle anatomy and tone. This allows the athlete to improve the quality of contraction of agonist muscles (through improved neuromuscular facilitation) and ensure greater relaxation of antagonist muscles during muscular training. He or she can also relax more deeply between efforts, thus allowing better quality training. In addition, mental

imagery techniques can be used to improve technique both in the weight room and on the running track. Psychological methods for modifying perception of fatigue can help endurance athletes cope with high-volume training.

Enhancing motor skill development

The usefulness of psychological techniques to develop skill levels is broadly acknowledged but less widely practiced. Skills must be acquired, maintained and often added together in sequences (e.g. in gymnastics routines or field events). Each of these aspects can be enhanced with mental training, particularly by mental imagery, control of arousal level, adherence to routines and injury prevention.

Mental imagery allows the athlete to perform multiple practises of a motor skill. In skills that are physically demanding, it allows the performer to rehearse a skill without risking technique faults through fatigue or suffering overuse injury.

Skills need to be practiced perfectly. Maintenance of an optimum arousal level permits high-quality skill training. Injury prevention permits uninterrupted training. The psychological factors influencing injury prevention have been discussed in Chapter 6.

Developing a specific routine helps to make skills, such as serving at tennis or shooting from the foul line in basketball, 'automatic'. The routine should encourage a full-flowing natural action, as opposed to a tense, jerky or 'wooden' movement. Use of a routine ensures that exactly the same psychomotor pattern is being trained. This improves the reproducibility of the technique, making it less vulnerable to change at critical times.

Sometimes, players find that they are unable to perform a skill they had previously mastered (e.g. the 'yips' in putting). In this situation, they must consider whether the problem is due to an inappropriate mental state or a technique problem.

Facilitating rehabilitation

After major injury many sportspeople have a fear of reinjury[13] and, thus, mental skills may help them to rehabilitate effectively.[14–16] Injured players can use cognitive imagery to learn and properly perform the rehabilitation exercises. They may employ motivational imagery for goal-setting (e.g. imagine being fully recovered), to help maintain concentration and to retain a positive attitude. Imagery can help manage pain in a variety of ways. For example, imagery can help the sportsperson practice dealing with expected pain, distract the person from the pain, imagine the pain dispersing, and also to block the pain. Players may employ positive and accurate visual and kinesthetic images.[17] It is helpful if clinicians understand the benefits of imagery in athletic injury rehabilitation as they are ideally placed to encourage injured athletes to use this adjuvant therapy.[14]

The roles of a sports psychologist in a team

Sporting performance will be determined by the effectiveness of the competitors (the on-field team) and the effectiveness of the coaches and other officials (the off-field team). How well these groups work together will usually significantly influence on-field outcome. Members of the sports medicine team must remember that they are responsible to the coach. They operate within the coach's parameters while adhering to appropriate professional ethics.

On-field team

The psychologist can assist in fostering good team dynamics as well as helping individual players maximize their mental skills by working on a one-to-one basis.

Team dynamics

The cliché that 'a champion team will beat a team of champions' emphasizes the importance of group dynamics. Positive group dynamics can only be achieved if players feel comfortable with their role in the team. Problems can arise when players are uncertain about their roles or have, for example, a 'lesser' role in their representative team compared with their club team.

These problems can be addressed by counseling, goal-setting and modification of psychological attributes if necessary. Although the coach will talk to the athlete, it is often difficult for the athlete to be totally frank about his or her feelings to the coach. Furthermore, the problem may linger in the player's mind (and be affecting performance) long after the coach has forgotten about the episode. The sports psychologist is in a position to counsel the athlete over a period.

Goal-setting is a way of minimizing the frustration of unrealistic expectations. A player who normally shoots 30 points in 40 minutes of club basketball may, at international level, come off the bench for a total of 20 minutes, and make 10 points and three assists. The player may need some specific modification of his or her psychological attributes to make him or her more team-oriented rather than self-oriented.

Goal-setting can also be used at the team level with the use of round table discussions of team goals. This allows all players to have input into team priorities and it can reinforce the sense of team achievement when goals are met. Many successful teams commit team goals—goals that are generated from the coaching staff or from the players or, often, by mutual agreement—to paper at their pre-game preparation. These goals can then be evaluated after competition.

Off-field team

The off-field team will vary from a coach and manager for small sporting teams to one including coach, assistant coaches, managers, medical and paramedical staff, sports science personnel and a sports psychologist for elite teams. At major games, the entire mission makes up an off-field team. It is vital for this off-field group to work together closely and to synchronize what may be conflicting demands. This requires long-term planning (e.g. four years, one year, several months ahead) as well as short-term planning (e.g. weeks, days ahead).

Meetings

As the psychologist is trained to facilitate communication and organization, he or she can ensure effective cooperation among the off-field team. The psychologist often has the role of ensuring daily or second-daily meetings when a team is traveling so that matters such as training, meal times, pre- and post-game analyses, and free time are all scheduled. Often the psychologist is in the best situation to help individuals resolve conflicts that exist within both the off-field and the on-field team without significant confrontation.

Definition of roles

The off-field team must be clearly aware of responsibilities and it can be useful to list these formally so that nothing is overlooked and no tasks duplicated.

Sports psychologist's role with the coach

The coach needs someone to talk to. Usually, elite coaches have excellent sporting 'instinct' but this can be honed by further education. Examples of personal development skills that a coach can find useful include: how to plan meetings; how to communicate with players in meetings and individually; when to talk to players; how much to say at a pre-game address; as well as how to provide positive and negative feedback.

Coaches suffer considerable mental pressure without the release of physical activity enjoyed by the players. Coaches should consider remaining physically fit to help control tension. They need to operate in the optimum arousal level, just as players do. This makes them more comfortable and helps players remain in the zone—players often tend to mirror the coach's arousal level.[18] It may also prevent them from being over-impulsive and perhaps inappropriately berating a player or a referee.

Recommended Reading

Andersen M, Kolt G. *Psychology in the Physical and Manual Therapies.* Edinburgh: Churchill Livingstone, 2004.

Blundell N. *So you Want to be a Tennis Pro?* Melbourne: Lothian, 1995.

Gardner FL, Moore SE. *Clinical Sport Psychology.* Champaign, IL: Human Kinetics, 2006.

Herrigel E. *Zen in the Art of Archery.* London: Random House, 1999.

Jackson SA, Csikszentmihalyi M. *Flow in Sports.* Champaign, IL: Human Kinetics, 1999.

Kolt G, Snyder-Mackler L. *Psychology of Injury and Rehabilitation in Physical Therapies in Sports and Exercise.* Edinburgh: Churchill Livingstone, 2003.

Taylor J, Wilson GS. *Applying Sport Psychology.* Champaign, IL: Human Kinetics, 2005.

References

1. Pain MA, Harwood CG. Knowledge and perceptions of sport psychology within English soccer. *J Sports Sci* 2004; 22: 813–26.

2. Kolt G, Spetch L. Adherence to sport injury rehabilitation: implications for sports medicine providers and researchers. *Phys Ther Sport* 2001; 2: 80–90.

3. Hammermeister J, VonGuenthner S. Sport psychology: training the mind for competition. *Curr Sports Med Rep* 2005; 4: 160–4.

4. Sugiyama T, Inomata K. Qualitative examination of flow experience among top Japanese athletes. *Percept Mot Skills* 2005; 100: 969–82.

5. Thelwell RC, Maynard IW. Anxiety-performance relationships in cricketers: testing the zone of optimal functioning hypothesis. *Percept Mot Skills* 1998; 87: 675–89.

6. Vergeer I. Exploring the mental representation of athletic injury: a longitudinal case study. *Psychol Sport Exerc* 2006; 7: 99–114.

7. Galambos SA, Terry PC, Moyle GM, et al. Psychological predictors of injury among elite athletes. *Br J Sports Med* 2005; 39: 351–4.

8. Ekenman I, Hassmen P, Koivula N, et al. Stress fractures of the tibia: can personality traits help us detect the injury-prone athlete? *Scand J Med Sci Sports* 2001; 11: 87–95.

9. Kjellgren A, Sundequist U, Norlander T, et al. Effects of flotation-REST on muscle tension pain. *Pain Res Manag* 2001; 6: 181–9.

10. Jacobs GD, Heilbronner RL, Stanley JM. The effects of short term flotation REST on relaxation: a controlled study. *Health Psychol* 1984; 3: 99–112.

11. Crust L. Carry-over effects of music in an isometric muscular endurance task. *Percept Mot Skills* 2004; 98: 985–91.

12. Crust L, Clough PJ, Robertson C. Influence of music and distraction on visual search performance of participants with high and low affect intensity. *Percept Mot Skills* 2004; 98: 888–96.

13. Kvist J, Ek A, Sporrstedt K, et al. Fear of re-injury: a hindrance for returning to sports after anterior cruciate ligament reconstruction. *Knee Surg Sports Traumatol Arthrosc* 2005; 13: 393–7.

14. Driediger M, Hall C, Callow N. Imagery use by injured athletes: a qualitative analysis. *J Sports Sci* 2006; 24: 261–72.

15. Gutkind S. Using solution-focused brief counselling to provide injury support. *Sport Psychol* 2004; 18: 75–88.

16. Podlog L, Eklund RC. Assisting injured athletes with the return to sport transition. *Clin J Sport Med* 2004; 14: 257–9.

17. Vergeer I, Roberts J. Movement and stretching imagery during flexibility training. *J Sports Sci* 2006; 24: 197–208.

18. Baker J, Cote J, Hawes R. The relationship between coaching behaviours and sport anxiety in athletes. *J Sci Med Sport* 2000; 3: 110–19.

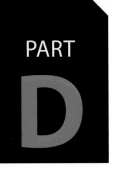

PART
D

Special Groups of Participants

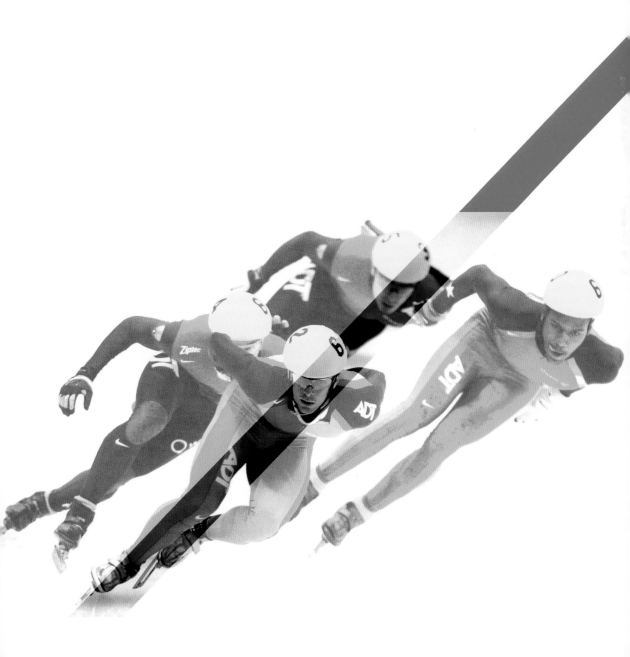

The Younger Athlete

WITH NICOLA MAFFULLI AND MERZESH MAGRA

CHAPTER

40

Sports medicine care for the younger athlete provides a number of challenges to the sports medicine clinician:

1. appropriate management of musculoskeletal conditions
2. assessment and advice regarding the risks and benefits of exercise in children with chronic illness
3. the question of 'How much sport is too much?'
4. advice regarding the nutritional needs of the growing child
5. encouragement of appropriate behavior of parents and coaches.

Each of these aspects of sports medicine is discussed in this chapter.

Management of musculoskeletal conditions

Younger athletes suffer many of the same injuries as their adult counterparts. However, there are also some significant differences in the type of injuries sustained by children and adolescents because of the differences in the structure of growing bone compared with adult bone. The different components of growing bone are indicated in Figure 40.1.

Anatomical differences between adult and growing bone

The differences between adult and growing bone (Fig. 40.2) are summarized below.

1. The articular cartilage of growing bone is a thicker layer than in adult bone and can remodel.

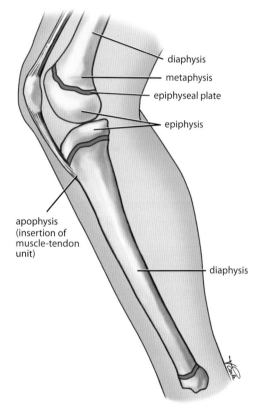

Figure 40.1 Different parts of the growing bone—the metaphysis, epiphysis, diaphysis, apophysis and articular cartilage

2. The junction between the epiphyseal plate and the metaphysis is vulnerable to disruption, especially from shearing forces.

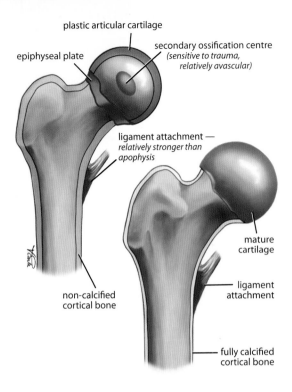

plastic articular cartilage

epiphyseal plate

secondary ossification centre
*(sensitive to trauma,
relatively avascular)*

ligament attachment —
*relatively stronger than
apophysis*

mature
cartilage

non-calcified
cortical bone

ligament
attachment

fully calcified
cortical bone

Figure 40.2 Contrasting features of growing bone (left) and adult bone (right)

3. Tendon attachment sites—apophyses—are cartilaginous plates that provide a relatively weak cartilaginous attachment, predisposing to the development of avulsion injuries.
4. The metaphysis of long bones in children is more resilient and elastic, withstanding greater deflection without fracture. Thus, children tend to suffer incomplete fractures of the greenstick type, which do not occur in adults.
5. During rapid growth phases, bone lengthens before muscles and tendons are able to stretch correspondingly and before the musculotendinous complex develops the necessary strength and coordination to control the newly lengthened bone. This may lead to muscle and tendon injuries,[1] although this is being disputed.[2] Growth temporarily reduces coordination[3] and this manifests as awkwardness in movement patterns while playing sport.

As a result of these differences, a particular mechanism of injury may result in different pathological conditions in the younger athlete compared with the mature adult. The younger athlete is more likely to injure cartilage and bone or completely avulse an apophysis than to have a significant ligament sprain. Some examples of different injuries in children and adults that are the result of similar mechanisms are shown in Table 40.1.

In children, traumatic injuries may result in fractures of the long bones or the growth plates. Strong, incoordinate muscle contractions are more likely to lead to an avulsion fracture at the site of attachment of the muscle or tendon rather than a tear of the muscle or tendon itself.

The osteochondroses are a group of conditions affecting the growth plates. Although the etiology of the osteochondroses is not well understood, non-articular osteochondroses may well be related to overuse (Table 40.2).

Each of the following common pediatric injury presentations are discussed in this chapter:

1. acute fractures
2. shoulder pain
3. elbow pain
4. wrist pain
5. back pain or postural abnormality
6. hip pain
7. knee pain
8. painless abnormalities of gait
9. foot pain.

Acute fractures

Fractures occur in the young athlete due to the line of weakness between the epiphyseal plate and the formed bone, and the relative weakness of apophyseal cartilage compared with the musculotendinous complex. Three types of fractures are seen in the younger athlete:

1. metaphyseal fractures
2. growth plate fractures
3. avulsion fractures.

Metaphyseal fractures

Metaphyseal fractures occur especially in the forearm and lower leg. The most common type of fracture seen is a buckling of one side of the bone. This incomplete fracture is often referred to as a greenstick fracture. Most fractures of the shaft of long bones that do not involve growth plates can be treated by simple immobilization and will heal quickly, usually within three weeks. Occasionally, angular or rotational deformity is present and requires open reduction and internal fixation.

Table 40.1 Comparison of injuries that occur with similar mechanisms in children and adults

Site	Mechanism	Injury in adult	Injury in child
Thumb	Valgus force as in 'skier's thumb'	Sprain of ulnar collateral ligament	Fracture of proximal phalangeal physis (usually Salter–Harris type III)
Distal interphalangeal joint of finger	Hyperflexion injury	Mallet finger	Fracture of distal phalangeal epiphysis (type II or III)
Hand	Punching injury as in boxing	Fracture of metacarpal head	Fracture of metacarpal epiphysis (type II)
Shoulder	Fall on point of shoulder	Acromioclavicular joint sprain	Fracture of distal clavicle epiphysis
Shoulder	Abduction and external rotation force	Dislocated shoulder	Fracture of proximal humeral epiphysis (type I or II)
Thigh/hip	Acute flexor muscle strain or extensor strain	Quadriceps strain or hamstring strain	Apophyseal avulsion of anterior inferior iliac spine or ischial tuberosity
Knee	Overuse injury	Patellar tendinopathy	Osgood-Schlatter lesion or Sinding-Larsen–Johansson lesion
Knee	Acute trauma (e.g. skiing) injury	Meniscal or ligament injury	Fractured distal femoral or proximal tibial epiphysis, avulsion of tibial spine
Heel	Overuse	Achilles tendinopathy	Sever's lesion

Table 40.2 Types of osteochondrosis

Type	Condition	Site
Articular	Perthes' disease Kienböck's lesion Kohler's lesion Freiberg's lesion Osteochondritis dissecans	Femoral head Lunate Navicular Second metatarsal Medial femoral condyle, capitellum, talar dome
Non-articular	Osgood-Schlatter lesion Sinding-Larsen–Johansson lesion Sever's lesion	Tibial tubercle Inferior pole of patella Calcaneus
Physeal	Sheuermann's lesion Blount's lesion	Thoracic spine Proximal tibia

Growth plate fractures

Fractures of the growth plate are of particular concern because of the dangers of interruption to the growth process via injury to the cells in the zone of hypertrophy. Growth plate fractures are classified according to Salter and Harris (Fig. 40.3). Salter–Harris types I and II fractures usually heal well. Type III and IV fractures involve the joint surface as well as the growth plate and have a high complication rate. If these fractures are not recognized, they could produce permanent injury to the growth plate, resulting in growth disturbances. When recognized, accurate anatomical reduction must be performed to reduce the possibility of interference in growth and to minimize the possibility of long-term degenerative change. However, occasionally the initial insult can produce permanent growth arrest despite subsequent anatomical reduction.

The common sites of growth plate fractures in the younger athlete with recommended management and potential complications are shown in Table 40.3.

It is most important to recognize an epiphyseal fracture. Radiographs should be obtained of both

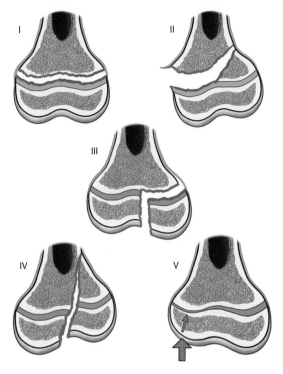

Figure 40.3 Salter–Harris classification of growth plate fractures

limbs (for comparison) if clinical features suggest growth plate injury. A normal radiograph does not exclude a growth plate fracture. A history of severe rotational or shear force with accompanying localized swelling, bony tenderness and loss of function should be regarded as a growth plate fracture. If there is any doubt regarding the diagnosis or management of these injuries, specialist orthopedic referral is mandatory.

Avulsion fractures

Avulsion fractures occur at the attachments of ligaments or, more commonly, large tendons to bones. One site of an avulsion fracture at a ligamentous attachment is at the attachment of the anterior cruciate ligament to the tibia. An acute rotational injury to the knee may present with the symptoms and signs of an anterior cruciate ligament tear. Instead of the in-substance tear common in adults, the more common injury in children is avulsion of the tibial spine or distal femoral attachment. Radiographs should be performed in all cases of acute knee injuries accompanied by hemarthrosis. Management involves surgical reattachment of the avulsed fragment and ligament.

More commonly, avulsion fractures occur at the apophyseal attachment of large musculotendinous units. The common sites are at the attachment of the:

- sartorius muscle to the anterior superior iliac spine
- rectus femoris muscle to the anterior inferior iliac spine
- hamstring muscles to the ischial tuberosity
- iliopsoas tendon to the lesser trochanter of the femur.

In the younger athlete, these fractures are the equivalent of acute muscle strain in the adult. Instead of a tear of the muscle fibers in the mid-substance of the muscle or at the musculotendinous junction, the tendon is pulled away with its apophyseal attachment. This is confirmed on plain radiographs (Fig. 22.12).

Management of avulsion fractures is identical to that for grade III tears of the muscle. It involves initial reduction of the pain and swelling, restoration of full range of motion with passive stretching and

Table 40.3 Management and possible complications of growth plate fractures in young athletes

Site	Management	Potential complications
Distal radius fracture	Cast immobilization (3–4 weeks)	Not recognized, growth disturbance
Supracondylar fracture of the elbow	Sling (3 weeks)	Vascular compromise of brachial artery, median nerve damage, malalignment
Distal fibular fracture	Cast, non-weight-bearing (4–6 weeks)	Growth disturbance can occur up to 18 months later
Distal tibial fracture	Cast, non-weight-bearing (4–6 weeks)	Premature closure of physis can lead to angulation and leg length discrepancy
Distal femur fracture	Anatomical reduction	Greater incidence of growth discrepancies than in other fractures, Salter–Harris type I and II fractures must be observed closely

active range of motion exercises as symptoms settle as well as a graduated program of muscle strengthening. Any biomechanical abnormalities that may have predisposed the athlete to this injury should be corrected. Reattachment of the avulsed fragment is rarely necessary.

Shoulder pain

Acute trauma to the shoulder may result in fracture of the proximal humerus, the clavicle, the acromion or the coracoid process. Dislocation of the glenohumeral joint is common in the adolescent but uncommon in the younger child. Dislocations in adolescents are associated with a high incidence of recurrence and development of post-traumatic instability. The management of acute dislocation of the shoulder is discussed in Chapter 17.

Overuse injuries around the shoulder are common in young athletes involved in throwing sports, swimming and tennis. A stress fracture of the proximal epiphyseal plate is seen in young throwers and has been termed 'Little Leaguer's shoulder'. Radiographs reveal widening of the epiphyseal line, followed at a later stage by evidence of new bone formation.

Shoulder impingement is also seen in the younger athlete. In the young athlete involved in throwing sports, the impingement is usually secondary to atraumatic instability, which develops because of repetitive stress to the anterior capsule of the shoulder joint at the end range of movement (Chapter 17). Impingement and rotator cuff tendinopathy also occur in swimmers where excessive internal rotation causes a tendency to impinge. The etiology of these problems in throwers and swimmers is discussed in Chapter 5.

Elbow pain

Delineating injury patterns to the elbow in children can be challenging, given the cartilaginous composition of the distal humerus and the multiple secondary ossification centers which appear and unite with the epiphysis at defined ages. The pitching motion in baseball, serving in tennis, spiking in volleyball, passing in American football, and launching in javelin throwing can all produce elbow pathology caused by forceful valgus stress, with medial stretching, lateral compression and posterior impingement. The valgus forces generated during the acceleration phase of throwing (Chapter 5) result in traction on the medial elbow structures and compression to the lateral side of the joint. This may injure a number of structures on the medial aspect of the joint. Injuries include chronic apophysitis of the medial epicondyle, chronic strain of the medial (ulnar)

collateral ligament or avulsion fracture of the epiphysis. The ulnar nerve may also be damaged.

The lateral compressive forces may damage the articular cartilage of the capitellum or radial head. The long-term sequelae of these repetitive valgus forces include bony thickening, loose body formation and contractures.

Flexion contractures can occur because of repeated hyperextension. The majority of these contractures are relatively minor (<15°). Significant contractures (>30°) should be treated with active and active-assisted range of motion exercises accompanied by a lengthy period of rest (e.g. three months).

Osteochondritis dissecans of the capitellum is also seen in pitchers and, more commonly, in gymnasts. Osteochondritis dissecans is a localized area of avascular necrosis on the anterolateral aspect of the capitellum. Initially, the articular surface softens and this may be followed by subchondral collapse and formation of loose bodies in the elbow. The early stages of osteochondritis dissecans may respond well to rest. Surgery is required to remove loose bodies. Joint debridement is usually performed at the same time. The results of surgical management of this condition are variable.

The younger child (under 11 years) may develop Panner's lesion. This self-limiting condition is characterized by fragmentation of the entire ossific center of the capitellum. Loose bodies are not seen in Panner's lesion and surgery is not required.

Ensuring adolescents have adequate rest between training sessions and that sporting technique is correctly coached and monitored by experts can prevent these injuries.

Wrist pain

Acute wrist pain can occur because of a fracture. The scaphoid bone is the most commonly affected bone. Dorsal wrist pain is commonly seen in gymnasts where pain is aggravated by weight-bearing with the wrist extended. The gymnast complains of tenderness over the dorsum of the hand and perhaps swelling. Examination findings are usually consistent with local injury. The most likely cause is a stress injury to the distal radial or distal ulnar growth plates. Longstanding injuries are associated with typical radiographic changes, including widening, irregularity, haziness or cystic changes of the growth plate. Acute growth plate slippage or fractures of the distal epiphyses are occasionally seen. Other causes of dorsal wrist pain include capsule sprain, a tear of the triangular fibrocartilage complex and stress fractures.

Management of the younger gymnast with dorsal wrist pain includes relative rest, splinting, electrotherapeutic modalities and NSAIDs. Strengthening of the wrist flexors may also be useful in association with tape and pads to decrease hyperextension of the wrist.

Kienböck's lesion of the wrist (Chapter 19) is an osteochondrosis of the lunate bone. It occurs generally in older patients (20 years old) and rarely in adolescents.

Back pain and postural abnormalities

Younger athletes may present with pain or postural abnormalities such as 'curvature' of the spine (or both).

Low back pain

Common causes of back pain in the younger athlete are similar to those in the mature adult. Minor soft tissue injuries to the intervertebral disk, the apophyseal joints and associated ligaments and muscle strains in the paravertebral muscles usually respond well to reduction in activity. Manipulative treatment in the management of these conditions in the younger athlete is probably contraindicated.

There are a number of other possible causes of low back pain in the younger athlete:

- spondylolysis
- spondylolisthesis
- vertebral end-plate fracture
- atypical Scheuermann's lesion (vertebral apophysitis)
- conditions not to be missed
  — tumor (osteogenic sarcoma)
  — infection (diskitis).

Stress fractures of the pars interarticularis (spondylolysis) may occur in the younger athlete, particularly because of repeated hyperextension of the lumbar spine. These injuries are typically seen as a result of ballet, gymnastics, diving, volleyball, fast bowling in cricket and serving in tennis. The management of this condition is discussed in Chapter 21. The amount of hyperextension activity must be reduced and this may involve some alteration in technique.

There is considerable debate whether these defects in the pars interarticularis are congenital or acquired. They are probably acquired, even though this may occur at an extremely young age. A fibrous union develops across the defect and this is susceptible to injury. The presence of a pars interarticularis defect does not automatically mean that this is the cause of the patient's pain. Radioisotopic bone scan or MRI may confirm that the pars interarticularis defect is the site of an acute fracture.

Severe disk injuries and tumors are occasionally seen in the lumbar spine of the adolescent athlete. Biomechanical abnormalities such as leg length discrepancy, pelvic instability and excessive subtalar pronation may also indirectly lead to low back pain and require correction if present.

Postural abnormalities

The commonest postural abnormality of the spine in the younger athlete is excessive kyphosis of the spine due to an osteochondrosis (Scheuermann's lesion). This condition occurs typically in the thoracic spine but is also seen at the thoracolumbar junction. Children can present with acute pain. It usually presents in later years as an excessive thoracic kyphosis in association with a compensatory excessive lumbar lordosis.

The typical radiographic appearance of Scheuermann's lesion is shown in Figure 40.4. This demonstrates irregularity of the growth plates of the vertebrae. The radiological diagnosis of Scheuermann's lesion is made on the presence of wedging of 5° or more at three adjacent vertebrae.

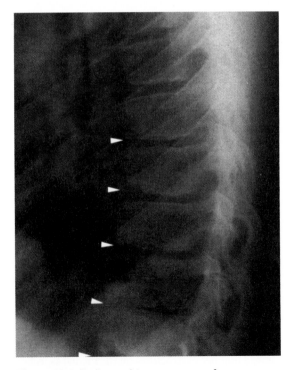

Figure 40.4 Radiographic appearance of Scheuermann's lesion

Management is aimed at preventing progression of the postural deformity and involves a combination of joint mobilization, soft tissue therapy to the thoracolumbar fascia, stretching of the hamstring muscles and abdominal muscle strengthening. A brace may be worn to decrease the thoracic kyphosis and lumbar lordosis. Surgery may be indicated if the kyphosis is greater than 50° or if signs of spinal cord irritation are present.

Hip pain

Hip pain is a more common presenting symptom in the younger athlete than the mature adult. The causes of hip pain in the younger athlete are shown in Figure 40.5. There are a number of possible causes of persistent hip pain and decreased range of motion in the younger athlete.

Apophysitis

A number of large musculotendinous units attach around the hip joint. Excessive activity can result in a traction apophysitis at one of these sites, usually the anterior inferior iliac spine at the attachment of the rectus femoris, the anterior superior iliac spine at the attachment of the sartorius, or the iliopsoas attachment to the lesser trochanter. Management involves a reduction in activity and attention to any predisposing factors such as muscle tightness. These conditions will always resolve.

Perthes' disease

Perthes' disease is an osteochondrosis affecting the femoral head. It presents as a limp or low-grade ache in the thigh, groin or knee. On examination there may be limited abduction and internal rotation of the hip. Perthes' disease is usually unilateral. It typically affects children between the ages of 4 and 10 years, is more common in males, and may be associated with delayed skeletal maturation. Radiographs vary with the stage of the disease but may show increased density and flattening of the femoral capital epiphysis (Fig. 40.6).

Management consists of rest from aggravating activity and range of motion exercises, particularly to maintain abduction and internal rotation. The age of the child and the severity of the condition will affect the intensity of the management. Rest, the use of a brace, and even surgery may be required. Recently, arthroscopic chondroplasty and loose body excision has shown good short-term results.[4]

The condition usually resolves and return to sport is possible when the athlete is symptom-free and radiographs show some improvement. The main long-term concern is the development of osteoarthritis due to irregularity of the joint surface.

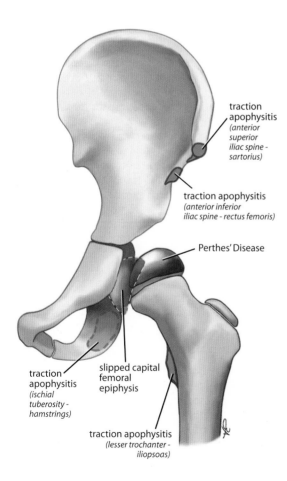

traction apophysitis
(anterior superior iliac spine - sartorius)

traction apophysitis
(anterior inferior iliac spine - rectus femoris)

Perthes' Disease

traction apophysitis
(ischial tuberosity - hamstrings)

slipped capital femoral epiphysis

traction apophysitis
(lesser trochanter - iliopsoas)

Figure 40.5 Causes of hip pain in children

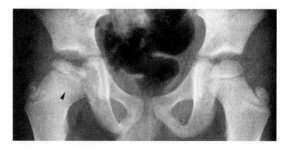

Figure 40.6 Radiographic appearance of Perthes' disease

Slipped capital femoral epiphysis

A slipped capital femoral epiphysis may occur in older children, particularly between 12 and 15 years. This is similar to a Salter–Harris type I fracture. It occurs typically in overweight boys who tend to be late maturers. The slip may occur suddenly or, more commonly, as a gradual process. There is sometimes associated pain, frequently in the knee, but the most common presenting symptom is a limp.

Examination reveals shortening and external rotation of the affected leg. Hip abduction and internal rotation are reduced. During flexion the hip moves into abduction and external rotation. Radiographs show widening of the growth plate and a line continued from the superior surface of the neck of the femur does not intersect the growth plate (Fig. 40.7). Bilateral involvement is common. Slips are a matter of considerable concern because they may compromise the vascular supply to the femoral head and lead to avascular necrosis. These require orthopedic assessment. A gradually progressing slip is an indication for surgery. An acute severe slip occurs occasionally. This is a surgical emergency.

Irritable hip

'Irritable hip' is common in children but should be a diagnosis of exclusion. The child presents with a limp and pain that may not be well localized. Examination reveals painful restriction of motion of the hip joint, particularly in extension and/or abduction in flexion. In the majority of cases, a specific cause is never identified and the pain settles after a period of bed rest and observation. Radiographs, bone scanning and blood tests are usually normal, and the child is treated with rest.[5]

Knee pain

Knee pain, especially anterior knee pain, is a common presentation in the younger athlete. The common causes of anterior knee pain are:

- Osgood-Schlatter lesion
- Sinding-Larsen–Johansson lesion
- patellofemoral joint pain (Chapter 28)
- patellar tendinopathy (Chapter 28)
- referred pain from the hip.

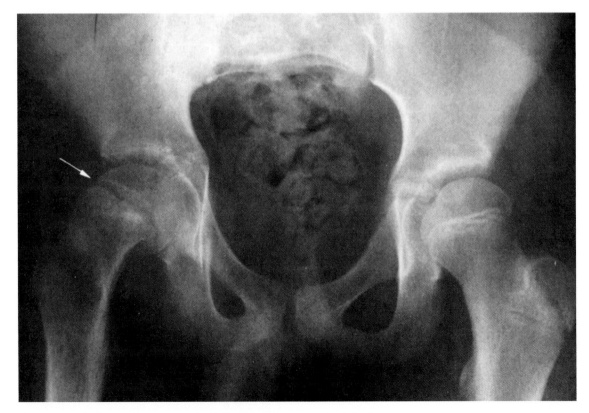

Figure 40.7 Radiographic appearance of slipped capital femoral epiphysis

Osgood-Schlatter lesion

Osgood-Schlatter lesion is an osteochondritis that occurs at the growth plate of the tibial tuberosity. Repeated contraction of the quadriceps muscle mass may cause softening and partial avulsion of the developing secondary ossification center.

This condition is extremely common in adolescents at the time of the growth spurt. It is usually associated with a high level of physical activity, especially in sports involving running and jumping, such as basketball, football or gymnastics. Pain around the tibial tuberosity is aggravated by exercise.

Examination reveals tenderness over the tibial tuberosity (Fig. 40.8). There may be associated tightness of the surrounding muscles, especially the quadriceps. The presence of excessive subtalar pronation may predispose to the development of this condition.

The diagnosis of Osgood-Schlatter lesion is clinical and radiographs are usually not required. In cases of severe anterior knee pain with more swelling than expected, a radiograph may be indicated to exclude bony tumor. Although all bone tumors are rare, the knee is a site of osteogenic sarcoma in the 10–30 year age group. The typical radiographic appearance of Osgood-Schlatter lesion is shown in Figure 40.9.

Osgood-Schlatter lesion is a self-limiting condition that settles at the time of bony fusion of the tibial tubercle. Its long-term sequel may be a thickening and prominence of the tubercle. Occasionally, a separate fragment develops at the site of the tibial tubercle. Athletes and parents need to understand the nature of the condition as symptoms may persist for up to two years.

Management of this condition requires activity modification. While there is no evidence that rest accelerates the healing process, a reduction in activity will reduce pain. As this condition occurs in young athletes with a high level of physical activity, it may be useful to suggest they eliminate one or two of the large number of sports they generally play. There is no need to rest completely. Pain should be the main guide as to the limitation of activity.

Symptomatic management includes applying ice to the region. A trial of local electrotherapy may be warranted but should be ceased if there is no noticeable improvement within two or three treatments as it is unhelpful in many cases.

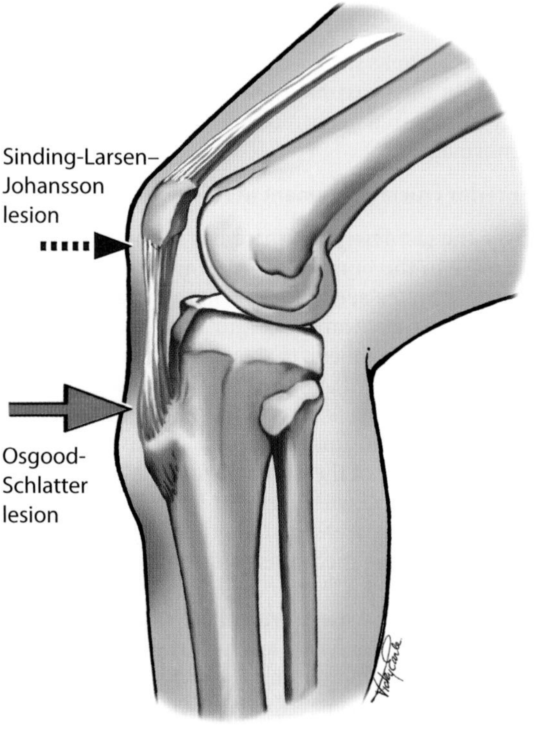

Sinding-Larsen–
Johansson
lesion

Osgood-
Schlatter
lesion

Figure 40.8 Sites of the Osgood-Schlatter lesion (distal) and the Sinding-Larsen–Johansson lesion (proximal)

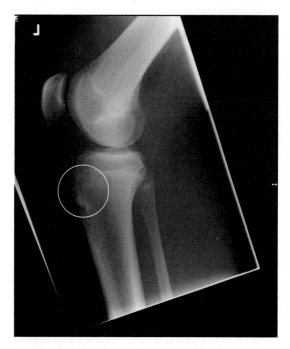

Figure 40.9 Radiographic appearance of Osgood-Schlatter lesion

Tightness of the quadriceps muscles may predispose to this condition. The athlete should commence a stretching program and, if possible, some soft tissue therapy to the quadriceps muscle. Muscle strengthening can be introduced as pain allows.

Correction of any predisposing biomechanical abnormality, such as excessive subtalar pronation, is necessary. Neither injection of a corticosteroid agent nor surgery is required. Very occasionally, the skeletally mature person may continue to have symptoms due to non-union. The separate fragment should then be excised.

Sinding-Larsen–Johansson lesion

This is a similar condition to Osgood-Schlatter lesion. It affects the inferior pole of the patella at the superior attachment of the patellar tendon (Fig. 40.8). It is much less common than Osgood-Schlatter lesion but the same principles of management apply.

Patellar tendinopathy

Although symptomatic tendinopathy was thought to be rare in children, there is now evidence that patellar tendinopathy is prevalent in junior basketball players.[6, 7] Management is as per tendinopathy in adults, although healing may be quicker in the adolescent years.

Referred pain from the hip

Conditions affecting the hip, such as a slipped capital femoral epiphysis or Perthes' disease, commonly present as knee pain. Examination of the hip joint is mandatory in the assessment of any young athlete presenting with knee pain.

Less common causes of knee pain

Osteochondritis dissecans may affect the knee. This generally presents with intermittent pain and swelling of gradual onset. Occasionally, it may present as an acute painful locked knee. This acute presentation is associated with hemarthrosis and loose body formation. Radiographs may reveal evidence of a defect at the lateral aspect of the medial femoral condyle. Osteochondritis dissecans requires orthopedic referral for possible fixation of the loosened fragment or removal of the detached fragment.

In juvenile rheumatoid arthritis (Still's disease) of the knee, there is persistent intermittent effusion with increased temperature and restricted range of motion. There may be a family history of rheumatoid arthritis. Investigation requires serological examination, including measuring the level of rheumatoid factor and the erythrocyte sedimentation rate and, if

indicated, serological examination of joint aspirate. The child's activity should be adapted to avoid using the painful joints while exercising other body parts and promoting cardiovascular fitness.

A differential diagnosis in pediatric arthritis that is relatively rare but is increasing in the developed world is acute rheumatic fever.[8] As there may be no history of sore throat and carditis may be silent, the diagnosis can only be made if the practitioner maintains an index of suspicion for this condition. Investigations should include markers of inflammation (erythrocyte sedimentation rate, C-reactive protein), serology for streptococci (anti-streptolysin-O titer, anti-DNase B titers) and echocardiography. Penicillin and aspirin (ASA) taken orally remain the mainstays of management.

A partial diskoid meniscus may cause persistent knee pain and swelling in the adolescent athlete. There is usually marked joint line tenderness. Arthroscopy may be diagnostic and therapeutic. A complete diskoid meniscus is characterized by a history of clunking in the younger child (4 years).

Adolescent tibia vera (Blount's disease) is an uncommon osteochondrosis that affects the proximal tibial growth plate. It usually affects tall, obese children around the age of 9 years. It is generally unilateral and radiographs show a reduced height of the medial aspect of the proximal tibial growth plate. Surgery may be required to correct any resultant mechanical abnormality.

Anterior cruciate ligament (ACL) injuries

Over the last few years there has been an apparent increase in the number of ACL injuries reported in young athletes secondary to higher participation levels, greater awareness and improved imaging modalities. It is difficult to ascertain the true incidence and prevalence of ACL injuries in young athletes because of the lack of documentation of skeletal maturity and the ambiguity in diagnosis.[9] There is a preponderance of these injuries in girls because of a smaller ACL size with a smaller intercondylar notch of the femur, decreased strength and conditioning, different playing mechanisms during play, and anatomical alignment.[10]

ACL injuries usually present with an acute history of a 'pop' in the knee, with an inability to return to play, followed by swelling in the knee within 6–12 hours. Children with chronic ACL insufficiency will present with functional instability in the knee when pivoting. The anterior drawer and Lachmann's tests are usually positive. Caution must be taken in interpreting the findings of these tests given the inherent laxity present in the pediatric knee. Thus, before reaching a clinical diagnosis, the contralateral knee should be examined. MRI scans of the knee should be undertaken to confirm the diagnosis of ACL injuries and to rule out the presence of any associated meniscal tears. MRI is not a substitute for a good history and physical examination, and imaging should only be used to correlate the findings of clinical examination.

The management of ACL injuries in the younger athlete is still controversial. Non-operative management is usually reserved for younger children who have not yet reached skeletal maturity (Tanner stage 1 and 2). However, non-operative management has a poor outcome.[11, 12] Surgery is usually performed in children who are either non-compliant to conservative management, or in those demonstrating functional instability with activities of daily living. When the child has associated meniscal pathology, ACL surgery is strongly recommended irrespective of the child's Tanner stage.[9] In skeletally immature children, physeal sparing combined with intra-articular and extra-articular reconstruction of the ACL using autologous iliotibial band graft has shown promising results.[13]

Painless abnormalities of gait

It is common for a child to present with an abnormality of gait. The child is usually brought in by a parent who has noticed an unusual appearance of the lower limb or an abnormal gait either while walking or running. The child may complain of foot pain (see below). However, in many instances, the abnormal gait is painless.

It is not sufficient to say that the child will 'grow out of it'. The child requires a thorough biomechanical assessment, which may reveal a structural abnormality. The most common biomechanical problems in children are rotational abnormalities originating from the hip and the tibia causing either in-toed or out-toed gait.

If the child is asymptomatic and biomechanical abnormalities are not marked, no treatment is indicated. If abnormalities are marked or if the child is symptomatic, management may involve the use of braces or night splints when the child is very young. In the older child, orthoses can be used to compensate for the deformity.

Foot pain

Foot pain of gradual onset is a common presenting symptom in the younger athlete. The causes of foot pain are either related to abnormal biomechanics or the development of an osteochondrosis. Examination of younger athletes with foot pain requires precise determination of the site of maximal tenderness.

Sever's lesion

Sever's lesion or calcaneal apophysitis is a traction apophysitis of the insertion of the Achilles tendon to the calcaneus which typically occurs between the ages of 7 and 10 years. This is the second most common osteochondrosis seen in the younger athlete after Osgood-Schlatter lesion. As with Osgood-Schlatter lesion, Sever's lesion is often present at a time of rapid growth during which muscles and tendons become tighter as the bones become longer.

The patient complains of activity-related pain and examination reveals localized tenderness and swelling at the site of insertion of the Achilles tendon. There may be tightness of the gastrocnemius or soleus muscles, and dorsiflexion at the ankle is limited. Biomechanical examination is necessary. Radiographic examination is usually not required except in persistent cases.

Management consists of activity modification so that the child becomes pain-free. The patient should be advised that the condition will always settle, usually within six to 12 months, but occasionally symptoms will persist for as long as two years. A heel raise should be inserted in shoes. Stretching of the calf muscles is also advisable. Any biomechanical abnormalities should be corrected. Orthoses may be required. Strengthening exercises for the ankle plantarflexors should be commenced when pain-free and progressed as symptoms permit. Corticosteroid injections and surgery are contraindicated in this condition.

Tarsal coalitions

Congenital fusions of the bones of the foot may be undetected until the child begins participation in sports. The most common form is a bony or cartilaginous bar between the calcaneus and navicular bone. The second most common coalition is between the calcaneus and talus. Calcaneocuboid coalition is the least common form. There is often a family history. The adolescent may present with midfoot pain, after recurrent ankle sprains or after repetitive running and jumping. The pain may be associated with a limp.

Examination reveals restriction of subtalar joint motion. There may be a rigid flat foot deformity. Radiographs taken at 45° oblique to the foot may confirm the diagnosis, but if these are normal and clinical suspicion persists, a CT scan or MRI should be obtained.

Management may require orthotic therapy. Surgical excision may be necessary in a young patient with severe symptoms or after failure of conservative therapy. The cartilaginous bar may recur after surgery.

Köhler's lesion

Köhler's lesion is a form of osteochondrosis affecting the navicular bone in young children, especially between the ages of 2 and 8 years. The child complains of pain over the medial aspect of the navicular bone and often develops a painful limp. Tenderness is localized to the medial aspect of the navicular bone. Radiographs reveal typical changes of increased density and narrowing of the navicular bone. Management in a walking cast for six weeks may accelerate relief of the symptoms. Orthoses should be used if biomechanical abnormalities are present.

Apophysitis of the tarsal navicular bone

Pain on the medial aspect of the tarsal navicular bone in the older child may result from a traction apophysitis at the insertion of the tibialis posterior tendon to the navicular. This condition is often associated with the presence of an accessory navicular (Fig. 35.13) or a prominent navicular tuberosity. Management involves modification of activity, local electrotherapy and NSAIDs, with orthoses to control excessive pronation if this is present.

Apophysitis of the fifth metatarsal

A traction apophysitis at the insertion of the peroneus brevis tendon to the base of the fifth metatarsal is occasionally seen. Examination reveals local tenderness and pain on resisted eversion of the foot. Management consists of modification of activity, stretching and progressive strengthening of the peroneal muscles.

Freiberg's lesion

Freiberg's lesion is an osteochondrosis causing collapse of the articular surface and adjacent bone of the metatarsal head. The second metatarsal is most commonly involved (especially in ballet dancers), the third occasionally and the fourth rarely. It occurs most frequently in adolescents over the age of 12 years.

Standing on the forefoot aggravates pain. The head of the second metatarsal is tender and there is swelling around the second metatarsal joint. Radiographs reveal a flattened head of the metatarsal with fragmentation of the growth plate. However, these changes may lag well behind the symptoms. Radioisotopic bone scan and MRI are more sensitive investigations.

If Freiberg's lesion is diagnosed early, management with activity modification, padding under the second metatarsal and footwear modification to reduce the

pressure over the metatarsal heads may prove successful. If the symptoms persist surgical intervention may be necessary.

Other considerations in the younger athlete

Physiological differences between the younger and the mature athlete may predispose the younger athlete to injury. Depending on the child's age, lack of motor skills may place him or her at a greater risk of injury.[14] The adolescent athlete is more susceptible to injury than the prepubescent athlete because of the circulating androgens that result in greater mass, speed and power. This, combined with the impulsive and reckless attitude typically seen in teenagers, may increase the risk of injury.[10] Growing children vary greatly in size and therefore may not have access to appropriately sized protective equipment.

Children with chronic illness

Children with chronic diseases have traditionally been discouraged from physical activity. However, physical activity has marked physical and psychological benefits for children with chronic disease.

Asthma

Children with asthma should be encouraged to join their peers in all activities but should always be permitted to stop exercising or use medications when they feel the need. When proper precautions are taken, asthma is not a barrier to participating and competing in sporting activities. In 1975, Fitch reported that there had been gold medalists with asthma in all the Olympics since 1956.[15] Swimming improves symptoms and quality of life, and reduces the need for medication in asthmatic children compared with non-exercising control patients.[16] It is important that the asthmatic child informs the coach and has appropriate medication readily available while playing sport. Asthma is discussed further in Chapter 46.

Cystic fibrosis

Cystic fibrosis, an inherited condition that affects the glandular secretions of the lungs, the pancreas and sweat, is the most common chronic lung disease in children. Secretions of mucus obstruct the small airways and, thus, interfere with respiration and predispose to infection. Exercise performance deteriorates proportionately to the extent of lung damage.

In cases of cystic fibrosis, the sodium and chloride concentration in sweat is three to five times the normal level. Prolonged exercise, particularly in hot humid conditions, can result in excessive loss of salt and water, making the child more susceptible to heat illness and dehydration.

Regular exercise is of great benefit to children with cystic fibrosis. Exercise helps clear mucus from the lungs, increases respiratory muscle endurance (often above that of normal children), decreases airway resistance and improves exercise performance.

The child should be allowed free access to salty foods to replace lost salt and avoid large fluid intake without added salt. The more severely affected child who may have heart problems secondary to lung disease should avoid intense exercise.

Diabetes mellitus

General guidelines for people with diabetes who wish to exercise are discussed in Chapter 48 and these apply to children. Most importantly, diabetes can be controlled, and diabetic individuals are able to participate in regular physical activity.[17]

For exercise of prolonged duration, the child will usually have to adjust both diet (by consuming more carbohydrate) and insulin (by decreasing dosage). Otherwise, hypoglycemia may occur during or after exercise. Experience, combined with medical advice, will allow appropriate adjustments to diet and insulin dosage to be made. Both the child and the coach or teacher should have a supply of sugar available at all times.

Cardiovascular disease

In children with cardiovascular disease, ill-advised activity can have severe, even fatal, consequences. A family history of childhood cardiac deaths or a 'heart murmur' requires medical assessment. Where serious cardiac conditions are suspected, a specialist cardiology assessment may be necessary (Chapter 45).

Symptoms and signs that should always alert parents, coaches and teachers to the necessity for further assessment include:

- undue shortness of breath
- chest pains with exertion
- fainting, dizziness or light-headedness with exertion
- undue fatigue
- cyanosis of the mouth and tongue with exercise.

Hemophilia

Hemophilia is an inherited disorder of blood clotting. Thus, relatively minor trauma can cause bleeding either externally or, more commonly, into muscles, joints or other organs. Such hemorrhages may result in joint damage, muscle wasting and contractures that impair muscle and joint function.

Management of the child with hemophilia requires minimizing the risk of trauma and early access to blood products if bleeding occurs. Contact sports such as football, skateboarding and boxing should be avoided.

Epilepsy

Epilepsy is discussed in Chapter 49. If a child has epilepsy, it is important for coaches to obtain information from the child's parents or doctor about their seizures, medications and any necessary restrictions on activity.

How much is too much?

Officials, coaches, teachers and parents must be aware of the individual variations that occur in the physical, physiological and psychological capacities of young athletes. It is not appropriate to take a recipe book approach to training the young athlete.

Prior to puberty, children should be encouraged to participate in a variety of activities so that general skills can be developed and all facets of athletic performance enhanced. Specialization at a young age is to be avoided. Overexposure during the important development years may cause a long-term aversion to sports. Some practical guidelines for those supervising general children's sports are listed below.

1. All coaches should gain accreditation by attending coaching courses.
2. Coaching programs must be individually tailored to the child, taking into account:
   (a) physical maturation
   (b) skill level
   (c) ability to learn new skills
   (d) enthusiasm
   (e) the presence of physical limitations (including injury).
3. Coaches or someone involved in the club or school should have a basic first-aid knowledge.
4. Any child complaining of pain, tenderness, limitation of movement or disability should be promptly referred for management by an appropriately qualified clinician.
5. Children playing sports should wear suitable clothing, footwear and protective equipment.

6. A responsible adult should ensure that sunburn, dehydration and heat stroke do not occur.
7. Warm-up and stretching should be encouraged before all training or competition.
8. Equipment should be maintained in good, safe working condition.
9. Training should be conducted on a variety of surfaces.
10. The frequency, duration and intensity of both training and competition should be monitored (see below).

As children develop, their physiological make-up changes so that different training regimens are required for different ages. We present general and sport-specific guidelines for training and competing in several popular activities. These suggestions comply with the position statement on physical training in children and adolescents of the International Federation of Sports Medicine (FIMS).[18] The recommended training frequency should take into account all other sports activities that the child plays. There are no strict rules as there is considerable variation between children.

General guidelines

1. Detailed pre-participation medical examination for children before admission into competitive sport.
2. Adequate medical coverage at sporting events.
3. Coaches should know the biological, physical and social problems related to child development, and be able to apply this knowledge in coaching.
4. Responsibility for the child's overall development must take precedence over training and competition requirements.
5. 'Training for maximum performance' at an early age should be condemned on medical and ethical grounds.
6. Children should be exposed to a wide variety of sporting activities to ensure that they identify the sport(s) that best meet their needs, interest, body build and physical capacities. Early specialization should be discouraged.
7. Besides the chronological age of participants, maturity, body size, skill and gender should be taken into account.
8. Proper equipment and field/surface playing conditions must be provided.
9. Planned training sessions should be tailored to the age of the participants to minimize the risk of injury.

Long distance running

The recommended maximum competition distances for children of various ages are shown in Table 40.4. The weekly training distance should not be more than twice the recommended maximum competition distance. Races up to 10 km in length can be undertaken on a weekly basis. Races over 10 km in length require longer recovery periods. Training frequency for those up to 14 years should not exceed three times per week. Those aged 15 years can train up to five times per week.

Young athletes should wear good quality, well-fitted running shoes. Specific racing shoes (e.g. spikes) may be used for track and cross-country racing for children over 10 years of age.

Sprints

Training frequency for those up to 14 years should not exceed three times per week. Those aged 15 years can train up to five times per week. The duration of each session should not exceed 1.5 hours, including a warm-up and stretching component. The young athlete should avoid training on hard surfaces such as bitumen or concrete and use a variety of surfaces such as grass, dirt or parklands to reduce the impact of training on the growing body.

Throwing events (shot put, discus, javelin, hammer)

Injuries can be avoided in throwing events if the correct technique is developed for each throwing discipline. Close supervision is required in training and competition. Suggested guidelines for throwing events are listed below.

1. No more than three training sessions per week.
2. Each session should not exceed 1.5 hours, including warm-up.

Table 40.4 Recommended maximum running distance at different ages

Age (years)	Distance (km)
Under 9	3
9–11	5
12–14	10
15–16	Half marathon (21.1)
17	30
18	Marathon (42.2)

3. The total number of throws permitted for each session should not exceed 20 for athletes up to 14 years and 40 for those between 15 and 18 years.

Javelin throwing is more demanding than shot put, so training repetitions should be reduced by one-third.

Jumping events (long jump, triple jump, high jump, pole vault)

Training frequency and duration should follow the guidelines listed below.

1. Each session should be no longer than 1.5 hours, including warm-up.
2. Athletes up to 14 years should not perform more than three sessions per week with a maximum of 10 jumps per session.
3. Athletes of 15–18 years should not perform more than five sessions per week with a maximum of 20 jumps per session.

Gymnastics

Boys and girls from a range of ages can compete on a variety of levels in this sport. The number of hours spent training per week depends on the number of years of training the gymnast has already undertaken. Recreational gymnasts and low-level competitive club gymnasts generally train 2 hours per week. Intermediate competitive stage and national gymnasts train up to 15 hours per week, while international level gymnasts often train between 20 and 30 hours per week. This group is at a particular risk of overuse injury. As a result of the high levels of activity and the importance of maintaining a low body fat level, young female gymnasts are at risk of the development of menstrual irregularities (e.g. delayed menarche, amenorrhea), delayed maturation, eating disorders and stress fractures. It is important that coaching is of extremely high quality and that the athletes' programs are appropriate to their maturational development and gymnastic ability. Although it was thought that gymnastics could lead to growth retardation, recent data suggest that this is not the case.[19, 20]

Swimming

Guidelines for the development of training programs designed for young swimmers are shown in Table 40.5.

Resistance training

Resistance training (also known as weight training or strength training) involves using resistance to increase muscle strength, power and endurance. It involves the use of free weights, weight machines, elastic bands or body weight. It is generally used to complement other aspects of sports training. Weightlifting, on the other hand, is the sport of lifting maximal weights through various set ranges of motion.

A well-organized, resistance training program can be beneficial to children of pre-adolescent ages. Acute injuries can be prevented through proper supervision, correct technique and attention to program variables.

While there is support for weight training, it is universally accepted that weightlifting by children should be avoided because of the high potential for injury when lifting maximal amounts at high speeds. The benefits of weight training for children are listed below.

1. Strength gains. Children of all maturity stages are capable of making significant strength gains and positive increases in muscle function following short-term weight training. Strength gains are lost six to eight weeks after stopping training. This is prevented by maintenance exercises.
2. Self-image. Psychological benefits, such as improved self-esteem and body image, occur with strength training.
3. Introduction to coaching techniques. Supervised strength training provides exposure to appropriate coaching techniques that may be useful in adult life.

The risk of injury through weight training is often emphasized. If, however, correct training and supervision principles are applied, accidents can be avoided. Most reported injuries in children occur during unsupervised sessions and when attempting a maximal lift.

Blackouts have also been reported occurring in children lifting maximum weights, with incorrect breathing techniques. There have been no such reports with a properly executed resistance training program.

Guidelines for resistance training

These guidelines incorporate the International Federation of Sports Medicine, British Association of Sport and Exercise Sciences, and American Academy of Pediatrics guidelines on resistance training in children.[21–23]

Table 40.5 The progressive development of the swimmer

Age (years)	Frequency and duration	Development	Activities	Competition
3–4	Whenever in bath, pool, beach, etc.	Confidence in water Ability to submerge and open eyes An extension of the playground	Blowing bubbles, looking underwater, jumping in to Mum or Dad and kicking on front or back with help from parent	Not relevant
5–7	Two 20-minute lessons a week (two to six persons in a group, warm waist-high water)	Basic water skills and stroke technique— aim at 25 m front and back crawl and also symmetrical breaststroke	Learn to dive, float, kick and dog paddle, with the help of kick-boards and other teaching aids Work up to basic strokes being taught	Not relevant
8–9	Two to three sessions per week of 45 minutes	Learn more advanced skills and technique with aim of swimming 25–50 m using basic strokes	Introduce turns, bent arm backstroke and whipkick breaststroke, using training clock for rest and departure intervals and working in groups to promote cooperation	Join swimming club for self-improvement and fun
10–12	Three to five sessions per week of 60–90 minutes	Introduction to competition and strengthen stroke technique	Introduce butterfly and increase training distance to 500 m with some 2000 m Use relay changeovers	Highest level of competition possible—school, intra- or inter-club or state level to promote group rather than individual participation
13–16	Five to nine sessions per week of 90–120 minutes Gear training to seasonal program of competition, peaking for one or two events	Maximize opportunities to develop all strokes over various distances	Maintain a 'mixed bag' of training with long distance workouts with all strokes Introduce strength training with own body weight and light weights together with stretching	Competition at high levels (i.e. regional, state, national if qualified)

Adapted from: Sports Medicine Australia. *Safety Guidelines for Children in Sport and Recreation*. Canberra: Sports Medicine Australia, 1997.

Resistance training programs should primarily focus on maintaining positive physiological, psychological and sociological welfare and health of the young athlete. Performance achievement should be secondary. Resistance training programs should not be implemented without the supervision of a certified strength and conditioning professional. The correct technique must be taught for each exercise. The size of the exercise equipment should correspond to the size of the child and routine safety inspections should be carried out. High training intensities should be avoided. Maximal intensities should not be performed before the child reaches 16 years of age or Tanner stage 5. There should be a gradual progression in training intensity. Resistance training should supplement rather than replace other forms of physical activity. All exercises should be performed in a controlled manner throughout a full range of motion. Fast, sudden and ballistic movements should be avoided. All training sessions should be preceded by stretching and followed by stretching and a cool-down period.

To introduce the athlete to specific strength training exercises, it is recommended that no load (resistance) be used initially. Later, once the athlete has mastered the exercise skill, gradual loads can be introduced. If the athlete's technique begins to break down, the load must be reduced to a point at which a proper technique is restored.

The maximum number for formal training sessions per week, including resistance training, for children up to 12 years of age should be three, each having a duration of no longer than 90 minutes. For elite athletes, the total training load may vary according to the sport and level of competition. However, resistance training should never exceed three sessions per week.

A typical 60 minute training session would consist of warm-up, 20 minutes of resistance training, 20 minutes for a run, cycle or swim and 20 minutes of soccer, gymnastics or basketball followed by a cool-down.

Training should be directed to high repetitions and low loads involving all muscle groups through a full range of movement at each joint. Weights/resistance should be less than 80% of the individual's one repetition maximum. When eight to 15 repetitions can be performed, more weight can be added in small increments. Certain exercises that are not considered safe are listed below.

Potentially dangerous resistance exercises

1. Bouncing squats. Bouncing out of the bottom position in the squat can cause knee damage and muscle strains.
2. Squat with knees tilting or rotating inwards. This can cause shearing pressures on the knees.
3. Standing presses with back flexion, extension or rotation. Increased lordosis of the lumbar spine may place excessive loading on the spine. This may be temporarily lessened in the seated position; however, this has the disadvantage of not developing the structural muscles of the lower back needed to carry out the exercise successfully.
4. Bench press with hips raised off bench. Although often seen with experienced power lifters, this places excessive load on the hyperextended back.
5. Straight arm pullovers. These result in greater strain on the rotator cuff than the safer, bent-arm version.
6. Rapid lumbar hyperextensions. These can strain muscles and injure joints.
7. Squatting/jerking in running shoes. Running shoes provide inadequate lateral stability for this exercise.
8. Full range of motion with rubber bands. Resistance with rubber bands increases proportionately with degree of stretch, which often leads to maximal force on a muscle at a point that is weaker than in its mid-range position and predisposing it to injury.

Nutrition for the younger athlete

At no time in life is nutrition more important than in childhood and adolescence. This is a time of rapid growth and, frequently, high levels of activity. Eating and drinking practises established at this stage often form the foundation of dietary habits practiced through life.

It is also a time of nutritional risk. Adolescents have a tendency to skip meals, snack frequently and rely heavily on fast foods. Girls, more so than boys, may become obsessed with achieving a slim figure.

One area of major concern has been the increased pressure on young, elite athletes to aim to achieve low levels of body fat, particularly where extreme thinness is prized (e.g. ballet dancing, gymnastics, endurance running). Eating disorders such as anorexia nervosa and bulimia may be more common in some of these sports than in a control population. These disorders are most commonly seen in adolescence. Inadequate nutrition affects growth and maturation (Chapter 37).

Energy

Children and adolescents involved in sport have high energy requirements. During the growth spurt, children engaging in physically demanding sports may find it difficult to satisfy their energy needs. This may be due to a small stomach capacity, poor appetite or food being a low priority. Fortunately, adolescents are great snackers. For some, snacks may provide the majority of their energy needs. Therefore, it is vital that these snacks are highly nutritious but low in fat.

Snack ideas for young athletes

- Wholemeal (whole-wheat) dry biscuits topped with:
  — a slice of low-fat cheese and tomato
  — peanut butter and celery strips
  — honey and banana
  — ricotta cheese and dried figs
- Wholegrain toast topped with ricotta cheese and jam
- Toasted English muffin spread with golden syrup/maple syrup
- Fruit loaf
- Pita bread (toasted) with 'healthy' dips (e.g. yoghurt and cucumber)
- Warm tacos with hummus and salad
- Frozen banana
- Fresh fruit salad

- Half rockmelon (cantaloupe) filled with blueberries
- Frozen yoghurt
- Low-fat muesli bar
- Baked apple
- Low-fat fruit yoghurt
- Low-fat ice-cream with fresh or frozen berries
- Milk smoothies—blend low-fat milk and yoghurt with fruit
- Baked custard (made with low-fat milk)
- Low-fat 'creamy rice'
- Baked potato topped with flavored cottage cheese
- Rice salad
- Pumpkin soup and toast
- Baked beans with wholemeal toast
- Wholemeal pancakes with stewed apple and cinnamon or maple syrup
- Corn on the cob with freshly ground black pepper
- Boiled noodles
- Raisin bread with honey

Protein

During childhood and adolescence, protein needs per kilogram of body weight are higher than at later stages of life. This is due to the increased needs of growth.

In the case of athletes, exact protein requirements remain controversial (Chapter 37). However, it is now widely accepted that exercise does increase protein requirements. A protein intake of 2.0 g/kg of body weight per day is recommended for children and adolescents. Providing the total daily energy intake is adequate and protein represents 12% of the total energy, it seems unlikely that young athletes will not meet their protein needs. Good sources of protein are lean meat, low-fat cheese, chicken without skin, milk, fish, legumes, rice, eggs, nuts and seeds.

Carbohydrates

The benefits of a high-carbohydrate diet on athletic performance have been well documented (Chapter 37). However, young athletes may have difficulty in eating enough to fulfill their requirements. In most cases, it is necessary to incorporate some refined carbohydrates such as sugar in the diets of young athletes to help meet their energy needs.

A very-high-carbohydrate diet is not recommended for children and adolescents as it may reduce protein intake. This may be detrimental to growth and development in the long term. Good sources of carbohydrates are rice, pasta, breads and cereals, fruit, starchy vegetables and legumes.

Fat

The fat intake of most schoolchildren is 40% of their energy needs. All children should be encouraged to reduce their fat intake to less than 30% of their total energy intake.

Vitamins and minerals

Vitamin deficiencies will adversely affect athletic performance. Certain diets may not provide adequate vitamin supplies. Diets that include excessive consumption of simple sugars may not only result in an inadequate intake of energy but may result in vitamin deficiencies, especially the B group. B group vitamins are needed for the conversion of sugar to energy. As simple sugars do not supply B group vitamins, excessive intake may exhaust the body's store.

While indiscriminate use of vitamin supplements in athletes should be discouraged, especially in the absence of dietary change, supplements may be appropriate for vulnerable groups of young athletes (e.g. those on low-energy diets) or those who exhibit signs of possible vitamin deficiency (e.g. excessive tiredness). Two minerals, calcium and iron, are particularly important for the young athlete.

Calcium

Aside from pregnancy and lactation, calcium requirements are highest during childhood and adolescence.[24] Calcium is required for the formation of bones and is essential for nerve and muscle function, blood clotting and hormonal regulation. Although the body can increase calcium retention when intake is low, an inadequate calcium intake may compromise attainment of peak bone mass and, thus, increase the risk of osteoporosis.

Girls tend to be particularly at risk of inadequate calcium intake. This is at a time when it is essential for females to develop peak bone mass. The combination of inadequate calcium and amenorrhea, often found in athletic girls, may increase the long-term risk of osteoporosis. The recommended daily intakes of calcium at various ages are shown in Table 37.10. The calcium content of common foods is shown in Table 37.11.

Iron

Iron deficiency, with or without anemia, is known to have a deleterious effect on athletic performance. Female athletes are at greater risk of iron deficiency because of increased iron losses through menstruation, in addition to the gastrointestinal, bladder and sweat losses, and decreased iron absorption common to all athletes.

Management of iron deficiency in athletes consists of regular screening (including serum ferritin levels), nutrition education and, in some cases, iron supplementation. Recommendations regarding iron intake are found in Chapter 37.

Thermoregulation and hydration

Exercising children are not as efficient as adults when it comes to thermoregulation. The thermoregulatory disadvantages faced by children when compared to adults are due to the following:[25]

- Children gain heat faster from the environment because of their greater surface area-to-body mass ratio compared to adults.
- Children produce more heat per mass unit than adults during activities that involve walking or running.
- The sweating capacity of children is considerably lower than adults, which reduces their ability to dissipate body heat by evaporation.
- Children acclimatize to exercising in hot weather at a slower rate than adults.

Maintenance of adequate hydration helps to prevent heat stress. During exercise, children may fail to ingest sufficient fluid to prevent dehydration because they often do not feel the urge to drink enough to replenish the fluid loss before or following exercise.[26] Thus, attention to adequate hydration is essential. All these factors combine to increase the risk of heat illness in children. The recommended fluid intakes for children of various ages are shown in Table 40.6. Water appears to be the best fluid. Further guidelines for the prevention of heat illness are contained in Chapter 53.

Table 40.6 Sports Medicine Australia guidelines for fluid replacement (water) for children and adolescents[a][27]

Age (years)	Time (min)	Volume (mL)
~15	45 (before exercise)	300–400
	20 (during exercise)	150–200
	As soon as possible after exercise	Liberal until urination
~10	45 (before exercise)	150–200
	20 (during exercise)	75–100
	As soon as possible after exercise	Liberal until urination

(a) In hot environments fluid intake may need to be more frequent.

Body image

Body image is an important issue for adolescents as physical and emotional changes occurring during this time accentuate self-consciousness about the body.[28] Body image concerns are not only confined to females but may also affect males who feel pressure to attain the ideal male body—masculine muscular physique.

These concerns about body image often translate to poor eating practises and disordered eating.[29] As many as 63% of girls and 16% of boys have dieted at least once and many claim to have used extreme methods.[30] For adolescent athletes, body image issues add to the many factors that may contribute to disordered eating patterns. These include: pressure to optimize performance; pressure to meet unrealistic body weight and fat goals; societal expectations; and established norms for certain sports that may influence athletes to attain a certain body shape.[31]

Obesity

Many studies show that obesity is not to be simply equated with overeating.[32] In fact, obese children often eat fewer calories than their lean counterparts. However, obese children do exhibit low levels of spontaneous activity.[33] Regular moderate activity for an hour a day can raise energy expenditure by 20%. This will contribute to weight loss. An exercise program for obese children should emphasize:

- enjoyment to ensure the child continues with physical activity
- regular, moderate exercise of up to 1 hour per day
- total time of activity per day rather than speed or performance
- caution with exercise in the heat since obese children tolerate heat poorly and adapt slowly to changes of temperature
- adequate fluid intake during exercise in the heat.

The 'ugly parent' syndrome

Although parents generally aspire to provide the best sporting experience for their children, it does not always turn out that way. Parental interference and pressure are among the main reasons that children (and coaches) drop out of sport. Children competing under excessive parental pressure may display physical ailments ranging from headaches to stomach aches and muscle pains. In addition, stress may cause sleep disturbances, emotional volatility, fatigue and prolonged depression. Guidelines for parents supporting their child's sporting interest are shown below.

1. Encourage children to participate if they are interested. However, if a child is not willing, do not force him or her.
2. Focus upon the child's efforts and performance rather than on the overall outcome of the event. This assists the child in setting realistic goals related to his or her ability by reducing the emphasis on winning.
3. Teach children that an honest effort is as important as victory, so that the result of each game is accepted without undue disappointment.
4. Encourage children to always participate according to the rules and settle disagreements without resorting to hostility or violence.
5. Never ridicule a child for making a mistake or losing a competition.
6. Remember that children are involved in organized sports for their own enjoyment, not for their parents' enjoyment.
7. Remember that children learn best from example. Applaud good play by all teams.
8. Respect officials' decisions and teach children to do likewise.
9. If you disagree with an official, raise the issue through the appropriate channels rather than questioning the official's judgment and honesty in public. Remember, most officials volunteer their time and effort to help children.
10. Support all efforts to remove verbal and physical abuse from sporting activities.
11. Recognize the value and importance of volunteer coaches. They give their time and resources to provide recreational activities for the children.
12. Respect the rights, dignity and worth of every young person regardless of their gender, ability, cultural background or religion.

Coaches' role

Coaches may have long-lasting positive influences on a child's enjoyment of sport. Unfortunately, many children feel ignored by coaches, are never given instructions about their faults, and never made aware of their progress.[34-36] It must be remembered that for a number of children, experience in a particular sport will be brief and the coach should aim to make the child the better for it. A code of behavior to assist coaches in achieving a beneficial influence on their athletes is listed below.

1. Be reasonable in demands on young players' time, energy and enthusiasm.
2. Teach players that rules of the sport are mutual agreements that no one should evade or break.
3. Whenever possible, group players to give a reasonable chance of success.
4. Avoid overplaying the talented players. The 'just average' players need and deserve equal time.
5. Remember that children participate for fun and enjoyment and that winning is only part of their motivation. Never ridicule or yell at children for making mistakes.
6. Ensure that equipment and facilities meet safety standards and are appropriate to the age and ability of the players.
7. Take into consideration the maturity level of the children when scheduling and determining the length of practise times and competition.
8. Develop team respect for the ability of opponents as well as for the judgment of officials and opposing coaches.
9. Follow the advice of a sports medicine practitioner when determining when an injured player is ready to recommence training or competition.
10. Remain informed of sound coaching principles and the principles of growth and development of children.
11. Avoid use of derogatory language based on gender.

Recommended Reading

Australian Sports Commission. *Codes of Behaviour for Children's Sports.* Canberra: ASC, 1991.

Australian Sports Medicine Federation. *Guidelines in Children's Sport.* Canberra: ASMF, 1989.

Bass S, Inge K. Nutrition for special populations: children and young athletes. In: Burke L, Deakin V, eds. *Clinical Sports Nutrition.* 3rd edn. Sydney: McGraw-Hill, 2006.

Caine DJ, Maffulli N. *Epidemiology of Pediatric Sports Injuries. Individual Sports.* Basel: Karger, 2005.

Chan KM, Micheli LJ. *Sports and Children.* Hong Kong: Williams & Wilkins, 1998.

Maffulli N. *Color Atlas and Text of Sports Medicine in Childhood and Adolescence.* London: Mosby-Wolfe, 1995.

Maffulli N, Bruns W. Injuries in young athletes. *Eur J Pediatr* 2000; 159: 59–63.

Maffulli N, Caine DJ. *Epidemiology of Pediatric Sports Injuries. Team Sports.* Basel: Karger, 2005.

References

1. Micheli LJ, Fehlandt AF Jr. Overuse injuries to tendons and apophyses in children and adolescents. *Clin Sports Med* 1992; 11(4): 713–26.

2. Feldman D, Shrier I, Rossignol M, Abenhaim L. Adolescent growth is not associated with changes in flexibility. *Clin J Sport Med* 1999; 9(1): 24–9.

3. Malina RM. Physical growth and biological maturation of young athletes. *Exerc Sport Sci Rev* 1994; 22: 389–433.

4. Kocher MS, Kim YJ, Millis MB, et al. Hip arthroscopy in children and adolescents. *J Pediatr Orthop* 2005; 25(5): 680–6.

5. Maffulli N, Bruns W. Injuries in young athletes. *Eur J Pediatr* 2000; 159(1–2): 59–63.

6. Cook JL, Khan KM, Kiss ZS, Griffiths L. Patellar tendinopathy in junior basketball players: a controlled clinical and ultrasonographic study of 268 patellar tendons in players aged 14–18 years. *Scand J Med Sci Sports* 2000; 10(4): 216–20.

7. Cook JL, Kiss ZS, Khan KM, Purdam CR, Webster KE. Anthropometry, physical performance, and ultrasound patellar tendon abnormality in elite junior basketball players: a cross-sectional study. *Br J Sports Med* 2004; 38(2): 206–9.

8. Williamson L, Bowness P, Mowat A, Ostman-Smith I. Difficulties in diagnosing acute rheumatic fever—arthritis may be short lived and carditis silent. *BMJ* 2000; 320: 362–5.

9. Paletta GA Jr. Special considerations. Anterior cruciate ligament reconstruction in the skeletally immature. *Orthop Clin North Am* 2003; 34(1): 65–77.

10. Adirim TA, Cheng TL. Overview of injuries in the young athlete. *Sports Med* 2003; 33(1): 75–81.

11. Kannus P, Jarvinen M. Knee ligament injuries in adolescents. Eight year follow-up of conservative management. *J Bone Joint Surg Br* 1988; 70B(5): 772–6.

12. Mizuta H, Kubota K, Shiraishi M, Otsuka Y, Nagamoto N, Takagi K. The conservative treatment of complete tears of the anterior cruciate ligament in skeletally immature patients. *J Bone Joint Surg Br* 1995; 77B(6): 890–4.

13. Kocher MS, Garg S, Micheli LJ. Physeal sparing reconstruction of the anterior cruciate ligament in skeletally immature prepubescent children and adolescents. *J Bone Joint Surg Am* 2005; 87A(11): 2371–9.

14. Harris S. Readiness to participate in sports in care of the young athlete. In: Sullivan JA, Anderson SJ, eds. *Care of the Young Athlete.* Rosemont, IL: American Academy of Orthopaedic Surgeons, 2000: 19–24.

15. Fitch KD. Exercise-induced asthma and competitive athletics. *Pediatrics* 1975; 56(5 Part 2 suppl.): 942–3.

16. Huang SW, Veiga R, Sila U, Reed E, Hines S. The effect of swimming in asthmatic children—participants in a swimming program in the city of Baltimore. *J Asthma* 1989; 26(2): 117–21.

17. Dorchy HPJ. Juvenile diabetes and sports. In: Bar-Or O, ed. *Encyclopedia of Sports Medicine.* Oxford: Blackwell Scientific, 1996: 455–79.

18. International Federation of Sports Medicine (FIMS). Position statement: excessive physical training in children. In: Chan KM, Micheli LJ, eds. *Sports and Children.* Hong Kong: Williams & Wilkins, 1998: 271–6.

19. Peltenburg AL, Erich WB, Zonderland ML, et al. A retrospective growth study of female gymnasts and girl swimmers. *Int J Sports Med* 1984; 5(5): 262–7.

20. Bass S, Bradney M, Pearce G, et al. Short stature and delayed puberty in gymnasts: influence of selection bias on leg length and the duration of training on trunk length. *J Pediatr* 2000; 136: 149–55.

21. International Federation of Sports Medicine (FIMS). Position statement: resistance training for children and adolescents. In: Chan KM, Micheli LJ, eds. *Sports and Children.* Hong Kong: Williams & Wilkins, 1998: 265–70.

22. Stratton G, Jones M, Fox KR, et al. BASES position statement on guidelines for resistance exercise in young people. *J Sports Sci* 2004; 22(4): 383–90.

23. Bernhardt DT, Gomez J, Johnson MD, et al. Strength training by children and adolescents. *Pediatrics* 2001; 107(6): 1470–2.

24. Bailey DA, Martin AD, McKay HA, Whiting SJ, Mirwald R. Calcium accretion in girls and boys during puberty: a longitudinal analysis. *J Bone Miner Res* 2000; 15: 2245–50.

25. Malina RM, Bouchard C, Bar-Or O. *Growth, Maturation and Physical Activity.* 2nd edn. Champaign, IL: Human Kinetics, 2004: 267–73.

26. Walker SM, Casa DJ, Levreault ML, et al. Children participating in summer sports camps are chronically dehydrated. *Med Sci Sports Exerc* 2004; 36(suppl. 5): 180–1.

27. Sports Medicine Australia. *Safety Guidelines for Children in Sport and Recreation.* Canberra: SMA, 1997.

28. Baum AL. Young females in the athletic arena. *Child Adolesc Psychiatr Clin N Am* 1998; 7(4): 745–55, viii.

29. Neumark-Sztainer D, Story M, Perry C, Casey MA. Factors influencing food choices of adolescents: findings from focus-group discussions with adolescents. *J Am Diet Assoc* 1999; 99(8): 929–37.

30. Gibbons K, Wertheim E, Paxton S, Petrovich J, Szmukler G. Nutrient intake of adolescents and its relationship to desire for thinness, weight loss behaviours, and bulimic tendencies. *Aust J Nutr Diet* 1995; 52(2): 69–74.

31. Van de Loo DA, Johnson MD. The young female athlete. *Clin Sports Med* 1995; 14(3): 687–707.

32. Gortmaker SL, Dietz WH Jr, Sobol AM, Wehler CA. Increasing pediatric obesity in the United States. *Am J Dis Child* 1987; 141(5): 535–40.

33. Gortmaker SL, Must A, Sobol AM, Peterson K, Colditz GA, Dietz WH. Television viewing as a cause of increasing obesity among children in the United States, 1986–1990. *Arch Pediatr Adolesc Med* 1996; 150(4): 356–62.

34. Ogilvie BC, Tofler IR, Conroy DE, Drell MJ. Comprehending role conflicts in the coaching of children, adolescents, and young adults. Transference, countertransference, and achievement by proxy distortion paradigms. *Child Adolesc Psychiatr Clin N Am* 1998; 7(4): 879–90.

35. Libman S. Adult participation in youth sports. A developmental perspective. *Child Adolesc Psychiatr Clin N Am* 1998; 7(4): 725–44, vii.

36. Kamm RL. A developmental and psychoeducational approach to reducing conflict and abuse in little league and youth sports. The sport psychiatrist's role. *Child Adolesc Psychiatr Clin N Am* 1998; 7(4): 891–918.

Women and Activity-Related Issues Across the Lifespan

WITH KIM BENNELL AND JULIA ALLEYNE

An approach to women's health issues can be applied to sports medicine to identify the areas of concern to females as they progress through the life cycle. Women's health is best understood by describing what is more common, more severe and/or exclusive to women as a basis for identifying areas of clinical and research needs. For example, osteoporosis is more common in women but not limited to women, whereas pregnancy is exclusive to women. Understanding women's health means developing assessment tools that are specific to the anatomical and physiological differences of women as well as understanding the gender differences that roles, society and opportunity play in providing a woman with an optimal sport environment.

Many areas of sports medicine and exercise play a role in achieving optimal performance. Health issues related to the menstrual cycle, exercise and pregnancy, and changes at the menopause are examples of the effect the female hormonal physiology has on sport performance. Female sports participants have a two- to eightfold greater risk of anterior cruciate ligament ruptures (ACL) than male counterparts engaged in the same activities (Fig. 41.1). That issue, and strategies for prevention of that injury, are covered in Chapter 27.

Similarities and differences between the sexes

Although differences exist between the sexes, there are far more similarities between males and females of the human species than males and females in many other species. A number of the differences between males and females can be related to the increased average

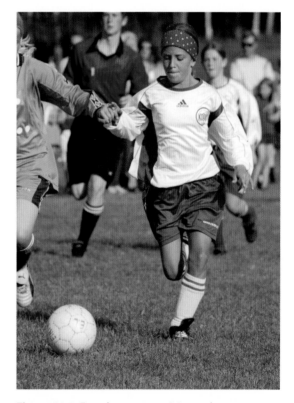

Figure 41.1 Female sports participants have a two- to eightfold greater risk of ACL rupture than male counterparts undertaking the same activities (see Chapter 27)

size of the male. When corrections are made for size, the differences are markedly reduced or abolished. Differences between the sexes will be considered in four different areas:

1. skeletal structure
2. body composition
3. physiology
4. training effects.

Prior to puberty, there is little difference between males and females. Females tend to reach puberty at a slightly earlier age (9–13 years) than males (10–14 years).

Skeletal differences

Bony growth is similar in males and females until approximately 9 or 10 years of age. Girls tend to commence their adolescent growth spurt around the age of 11 years and surge ahead of boys in height and weight. Boys begin their adolescent growth spurt, on average, two years later, around the age of 13 years. The rate of linear growth in girls usually decelerates with menarche (beginning of menstruation), between 12 and 14 years. After menarche, girls will usually gain approximately 5 cm (2.5 in.) and reach their maximal height by 16 or 17 years. The growth spurt in boys usually occurs between 12 and 15 years and full maturation may not occur until 20–21 years of age.

The pattern of body weight development is similar to that of height. The earlier growth spurt gives females an increased weight in the early teenage years. However, by 15 years of age, boys' weight usually exceeds that of girls. At full sexual maturity, the male outweighs the female by approximately 11 kg (24 lb). This is due to additional bone and muscle mass.

A substantial amount of bone mineral is accumulated during the growing years, particularly in adolescence. In fact, as much bone mineral is laid down during the adolescent years as most people will lose during their entire adult lives.[1] The timing of peak gains in bone accrual occurs approximately one year after the age of peak linear growth and is earlier in girls than boys, consistent with the earlier onset of sexual maturation in girls. This dissociation between linear growth and bone mineral accrual suggests a transient period of relative weakness during the adolescent growth spurt[2] and may partially explain the increase in fractures seen in children around the time of peak linear growth.[3] Women, on average, have a smaller peak bone mass than men because their skeletons are physically smaller. However, a gender difference in bone density is not nearly as clear-cut and probably varies from site to site.[4]

Males usually have wide shoulders and narrow hips, whereas a female generally has a wide pelvis in relation to the width of her shoulders. Because the woman is shorter and has a wider pelvis, she has a lower center of gravity and possibly greater stability. This may lead to improved balance.

The wider pelvis leads to an increased inward slant of the thigh and, therefore, an increased Q angle at the knee (Chapter 28). Women have shorter limbs, especially the upper arm, and thus have less lever action with a resultant loss of power. Females have an increased carrying angle at the elbow.

Body composition

Women's average body fat composition is approximately 26% compared with that of men of 14%. Women have lower lean body mass, indicating less muscle mass. The greater muscle mass in males is due to the predominant effect of the androgenic hormones, whereas estrogen, which is the predominant hormone in females, results in increased body fat. In males, the subcutaneous fat is found mainly in the abdominal and upper regions of the body, whereas the female has a greater concentration of body fat in the hips and thighs.

Physiological differences

There are significant differences between the sexes in the cardiovascular system. The female has a smaller heart size and therefore a reduced stroke volume. This results in reduced blood flow to the muscles with each heart beat at a given level of work compared with in the male. This may be compensated for by an increase in heart rate. A woman's heart rate may be 5 beats per minute faster than a man's at an equal exercise load. Men are able to deliver a 30% higher maximal cardiac output. This appears to be related to larger heart volume as maximal heart rate is similar.

The female has a smaller thorax than the male and this results in a smaller vital capacity, residual volume and, therefore, total lung capacity. Females have a lower basal metabolic rate, the rate of conversion of food to energy under conditions of total rest. This appears to be related to the greater lean body mass of the male and the greater proportion of adipose tissue in the female. When basal metabolic rate is calculated in terms of lean muscle mass rather than body surface area, the difference disappears.

Absolute VO_{2max} values (a measure of aerobic fitness) are typically 40% higher in men than women. When expressed per kilogram of body weight, this difference is reduced to 20%. When expressed relative to fat-free instead of total body weight, the sex difference in VO_{2max} is further reduced to 10% or less.

Females tend to have fewer red blood cells with a reduced hemoglobin level per red cell. This leads to a lowered oxygen-carrying capacity.

The male has a larger muscle mass due to the effect of the androgenic hormones but there is no difference in the relative percentages of slow-twitch and fast-twitch fibers. The difference in muscle mass is due to the increased size of the various muscle fibers. Some physiological differences between the sexes are shown in Table 41.1.

Training and performance

Females are, on average, only two-thirds as strong as males. Strength is related both to the number of muscle fibers recruited and to the absolute size of the muscle fibers. Males are stronger than females because of their increased muscle mass. When correction is made for this difference in muscle mass, the difference in strength disappears. In other words, per unit of muscle mass, the female is as strong as the male.

When males perform strength training, they develop increased strength and increased muscle size due to hypertrophy of the muscles. This hypertrophy is due to the effect of testosterone. Females performing strength training gain increased strength with relatively less muscle hypertrophy. Females may gain as much strength, relatively, as males with appropriate training. There is no increased risk in strength training for females compared with males.

In endurance sports, performances by females lag behind performances by males by between 5% and 15%. This is probably related to the differences in body size and body composition.[5]

As stated, the Vo_{2max} of males is, on average, 40% greater than in females. This may be reduced to approximately 20% by considering the Vo_{2max}/kg body weight and to approximately 10% by considering the Vo_{2max}/kg lean body weight. Therefore, the extra body fat in females probably accounts for about 75% of the difference in endurance performance. The remaining difference is attributed to the higher cardiac output produced by males than females due to the greater heart size and to their increased amount of hemoglobin, which enables them to have an increased oxygen-carrying capacity.

Physiology of the menstrual cycle

A normal menstrual cycle varies between 23 to 35 days but an average cycle lasts 28 days. It is regulated by the hypothalamus, which produces gonadotrophin-releasing hormone (GnRH) to stimulate the pituitary hormones. The first half of the cycle, known as the follicular phase, is characterized by an increase in follicle-stimulating hormone (FSH), which results in estrogen production by the ovaries. These hormones stimulate the formation of the primary follicle and proliferative growth of the uterine lining. The follicular phase ends with rupture of the follicle and release of the ovum approximately 14 days before the next menstrual bleed begins. The luteal phase, also lasting about 14 days, is marked by a surge in luteinizing hormone (LH) triggered by rising levels of estrogen. A resulting increase in progesterone stimulates maturation of the follicle and ovulation. If fertilization does not occur, luteal function declines and a rapid decrease in estrogen and progesterone leads to menstruation. The female sex hormones exert a range of effects on many metabolic, thermoregulatory, cardiovascular

Table 41.1 Some physiological differences between the sexes from the female perspective in relation to exercise performance

Difference	Result
Lower blood volume Fewer red blood cells (~6%) Less hemoglobin (~15%)	Lower total oxygen-carrying capacity of blood
Smaller heart	Higher heart rate, smaller stroke volume
Lower maximum cardiac output	Lower maximum aerobic capacity (20%)
Smaller thorax	Lower vital capacity, lower tidal volume, lower residual volume, lower maximal breathing capacity
Less lung tissue	Lower minute ventilation
Less muscle mass (fewer fibers and smaller fibers)	40% less upper body strength; when strength expressed relative to lean body mass, no difference in some instances

and respiratory parameters that may influence athletic performance.[6] These are summarized in the boxes below.

Actions of estrogen

Effects on cardiovascular system

- Altered plasma fibrinolytic activity and platelet aggregation—increase in thrombosis.
- Decreased total cholesterol and low-density lipoprotein levels and increased high-density lipoprotein levels—protection against atherosclerosis.
- Vasodilatory effect on vascular smooth muscle.

Effects on regulation of substrate metabolism

- Increased intramuscular and hepatic glycogen storage and uptake—possibly increased endurance performance.
- Glycogen-sparing effect through increased lipid synthesis, muscle lipolysis and greater use of free fatty acids.
- Decreased insulin-binding capacity— decreased glucose tolerance and insulin resistance.

Other effects

- Deposition of fat in breasts, buttocks and thighs.
- Increased blood pressure.
- Increased calcium uptake in bone.
- Change in neurotransmitters—possible improved cognitive function and memory.

Actions of progesterone

- Increased core body temperature of 0.3–0.5°C (0.5–0.9°F).
- Increased minute ventilation.
- Augmented ventilatory response to hypoxia and hypercapnia.
- Postovulatory fluid retention via effects on aldosterone and the renin–angiotensin system.
- Actions on insulin receptors leading to peripheral insulin resistance.
- Metabolic effects resulting in a greater dependence on fat as a substrate.

Effect of the menstrual cycle on performance

The measurement of athletic performance is difficult and encompasses physical fitness (aerobic fitness, anaerobic fitness, muscle strength, flexibility, body composition) as well as neuromotor, cognitive and psychological factors. There is some anecdotal evidence from athletes that performance may be negatively affected during the pre-menstrual or menstrual phases. However, the results of studies vary probably because of methodology issues, including different aspects of performance assessed as well as considerable inter- and intra-individual variation in both hormone levels and response.[7] Overall, most research has failed to find a link between fluctuations in female reproductive hormones throughout the menstrual cycle and muscle contractile characteristics or determinants of maximal oxygen consumption, suggesting that performance in strength-specific sports and intense anaerobic/aerobic sports is not affected.[8] For prolonged exercise performance, some research has found a higher cardiovascular strain in the mid-luteal phase and a reduced time to exhaustion in hot conditions.[8] Practical implications may be that endurance performance may be reduced if training in hot climates during the luteal phase, although further research needs to corroborate these findings. There has been less research about whether aspects of neuromotor control may be affected, although a recent study reported reduced knee kinesthesia during the luteal phase.[9]

Dysmenorrhea

Dysmenorrhea is the term used to describe the painful, uterine cramps experienced by many women during menstruation. It affects the majority of women in some form or other, with two peaks of incidence in the teenage years and later in the 30s age group. The majority of women report mild symptoms that have minimal effects on their lifestyle. They are treated with simple analgesics or, frequently, no medication at all.

Many women suffer from moderate or severe dysmenorrhea with extremely painful cramping sensations for the first day or two of menstruation. These patients often have associated heavy menstrual flow. In an athlete, these symptoms may adversely affect training or competition.

It seems that women who exercise have a reduced incidence of dysmenorrhea. This may be due to exercise-related hormonal effects on the lining of the uterus or increased levels of circulating endorphins.

Athletes suffering from dysmenorrhea may benefit from simple analgesics, prostaglandin inhibitors such as mefenamic acid (250 mg 6 hourly) or naproxen (500 mg twice a day) commencing 24 hours prior to the expected onset of menses, or the oral contraceptive pill.

Pre-menstrual syndrome

The pre-menstrual syndrome is defined as the presence of emotional and/or physical symptoms occurring cyclically, commencing some days prior to menstruation and disappearing with the onset of menstruation. Symptoms may include anxiety, depression, mood swings, headaches, fluid retention, breast soreness and breast enlargement. Exercise may reduce the severity of pre-menstrual symptoms.

For an athlete, the most distressing symptoms are those relating to fluid retention. A diuretic agent can be taken; however, this may lead to dehydration in the athlete and should be avoided if possible. Most diuretics are banned by the International Olympic Committee (Chapter 61). Treatments of pre-menstrual syndrome that are supported with evidence, particularly in cases with severe symptoms, include consumption of soy isoflavones,[10] selective serotonin reuptake inhibitors,[11] a low dose oral contraceptive with drospirenone[12] and luteal phase dosing with paroxetine controlled release.[13]

Manipulation of the menstrual cycle

Women who are, or perceive that they are, adversely affected during the pre-menstrual and/or menstrual phases may wish to manipulate their menstrual cycle to avoid that stage of the cycle coinciding with a major event. This manipulation should be reserved for major activities and should not be used on a regular basis.

The most effective means of manipulating the cycle is by the use of the oral contraceptive pill (OCP). This can be done in one of two ways. The OCP can be ceased 10 days prior to the planned activity, which will usually induce a withdrawal bleed. The pill can either be resumed at the end of menstruation or following the completion of the sporting event. If this method is used, suppression of ovulation may fail and additional barrier methods of contraception (e.g. condoms) must be used until two weeks after recommencing the pill. Alternatively, the athlete may omit the seven day tablet-free interval (or sugar pills) and continue taking the OCP throughout the sporting event to prevent menstruation occurring prior to or during the event. This method is simpler to use with monophasic pills than with triphasic pills. In view of this, monophasic OCPs may be more appropriate than triphasic OCPs for use by athletes who wish to manipulate their menstrual cycles. For those who do not wish to use the pill, a menstrual bleed can be induced 10 days prior to the event with administration of a progesterone derivative for 10 days duration, finishing the course 10 days prior to the event.

Injectable progesterone as medroxyprogesterone acetate is a form of contraception that eliminates menstrual bleeding in most women and only requires administration every three months. However, recent studies[14, 15] have confirmed that progesterone-only contraception is associated with a greater risk of pre-menopausal osteoporosis.

Menstrual irregularities associated with exercise

Exercise is associated with disorders of the menstrual cycle, such as delayed menarche, luteal dysfunction and amenorrhea.

Delayed menarche

The average age of menarche is between 12 and 13 years. Menarche, or the onset of menstrual bleeding, usually occurs one to two years after the commencement of the pubertal growth spurt in girls. The exact mechanisms determining the timing of menarche are not known, although genetic factors play an important role.

It has been observed that the age of menarche appears to be correlated with athletic performance, that is, high-performance athletes tend to have had a later age of menarche than the normal population.[16] These high-performance athletes fall into two groups—a group that commenced intense physical training prior to menarche and a group that commenced training after menarche. The presence of a delayed onset of menarche in both groups indicates that there may be a combination of factors causing this condition.

Intense training in pre-menarcheal years, as occurs commonly in ballet dancers and gymnasts, is associated with a delayed onset of menarche. This association does not necessarily imply cause and effect. It may be that thinness, which may occur as a result of intense training, may be the most important factor preventing the onset of menses.[16] The combination of intensive exercise and low body weight may affect the hypothalamic secretion of hormones, thus delaying the onset of menarche. While breast development and menarche are delayed in this group of intensively exercising pre-pubertal athletes, the development of pubic hair is not delayed.

The observation that high-performance female athletes give a history of delayed onset of menarche, even without a history of intense training prior to menarche, suggests that delayed menarche may confer some athletic advantage. Athletes may inherit a tendency for a slower rate of maturation. Late maturation may lead to prolonged bony growth due to delayed closure of the epiphyseal growth plates. Late maturity is associated with longer legs, narrower hips, less weight per unit height and less relative body fat than the early maturer. These factors would be advantageous to athletic performance. There may also be a sociological component to this process. Current research emphasizes the primary role of constitutional factors in the selection process of athletes at relatively young ages.[17] The management of the girl with delayed menarche is discussed later in this chapter.

Whether delayed menarche has clinical consequences is unclear. A later age of menarche has been found to be associated with a lower rate of bone mineral accretion during adolescence and hence decreased peak bone mass.[18] This could have implications for the risk of osteoporotic fractures in later life. There have also been some reports of a greater incidence of stress fractures in athletes with delayed menarche,[18, 19] although this is not necessarily a consistent finding.[20]

Luteal phase defects

Abnormal luteal function is common among athletes.[21] The luteal phase extends from the time of ovulation to the onset of menstruation. It is normally associated with high levels of estrogen and progesterone and its normal length is 14 days. A shortened luteal phase of less than 10 days is commonly found in exercising women. This is usually associated with lower than normal levels of progesterone during the luteal phase of the cycle and anovulatory cycles. This abnormality of the luteal phase is often not recognized as women still menstruate regularly and it may be associated with a slightly prolonged follicular phase resulting in normal or near-normal lengths of the menstrual cycle (28 days). This condition may only be recognized by plotting the basal body temperature, which fails to show the expected rise seen in a normal luteal phase, or using commercially available urine test kits which can detect the surge of LH preceding ovulation. Low progesterone levels in the luteal phase of the cycle may also be an indicator of luteal phase defect.

There appears to be a direct relationship between the amount of exercise and the development of luteal phase defects.[22, 23] It is uncertain whether this luteal insufficiency is a stage in a continuum of menstrual cycle irregularity proceeding to oligomenorrhea or amenorrhea, or whether it is a separate entity. The main effect of luteal phase defects is infertility or subfertility as well as spontaneous habitual miscarriage. There have also been reports of bone loss associated with luteal phase defects. Several studies found that recurrent short luteal phase cycles and anovulation were associated with spinal bone loss of approximately 2–4% per year in physically active women.[24]

Oligomenorrhea and amenorrhea

Oligomenorrhea (irregular menstruation, three to six cycles per year) and amenorrhea (absent menstruation, fewer than three cycles per year or no cycles for the past six months) are prevalent in the sporting population. The incidence of these conditions in athletes is between 10% and 20%, while the incidence in the general population may be about 5%.[25–27] The incidence in runners and ballet dancers has been found to be particularly high compared with swimmers and cyclists. It is thought that as many as 50% of competitive distance runners have reduced or absent periods. Menstrual disturbances have also been found to be higher in sports emphasizing leanness.[16] Oligomenorrhea and amenorrhea are associated with a disruption of the hypothalamic–pituitary–ovarian axis, which manifests itself as low amplitude, irregular and infrequent LH pulsatility and low levels of estrogen and progesterone. This is known as hypothalamic amenorrhea. Other neuroendocrine abnormalities associated with oligomenorrhea and amenorrhea include lower levels of thyroid hormones, insulin-like growth factor-1 and leptin (expressed mainly in adipose tissue), together with an increase in stress hormones (cortisol).

Causes of exercise-associated menstrual cycle irregularities

The etiology of exercise-associated menstrual cycle irregularity appears to be related to 'energy drain'—the phenomenon of a calorie deficit. Restricted energy availability as a result of reduced energy intake and/or increased energy expenditure leads to low leptin levels[28] and stimulates compensatory mechanisms such as weight loss, metabolic hormone alterations, or energy conservation that subsequently cause a central suppression of reproductive function and concomitant hypoestrogenism.[29] A summary of the causes of menstrual cycle irregularities is shown in Figure 41.2. Other factors that have been implicated are discussed briefly below.

Low body fat

There is a clear association between a reduced amount of body fat and the incidence of menstrual cycle irregularity. This is not to say that there is a critical level of body fat below which menstrual cycle irregularities develop, as was once thought. There is considerable individual variation and there may be a critical level in each individual. Numerous examples have been reported where amenorrheic athletes have increased their percentage body fat for some reason (e.g. reduction in activity or injury) and normal menstruation has resumed.

Psychological stress

Psychological stress can affect hypothalamic function. Many athletes suffer high levels of psychological stress either related to their sporting activity or to outside factors such as work, family or relationships.

Psychological stress may be a contributory factor in the development of menstrual irregularities in athletes but, as yet, there is no convincing evidence from the few studies carried out.

Level of exercise

There appears to be a relationship between menstrual irregularities and the level of exercise performed. The level of exercise may be the total amount of exercise or the intensity of the exercise.

As mentioned previously, normal menstruation often resumes with cessation of the athletic activity due to injury, retirement or a reduction of exercise during a pre-competition taper or in the off-season. Frequently, menstruation will cease again on resumption of the previous level of exercise.

The level of exercise is most likely related to menstrual disturbances via its contribution to an energy imbalance. The higher the level of exercise performed, the greater the energy utilized. It is also feasible that exercise, as a form of stress, may have a direct effect on the hypothalamus or, alternatively, have its effect through the actions of one or more of the hormones whose levels are elevated by exercise. Hormones that are elevated during exercise and may affect the hypothalamus are cortisol and the opioid peptides. Cortisol levels increase with exercise. This may be associated with increased corticotropin and corticotropin-releasing hormone (CRH). It is possible that CRH may inhibit the secretion of LH from the pituitary gland. Opioid peptides, such as beta-endorphins, are elevated with exercise and may have a negative feedback effect on the hypothalamus.

'Immature' reproductive system

The above factors may all interact to affect hypothalamic and pituitary function in athletes. Why, then, do only certain athletes develop menstrual cycle irregularities? It may be that certain women have a susceptibility to develop these irregularities, possibly associated with immaturity of the reproductive system. This may explain why the incidence of menstrual cycle irregularities is more common in younger women, women who have not been pregnant, women with a history of menstrual irregularity and those with a history of delayed menarche.

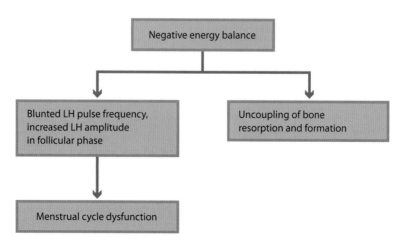

Figure 41.2 The causes of menstrual cycle irregularities

Complications of exercise-associated menstrual cycle irregularities

There are two major problems associated with menstrual cycle irregularities. These are:

1. reduced fertility
2. reduced bone mass.

Reduced fertility

There is an increased incidence of reduced fertility among intensely exercising females compared with their sedentary counterparts. Anovulatory cycles are common in athletes and may be associated with amenorrhea, oligomenorrhea or luteal phase defects, and may even occur in normally menstruating athletes. A good indication that ovulation has occurred in a particular cycle is the presence of either pre-menstrual symptoms at the end of the cycle or ovulation pain mid cycle. Ovulation may be confirmed by measuring the basal body temperature. This rises between 0.2°C and 0.6°C (0.36°F and 1.04°F) at the time of ovulation and remains elevated during the luteal phase. It may also be confirmed using commercially available urine dipsticks which detect the surge of LH just prior to ovulation.

The athlete should not automatically assume that because she has been amenorrheic for some time that she is necessarily infertile. There have been many examples of athletes with long histories of amenorrhea becoming pregnant. The cause of their amenorrhea then becomes pregnancy rather than exercise and often the first the athlete knows about the pregnancy is an unexplained poor athletic performance or an increase in abdominal girth.

If pregnancy is desired, ovulation and a normal menstrual cycle can usually be induced by reducing the level of exercise or increasing the level of body fat. If this does not induce ovulation, the athlete should be referred for gynecological assessment and, if necessary, induction of ovulation by pharmacological means.

Reduced bone mass

The detrimental effects of athletic amenorrhea on bone mass were first identified in the 1980s.[30–33] Since then, numerous others have shown lower axial bone density in athletes with amenorrhea or oligomenorrhea compared with their eumenorrheic counterparts.[31, 34–36] Appendicular bone density may also be affected,[36–38] but this has been a less consistent finding. Thus, in athletes, exercise-induced osteogenic benefits are lessened when training is associated with menstrual dysfunction,[39] particularly at trabecular bone sites. However, it appears that some sports that apply high loads to bone (such as gymnastics) may be able to partly offset the negative skeletal effects of amenorrhea.[40]

Bone is lost rapidly in the first two or three years following menstrual disturbances at a rate of approximately 4% per year. After the first few years, the rate of loss continues at a slower rate. This is an important consideration in the treatment of amenorrheic athletes.

Osteoporosis is one of the components of the so-called 'female athlete triad', which was coined to represent a syndrome of disordered eating, amenorrhea and osteoporosis and thought to be common in athletes. However, a recent Norwegian study of the prevalence of the triad found that fewer than 5% of elite female athletes met all the triad criteria and that this prevalence was comparable to that seen in normally active girls and young women.[41] When evaluating the presence of two of the components of the triad, prevalence ranged from 5.4% to 26.9% in the athletes. This implies that a significant proportion of female athletes suffer from components of the triad rather than the triad itself and that this is not just confined to elite athletes. It has also been suggested that osteopenia is the likely effect of disordered eating on bone; osteoporosis is rare in this group of active women.[42]

The mechanisms responsible for the deleterious effects of menstrual disturbances on bone density are probably multifactorial. Previously, the main cause was thought to be low circulating estrogens. Compared with their eumenorrheic counterparts, amenorrheic athletes have significantly lower plasma estradiol levels, resembling those of post-menopausal women.[31, 43, 44] However, this primary mechanism for bone loss is now questioned.[45] Evidence for this is related to findings of bone turnover studies[46] and to the fact that amenorrheic athletes appear to be less responsive to estrogen therapy[47–50] than women with ovarian failure. The post-menopausal state is characterized by increased bone turnover with an excess of bone resorption.[51] Conversely, the pattern of bone remodeling in amenorrheic athletes is atypical of an estrogen-deficient state, with either no change[44, 52] or an apparent reduction in bone turnover and reduced bone formation.[53] Other work now suggests that undernutrition and its metabolic consequences (reduced levels of insulin-like growth factor-1 and leptin) may underlie the bone remodeling imbalance and bone loss in active amenorrheic women.[46, 54, 55]

A recent experiment showed that bone formation is impaired at much higher levels of energy availability than is bone resorption[56] and at levels that may not manifest as amenorrhea.

Reduction in bone mass in athletes is particularly important for two reasons. In the short term, there is a possible increased susceptibility of these athletes to the development of stress fractures and, in the long term, the risk of osteoporosis in later life.

Stress fractures

Stress fractures occur in males and in normally menstruating females; however, it seems that the incidence of stress fractures in amenorrheic females is higher than in normally menstruating females.[19, 57–61] This could be related to lower bone density as studies have found that female athletes who developed stress fractures had lower bone density than those who did not.[19, 59, 62] However, bone density may not necessarily be lower than that of less active non-athletes, which suggests that the level of bone density required by physically active individuals for short-term bone health may be greater than that required by the general population. Another mechanism by which menstrual disturbances could increase the risk of stress fracture is via alterations in bone formation independent of reductions in bone density. Athletes with menstrual disturbances also often present with other factors, such as low calcium intake,[26] greater training load and lower body fat or body mass index,[55, 63] all of which could impact upon stress fracture development.

Post-menopausal osteoporosis

The second possible consequence of a reduction in bone mass is that it may increase the susceptibility of these athletes to the development of post-menopausal osteoporosis if bone loss cannot be reversed once menses return. The most important means of prevention of post-menopausal osteoporosis is the attainment of a high peak bone mass. Peak bone mass, which is usually attained around the late teens–early twenties, is dependent upon a number of interrelated factors, including genetics, nutrition (especially calcium intake and energy balance), exercise and hormonal status.

The reversibility of bone loss observed with amenorrhea has been a concern due to the long-term consequences on bone mass. Drinkwater et al. followed-up athletes with amenorrhea 15 months after they regained menses and showed a 6% increase in vertebral bone density.[64] The resumption of menses was also associated with an increase in body weight and a reduction in exercise level. However, it was later reported[65] that the gain ceased after two years, suggesting that bone mass may never fully recover. Other authors have also showed that, despite resumption of menses, previously irregularly menstruating runners still have reduced vertebral bone mass compared with regularly menstruating runners.[18, 66, 67] A history of menstrual irregularity is therefore detrimental to the attainment and maintenance of peak bone mass.

Treatment of exercise-associated menstrual cycle irregularities

When a woman presents with menstrual cycle irregularities, including amenorrhea, oligomennorhea and menstrual cycle length disorders, the physician should take a history (including dietary intake, Chapter 37), complete a focused physical examination and investigate the serum hormonal profile. If menstrual dysfunction is identified and linked to low body weight or increased exercise intensity (i.e. energy imbalance[68]), treatment aims to normalize nutritional intake and provide a better balance of training, exercise intensity and recovery strategies. This should be monitored and supported through education and review of training logs for at least a six-month period prior to initiation of the OCP for menstrual dysfunction. It is quite common that the menstrual cycle can remain irregular despite an increased number of cycles over the first year. A key clinical indicator of recovery is the patient reporting greater energy and more consistent performance.

Contraception

Contraceptive methods used by athletes include the oral contraceptive pill, barrier methods (e.g. condom and diaphragm), intrauterine devices (IUDs) and a variety of other methods including the rhythm method, basal body temperature and mucus method.

Oral contraceptive pill

With the introduction of low-dose pills with few side-effects and seemingly no adverse effects on performance, athletes use of the OCP has increased. The OCP can be administered safely from the age of 16 years or three years post menarche. OCPs have numerous beneficial effects for the athlete apart from contraception and cycle control, including a reduction in dysmenorrhea, pre-menstrual syndrome, menorrhagia and iron-deficiency anemia secondary to excessive monthly blood loss.[6] Women taking the

OCP have a decreased frequency of dysfunctional uterine bleeding, ovarian cysts, pelvic inflammatory disease, benign breast disease and ectopic pregnancies. The risks of ovarian and endometrial cancers are also reduced.

Initial high-dose pills were associated with a high incidence of side-effects, such as weight gain, that were unacceptable to athletes. Studies also suggested a possible diminution of performance, especially endurance performance, associated with use of the OCP.

The advent of low-dose pills has meant a reduction in side-effects. Most population studies indicate no overall effect on body weight while taking the OCP,[69, 70] although individual responses to the hormones may involve some weight gain either due to fluid retention or possibly appetite stimulation. Athletes should be counseled about the misconception of weight gain as an inevitable consequence of OCP use. There is also no convincing evidence that the OCP affects performance.[71–74]

The risk of breast cancer and cervical cancer may be higher in users of the OCP, although this is still controversial.

The OCP may be used in the monophasic form as a constant daily dose or in the triphasic form with variable dosages throughout the cycle.

The OCP also enables the athlete to manipulate her periods to avoid a major event coinciding with the pre-menstrual or menstrual period. If this is to be done, a monophasic pill should be used.

Evidence-based guidelines recommend that there are two prerequisites for safe screening for potential OCP users:

1. a careful personal and family medical history with particular focus on cardiovascular risk factors
2. an accurate blood pressure measurement.[75]

Absolute contraindications to estrogen therapy include cerebrovascular accident, coronary occlusion, thromboembolitic disorder, impaired liver function, estrogen-dependent neoplasia, undiagnosed vaginal bleeding and carcinoma of the breast. Relative contraindications include hypertension, abnormal glucose tolerance, hyperlipidemia, renal, hepatic or gallbladder disease, migraine headaches, depression and recent major elective surgery.[6]

Barrier methods have always been popular with athletes. The diaphragm has virtually no side-effects and when correctly fitted can be worn comfortably during exercise. The condom has had a recent resurgence in popularity due to the prevalence of the acquired immunodeficiency syndrome (AIDS)

and other sexually transmitted infections. The effectiveness of the condom is increased if it is used in conjunction with a spermicidal cream or gel. Barrier methods are generally not as reliable as the OCP or the IUD but are more reliable than the rhythm or withdrawal method.

IUDs have the advantage of being placed in situ rather than having to be reapplied as in barrier methods. There is no hormonal interference but side-effects such as increased dysmenorrhea and heavy bleeding may occur. Infections are a serious but uncommon side-effect. Recent adverse publicity regarding IUDs has resulted in a reduction in their use.

Other methods, such as the rhythm method, basal body temperature and mucus method, are widely used and have the advantage of being 'natural' forms of birth control. The increased incidence of menstrual cycle irregularities in athletes, however, may reduce the reliability of these methods. The use of injectable depot medroxyprogesterone acetate should be avoided as it may lead to amenorrhea, lower estrogen levels and decrease bone mineral density.[76]

Exercise and pregnancy

Research supports the prescription of exercise during pregnancy as an effective tool for improving general emotional well-being, maintaining optimal weight management and controlling blood glucose levels. The Par-Med X is a validated screening tool to assess readiness for physical activity and screen for contraindications while providing current exercise education. The current guidelines for exercise prescription during pregnancy refer to low-risk, single pregnancies[77] and these are detailed below, after a discussion of the possible risks of exercise in pregnancy.

Potential risks of maternal exercise to the fetus

The potential risks of maternal exercise to the fetus include:

- fetal injury
- fetal distress
- intrauterine growth retardation
- prematurity
- fetal malformations.

Direct trauma to the fetus is rare but may occur in the second and third trimester when the uterus lies in the abdomen. For this reason, contact sports or sports with a high risk of collision should be avoided after the first trimester.

Changes in fetal heart rate may occur in response to exercise, although this seems to be related to gestational age and the duration, intensity and type of exercise. Changes in fetal heart rate may be due to relative hypoxia caused by a decreased uterine blood flow during exercise. Uterine blood flow increases significantly during pregnancy but is postulated to be reduced during exercise due to shunting of blood away from the splanchnic organs to the exercising muscles. However, blood flow to the uterus during exercise is maximal at the area of attachment of the placenta, therefore minimizing the hypoxic effect on the fetus. Generally, increases in fetal heart rate of between 10 and 30 beats per minute are found following maternal exercise.[78] Occasionally, bradycardia (slowing of the heart rate) is observed.[79] The clinical significance of fetal tachycardia or bradycardia is uncertain.

The average birthweight of babies whose mothers have exercised intensively and very frequently during pregnancy is lower than that of babies born to sedentary mothers.[80] There do not appear to be any short- or long-term adverse sequelae as a result of this difference in weight between groups. There is a theoretical risk of premature labor associated with maternal exercise due to increased levels of noradrenalin (norepinephrine), which may cause increased uterine irritability and subsequent premature labor. This has not been observed in practise.

The other major area of concern for the health of the fetus with maternal exercise is the risk of hyperthermia. Animal data suggest that a core temperature in excess of 39°C (102°F) may result in neural tube defects in the fetus. This malformation is the result of failure of closure of the neural tube, a process that occurs approximately 25 days after conception. This has not been confirmed in humans. Pregnant women, however, should avoid hyperthermia during the first weeks of their pregnancy. Moderate exercise in normal environmental conditions results in minimal increases in core temperature.

Risks to the mother

The pregnant woman shows an increased susceptibility to musculoskeletal injuries, especially the development of pain in the low back, sacroiliac region or pubic symphysis. The mechanism of the development of low back and pelvic girdle pain in the pregnant woman probably relates to a combination of factors, including a change in the center of gravity upwards and forwards associated with forward tilting of the pelvis, an increase in lumbar lordosis and loosening of ligaments associated with increased levels of the hormone relaxin.[81]

The incidence of low back pain can be reduced by careful attention to posture and avoidance of sudden movements, as well as strengthening of the abdominal and back muscles. Pelvic girdle pain can be reduced by advice on posture, use of a sacroiliac belt, stabilizing exercises and acupuncture.[82, 83] Another possible problem affecting the pregnant woman is hypotension. Postural hypotension results from prolonged standing whereby there is a decrease in cardiac output due to slowed venous return. Supine hypotension can occur with lying or exercising in the supine position. In the supine position, the uterus compresses the major blood vessels, resulting in reduced blood return to the heart and hypotension.

Advantages of exercise during pregnancy

The advantages of exercise during pregnancy relate more to the general physical and psychological well-being of the mother rather than to any effects on the pregnancy itself.

Women who exercise prior to pregnancy and continue to do so in pregnancy weigh less, gain less weight and deliver slightly smaller babies than sedentary women. Increased fitness may enable women to cope better with labor. There is no evidence that women who have exercised during pregnancy have a shorter or easier labor. Even overweight pregnant women who commence an aerobic exercise program can reap beneficial effects on fitness levels throughout pregnancy.[84]

Exercise during pregnancy is also valuable for the prevention and treatment of illnesses such as gestational diabetes. The activation of large groups of muscles allows for an improved glucose utilization by simultaneously increasing insulin sensitivity.[77] Even though data are sparse, it appears that women who engage in recreational physical activity during pregnancy have an approximately 50% reduction in the risk of gestational diabetes compared with inactive women. Active women also have an approximately 40% reduction in risk of pre-eclampsia.[85–87]

Contraindications to exercise during pregnancy

Exercise is contraindicated in women with any serious or potentially serious complication of pregnancy. A list of these contraindications is shown in the box on page 760.[88]

Guidelines for exercise during pregnancy

The majority of women are able to perform exercise during pregnancy to benefit their health and

Contraindications to aerobic exercise during pregnancy[a][88]

Absolute contraindications

- Hemodynamically significant heart disease
- Restrictive lung disease
- Incompetent cervix/cerclage
- Multiple gestations at risk of premature labor
- Persistent 2nd or 3rd trimester bleeding
- Placenta previa after 26 weeks of gestation
- Premature labor during the current pregnancy
- Ruptured membranes
- Pre-eclampsia/pregnancy-induced hypertension

Relative contraindications

- Severe anemia
- Unevaluated maternal cardiac arrhythmia
- Chronic bronchitis
- Poorly controlled type 1 diabetes
- Extreme morbid obesity
- Extreme underweight (BMI ≤ 12)
- History of extremely sedentary lifestyle
- Intrauterine growth restriction in current pregnancy
- Poorly controlled hypertension
- Orthopedic limitations
- Poorly controlled seizure disorder
- Poorly controlled hyperthyroidism
- Heavy smoker

(a) Additional contraindications should be left for the physician to individualize.

---

well-being. Serious athletes who wish to continue intense training during pregnancy should be counseled on an individual basis. In most cases, providing the pregnancy progresses normally, they will be able to maintain a reasonably high level of training until discomfort forces them to reduce their training, usually around the sixth month. Guidelines for exercise during pregnancy are listed below.[88, 89]

1. Accumulate 30 minutes or more of moderate exercise between three to five times a week. If a woman has been sedentary prior to pregnancy, then new exercise regimens should be avoided until the second trimester. All exercise should be gradually introduced and self-paced in low-impact aerobic forms.
2. Avoid exercise in the supine position after the first trimester.
3. Avoid exercise in hot weather.
4. It is recommended that an additional 1256 kJ (300 kcal) of nutrition be consumed for every exercise session, including 230 mL (8 oz) of fluid intake.
5. Perform a good warm-up and cool-down.
6. Avoid excessive or ballistic stretching.
7. Wear a firm supportive bra.
8. Cease activity immediately if any abnormal symptoms develop, such as pain, uterine contractions, vaginal bleeding or leakage of amniotic fluid, dizziness or faintness, shortness of breath, palpitations or tachycardia, nausea or vomiting, pins and needles, numbness or visual disturbances.

Type of exercise

There is no one recommended type of exercise during pregnancy. Readers are referred to published guidelines for safe exercise during pregnancy.[88, 90, 91] The pregnant woman should continue performing the exercise she enjoys most unless she wishes to change for reasons of comfort, such as changing from jogging to water exercises late in pregnancy.

Jogging is an extremely popular form of exercise and may be continued but not commenced during pregnancy. Many pregnant women will reduce the distance run during pregnancy, particularly in the later stages. Care must be taken to avoid exercise in hot and humid conditions and close attention should be paid to fluid intake. Running on softer surfaces and wearing running shoes with adequate support will reduce the impact of jogging and may prevent musculoskeletal injuries, particularly sacroiliac joint strain.

Aerobics classes may be continued but modification of certain exercises may be required. Exercises involving lying supine or hyperextension of the lumbar spine should be avoided. Low-impact aerobics is preferable to high-impact aerobics during pregnancy. Bouncing or ballistic movements should be avoided. Yoga is an excellent means of maintaining flexibility and relaxation. Excessive stretching should be avoided because the hormone relaxin loosens ligaments.

Cycling has the advantage of being a non-weight-bearing activity. In the middle and later stages of pregnancy, it may be advisable to use a stationary bike because of balance problems caused by the shift in the center of gravity. Cycling should be avoided in high temperatures or humidity.

Water activities are popular during pregnancy because of the support provided by the buoyancy of the water. Swimming, walking or running in the water and water aerobics are all excellent forms of exercise during pregnancy.

Pelvic floor exercises are important to provide women with a good understanding of the function of the pelvic floor and its vital role in continence, structural support of the pelvic organs and sexual satisfaction. They are also important to create an awareness of the muscle group so that women can increase their control over the pelvic floor and their ability to relax it during the second stage of labor.[86]

Trunk stability is of prime importance during pregnancy and in the postnatal period due to increased load of the fetus on the spine, decreased strength of the rectus abdominis and the postural changes.[86] Exercises concentrating specifically on the internal obliques and transversus abdominis should be performed. If a diastasis of the abdominal muscles occurs (separation of the rectus abdominis), physical activities that increase the visible herniation should be avoided. The diastasis generally corrects itself over time after delivery.

Certain sports such as parachute jumping should be avoided during pregnancy. Anecdotal and survey evidence suggests that shallow scuba diving not requiring decompression (in less than 10 m [30 ft] in which the risk of venous air embolism is low) is not associated with an abnormal outcome unless it is frequent and occupationally related.[92, 93] Contact sports or those involving a high risk of collision are not recommended. Water skiing is also not recommended due to potential trauma during a fall and vaginal douching. Exercising at high altitudes above 3000 m (10 000 ft) may not be wise due to the fact that the rates of pregnancy complications are much higher and birthweights lower at these altitudes.[94] At moderate altitudes, there have been no reports of injury, pregnancy complications or losses associated with exercise at altitude (e.g. skiing, running, hiking, mountain biking).[93]

Weight training may be continued by the experienced athlete but heavy weights should be avoided. Concentration on high repetition, low weight exercises is advisable. During training the Valsalva maneuver should be avoided. The American College of Obstetricians and Gynecologists' warning signs for a pregnant woman to terminate exercise are listed in the box below.

Post-partum exercise

After a normal vaginal delivery, gentle exercises such as walking or stretching may be commenced as early as the mother is comfortable. The changes invoked by pregnancy may take some time to return to normal,

> ### Warning signs for a pregnant woman to terminate exercise[88]
>
> - Vaginal bleeding
> - Dyspnea prior to exertion
> - Dizziness
> - Headache
> - Chest pain
> - Muscle weakness
> - Calf pain or swelling (until deep venous thrombosis is ruled out)
> - Preterm labor
> - Decreased fetal movement
> - Amniotic fluid leakage

so care should be taken in the first six weeks after delivery to avoid sudden high impact or contact. Avoidance of excessive stretching or lifting is advisable in this period.

After a Cesarean section, strenuous activity should be avoided for six weeks and heavy weight training for 12 weeks. Attention should be paid to pelvic floor muscle strength and this needs to be adequate for the activity that the athlete will return to.

Lactating women need to pay special attention to adequate fluid and energy intake. A good supportive bra is also important for exercise during this period. Lactation and exercise can be successfully combined without any disruption of milk production or flow.

Menopause

Menopause is defined as the time of cessation of menstruation. The exact timing of menopause can only be determined retrospectively as a period of 12 months must occur without any evidence of menstruation. The time of hormonal change before and after the menopause is technically known as the climacteric but more popularly referred to as the perimenopause. This is associated with a gradual reduction in endocrine function of the ovarian follicle, which commences some years before the actual menopause. The average age of menopause in women in Western societies is approximately 50 years.

The changes of the menopause and perimenopause are due to the decreased ability of the ovaries to respond to stimulation by the pituitary gonadotropins. The alteration in ovarian function initially causes dysfunctional (irregular) uterine bleeding in the premenopausal stage. Hormone-dependent symptoms such as hot flushes and vaginal dryness are also associated with a decrease of estrogen production and may occur prior to and around the time of menopause. Some time after the menopause, symptoms of chronic estrogen deprivation may occur, such as chronic atrophic vaginitis and urinary incontinence.

With the steadily increasing life expectancy in most Western societies, increased attention is being paid to the problems of the menopause and the post-menopausal years. A woman who reaches the age of 65 years can now expect to live into her 80s. A steadily increasing percentage of the population will be in the post-menopausal years. There are two major health concerns related to the hormonal changes occurring around the time of menopause. These are an increased incidence of osteoporosis and coronary heart disease.

Osteoporosis

Osteoporosis is a major health problem in Western societies. Its major complications—fractures, especially of the spine, neck of the femur and wrist—are associated with a high morbidity and mortality. Diagnostic criteria have been established by the World Health Organization based on bone mineral density (BMD) from dual-energy X-ray absorptiometry[95] and are shown in Table 41.2.

To reduce the risk of osteoporosis, women need to acquire as much bone mass as possible prior to menopause and reduce the rate at which bone is lost after menopause. Reducing the risk of falling will also reduce the likelihood of fracture. Women attain their peak bone mass during the second decade of life. From then until the time of menopause, there is a very slow rate of bone loss. This is accelerated at menopause and for a few years following the menopause may be as high as 5% per year. Later, the rate slows again.

Maximizing bone mass

The greater the bone mineral content at the time of peak bone mass, the more bone an individual can afford to lose. Thus, the period of early adolescence is a window of opportunity to maximize bone mass.

While genetic factors are an important contributor to peak bone mass, there are a number of ways in which women can maximize their bone mass.

Animal studies have demonstrated that bone responds best to activities that generate high strain magnitudes, high strain rates, and strains that are different to what the bone is normally accustomed to. Fewer loading cycles are needed and better responses are gained if the loading bout is broken up with rest intervals in between.[96] Thus, a variety of weight-bearing, high-impact activities should be encouraged (Table 41.3). Even a modest amount of jump training per se[97] or incorporated into the school curriculum can have beneficial effects on bone density.[98] Based on the principal of breaking the load up into smaller bouts, 10 jumps three times a day when the school bell rang was found to improve bone density.[98] Non-weight-bearing exercise such as swimming or cycling has not been shown to be effective.

The effects of exercise on bone appear to be maximized with adequate calcium intake. Studies have shown that in adolescents, exercise together with calcium supplementation was more effective than exercise alone.[99, 100] It is thought that the period from early childhood to young adulthood is important for calcium intake. It is recommended that a daily intake of 1200 mg of calcium be consumed during that time.

Excessive exercise associated with energy imbalance and menstrual irregularity may have a negative effect on bone mass as discussed previously. Lengthy periods of bed rest should be avoided if possible. Loss of bone mass associated with bed rest is thought to be approximately 4% per month. Reversal of this bone loss takes a relatively longer period of time. Smoking and excessive alcohol consumption are also detrimental to bone health.

Minimizing bone loss

The second principle of prevention of osteoporosis is to reduce the rate at which bone is lost after menopause. As bone is lost more rapidly in the

Table 41.2 Diagnostic criteria for osteoporosis

Classification	Dual-energy X-ray absorptiometry result
Normal	BMD greater than 1 standard deviation (SD) below the mean of young adults (T score: >–1)
Osteopenia	BMD between 1 and 2.5 SD below the mean of young adults (T score: –1 to –2.5)
Osteoporosis	BMD more than 2.5 SD below the mean of young adults (T score: <–2.5)
Severe or established osteoporosis	BMD more than 2.5 SD below the mean of young adults plus one or more fragility fractures

Table 41.3 Recommendations for exercise prescription for bone health in children and adolescents, and adults[a]

Exercise prescription	Children and adolescents	Adults
Mode	Impact activities (e.g. gymnastics, plyometrics, jumping) and moderate intensity resistance training; participation in sports that involve running and jumping (e.g. soccer, basketball)	Weight-bearing endurance activities (e.g. tennis, stair climbing, jogging, at least intermittently during walking); activities that involve jumping and resistance training
Intensity	High in terms of bone loading forces; for safety reasons, resistance training should be <60% of 1 repetition maximum	Moderate to high in terms of bone loading forces
Frequency	At least 3 times per week	Weight-bearing endurance activities 3–5 times per week; resistance exercises 2–3 times per week
Duration	10–20 minutes (2 times per day may be more effective)	30–60 minutes per day of a combination of activities

(a) American College of Sports Medicine. Position stand. Physical activity and bone health. 2004. Available online: <http://www.acsm-msse.org/pt/re/msse/positionstandards>.

years immediately after menopause, it is important to institute measures to reduce the loss of bone prior to or at the time of menopause. A variety of moderate-impact exercises and strength training has been shown to reduce the rate of loss of bone mass in the post-menopausal period[101, 102] even in those with low bone density.[103] Walking programs of up to a year have generally not been effective in preventing bone loss in healthy ambulant individuals. This is not surprising as walking does not impart high loading forces onto bone, nor does it represent a unique loading stimulus. However, this does not exclude the possibility that long-term habitual walking for many years helps to preserve bone mass. Exercise guidelines are shown in Table 41.3. Smoking and excessive alcohol should be avoided.

An adequate calcium intake is considered essential for the positive effects of exercise to occur. In post-menopausal women, greater calcium intake is needed to retain calcium balance because of increased urinary calcium losses associated with low estrogen levels.[104, 105] The recommended daily intake of calcium in post-menopausal women is 1200 mg per day. However, evidence from a recent Cochrane review states that calcium supplementation alone has a small positive effect on bone density. The data show a trend towards a reduction in vertebral fractures, but it is unclear if calcium supplementation reduces the incidence of non-vertebral fractures.[105]

Vitamin D is also important for bone health. Vitamin D is obtained through the skin via sunlight and thus vitamin D deficiency can be a problem in particular climates and in those whose exposure to

sunlight is minimal. Oral vitamin D supplementation of 700–800 IU/day appears to reduce the risk of hip and any non-vertebral fractures in ambulatory or institutionalized elderly persons. An oral vitamin D dose of 400 IU/day is insufficient for fracture prevention.[106]

Reducing falls risk

Falling is an important risk factor for fracture and risk of falling increases rapidly with age.[107] One in three individuals over the age of 65 years will suffer a fall each year. Risk factors for falling include visual impairment, neurological and musculoskeletal disabilities, muscle weakness, certain medications, postural hypotension, poor balance, environmental hazards, cognitive impairments and stumbling gait. Assessment and treatment of modifiable factors should be included to reduce the risk of osteoporotic fracture,[108] including the implementation of proprioceptive and balance training combined with toning programs.

Exercise may reduce falls as high levels of habitual activity in the elderly are associated with a lower prevalence of many of these risk factors.[109, 110] The types of exercise found to be effective for reducing falls and falls risk include balance and strengthening activities[111] and Tai Chi[112] and these are detailed in Chapter 55.

Pharmacotherapy

Various medications are effective in reducing fracture rates among osteoporotic women (and men).[113] The first-line therapy of post-menopausal osteoporosis is bisphosphonates.[114] Other effective treatments include selective estrogen receptor modulators (SERMS) and parathyroid hormone (PTH). Bisphosphonates halve the risk of osteoporotic fracture, including hip fracture. Patients at risk of vitamin D deficiency on the basis of low 25-hydroxyvitamin D levels should be given oral vitamin D in the order of 800 IU daily. Selective estrogen modulators include raloxifene, which can prevent vertebral fractures. Side-effects of raloxifene include hot flushes and muscle cramps. Thus, it is most popular among those women well beyond the menopause who may be less likely to have recurrence of hot flushes.

The use of estrogen therapy in the post-menopausal woman has reduced in light of the results of the Women's Health Initiative (WHI), a trial of post-menopausal hormone replacement therapy. In May 2002, the trial was interrupted earlier than expected. The studied hormonal formulation was the association of conjugated equine estrogens and medroxyprogesterone. The reason for termination was an increased risk of breast cancer and myocardial infarction in the hormone-therapy group. Later, reports confirmed that this type of hormone replacement therapy should not be used for the primary prevention of coronary heart disease. There is an increased risk of venous thromboembolism with post-menopausal estroprogestative replacement. This risk does not seem to exist with transdermal estrogens. The other WHI findings concerned the lack of protection against dementia and cognitive decline. Despite these adverse events, the treatment reduced osteoporotic hip fractures and colorectal cancers. In April 2004, the estrogen-only arm of the same WHI study was also prematurely interrupted because of an increase in the incidence of stroke.

Coronary heart disease

There appears to be an increased risk of coronary artery disease in women after menopause. In particular, the severity of coronary artery disease appears to increase as evidenced by an increase in the presentation of myocardial infarction and sudden death but no change in the frequency of patients presenting with angina. This increase in coronary artery disease may be due to the observed increases in total plasma cholesterol levels and a decrease in high-density lipoprotein cholesterol levels.

Physical activity appears to have an effect in reducing the risk of coronary heart disease in post-menopausal women. As little as 30 minutes of moderate-intensity activity per day can result in risk reductions. Protective mechanisms of physical activity include the regulation of body weight; the reduction of insulin resistance, hypertension, atherogenic dyslipidemia, and inflammation; and the enhancement of insulin sensitivity, glycemic control, and fibrinolytic and endothelial function.[115] Women with coronary artery disease, peripheral vascular disease or diabetes mellitus must be considered individually when prescribing exercise and a pre-participation medical evaluation is recommended.[116]

Aerobic fitness

For many years aerobic fitness was thought to steadily decrease with age. It was also thought that this decrease was accelerated at the onset of menopause. It now appears that any decrease in aerobic fitness is related more to a decrease in activity than age. Post-menopausal women are able to increase their aerobic fitness as measured by VO_{2max}. The less fit the woman is prior to the commencement of exercise, the greater the gain in aerobic fitness.

Stress urinary incontinence

This is a common problem for the adult female athlete, especially after menopause and with high-impact activities.[117] There is a positive correlation between incontinence and the number of vaginal deliveries a woman has had. Pelvic floor muscle rehabilitation can be taught by specialized physiotherapists.

Exercise guidelines

Women should be encouraged to continue, resume or commence exercise in the post-menopausal period. For those wishing to commence an exercise program, a comprehensive pre-exercise evaluation is necessary. A thorough history and examination should be performed, paying particular attention to cardiovascular risk factors. Blood measurements of hemoglobin, glucose, electrolyte and cholesterol levels may also be performed. An exercise ECG/EKG should be performed prior to commencing an exercise program in the presence of abnormal symptoms (e.g. chest pain) or cardiovascular risk factors (e.g. strong family history).

It is important to tailor the exercise for the individual, taking into consideration fitness level, associated medical problems and, most importantly, individual enjoyment. The American College of Sports Medicine position stands on exercise and physical activity for older adults[118] and exercise and osteoporosis[119] provide information about exercise prescription in this age group. Exercise involving large muscle groups, such as walking, swimming, cycling or dancing, is recommended together with balance exercises. For a positive health benefit, exercise should be performed between three and five times per week for a period of 20 minutes each. The patient should aim to attain a heart rate equivalent to 70% of the maximum heart rate, which can be calculated by subtracting the patient's age from 220. Some form of weight-bearing exercise should be included. Progressive strength training is also important to prevent the muscle weakness that is a universal characteristic of advancing age. It has been shown that given an adequate training stimulus, older women (and men) show similar or greater strength gains as a result of strength training compared with young individuals.[120] Each work-out should consist of up to 15 repetitions of eight to 10 different exercises that train the major muscle groups (see Chapter 55). Sets of one to two can be performed, two or three times per week. The weight lifted should be up to 85% of one repetition maximum.[121, 122] An appropriate warm-up and warm-down should be performed and attention should be paid to good quality shoes and equipment as well as personal safety.

Risks of exercise

The main concern of exercise in this age group is cardiovascular disorders, such as angina, myocardial infarction and sudden death. Careful clinical assessment is required prior to the commencement of an exercise program. The patient must be counseled to cease activity immediately and report to her doctor if any abnormal symptoms such as chest pain, irregular heart beats, dizziness, shortness of breath or excessive fatigue should occur. The majority of people who have a serious cardiovascular episode (e.g. myocardial infarction) while exercising have experienced previous symptoms that they have ignored.

The other problem associated with exercise in this age group is musculoskeletal injuries, often as a result of a fall. Care should be taken to ensure a suitable environment for exercise with a level terrain and adequate light, as well as wearing appropriate supportive shoes to reduce the possibility of falls.

The breast

The breast is composed primarily of fatty tissue. Breast size and shape is largely determined by genetic predisposition but may be affected by general weight loss or weight gain. Breast changes are common in the pre-menstrual period, where the breast may increase in size up to 40%.

Trauma

Breast trauma is not common but a contusion may occur as a result of a direct blow from a ball, racquet or opponent. This contusion is associated with bleeding and swelling. It should be treated with ice, analgesics and support. Occasionally, a deep hematoma will require aspiration. There is no evidence that trauma to the breast causes tumors.

Nipple problems

'Runners' nipples' is a common condition in which the nipples are irritated and abraded by rubbing against clothing during prolonged activity. This condition is actually more common in males than females and is more likely to occur in cold weather where the nipple is more prominent and harder. It may be prevented by the use of petroleum jelly, tape over the nipples or a seamless bra (Table 41.4).

Cyclists also commonly develop nipple problems as a result of a combination of perspiration and cold. This can be prevented by the use of appropriate clothing, especially a wind-breaking material over the chest.

Sports bras

Excessive movement of the breasts, particularly in an up and down motion, occurs during exercise. This may lead to pain and discomfort and affect sports performance. A number of specialized sports bras are now available.

Sports bras should give support from above, below and the sides. They should be made of a material that is firm, mostly non-elastic, non-abrasive and has good absorptive quality. The straps should be of non-stretch material and, ideally, criss-crossed or Y-shaped at the back. There should be no seams or ridges in the nipple area and no fasteners or hooks. The sports bra should be individually fitted and be comfortable both at rest and with vigorous activity. There should also be provision for the insertion of padding for use in contact sports.

Various degrees of padding can be added to the bra. In certain sports, such as martial arts and football, a plastic cup bra may be placed over the normal sports bra. Protective chest pads should be worn in softball and hockey.

Table 41.4 Recommendations for breast care in sport

Issue	Garment solution	Healthcare practitioner role
Increased physical activity	Advise garment suited to type of exercise: • impact: supportive, compression, seamless, sweat absorbent • endurance: ventilated, scapular reinforcement, porous fabric • contact: protective padding	Advise exercise for health: • include bra advice in addressing active wear issues • awareness that chaffing, bruising, irritation and pain are not normal and should be addressed • refer to physician if further evaluation is required
Bruising: • shoulder strap • anterior breast	• Wider shoulder straps, can add strap pads • Less anterior compression, separate cup style may help	Address the contact component of sport: • technique changes • shell chest protectors • game conduct
Nipple chaffing	Seamless cups: • ensure proper size and fit • sweat-absorbent material	Hygiene issues: • dry nipples (change out of sweaty or wet garments) • air dry after showering • use moisturizers such as vitamin E cream or lanolin • use lubricants such as Body Glide or Vaseline • educate on signs of infection
Controlling breast movement	Compression style garment: • full figure support • Spandex body suit for additional support • proper sizing and fit	Advise on proper posture: • rhomboid and scapular stabilization strengthening to reduce forward posture • gait and footwear to ensure correct movement patterns

Environmental factors

The main gender difference in hot conditions is an increased sweat rate in males in a humid environment. There appears to be no difference in heat acclimatization between the genders.

The basal body temperature is increased following ovulation. This increase in temperature after ovulation results in an increase in the threshold core temperature for both sweating and cutaneous vasodilation. However, there is no evidence of a change in exercise tolerance to heat in the different phases of the menstrual cycle.

A larger ratio of surface area to mass should disadvantage the female in colder environments. However, the female's greater proportion of body fat and its location in the subcutaneous fat layer provides good insulation and probably counteracts the effect of the large surface area. Females have been shown to have a lower skin temperature in cold environments but no difference is noted with rectal temperature, probably due to the insulation effect.

Nutrition

The nutritional requirements of female athletes are similar to those of their male counterparts (Chapter 37). The two main exceptions are iron and calcium.

The incidence of iron deficiency among female athletes is particularly high.[123] The factors that may contribute to iron deficiency are discussed in Chapter 37. Females have an added susceptibility to iron deficiency because of their low iron stores and loss of iron through menstrual blood loss. This is compounded by a frequently inadequate iron intake when female athletes are on low-energy diets.[124, 125] Females who do not eat red meat are particularly likely to develop iron deficiency.

The most common presenting symptom of iron deficiency is tiredness or impaired performance (Chapter 52). Any athlete who presents complaining of tiredness or impaired performance should be suspected of iron deficiency. This is particularly likely if the female athlete is an endurance athlete and does not eat red meat. Anemia may occasionally be present but, more commonly, depletion of iron stores as measured by low serum ferritin levels is the cause of the athlete's symptoms (Chapter 37).

The importance of calcium has been mentioned previously in this chapter, both in the management of the amenorrheic athlete and in relation to osteoporosis. A high calcium intake in the adolescent and young adult years appears to be particularly important in maximizing peak bone mass, while an adequate calcium intake in the post-menopausal years is necessary for the benefits of exercise to occur. Calcium intake is discussed fully in Chapter 37.

Another nutritional concern is the apparent inadequate energy intake of many female athletes when compared to their energy expenditure. The 'energy drain' hypothesis has been put forward as a mechanism for the development of menstrual disturbances.

Eating disorders

There has been considerable discussion regarding the relationship between eating disorders and intense athletic activity. While a direct relationship is unlikely, the emphasis on thinness and reduction in body fat in particular sports, such as gymnastics, endurance running and ballet dancing, may lead to an increased incidence of eating disorders in susceptible individuals.[126] Pressure from coaches, parents or fellow competitors regarding ideal body shape may lead to abnormal eating patterns. Other psychological risk factors include low self-esteem, poor coping skills, perfectionism, obsessive–compulsive traits and anxiety.

Disordered eating occurs on a spectrum that can range from restrictive eating patterns to pathological weight control measures to classic eating disorders such as anorexia nervosa and bulimia nervosa. Clinicians should have a high index of suspicion of the presence of eating disorders in young females who appear excessively thin, who have a distorted body image (i.e. they are convinced they are too fat when in fact they are extremely thin) or who present with amenorrhea. Amenorrhea related to anorexia nervosa seems to have a more marked effect on reduction of bone density than does exercise-associated amenorrhea.[127, 128] Patients presenting with unusual stress fractures, such as fractures of the pubic ramus, may have severely reduced bone density secondary to anorexia nervosa. A comprehensive evaluation should include assessment of exercise behaviors, nutritional intake, weight control measures, psychological factors and laboratory or diagnostic testing as appropriate. The management of eating disorders such as anorexia nervosa and bulimia can be difficult and may require specialized expertise involving a multidisciplinary approach.

Injuries

Injuries to the female genital organs occur occasionally. Vulval contusions and lacerations can occur from direct trauma, especially in gymnastics. These should be treated with the application of ice and surgical repair of the laceration if necessary.

Some concerns have been expressed about the dangers of water-skiing for females. Forceful vaginal douching may occur and occasionally lead to pelvic infection. The wearing of tight-fitting wetsuit pants should be mandatory for all female water-skiers.

Three musculoskeletal injuries that may occur more frequently in females are stress fractures, patellofemoral pain (Chapter 28) and anterior cruciate ligament injuries.

It has been noted in Chapter 27 that stress fractures occur more frequently in amenorrheic women than in those who are menstruating normally. The exact mechanism of the development of stress fractures in amenorrheic women is uncertain and may not necessarily be related to low bone density. However, menstrual status should be assessed in all female athletes who present with stress fractures. A bone density measurement should be considered in these athletes.

Females have a two to eight times greater predisposition to anterior cruciate ligament rupture than males. There are many theories as to why this difference in injury rate exists. These include intrinsic factors, such as joint laxity, hormonal influences, limb alignment, notch dimensions and ligament size, as well as extrinsic factors, such as type of sport, conditioning and equipment.[129] The reader is directed to Chapter 27 for a detailed discussion of this problem and preventive strategies.

Recommended Reading

Davies GA, Wolfe LA, Mottola MF, MacKinnon C. Joint SOGC/CSEP clinical practice guideline: exercise in pregnancy and the postpartum period. *Can J Appl Physiol* 2003; 28(3): 330–41.

DiPietro L, Stachenfeld NS. The myth of the female athlete triad. *Br J Sports Med* 2006; 40(6): 490–3.

Loucks AB, Verdun M. Energy availability, not body fatness, regulates reproductive function in women. *Exerc Sport Sci Rev* 2003; 31: 144–8.

Olsen, OE, Myklebust G, Engebretsen L, et al. Exercises to prevent lower limb injuries in youth sports: cluster randomised controlled trial. *BMJ* 2005; 330(7489): 449–56.

Recommended Websites

American College of Sports Medicine. Position stand. Exercise and hypertension. 2004. Available online: <http://www.acsm-msse.org/pt/re/msse/positionstandards>.

American College of Sports Medicine. Position stand. Physical activity and bone health. 2004. Available online: <http://www.acsm-msse.org/pt/re/msse/positionstandards>.

American College of Sports Medicine. Position stand. Exercise and physical activity for older adults. 1998. Available online: <http://www.acsm-msse.org/pt/re/msse/positionstandards>.

References

1. Bailey DA, Martin AD, McKay HA, Whiting SJ, Mirwald R. Calcium accretion in girls and boys during puberty: a longitudinal analysis. *J Bone Miner Res* 2000; 15: 2245–50.

2. Bailey DA, Wedge JH, McCulloch RG, Martin AD, Bernhardson SC. Epidemiology of fractures of the distal end of the radius in children as associated with growth. *J Bone Joint Surg Am* 1989; 71A(8): 1225–31.

3. Faulkner RA, McCulloch RG, Fyke SL, et al. Comparison of real and estimated volumetric bone mineral density values between older men and women. *Osteoporosis Int* 1995; 5(4): 271–5.

4. Wang Q, Alen M, Nicholson P, et al. Growth patterns at distal radius and tibial shaft in pubertal girls: a 2-year longitudinal study. *J Bone Miner Res* 2005; 20(6): 954–61.

5. Cheuvront SN, Carter R, Deruisseau KC, Moffatt RJ. Running performance differences between men and women: an update. *Sports Med* 2005; 35(12): 1017–24.

6. Frankovich RJ, Lebrun CM. Menstrual cycle, contraception, and performance. *Clin Sports Med* 2000; 19(2): 251–71.

7. Constantini NW, Dubnov G, Lebrun CM. The menstrual cycle and sport performance. *Clin Sports Med* 2005; 24(2): e51–e82, xiii–xiv.

8. Janse de Jonge XA. Effects of the menstrual cycle on exercise performance. *Sports Med* 2003; 33(11): 833–51.

9. Friden C, Hirschberg AL, Saartok T, Renstrom P. Knee joint kinaesthesia and neuromuscular coordination during three phases of the menstrual cycle in moderately active women. *Knee Surg Sports Traumatol Arthrosc* 2006; 14(4): 383–9.

10. Bryant M, Cassidy A, Hill C, Powell J, Talbot D, Dye L. Effect of consumption of soy isoflavones on behavioural, somatic and affective symptoms in women with premenstrual syndrome. *Br J Nutr* 2005; 93(5): 731–9.

11. Wyatt KM, Dimmock PW, O'Brien PM. Selective serotonin reuptake inhibitors for premenstrual syndrome. *Cochrane Database Syst Rev* 2002; 4: CD001396.

12. Yonkers KA, Brown C, Pearlstein TB, Foegh M, Sampson-Landers C, Rapkin A. Efficacy of a new low-dose oral contraceptive with drospirenone in premenstrual dysphoric disorder. *Obstet Gynecol* 2005; 106(3): 492–501.

13. Steiner M, Hirschberg AL, Bergeron R, Holland F, Gee MD, Van Erp E. Luteal phase dosing with paroxetine controlled release (CR) in the treatment of premenstrual dysphoric disorder. *Am J Obstet Gynecol* 2005; 193(2): 352–60.

14. Wanichsetakul P, Kamudhamas A, Watanaruangkovit P, Siripakarn Y, Visutakul P. Bone mineral density at various anatomic bone sites in women receiving combined oral contraceptives and depot-medroxyprogesterone acetate for contraception. *Contraception* 2002; 65(6): 407–10.

15. Rome E, Ziegler J, Secic M, et al. Bone biochemical markers in adolescent girls using either depot medroxyprogesterone acetate or an oral contraceptive. *J Pediatr Adolesc Gynecol* 2004; 17(6): 373–7.

16. Torstveit MK, Sundgot-Borgen J. Participation in leanness sports but not training volume is associated with menstrual dysfunction: a national survey of 1276 elite athletes and controls. *Br J Sports Med* 2005; 39(3): 141–7.

17. Thomis M, Claessens AL, Lefevre J, Philippaerts R, Beunen GP, Malina RM. Adolescent growth spurts in female gymnasts. *J Pediatr* 2005; 146(2): 239–44.

18. Warren MP, Brooks-Gunn J, Fox RP, Holderness CC, Hyle EP, Hamilton WG. Osteopenia in exercise-associated amenorrhea using ballet dancers as a model: a longitudinal study. *J Clin Endocrinol Metab* 2002; 87(7): 3162–8.

19. Bennell KL, Malcolm SA, Thomas SA, et al. Risk factors for stress fractures in track and field athletes. A twelve-month prospective study. *Am J Sports Med* 1996; 24(6): 810–18.

20. Loud KJ, Gordon CM, Micheli LJ, Field AE. Correlates of stress fractures among preadolescent and adolescent girls. *Pediatrics* 2005; 115(4): e399–e406.

21. De Souza MJ. Menstrual disturbances in athletes: a focus on luteal phase defects. *Med Sci Sports Exerc* 2003; 35(9): 1553–63.

22. Prior JC, Vigna YM. Ovulation disturbances and exercise training. *Clin Obstet Gynecol* 1991; 34(1): 180–90.

23. Williams NI, Bullen BA, McArthur JW, Skrinar GS, Turnbull BA. Effects of short-term strenuous endurance exercise upon corpus luteum function. *Med Sci Sports Exerc* 1999; 31(7): 949–58.

24. Petit MA, Prior JC, Barr SI. Running and ovulation positively change cancellous bone in premenopausal women. *Med Sci Sports Exerc* 1999; 31(6): 780–7.

25. Malina RM, Spirduso WW, Tate C, Baylor AM. Age at menarche and selected menstrual characteristics in athletes at different competitive levels and in different sports. *Med Sci Sports Exerc* 1978; 10(3): 218–22.

26. Kaiserauer S, Snyder AC, Sleeper M, Zierath J. Nutritional, physiological, and menstrual status of distance runners. *Med Sci Sports Exerc* 1989; 21(2): 120–5.

27. Nattiv A, Puffer JC, Green GA. Lifestyles and health risks of collegiate athletes: a multi-center study. *Clin J Sport Med* 1997; 7(4): 262–72.

28. Chan JL, Mantzoros CS. Role of leptin in energy-deprivation states: normal human physiology and clinical implications for hypothalamic amenorrhoea and anorexia nervosa. *Lancet* 2005; 366(9479): 74–85.

29. De Souza MJ, Williams NI. Beyond hypoestrogenism in amenorrheic athletes: energy deficiency as a contributing factor for bone loss. *Curr Sports Med Rep* 2005; 4(1): 38–44.

30. Cann CE, Martin MC, Genant HK, Jaffe RB. Decreased spinal mineral content in amenorrheic women. *JAMA* 1984; 251(5): 626–9.

31. Drinkwater BL, Nilson K, Chesnut CH 3rd, Bremner WJ, Shainholtz S, Southworth MB. Bone mineral content of amenorrheic and eumenorrheic athletes. *N Engl J Med* 1984; 311(5): 277–81.

32. Linnell SL, Stager JM, Blue PW, Oyster N, Robertshaw D. Bone mineral content and menstrual regularity in female runners. *Med Sci Sports Exerc* 1984; 16(4): 343–8.

33. Marcus R, Cann C, Madvig P, et al. Menstrual function and bone mass in elite women distance runners. Endocrine and metabolic features. *Ann Intern Med* 1985; 102(2): 158–63.

34. Rutherford OM. Spine and total body bone mineral density in amenorrheic endurance athletes. *J Appl Physiol* 1993; 74(6): 2904–8.

35. Micklesfield LK, Lambert EV, Fataar AB, Noakes TD, Myburgh KH. Bone mineral density in mature premenopausal ultramarathon runners. *Med Sci Sport Exerc* 1995; 27(5): 688–96.

36. Tomten SE, Falch JA, Birkeland KI, Hemmersbach P, Hostmark AT. Bone mineral density and menstrual irregularities. A comparative study on cortical and trabecular bone structures in runners with alleged normal eating behavior. *Int J Sports Med* 1998; 19(2): 92–7.

37. Pettersson U, Stalnacke B, Ahlenius G, Henriksson-Larsen K, Lorentzon R. Low bone mass density at multiple skeletal sites, including the appendicular skeleton in amenorrheic runners. *Calcif Tissue Int* 1999; 64(2): 117–25.

38. To WW, Wong MW, Lam IY. Bone mineral density differences between adolescent dancers and non-exercising adolescent females. *J Pediatr Adolesc Gynecol* 2005; 18(5): 337–42.

39. Morris FL, Payne WR, Wark JD. The impact of intense training on endogenous estrogen and progesterone concentrations and bone mineral acquisition in adolescent rowers. *Osteoporosis Int* 1999; 10(5): 361–8.

40. Robinson TL, Snow-Harter C, Taaffe DR, Gillis D, Shaw J, Marcus R. Gymnasts exhibit higher bone mass than runners despite similar prevalence of amenorrhea and oligomenorrhea. *J Bone Miner Res* 1995; 10(1): 26–35.

41. Torstveit MK, Sundgot-Borgen J. The female athlete triad exists in both elite athletes and controls. *Med Sci Sports Exerc* 2005; 37(9): 1449–59.

42. Khan KM, Liu-Ambrose T, Sran MM, Ashe MC, Donaldson MG, Wark JD. New criteria for 'female athlete triad' syndrome? *Br J Sports Med* 2002; 36: 10–13.

43. Myerson M, Gutin B, Warren MP, Wang J, Lichtman S, Pierson RN Jr. Total body bone density in amenorrheic runners. *Obstet Gynecol* 1992; 79(6): 973–8.

44. Hetland ML, Haarbo J, Christiansen C, Larsen T. Running induces menstrual disturbances but bone mass is unaffected, except in amenorrheic women. *Am J Med* 1993; 95(1): 53–60.

45. Zanker CL. Bone metabolism in exercise associated amenorrhoea: the importance of nutrition. *Br J Sports Med* 1999; 33(4): 228–9.

46. Zanker CL, Swaine IL. Relation between bone turnover, oestradiol, and energy balance in women distance runners. *Br J Sports Med* 1998; 32(2): 167–71.

47. Hergenroeder AC. Bone mineralization, hypothalamic amenorrhea, and sex steroid therapy in female adolescents and young adults. *J Pediatr* 1995; 126(5 Part 1): 683–9.

48. Hergenroeder AC, Smith EO, Shypailo R, Jones LA, Klish WJ, Ellis K. Bone mineral changes in young women with hypothalamic amenorrhea treated with oral contraceptives, medroxyprogesterone, or placebo over 12 months. *Am J Obstet Gynecol* 1997; 176(5): 1017–25.

49. Rickenlund A, Carlstrom K, Ekblom B, Brismar TB, Von Schoultz B, Hirschberg AL. Effects of oral contraceptives on body composition and physical performance in female athletes. *J Clin Endocrinol Metab* 2004; 89(9): 4364–70.

50. Braam LA, Knapen MH, Geusens P, Brouns F, Vermeer C. Factors affecting bone loss in female endurance athletes: a two-year follow-up study. *Am J Sports Med* 2003; 31(6): 889–95.

51. Prince RL, Dick I, Devine A, et al. The effects of menopause and age on calcitropic hormones: a cross-sectional study of 655 healthy women aged 35 to 90. *J Bone Miner Res* 1995; 10(6): 835–42.

52. Stacey E, Korkia P, Hukkanen MV, Polak JM, Rutherford OM. Decreased nitric oxide levels and bone turnover in amenorrheic athletes with spinal osteopenia. *J Clin Endocrinol Metab* 1998; 83(9): 3056–61.

53. Zanker C, Swaine I. Bone turnover in amenorrheic eumenorrheic women distance runners. *Scand J Med Sci Sports* 1998; 8: 20–6.

54. Thissen JP, Ketelslegers JM, Underwood LE. Nutritional regulation of the insulin-like growth factors. *Endocr Rev* 1994; 15(1): 80–101.

55. De Souza MJ, Miller BE, Loucks AB, et al. High frequency of luteal phase deficiency and anovulation in recreational women runners: blunted elevation in follicle-stimulating hormone observed during luteal-follicular transition. *J Clin Endocrinol Metab* 1998; 83(12): 4220–32.

56. Ihle R, Loucks AB. Dose–response relationships between energy availability and bone turnover in young exercising women. *J Bone Miner Res* 2004; 19(8): 1231–40.

57. Carbon R, Sambrook PN, Deakin V, et al. Bone density of élite female athletes with stress fractures. *Med J Aust* 1990; 153: 373–6.

58. Frusztajer NT, Dhuper S, Warren MP, Brooks-Gunn J, Fox RP. Nutrition and the incidence of stress fractures in ballet dancers. *Am J Clin Nutr* 1990; 51(5): 779–83.

59. Myburgh KH, Hutchins J, Fataar AB, Hough SF, Noakes TD. Low bone density is an etiologic factor for stress fractures in athletes. *Ann Intern Med* 1990; 113(10): 754–9.

60. Kadel NJ, Teitz CC, Kronmal RA. Stress fractures in ballet dancers. *Am J Sports Med* 1992; 20(4): 445–9.

61. Tomten SE. Prevalence of menstrual dysfunction in Norwegian long-distance runners participating in the Oslo Marathon games. *Scand J Med Sci Sports* 1996; 6(3): 164–71.

62. Vinther A, Kanstrup IL, Christiansen E, et al. Exercise-induced rib stress fractures: influence of reduced bone mineral density. *Scand J Med Sci Sports* 2005; 15(2): 95–9.

63. Rosetta L, Harrison GA, Read GF. Ovarian impairments of female recreational distance runners during a season of training. *Ann Hum Biol* 1998; 25(4): 345–57.

64. Drinkwater BL, Nilson K, Ott S, Chesnut CH 3rd. Bone mineral density after resumption of menses in amenorrheic athletes. *JAMA* 1986; 256(3): 380–2.

65. Drinkwater BL, Bruemner B, Chesnut CH 3rd. Menstrual history as a determinant of current bone density in young athletes. *JAMA* 1990; 263(4): 545–8.

66. Keen AD, Drinkwater BL. Irreversible bone loss in former amenorrheic athletes. *Osteoporosis Int* 1997; 7(4): 311–15.

67. Micklesfield LK, Reyneke L, Fataar A, Myburgh KH. Long-term restoration of deficits in bone mineral density is inadequate in premenopausal women with prior menstrual irregularity. *Clin J Sport Med* 1998; 8(3): 155–63.

68. Loucks AB, Verdun M. Energy availability, not body fatness, regulates reproductive function in women. *Exerc Sports Sci Rev* 2003; 31: 144–8.

69. Dusterberg B, Ellman H, Muller U, Rowe E, Muhe B. A three-year clinical investigation into efficacy, cycle control and tolerability of a new low-dose monophasic oral contraceptive containing gestodene. *Gynecol Endocrinol* 1996; 10(1): 33–9.

70. Rosenberg M. Weight change with oral contraceptive use and during the menstrual cycle. Results of daily measurements. *Contraception* 1998; 58(6): 345–9.

71. Lynch NJ, Nimmo MA. Effects of menstrual cycle phase and oral contraceptive use on intermittent exercise. *Eur J Appl Physiol Occup Physiol* 1998; 78(6): 565–72.

72. De Bruyn-Prevost P, Masset C, Sturbois X. Physiological response from 18–25 years women to aerobic and anaerobic physical fitness tests at different periods during the menstrual cycle. *J Sports Med Phys Fitness* 1984; 24(2): 144–8.

73. Lebrun CM. Effect of the different phases of the menstrual cycle and oral contraceptives on athletic performance. *Sports Med* 1993; 16(6): 400–30.

74. Bryner RW, Toffle RC, Ullrich IH, Yeater RA. Effect of low dose oral contraceptives on exercise performance. *Br J Sports Med* 1996; 30(1): 36–40.

75. Hannaford PC, Webb AM. Evidence-guided prescribing of combined oral contraceptives: consensus statement. An International Workshop at Mottram Hall, Wilmslow, UK, March, 1996. *Contraception* 1996; 54(3): 125–9.

76. Scholes D, LaCroix AZ, Ichikawa LE, Barlow WE, Ott SM. Change in bone mineral density among adolescent women using and discontinuing depot medroxyprogesterone acetate contraception. *Arch Pediatr Adolesc Med* 2005; 159(2): 139–44.

77. Hartmann S, Bung P. Physical exercise during pregnancy—physiological considerations and recommendations. *J Perinat Med* 1999; 27(3): 204–15.

78. Clapp JF 3rd, Little KD, Capeless EL. Fetal heart rate response to sustained recreational exercise. *Am J Obstet Gynecol* 1993; 168(1 Part 1): 198–206.

79. Bung P, Huch R, Huch A. Maternal and fetal heart rate patterns: a pregnant athlete during training and laboratory exercise tests; a case report. *Eur J Obstet Gynecol Reprod Biol* 1991; 39(1): 59–62.

80. Clapp JF 3rd, Capeless EL. Neonatal morphometrics after endurance exercise during pregnancy. *Am J Obstet Gynecol* 1990; 163(6 Part 1): 1805–11.

81. Rungee JL. Low back pain during pregnancy. *Orthopedics* 1993; 16(12): 1339–44.

82. Elden H, Ladfors L, Olsen MF, Ostgaard HC, Hagberg H. Effects of acupuncture and stabilising exercises as adjunct to standard treatment in pregnant women with pelvic girdle pain: randomised single blind controlled trial. *BMJ* 2005; 330(7494): 761.

83. Nilsson-Wikmar L, Holm K, Oijerstedt R, Harms-Ringdahl K. Effect of three different physical therapy treatments on pain and activity in pregnant women with pelvic girdle pain: a randomized clinical trial with 3, 6, and 12 months follow-up postpartum. *Spine* 2005; 30(8): 850–6.

84. Santos IA, Stein R, Fuchs SC, et al. Aerobic exercise and submaximal functional capacity in overweight pregnant

women: a randomized trial. *Obstet Gynecol* 2005; 106(2): 243–9.

85. Dempsey JC, Butler CL, Williams MA. No need for a pregnant pause: physical activity may reduce the occurrence of gestational diabetes mellitus and preeclampsia. *Exerc Sport Sci Rev* 2005; 33(3): 141–9.

86. Horsley K. Fitness in the child-bearing years. In: Sapsford R, Bullock-Saxton J, Markwell S, eds. *Women's Health. A Textbook for Physiotherapists*. London: WB Saunders, 1998: 168–91.

87. Weissgerber TL, Wolfe LA, Davies GA. The role of regular physical activity in preeclampsia prevention. *Med Sci Sports Exerc* 2004; 36(12): 2024–31.

88. ACOG Committee opinion. Number 267, January 2002: exercise during pregnancy and the postpartum period. *Obstet Gynecol* 2002; 99(1): 171–3.

89. American College of Sports Medicine. *ACSM's Guidelines for Exercise Testing and Prescription*. 7th edn. Hagerstown, MD: Lippincott Williams & Wilkins, 2005.

90. De Cree C. Safety guidelines for exercise during pregnancy. *Lancet* 1998; 351(9119): 1889–90.

91. Davies GA, Wolfe LA, Mottola MF, MacKinnon C. Joint SOGC/CSEP clinical practice guideline: exercise in pregnancy and the postpartum period. *Can J Appl Physiol* 2003; 28(3): 330–41.

92. Camporesi EM. Diving and pregnancy. *Semin Perinatol* 1996; 20(4): 292–302.

93. Clapp JF 3rd. Exercise during pregnancy. A clinical update. *Clin Sports Med* 2000; 19(2): 273–86.

94. Jensen GM, Moore LG. The effect of high altitude and other risk factors on birthweight: independent or interactive effects? *Am J Public Health* 1997; 87(6): 1003–7.

95. Kanis JA, Melton LJ 3rd, Christiansen C, Johnston CC, Khaltaev N. The diagnosis of osteoporosis. *J Bone Miner Res* 1994; 9(8): 1137–41.

96. Turner CH, Robling AG. Designing exercise regimens to increase bone strength. *Exerc Sport Sci Rev* 2003; 31(1): 45–50.

97. Kato T, Terashima T, Yamashita T, Hatanaka Y, Honda A, Umemura Y. Effect of low-repetition jump training on bone mineral density in young women. *J Appl Physiol* 2006; 100: 839–43.

98. McKay HA, MacLean L, Petit M, et al. 'Bounce at the Bell': a novel program of short bouts of exercise improves proximal femur bone mass in early pubertal children. *Br J Sports Med* 2005; 39(8): 521–6.

99. Courteix D, Jaffre C, Lespessailles E, Benhamou L. Cumulative effects of calcium supplementation and physical activity on bone accretion in premenarchal children: a double-blind randomised placebo-controlled trial. *Int J Sports Med* 2005; 26(5): 332-8.

100. Iuliano-Burns S, Saxon L, Naughton G, Gibbons K, Bass SL. Regional specificity of exercise and calcium

during skeletal growth in girls: a randomized controlled trial. *J Bone Miner Res* 2003; 18(1): 156–62.

101. Kerr D, Morton A, Dick I, Prince R. Exercise effects on bone mass in postmenopausal women are site-specific and load-dependent. *J Bone Miner Res* 1996; 11(2): 218–25.

102. Engelke K, Kemmler W, Lauber D, Beeskow C, Pintag R, Kalender WA. Exercise maintains bone density at spine and hip EFOPS: a 3-year longitudinal study in early postmenopausal women. *Osteoporosis Int* 2006; 17(1): 133–42.

103. Korpelainen R, Keinanen-Kiukaanniemi S, Heikkinen J, Vaananen K, Korpelainen J. Effect of impact exercise on bone mineral density in elderly women with low BMD: a population-based randomized controlled 30-month intervention. *Osteoporosis Int* 2006; 17(1): 109–18.

104. Delaney MF. Strategies for the prevention and treatment of osteoporosis during early postmenopause. *Am J Obstet Gynecol* 2006; 194(2 suppl.): S12–S23.

105. Shea B, Wells G, Cranney A, et al. Calcium supplementation on bone loss in postmenopausal women. *Cochrane Database Syst Rev* 2004; 1: CD004526.

106. Bischoff-Ferrari HA, Willett WC, Wong JB, Giovannucci E, Dietrich T, Dawson-Hughes B. Fracture prevention with vitamin D supplementation: a meta-analysis of randomized controlled trials. *JAMA* 2005; 293(18): 2257–64.

107. Nguyen TV, Eisman JA, Kelly PJ, Sambrook PN. Risk factors for osteoporotic fractures in elderly men. *Am J Epidemiol* 1996; 144(3): 255–63.

108. Kannus P, Sievanen H, Palvanen M, Jarvinen T, Parkkari J. Prevention of falls and consequent injuries in elderly people. *Lancet* 2005; 366(9500): 1885–93.

109. Henderson NK, White CP, Eisman JA. The roles of exercise and fall risk reduction in the prevention of osteoporosis. *Endocrinol Metab Clin North Am* 1998; 27(2): 369–87.

110. Gillespie LD, Gillespie WJ, Robertson MC, Lamb SE, Cumming RG, Rowe BH. Interventions for preventing falls in elderly people. *Cochrane Database Syst Rev* 2003; 4: CD000340.

111. Liu-Ambrose T, Khan KM, Eng JJ, Janssen PA, Lord SR, McKay HA. Resistance and agility training reduce fall risk in women aged 75 to 85 with low bone mass: a 6-month randomized, controlled trial. *J Am Geriatr Soc* 2004; 52(5): 657–65.

112. Li F, Harmer P, Fisher KJ, McAuley E. Tai Chi: improving functional balance and predicting subsequent falls in older persons. *Med Sci Sports Exerc* 2004; 36(12): 2046–52.

113. Hauselmann HJ, Rizzoli R. A comprehensive review of treatments for postmenopausal osteoporosis. *Osteoporosis Int* 2003; 14(1): 2–12.

114. Papapoulos SE, Quandt SA, Liberman UA, Hochberg MC, Thompson DE. Meta-analysis of the efficacy of alendronate

for the prevention of hip fractures in postmenopausal women. *Osteoporosis Int* 2005; 16(5): 468–74.

115. Bassuk SS, Manson JE. Epidemiological evidence for the role of physical activity in reducing risk of type 2 diabetes and cardiovascular disease. *J Appl Physiol* 2005; 99(3): 1193–204.

116. Armen J, Smith BW. Exercise considerations in coronary artery disease, peripheral vascular disease, and diabetes mellitus. *Clin Sports Med* 2003; 22(1): 123–33, viii.

117. Bo K. Urinary incontinence, pelvic floor dysfunction, exercise and sport. *Sports Med* 2004; 34(7): 451–64.

118. American College of Sports Medicine. Position stand. Exercise and physical activity for older adults. *Med Sci Sports Exerc* 1998; 30(6): 992–1008.

119. Kohrt WM, Bloomfield SA, Little KD, Nelson ME, Yingling VR. American College of Sports Medicine position stand: physical activity and bone health. *Med Sci Sports Exerc* 2004; 36(11): 1985–96.

120. Miszko TA, Cress ME. A lifetime of fitness. Exercise in the perimenopausal and postmenopausal woman. *Clin Sports Med* 2000; 19(2): 215–32.

121. Evans WJ. Exercise training guidelines for the elderly. *Med Sci Sports Exerc* 1999; 31(1): 12–17.

122. Feigenbaum MS, Pollock ML. Prescription of resistance training for health and disease. *Med Sci Sports Exerc* 1999; 31(1): 38–45.

123. Fogelholm M. Indicators of vitamin and mineral status in athletes' blood: a review. *Int J Sport Nutr* 1995; 5(4): 267–84.

124. Ronsen O, Sundgot-Borgen J, Maehlum S. Supplement use and nutritional habits in Norwegian elite athletes. *Scand J Med Sci Sports* 1999; 9(1): 28–35.

125. Ziegler PJ, Nelson JA, Jonnalagadda SS. Nutritional and physiological status of U.S. national figure skaters. *Int J Sport Nutr* 1999; 9(4): 345–60.

126. Johnson C, Powers PS, Dick R. Athletes and eating disorders: the National Collegiate Athletic Association study. *Int J Eat Disord* 1999; 26(2): 179–88.

127. Grinspoon S, Miller K, Coyle C, et al. Severity of osteopenia in estrogen-deficient women with anorexia nervosa and hypothalamic amenorrhea. *J Clin Endocrinol Metab* 1999; 84(6): 2049–55.

128. Soyka LA, Grinspoon S, Levitsky LL, Herzog DB, Klibanski A. The effects of anorexia nervosa on bone metabolism in female adolescents. *J Clin Endocrinol Metab* 1999; 84(12): 4489–96.

129. Harmon KG, Ireland ML. Gender differences in noncontact anterior cruciate ligament injuries. *Clin Sports Med* 2000; 19(2): 287–302.

The Older Person who Exercises

WITH JACK TAUNTON, WENDY COOK AND JACQUELINE CLOSE

CHAPTER

42

Increasing numbers of older people perform regular physical activity that ranges from recreational walking and swimming or lawn bowls, to vigorous and/or competitive activity. The Veterans or Masters sports movements have grown rapidly and now provide competition at local, national and international levels for an increasing number of older athletes.[1] Although the variability in health and functional status among those of a similar age makes defining 'older' by chronology difficult, some authors consider those aged 75 years or more as differing from younger persons in key factors, including the prevalence of asymptomatic coronary artery disease and physical limitations preventing most in this age group from engaging in vigorous high-intensity aerobic training.[2]

The physiology of aging is outside the scope of this book but is well described elsewhere.[3] We focus on the epidemiological and mechanistic evidence for the considerable physiological and psychological benefits of exercise in the older person. However, there are certain risks associated with exercise for older people that can be minimized by adequate medical screening as well as an awareness of, and appropriate response to, warning symptoms. Finally, we comment on the potential interactions between medications commonly used by the elderly and exercise. For guidance to prescribe an exercise program in the elderly, the reader is directed to Chapter 55.

The benefits of physical activity in the elderly

Physical activity benefits all body organs as well as the psyche.[1, 2, 4–8] The most dramatic benefits have been found in the cardiovascular system.[9, 10] Exercise interventions in older patients with coronary heart disease decreased morbidity, mortality and symptoms, and reduced cardiac rehospitalizations.[10]

Numerous mechanisms may contribute to these benefits.[11] Increased demand on the myocardium improves oxygen utilization. Capillaries dilate and multiply to improve the delivery of oxygen and other nutrients to muscles. The myoglobin content of muscle is increased, thus improving the transfer of oxygen from the red blood cells to muscle cells. Inside the cell, the number of mitochondria increases, enhancing aerobic metabolism. There is also an increase in the glycogen storage sites of muscle. Exercise tends to lower the resting heart rate and the resultant increased diastolic time allows improved coronary blood flow. Stroke volume increases.

Exercise also has an effect on blood lipid levels, raising levels of high-density lipoprotein cholesterol, the 'cardioprotective' lipid, and lowering levels of low-density lipoprotein cholesterol. Exercise lowers blood pressure[12] and reduces obesity. A combination of these two factors, in addition to the reduction in cholesterol, decreases the risk of ischemic heart disease.

Exercise may also improve exercise tolerance in older people with chronic obstructive pulmonary disease.[13] They will also benefit from the associated benefits of aerobic fitness. Exercise may improve blood sugar control in people with diabetes by decreasing insulin resistance, and may reduce the need for medication.

Resistance training and high-impact activities help maintain bone mass in the elderly.[14] An exercise program may also be beneficial for older people with osteoarthritis by improving joint mobility and increasing muscle strength.[15] Exercise in the form of strength and balance training has been shown to reduce an older person's risk of falling.

BRUKNER AND KHAN, CLINICAL SPORTS MEDICINE 3E REV, McGRAW-HILL PROFESSIONAL

Along with the physical benefits of exercise, the older athlete benefits from improved sleep,[16] cognitive function[17, 18] and mood. The muscle control and weight loss associated with exercise may lead to improvements in body image and reverse the elderly person's fear of activity.[19]

Exercise reduces anxiety in elderly patients, especially in those recovering from illness. Exercise can lessen depressive symptoms[20] and perhaps even reduce the risk of developing depression.[21]

Risks of exercise in the elderly

The risks associated with a sedentary lifestyle are well known although difficult to quantify objectively and compare with the risks associated with exercise in later years. Underlying co-morbidity is often cited as a reason to preclude exercise despite the overwhelming evidence to support the benefits of exercise in many common and chronic diseases. From a safety standpoint, clinicians prescribing exercise for older people are concerned that exercise may induce myocardial ischemia and, in turn, precipitate myocardial infarction or sudden death. Gill and colleagues have provided recommendations regarding precautions that can be taken to minimize the risk of serious adverse cardiac events among previously sedentary older persons who do not have symptomatic cardiovascular disease and are interested in starting an exercise program.[2]

Reducing the risks of exercise

Before starting an exercise program, all older persons should have a complete history and physical examination performed by a physician. Contraindications to exercise outside of a monitored environment include: myocardial infarction within six months, angina or physical signs and symptoms of congestive heart failure, and a resting systolic blood pressure of 200 mmHg or higher. A functional test of cardiac capacity is to ask the patient to walk 15 m (50 ft) or climb a flight of stairs.[2] A resting ECG/EKG should be reviewed for new Q waves, ST segment depressions or T-wave inversion. Persons who have features of cardiovascular disease should be referred for appropriate management. If the patient has no overt cardiovascular disease, and no other medical or orthopedic contraindications to exercise, he or she can begin a low-intensity exercise program as discussed below.[2] Adhering to the principles outlined in Chapter 6 reduces the risk of injury.

Exercise prescription for the older individual

Inactive older people

For older adults who undertake no physical activity, the first goal of exercise prescription is simply to reduce the time spent sitting. Thus, the action plan might be to reduce the amount of time spent watching television. Other suggestions include parking further away at malls and shopping centers, taking the stairs instead of the elevator, or taking a brief walk several times a day. It is wise to suggest exercises that are functional and relevant to the individual and are incorporated into daily activities. The aphorism 'start low, go slow' applies in this population as it does in exercise prescription in general. The practitioner should set easily attainable short-term goals and increase time spent performing moderate activities by no more than 5% per week. The eventual goal is to accumulate 30 minutes a day of moderately intense physical activity on most days of the week.

Generally active older people

For older people who are generally active, begin by increasing the volume of aerobic exercise or resistance training. Aerobic exercises that are particularly attractive to older individuals are cycling on a stationary bicycle, brisk walking, swimming and water aquatics. The person should warm up (e.g. slow walking) for 5 minutes and stretch slowly for 5–10 minutes before exercising at a moderate level—one at which a conversation can be easily maintained. The cool-down after the exercise session should be by walking slowly and stretching for about 15 minutes. The person about to undertake resistance training should also perform a warm-up and stretch first. Free weights and commercially available equipment are both suitable for the older person exercising. Proper breathing consists of exhaling during the lift for 2–4 seconds followed by inhaling during the lowering of the weight for 4–6 seconds, working through the entire range of motion (or as tolerated for those with arthritis). The Valsalva maneuver should be avoided, particularly in the elderly who are more prone to postural hypotension and syncope than their younger counterparts. The lifts should be separated by 2 seconds of rest. The goal is to perform one or two sets of eight to 15 repetitions per set with 1–2 minutes of rest between sets. The patient should aim to lift a weight that is 70–80% of a one repetition maximum or the most that he or she can lift through a full range of motion at one time. The resistance should be increased no more frequently than monthly. Strength exercises should be followed by a cool-down and a stretch. The principles of follow-up and praise for progress, as outlined in the general introduction to exercise prescription, apply particularly to seniors, who may feel less confident about their capacity for activity. Current evidence suggests that participants who undertake this type of program twice weekly or more obtain benefits. Only the very unfit benefit from a once-weekly program.[22]

Interaction between medication and exercise in the older person

As most older persons have at least one chronic medical condition, and many have multiple chronic conditions, medication use is prevalent. There are certain problems associated with exercise and some of these drugs.

Medications affecting the renin–angiotensin system

Drugs affecting the renin-angiotensin system, such as angiotensin-converting enzyme (ACE) inhibitors and angiotensin II receptor blockers, lower peripheral vascular resistance. They are widely used to treat hypertension, systolic heart failure and chronic kidney disease. These drugs are suitable for the hypertensive athlete as they do not limit maximal oxygen uptake. Although the risk of dehydration among young people may have been over-represented in recent years (Chapter 53), older people who are taking these medications may have an increased susceptibility to the effects of exercise-related dehydration. The vasodilator effect may combine with fluid losses to cause hypotension and dizziness.

Beta-blockers

Beta-blockers are used to treat hypertension, angina, tremor and migraine but they may be less effective in older people than in middle-aged patients. These drugs are often prescribed after acute myocardial infarction. Beta-blockers reduce cardiac rate and output and attenuate the normal physiological response to exercise. The lack of tachycardia induced by exercise bothers some people—they dislike the absence of the 'adrenalin surge'. Older athletes who are taking beta-blockers will have a restricted exercise capacity, particularly in endurance events. Side-effects range from postural hypotension, asthma, excessive

tiredness, impotence, hyerkalemia and lethargy to exacerbating peripheral vascular disease and the potential of masking hypoglycemia in people with diabetes taking older non-selective agents.

Diuretics

Systematic reviews and clinical guidelines suggest that thiazide diuretics should be the first-line therapy for hypertension.[23] Diuretics are used in the treatment of heart failure and fluid retention to increase urinary excretion of excess salt and fluid. Older athletes who exercise in warm-to-hot conditions and take diuretics are at a particular risk of dehydration. Side-effects of thiazide diuretics include increased blood sugar levels[24] and increased uric acid levels, which can be sufficient to precipitate gout. Side-effects of thiazide diuretics include increased blood sugar levels and increased uric acid levels in those with gout. A combination of antihypertensive medication and vigorous exercise with associated dehydration may decrease the intravascular volume and cause postural hypotension, which may manifest itself as light-headedness or fainting. Prevention includes maintaining adequate hydration and avoiding standing still immediately after exertion. Alternatively, other medications may be available.

By definition, diuretics lead to increased fluid excretion through the renal tract and the diuresis occurs in relatively close proximity to oral ingestion. Older exercise participants attending classes or undertaking exercise outdoors may wish to delay the intake of their diuretic until after exercise to avoid the need to urinate excessively. This should be undertaken in consultation with their medical practitioner.

Other cardiac drugs

Calcium-channel blockers and nitrates (glyceryl trinitrate [nitroglycerin]) are used to treat hypertension and angina. They may impair cardiac output in exercise and cause peripheral vasodilatation, thus reducing performance. Peripheral venous pooling and the vasodilatation can lead to postural hypotension, particularly during the cool-down period of exercise. These side-effects should, however, be weighed up against the fact that this drug may have a direct effect on improving exercise tolerance by improving blood flow to the heart. Antiarrhythmic drugs may also reduce cardiac output.

Non-steroidal anti-inflammatory drugs

NSAIDs are commonly used for the treatment of arthritis and musculoskeletal problems in the older athlete. Serious side-effects of these medications include hypertension, fluid retention and the development of peptic ulceration. These drugs can impair renal function among older people. The risk of cardiac events in those taking certain NSAIDs was discussed in Chapter 10. The drugs should be used cautiously in the elderly and discontinued if the patient complains of adverse effects. NSAIDs should not be prescribed to athletes with a history of a bleeding disorder or those taking anticoagulants. To minimize the risk of gastric irritation, these medications should be taken with food or an acid-lowering medication (Chapter 10). Topical anti-inflammatory medications may be a useful alternative.

Medications affecting the central nervous system

Medications such as the long-acting benzodiazepines, including nitrazepam and diazepam, as well as the shorter-acting oxazepam, temazepam and lorazepam may affect fine motor skills, coordination and reaction time, and thermoregulation. This may lead to an increased risk of injury, especially in contact sports. Often, people who commence exercise can reduce their need for these medications.

Insulin and oral hypoglycemic drugs

The dosages of insulin and the oral hypoglycemic drugs may need to be reduced prior to exercise to avoid hypoglycemia (Chapter 48). Early symptoms of insulin resistance in older people can be postprandial hyperglycemia. Close monitoring of glycemic control and symptoms during exercise is necessary when initiating an exercise regimen in order to minimize the risk of hypoglycemia during exercise.

Recommended Reading

American Thoracic Society; American College of Chest Physicians. ATS/ACCP statement on cardiopulmonary exercise testing. *Am J Respir Crit Care Med* 2003; 167(2): 211–77. Erratum in *Am J Respir Crit Care Med* 2003; 167: 1451–2.

Christmas C, Andersen RA. Exercise and older patients: guidelines for the clinician. *J Am Geriatr Soc* 2000; 48: 318–24.

Cunningham GO, Michael YL. Concepts guiding the study of the impact of the built environment on physical activity for older adults: a review of the literature. *Am J Health Promot* 2004; 18(6): 435–43.

Gill TM, DiPietro L, Krumholz HM. Role of exercise stress testing and safety monitoring for older persons starting an exercise program. *JAMA* 2000; 284(3): 342–9.

Hirvensalo M, Heikkinen E, Lintunen T, Rantanen T. Recommendations for and warnings against physical activity given to older people by health care professionals. *Prev Med* 2005; 41(1): 342–7.

Huang G, Gibson CA, Tran ZV, Osness WH. Controlled endurance exercise training and VO_{2max} changes in older adults: a meta-analysis. *Prev Cardiol* 2005; 8(4): 217–25.

Huang G, Shi X, Davis-Brezette JA, Osness WH. Resting heart rate changes after endurance training in older adults: a meta-analysis. *Med Sci Sports Exerc* 2005; 37(8): 1381–6.

Kramer AF, Bherer L, Colcombe SJ, Dong W, Greenough WT. Environmental influences on cognitive and brain plasticity during aging. *J Gerontol A Biol Sci Med Sci* 2004; 59(9): M940–57.

Netz Y, Wu MJ, Becker BJ, Tenenbaum G. Physical activity and psychological well-being in advanced age: a meta-analysis of intervention studies. *Psychol Aging* 2005; 20(2): 272–84.

Peel NM, McClure RJ, Bartlett HP. Behavioral determinants of healthy aging. *Am J Prev Med* 2005; 28(3): 298–304.

Singh NA, Stavrinos TM, Scarbek Y, Galambos G, Liber C, Fiatarone Singh MA. A randomized controlled trial of high versus low intensity weight training versus general practitioner care for clinical depression in older adults. *J Gerontol A Biol Sci Med Sci* 2005; 60(6): 768–76.

Stiggelbout M, Popkema DY, Hopman-Rock M, de Greef M, van Mechelen W. Once a week is not enough: effects of a widely implemented group based exercise programme for older adults; a randomised controlled trial. *J Epidemiol Community Health* 2004; 58(2): 83–8.

Tessari P. Changes in protein, carbohydrate, and fat metabolism with aging: possible role of insulin. *Nutr Rev* 2000; 58: 11–19.

References

1. Galloway MT, Jokl P. Aging successfully: the importance of physical activity in maintaining health and function. *J Am Acad Orthop Surg* 2000; 8(1): 37–44.

2. Gill TM, DiPietro L, Krumholz HM. Role of exercise stress testing and safety monitoring for older persons starting an exercise program. *JAMA* 2000; 284(3): 342–9.

3. Timiras PS, ed. *Physiological Basis of Aging and Geriatrics.* 3rd edn. Boca Raton, FL: CRC Press, 2003.

4. Christmas C, Andersen RA. Exercise and older patients: guidelines for the clinician. *J Am Geriatr Soc* 2000; 48(3): 318–24.

5. Daley MJ, Spinks WL. Exercise, mobility and aging. *Sports Med* 2000; 29(1): 1–12.

6. Curl WW. Aging and exercise: are they compatible in women? *Clin Orthop* 2000; 372: 151–8.

7. Singh MA. Exercise and aging. *Clin Geriatr Med* 2004; 20(2): 201–21.

8. Lee IM, Sesso HD, Oguma Y, Paffenbarger RS Jr. The 'weekend warrior' and risk of mortality. *Am J Epidemiol* 2004; 160(7): 636–41.

9. American College of Sports Medicine. Position statement. The recommended quantity and quality of exercise for developing and maintaining cardiorespiratory and muscular fitness in healthy adults. *Med Sci Sports Exerc* 1990; 22: 265–74.

10. Ades PA, Coello CE. Effects of exercise and cardiac rehabilitation on cardiovascular outcomes. *Med Clin North Am* 2000; 84(1): 251–65, x–xi.

11. Booth FW, Gordon SE, Carlson CJ, Hamilton MT. Waging war on modern chronic diseases: primary prevention through exercise biology. *J Appl Physiol* 2000; 88(2): 774–87.

12. Young DR, Appel LJ, Jee S, Miller ER. The effects of aerobic exercise and T'ai Chi on blood pressure in older people. Results of a randomized trial. *J Am Geriatr Soc* 1999; 47: 277–84.

13. Ries AL, Make BJ, Lee SM, et al. The effects of pulmonary rehabilitation in the national emphysema treatment trial. *Chest* 2005; 128(6): 3799–809.

14. Kohrt WM, Ehsani AA, Birge SJ. Effects of exercise involving predominantly either joint-reaction or ground-reaction forces on bone mineral density in older women. *J Bone Miner Res* 1997; 12: 1253–61.

15. Messier SP, Royer TD, Craven TE, O'Toole ML, Burns R, Ettinger WH Jr. Long-term exercise and its effect on balance in older, osteoarthritic adults: results from the Fitness, Arthritis, and Seniors Trial (FAST). *J Am Geriatr Soc* 2000; 48(2): 131–8.

16. Li F, Fisher KJ, Harmer P, Irbe D, Tearse RG, Weimer C. Tai chi and self-rated quality of sleep and daytime sleepiness in older adults: a randomized controlled trial. *J Am Geriatr Soc* 2004; 52(6): 892–900.

17. Kramer AF, Colcombe SJ, McAuley E, Scalf PE, Erickson KI. Fitness, aging and neurocognitive function. *Neurobiol Aging* 2005; 26 (suppl. 1): 124–7.

18. Colcombe S, Kramer AF. Fitness effects on the cognitive function of older adults: a meta-analytic study. *Psychol Sci* 2003; 14(2): 125–30.

19. Sattin RW, Easley KA, Wolf SL, Chen Y, Kutner MH. Reduction in fear of falling through intense tai chi exercise training in older, transitionally frail adults. *J Am Geriatr Soc* 2005; 53(7): 1168–78.

20. Singh NA, Stavrinos TM, Scarbek Y, Galambos G, Liber C, Fiatarone Singh MA. A randomized controlled trial of high versus low intensity weight training versus general practitioner care for clinical depression in older adults. *J Gerontol A Biol Sci Med Sci* 2005; 60(6): 768–76.

21. Salminen M, Isoaho R, Vahlberg T, Ojanlatva A, Kivela SL. Effects of a health advocacy, counselling, and activation programme on depressive symptoms in older coronary heart disease patients. *Int J Geriatr Psychiatry* 2005; 20(6): 5528.

22. Stiggelbout M, Popkema DY, Hopman-Rock M, de Greef M, van Mechelen W. Once a week is not enough: effects of a widely implemented group based exercise programme for older adults; a randomised controlled trial. *J Epidemiol Community Health* 2004; 58(2): 83–8.

23. Tu K, Campbell NR, Duong-Hua M, McAlister FA. Hypertension management in the elderly has improved: Ontario prescribing trends, 1994 to 2002. *Hypertension* 2005; 45(6): 1113–18.

24. Mason JM, Dickinson HO, Nicolson DJ, Campbell F, Ford GA, Williams B. The diabetogenic potential of thiazide-type diuretic and beta-blocker combinations in patients with hypertension. *J Hypertens* 2005; 23(10): 1777–81.

The Disabled Athlete

CHAPTER

43

WITH NICK WEBBORN

Participation in sports by people with disabilities made significant increases over the latter half of the last century. In 1948, 16 competitors took part in the first Stoke Mandeville Games, a sporting competition for people with disabilities. Today, over 4000 athletes from more than 130 countries compete in the summer Paralympic Games.

In this chapter we provide a brief historical perspective and discuss the challenges that people with disability face to achieve the health benefits of physical activity. We discuss common clinical concerns of the person with various major disabilities (e.g. spinal cord injury, amputation, cerebral palsy). We outline the classification system that categorizes persons with disabilities to permit fair competition. The chapter finishes with three practical and specific issues—winter sports for disabled persons, anti-doping and travel with teams.

Historical perspective

At the start of the 19th century sports participation among people with disabilities was very limited. With the advent of two World Wars, many young men were living in society with a wide range of serious injuries. These disabled men needed to be integrated back into society and part of the rehabilitation process included involving them in sporting activity.

A most significant figure in the history of disability sport was Sir Ludwig Guttman, who ran the Spinal Injuries Unit at Stoke Mandeville Hospital in England. He introduced sporting activity as part of the rehabilitation process for those with spinal cord injury. On the opening day of the 1948 Olympic Games in London, he arranged an archery contest on the lawns of the hospital between two spinal injury units. Thus began the Stoke Mandeville Games; four years later, the games became the International Stoke Mandeville Games with the inclusion of a team of spinally injured patients from Holland.

Guttman believed that 'by restoring activity in mind and body—by instilling self-respect, self-discipline, a competitive spirit and comradeship—sport develops mental attitudes that are essential for social reintegration'. The inclusion of other sports such as athletics, swimming, table tennis and basketball increased the diversity of opportunities for people with disabilities. Participation improved slowly and in 1960 the International Stoke Mandeville Games were held in Rome after the Olympic Games with a plan to hold these quadrennial games in the Olympic Games host city where possible. In 1976 people with vision impairment and limb deficiencies were included and those with cerebral palsy joined in 1980.

Initially the term Olympics for the Disabled was used but this was not acceptable to the International Olympic Committee (IOC) and in 1985 the term Paralympic was devised to describe a games 'parallel to the Olympics' (not 'paraplegic', a common misconception). In 1989, the International Paralympic Committee (IPC) was formed and since that time the games have truly been the Paralympic Games; cities bid to host the Olympics and Paralympic Games together. In the 11-day Athens 2004 Paralympic Games, 4000 athletes represented 142 countries and competed before 800 000 spectators.

The different disability groups are organized by a variety of national and international organizations. The IPC is the international representative body for elite sports for athletes with disabilities, which are primarily physical disabilities but also include visual impairment. The International Sports Federation for

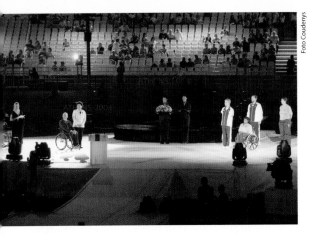

Figure 43.1 The Athens 2004 Paralympic Games closing ceremony

Persons with Intellectual Disability (INAS-FID) is affiliated with the IPC and represents solely elite athletes with intellectual disabilities. The Special Olympics is an organization for people with a full range of intellectual disability and focuses on participation at all ability levels. Its motto is 'Let me win. But if I cannot win, let me be brave in the attempt'. Hearing-impaired athletes participate in the 'Deaflympics' organized by the international organization Comité International Sports des Sourds (CISS).

Health benefits of physical activity

The health benefits of physical activity are well known[1] but people with disabilities have fewer opportunities to participate in regular physical activity for reasons that include physiological restrictions associated with the disability and access to facilities, as well as sociocultural factors. Obesity affects the disabled;[2] on the other hand, disabled people who are regularly physically active have fewer healthcare costs, including fewer visits to physicians and hospitalizations, than their inactive counterparts. In addition to the musculoskeletal benefits of regular physical activity, social and psychological benefits include improvement in self-esteem and social integration.

It is challenging for a person with a disability to perform a sufficient intensity of exercise to optimize health benefits. For example, the person using a standard wheelchair will find it difficult to push with sufficient intensity to raise the heart rate and blood pressure to the level required to significantly reduce coronary risk factors and prevent type 2 diabetes.

Thus, other modes of exercise are needed to provide more intense and prolonged activity. An activity such as hand cycling can permit higher intensity exercise but requires more expensive equipment. Another approach to greater duration and intensity of exercise is to use functional electrical stimulation of paralyzed muscles. For example, this can be used on a paralyzed leg to permit a rowing action. It is evident that this requires more expensive special equipment.

Choosing a suitable sport

The clinician who advises a disabled person about sport choices should realize that people with disabilities take part in a wide range of sports. For some sports, such as swimming, the rules and facilities require little or no adaptation. Other sports have modified equipment or rules to accommodate persons with disability (e.g. wheelchair basketball). Certain sports have been developed with specific disability groups in mind, for example, goalball, a court-based ball sport developed for the visually impaired, or boccia, an adaptation of boules for people with severe cerebral palsy. Today, people with disabilities engage in all sports—even high-risk activities such as mountain climbing and diving.

The sports available to people with disabilities depend on a variety of aspects that includes access to facilities and equipment, coaching and local competition. For some disabled people, sport is a way of obtaining physical activity for health benefit or disease modification, whereas others may be aspiring towards elite events such as Paralympic Games (Table 43.1).

Competitive sports have certain physiological requirements such as aerobic or anaerobic fitness, skill or strength. Some sports include a risk of trauma. Not all sports, however, need to be organized or competitive—the focus may be on building self-esteem and facilitating social benefits.

Factors that influence the athlete's decision may include:

- personal preference—enjoyment and achievement foster participation
- characteristics of the sport—physiological demands, coordination requirements, collision potential, preference for team or individual sport
- medical condition of the individual—exercise may be beneficial or detrimental to the disability
- cognitive ability and social skills—these determine whether a person can follow rules and interact with others

Table 43.1 Sports of the 2004 and 2006 Paralympic Games

Summer (2004)	Winter (2006)
Archery	Biathlon
Athletics	Cross-country (Nordic) skiing
Basketball	Downhill (Alpine) skiing
Boccia	Sledge hockey
Cycling	Wheelchair curling
Equestrian	
Fencing	
Football (CP, VI)	
Goalball	
Judo	
Power lifting	
Sailing	
Shooting	
Swimming	
Table tennis	
Wheelchair tennis	
Volleyball	
Wheelchair rugby	

CP = cerebral palsy; VI = visually impaired.

- facilities for training and competition
- availability of coaching and support staff
- availability of equipment—this may be expensive (e.g. specialist wheelchairs are used in road racing, wheelchair tennis, rugby and basketball; prosthetics aids for amputees for sprinting).

For elite competition (e.g. the Paralympic Games) athletes are categorized as having:

1. a physical disability
2. visual impairment or
3. intellectual impairment.

Some sports are designed for one disability group (e.g. those with tetraplegia in wheelchair Rugby), whereas other sports (e.g. swimming) have competitions for all disability groups categorized by disability. In the following sections we discuss each of these categories in turn.

The sportsperson with a physical disability

To permit fair competition, persons with physical disabilities are subcategorized into those with:

1. spinal cord injury, either congenital or acquired
2. limb deficiency or amputation
3. cerebral palsy

4. 'Les Autres'—physical disabilities such as muscular dystrophies, syndromic conditions and ankylosis or arthritis of major joints that do not fit within the other three categories.

The sports clinician needs to be familiar with the different sports risks, and capacities, of each disability group.

Spinal cord injury and sports medicine

The spinal cord lesion may be a congenital lesion such as spina bifida, or an acquired lesion through disease or trauma. Of those with a traumatic spinal cord injury, approximately 80% are men and the majority of these are aged between 16 and 30 years. Most spinal cord injuries occur as a result of motor vehicle accidents but about 15% occur during sporting activity. The sports where spinal cord injury is more likely and, thus, require vigilant prevention efforts include equestrian activities, gymnastics and trampolining, rugby union, American football and skiing. Spinal cord injury databases usually include 'diving' into shallow water (often under the influence of alcohol) as a 'sporting injury'.

Sports-related spinal cord injuries can result in paraplegia or quadriplegia with different degrees of completeness. There are approximately equal percentages of complete and incomplete quadriplegias and paraplegias. Although the loss of motor function in spinal cord injury is immediately apparent to the observer, sensory impairment also has a major impact with loss of light touch, proprioception or pain sensation. Also, autonomic dysfunction alters thermoregulation and impairs bladder and bowel function.[3] A high thoracic spinal injury, around T1–4, causes sympathectomy of the myocardium, which reduces the maximal heart rate to between 110–130 beats per minute.[4] This means that training intensity scales that rely on percentages of heart rate maximum or heart rate reserve are inappropriate but rating of perceived exertion (Borg scale) remains useful.[5]

Overall, exercise prescription in persons with spinal cord injury does not vary dramatically from the advice offered to the general population.[6–8] Systems of functional electrical stimulation activate muscular contractions within the paralysed muscles of some persons with spinal cord injury. Coordinated patterns of stimulation allow purposeful exercise movements, including recumbent cycling, rowing[9, 10] and upright ambulation. Exercise activity in persons with spinal cord injury is not without risks that relate to systemic dysfunction such as autonomic dysreflexia, low bone mass[11] and altered geometry,[12] joint contractures and problems with thermoregulation (see below). Persons with spinal cord injury can benefit greatly by participation in exercise activities,[13] but those benefits can be enhanced and the relative risks may be reduced with accurate classification of the spinal injury.

Thermoregulation—vulnerability to heat and cold

People with spinal cord injury are vulnerable to heat injury[14] due to a reduction in peripheral receptor and cooling mechanisms; sweating is impaired below the level of the spinal injury. Thus, athletes need to hydrate appropriately and acclimatize where possible. There is evidence that cooling and pre-cooling strategies offset the risk of heat illness and enhance endurance of performance.[15]

There is also an increased inability to maintain body temperature in a cold environment because of lack of sensory input and shivering response. Thus, adequate preventive measures, including appropriate clothing, are particularly important for the person with disabilities. The reader is also directed to Chapters 53 and 54, relating to exercising in hot and cold climates, for more information.

Pressure sores due to insensible skin

The insensible areas of skin below the level of the lesion are susceptible to unnoticed skin abrasions or pressure sores from prolonged sitting. Once established, a pressure sore can entail many weeks or months out of normal activities for the individual. The keys to prevention are regular inspection of the skin after activity, looking for telltale red areas and abrasions.

Autonomic dysreflexia

An injury such as a fracture below the level of the lesion may not result in the normal pain response but may trigger a phenomenon known as autonomic dysreflexia. This can be caused by any nociceptive input below the level of the lesion, such as a blocked catheter causing bladder distension, constipation, urinary calculi or ingrowing toenails. The nociceptive stimulus results in inappropriate levels of noradrenalin (norepinephrine) being secreted, producing hypertension, sweating and skin blotching above the level of the lesion and a pounding headache. Case reports have documented hypertension severe enough to cause cerebral hemorrhage, fits and death. Thus, the condition is a medical emergency with urgent attention to removing the nociceptive stimulus and reducing blood pressure with medication such as sublingual nifedipine.

Some wheelchair athletes have found that when they were in the dysreflexic state while exercising it appeared to reduce their rating of perceived exertion for performing a given intensity of exercise. Hence some athletes started to induce this state intentionally to improve their performance by as much as 10%. The technique became known as 'boosting'.[16] In 1994, inducing the dysreflexic state was considered doping and was banned by the IPC. However, as the condition may occur without intent and the athletes cannot be assessed during competition, boosting was removed as a doping method. Athletes may, however, have their blood pressure taken in a pre-competition setting and if a systolic blood pressure is 180 mmHg or greater, then they may be removed from competition on safety grounds. No sanction is imposed but the athlete is unable to compete in that event.

Osteopenia

The paralysis and consequent immobility also results in progressive loss of bone mineral density causing osteopenic or osteoporotic changes in the lower limbs and spine. This may result in fractures caused by minimal trauma or from impact collisions in sports such as ice sledge hockey or a fall from a chair in basketball. The sports clinician needs to raise her or his index of suspicion for fractures as mechanisms of injury that would normally be benign may cause fracture in the wheelchair athlete. Even though the limbs are not used for ambulation, fracture healing is important as persistent deformity may result in increased difficulty with transferring to and from the chair and performing activities of daily living.

Overuse shoulder injuries

In addition to trauma, the musculoskeletal system is also prone to overuse injuries. Upper limb injuries are common among wheelchair users because of repetitive use of the arms for propulsion as well as transferring in and out of the chair. Shoulder pain is a common presenting symptom in wheelchair users, but whether such shoulder pain is more common in sedentary wheelchair users than among those who are regularly active remains unclear. Nevertheless, in sports such as swimming or those involving overhead activities (e.g. tennis), the person with disability is prone to additional sport-specific risk factors for shoulder injuries.

Shoulder pain may be referred from the cervical or thoracic spine because of the underlying spinal pathologies. Factors such as scoliosis, poor seating position and muscle imbalance that results from pushing techniques may all contribute to alterations in scapula stabilization and abnormal patterns of movement (Chapter 17).

The sportsperson with a limb deficiency

Limb deficiencies may be congenital or acquired and persons may compete with or without a prosthesis, or in a wheelchair. A single leg amputee has jumped over 2 m (6 ft) in the high jump. Some amputee athletes use a wheelchair to play sports such as tennis and basketball. These athletes have full muscular strength and proprioceptive capability, which may not be the case for their spinal cord injured counterparts. This is further discussed under classification.

A lower limb amputee who uses a prosthetic limb for running can now avail him or herself with equipment that enhances performance. The flexible carbon fiber lower portion of the prosthesis now absorbs and returns energy to the runner in much the same way as the human Achilles tendon does. The 100 m sprint time is now about 11 seconds. Advances in technologies permit control of the swing of the prosthetic knee to aid sporting performance and also day-to-day life. Microprocessor technology is used to detect movement patterns and the joint can be programmed from a laptop computer to adapt to different situations.[17] Upper limb adaptations can be useful in sports such as lawn bowls or equestrian riding or target sports such as archery.

Despite the benefits of these technologies, they remain expensive and the impact of running at these speeds on the residual limb can result in skin chaffing, abrasion and bone bruising. Thus, the residual limb must be inspected regularly and cared for diligently to avoid injury. Because the prosthetic limb is shorter than the unaffected limb to allow it to swing through, there is a side-to-side discrepancy that may cause pelvic or low back pain.

The sportsperson with cerebral palsy

Cerebral palsy is a complex condition characterized by a variety of movement disorders. It is a 'non-progressive but not unchanging disorder of movement or posture due to an insult or anomaly of the developing brain'. Classification often occurs by the number of affected limbs, for example, diplegia, hemiplegia or monoplegia, or alternatively by the type of movement disorder. This may be a spastic cerebral palsy with increased tone, choreo-athetoid cerebral palsy with large amounts of involuntary movement and poor coordination, a hypotonia or a mixture of these patterns. This may result in classifying a particular person's disability with terms such as a 'spastic diplegia'. Approximately 50% of people participating in Paralympic sports with cerebral palsy will do so in a wheelchair, with the others being ambulant.

Cerebral palsy is also commonly associated with a variety of other problems as well as movement impairment. These include epilepsy, visual defects, deafness and intellectual impairment, and they can occur in combination.

Muscle spasticity presents a variety of problems. It may cause discomfort and poor posture that may predispose the athlete to other injuries. We note that spasticity may provide joint stabilization and excessive stretching of these muscles may inhibit performance, particularly in the ambulant athlete who uses the tone in function. Thus, although flexibility exercises are performed to maintain range of motion in joints, the timing of this relative to competition needs to be reviewed with each individual athlete.

The sportsperson with visual impairment

Visually impaired athletes can take part in a variety of sports with different degrees of adaptation of the sport. For example, in judo, the competitors start by holding on to each other's tunic. In athletics, a guide runner will run alongside the visually impaired athlete, sometimes attached by a cord or leash. Some sports such as goalball have been developed specifically for the visually impaired. This court-based sport has a large goal and is played with a ball with a bell. Players on one side hurl the ball towards the opponent's goal and the opponents hear where the ball is going and try to block it entering their goal. In swimming, a method is used to indicate to the swimmers when they are approaching the end of the lane to initiate a turn or to finish and this is achieved by tapping them on the head or shoulders as they approach the end using a long stick with a padded end.

Athletes are classified by an accredited ophthalmologist according to three levels of visual impairment: B1, B2 or B3.

1. B1: athletes have either a total absence of perception of light in both eyes or some perception of light but are unable to recognize the form of a hand at any distance and in any direction
2. B2: athletes have the ability to recognize the form of a hand to a visual acuity of 2/60 and/or a visual field of less than 5°
3. B3: athletes have a visual acuity of above 2/60 to a visual acuity of 6/60 and/or a visual field of more than 5° and less than 20°.

Visual impairment may result in alterations in gait that may cause overuse injuries. Athletes with a visual impairment are also subject to collisions and falls.

The sportsperson classified as 'Les Autres'

This group of athletes consists of people with physical impairments that do not fit into any other particular physical disability category. Numerous rare syndromic conditions cause physical restrictions and, as is common with syndromic conditions, there may be a variety of concurrent medical problems other than the physical limitation. It is important that the clinician serving any of these athletes be familiar with the other aspects of the condition. For example, Stickler syndrome affects collagen synthesis and is a congenital condition associated with myopia, retinal detachment, cataracts and glaucoma. The athlete, therefore, may be competing in a visually impaired category but the collagen abnormality will result in hypermobility of joints, poor healing and the risk of early onset of osteoarthritis.

Athletes with an intellectual disability may also have coexisting medical conditions depending on the cause of the impairment. For example, following head injury there may be epilepsy, or there may be heart disease in a person with Down syndrome. As with any care of any sporting team, a key component is preparation and the clinician should ensure that adequate medical records or information regarding athletes' past medical history is available.

Classification

The traditional system of classification for physical disabilities was based on a medical model. There is now an increasing push away from purely medical criteria towards functional performance and sport-specific testing.

The medical model classified athletes by their disability. For example, athletes with a similar level of spinal cord injury were grouped and would compete against each other; this resulted in multiple races within each event (e.g. 100 m sprint). Then some sports started to move to a more functional classification so that athletes of different disability groups were classified according to factors such as muscle strength, range of motion and proprioception and also dynamically by sport performance. For example, a single race may contain competitors with paraplegia, cerebral palsy and multiple limb deficiencies. This approach has led to improved competition, fewer classes, and improved public understanding of the sports.

Some sports (e.g. basketball) use a system to encourage athletes with different levels of disability to play together. This means that people with tetraplegia, paraplegia or an amputation can play together as a team. It uses a points system where athletes are awarded points according to their degree of disability, with eight classes from 1 point going up in half points to 4.5 points; a higher classification number represents a greater ability to perform basketball-specific skills. The coach is only allowed players who contribute a maximum of 14 points on the court at any one time. The classification includes sport-specific tests such as shooting, passing, pushing and dribbling rather than any medical examination of muscle function. This allows on-court assessment during practise and competition to verify the players' capability. The process of classification is evolving in all sports to seek the fairest and most sport-specific way to classify for each individual sport.

Athletes with an intellectual impairment have been included at the elite level of competition since 1989 but verification of the classification has proven challenging. The Sydney 2000 Paralympics included events for athletes with an intellectual disability and the Spanish team won the gold medal. It was later discovered, however, that 10 of the 12 players had no learning difficulties. The team was stripped of its title and the scandal led to the IPC scrapping the 'athletes with an intellectual disability' category on the grounds that athlete eligibility was too difficult. New criteria for intellectual disability have been adopted and it is hoped that this new classification system will again allow athletes with intellectual disability to participate in the Paralympic Games.

To qualify as intellectually impaired, an athlete must:

1. have significant impairment of intellectual functioning as indicated by a full scale score of 75 or lower on an internationally recognized and professionally administered IQ test
2. show significant limitations in adapted behavior as expressed in conceptual, social and practical adapted skills—this includes communication difficulties, problems with self-care and social and interpersonal skills; the limitations in adapted behavior can be established with the use of standardized measures that have been referenced against the general population
3. have had evidence of intellectual disability during the developmental period—from conception to age 18 years.

These requirements are necessary for athletes undertaking elite sport and not for the Special Olympics.

A practical implication for the sports clinician working with the intellectually disabled is that consent to medical treatment should be agreed with the guardian or parent.

Adapting performance testing and training for disabled athletes

Within able-bodied sport, there are well-established physiological profiles and scientific literature on the performance capability of athletes. Within disability sport, research has been limited.[18] A challenge in disabled sport is that physiological responses to exercise vary in different athletes. For example, heart rate response differs between paraplegic and quadriplegic athletes because the maximal heart rate is restricted in the quadriplegic athlete.[19, 20] People with cerebral palsy have different capacities to clear lactate because of hypertonia.

The base of knowledge within disability sport has traditionally come from the rehabilitation or exercise therapy setting rather than from performance and so the base of knowledge focuses on this aspect rather than on elite sport performance. There has also been limited exposure to good-quality coaching. All these factors lead to difficulties in performance profiling.

Methods of assessment of fitness also need to be different. Arm crank ergometry has been used for wheelchair users but is not specific to the normal action used in propelling a wheelchair. Wheelchair-usable treadmills and roller systems are available for assessing aerobic capacity. Wheelchair propulsion is akin to cycling and running and so Vo_{2max} peak measures are usually expressed as liters per minute. Modifications to field tests that serve athletes with a disability include a multistaged 'shuttle' fitness test adapted to and performed around an octagonal circuit to avoid the abrupt forwards and backwards turning that would be required in a regular 'shuttle' run.[21]

The standard principles of strength training need to be adapted according to the disability. The wheelchair user may be unable to stabilize the trunk to perform the action, or the equipment needs to be adapted to allow the exercise to take place. Although there has been concern that athletes with cerebral palsy may suffer increased muscle tone effects from strength training, there seems to be little evidence for this in practise. The standard principles of biomechanics also need to be re-examined where, for example, stroke technique in swimming, symmetry of running,[22] or javelin throwing techniques must be re-evaluated in the light of the disability. Efforts can be made to improve streamlining in the water or to improve range of motion in a joint, for example, but normal models of 'correct technique' may have to be re-evaluated.

Winter sports and common injuries

Winter sports exist in a variety of disciplines for people with disabilities and participation can include the competitive Paralympic level (Table 43.1). The Alpine events can be for the visually impaired, spinally injured or the limb-deficient athlete. Guide skiers are used for the visually impaired and a sitting monoski is used for paraplegic athletes.

Standing athletes are at risk of the usual skiing injuries (e.g. head injury or ACL rupture). In the sitting classes, small outriggers are used with a ski on the end to control the ski so forceful impact landing on the outrigger can cause wrist fracture or shoulder injury. The cross-country events are associated with overuse injuries and the sit-skier may suffer shoulder and elbow problems. Biathlon (skiing and shooting) can be performed by the visually impaired using a sighting mechanism that utilizes an audible signal with increasing tone as the competitor points towards the center of the target.

Sledge hockey is an adapted form of ice hockey. Competitors sit on the sledge and skate by pushing two sticks, which are also used to strike the puck. A variety of disability groups participate in this sport as there are only minimal disability entry criteria. Injuries occur by direct contact between players, use of the stick (intentionally or accidentally) or by being hit by the puck. As mentioned above, athletes with spinal cord injury-induced low bone mass are susceptible to fracture in this sport. Wheelchair curling was introduced to the Paralympic Winter Games in Torino in 2006 and caused few injuries.

Anti-doping issues

The IOC is a signatory to the World Anti-Doping Code (Chapter 61). The list of prohibited substances is the same for Paralympic athletes as for able-bodied athletes. Because of the nature of athletes' disabilities, it is more likely that they may need to take medications on the prohibited list to manage medical conditions. To do this, they must complete a therapeutic use exemption (TUE) application process that is outlined in Chapter 61. A successful application has to meet the same criteria as for able-bodied athletes:

1. that the athlete would experience a significant impairment to health if the prohibited substance or method was to be withheld in the course of treating an acute or chronic medical condition
2. that the therapeutic use of the prohibited substance would not produce additional enhancement of performance other than that which might be anticipated by a return to a state of normal health
3. that there are no reasonable therapeutic alternatives to the use of the prohibited substance or method
4. that the necessity for the use of the prohibited substance or method is not as a consequence of prior non-therapeutic use of the prohibited substance.

There are some differences to the sample collection process which will vary according to the disability. Athletes who use intermittent catheterization are permitted to use their own catheter to collect the urine sample. For athletes who use a condom and leg bag drainage system, the contents of the leg bag must first be emptied, and a fresh sample of urine collected. This is to avoid the potential for inserting a 'clean' sample of urine into the leg bag prior to competition.

Athletes who are visually impaired receive help to complete forms and are supervised by their own observer in the sample collection process. The athlete's representative observes the Doping Control Officer during the sample collection process to ensure that there is no tampering of the sample during the collection process. Athletes with an intellectual disability need to be accompanied by a representative who understands the process.

Disability sport does not appear to be rife with the abuse of prohibited substances. However, as in able-bodied sport, power lifting has been tainted by anabolic steroid use. Understandably, there have been claims of inadvertent use of diuretics or beta-blockers to treat hypertension. It is challenging for athletes to be aware of the anti-doping restrictions on medication used to manage their medical conditions; this population requires particularly skilled sports medicine care.

Travel with teams

Although Chapter 59 is devoted to travel with teams, athletes with disability have specific needs. Firstly, the simple logistics of boarding a team of wheelchair users on and off an aircraft takes additional time and may require lifting and handling. Toileting on board aircraft using a small-wheeled aisle chair is difficult and is likely to decrease the fluid intake of wheelchair users, leading to dehydration. Transportation at the destination needs to be accessible so the team clinician should aim to be familiar with the accessibility of toilets, rooms and sports facilities in advance if at all possible.

Prolonged sitting without the use of the normal pressure cushion may result in pressure areas on the skin. Athletes should try to take pressure-relieving measures during the journey and check pressure areas on arrival. The risk of deep venous thrombosis exists for all long-haul passengers but there are no data to suggest that athletes with disabilities are any more prone to this than those with comparable medical problems. After such trips, dependent edema can be a particular problem among individuals who do not have the capacity to use the active muscle pump. Compression stockings can be appropriate.

Recommended Reading

Dodd KJ, Taylor NF, Damiano DL. A systematic review of the effectiveness of strength-training programs for people with cerebral palsy. *Arch Phys Med Rehabil* 2002; 83(8): 1157–64.

Myslinski MJ. Evidence-based exercise prescription for individuals with spinal cord injury. *J Neurol Phys Ther* 2005; 29(2): 104–6.

Nash MS. Exercise as a health-promoting activity following spinal cord injury. *J Neurol Phys Ther* 2005; 29(2): 87–103, 106.

Webborn AD. 'Boosting' performance in disability sport. *Br J Sports Med* 1999; 33(2): 74–5.

Webborn N, Price MJ, Castle PC, Goosey-Tolfrey VL. Effects of two cooling strategies on thermoregulatory responses of tetraplegic athletes during repeated intermittent exercise in the heat. *J Appl Physiol* 2005; 98(6): 2101–7.

Recommended Website

The website of the International Classification of Functioning, Disability and Health provides the World Health Organization policy that relates to disability and health: <http://www3.who.int/icf/icftemplate.cfm>

References

1. Booth FW, Gordon SE, Carlson CJ, Hamilton MT. Waging war on modern chronic diseases: primary prevention through exercise biology. *J Appl Physiol* 2000; 88(2): 774–87.

2. Bertoli S, Battezzati A, Merati G, et al. Nutritional status and dietary patterns in disabled people. *Nutr Metab Cardiovasc Dis* 2006; 16(2): 100–12.

3. Schmid A, Schmidt-Trucksass A, Huonker M, et al. Catecholamines response of high performance wheelchair athletes at rest and during exercise with autonomic dysreflexia. *Int J Sports Med* 2001; 22(1): 2–7.

4. Dela F, Mohr T, Jensen CM, et al. Cardiovascular control during exercise: insights from spinal cord-injured humans. *Circulation* 2003; 107(16): 2127–33.

5. Hopman MT, Houtman S, Groothuis JT, Folgering HT. The effect of varied fractional inspired oxygen on arm exercise performance in spinal cord injury and able-bodied persons. *Arch Phys Med Rehabil* 2004; 85(2): 319–23.

6. Jacobs PL, Nash MS. Exercise recommendations for individuals with spinal cord injury. *Sports Med* 2004; 34(11): 727–51.

7. Nash MS. Exercise as a health-promoting activity following spinal cord injury. *J Neurol Phys Ther* 2005; 29(2): 87–103, 106.

8. Myslinski MJ. Evidence-based exercise prescription for individuals with spinal cord injury. *J Neurol Phys Ther* 2005; 29(2): 104–6.

9. Wheeler GD, Andrews B, Lederer R, et al. Functional electric stimulation-assisted rowing: increasing cardiovascular fitness through functional electric stimulation rowing training in persons with spinal cord injury. *Arch Phys Med Rehabil* 2002; 83(8): 1093–9.

10. Halliday SE, Zavatsky AB, Hase K. Can functional electric stimulation-assisted rowing reproduce a race-winning rowing stroke? *Arch Phys Med Rehabil* 2004; 85(8): 1265–72.

11. Shields RK, Dudley-Javoroski S, Law LA. Electrically induced muscle contractions influence bone density decline after spinal cord injury. *Spine* 2006; 31(5): 548–53.

12. Giangregorio LM, Craven BC, Webber CE. Musculoskeletal changes in women with spinal cord injury: a twin study. *J Clin Densitom* 2005; 8(3): 347–51.

13. de Groot PC, Hjeltnes N, Heijboer AC, Stal W, Birkeland K. Effect of training intensity on physical capacity, lipid profile and insulin sensitivity in early rehabilitation of spinal cord injured individuals. *Spinal Cord* 2003; 41(12): 673–9.

14. Webborn AD. Heat-related problems for the Paralympic Games, Atlanta. *Br J Ther Rehabil* 1996; 3: 429–36.

15. Webborn N, Price MJ, Castle PC, Goosey-Tolfrey VL. Effects of two cooling strategies on thermoregulatory responses of tetraplegic athletes during repeated intermittent exercise in the heat. *J Appl Physiol* 2005; 98(6): 2101–7.

16. Webborn AD. 'Boosting' performance in disability sport. *Br J Sports Med* 1999; 33(2): 74–5.

17. Agarwal S, Triolo RJ, Kobetic R, et al. Long-term user perceptions of an implanted neuroprosthesis for exercise, standing, and transfers after spinal cord injury. *J Rehabil Res Dev* 2003; 40(3): 241–52.

18. Tasiemski T, Bergstrom E, Savic G, Gardner BP. Sports, recreation and employment following spinal cord injury—a pilot study. *Spinal Cord* 2000; 38(3): 173–84.

19. Bhambhani Y. Physiology of wheelchair racing in athletes with spinal cord injury. *Sports Med* 2002; 32(1): 23–51.

20. van der Woude LH, Bouten C, Veeger HE, Gwinn T. Aerobic work capacity in elite wheelchair athletes: a cross-sectional analysis. *Am J Phys Med Rehabil* 2002; 81(4): 261–71.

21. Vanderthommen M, Francaux M, Colinet C, et al. A multistage field test of wheelchair users for evaluation of fitness and prediction of peak oxygen consumption. *J Rehabil Res Dev* 2002; 39(6): 685–92.

22. Burkett B, Smeathers J, Barker T. Walking and running inter-limb asymmetry for Paralympic trans-femoral amputees: a biomechanical analysis. *Prosthet Orthot Int* 2003; 27(1): 36–47.

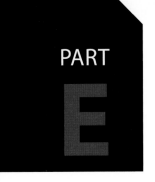

PART E

Management of Medical Problems

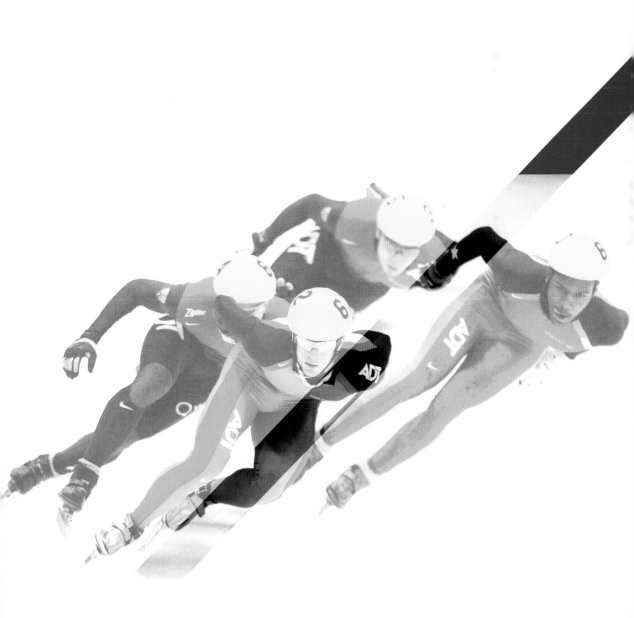

Sport and Exercise-Associated Emergencies: On-Site Management

WITH GARTH HUNTE

Life- or limb-threatening sport and exercise-associated emergencies require rapid assessment, intervention and transportation to definitive care. Hence, although such events are uncommon, the sports medicine practitioner must be prepared. It is incumbent on any on-site provider to anticipate, train and rehearse for these emergencies. Principles of management include:

- a team approach
- advance preparation
- rapid assessment
- timely life- and limb-saving interventions
- early transportation to an appropriate level medical facility
- regular reassessment.

We aim to help the sports medicine practitioner prepare for on-site management of emergencies. This chapter reviews the sideline or field management of sport and exercise-associated emergencies and summarizes the sequence of priorities to be followed when assessing and treating a severely ill or injured athlete. The emphasis is on trauma, but other threats to life and limb, including anaphylaxis, are also briefly reviewed.

Preparation

Successful initial management of sport and exercise-associated emergencies requires anticipation and thorough preparation. Preparation includes personnel, training and equipment consistent with the potential severity of illness and injury associated with the sport or activity, the environment and the participant population. For example, on-site coverage of high-velocity and contact or collision sports will

require preparation for potentially severe traumatic injuries, whereas coverage of citizen endurance events will require preparation for exercise-associated collapse, including thermal injury and sudden cardiac arrest.

Personnel and training

The minimum requirement should be the presence at all sporting events of someone with formal first-aid and cardiopulmonary resuscitation (CPR) training. Everyone should learn first aid and CPR, and coaches, parents and competitors should be encouraged to receive appropriate training. First aid, however, should not delay activation of local emergency medical services (EMS) or other medical assistance when required. Brief, accurate and organized communication with EMS should be initiated early, and a working mobile phone or radio communication with local emergency contacts should be available on-site. Advance contact with local EMS providers or hospital emergency departments is prudent if the nature of the activity or the size of the population involved increases the likelihood of a life- or limb-threatening event.

The initial responders to an emergency should be comfortable with primary airway management, manual in-line stabilization of the cervical spine, hemorrhage control and CPR. Additional training, such as lifesaving, industrial or wilderness first aid, or pre-hospital trauma life support would be advantageous. One practitioner, preferably a physician trained in sports medicine, emergency medicine, and/or advanced cardiac and trauma life support (ACLS/ATLS), should be identified as the leader of the team in advance of the event.

Standard protocols and communication pathways for such procedures as assessment and removal of an injured athlete from the field of play, assessment of the concussed or unconscious athlete, and assessment and protection of an athlete with possible spinal injury should be rehearsed with the team of providers before the start of the season and at regular intervals. This will help ensure that in a situation of true emergency each member of the team knows what to do.

Equipment

Specific equipment that is useful in sporting emergencies includes defibrillators, airway and ventilation adjuncts, spinal boards, and devices that aid immobilization of injured parts.

Universal precautions

Every practitioner must be protected against exposure to an injured athlete's blood or other body fluids. This requires a mask (for mouth-to-mask resuscitation, see below), eye protection and gloves.

Airway and ventilation adjuncts

A patent and protected conduit for gas exchange is the first priority. Oropharyngeal and/or naso-pharyngeal airway devices, a mouth-to-mask device, and a commercially prepared cricothyrotomy kit should be readily available. A 14-gauge catheter-over-needle device will allow for needle decompression of a tension pneumothorax or needle criocothyrotomy if high-pressure equipment for transtracheal jet ventilation is available. A supplemental oxygen supply with an adjustable flow rate, a bag-valve-mask

delivery system, and portable suction (Fig. 44.1) should also be accessible.

Automatic external defibrillator

Early defibrillation is the most important factor affecting survival in out-of-hospital cardiac arrest. Although automatic external defibrillators (AEDs) (Fig. 44.2) are easy to use and have become smaller and more affordable, the role of AEDs in the high school and university athletic setting is still evolving.[1] The most common reported causes of death in athletes less than 35 years of age with cardiac arrest include structural heart disease (e.g. hypertrophic cardiomyopathy) or commotio cordis, rather than coronary artery disease. Despite evidence of a public health benefit with AED placement in sporting venues and fitness or training facilities with a large population of participants or a local EMS call-to-shock interval of greater than 5 minutes, the role, efficacy and optimal placement of AEDs for resuscitation of young athletes has not been determined.

Spinal immobilization

Although there is insufficient evidence to support standards and guidelines for pre-hospital spinal

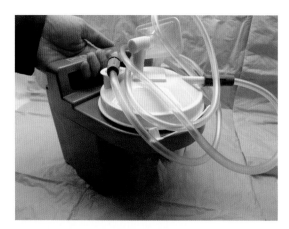

Figure 44.1 Portable suction device

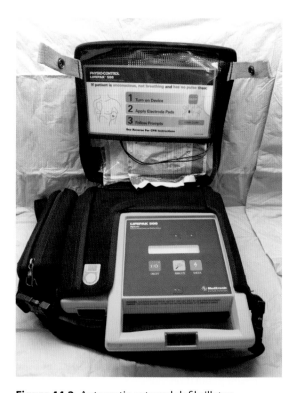

Figure 44.2 Automatic external defibrillator

immobilization following trauma, all trauma patients with evidence of a spinal column injury or a mechanism of injury with the potential to cause a spinal column injury should be immobilized at the scene and during transport. The combination of an appropriately sized or adjusted semi-rigid cervical collar and lateral support on a backboard with straps at the shoulders and pelvis is effective in limiting motion of the spine. Split-scoop stretchers permit spinal immobilization and transportation without log rolling or lifting, while use of a vacuum mattress will help reduce the discomfort of lying on a rigid backboard for a prolonged period of time. Pre-hospital clearance of a spinal injury is discussed below.

Splints

Appropriate splints and slings are necessary for emergency immobilization of fractures and/or dislocations of the extremities. Compression bandages, sterile gauze and saline are required to assist with control of bleeding and swelling and for initial wound care.

Medication

At a minimum, emergency drugs for the immediate treatment of anaphylaxis, hypoglycemia and asthma exacerbation should be available on-site. Adrenalin (epinephrine) pre-packaged in a 1:1000 dilution (e.g. EpiPen) is recommended for the initial management of anaphylaxis. Glucagon (1 mg given subcutaneously, intramuscularly or intravenously), oral glucose paste (50 g) or intravenous (IV) dextrose (D50) should be readily available to treat documented hypoglycemia in patients over 20 kg; for children under 20 kg or less than 12 years of age, the recommended dose is reduced by half. Glucagon can also be used for those patients with anaphylaxis who are taking a beta-blocker and do not respond to adrenalin (epinephrine). A short-acting beta-agonist with spacer device would be prudent to have on hand for treatment of acute asthma exacerbations. Other medications, such as aspirin (ASA), glyceryl trinitrate (nitroglycerin), ACLS drugs and intravenous fluids should be considered depending on the situation and population involved.

Other equipment

A glucose monitor is advised if any athlete is known to have diabetes or the population is unknown. Other equipment will depend on the specifics of the sport or activity. For example, a screwdriver should be on hand to help release helmets if facemasks are being worn. In situations where a thermal injury may occur, such as endurance events, a means of rapid cooling or warming should be available.

Approach to the acutely ill or injured athlete

Although discussed in sequence, assessment and resuscitation is ideally and most appropriately accomplished in parallel by a coordinated team. This approach requires advance preparation, appointment of a team leader, effective communication, and orchestration of roles and tasks. The kinetic energy generated in the forces and motion involved in high-velocity recreational activities and contact sports can produce significant injuries. Knowledge of injury mechanism and a rapid but complete physical examination will help ensure occult injuries are not overlooked. In particular, the speed of a projectile or victim, impact with stationary objects, the use of protective equipment, and information provided by witnesses should be sought. Blunt injuries of the abdomen or chest may only be suggested by history; likewise, high-velocity deceleration injuries should heighten suspicion for tears of the thoracic aorta or capsular tears of solid intra-abdominal organs. Some medications, such as steroids or beta-blockers, may alter the physiological response to injury and obscure typical physical findings. Some key diagnoses to consider in the sporting emergency are listed in Table 44.1.

In brief, the approach consists of the following:

1. Establishment of scene safety.
2. A rapid primary survey with resuscitation and immediate treatment of life- and limb-threatening problems.
3. A detailed secondary survey.
4. Initiation of definitive care based on the secondary survey.

Scene safety

The first priority is establishing scene safety. Threats to scene safety might include unstable environmental conditions, such as avalanche hazards or falling rock, water hazards, fire or electrical hazards and must be dealt with prior to approaching the patient.

Primary survey

Life- and limb-threatening problems are rapidly identified in the primary survey and resuscitation initiated in conjunction with the assessment. Care of the airway, cardiopulmonary resuscitation and other direct life- or limb-saving maneuvers, such as needle decompression of a tension pneumothorax, stabilization of a flail chest segment, or direct compression of an active hemorrhage, are performed as soon as the

Table 44.1 Causes of exercise-associated emergencies

Traumatic	Non-traumatic
Head injury	Cardiac
Severe	Coronary artery disease
Minor (Chapter 13)	Arrhythmia
Spinal cord injury	Congenital abnormality
Cervical	Hypertrophic
Thoracic	cardiomyopathy
Lumbar	Hyperthermia
Thoracic injury	Hypothermia
Flail chest	Cerebrovascular accident
Hemothorax	Hypoglycemia
Tension pneumothorax	Hyponatremia
Cardiac tamponade	Respiratory
Cardiac contusion	Asthma
Abdominal injury	Spontaneous
Ruptured viscus (e.g.	pneumothorax
liver, spleen, kidney,	Pulmonary embolism
bladder, pancreas,	Allergic anaphylaxis
bowel)	Drugs
Multiple fractures	Cocaine, morphine
(particularly femoral	Other
or pelvic fractures)	Vasovagal (fainting)
Blood loss	Postural hypotension
	Blood pooling post
	exercise
	Hyperventilation
	Hysteria

problem is identified. The time-honored and widely followed ABCDE protocol includes:

Airway maintenance with cervical spine (C-spine) control
Breathing
Circulation and hemorrhage control
Disability/drugs—assessment of neurological status
Expose the patient, but protect against hypothermia

The primary survey begins with a general impression of the athlete's overall condition. If the athlete is alert and talking in a normal voice, and has no complaint of neck pain or evidence of hemorrhage, the primary survey is complete. Failure to respond, or evidence of a major injury demands a rapid, efficient assessment and timely intervention, often while en route to an appropriate medical facility. The goal is to establish quickly if the athlete is presently or imminently in a critical condition, to decide early if additional resources are required, and to minimize scene time. Responders should call for help as soon as they are aware that the athlete has a life- or limb-threatening condition.

Airway with cervical spine protection

The airway is the first priority. A patent and protected conduit for gas exchange must be maintained for oxygenation and ventilation. A quick assessment is made by looking for chest wall motion and listening and feeling for air movement at the mouth. Clearing foreign debris or teeth with suction, a finger sweep and/or lifting the mandible with a jaw thrust may be required to establish patency. Manual in-line stabilization of the neck should be initiated during opening of the airway to protect the athlete's spine from unnecessary movement.

The jaw thrust maneuver is performed by grasping the angles of the jaw (one hand on each side) and displacing the mandible forward (Fig. 44.3). Since the jaw thrust maneuver does not hyperextend the neck, it is the method of choice for a trauma victim with a potential cervical spine injury.

Airway adjuncts

Inability to open or maintain airway patency requires an attempt with an oropharyngeal or nasopharyngeal airway. An oral airway should only be used if the athlete is unconscious and the gag reflex is absent. It is inserted into the mouth behind the tongue and can be facilitated by using a tongue blade. An alternative technique is to insert the oral airway in the upside down position with its concavity upwards. When the soft palate is encountered the airway is rotated 180° and slipped over the tongue. Care must be taken not to push the tongue backwards and thereby block, rather than clear, the airway.

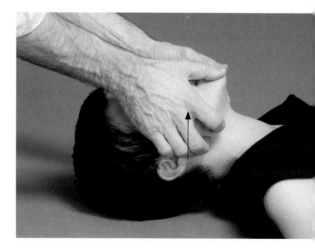

Figure 44.3 Jaw thrust maneuver to open the airway of an individual with a suspected cervical spine injury

A nasal airway is pliable tube that is often tolerated in patients with an intact gag reflex. Passage of a nasal airway will be made easier by lubricating the tip and inserting it into the most patent nostril, parallel to the palate, and with a gentle rotation. This simple device allows air to bypass upper airway obstruction caused by the tongue and/or decreased pharyngeal muscle tone, but may cause hemorrhage from the nasal passage.

Should efforts to obtain a patent airway continue without success using these airway adjuncts, then advanced airway interventions, such as appropriate placement of an endotracheal tube, esophageal tracheal Combitube (Fig. 44.4) or laryngeal mask airway should be attempted as soon as possible. It behooves the sports medicine provider to undertake training and practice with one of these advanced techniques and to become comfortable with their use. Training courses such as ACLS, ATLS or The Difficult Airway Course are examples of curricula that cover advanced airway techniques. Additional resources should be accessed early when the situation exceeds the capabilities of the local providers. If trained personnel or equipment for an advance airway are lacking, or an attempted trial is unsuccessful, then a surgical airway will be necessary (see below).

Advanced airway management

Conditions that demand advanced airway management prior to the onset of frank compromise of the airway or gas exchange include severe head injury (Glasgow Coma Scale <8 [see Table 44.2]), injuries associated with potential airway obstruction such as penetrating neck trauma, upper airway burns and anaphylaxis with upper airway edema, thoracic injuries with ventilatory compromise, inability to establish or protect the airway, and respiratory failure or arrest. Early, definitive airway management with endotracheal intubation is preferred. Failure to act early with neck trauma, burns or edema may lead to complete upper airway obstruction. Advanced airway management should not delay transport and should be accomplished en route to hospital if possible.

Endotracheal intubation

Endotracheal intubation allows for protection of a patent airway and gives access for positive pressure ventilation and pulmonary toilet. Successful, atraumatic endotracheal intubation requires training, experience and regular practise. It is incumbent on anyone undertaking intubation of a patient to have assessed for and be prepared for a difficult airway, and to have a well thought out plan for the potential 'can't

intubate, can't ventilate' scenario. The head should be maintained in a neutral position with in-line immobilization applied by an assistant. The method of choice is the method the provider is most comfortable and competent with and can accomplish in a timely fashion. In previous years, blind nasotracheal intubation was advocated, however, this technique has a significant complication rate, is contraindicated in maxillofacial trauma, and should only be considered in special circumstances, particularly when oral access is limited (e.g. angioedema). Orotracheal intubation with in-line immobilization and rapid sequence induction is now the modality of choice.

Attempts at endotracheal intubation without adequate training, experience and preparation in a patient who is obtunded, combative and potentially head injured are to be avoided. Traumatic attempts at endotracheal intubation without appropriate pharmacological preparation increase intracranial pressure, stress the cardiovascular system, can injure the upper airway, can induce laryngospasm or aspiration of the stomach contents, and unnecessarily place the patient at risk. An intubation attempt is optimized by:

1. utilizing oximetric, cardiac and blood pressure monitoring
2. providing pre-oxygenation with four vital capacity breaths
3. having immediate access to working suction
4. confirming the laryngoscope has a working bulb and an appropriately sized blade
5. the use of appropriate pre-medications when indicated (e.g. fentanyl)
6. allowing time for pre-treatment medications to work
7. patient positioning (sniffing position if no cervical spine injury)
8. performing a rapid sequence induction with an induction agent, cricoid pressure and a short-acting neuromuscular blocking agent (e.g. suxamethonium [succinylcholine])
9. intubating under controlled conditions.

If a difficult airway is anticipated, then neuromuscular blocking agents and excessive sedation should be avoided unless the glottis has been visualized on an awake laryngoscopy using titrated light sedation and topical anesthesia. The potential for converting a suboptimal airway into no airway must be considered whenever neuromuscular blocking agents are utilized. However, deep sedation without a neuromuscular blocking agent should also be avoided as it offers suboptimal intubating conditions and has neither the success nor low complication rate of either a properly performed rapid sequence induction or an awake intubation.

An appropriately sized endotracheal tube should be selected and another endotracheal tube one-half to one full size smaller should be available. The endotracheal tube should not be forced, and care should be taken to avoid main-stem bronchial intubation. Confirmation of tube placement should be obtained by visualizing the vocal cords, auscultating over the apices and stomach, and monitoring or detecting end-tidal carbon dioxide. Once correct placement is confirmed, the endotracheal tube should be secured. Constant vigilance and continual reassessment is essential as the endotracheal tube may become displaced, kinked or obstructed with secretions.

Other devices including surgical airway

Options for the 'can't intubate, can't ventilate' scenario include a laryngeal mask airway, an esophageal tracheal Combitube (Fig. 44.4), retrograde intubation, transtracheal jet ventilation or a surgical airway (see below).

Inability to secure the airway by other means is the primary indication for a surgical airway. Blunt or penetrating neck trauma can make endotracheal intubation impossible due to edema of the glottis, a fractured larynx or crushing injury of the trachea (e.g. a hard-struck hockey puck strikes the neck), severe oropharyngeal or neck hemorrhage or laryngeal spasm. Cricothyrotomy or needle cricothyrotomy are preferred.

Surgical cricothyrotomy is performed by making a vertical or skin incision with a number 10 blade and extending the incision down to the cricothyroid membrane. The skin edges are then retracted and the cricothyroid membrane is incised transversely. The handle of the scalpel is then inserted and turned vertically to hold the membrane open while a hemostat is inserted on either side of the blade to gently enlarge the hole. The scalpel is then removed and a small tracheostomy tube is inserted. This technique is rapid, safe, relatively bloodless and relatively easy.

Percutaneous needle cricothyrotomy is indicated in children under the age of 12 because the cricoid cartilage provides the only circumferential support to the upper trachea in this age group. A 14-gauge catheter-over-needle is inserted into the trachea through the cricothyroid membrane, and the cannula connected to a high-flow oxygen source via a Y-connector. Intermittent ventilation may be achieved using a rhythm of 1 second on and 4 seconds off by placing the thumb over the open end of the Y-connector. The advantage of this maneuver is that it can provide adequate oxygenation for 30–45 minutes. The disadvantage of this procedure is that although some exhalation will occur, it is insufficient for complete ventilation: carbon dioxide will accumulate leading to a respiratory acidosis. Note that a 3 mL syringe fits a size 7 endotracheal tube adaptor and this can be connected to a 14-gauge needle to create an emergency cricothyrotomy kit.

A third option uses the percutaneous (Seldinger) technique to combine the needle cricothyrotomy approach with the insertion of a cuffed or uncuffed cricothyrostomy tube. A catheter-over-needle is introduced through the cricothyroid membrane until air is aspirated, and then the needle removed, leaving the catheter in place. A guide wire is then passed through the catheter, the catheter removed over the wire, and a dilator device with a cuffed or uncuffed tube passed over the wire through the cricothyroid membrane (Fig. 44.5). The dilator is then removed and the cricothyrostomy tube is left in the trachea. This

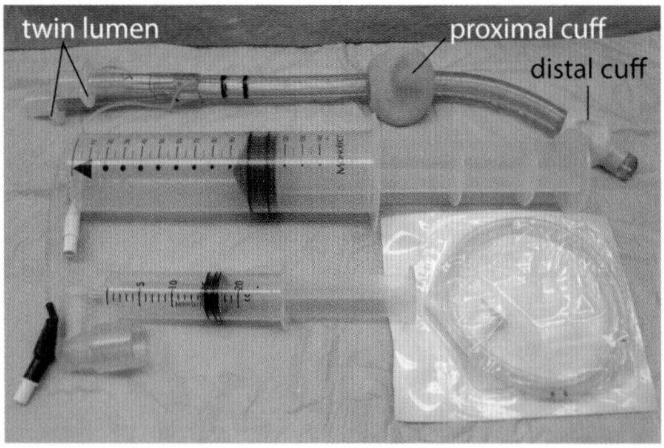

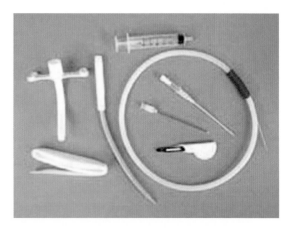

Figure 44.4 Esophageal tracheal Combitube—a twin lumen device for difficult airways

Figure 44.5 Cook Melker cricothyrotomy kit

Anaphylaxis

Reduced peripheral perfusion in anaphylaxis results from a widespread increase in vascular permeability and cardiovascular collapse secondary to an acute, abnormal systemic response. Early, definitive airway management, fluid resuscitation and pharmacological therapy comprise the initial approach. As previously noted, pre-emptive airway management can be lifesaving. Adrenalin (epinephrine) is the primary drug treatment of anaphylactic reactions and should be given as soon as anaphylaxis is recognized. An intramuscular (IM) injection of 0.3–0.5 mg (1:1000) should be given early to all patients with signs of a systemic reaction, particularly hypotension, airway swelling or difficulty breathing. Glucagon 1 mg IM can be given to patients who are unresponsive to adrenalin (epinephrine).

option provides the advantages of both techniques with few complications.

Breathing

Injuries to the chest may prevent adequate oxygenation and ventilation even in the presence of a patent airway. The patient's chest should be completely exposed to be sure that ventilation is adequate and symmetric. If there is no spontaneous breathing, the athlete needs to be artificially ventilated. This may be achieved by mouth-to-mask respiration, or by using a bag and mask device depending on availability and experience. It is advisable for practitioners to carry a mask. Supplemental oxygen should also be administered at high flow rates (10 L/min) if available. The trachea should be palpated for deviation and the presence of subcutaneous emphysema. Four life-threatening conditions—tension pneumothorax, open pneumothorax, flail segment and cardiac tamponade—should be systematically identified or excluded. Tension pneumothorax is relieved by inserting a 14-gauge intravenous catheter-over-needle through the second intercostal space at the mid-clavicular line on the affected side. Needle decompression, covering a sucking wound and stabilizing a flail segment will temporarily stabilize the patient until more definitive interventions are possible. A chest tube can be inserted later, depending on local resources and expertise. For prolonged trips and air transport it may be appropriate to secure chest decompression prior to transporting.

Circulation and hemorrhage control

Adequacy of circulation is best obtained initially by assessing skin color and capillary refill, and palpating the peripheral pulses for presence, strength and rate. In a normovolemic patient, capillary refill should occur within 2 seconds (the time it takes to say 'capillary refill'). Blood pressure measurement is unnecessarily time consuming and often inappropriately reassuring. As a rough guide, a palpable pulse is associated with the following minimum systolic pressures: radial, 80 mmHg; femoral, 70 mmHg; and carotid, 50 mmHg. Obvious blood loss should be identified and controlled with direct pressure. Tourniquets, hemostats and pneumatic splints are generally to be avoided because of their potential for tissue injury, negative effects on cellular metabolism and frequent inability to control bleeding. Redundant intravenous access should be established using two large-bore intravenous catheters (18 gauge or larger). However, intravenous access must not delay transport to a surgical facility and is often better established en route.

Cardiopulmonary resuscitation

Any traumatic injury or spontaneous collapse resulting in loss of consciousness requires a rapid primary assessment of the ABCs. If the airway is patent but spontaneous breathing is absent and a pulse cannot be felt, then CPR should be initiated without delay. Responders are encouraged to push hard, push fast, allow complete chest recoil after compression, and to minimize interruptions in chest compressions. For the victim with sudden collapse the lone responder should first call for help and an AED and then begin CPR using a cycle of 30 compressions to two respirations. The AED should be used when available to deliver a single shock before resuming CPR. Five cycles of CPR should be completed before the next shock is applied. If two responders are present and an advanced airway device is in place, then compressions should be delivered at 100 per minute without breaks for ventilation, while ventilation should be delivered at eight to 10 breaths per minute.[2] Updated guidelines for cardiac arrest are available in the 2005 American Heart Association Guidelines for CPR and Emergency Cardiovascular Care (available online at <www.americanheart.org>).

Disability (brief neurological examination)

A rapid neurological assessment is performed towards the end of the primary survey in order to assess whether the athlete is alert, responds to verbal stimulus, responds to painful stimulus, or is unconscious.

The simple mnemonic AVPU can be used to guide the assessment:

A alert
V responds to vocal stimuli
P responds to painful stimuli
U unresponsive

However, the Glasgow Coma Scale (GCS) is preferred for communication with others and should be documented (Table 44.2).

The presence of an asymmetrically enlarged pupil in a patient with a GCS less than 15 may represent an intracranial mass effect and should be managed by ensuring adequate oxygenation and ventilation during urgent transfer to a hospital with neurosurgical facilities. Definite capture of the airway with endotracheal intubation should be established en route in any patient with centrally caused focal or progressive neurological impairment, particularly those with a GCS less than 8. Motor function, pain response, deep tendon and plantar reflexes should be assessed and communicated to the emergency department at the destination as needed.

The box below lists the conditions that require urgent referral of the patient to a hospital with neurosurgical capabilities for further assessment.

> ## Indications for urgent referral of an injured athlete to a neurosurgical hospital for assessment
>
> - Prolonged loss of consciousness (more than 5 minutes)
> - Development of increasing headache, nausea and vomiting
> - Unequal pupils
> - Gradual increase in blood pressure or decrease in pulse rate
> - Convulsion
> - Changing neurological signs (changing signs means changing pathology)

If the primary survey suggests a possible spinal injury

Any unconscious athlete or any athlete who complains of numbness, weakness, paralysis or neck pain should be assumed to have cervical spine injury until proven otherwise.

Immobilization is best managed with the patient in the supine position on a firm, flat surface with the head and neck maintained in a neutral position by cervical in-line immobilization. If the athlete is wearing thick padding (e.g. American football, ice hockey), the neck will need to be supported to keep it in a neutral position relative to the padded body. If the patient has a suspected spinal injury, the helmet can remain in place during transport and removed in the controlled setting of an emergency department. The athlete should not be transported from the field of play until the ABCs and the spine have been stabilized.

The athlete with a seizure

The athlete who is having a seizure should be protected from further injury and placed in the recovery position. The ABCs should be assessed and stabilized. The cervical spine should be protected if the seizure is unwitnessed or occurs following trauma. First-time seizures and prolonged seizures require emergency evaluation.

Exposure during the primary survey

All clothing should be removed to allow for a careful examination and assessment of the entire patient, being careful to maintain core temperature by providing warm blankets or warming lights.

At completion of the primary survey a decision should be made regarding level of care required. Timely transport should be initiated and unnecessary delays avoided. A philosophy of 'load and go' is preferable if definitive surgical care is nearby. Prolonged transport, however, will dictate more extensive field resuscitation and stabilization in order to establish a secure airway, redundant large-bore vascular access,

Table 44.2 Glasgow Coma Scale

Eye opening (E)	Verbal response (V)	Motor response (M)
4 = spontaneous	5 = normal conversation	6 = normal
3 = to voice	4 = disoriented conversation	5 = localizes to pain
2 = to pain	3 = incoherent words	4 = withdraws to pain
1 = none	2 = no words, only sounds	3 = decorticate posture
	1 = none	2 = decerebrate posture
		1 = none

Total = E + V + M.

and chest decompression if required. These procedures are generally easier to perform prior to departure as limited space in either ground or air transport vehicles makes them that much more challenging. Constant vigilance for a change in the patient's status allows for early and potentially lifesaving intervention. The ABCs should be continually reassessed following any intervention or change in status. Remaining alert, anticipating problems and being prepared for rapid surgical intervention will offer the trauma victim the greatest chance of recovery.

Secondary survey

The secondary survey involves examination of the entire body from the top of the patient's head to the feet. The examination may be divided into anatomical regions or physiological systems, depending on the preference of the examiner, but must include a thorough assessment of the head and neck, including the eyes, ears, nose and mouth, the chest and abdomen, including the rectum and pelvis, the spine and extremities, and a neurological evaluation. A focused history and understanding of the mechanism of injury will help guide the search for associated injuries and comorbid complications that may not be apparent initially.

Head

The eyes should be re-evaluated for pupillary size, extraocular movements and visual fields. The fundi should also be assessed for hemorrhages, the lens for dislocation, the anterior chamber for blood, and the globe for evidence of a penetrating injury. The scalp, ear canal and tympanic membrane should be examined for evidence of bruising, blood or fluid.

Spine

The NEXUS low-risk criteria[3] (Table 44.3) and the Canadian C-spine rule[4] (Fig. 44.6) are sufficiently sensitive in the alert, stable, blunt-trauma patient without neurological deficit to assist the provider in determining which athlete does not require radiographic cervical spine assessment. However, in any other circumstance, adequate assessment of the cervical spine cannot be provided by physical examination alone. The patient's head and neck should be immobilized with manual in-line stabilization until an appropriately fitting semi-rigid collar with secure lateral support can be applied. The spine should be immobilized until an adequate radiographic and clinical assessment can be made. Log rolling of the patient to assess the back and thoracic and lumbar

Table 44.3 NEXUS low-risk criteria

The National Emergency X-Radiography Utilization Study Group (NEXUS) low-risk criteria[3]

- No midline cervical tenderness
- No focal neurological deficit
- Normal alertness
- No intoxication
- No painful, distracting injury

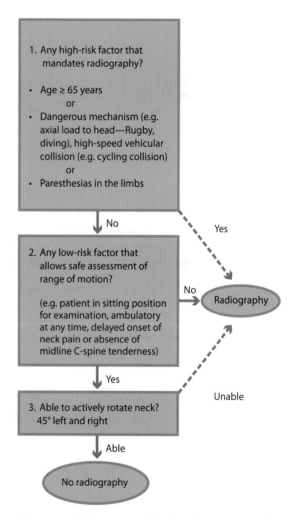

Figure 44.6 Adaptation of the Canadian C-spine rule for radiography for alert and stable trauma patients who may have suffered cervical spine injury in a sporting event

FROM STIELL IG, WELLS GA, VANDEMHEEN KL, ET AL. THE CANADIAN C-SPINE RULE FOR RADIOGRAPHY IN ALERT AND STABLE TRAUMA PATIENTS. *JAMA* 2001; 286(15): 1841–8

spine should only be undertaken by a well-coordinated and practiced team and should not delay transport to hospital.

Facial trauma

The management of dentoalveolar trauma is discussed in Chapter 15. Maxillofacial trauma can be treated after the patient is stabilized if not associated with airway compromise. An unconscious patient with maxillofacial trauma should be presumed to have a cervical spine fracture until proven otherwise.

Epistaxis

Most cases of epistaxis related to trauma can be controlled with direct pinching of the nostrils against the nasal septum for a period of at least 10 minutes. The posterior pharynx should be examined early to detect posterior bleeding. If there is a posterior bleed, then tamponade with an epistaxis balloon or Foley catheter will be required. A 12–16 French Foley catheter can be inserted into the nose along the floor of the nasopharynx until the tip is visible in the posterior pharynx. The balloon is slowly inflated with 15 mL of sterile water and pulled anteriorly until it is firmly against the posterior choanae. The catheter is then secured with either an umbilical clamp or a hemostat. Emergency follow-up with an ear, nose and throat specialist is required for all posterior bleeds.

The anterior nose should be packed in any episode of posterior epistaxis, or when an anterior bleed is unresponsive to pressure, topical vasoconstriction and attempted cautery. Patients with an anterior pack should be followed up within 48 hours and covered with amoxycillin (amoxicillin) or cephalexin to minimize the risk of sinusitis or toxic shock.

Chest

Blunt trauma to the chest wall may cause rib fractures, flail chest, pneumothorax, hemothorax, diaphragm rupture, myocardial contusion or cardiac tamponade. Deceleration injuries, sometimes seen in high-velocity activities such as motor sports and ski racing where athletes can come to a sudden, unplanned stop, can injure the aorta or pulmonary vessels. Circumferential burns may restrict chest expansion and impair ventilation, and release by escharotomy may be required. Applying gentle anterior/posterior or lateral pressure across the chest can help identify the presence of fractured ribs.

Auscultation and percussion of the lung fields may identify a hemothorax if breath sounds are reduced or if dullness is percussed over dependent areas of the chest. Conversely, reduced breath sounds and hyper-resonance in the apices or anterior chest may identify a pneumothorax. Distant heart sounds, distended neck veins and hypotension (Beck's triad) are indicative of cardiac tamponade.

If air or blood exists within the thoracic cavity it requires decompression with a needle (if under tension) and should eventually be drained by chest tube thoracostomy. Needle decompression of a tension pneumothorax is readily accomplished by inserting a large (14 gauge) needle into the second intercostal space along the mid-clavicular line on the affected side. This should result in an immediate rush of air out of the needle and stabilization of the patient. Needle decompression should be followed up by insertion of a chest tube if available, but this should not delay transport. A secure chest tube is preferred prior to air or prolonged ground transport.

Crushing and deceleration injuries of the chest may also result in cardiac contusion and/or cardiac tamponade. The classic features of cardiac tamponade (Beck's triad) may not be initially present or may be difficult to detect. However, tamponade should be suspected in any patient with a chest contusion, hemodynamic compromise without evidence of hemorrhage, and/or pulseless electrical activity with a fast, narrow QRS complex. The athlete will require urgent transport to an emergency department for possible cardiac ultrasound and pericardiocentesis.

Shock

Although shock related to trauma might be due to conditions other than blood loss, for example, obstructive shock (cardiac tamponade or tension pneumothorax, see above) or distributive shock (spinal cord injury, see below), a shock-like state associated with trauma is most often due to hemorrhage. The areas where life-threatening internal bleeding can occur include the chest, the abdomen, the pelvis and the femur. Controlling hemorrhage is the goal in hemorrhagic shock and urgent surgical intervention is required when direct vascular control of ongoing hemorrhage is not achievable. Resuscitation to normotension may worsen ongoing hemorrhage in some situations, particularly in penetrating trauma, and delay of aggressive fluid replacement until the onset of operative intervention may be more appropriate. This advice, however, is predicated on rapid access to a surgical facility and cannot be extrapolated to blunt trauma or situations of prolonged transport distances. Hence, it remains reasonable to establish intravenous access en route to a surgical facility and to initiate a bolus of crystalloid intravenous fluid.

Early signs of shock are subtle and may only include delayed capillary refill, relative tachycardia and anxiety. Systolic hypotension is a late sign and suggests that the compensatory mechanisms for increasing peripheral resistance and redistribution of circulation have exceeded their limits. The 'classic' signs of shock—pallor, clammy skin, confusion, tachycardia, hypotension and reduced urinary output—are more likely to present late during acute blood loss in a young, healthy endurance athlete. The presence of enhanced vagal tone, increased blood volume, cardiac reserve and peripheral circulation allow for much greater compensation. A 50% increase in pulse rate and equivalent decrease in pulse pressure, as might occur with a 25% reduction in blood volume (class II hemorrhage, see box below), is the difference between a blood pressure of 130/70 mmHg and a heart rate of 60 beats per minute (bpm), and a blood pressure of 115/90 mmHg and heart rate of 90 bpm. Such hemodynamic 'stability' belies compensatory mechanisms under stress. When these fail, vascular collapse can be sudden and dramatic. Failure to recognize ongoing hemorrhage delays aggressive pursuit of the source of bleeding with investigations or surgical exploration. A high index of suspicion, based on a suspected or known mechanism of injury, must be maintained.

Neurogenic shock is marked by bradycardia and hypotension, and is a form of distributive impairment. Ventricular performance and fluid volume are preserved but peripheral perfusion is inadequate secondary to loss of sympathetic input, unopposed vagal stimulation and poor vascular tone. The higher the spinal injury, and in particular those above T1, the more likely and more severe the resulting shock state. The diagnosis and treatment of neurogenic shock comes after the initial ABCs and accompanying resuscitation. It should be considered only after other causes of hypotension have been investigated and treated. Initial management remains rapid infusion of crystalloid and transportation to an acute medical facility.

Abdomen

Any abdominal or retroperitoneal injury is potentially dangerous, but the specific diagnosis is not as important as the recognition that an injury exists and surgical intervention may be required. In addition, the initial negative examination may belie the seriousness of the patient's condition and the need for continued re-evaluation must be emphasized.

The athlete who has sustained an injury to one or more abdominal organs may complain of severe pain and develop signs of shock, or may progress slowly over a period of hours. Shoulder pain may occur due to irritation of the diaphragm. The abdomen should be carefully palpated for tenderness and guarding. Increasing abdominal pain, evidence of guarding, signs of hemodynamic instability, or suspicion of an intra-abdominal injury all indicate a need for urgent transportation for surgical evaluation. Intravenous

Categorization of hemorrhagic shock

The American College of Surgeons proposes the following categorization of hemorrhagic shock:

Class I: 15% blood volume loss (750 mL in a 70 kg male)

This is minimal, uncomplicated hemorrhage, with no changes in heart rate, blood pressure or respiratory rate. Treatment is by crystalloid replacement in a 3:1 ratio (i.e. 3 L of crystalloid per liter of blood loss).

Class II: 15–30% blood volume loss (up to 1500 mL in a 70 kg male)

Tachycardia, tachypnea, anxiety, delayed capillary refill and decreased pulse pressure is usually present. Urinary output is only minimally affected. A 2 L bolus of crystalloid replaces the equivalent of approximately 600 mL of blood and is generally sufficient to restore hemodynamic stability. Blood replacement is not usually required and the remaining fluid deficit can be replaced with further crystalloid infusion.

Class III: 30–40% blood volume loss (up to 2000 mL in a 70 kg male)

Classic signs of shock are present with changes in mental status, significant fall in systolic blood pressure, and reduced urinary output. Blood transfusion/volume expansion is indicated.

Class IV: >40% blood volume loss (>2000 mL in a 70 kg male)

Hypotension is profound, urinary output is absent, and the patient is lethargic and near comatose. Immediate blood replacement and surgical intervention is necessary.

access should be established en route to hospital, and nothing further given by mouth.

Pelvic injuries

Athletes who sustain pelvic fractures are usually competing in high-velocity sports. If the integrity of the pelvic ring has been disrupted, there may be associated complications such as a ruptured bladder, ruptured urethra, rectal injury or internal hemorrhage. These injuries require urgent surgical management. The force required to fracture the pelvis is also likely to cause other significant injuries and should heighten suspicion. Clinical examination begins with gentle and careful anteroposterior and lateral compression of the pelvic ring to look for tenderness. Rocking force is unnecessarily painful and may increase hemorrhage. The urethral opening should be inspected for blood, and a rectal examination should be performed to assess rectal tone and the position of the prostate. A high-riding prostate suggests urethral disruption.

Pneumatic anti-shock garments, although once common, are now rarely used. In conjunction with the above resuscitative measures, they may still have benefit in the setting of unstable pelvic fractures. If used, they are inflated from the periphery towards the core until an adequate blood pressure response has been obtained. Likewise, the deflation process should be gradual while vital signs are monitored. Pneumatic anti-shock garments should be used with care. They act to increase afterload and do not autotransfuse pooled peripheral blood. There is no evidence that they improve survival in patients with hemorrhagic shock following trauma. Furthermore, they are contraindicated if pulmonary edema is present and should not be used if thoracic or diaphragmatic injuries, evisceration of abdominal contents, penetrating objects or pregnancy are present or suspected. Pressure changes can occur in the anti-shock garment and include rapid expansion in a warm room after being in a cold environment or rapid expansion in an unpressurized cabin of an aircraft at altitude.

Blunt trauma to the scrotum may rupture a testicle. An associated injury to the pampiniform plexus may cause massive swelling of the scrotum, making diagnosis of the ruptured testicle difficult. Cases of a ruptured testicle require surgical exploration and repair.

Extremity injuries

Injuries to the limbs may involve damage to the bones, joints, vessels or nerves. The initial management of an injured limb includes control of hemorrhage, prevention of further injury, and restoration of blood flow to the limb. In general, bleeding at the site of the injury should be controlled by direct pressure. Open wounds should be covered with sterile dressings as soon as possible.

The amount of hemorrhage following blunt trauma should not be underestimated. A closed femoral fracture can produce up to 2 L of blood loss, whereas a pelvic fracture can result in a blood loss of 3–4 L. Longitudinal traction of femoral fractures will help reduce blood loss and a pneumatic anti-shock garment may help temporize bleeding from a pelvic fracture by providing some stability. However, the application of the pneumatic anti-shock garment is secondary to the requirement for external pelvic fixation and is only potentially useful during transport.

Fractures of the extremities are detected visually or with palpation of tenderness. Angulated fractures are splinted as they lie unless there is neurovascular compromise. Closed angulated fractures of the femur are best straightened prior to splinting. Obtain satisfactory alignment by applying longitudinal traction to the distal part. If this is not achieved with one attempt, further attempts should only be made in hospital. The injured area should be splinted; rolled-up blankets, clothing, pillows, ski poles, oars, paddles or adjacent body parts can all be used as a splint. It is essential that the neurovascular status of a limb should be documented prior to and following any manipulation of a fracture or dislocation. Palpate distal pulses such as the dorsalis pedis and posterior tibial pulses of the leg and the radial and ulnar pulses of the arm. Note skin color, capillary return, temperature and sensation. Assess peripheral nerve function with specific motor and sensory testing (e.g. two-point discrimination is very useful).

Fracture–dislocations around the elbow, knee and ankle can be associated with vascular occlusion or disruption. Neurovascular status should be assessed and documented in all cases of joint dislocation before and after reduction and splinting of the injured limb. Trained personnel should attempt careful reduction as soon as possible. Evidence of vascular injury should be sought after elbow (Chapter 18) and knee dislocation (Chapter 27). Clinical assessment is not sufficient to determine that blood vessels remain intact, and further investigation should be considered. Popliteal artery injury occurs in approximately a third of knee dislocations and vascular integrity should be assessed by arteriography if suspicion exists.

Exposed bones and open wounds associated with suspected fractures should be covered using sterile saline-soaked dressings. Splint the fracture without attempting reduction unless there is neurovascular compromise. Do not push the protruding bone back into the wound. Transport the patient to hospital urgently for fracture management, antibiotic therapy and tetanus prophylaxis. Any patient with an open fracture should be kept nil by mouth to facilitate rapid surgical treatment, if needed.

Acute compartment syndrome should be considered and sought in any patient with an extremity injury marked by hematoma or edema. A conscious patient will complain of pain but severely injured or unconscious patients may not be able to communicate their distress. Hence, a heightened index of suspicion is required and, if in doubt, compartment pressures should be measured. Treatment requires immediate surgical decompression.

The most common site of acute compartment syndrome is the anterior compartment of the lower leg. Clinical features include persistent shin pain (greater than one would expect given the nature of the injury), swelling and pain on passive muscle stretch of the involved compartment. There may also be progressive loss of sensory and motor function. Paresthesia and numbness on the dorsum of the foot may accompany weakness of dorsiflexion of the ankle. Absence of pedal pulses is a late sign.

A *pulseless extremity* should be assessed by Doppler ultrasound. If circulation is compromised, then decompression of circumferential burns with escharotomy, and acute compartment syndrome by fasciotomy, should be achieved early. Vascular compromise secondary to joint dislocation should be relieved by longitudinal traction and attempted reduction with documentation of neurovascular status before and after any manipulation.

Traumatic amputations (e.g. fingertip) may cause substantial hemorrhage so the practitioner should apply pressure and elevate the extremity to minimize blood loss. The proximal stump should ideally be cleaned with sterile saline and dressed with sterile gauze. The amputated part should be wrapped in moist sterile gauze, sealed in a plastic bag and transported in an ice bath with the patient to a center where microsurgical reattachment could be performed if possible.

Neurological evaluation

The neurological examination includes repeat evaluation of the level of consciousness, assessment of recall and attention, examination of pupillary reactions, extraocular movements, and visual fields, and documentation of motor and sensory function in the extremities, of deep tendon reflexes, of cerebellar function, and of rectal tone. The GCS allows sequential monitoring and standardized communication and should be reported for each component of the score (e.g. E4 + V5 + M6 = 15) to ensure consistent evaluation. Any findings of paralysis or paresis suggest a major injury to the spinal cord or peripheral nervous system. Adequate immobilization using a long spinal board and a semi-rigid cervical collar with lateral support and secure straps to the head and torso must be provided. Padding behind the knees, between the legs and under the arms, and under the heels and head will make the potentially extended length of time immobilized less uncomfortable for the awake patient.

Any athlete with a head injury requires assessment of the ABCs. If the athlete is conscious or semi-conscious, the neurological examination commences with inspection of the player's facial expression, followed by assessment of their orientation, recall and attention, and observation of their gait: 'Hear them talk, see them walk, and look in their eyes'.

Any athlete with suspicion of a head injury should be removed from play and not allowed to resume activity until cleared by a physician knowledgeable in concussion management.

Definitive care and ongoing reassessment

If local providers and resources are unable to adequately manage the athlete's injuries, then early transport to a surgical facility, and ideally to the care of a physician accustomed to trauma, should be undertaken. Communication should be established between the sending and receiving physicians, and arrangements made for appropriate, timely transport. A secure, patent and protected airway, spinal immobilization, secure duplicate large-bore vascular access, chest decompression (if required), oximetry and cardiac monitoring, and trained personnel should be provided prior to transport or en route.

Continued reassessment and evaluation of response to treatment is important. A life-threatening problem that was not apparent initially may become apparent at a later time. Furthermore, the initial event may have been precipitated by an underlying medical problem, such as a cardiac dysrhythmia, myocardial infarction, seizure, intracranial hemorrhage, thermal injury, hypoglycemia, electrolyte abnormality, or a drug or toxin effect. Asking not only what, where, when and how the injury occurred but also *why* the injury occurred at this point in time may help decipher causes that were not initially recognized.

Documentation

A quick mnemonic used to assess the athlete's past history is AMPLE:

Allergies
Medications
Past illness
Last meal
Events surrounding the injury

It is easiest to obtain the history and document the information soon after the event. Additional personnel may be required to contact witnesses or relatives to obtain the necessary information. Confidentiality must be maintained.

Meticulous record keeping, including a chronological report with flow sheets, allows easy documentation of events and their treatment as they progress. In life-threatening emergencies consent for treatment is presumed; treatment should be given and formal consent for subsequent treatment obtained later.

Summary

Effective care of the severely ill or injured athlete demands advance planning and preparation, education of personnel, and team rehearsal. Knowledge of injury mechanism, heightened index of suspicion, aggressive resuscitation, vigilance and continual reassessment, and early access to appropriate surgical care will allow for the best possible outcome. Other causes of collapse in the athlete are described elsewhere in this book. They include concussion (Chapter 13), cardiac causes (Chapter 45), heat stroke (Chapter 53), hypothermia (Chapter 54), hyponatremia (Chapter 53) and drugs (Chapter 61).

Recommended Reading

Anon. Sideline preparedness for the team physician: consensus statement. *Med Sci Sports Exerc* 2001; 33(5): 846–9.

Hoffman JR, Mower WR, Wolfson AB, et al. Validity of a set of clinical criteria to rule out injury to the cervical spine in patients with blunt trauma. National Emergency X-Radiography Utilization Study Group. *N Engl J Med* 2000; 343(2): 94–9.

Hunte GS. Emergency treatment of life threatening conditions. In: Jackson R, ed. *Sport Medicine Manual*. 2nd edn. Laussanne: International Olympic Committee, 2000: 235–52.

Stiell IG, Wells GA, Vandemheen KL, et al. The Canadian C-spine rule for radiography in alert and stable trauma patients. *JAMA* 2001; 286(15): 1841–8.

References

1. Drezner JA. Practical guidelines for automated external defibrillators in the athletic setting. *Clin J Sport Med* 2005; 15(5): 367–9.

2. Hazinski MF, Nadkarni VM, Hickey RW, et al. Major changes in the 2005 AHA guidelines for CPR and ECC. Reaching the tipping point for change. *Circulation* 2005; 112(24 suppl.): IV206–11.

3. Hoffman JR, Mower WR, Wolfson AB, et al. Validity of a set of clinical criteria to rule out injury to the cervical spine in patients with blunt trauma. National Emergency X-Radiography Utilization Study Group. *N Engl J Med* 2000; 343(2): 94–9.

4. Stiell IG, Wells GA, Vandemheen KL, et al. The Canadian C-spine rule for radiography in alert and stable trauma patients. *JAMA* 2001; 286(15): 1841–8.

Cardiovascular Symptoms During Exercise

Cardiovascular presentations associated with exercise include palpitation, syncope and chest pain; a cardiac murmur may also be detected on physical examination. Given that in the United States alone cardiovascular diseases claim a life every 34 seconds,[1] these presentations demand accurate assessment.

This chapter updates the reader on some aspects of cardiovascular physiology and then details the approach to each of the clinical presentations mentioned above. We then discuss conditions that are of particular relevance in sports medicine, including hypertrophic cardiomyopathy, coronary artery disease and Marfan's syndrome. The chapter concludes with a discussion of the specialized cardiac investigations that aid diagnosis and, thus, may prevent serious cardiovascular events in exercise.

Cardiovascular changes with exercise

Certain structural and functional adaptations distinguish the heart of an athlete (the athletic heart syndrome) from the heart of the non-athlete[2] and this should be regarded as a normal physiological response to exercise. The heart responds to increased demand by increasing its rate and contractility. Structural adaptations occur after long-term increased demand, which may result from pressure overload, associated with resistance training, or volume overload, associated with endurance training.[3]

In response to chronic pressure overload (e.g. weightlifting and throwing athletes), there is an increase in septal and free wall ventricular thickness. In response to chronic volume overload (e.g. distance running athletes), the left ventricular end diastolic diameter increases with a proportional increase in the ventricular wall thickness. Athletes who combine weight training and endurance activities (e.g. cycling, rowing) have a cardiac structure that is between these two extremes.[3] These overload changes are shown in Figure 45.1. In keeping with the recent recognition of the benefits of resistance training for the cardiovascular system, the American Heart Association now recommends it as part of the exercise prescription for cardiovascular health.[4]

It is important that clinicians are able to distinguish between cardiovascular adaptations to exercise and cardiovascular changes that may suggest disease. The possible changes in physical examination findings in the cardiovascular system of athletes are shown in Table 45.1.

ECG/EKG (hereon referred to as ECG) changes are also seen in athletes.[5] These are summarized in Table 45.2. Athletes will usually have evidence of cardiac enlargement on chest X-ray. Echocardiogram findings will vary depending on the type of training performed, as mentioned above. Endurance athletes may also have false positive thallium stress scans (see p. 815).

Palpitation

The symptoms of palpitation in association with physical activity may be of no consequence but they may also be of concern, particularly if accompanied by exertional chest pain and/or syncope. Typically, however, variations in heart rhythm in athletes are benign and do not preclude participation in sport.

The athlete may use terms such as 'pounding', 'fluttering', 'flopping' and 'skipping' to describe palpitation.

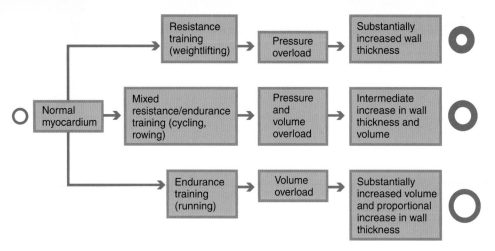

Figure 45.1 Cardiac adaptations to chronic exercise

Table 45.1 Findings on cardiovascular examination in athletes

Signs	Findings in athletes
Resting pulse rate	Decreased or normal
Jugular venous pressure	Normal
Blood pressure	Normal or decreased
Left ventricular size	Increased
Apex beat	Displaced laterally
Edema	Always abnormal
Heart sounds	
• First, second	Normal
• Third	Often occur ('physiological')
• Fourth	May occur in athletes but if present warrants cardiological assessment
Systolic murmurs	Frequent

Clinical approach

The mode of onset and offset of palpitation helps distinguish an underlying sinus tachycardia from other causes of tachycardia (ectopic tachycardias). The ectopic rhythms characteristically begin instantaneously, while sinus tachycardia has a more gradual onset and ends over seconds or minutes. The history should also include any previous episodes or symptoms (e.g. syncope or near-syncope, dizziness, chest pain or discomfort, seizures), recent medication or recreational drug use, eating disorders and a history

of congenital heart disease or previous cardiac surgery. The practitioner should ask if there is any family history of cardiac events including sudden death, arrhythmias or congenital cardiac conditions.

Other causes of palpitation include thyrotoxicosis, hypoglycemia, adrenalin (epinephrine)-producing tumor, fever and drugs. Palpitation can be associated with the use of tobacco, caffeinated products, alcohol, adrenalin (epinephrine), ephedrine, aminophylline (asthma) or thyroid medication.

The physical examination must not be limited to the cardiovascular system otherwise causes of arrhythmias such as thyrotoxicosis will be missed. If the patient is seen during an attack, carotid sinus massage can help diagnose supraventricular tachycardia. An ECG during an attack usually provides a definitive diagnosis. When this cannot be obtained, Holter (ambulatory) monitoring and exercise ECG testing can prove useful (see p. 814).

Management

The approach to management of the athlete presenting with palpitation is shown in Figure 45.2. A task force of cardiologists has published comprehensive guidelines for the management of specific arrhythmias in athletes[6, 7] and we recommend a specialist cardiologist assess any athlete with palpitation who is proven to have an arrhythmia[6, 7] because treatment protocols and medications are updated regularly. The treatment of common arrhythmias is summarized in Tables 45.3 and 45.4.

The practitioner must determine whether or not an athlete has a structural lesion underlying the

Table 45.2 Electrocardiograph changes seen in athletes

ECG finding	Normal population (%)	Athletes (%)
Sinus bradycardia	24	50–80
Sinus arrhythmia	2–20	14–70
First-degree atrioventricular block	<1	6–33
Second-degree atrioventricular block	<0.1	0.1–10
Third-degree atrioventricular block	<0.001	0.02
Atrial fibrillation	0.004	0.06
Premature ventricular contractions (>5 per hour)	43	33
Runs of ventricular tachycardia	6.5	0
Left ventricular hypertrophy (on ECG)	<0.1	14–85
Repolarization abnormalities (ST segment elevation)	2	40–100

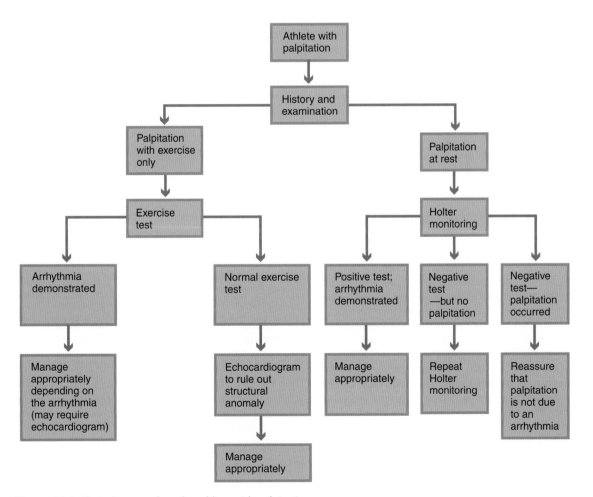

Figure 45.2 Clinical approach to the athlete with palpitation

Table 45.3 Treatment of cardiac arrhythmias that have a regular heart rate

Diagnosis	Underlying cause	Treatment	Sports participation (guidelines only)
Sinus tachycardia	Anxiety, fever, anemia, thyrotoxicosis	Treat underlying disease if present, exclude structural abnormality	Generally full
Supraventricular tachycardia	None (60%), drugs, tobacco, caffeine, Wolff–Parkinson–White syndrome, thyrotoxicosis	Valsalva maneuver, carotid sinus massage, verapamil, adenosine	Athletes whose symptoms are controlled and who have no structural abnormality can participate in all sports
Wolff–Parkinson–White syndrome	Atrioventricular bypass tract	Pharmacological, including calcium channel blockers, quinidine, flecainide. Surgical ablation of abnormal bypass tracts	Athletes over 20 years who are free of structural heart disease, palpitation and tachycardias can participate in all competitive sports after appropriate work-up
Sinus bradycardia	Physiological, acute myocardial infarction, hypothyroidism, hypothermia, sinoatrial node disease	Nil if asymptomatic; treat underlying disease if present	Full sports participation if physiological or underlying condition is treated
Atrial flutter	May be caused by structural heart disease	Beta-blockers, calcium antagonist, other cardiac drugs, DC cardioversion	When rhythm is controlled with pharmacotherapy, participation is permitted in low-intensity sports. Successful control for 3–6 months permits return to all competitive sports if there is no structural abnormality

palpitation and arrhythmia. Even if the arrhythmia can be controlled, a structural heart abnormality may preclude full athletic participation, depending on the nature of the lesion. For example, persons with the congenital long QT syndrome, a cause of ventricular tachycardia, should be excluded from competitive sports because of the risk of sudden death.[6, 7]

Note that beta-blockers, a common therapy for arrhythmia, are not well tolerated by athletes as they reduce exercise tolerance. Furthermore, beta-blockers are on the World Anti-Doping Agency's list of banned substances in certain sports (Chapter 61) because they cause a lengthening of diastole, which is an advantage in precision sports such as shooting.

Syncope

Syncope is defined as a generalized weakness of muscles, with loss of postural tone, inability to stand upright and a loss of consciousness. The term faintness, or presyncope, refers to lack of strength with a sensation of impending loss of consciousness. At the beginning of a syncopal attack the patient is usually in the upright position. Nausea and sometimes vomiting may accompany these symptoms. There is a striking pallor or ashen gray color of the face and very often the face and body are bathed in cold perspiration. When there is time, the patient may take protection against injury; sometimes syncope occurs suddenly and without warning.

Table 45.4 Treatment of cardiac arrhythmias that have an irregular heart rate

Diagnosis	Underlying cause	Treatment	Sports participation (guidelines only)
Atrial fibrillation	Thyrotoxicosis, alcohol, illicit drugs, myocardial ischemia, pericarditis, digoxin	Digoxin, intravenous verapamil, beta-blockers, treat underlying disease, DC cardioversion	If there is no structural heart disease, participation is permitted if the ventricular rate in exercise can reach the expected rate of sinus tachycardia. If structural heart disease is present, recommendation depends on the lesion present. If taking anticoagulants, should not participate in contact sports because of risk of bleeding complications
Premature ventricular complexes	None (50%), stress, caffeine, sleep deprivation, alcohol, ischemia, digoxin, cardiomyopathy, low serum potassium concentration	Treat cause as appropriate	In the absence of symptoms and structural heart disease, athletes may participate in all activities.[6, 7] Restrict to low-intensity sport when rhythm worsens with exercise or when structural heart disease is present
Ventricular tachycardia	Generally structural, most commonly ischemic heart disease, cardiomyopathy, metabolic disturbances, drug toxicity, prolonged QT syndrome	Specialist assessment mandatory and may include cardiac catheterization and electrophysiological study	If no structural lesion, no sports participation for 6 months following the last episode; monitor clinically. If structural heart disease is present, low-intensity sports only as long as there are no recurrences[6]

Syncope may be due to reduced cerebral blood flow, alteration of blood physiology or cerebral events. Cerebral blood flow is reduced by loss of vasoconstrictor mechanisms (e.g. postural hypotension), loss of circulating blood volume (e.g. blood loss), mechanical obstruction of venous return (e.g. Valsalva maneuver in weightlifting), reduced cardiac output and arrhythmias. Syncope is more likely to occur with normal cerebral blood flow if the blood itself is altered (e.g. anemia, hypoglycemia). Syncope can also arise from cerebral events (e.g. cerebral ischemic attacks, emotional disturbances).

In an athlete with syncope, the sports medicine practitioner must determine whether the syncope occurred during or after sport.[8,9] If syncope occurs immediately the athlete stops being active, such as at the end of an endurance event, syncope is likely to be due to the pooling of blood in the lower limbs in the absence of muscular contraction to pump the blood back to the heart.[8,9] This sudden reduction in blood pressure is a common cause of syncope and has been labeled as exercise-associated collapse (Chapter 53). The athlete should be placed in a head-down position with the legs and pelvis elevated and he or she will most likely recover quickly and spontaneously.[9] Although this is a benign condition, other causes of syncope should be excluded by clinical assessment. There is no indication for routine investigation of this syncope.

If, on the other hand, an athlete has one or more syncopal attacks during sporting activities, it may indicate a serious medical problem. These patients should be thoroughly assessed by taking a history, physical examination and appropriate investigations.

> **KEY FACT** It is important to note that syncope while exercising indicates a serious medical problem.

History

Once the athlete is stabilized (Chapter 44), it is essential to inquire about the following risk factors for cardiac disease:

- a family history of cardiac events in first- and second-degree relatives at an age younger than 65 years
- diabetes mellitus
- a history of valvular disease, including rheumatic fever
- hypercholesterolemia, hypertension, smoking.

The patient should be asked about chest pain, palpitation, unusual shortness of breath with exercise, or previous episodes of light-headedness, dizziness or collapse.

Examination

Even in the presence of significant structural cardiac abnormality, examination may be normal. Cardiovascular examination focuses on the nature of the carotid pulse for valvular disease, and the quality of the apex beat and auscultation for heart sounds and murmurs. If a murmur is present, it should be tested with the patient performing the Valsalva maneuver and also a squat (see below). These clinical tests are aimed at detecting hypertrophic cardiomyopathy and valvular disease.

Investigations

Investigations should include chest X-ray, ECG, exercise stress test and echocardiogram, which are discussed later in this chapter. Although supraventricular tachycardia is uncommonly associated with syncope, patients with Wolff–Parkinson–White syndrome are susceptible to syncope and this may need investigation with electrophysiological studies (see p. 816) to define

the mechanism and pathway of the tachycardia.[10] Tilt table testing may be used to assess the athlete's susceptibility to further syncopal episodes.

Heart murmur

Heart murmurs occur in both normal and athletic populations. In the case of an athlete, a heart murmur is usually detected as part of a screening examination (Chapter 57). The clinician must determine whether the heart murmur is 'innocent' or significant.

An innocent flow murmur is usually a short systolic murmur that can be differentiated from the murmur of aortic stenosis, which produces a harsh crescendo–decrescendo murmur radiating to the neck. Diastolic murmurs are always pathological and require further investigation. The more common causes of heart murmurs are shown in Table 45.5. An uncommon cause of heart murmurs with potentially serious complications for the athlete is hypertrophic cardiomyopathy. The clinical approach to the athlete with a heart murmur is shown in Figure 45.3.

Chest pain

The diagnosis and treatment of the athlete with chest pain of musculoskeletal origin has been discussed in Chapter 20. Although musculoskeletal causes, including referred pain from the thoracic spine, are common in young athletes, the practitioner must consider the possibility of a cardiac or pulmonary cause. Chest pain can originate in a number of structures, including the myocardium, pericardium, great vessels, esophagus, lungs, chest wall, thoracic spine and breast. The main differentiating features between

Table 45.5 Causes of heart murmurs

Timing of the murmur	Cause
Systolic	Normal 'flow' murmur
	Aortic sclerosis
	Aortic stenosis
	Hypertrophic cardiomyopathy
	Pulmonary stenosis
	Atrial septal defect
	Ventricular septal defect
	Mitral incompetence
Diastolic	Aortic incompetence
	Mitral stenosis
Continuous	Coarctation of the aorta
	Patent ductus arteriosus

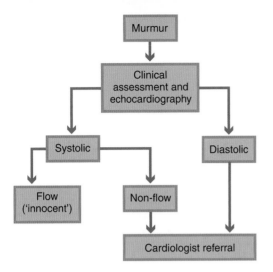

Figure 45.3 Clinical approach to the athlete with a heart murmur

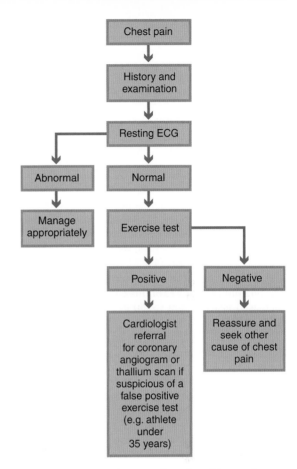

Figure 45.4 Clinical approach to the athlete with chest pain of suspected cardiac origin

pain originating from the thoracic spine and chest pain from myocardial ischemia have been described in Table 20.3.

Important cardiac causes of chest pain include coronary artery disease, aortic stenosis, hypertrophic cardiomyopathy and acute pericarditis. Vascular causes of chest pain, such as aortic dissection and pulmonary embolism, although rare, have occurred even in young athletes.

The clinical approach to the patient with chest pain of suspected cardiac origin[11] is shown in Figure 45.4. If coronary artery disease is detected, treatment may be medical or surgical depending on the extent of the disease. If coronary artery disease is not detected, the patient should be reassured and the practitioner should perform a thorough examination of the respiratory, gastrointestinal and musculoskeletal systems, paying particular attention to the thoracic spine.

Sudden cardiac death

Sudden cardiac death related to exercise is uncommon but it is perhaps the single biggest challenge to sports medicine practitioners.[12, 13] Although the overall risk of sudden death due to cardiac causes is substantially reduced in those who exercise regularly,[14,15] the risk is temporarily increased during exercise. Recent prospective studies suggest this increase is very slight in most individuals.[16]

The likelihood of any particular condition being the cause of the sudden death varies according to the age of the athlete. It is convenient to divide athletes

into two groups—those under the age of 35 years and those over 35 years. Most young athletes who die suddenly show evidence of a structural congenital cardiovascular lesion, most commonly hypertrophic cardiomyopathy (Table 45.6). Coronary artery disease is the leading cause of sudden death in athletes over the age of 35 years. Other less common causes in that age category are mitral valve prolapse, acquired valve disease and hypertrophic cardiomyopathy.

Hypertrophic cardiomyopathy

Hypertrophic cardiomyopathy (HCM) is generally regarded as the most common cause of sudden cardiac death in athletes, accounting for 36% of deaths in one study.[17] HCM is a primary disease of cardiac muscle, characterized by a hypertrophied but non-dilated left ventricle. It occurs in up to two per 1000 of the general population and is a primary and familial cardiac

Table 45.6 Causes of sudden death of cardiac origin of athletes under the age of 35 years

Common	Less common
Hypertrophic cardiomyopathy	Myocarditis
Congenital coronary artery anomalies	Mitral valve prolapse
Aortic rupture (e.g. Marfan's syndrome)	Aortic stenosis
	Arrhythmogenic right ventricular dysplasia
	Conduction abnormalities, including Wolff–Parkinson–White syndrome
	Prolonged QT syndrome
	Dilated cardiomyopathy
	Coronary artery disease

malformation with a heterogeneous expression and a diverse clinical course for which disease-causing mutations in 10 genes encoding sarcomeric and regulatory proteins have been reported.[18]

There are two types of HCM, the obstructive type and the much more common non-obstructive type. The anatomical features of this condition include an increased heart weight (>360 g) and asymmetrical ventricular wall thickening.

Unfortunately, sudden death is frequently the first indication of the presence of HCM. About 90% of deaths in athletes caused by HCM occur in males, which partly reflects higher participation rates and more intense activity levels. About 60% of athletes were high school age at the time of death.[18] Most athletes had been symptom free and not suspected of having cardiovascular disease. Sudden collapse was usually associated with exercise, predominantly in the late afternoon or early evening.

In those who had prodromal symptoms, the most prominent were exertional dyspnea (the most common symptom), chest pain, palpitation as well as presyncope and syncope. In patients with associated obstruction to left ventricular flow (the obstructive type of HCM), the diagnosis may be suggested by a characteristic rapid, jerky upstroke of the carotid pulse, a double or triple apex beat and the presence of a systolic cardiac murmur that increases in intensity during the Valsalva maneuver or while standing and decreases with squatting. There may be a fourth heart sound. A number of patients with HCM have typical clinical findings at rest; however, the majority have no symptoms because they either have no, or minimal, obstruction to left ventricular outflow at rest. The sensitivity of physical examination is therefore relatively low.

Patients with HCM generally have ECG evidence of left ventricular hypertrophy, ST segment and T wave abnormalities, and occasionally prominent Q waves. Although the ECG changes are not specific for this condition, a normal ECG makes the diagnosis of

hypertrophic cardiomyopathy unlikely. Chest X-ray may demonstrate an enlarged heart but most patients with hypertrophic cardiomyopathy have normal chest X-rays.

Echocardiography is the investigation of choice in cases of HCM. A hypertrophied, non-dilated left ventricle in the absence of other diseases strongly suggests the diagnosis of HCM. The HCM disease spectrum has been characterized by considerable diversity of patterns and extent of left ventricular hypertrophy. While the anterior ventricular septum is usually the predominant region of hypertrophy, virtually all patterns of left ventricular hypertrophy occur in HCM. For example, although many patients show diffusely distributed hypertrophy, about 30% demonstrate localized wall thickening confined to only one left ventricle segment.

Absolute thickness of the left ventricle wall is nearly always greater than 15 mm (0.6 in.) but varies greatly, with the average being 21–22 mm (1 in.). Some patients, however, show only a mild increase up to 15 mm (0.6 in.), including a few genetically affected individuals with normal thickness (<12 mm [0.5 in.]). Wall thicknesses of 13–15 mm (0.5–0.6 in.) represent a 'gray zone' of diagnostic uncertainty. Patterns of wall thickening in HCM are often strikingly heterogeneous, involving non-contiguous left ventricle segments. Transitions between thickened areas and regions of normal thickness are often sharp and abrupt.[18] Echocardiography may also reveal marked systolic anterior motion of the mitral valve and mid-systolic closure of the aortic valves. There is normal or increased systolic contractility.

Differentiating between HCM and athlete's heart

The septal thickness in cases of 'athlete's heart' rarely exceeds 15 mm (0.6 in.), whereas in cases of HCM the septum is usually at least 15 mm (0.6 in.) thick,[17] although in some young athletes, wall thicknesses of

13–15 mm (0.5–0.6 in.) are consistent with a relatively mild morphological expression of HCM and may be difficult to distinguish from physiological left ventricular hypertrophy (athlete's heart).

An enlarged left ventricle end-diastolic cavity dimension (>55 mm [>2 in.]) is present in more than one-third of highly trained elite male athletes.[18] Conversely, the diastolic cavity dimension is small (<45 mm [<1.8 in.]) in most patients with HCM.

An abnormal Doppler transmitral flow-velocity pattern strongly supports the diagnosis of HCM, while a normal Doppler study is compatible with either HCM or athlete's heart.[18] Elite athletes with left ventricular hypertrophy may show a reduction in wall thickness of about 2–5 mm (0.1–0.2 in.) with three months of deconditioning. A decrease such as this would be inconsistent with pathological hypertrophy and HCM.

In athletes in whom the distinction between HCM and athlete's heart cannot be achieved by other methods, echocardiographic screening of family members may resolve the diagnosis as the presence of HCM in a relative is strong evidence for HCM.

Eligibility for sport

Although not all patients with HCM incur the same risk for sudden death, differentiating subgroups with disparate risks has proven challenging. The 26th Bethesda Conference recommended that 'athletes with the unequivocal diagnosis of HCM should not participate in most competitive sports, with the possible exception of those of low intensity. This recommendation includes those athletes with or without symptoms and with or without left ventricular outflow obstruction' (Table 45.7).[6] Patients with HCM judged to be at high risk should be considered for implantation of a cardioconverter defibrillator.[19]

Marfan's syndrome

Marfan's syndrome, a genetic disorder of the connective tissues, has an autosomal dominant inheritance caused by mutations in the gene for the fibrillin-1 protein. The prevalence of Marfan's syndrome in the general population is estimated at two to three in

Table 45.7 26th Bethesda Conference Guidelines for athletic participation for selected cardiovascular abnormalities

Cardiovascular abnormality	Guideline for exclusion
Hypertrophic cardiomyopathy	Exclusion from most competitive/non-competitive sports with possible exception of low-intensity sports, regardless of medical treatment, absence of symptoms, or implantation of defibrillator
Coronary artery abnormalities	Exclusion from all competitive sports. Participation may be considered 6 months after surgical correction and after exercise stress testing
Arrhythmogenic right ventricular dysplasia	Exclusion from all competitive sports
Mitral valve prolapse	Exclusion if history of syncope associated with arrhythmia, family history of mitral valve prolapse and sudden death, documented arrhythmia, or moderate-to-severe mitral regurgitation
Marfan's syndrome	Exclusion from contact sports. Patients with aortic regurgitation and marked dilatation of the aorta are excluded from all competitive sports. Others may participate in low-intensity sports, with biannual echocardiography
Long QT syndrome	Exclusion from all competitive sports
Myocarditis	Athletes with a history of myocarditis in previous 6 months banned from all competitive sports
Wolff–Parkinson–White syndrome	Patients with normal exercise testing +/– electrophysiological study may be eligible for participation in all sports
Coronary artery disease	Individual risk assessment based upon ejection fraction, exercise tolerance, presence of inducible ischemia or arrhythmias, and presence of hemodynamically significant coronary stenoses on angiography

10 000. Family history is negative in approximately one-third of patients with Marfan's syndrome and presumed to be due to a new mutation.[20]

Affected individuals have multisystem involvement including the cardiovascular (heart and aorta), ocular and musculoskeletal systems. Aortic root aneurysm rupture or dissection is the most common cause of sudden death. Mutation of the fibrillin gene results in abnormal structural integrity of the ascending aorta. The aortic root dilatation starts at the sinuses of Valsalva and extends distally. The common clinical features are tall stature, wide arm span, pectus excavatum chest deformity, myopia, hypermobile joints and a cardiac murmur. Mitral valve prolapse and regurgitation typically occur when Marfan's syndrome manifests in infancy.

The diagnosis depends on the presence of major criteria in a number of organ systems. If a primary relative has Marfan's syndrome, the diagnosis is likely if two organ systems are involved with at least one major manifestation, such as lens dislocation, cystic medial necrosis of the aorta resulting in aortic dilatation/aortic dissection, or the central nervous system abnormality, dural ectasia.

To make the diagnosis in the absence of a family history, skeletal features are required in addition to two of the major manifestations listed above. The skeletal features of Marfan's syndrome include a high arched palate, long tubular bones, wide arm span and hyperflexible joints. Note that these skeletal 'abnormalities' may provide a benefit in sports such as basketball and volleyball, so clinicians covering sports with tall athletes should maintain an index of suspicion for this condition.

Investigations that may be helpful in the athlete with suspected Marfan's syndrome include chest X-ray (which may occasionally suggest aortic dilatation) and, more importantly, echocardiography. This should be performed whenever there is clinical suspicion of Marfan's syndrome. Magnetic resonance angiography (MRA) is becoming used more widely as an efficient means of imaging the aortic arch.

If the diagnosis is suspected, the athlete should be referred to appropriate subspecialists, as definitive diagnosis is not straightforward, particularly when there is no family history. The complexity of diagnosis arises because the entire list of manifestations of Marfan's syndrome is lengthy and conditions such as homocystinuria and Ehlers-Danlos syndrome mimic Marfan's syndrome.

The athlete with Marfan's syndrome with aortic dilatation should avoid vigorous activities. Cardiovascular abnormalities cause death in 95% of cases. If no aortic dilatation is present, sport should be limited to low-intensity activities.

When the aorta is involved, the primary goal of therapy is to slow or prevent progressive dilatation of the aortic root. The mainstay of treatment is with beta-blockers and regular echocardiography to detect progressive dilatation. Early surgical intervention for aortic and mitral valve replacement is warranted when the disease has progressed.[21]

Coronary artery disease

Coronary artery disease is the most common cause of exercise-related deaths in those aged over 35 years and an infrequent cause of sudden death in athletes under that age. Typical symptoms of coronary artery disease include classic angina (a pressure-type pain in the chest) or similar discomfort in the neck, jaws, shoulders, arms and back, precipitated by exercise, that disappears with the cessation of activity.

Nevertheless, prodromal symptoms are common prior to exercise-related deaths but are frequently ignored by the athlete, who considers the pain to be of musculoskeletal, rather than cardiac, origin.

Other significant cardiac conditions

Congenital anomalies of the coronary arteries

A number of congenital anomalies of the coronary arteries exist and may result in sudden death in athletes. The abnormality most often associated with sudden death in exercise is the anomalous origin of the left coronary artery from the right (anterior) sinus of Valsalva. The aberrant artery passes between the aorta and the right ventricular outflow tract, with a potential risk of compression, especially following exercise. Clinical recognition depends on careful evaluation of athletes with symptoms of exertional chest pain or syncope. Coronary angiography will confirm the diagnosis.

Arrhythmogenic right ventricular dysplasia

Arrhythmogenic right ventricular cardiomyopathy/dysplasia is a rare condition in most countries but appears to have an increased prevalence in the Veneto region of north-eastern Italy where it is the major cause of sudden death in young athletes.[22] The pathophysiology involves fibrofatty replacement of the right ventricular myocardium, producing an unstable substrate from which lethal arrhythmias may arise. Frequently the first manifestation of the disease is sudden death. Some patients complain of palpitations and syncope. Ventricular arrhythmias ranging from isolated premature ventricular beats to sustained ventricular tachycardia are the most common clinical presentation. Echocardiography may demonstrate right ventricular wall motion abnormalities or abnormal morphology.

Myocarditis

Myocarditis is an inflammatory process involving the myocardial wall, which can be precipitated by a number of bacterial, viral and other agents. Most cases of acute myocarditis are of viral origin and coxsackie B virus is the most commonly identified pathogen. The condition is important because it has been implicated in sudden cardiac death due to ventricular arrhythmia in athletes.[23] Clinical diagnosis relies on a recent history of myalgia, combined with chest pain, fatigue, dyspnea and palpitation. Congestive cardiac failure may develop. Arrhythmias and heart block may develop. When evaluating an athlete with an acute illness, a tachycardia out of proportion to other systemic features should alert the clinician to the possibility of myocarditis.

Diagnostic tests include erythrocyte sedimentation rate, C-reactive protein level and cardiac enzyme assay. ECG changes may be non-specific. Acute and convalescent antibody titers may yield a causative agent. An echocardiogram reveals diminished cardiac function.

Following myocarditis, the athlete should refrain from competitive sport for six months.[23] If clinical features are normal, ECG and echocardiography at rest and during exercise reveal cardiac function and dimensions are normal, and Holter monitoring shows that there are no arrhythmias with activities of daily living, the athlete may return to competition.[6]

Arrhythmia and conduction abnormalities

A number of rare abnormalities may occasionally cause sudden death in young athletes. These include congenital long QT syndrome, Wolff–Parkinson–White syndrome, idiopathic ventricular tachycardia and Brugada syndrome.

Congenital long QT syndrome is a familial disease characterized by a prolonged QT interval in the ECG, and cardiac symptoms (ranging from minor symptoms such as dizziness, to major events such as seizure, syncope and sudden death) result from the precipitation of ventricular tachyarrythmias.[24] The

incidence is estimated as one in 7000–17000 and usually the heart is completely normal on examination. Treatment with beta-blockers has been shown to reduce the incidence of syncope and sudden cardiac death, but athletes with this condition are advised to participate in low-intensity activities only.

Wolff–Parkinson–White syndrome is the result of an accessory pathway between the atrium and ventricle. ECG displays a short PR interval with a delta wave, and conduction of arrhythmias at supraphysiological rates (>300 beats/min). Treatment of symptomatic patients is with radiofrequency ablation. If athletes are free of symptoms three to six months after radiofrequency ablation, then they can resume sport with no limitations.[25]

Idiopathic ventricular tachycardia is a rare cause of sudden death that originates from one of the ventricular outflow tracts. It can also be treated with radiofrequency ablation and, following successful treatment, sport may be resumed.

Brugada syndrome, characterized by an ECG showing right bundle branch block and ST elevation in the right precordial leads, can be a marker of malignant arrhythmias and a rare cause of sudden death.[25]

Aortic stenosis

Aortic stenosis may be congenital, due to rheumatic inflammation of the aortic valve and, in the elderly, can result from calcific degeneration of the aortic cusps. This condition is an infrequent cause of sudden cardiac death. Patients with severe stenosis should avoid physical exertion, even if asymptomatic;[26] those with mild disease may compete in sports.[26]

Mitral valve prolapse

This condition affects 5% of the population and many athletes have trivial degrees of mitral regurgitation.[27] However, it can also be associated with sudden cardiac death[28] so it can be difficult for the sports medicine practitioner to manage athletes with this condition. We suggest clinicians investigate those patients with a positive family history of sudden death, as well as those with significant symptoms such as dizziness, syncope, palpitation and/or shortness of breath. Any physical findings suggesting a body habitus of Marfan's syndrome or that the murmur may be due to HCM also warrant further investigation, as does an abnormal ECG. The majority of athletes who do not meet any of those criteria may receive full clearance for sports participation and are at low risk for sudden cardiac death.[27]

Commotio cordis

Commotio cordis occurs when blunt force trauma is applied to the chest (usually via a projectile) that results in life-threatening ventricular arrhythmia. It is commonly seen in baseball, hockey, lacrosse, softball and after bodily impacts. Three determinants of such an event have been identified. These include relatively low-energy chest impact located directly over the heart, precise timing of the blow at a vulnerable period during the cardiac cycle, and a narrow compliant chest wall. The vulnerable period of the cardiac cycle that has been identified is a 15–30 ms interval just before the T wave peak.[29] When impact occurs during this repolarization period, transient complete heart block may be induced. In approximately 10% of individuals, collapse does not occur directly upon impact but may be preceded by several moments of relative wakefulness. The athlete may take a few steps, open his or her eyes, or speak before the final cardiac arrest occurs, suggesting a brief period of tolerated arrhythmia before circulatory collapse.[29]

Special cardiac investigations

Tests that are commonly used to aid with diagnosis in patients with cardiovascular symptoms and signs include echocardiography and exercise stress test. Less commonly used tests, particularly in athletes, are thallium scans, radionuclide ventriculography, Holter monitoring and electrophysiological testing. MRA is being used more widely.

Echocardiography

Cardiac structural abnormalities are the major cause of cardiac death in athletes under the age of 35 years and echocardiography is the most accurate non-invasive way to assess cardiac structure. Echocardiography uses ultrasound beams of between 2 and 10 megahertz (MHz). There are several modes of echocardiography to provide a range of data for the clinician. M-mode echocardiography provides an 'ice-pick-like' view of the heart; it detects structures in a one-dimensional linear array. Printing this out on a strip recorder, it provides a temporal dimension, similar to an ECG rhythm strip. Two-dimensional echocardiography images a wedge-shaped sector of the heart and allows a two-dimensional image to be constructed. Doppler echocardiography images blood flow within the heart and is particularly useful in detecting stenotic or regurgitant valves.

Echocardiography is the clinical test of choice for left ventricular hypertrophy and HCM. Thus, it is indicated in patients with presyncopal episodes, syncope,

shortness of breath, chest pain and a family history of sudden death or HCM. The test should also be considered when examination reveals a double systolic arterial pulse (bisferiens pulse), a prominent *a*-wave in the jugular venous pulse, a left ventricular heave, a crescendo–decrescendo mid-systolic murmur or a fourth heart sound; or if ECG indicates left ventricular hypertrophy, ST segment or T wave abnormalities, or Q waves. Echocardiography can be performed when the patient is exercising to detect subtle abnormalities of wall motion.[30, 31]

Exercise stress testing

Exercise stress testing on a treadmill is the most commonly used test to diagnose and evaluate coronary artery disease. It is also used in exercise medicine to measure functional capacity as part of the work-up for exercise prescription (e.g. after myocardial infarction, in patients with diabetes mellitus). The test is contraindicated in certain individuals (Table 45.8).

The test includes a baseline heart rate, blood pressure and ECG. The patient is then asked to exercise progressively according to a standard protocol and a physician monitors heart rate, blood pressure, symptoms and the ECG. It is important to terminate the exercise test as soon as any abnormalities occur. There are patient, physician and protocol end points for exercise testing (Table 45.9).[32]

Exercise testing does not have 100% sensitivity or specificity so it is not suitable as a screening test in a population where the pre-test probability of the disease is low.[33] For example, a positive test in a 55-year-old male with angina is associated with a 90% probability of disease but the same result in a 45-year-old asymptomatic male without risk factors is 90% likely to be a false positive! Therefore, determining guidelines as to who should undergo exercise testing remains challenging.

Exercise testing should be performed for any athlete complaining of chest pain or discomfort of possible cardiac origin or palpitation. It is also useful to assess functional capacity and prognosis in patients with coronary artery disease as these individuals will be involved in exercise rehabilitation programs. Whether or not exercise testing should be performed in those aged over 40 years who have been sedentary but plan to enter a vigorous exercise program remains a subject of debate.[34]

Both the American College of Sports Medicine and Sport Medicine Australia recommend that 'high-risk' individuals (i.e. men over 45 and women over 55, individuals with more than two cardiovascular

Table 45.8 Contraindications to exercise testing

Unstable or severe cardiac disorders	Non-cardiovascular disorders
Recent acute myocardial infarction	Active infections
Unstable angina	Severe emotional distress
Uncontrolled cardiac arrhythmias	Uncontrolled metabolic diseases (e.g. hyper/hypothyroidism,
Severe congestive cardiac failure	diabetes mellitus)
Severe aortic stenosis	Neuromuscular, musculoskeletal or arthritic conditions that
Acute myocarditis, pericarditis or endocarditis	preclude exercise
Dissecting aortic aneurysm	Other systemic conditions that would make exercise difficult
Recent pulmonary or systemic emboli	
Resting blood pressure >200/>120 mmHg	
Acute thrombophlebitis	

Adapted from Fardy PS, Yanowitz FG. *Cardiac Rehabilitation, Adult Fitness, and Exercise Testing*. Baltimore, MD: Williams & Wilkins, 1995: 156–244.

Table 45.9 End points for exercise testing

Patient-determined end points	Physician-determined end points	Protocol end points (submaximal tests)
Patient wants to stop	Patient appears unwell (e.g. ataxia, confusion, pallor)	Heart rate determined (e.g. 120 beats/min)
Significant chest discomfort	ECG end points: marked ST segment depression or elevation; new bundle branch block or atrioventricular junctional heart block; ventricular tachycardia or fibrillation; increasing frequency of premature ventricular complexes; supraventricular tachyarrhythmias	Workload determined (e.g. 5 metabolic equivalents)
Marked fatigue	Exertional hypotension (systolic BP falls below standing BP)	
Severe dyspnea	Systolic BP >250 mmHg	
Other limiting symptoms (e.g. dizziness, leg cramps, joint discomfort)	Diastolic BP >120 mmHg	
	Equipment failure	

BP = blood pressure.
Adapted from Fardy PS, Yanowitz FG. *Cardiac Rehabilitation, Adult Fitness, and Exercise Testing*. Baltimore, MD: Williams & Wilkins, 1995: 156–244.

risk factors, and those with known disease) undergo exercise stress testing before starting a *vigorous* exercise program.[35] However, the American College of Cardiology and the American Heart Association suggest that the use of screening exercise tests is not well established by evidence, and that the tests are a poor predictor of the major cardiac complications (myocardial infarction and sudden cardiac death) during exercise.[36] Routine exercise testing has not been shown to prevent exercise-related acute cardiac events and also yields a significant number of false-positive tests. A true positive exercise test requires the presence of a pre-existing hemodynamically significant coronary obstruction, whereas acute coronary events often involve plaque rupture and thrombosis at the site of previously unobstructive atherosclerotic plaque.[37] It is very rare for this to occur during *moderate intensity* activities such as brisk walking.

Thallium studies

Thallium-201 is the radionuclide most commonly used for the evaluation of myocardial perfusion. The radiolabeled substance is injected intravenously and accumulates in viable myocardial cells in proportion to myocardial blood flow. Areas of myocardium that are poorly vascularized take up less thallium and appear as relative defects. Over a period of hours, thallium washes out of cells with normal perfusion. Thus, defects that improve over time suggest reversible ischemia, whereas defects that persist suggest a non-viable myocardium (e.g. infarction).[33]

Radionuclide ventriculography

Radionuclide ventriculography, or 'gated cardiac blood pool scan', examines global and segmental cardiac function. The term 'gated' refers to the concept of collecting a series of images and using the ECG rhythm to superimpose all of the images at comparable times during the sequence of systole and diastole. The test can be used to calculate ejection fractions, volumes and filling rates. To obtain a more sensitive test of myocardial function, patients can be asked to exercise supine on a bicycle ergometer while undergoing this test. When the myocardium is diseased, wall motion abnormality will increase with exercise and the ejection fraction will decrease, rather than increase.

Holter monitors and event recorders

The most commonly used long-term ECG recording system is the Holter monitor, which is generally worn for 24 or 48 hours to record a continuous ECG. The ECG is then analyzed by an automated system that prints out selected strips for physician interpretation. Event recorders operate in a similar fashion but require the patient to trigger the recording.

Electrophysiological studies

Electrophysiological studies are performed by a cardiologist placing an electrode catheter via venous access into various intracardiac sites. The catheters record intracardiac electrograms and can deliver paced beats to induce arrhythmias if indicated. This approach is most likely to be used in the athletic individual to assess syncope but the diagnostic yield is only a small, but important, 10%. Given the invasive nature of these tests, electrophysiological studies are only indicated when patients have clear symptoms and remain undiagnosed after a comprehensive non-invasive assessment.

Prevention of sudden death

Screening asymptomatic patients under the age of 35 years for the presence of congenital heart disease cannot be justified. Theoretically, to prevent one sudden death in this group, it would be necessary to screen approximately 20 000 people.[28, 38] Therefore, screening must be selective (Chapter 56).

The American Heart Association focuses on the identification of historical and physical features associated with increased risk of sudden death.[39] These are shown in Table 45.10.

Brent Rich has suggested that the following clinical findings warrant referral to a cardiologist:[40]

- new systolic murmur greater than 3/6 intensity
- diastolic murmur
- sudden cardiac death in a first-degree relative
- exercise-induced or unexplained syncope, dyspnea or chest pain
- new onset arrhythmias
- first-degree relative with hypertrophic cardiomyopathy, Marfan's syndrome or unexplained cardiomyopathy
- significant family history of coronary artery disease
- prolonged recovery from viral or systemic disease
- exercise prescription for a sedentary individual with two or more cardiac risk factors.

It could be argued that following this recommendation will lead to a large number of referrals but we agree that if the practitioner has any doubt whatsoever when managing cardiac problems in athletes, over-referral is far preferable to under-referral.

Table 45.10 American Heart Association recommendations for pre-participation screening

Personal history
Exertional chest pain
Heart murmur
Easily fatigued
Syncope
Exertional dyspnea
Systemic hypertension
Family history
Premature sudden death
Heart disease in close relatives younger than 50 years of age
Physical examination
Heart murmur
Femoral pulses
Stigmata of Marfan's syndrome
Blood pressure measurement

Recommended Reading

Beckerman J, Wang P, Hlatky M. Cardiovascular screening of athletes. *Clin J Sport Med* 2004; 14(3): 127–33.

Crawford MH. Choosing the appropriate stress modality. A clinical cardiologist's perspective. *Cardiol Clin* 1999; 17: 597–606.

Kane SF, Oriscello RG, Wenzel RB. Electrocardiographic findings in sports medicine: normal variants and the ones that should not be missed. *Curr Sports Med Rep* 2005; 4: 68–75.

Maron BJ. Hypertrophic cardiomyopathy. Practical steps for preventing sudden death. *Physician Sportsmed* 2002; 30(1): 19–24.

Rich BSE, Havens SA. The athletic heart syndrome. *Curr Sports Med Rep* 2004; 3: 84–8.

Rizvi AA, Thompson PD. Hypertrophic cardiomyopathy: who plays and who sits. *Curr Sports Med Rep* 2002; 1: 93–9.

Robinson K. *Preventive Cardiology: A Guide for Clinical Practise.* Armonk, NY: Futura Publishing, 1998.

Rowland TW. Evaluating cardiac symptoms in the athlete. Is it safe to play? *Clin J Sport Med* 2005; 15(6): 417–20.

Thompson PD. Cardiovascular risks of exercise. Avoiding sudden death and myocardial infarction. *Physician Sportsmed* 2002; 29(4): 33–47.

Thompson P, Estes NA. Athlete's heart. In: Topol EJ, Califf RM, Isner J, et al., eds. *Textbook of Cardiovascular Medicine.* 2nd edn. Philadelphia: Lippincott Williams & Wilkins, 2002.

Vasamreddy CR, Ahmed D, Gluckman TY, et al. Cardiovascular disease in athletes. *Clin Sports Med* 2004; 23: 455–71.

Wen DY. Preparticipation cardiovascular screening of young athletes. An epidemiologic perspective. *Physician Sportsmed* 2004; 32(6): 23–30.

Wike J, Kernan M. Sudden cardiac death in the active adult: causes, screening and preventive strategies. *Curr Sports Med Rep* 2005; 4: 76–82.

References

1. American Heart Association. *Heart and Stroke Facts.* Dallas, TX: AHA Publication, 1992.

2. Montgomery H, Woods D. High intensity training and the heart. *Hosp Med* 1999; 60: 187–91.

3. Pluim BM, Zwinderman AH, van der Laarse A, et al. The athlete's heart. A meta-analysis of cardiac structure and function. *Circulation* 2000; 101: 336–44.

4. Pollock ML, Franklin BA, Balady GJ, et al. AHA Science Advisory. Resistance exercise in individuals with and without cardiovascular disease: benefits, rationale, safety, and prescription. An advisory from the Committee on Exercise, Rehabilitation, and Prevention, Council on Clinical Cardiology, American Heart Association: position paper endorsed by the American College of Sports Medicine. *Circulation* 2000; 101: 828–33.

5. Zehender M, Meinertz T, Keul J, et al. ECG variants and cardiac arrhythmias in athletes: clinical relevance and prognostic importance. *Am Heart J* 1990; 119: 1378–91.

6. Maron BJ, Isner JM, McKenna WJ. 26th Bethesda conference: recommendations for determining eligibility for competition in athletes with cardiovascular abnormalities. Task Force 3: hypertrophic cardiomyopathy, myocarditis and other myopericardial diseases and mitral valve prolapse. *J Am Coll Cardiol* 1994; 24: 880–5.

7. American Academy of Pediatrics. Cardiac dysrhythmias and sports. American Academy of Pediatrics Committee on Sports Medicine and Fitness. *Pediatrics* 1995; 95: 786–8.

8. Noakes TD. Why marathon runners collapse. *S Afr Med J* 1988; 73: 569–71.

9. Holtzhausen LM, Noakes TD. Collapsed ultraendurance athlete: proposed mechanisms and an approach to management. *Clin J Sport Med* 1997; 7: 292–301.

10. Martin JB, Ruskin J. Faintness, syncope, and seizures. In: Isselbacher KJ, Braunwald E, Wilson JD, et al., eds. *Harrison's Principles of Internal Medicine.* 13th edn. New York: McGraw-Hill, 1994: 90–6.

11. Lewis WR, Amsterdam EA. Chest pain emergency units. *Curr Opin Cardiol* 1999; 14: 321–8.

12. Maron BJ. Sudden death in young athletes. Lessons from the Hank Gathers affair. *N Engl J Med* 1993; 329: 55–7.

13. Garson A, Jr. Arrhythmias and sudden cardiac death in elite athletes. American College of Cardiology, 16th Bethesda Conference. *Pediatr Med Chir* 1998; 20: 101–3.

14. Wilson PWF. Physical activity and coronary heart disease. In: Robinson K, ed. *Preventive Cardiology: A Guide for Clinical Practise.* Armonk, NY: Futura Publishing, 1998: 51–67.

15. Blair SN, Kampert JB, Kohl HW, et al. Influences of cardiorespiratory fitness and other precursors on cardiovascular disease and all-cause mortality in men and women. *JAMA* 1996; 276: 205–10.

16. Morrey MA, Hensrud DD. Risk of medical events in a supervised health and fitness facility. *Med Sci Sports Exerc* 1999; 31: 1233–6.

17. Maron BJ, Shirani J, Poliac L, et al. Sudden death in young competitive athletes. Clinical, demographic, and pathological profiles. *JAMA* 1996; 276(3): 199–204.

18. Maron BJ. Hypertrophic cardiomyopathy. Practical steps for preventing sudden death. *Physician Sportsmed* 2002; 30(1): 19–24.

19. Maron BJ, Shen WK, Poliac LC, et al. Efficacy of implantable cardioconverter-defibrillators for the

prevention of sudden death in patients with hypertrophic cardiomyopathy. *N Engl J Med* 2000; 342(6): 365–72.

20. Salim MA, Alpert BS. Sports and Marfan syndrome. *Physician Sportsmed* 2001; 29(5): 80–93.

21. Glorioso J, Reeves M. Marfan syndrome: screening for sudden death in athletes. *Curr Sports Med Rep* 2002; 1: 67–74.

22. Corrado D, Basso C, Thiene G. Arrhythmogenic right ventricular cardiomyopathy: diagnosis, prognosis, and treatment. *Heart* 2000; 83: 588–95.

23. Bresler MJ. Acute pericarditis and myocarditis. *Emerg Med J* 1992; 24: 36–51.

24. Schulze-Bahr E, Monnig G, Eckardt L, et al. The long QT syndrome: considerations in the athletic population. *Curr Sports Med Rep* 2003; 2: 72–8.

25. Vasamreddy CR, Ahmed D, Gluckman TY, et al. Cardiovascular disease in athletes. *Clin Sports Med* 2004; 23: 455–71.

26. Cheitlin MD, Douglas PS, Parmley WW. 26th Bethesda conference: recommendations for determining eligibility for competition in athletes with cardiovascular abnormalities. Task Force 2: acquired valvular heart disease. *Med Sci Sports Exerc* 1994; 26(suppl.): S254–S260.

27. Maron BJ, Isner JM, McKenna WJ. Hypertrophic cardiomyopathy, myocarditis, and other myopericardial diseases and mitral valve prolapse. *Med Sci Sports Exerc* 1994; 26(suppl.): S261–S267.

28. Epstein SE. Sudden death and the competitive athlete. *J Am Coll Cardiol* 1986; 7: 220–30.

29. Lateef F. Commotio cordis: an underappreciated cause of sudden death in athletes. *Sports Med* 2000; 30: 301–8.

30. Armstrong GP, Griffin BP. Exercise echocardiographic assessment in severe mitral regurgitation. *Coron Artery Dis* 2000; 11: 23–30.

31. Ketteler T, Krahwinkel W, Godke J, et al. Stress

echocardiography: personnel and technical equipment. *Eur Heart J* 1997; 18(suppl. D): D43–D48.

32. Fardy PS, Yanowitz FG. *Cardiac Rehabilitation, Adult Fitness, and Exercise Testing.* Baltimore, MD: Williams & Wilkins, 1995: 156–244.

33. Gibson RS. The diagnostic and prognostic value of exercise electrocardiography in asymptomatic subjects and stable symptomatic patients. *Curr Opin Cardiol* 1991; 6: 536–46.

34. Brukner P, Brown W. Is exercise good for you? *Med J Aust* 2005; 183(10): 538–41.

35. Mahler DA, Froelicher VF, Miller NH. Health screening and risk satisfaction. In: Kenney WL, Humphrey RH, Bryant CX, eds. *ACSM's Guidelines for Exercise Testing and Prescription.* 5th edn. Philadelphia: Lippincott Williams & Wilkins, 1995: 12–26.

36. Gibbons RJ, Balady GJ, Beasley JW. ACC/AHA guidelines for exercise testing. *J Am Coll Cardiol* 1997; 30(11): 260–311.

37. Little WC, Constantinescu M, Applegate RJ, et al. Can coronary angiography predict the site of a subsequent myocardial infarction in patients with mild-to-moderate coronary artery disease? *Circulation* 1988; 78: 1157–66.

38. Lewis JF, Maron BJ, Diggs JA, et al. Preparticipation echocardiographic screening for cardiovascular disease in a large, predominantly black population of collegiate athletes. *Am J Cardiol* 1989; 64: 1029–33.

39. Maron BJ, Thompson PD, Puffer JC, et al. Cardiovascular pre-participation screening of competitive athletes. A statement for health professionals from the Sudden Death Committee (clinical cardiology) and Congenital Cardiac Defects Committee (cardiovascular disease in the young), American Heart Association. *Circulation* 1996; 94(4): 850–6.

40. Rich BS. Sudden death screening. *Med Clin North Am* 1994; 78: 267–88.

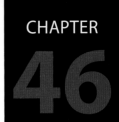
Respiratory Symptoms During Exercise

WITH KAREN HOLZER

The normal functioning of the respiratory system is critical to athletic performance. The integrity of this system results in the delivery of oxygen to the blood (and subsequently to exercising muscles) and the elimination of waste products such as carbon dioxide. Any dysfunction of these processes results in impaired performance. A number of medical conditions such as asthma and respiratory infections may affect performance.

Common respiratory symptoms

There are a number of symptoms with which an athlete may present that indicate the presence of respiratory disease. These include:

- shortness of breath (dyspnea)
- wheeze
- cough
- chest pain or tightness.

Shortness of breath and wheeze

Some degree of breathlessness (dyspnea) is a normal physiological response to exercise. Often occurring during intense exercise, it may represent the reaching of maximal exercise and ventilatory capacity. However, an individual complaining of excessive shortness of breath, chest tightness and/or wheezing, particularly during rest or low-intensity exercise, may be suffering from a respiratory or cardiac condition.

Breathlessness is a subjective symptom that can be defined as an increased difficulty in breathing. Despite the frequency of this complaint, the exact physiological mechanism is unknown. The most important cause

from an athletic point of view is asthma (exercise-induced bronchospasm [EIB]), which is discussed on page 821. In the older athlete, especially with a history of smoking, chronic obstructive pulmonary disease (COPD) or cardiac ischemia should be considered. Dyspnea may be classified clinically as acute, chronic or intermittent (see box).

Causes of dyspnea in athletes
Acute
Asthma
Cardiac
Infections
Spontaneous pneumothorax
Pulmonary embolism (rare)
Aspiration of foreign body (can occur in athletes with dental prosthesis or those who chew gum)
Chronic
Asthma
COPD
Cardiac dysfunction—cardiac failure, ischemia, valvular
Anemia
Metabolic disorders (e.g. diabetes mellitus)
Pulmonary dysfunction
Obesity
Intermittent
Asthma (most likely)
Left ventricular dysfunction
Mitral stenosis
Psychological

Examination of the patient together with the history of the dyspnea may indicate the likely cause of the dyspnea. It is important to remember that examination of both the patient with EIB or cardiac ischemia may be normal at rest.

Respiratory function tests (e.g. spirometry) are required to further assess dyspnea. Spirometry pre and post bronchodilator should be performed, and if required a bronchial provocation challenge test performed. If a cardiac cause is suspected, an exercise ECG/EKG and echocardiogram are required. A chest X-ray is essential to assess for a respiratory tract infection, cardiac failure, carcinoma, COPD and a pneumothorax. Blood tests, in particular the hemoglobin level and iron studies, may be required to exclude anemia or severe iron deficiency. Gastroscopy may be required to assess for gastroesophageal reflux. Psychological factors, such as anxiety, are considered once other diagnoses are excluded and may require further assessment.

Cough

Coughing is such a common symptom that its presence and severity may be underestimated by both patients and clinicians. From the clinical history it is important to determine the nature of the cough, whether the cough is acute or chronic, productive or non-productive, as well as the nature and color of any sputum. The timing of the cough, whether it occurs during the day or night and whether it occurs before or after exercise, is important. Any associated disease such as sinusitis or gastroesophageal reflux should also be noted. It is important to establish whether the patient is or has been a smoker or exposed to passive smoking.

From this clinical history the etiology of the cough may be established. A guide to the causes of acute and chronic cough is shown in Table 46.1.

The treatment of cough is more likely to succeed if a specific diagnosis is made and treated appropriately. The treatment of asthma and respiratory tract infections are discussed on pages 823 and 869. Non-specific treatment for cough (e.g. pholcodine, 10 mg 6 hourly) may be helpful when the symptoms are distressing. Perhaps more effective than any medication is an adequate explanation and reassurance when appropriate.

Chest pain or tightness

When considering respiratory symptoms, chest pain or tightness is not usually considered; however, many people with asthma may present with a

Table 46.1 Causes of cough

Acute	Chronic
Upper respiratory tract infection	Post-nasal drip
Asthma	Asthma
Bronchitis	Chronic bronchitis
Bronchogenic carcinoma	Gastroesophageal reflux
Foreign body inhalation	Post-infective cough
Left ventricular failure	Psychogenic
	Carcinoma
	Interstitial lung disease
	Benign tumors of the lung
	Drugs (e.g. ACE inhibitors)

ACE = angiotensin-converting enzyme.

subjective feeling of chest tightness alone. As well as the respiratory causes of chest tightness, there are other important and even life-threatening causes of chest tightness, such as cardiac ischemia. Hence, this symptom must be investigated appropriately.

The causes of chest pain are set out in Table 46.2. Successful treatment depends upon the correct diagnosis being made. Prompt investigation of patients with this symptom is essential because of a number of potentially life-threatening causes.

Investigation of the athlete with chest pain or tightness is very similar to that of the athlete with dyspnea, as mentioned above, and may include chest X-ray, spirometry, bronchial provocation challenge tests, exercise ECG/EKG, echocardiogram, blood tests or gastroscopy. The investigations should be guided by the history and examination findings.

Asthma

Asthma is a chronic inflammatory disorder of the airways in which many inflammatory cells and cellular elements play a role, in particular, mast cells, eosinophils, T lymphocytes, macrophages, neutrophils

Table 46.2 Causes of chest pain or tightness in the athlete

Common causes	Conditions not to be missed
Asthma	Cardiac ischemia
Exercise-induced bronchoconstriction	Carcinoma
Infection	Interstitial lung disease
Chest wall injuries	Herpes zoster (shingles)
Referred pain from thoracic spine	

and epithelial cells. In susceptible individuals, this inflammation causes recurrent episodes of widespread but variable airflow obstruction that is usually reversible, either spontaneously or with treatment. The inflammation also causes an increase in existing bronchial hyperresponsiveness to a variety of stimuli. Common stimuli or triggers include upper respiratory tract infections, cigarette smoke, exercise, inhaled allergens (e.g. dust mite, pollens), emotional triggers (e.g. stress, laughter), changes in temperature and weather, and environmental factors (e.g. dust, bush fires, pollution).

Epidemiology

The incidence and prevalence of asthma reported depends on the age of the population studied, the nature of the population and the criteria used for diagnosis. Asthma is more prevalent in developed countries, and it is thought by some that the 'clean' lifestyle in these countries may contribute. Although 20–30% of people have experienced wheezing in the last 12 months, this is usually transient in response to a viral infection. Australia has the second highest prevalence of current established asthma in the world, with a prevalence of 12%. New Zealand has the highest prevalence at 15%, while in the United Kingdom and the United States the prevalences are 9% and 7% respectively. In Australia, 1 in 4 children, 1 in 7 adolescents and 1 in 10 adults have current established asthma. Asthma is more common in children than adults, with over half the cases developing in childhood and another third before the age of 40. Genetic factors are thought to play a role.

Clinical features

The characteristic symptoms of asthma are:

1. cough—dry, irritating and persistent, often worse in the early morning or late at night
2. wheeze
3. shortness of breath
4. chest tightness.

However, since the degree of airway narrowing and obstruction varies with the condition and treatment, the symptoms can also vary from being absent, to low grade and occasional through to severe and persistent. The symptoms are usually reversible, either spontaneously or with treatment.

 The absence of a wheeze does not exclude the diagnosis of exercise-induced bronchoconstriction.

Types of asthma

Historically, a distinction was made between intrinsic (non-allergic) and extrinsic (allergic) asthma in the International Disease Classification. This distinction is now rarely applied as it has been shown that the two types of asthma share many of the same pathological features.

Most existing guidelines classify patients with asthma as having intermittent or persistent asthma based on the severity of asthma, as determined by the patient's symptoms and spirometry before treatment is commenced. Importantly, the classification may change with time and a severe episode of asthma may occur in any of the groups.[1] The current classification of asthma is outlined below.

1. Mild intermittent asthma:
   - Symptoms occur less than twice a week and are not present between asthma episodes
   - Asthma episodes are brief (few hours to a few days) and may vary from mild to severe
   - Night-time symptoms occur less than twice a month
   - Spirometry when not having an asthma episode is 80% or greater than predicted, and the peak expiratory flow rate (PEFR) varies little from morning to afternoons
2. Mild persistent asthma:
   - Symptoms occur more than twice a week but less than once a day
   - Asthma episodes interfere with daily activities
   - Night-time symptoms occur more than twice a month
   - Spirometry when not having an asthma episode is 80% or greater than predicted, and the PEFR varies little from morning to afternoons
3. Moderate persistent asthma:
   - Symptoms occur daily and inhaled short-acting asthma medications are used every day
   - Episodes interfere with daily activities, and occur more than twice a week and last for days
   - Night-time symptoms occur more than once a week
   - Spirometry is abnormal, and is more than 60% but less than 80% of predicted value; the PEFR varies more than 30% between morning and afternoon readings
4. Severe persistent asthma:
   - Symptoms occur all the time during the day

- Daily physical activities are limited
- Asthma episodes occur frequently
- Night-time symptoms occur frequently
- Spirometry is abnormal and less than or equal to 60% of predicted value; the PEFR varies more than 30% between morning and afternoon readings

Precipitating factors

Airway inflammation appears to be an important factor leading to the development of increased airway reactivity. A series of immunological and cellular events occurs in response to airway 'triggers'. Mast cell degranulation occurs, resulting in the release of a number of mediators such as histamine, prostaglandins, leukotrienes and cytokines, with a subsequent influx of inflammatory cells into the airways. As a consequence, inflammation of the airways results, with mucosal edema due to the increased permeability of the airway epithelium, mucus production, and contraction of the airway smooth muscle, the cumulative result being narrowing of the airways, which is the pathophysiological hallmark of asthma. Neurological factors, possibly mediated by the autonomic nervous system via the action of neuropeptides, have also been shown to play a role. This bronchial hyperreactivity may persist and become permanent.

Bronchial hyperreactivity may occur in response to specific stimuli, such as house dust mite (*Dermatophagoides pteronyssinus*) or fungal spores (e.g. *Aspergillus fumigatus*). It may also occur in response to non-specific stimuli such as cold, dust, smoke and exercise. The role of food allergy in asthma remains controversial. Food intolerance does not necessarily indicate an allergic mechanism. Most cases of asthma induced by specific food intolerance are evident from a carefully taken history, so elaborate exclusive diets are not warranted and have generally been disappointing. Skin prick tests and radioallergosorbent tests (RAST) may be helpful in confirming the patient's atopic status and also in establishing certain allergies (e.g. to house dust mite) but have no role in the diagnosis of 'food allergies'.

Drugs may be implicated in the production of asthma, especially beta-blocking agents and prostaglandin inhibitors such as aspirin (ASA) and NSAIDs. Occasionally, drugs used to treat asthma such as ipratropium bromide have been responsible for provoking bronchoconstriction.

Psychological factors also can induce asthmatic episodes, although they do not produce asthma in subjects without underlying airway reactivity. Therefore, stress and emotional disturbance need to be taken into account in the overall management of asthmatic patients.

Risk factors

The main risk factors for the development of and worsening of asthma are:

1. *Genetic predisposition.* Atopy is characterized by the body's production of immunoglobulin E (IgE) after exposure to common environmental allergens. A person with high levels of IgE in the blood is more likely to have an allergic response when exposed to certain allergens in the environment. If a person has a parent with asthma, he or she is three to six times more likely to develop asthma.
2. *Environmental exposures.* The US Institute of Medicine[2] studied components in the environment that affected both the development of asthma and the exacerbation of the symptoms in someone who already has the disease. These are outlined below.
   (a) Causal relationship between exposure to and the *development of asthma* in susceptible children in regards to:
      - house dust mite
      - environmental tobacco smoke—both prenatal exposure to maternal smoking and environmental exposure after birth
      - cockroach allergen
      - respiratory syncytial virus
   (b) Four exposures are considered causes of *asthma exacerbations*:
      - cat
      - cockroach
      - house dust mite
      - environmental tobacco smoke
   (c) Four additional exposures are associated with *worsening of the disease*:
      - dog allergen
      - fungi or moulds
      - rhinoviruses
      - high level of nitrous oxides

Asthma management

The general principles of asthma management are listed below.

1. Asthma is an inflammatory disease and treatment should be primarily directed against this inflammatory component.
2. Bronchodilators should be used for the relief of symptoms only. Increased use of

bronchodilators indicates the need for increased anti-inflammatory treatment.

3. Recognition of symptoms and objective assessment of airflow obstruction by regular peak flow rate measurements are essential for optimal asthma management.

4. The patient must take responsibility for the initial assessment and treatment of worsening asthma through the use of a predetermined self-management plan.

The assessment of the severity of an asthma attack may be affected by the speed of onset of the attack. In some cases, severe episodes can occur within minutes with little or no warning. All patients should be educated to respond appropriately if they fail to obtain relief from their usual treatment or if peak flow rates fall significantly.

The patient's inability to assess and appreciate the severity of an asthma attack can result in a delay in commencing appropriate treatment. This occurs because patients determine the severity of their asthma by symptoms alone. Symptoms are a poor indicator of severity. Patients can assess airway function themselves on a regular basis with the use of a peak flow meter (Fig. 46.1).

While it is impossible to lay down strict criteria for hospital admission, the severity of the attack and the previous history of response to treatment are the main guides. Continued observation is essential once admitted.

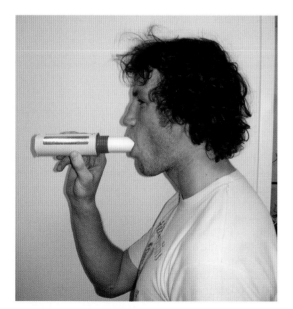

Figure 46.1 Peak flow meter

Exercise-induced bronchospasm

Exercise-induced asthma (EIA) or exercise-induced bronchospasm (EIB) is described as a transitory increase in airway resistance that occurs following vigorous exercise.[3]

Epidemiology

Although EIB occurs mainly in those with clinically recognized asthma—in 80% of asthmatics not taking inhaled corticosteroids and in 50% of those that do—it has also recently been documented in healthy asymptomatic persons. Such studies include those performed in schoolchildren, defense force recruits, highly trained athletes and skaters. In one study performed, 10% of Australian schoolchildren with no suggestive history of asthma were found to have EIB.[4] The prevalence of EIB in the total Australian population is thought to be 12%, with equal distribution in both sexes. In elite athletes the prevalence has also been shown to be significant.

The prevalence of EIB in elite athletes has progressively increased over the years. In the 1976 and 1980 Summer Olympic games, 9.7% and 8.5% respectively of the Australian Olympic athletes reported asthma in a physical examination.[5] However, in the 2000 Australian Summer Olympic team 21% of the athletes reported asthma or EIB.[6] Similarly, in the 1984 US Summer Olympic team, 11% reported on a medical history that they had asthma,[7] whereas in the 1996 Summer Olympic Games, 17% of the athletes had asthma, as defined by athlete-reported use of medication and/or previous diagnosis of asthma by a physician.[8] A similar high prevalence of EIB was seen in the 1998 US Winter Olympic team; 22% had asthma defined as athlete-reported use of asthma medication and/or previous diagnosis of asthma by a physician.[9] The occurrence of asthma was highest in athletes performing in endurance sports, such as cycling, running, rowing and triathlons, in swimming and in winter sports such as cross-country skiing and figure skating.

Pathophysiology

In most cases, bronchoconstriction does not occur during the first few minutes of exercise but rather begins during the first few minutes of recovery. Two separate theories have been proposed to explain how the airway is protected from bronchoconstriction during exercise but is susceptible after exercise. In both theories, the primary stimulus for bronchoconstriction is the evaporation of water lining the airways secondary to the increased level of ventilation.

Gilbert and McFadden have suggested that airway cooling during exercise and subsequent warming, with reactive hyperemia of the airway tissues after exercise, is responsible for the major component of the post-exercise bronchoconstriction.[10] In an alternative hypothesis, the osmotic hypothesis, Anderson has suggested that it is the increased osmolarity of the airway tissues subsequent to the evaporation of water that occurs with hyperventilation that results in mast cell degranulation and the release of bronchoconstrictor mediators.[11]

Over recent years the osmotic hypothesis has gained popularity as a number of subsequent studies have shown that it is changes in the inspired air water content but not temperature during exercise and recovery that modify the magnitude of EIA.[12, 13] Furthermore, bronchoconstriction may be induced by inhaling hypotonic and hypertonic aerosols of saline solution, dextrose and urea.[14–16]

The protection against bronchoconstriction throughout the exercise period has been attributed to the bronchodilating effect of circulating catecholamines;[17] however, this explanation fails to account for why the bronchoconstriction associated with eucapnic voluntary hyperpnoea (EVH) is often delayed until ventilation returns to normal. In an alternative explanation, it is thought that the increased tidal volume during exercise exerts a protective effect on the airways, similar to the bronchodilating effects of a single deep inspiration.

Etiology

The actual etiology of EIB in elite athletes appears to vary depending on the type of sport that the athlete is involved in and regularly performs. EIB is thought to develop as a consequence of injury to the airways secondary to exposure of the airways to large volumes of cold air, allergens, pollens, pollutants, smoke or dust. Elite athletes may increase their ventilation during intense exercise to up to 200 L/min, and thus the load of such substances delivered to the airways may be extremely large.

In summer athletes it has been proposed that exposure to and inhalation of allergens play a major role in the development of EIB,[18–21] in winter athletes, inhalation of cold air[22] and in swimmers, inhalation of the gases of chlorine and its metabolites, which form a layer on the water surface of all pools.[23]

Clinical features

During exercise, flow rates and volumes actually improve in many subjects, in both those with and without EIB. When exercise is continued for 6–8 minutes, the flow rates begin to fall in those with EIB. The lowest rates are usually, but not always, observed 5–12 minutes following exercise cessation. It is the falling flow rates and volumes that is characteristic of the 'asthmatic response'.

Siblings of asthmatics, hay fever sufferers and patients with cystic fibrosis may also increase their flow rates during exercise, but only those with EIB show a reduction in excess of 10% after cessation of exercise.[24] When establishing a history of EIB, it is important to confirm that the patient had symptoms after exercise ceased, not only during exercise.

Most athletes with mild EIB recover spontaneously within minutes or soon after treatment with a bronchodilator; however, more severe bronchoconstriction may persist for up to an hour without treatment. In 50% of athletes who suffer from EIB, there is a period after an episode of bronchoconstriction where further exercise is followed by either less severe or no bronchoconstriction at all. This 'refractory period' may persist for up to 4 hours following the initial episode of EIB.

Diagnosis

A clinical suspicion of EIB may be indicated by symptoms of:

- shortness of breath
- chest tightness
- wheeze
- a dry cough post exercise
- poor performance
- fatigue.

Often the symptoms are made worse when exercising during the pollen season, indoors or in the cold air. A firm diagnosis of EIB, however, cannot be made on symptoms alone as these have been shown to be poor indicators of EIB. A number of studies have shown that a diagnosis based purely on a history of exercise-related respiratory symptoms has a high level of misdiagnosis, both over- and under-diagnosis.[25, 26] Diagnosis thus depends on demonstrating a deterioration in lung function, in particular the forced expiratory volume in 1 second (FEV_1), measured by lung spirometry (Figs 46.2, 46.3) following a recognized bronchial provocation challenge test. Previously, reductions in PEFR or forced expiratory flow (FEF_{25-75}) were also accepted,

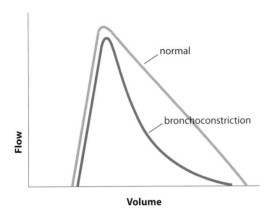

Figure 46.2 Flow volume graph showing normal and bronchconstriction pattern

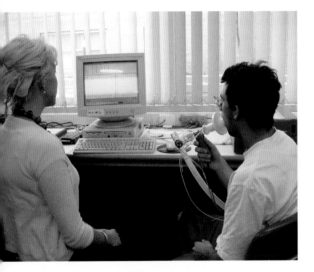

Figure 46.3 Lung spirometry

but these are now discouraged due to problems with reliability and reproducibility.

Over recent years the accurate diagnosis of asthma or EIB has become crucial in elite athletes. The International Olympic Committee-Medical Commission (IOC-MC) and other major sporting bodies require objective evidence of asthma or EIB for athletes to be permitted to use asthma medications, in particular both short- and long-acting inhaled beta-2 agonists. Furthermore, the World Anti-Drug Agency (WADA) requires that abbreviated Therapeutic Use Exemption forms (TUEs) be submitted for a number of commonly used asthma medications, including inhaled beta-2 agonists and inhaled corticosteroids for all athletes at state level or above.

Bronchial provocation challenge tests

The challenge tests are classified as being either direct or indirect.

Direct challenge tests

Direct challenge tests, otherwise known as the pharmacological challenge tests, involve the administration of increasing doses of a drug, usually histamine or methacholine, which acts directly on the airway smooth muscle receptors to elicit bronchoconstriction. The main problem with this type of challenge test is that although they have a high sensitivity for detecting bronchial hyperresponsiveness, they have a low specificity for EIB, as both healthy subjects and those with other lung diseases may also have a positive response. Another disadvantage is that direct challenge tests, in contrast to indirect challenge tests, cannot be used to assess the response of a patient to treatment.

Indirect challenge tests

Indirect challenge tests act indirectly by provoking mast cell degranulation and thus the release of mediators, which then act on the receptors to elicit narrowing of the airways. They have been found to have both a high sensitivity and specificity for EIB.

1. *Exercise challenge test*. This involves exercising the patient on the exercise bike or treadmill for a minimum of 4 minutes, but preferably for up to 8 minutes, at an intensity sufficient to raise ventilation to approximately 50% of the predicted maximum voluntary ventilation for the duration of the exercise. This test has the disadvantage that in elite athletes a sufficient level of ventilation cannot be achieved.[27]

2. *Eucapnic voluntary hyperpnea challenge test* (Fig. 46.4). This test requires the voluntary hyperventilation of dry air containing 4.9% carbon dioxide. One of two protocols may be used. The progressive protocol involves the patient ventilating at each of 30%, 60% and 90% of his or her maximum voluntary ventilation for a period of 3 minutes. The steady state protocol involves the patient ventilating at 80% maximum voluntary ventilation for 6 minutes. The progressive protocol is recommended for clinically recognized asthmatics, while the steady state protocol is recommended for asymptomatic subjects, elite athletes, defense force recruits and persons with no recent history of asthma or in those in whom no airway narrowing was elicited in the progressive

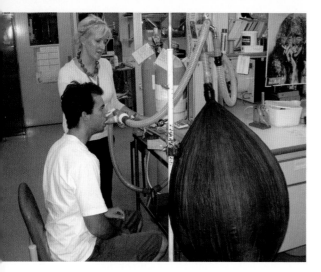

Figure 46.4 Eucapnic voluntary hyperpnoea challenge test

protocol. This challenge test is the current gold standard for the diagnosis of EIB.[27, 28]

3. *Hyperosmolar saline challenge test.* This test requires the administration of increasing doses of inhaled 4.5% saline, which is thought to increase the osmolarity of the airways and, in susceptible individuals, leads to mast cell degranulation and release of mediators. These mediators then act to provoke airway narrowing. After each dose of saline, measurements of lung function are recorded. The test is aborted when the lung function falls by greater than 15% from pre-testing levels or when the full dose of 22 mL is reached. The response is said to be mild when the dose causing a fall of 15% is greater than 6 mL, moderate at 2.1–6.0 mL and severe at less than 2 mL. This test is particularly valuable for assessing a subject's suitability for scuba diving.[27]

4. *Mannitol challenge test.* Similar to the hyperosmolar challenge test, this test requires the administration of doubling doses of inhaled mannitol, which acts to increase the osmolarity of the airways, thus leading to mast cell degranulation and subsequent airway narrowing in those with bronchial hyperresponsiveness. Again after each dose, airway function is measured. The test is continued until a greater than 15% fall in lung function occurs or a cumulative dose of 635 mg of mannitol is given This test has been shown to have a high sensitivity and specificity for the diagnosis of EIB in athletes.[29] This test has the advantages of

not being laboratory dependent, unlike those above, being safe, not time consuming and inexpensive.[30] It is currently available only in specialized centers.

Each of the above challenge tests involves the measurement of lung function, in particular the FEV_1, PEFR or FEF_{25-75} for up to 20 minutes following the challenge. The FEV_1 is the most sensitive and reliable measure of lung function, and is universally accepted. The FEF_{25-75}, which measures the flow through the mid portions of the vital capacity, was previously considered important in the diagnosis of EIB; however, similar to the PEFR, it has been shown to have high variability and to be dependent on the vital capacity, which can change from pre to post exercise. Thus, the diagnosis of EIB based on changes in the PEFR or FEF_{25-75} is neither recommended nor accepted by major sporting bodies. Depending on the type of challenge test, the accepted fall in the FEV_1 for a positive challenge varies from 10% to 20% and must occur within a specified period following the administration of the challenge dose, or within a specific cumulative dose of administered agent. The IOC-MC accepts a fall of 10% in FEV_1 from baseline for the EVH and exercise challenge tests, both in the field and laboratory, of 15% for the hypertonic saline challenge test and of 20% for the methacholine challenge test (Table 46.3).

It is important on the day of testing that patients not undertake any form of exercise prior to the challenge, and that they withhold their usual asthmatic medication, the duration depending on the type of medication.

The severity of the EIB can be assessed either by the percentage fall in the FEV_1 in response to a standard challenge (e.g. exercise or hyperventilation) (Table 46.4) or the dose of an agent required to induce a

Table 46.3 Diagnostic criteria for EIB as guided by the IOC-MC

Bronchial provocation challenge test	Change in FEV_1 from baseline values
Post bronchodilator	Increase by ≥12%
EVH challenge	Decrease by ≥10%
Laboratory exercise challenge	Decrease by ≥10%
Field exercise challenge	Decrease by ≥10%
Methacholine challenge	Decrease by ≥20%
Hypertonic saline challenge	Decrease by ≥15%

15% fall in FEV_1 (e.g. hypertonic saline or mannitol) (Table 46.5).

The factors influencing the severity of EIB are:[31]

1. type of exercise—endurance sports, cold weather sports and swimming (Table 46.6)
2. duration of exercise
3. intensity of exercise—in general, the more strenuous the exercise, the more likely EIB will occur
4. environmental factors:
   (a) cold more than warm
   (b) dry more than humid
   (c) air pollutants (e.g. sulfur dioxide and ozone)
5. interval since last episode of EIB (refractory period)
6. underlying bronchial hyperreactivity.

Treatment

The treatment of EIB is summarized in the flow chart given in Figure 46.5.

Non-pharmacological treatment

Most principles of non-pharmacological treatment are based on the theory that the primary stimulus for EIB is the respiratory water loss.

Masks

Masks capture some of the heat and water on expiration so that it is inhaled in the next inspiration. They have been found to be successful in reducing the severity of EIB.[32]

Nose breathing

Nose breathing during exercise has a similar effect to that of wearing masks.[33] However, nose breathing is not effective in everyone or during vigorous exercise. In addition, in some athletes the nasal mucosa is as sensitive as the lower airways, leading to nasal stuffiness, increased secretions and sneeze.

Table 46.4 Severity of EIB—exercise/hyperpnea challenge test

Severity	Fall in FEV_1
Mild	10–25%
Moderate	25.1–50%
Severe	>50%

Table 46.5 Severity of EIB—hypertonic saline challenge test

Severity	Saline (mg)
Mild	>6
Moderate	2.1–6.0
Severe	<2.1

Table 46.6 Sports likely to be associated with EIB

Middle/long-distance running
Cross-country skiing
Figure skating
Swimming
Aerobics
Cycling
Dancing
Basketball
Soccer
Rugby

Exercise training

The results of exercise training have been controversial. Training has been shown to increase the threshold at which EIB occurs.[34] There are a few reports of a reduced severity in EIB symptoms post training, but the majority of studies demonstrate no change in the occurrence or degree of EIB.[35, 36]

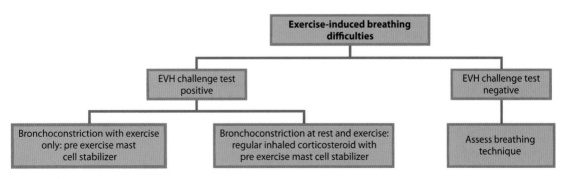

Figure 46.5 Management of exercise-induced bronchospasm

Warm-up

Both submaximal work and short sprints have been shown to facilitate marked reductions in EIB for subsequent exercise.[37–39] It is felt that such warm-ups increase bronchial blood flow and thus improve water delivery to the airways.

Refractory period

The refractory period occurs after exercise in more than 50% of subjects and may be used to lessen the severity of EIB.[40] The exact mechanism whereby a person becomes refractory is not known but may be secondary to an improved delivery of water to the airways during the second episode of exercise. This effect is short-lived (a few hours) and can be inhibited by the use of NSAIDs.

Pharmacological treatment

Sodium cromoglycate (cromolyn)

Sodium cromoglycate (cromolyn) is a prophylactic aerosol medication administered in a dose of 20–40 mg, 5–10 minutes prior to exercise. Its mode of action is thought to be that of stabilization of the basement membrane of the mast cell, preventing the release of the mediators for EIB. It also acts to decrease vagal nerve afferent activity. It is most effective within 2 hours of administration and has been shown to prevent both the early- and late-phase asthmatic reactions. It has no bronchodilating effects so cannot be used in the treatment of acute symptoms. It has minimal side-effects.[41]

Nedocromil sodium

Like sodium cromoglycate, nedocromil sodium has a membrane-stabilizing effect, preventing the release of mediators from mast cells and other inflammatory cells. It is administered in an inhaled dose of 4 mg, 5–10 minutes prior to exercise, with a duration of action of up to 4 hours. It, too, is effective in preventing the early- and late-phase asthmatic reactions but it is ineffective when used to treat acute symptoms.[42–44] Although it has minimal side-effects, some patients do complain of the taste of this medication.

Beta-2 agonists

Inhaled beta-2 agonists are the most effective drugs available for the relief of acute asthma symptoms. They induce bronchodilation, prevent the release of mediators from mast cells, and modify the effects of the mediators on both the contractility of smooth muscle and the permeability of mucosal cells. Although it is effective in providing rapid symptomatic improvement to EIB, it has been found that regular use of beta-2 agonists actually leads to tolerance to the effects of these medications and may result in a reduction in baseline lung function, poor asthma control in addition to increased bronchial hyperresponsiveness.[45] Two main types of beta-2 agonists are available:

1. Short-acting agents (e.g. salbutamol [albuterol], terbutaline). These agents have a rapid onset of action, usually within 5 minutes, with peak bronchodilation occurring within 15 minutes. Duration of action varies but effectiveness against EIB usually lasts 3–6 hours. These agents are the gold standard for the treatment of symptoms of EIB but are not recommended for use in the prevention of EIB.

2. Long-acting agents (e.g. salmeterol, formoterol). These agents have a slower onset of action and, as such, cannot be used in the treatment of symptoms of EIB. The onset of action usually occurs within 20 minutes and the duration of action is at least 12 hours. Formoterol has been shown to induce bronchodilation at both 15 minutes and 4 hours post-administration.[46] In addition to the above complications associated with regular use of beta-2 agonists, salmeterol has the additional problem of a reduction in the acute bronchoprotection against EIB.[47]

Leukotriene antagonists

Leukotrienes are potent bronchoconstrictors that also act to stimulate bronchial secretion of mucus and increase venopermeability, leading to airway edema. They are present in the airways of asthmatics but not normal subjects. Leukotriene antagonists (montelukast, zafirlukast) given orally prior to exercise attenuate the bronchoconstrictor and inflammatory response that would otherwise occur in response to the exercise.[48] One study showed that montelukasts provided superior protection compared with inhaled salmeterol, a long-acting beta-2 agonist.[49]

Inhaled corticosteroids

Inhaled corticosteroids improve asthma symptoms by reducing airway inflammation and bronchial hyperreactivity. They do not have an immediate bronchodilator effect and are not effective if used as prophylaxis just prior to exercise. The main role of corticosteroids is that of a maintenance therapy to help control asthma, but in doing so they also act to reduce bronchial responsiveness to exercise, thereby reducing the propensity for EIB. They are often used on a regular basis, with sodium cromoglycate (cromolyn) or nedocromil sodium given prior to exercise.

Inhaled corticosteroids have been shown to reduce the incidence and severity of EIB.[50, 51] The main side-effects are oral candidiasis and dysphonia, both of which can be reduced by rinsing the mouth following administration.[47]

Theophylline

The role of theophylline in the management of asthma has changed profoundly over recent years as research into the inflammatory etiology of asthma has led to the development of medications aimed to minimize this inflammation. Theophylline should not be used as intermittent prophylaxis for EIB as it is not a potent bronchodilator. In addition, the intermittent use increases the likelihood of adverse side-effects such as headaches, nausea, vomiting, tachycardia and central nervous system stimulation. The use of theophylline is, therefore, now limited to those with moderate–severe chronic asthma not controlled by main-line anti-asthmatic medications.

Treatment model

It is important to note that some drugs used to treat asthma are banned by the World Anti-Doping Agency (Chapter 61). In athletes subject to drug-testing procedures, clinicians are urged to check current banned drug listings. A treatment model for those athletes with EIB is shown in Table 46.7. In athletes who are prone to developing EIB, the regular use of medication prior to exercise is advised.

Conditions that may mimic EIB

Vocal cord dysfunction

Vocal cord dysfunction (VCD) is a psychogenic disorder of breathing, resulting in exercise-induced breathing difficulties. During normal breathing the true vocal cords abduct during inspiration and expiration; however, during VCD, the true vocal cords adduct inappropriately during inspiration, resulting in airflow obstruction. Less commonly, severe narrowing of the vocal cords may occur during expiration.

The condition commonly occurs in 20–40 year old women, although it may also occur in men and adolescents. Although in some situations it is related to an underlying psychiatric illness, such as generalized anxiety, depression, post-traumatic stress disorder or a history of sexual abuse, in many cases there is no underlying psychological condition.

Clinical features

The classic symptoms of VCD commonly occur during exercise and resolve within 5 minutes of cessation. They consist of a marked throat tightness or choking, in conjunction with severe dyspnea and an inspiratory stridor—the hallmark feature of VCD. The symptoms are variable and not necessarily reproducible when exercising under identical conditions. Both acute or prophylactic treatment with inhaled beta-2 agonists is ineffective. The symptoms may be worse during times of stress or moderate-to-severe lethargy.

VCD should be considered in all athletes complaining of exercise-induced dyspnea, especially when either a diagnosis of EIB has been excluded or, alternatively, made but the athlete has failed to respond to appropriate treatment.

Investigations

The diagnosis of VCD is often one of exclusion. An appropriate bronchial provocation challenge test should be performed, preferably an EVH challenge test, to exclude underlying EIB. Ideally, reproduction of the symptoms during an exercise challenge or, in some situations, participation in normal competition is required as it is essential for the treating physician to witness the athlete when experiencing the symptoms. Typically the athlete struggles to breathe with rapid shallow breaths and a loud inspiratory stridor; the athlete often leans forward, complaining of severe tightness of the throat.

Table 46.7 Pharmacological treatment of EIB

Severity	Pre-exercise treatment	Regular treatment	Symptoms treatment
Mild	Sodium cromoglycate (cromolyn)/nedocromil sodium		Short-acting beta-2 agonist
Moderate	Sodium cromoglycate (cromolyn)/nedocromil sodium	Low-dose inhaled corticosteroids	Short-acting beta-2 agonist
Severe	Sodium cromoglycate (cromolyn) and/or nedocromil sodium	Higher dose inhaled corticosteroids	Short-acting beta-2 agonist

Spirometry should be performed at the time of symptoms, when a flattening or truncation of the inspiratory limb of the flow-volume loop is usually seen.[52] However, in some cases, spirometry may miss the diagnosis.[53]

 In a patient with some of the symptoms of EIB but with a normal EVH, the diagnosis of vocal cord dysfunction should be considered, especially in a young female.

Direct laryngoscopy is required to exclude other causes of upper airway obstruction such as vocal cord paralysis, glottic or tracheal stenosis, laryngeal polyps and other laryngeal abnormalities. Although difficult, it is essential to perform direct laryngoscopy while the acute symptoms are present to visualize laryngeal closure.

Treatment

Treatment revolves around speech and relaxation therapy. It is essential that the speech therapist has experience with patients with VCD. The focus of speech therapy is on respiratory control and diaphragmatic breathing patterns. As the athlete gains control over breathing patterns, he or she may realize a sense of control of this condition and reduce the emotional stress associated with dyspnea.

Consultation with a psychologist is recommended to help the athlete to recognize and come to terms with stress. It is also important for the psychologist to assess for, and manage, any other underlying psychological condition.

Speech therapy, alone or in combination with other treatment interventions, has proven to be successful in reducing or eliminating the paroxysms of wheezing, stridor and dyspnea.[54] With appropriate treatment, nearly all athletes who have VCD should be able to exercise and compete unimpeded.[55]

Exercise-induced hyperventilation

Exercise-induced hyperventilation is a common condition occurring in both those athletes with underlying EIB and those without. Often during intense exercise the athlete loses control of his/her breathing, resulting in rapid shallow breaths—the abdominal muscles are not used. The patient typically presents with shortness of breath and throat tightness occurring while exercising, resolving immediately with rest. Bronchial provocation challenge tests, preferably an EVH challenge test, should be performed to exclude underlying

Table 46.8 Comparative features of exercise-induced bronchoconstriction, vocal cord dysfunction and exercise-induced hyperventilation

Feature	EIB	VCD	Hyperventilation
During or after exercise	Worse in first 12 minutes following cessation of exercise	Worse during exercise. Resolves within 5 minutes of cessation	Worse during exercise. Resolves within 5 minutes of cessation
Reproducibility under controlled situations	Reproducible	Often not reproducible	Often not reproducible
Classic symptoms	Chest tightness Dyspnea Cough Expiratory wheeze	Throat tightness/choking Dyspnea Inspiratory stridor	Throat tightness Dyspnea
Site of tightness	Chest	Throat	Throat
Bronchial provocation challenge tests	Abnormal	Normal	Normal
Spirometry	May be abnormal at rest	Normal at rest, abnormal during episode	Normal at all times
Laryngoscopy	Normal	Abnormal	Normal
Effect of beta-2 agonists	Prophylactic—prevents episode Therapeutic—resolves symptoms	Prophylactic—nil effect Therapeutic—nil effect	Prophylactic—nil effect Therapeutic—nil effect
Symptoms outside exercise	May be present	Absent	Absent

EIB, or in those with known EIB not responding to treatment, the challenge test should be performed while on medication to confirm adequate control with the medication. An exercise challenge test should be performed to allow the treating physician to assess the athlete while he or she is experiencing the symptoms. Laryngoscopy is required to exclude VCD.

Treatment involves educating the athlete to breathe, especially during times of stress or intense exercise. Consultation with a psychologist with experience in this area is essential. Training is required and appropriate exercises are given. Concentration on the use of abdominal muscles during breathing is required. Principles similar to the Butyeko method of breathing may be used.

Sinus-related symptoms

Sinusitis is a common disorder in both athletes and non-athletes. While acute infections are easily diagnosed, chronic sinusitis may be far more subtle in its presentation. The paranasal sinuses are air-filled spaces within the skull that communicate with the nose. Most commonly, the maxillary sinus is affected.

Clinical features of acute sinusitis may include facial pain, headache, toothache, post-nasal drip, cough, rhinorrhea, nasal obstruction, pyrexia and epistaxis. It is important to establish whether these symptoms are evidence of infective sinusitis or, alternatively, inflammation that is causing pain in the absence of infection. Inflammatory sinus pain may accompany acute exacerbations of rhinitis and is often short-lived. Features of chronic sinusitis are vague facial pain, post-nasal drip, cough, nasal obstruction, dental pain, malaise and halitosis.

General and local factors may predispose towards sinusitis. General factors include diabetes, immune deficiency, mucus abnormalities and disturbances in cilia function. Specific or local factors that may predispose athletes to this condition include anatomical deformities, polyps, foreign bodies, dental infections, cigarette smoking, barotrauma and local tumors. Failure to respond to therapy or recurrent episodes should prompt the search for a complicating condition (e.g. fracture, tumor or other abnormality).

When investigating these patients, assessment may be difficult due to the degree of edema. This may obscure the relevant abnormality. Full examination sometimes must be delayed until treatment has been effective. The use of plain X-rays should be interpreted with caution since up to 1 cm (0.5 in.) of mucoid thickening may be regarded as normal. In children, a number of developmental changes also make radiological interpretation almost impossible. Useful findings that may be seen on plain X-ray include the presence of a fluid level and/or opacification of a sinus. CT scan will provide additional information. In the patient with infective sinusitis, microbiological culture of nasal pus may be useful; however, the presence of normal bacterial flora makes interpretation difficult. Approximately 50% of infections are due to *Hemophilus influenzae* or *Streptococcus pneumoniae* but there are a variety of other organisms that may play a role, including *Branhamella catarrhalis* (most common organism in children) and other mixed oral anaerobes.

Management of sinusitis

The principles of management of sinusitis are, firstly, appropriate antibiotic therapy, secondly, the establishment of sinus drainage through the release of obstruction and the stimulation of mucus flow and, thirdly, the control of any predisposing factors. The antibiotic of first choice is amoxycillin (amoxycillin), either used alone or in combination with clavulanic acid. Penicillin-allergic patients should use cefaclor, cotrimoxazole or doxycycline. If a dental infection is the primary source, then anaerobic cover should be added (e.g. metronidazole).

Systemically administered decongestants, including pseudoephedrine, are of some value in the treatment of acute sinusitis. However, a topical decongestant is more effective and will have fewer systemic side-effects. Antihistamines usually slow mucociliary function but may have a role, especially if sinusitis is the result of nasal allergy. The use of topical steroids is widely advocated in the acute situation but there is often a latent period before these are effective. The maintenance of hydration in the treatment of these patients is critical and there may well be a role for surgery in either the acute or chronic condition where there is an anatomical deformity, polyps or a failure to respond to medical treatment.

Other exercise-related conditions

Exercise-induced anaphylaxis

Approximately 500 cases of exercise-induced anaphylaxis have been reported, mostly occurring in athletes.[56, 57] Numerous attacks may occur before the diagnosis is correctly made.

The condition is characterized by a sensation of warmth, pruritis, cutaneous erythema, angioedema, urticaria (greater than 1 cm [0.5 in.] diameter), upper respiratory tract obstruction and, occasionally, vascular collapse. It is considered a distinct entity from other exertion-related phenomena.

Risk factors include:

- previous atopic history (50%)
- family atopic history (67%)
- food ingestion (e.g. shellfish, celery, nuts, alcohol)
- weather conditions (e.g. heat, high humidity)
- drug ingestion (e.g. aspirin [ASA], NSAIDs).

The management of this condition involves:

1. prevention through modification of the exercise program to:
   (a) decrease intensity
   (b) avoid exercise during warm and humid days
   (c) stop exercise at the earliest sign of itching
   (d) avoid meals 4 hours before exercise
2. drugs/therapy
   (a) antihistamines
   (b) cromoglycate (cromolyn)
   (c) adrenalin (epinephrine)—should have an injection available
   (d) pre-treatment does not prevent onset.

Cholinergic urticaria

This condition is an exaggerated cholinergic response to rapid elevation of the core body temperature through a mechanism such as exercise (most commonly), hot showers, fever or anxiety.[58] It is characterized by generalized flushing, tan urticarial rash and pruritus. Generally, the urticarial papules appear first within 10 minutes of starting exercise on the neck or upper thorax and spread to the limbs.[59] Systemic reactions such as syncope, abdominal pain and wheezing are rare. Cholinergic symptoms such as lacrimation, salivation and diarrhea may be observed. Recovery usually occurs spontaneously in 2–4 hours provided there are no systemic symptoms.[58] Antihistamines are generally used in treatment (e.g. hydroxyzine, 250 mg/day or cyproheptadine, 4 mg/day).

Exercise-induced angioedema

Angioedema is a non-itchy swelling occurring in the deep dermis and subcutaneous tissue. Although angioedema can affect any body region, it tends to involve the face and oral region. Occasional visceral manifestations occur. Attacks may be life-threatening if the airway is involved. Frank asthmatic attacks rarely occur in the setting of exercise-induced angioedema.[60]

Prevention may be achieved with modification of the exercise program and/or the use of antihistamines (e.g. diphenhydramine). The selective histamine H_2-receptor blockers (e.g. cimetidine) have been used in the treatment of this condition.

Recommended Reading

Holzer K, Brukner P, Douglass J. Evidence-based management of exercise-induced asthma. *Curr Sports Med Rep* 2002; 1: 86–92.

Langdeau J-B, Boulet L-P. Prevalence and mechanisms of development of asthma and airway hyperresponsiveness in athletes. *Sports Med* 2001; 31(8): 601–16.

Pope JS, Koenig SM. Pulmonary disorders in the training room. *Clin Sports Med* 2005; 24: 541–64.

Rundell KW, Jenkinson DM. Exercise-induced bronchospasm in the elite athlete. *Sports Med* 2002; 32(9): 583–600.

Rundell KW, Wilber RL, Lemanske RF Jr. *Exercise-Induced Asthma.* Champaign, IL: Human Kinetics Publishers, 2002.

Shepard RJ. Does cold air damage the lungs of winter athletes? *Curr Sports Med Rep* 2004; 3: 289–91.

Storms WW. Review of exercise-induced asthma. *Med Sci Sports Exerc* 2003; 35(9): 1464–70.

References

1. National Institutes of Health. *Practical Guide for the Diagnosis and Management of Asthma*. Bethesda, MD: NIH Publication, 1997.

2. Institute of Medicine. *Clearing the Air: Asthma and Indoor Air Exposure*. Washington, DC: National Academy of Press, 2000.

3. Anderson SD. Exercise-induced asthma. In: Middleton E, Reed C, Ellis E, et al., eds. *Allergy: Principles and Practice*. 4th edn. St Louis: CV Mosby, 1993: 1343–67.

4. Anderson S. Exercise-induced asthma. In: Carlsen K-H, Ibsen T, eds. *Exercise-Induced Asthma and Sports in Asthma*. Copenhagen: Munksgaard Press, 1999: 11–17.

5. Fitch KD. Management of allergic Olympic athletes. *J Allergy Clin Immunol* 1984; 73: 722–7.

6. Corrigan B, Kazlaukas R. Medication use in athletes selected for doping control at the Sydney Olympics (2000). *Clin J Sport Med* 2003; 13: 33–40.

7. Voy RO. The US Olympic committee experience with exercise-induced bronchospasm, 1984. *Med Sci Sports Exerc* 1986; 18(3): 328–30.

8. Weiler JM, Layton T, Hunt M. Asthma in United States

Olympic athletes who participated in the 1996 summer games. *J Allergy Clin Immunol* 1998; 102(5): 722–6.

9. Weiler JM, Ryan EJ 3rd. Asthma in United States Olympic athletes who participated in the 1998 Olympic winter games. *J Allergy Clin Immunol* 2000; 106(2): 267–71.

10. Gilbert IA, McFadden ER. Airway cooling and rewarming. The second reaction sequence in exercise-induced asthma. *J Clin Invest* 1992; 90: 699–704.

11. Anderson SD. Is there a unifying hypothesis for exercise-induced asthma? *J Allergy Clin Immunol* 1984; 73: 660–5.

12. Godfrey S, Bar-Yishay E. Exercise-induced asthma revisited. *Respir Med* 1993; 87: 331–44.

13. Argyros GJ, Phillips YY, Rayburn DB, et al. Water loss without heat flux in exercise-induced bronchospasm. *Am Rev Respir Dis* 1993; 147: 1419–24.

14. Schmidt A, Bundgaard A. Exercise-induced asthma after inhalation of aerosols with different osmolarities. *Eur J Respir Dis Suppl* 1986; 143: 57–61.

15. Anderson SD, Smith CM. Osmotic challenges in the assessment of bronchial hyperresponsiveness. *Am Rev Respir Dis* 1991; 143: S43–S46.

16. Burge PS, Harries MG, Lam WK, et al. Occupational asthma due to formaldehyde. *Thorax* 1985; 40: 255–60.

17. Godfrey S. Exercise-induced asthma. In: Barnes PJ, Grunstein MM, Leff AR, et al., eds. *Asthma*. Philadelphia: Lippincott-Raven, 1997: 1105–20.

18. Boulet L-P, Turcotte H, Laprise C. Comparative degree and type of sensitisation to common indoor and outdoor allergens in subjects with allergic rhinitis and/or asthma. *Clin Exp Allergy* 1997; 27: 52–9.

19. Helenius IJ, Tikkanen HO, Haahtela T. Association between type of training and risk of asthma in elite athletes. *Thorax* 1997; 52: 157–60.

20. Holzer K, Anderson SD, Douglass J. Exercise in elite summer athletes: challenges for diagnosis. *J Allergy Clin Immunol* 2002; 110(3): 374–80.

21. Warner JO. Bronchial hyperresponsiveness, atopy, airway inflammation and asthma. *Pediatr Allergy Immunol* 1998; 9: 56–60.

22. Langdeau JB, Boulet LP. Prevalence and mechanisms of development of asthma and airway hyperresponsiveness in athletes. *Sports Med* 2001; 31(8): 601–16.

23. Drobnic F, Freixa A, Casan P, et al. Assessment of chlorine exposure in swimmers during training. *Med Sci Sports Exerc* 1996; 28(2): 271–4.

24. Anderson SD, Silverman M, Konig P, et al. Exercise-induced asthma. A review. *Br J Dis Chest* 1975; 69: 1–39.

25. Rundell KW, Im J, Mayers LB, et al. Self-reported symptoms and exercise-induced asthma in the elite athlete. *Med Sci Sports Exerc* 2001; 33(2): 208–13.

26. Holzer K, Douglass J, Anderson SD. Methacholine has a low sensitivity to identify elite athletes with a positive response to eucapnic voluntary hyperpnea and should

not be used to exclude potential exercise-induced bronchoconstriction. *Respirology* 2002; 7(suppl.): A28.

27. Anderson SD. Exercise-induced asthma. In: Kay AB, ed. *Allergy and Allergic Diseases*. Oxford: Blackwell Scientific Publications, 1997; 692–711.

28. Anderson SD, Argyros GJ, Magnussen H, et al. Provocation by eucapnic voluntary hyperpnoea to identify exercise induced bronchoconstriction. *Br J Sports Med* 2001; 35: 344–7.

29. Holzer K, Anderson SD, Chan H-K, et al. Mannitol as a challenge test to identify exercise-induced bronchoconstriction in elite athletes. *Am J Respir Crit Care Med* 2003; 167(4): 534–47.

30. Anderson SD, Brannan J, Spring J, et al. A new method for bronchial-provocation testing in asthmatic subjects using a dry powder of mannitol. *Am J Respir Crit Care Med* 1997; 156: 758–65.

31. Mahler DA. Exercise-induced asthma. *Med Sci Sports Exercise* 1993; 25(5): 554–61.

32. Nisar M, Spence DPS, West D, et al. A mask to modify inspired air temperature and humidity and its effect on exercise induced asthma. *Thorax* 1992; 47: 446–50.

33. Shturman-Ellstein R, Zeballos RJ, Buckley JM, et al. The beneficial effect of nasal breathing on exercise-induced bronchoconstriction. *Am Rev Respir Dis* 1978; 118: 65–73.

34. Fitch KD, Blitvich JD, Morton AR. The effect of running training on exercise-induced asthma. *Ann Allergy Asthma Immunol* 1986; 7: 90–4.

35. Welsh L, Kemp JG, Roberts RGD. Effects of physical conditioning on children and adolescents with asthma. *Sports Med* 2005; 35(2): 127–41.

36. Ram FS, Robinson SM, Black PN. Effects of physical training in asthma: a systematic review. *Br J Sports Med* 2000; 34(3): 162–7.

37. de Bisschop C, Guenard H, Desnot P, et al. Reduction of exercise-induced asthma in children by short, repeated warm ups. *Br J Sports Med* 1999; 33: 100–4.

38. Schnall RP, Landau LI. Protective effects of repeated short sprints in exercise-induced asthma. *Thorax* 1980; 35: 828–32.

39. McKenzie DC, McLuckie SL, Stirling DR. The protective effects of continuous and interval exercise in athletes with exercise-induced asthma. *Med Sci Sports Exerc* 1994; 26(8): 951–6.

40. Edmunds A, Tooley M, Godfrey S. The refractory period after exercise-induced asthma: its duration and relation to the severity of exercise. *Am Rev Respir Dis* 1978; 117: 247–54.

41. Anderson SD. Exercise-induced asthma: stimulus, mechanism, and management. In: Barnes PJ, Rodger I, Thomson NC, eds. *Asthma: Basic Mechanisms and Clinical Management*. London: Academic Press, 1988: 503–22.

42. Speelberg B, Verhoeff NPLG, van den Berg NJ, et al. Nedocromil sodium inhibits the early and late asthmatic response to exercise. *Eur Respir J* 1992; 5: 430–7.

43. Spooner C, Rowe BH, Saunders LD. Nedocromil sodium in the treatment of exercise-induced asthma: a meta-analysis. *Eur Respir J* 2000; 16(1): 30–7.

44. Spooner CH, Saunders LD, Rowe BH. Nedocromil sodium for preventing exercise-induced bronchoconstriction (Cochrane review). *Cochrane Database Syst Rev* 2002; 1: CD001183.

45. Bhagat R, Kalra S, Swystun A. Rapid onset of tolerance to the bronchoprotective effect of salmeterol. *Chest* 1995; 108: 1235–9.

46. Ferrari M, Balestreri F, Baratieri S, et al. Evidence of the rapid protective effect of formoterol dry-powder inhalation against exercise-induced bronchospasm in athletes with asthma. *Clin Invest Med* 2000; 67: 510–13.

47. Rupp NT. Diagnosis and management of exercise-induced asthma. *Physician Sportsmed* 1996; 24(1): 77–87.

48. Makker HK, Lau LC, Thomson HW, et al. The protective effect of inhaled leukotriene D_4 receptor antagonist ICI 204,219 against exercise-induced asthma. *Am Rev Respir Dis* 1993; 147: 1413–18.

49. Ferrari M, Segattini C, Zanon R, et al. Comparison of the protective effect of salmeterol against exercise-induced bronchospasm when given immediately before a cycloergometric test. *Respiration* 2002; 69(6): 509–12.

50. Henriksen JM, Dahl R. Effects of inhaled budesonide alone and in combination with low-dose terbutaline in children with exercise-induced asthma. *Am Rev Respir Dis* 1983; 128: 993–7.

51. Waalkans HJ, van Essen-Zandvliet EEM, Gerritsen J, et al. The effect of an inhaled corticosteroid (budesonide) on exercise-induced asthma in children. *Eur Respir J* 1993; 6: 652–56.

52. Newman KB, Mason III UG, Schmaling KB. Clinical features of vocal cord dysfunction. *Am J Respir Crit Care Med* 1995; 152(4 Pt 1): 1382–6.

53. Morris MJ, Deal L, Bean DR, et al. Vocal cord dysfunction in patients with exertional dyspnea. *Chest* 1999; 116(6): 1676–82.

54. Sullivan MD, Heywood BM, Beukelman DR. A treatment for vocal cord dysfunction in female athletes: an outcome study. *Laryngoscope* 2001; 111(10): 1751–5.

55. Newshaun KR, Claben DK, Miller DJ, et al. Paradoxical vocal cord dysfunction management in athletes. *J Athl Train* 2002; 37: 325–8.

56. Castells MC, Horan RS, Sheffer AL. Exercise induced anaphylaxis. *Clin Rev Allergy Immunol* 1999; 17: 413–24.

57. Castells MC, Horan RS, Sheffer AL. Exercise induced anaphylaxis. *Curr Allergy Asthma Rep* 2003; 3: 15–21.

58. Volcheck GW, Li JT. Exercise-induced urticaria and anaphylaxis. *Mayo Clin Proc* 1997; 72(2): 140–7.

59. Sweeney TM, Dexter WW. Cholinergic urticaria in a jogger: ruling out exercise-induced anaphylaxis. *Physician Sportsmed* 2003; 31(6): 32–6.

60. Leung AKC, Hedge HR. Exercise-induced angiodema and asthma. *Am J Sports Med* 1989; 17(3): 442–3.

Gastrointestinal Symptoms During Exercise

WITH CHRIS MILNE

Although moderate physical activity promotes several health benefits for the gastrointestinal tract,[1] frequent, high-intensity exercise can be associated with gastrointestinal symptoms, such as loss of appetite, heartburn, chest pain, belching, nausea, vomiting, abdominal cramps, urge to defecate, diarrhea and rectal bleeding. These symptoms may be divided into those relating to the upper and lower gastrointestinal tract, as shown in Table 47.1.

Physiological changes that alter gastrointestinal function during exercise include reduced blood flow to the abdominal viscera, gastrointestinal hormonal changes and alterations to gastric emptying rates and intestinal motility. Also, vigorous diaphragmatic movements, abdominal contractions and intestinal jarring can all cause abdominal symptoms.[2]

It must be remembered, however, that although the incidence of gastrointestinal symptoms is increased with exercise, the presence of symptoms in an athlete should not automatically be assumed to be solely related to exercise. Athletes as well as non-athletes suffer from common conditions such as hiatus hernia and peptic ulceration, inflammatory bowel disease, polyps and cancer. Clinical judgment is required to appreciate when these conditions must be considered in the athlete with gastrointestinal symptoms.

Upper gastrointestinal symptoms

Heartburn, reflux, nausea, vomiting and upper abdominal pain are the most common upper gastrointestinal tract symptoms related to exercise. Gastroesophageal reflux is a common complaint among athletes.[3] Twenty per cent of patients with established reflux consider exercise to be the major contributor to their symptoms. The mechanism by which exercise causes reflux is not well understood, as reflux is normally associated with relaxation of the lower esophageal sphincter; this has not been described with exercise. Reflux appears to be more common when exercise is performed after a meal. Importantly, exercise does not appear to have any effect on gastric acid secretion.

 The distinction between chest pain due to gastroesophageal reflux or esophageal muscular spasm and chest pain due to chest wall or cardiac causes may be difficult. Any athlete presenting with chest pain on exertion must be thoroughly assessed to exclude cardiac causes.

Much attention has been paid to the factors that may affect the gastric emptying rate (GER). Exercise at a very high intensity reduces the GER. However, exercise intensity does not appear to be a significant factor, as this level of exercise cannot be maintained for long. Increased volume in the stomach results

Table 47.1 Gastrointestinal symptoms associated with exercise

Upper gastrointestinal tract	Lower gastrointestinal tract
Heartburn	Cramping
Reflux	Urge to defecate
Nausea	Diarrhea
Vomiting	Rectal bleeding
Bloating	Flatulence
Epigastric pain	

in an initial rapid emptying, followed by a phase of reduced emptying once the volume of the stomach has decreased to about 30% of its initial content.

It was thought until recently that osmolality was an important factor in GER. While it is true that liquids empty more quickly than solids, there does not appear to be significant differences in the GER for liquids of different osmolality.[4, 5] Other factors that may be involved include gastrointestinal hormone levels, particle size, meal volume, dietary fiber, gastric acidity and the athlete's anxiety level.

Treatment

The treatment of upper gastrointestinal symptoms associated with exercise is aimed at reducing the contents of the stomach during exercise. This is achieved by avoiding solid foods for 3 hours before intense exercise. The pre-exercise meal should be high in carbohydrate and low in fat and protein.

If additional measures are required, the use of antacid medication, either in tablet or liquid form, may reduce the incidence of heartburn and upper abdominal pain associated with exercise. Antacids usually remain in the stomach for 30 minutes. If this is not sufficient, the use of histamine H_2-receptor antagonists, such as ranitidine and cimetidine, may occasionally be necessary. Also, many expert clinicians have found an effective treatment is domperidone 10–20 mg 1 hour before meals.

Gastrointestinal bleeding

A classic clinical account of the problem of gastrointestinal bleeding in athletes came from Australian marathoner, Derek Clayton, after he completed a world record marathon performance in 1969 (*Runners' World* May 1979, p. 72):

> Two hours later, the elation had worn off. I was urinating quite large clots of blood, and I was vomiting black mucus and had a lot of black diarrhea. I don't think too many people can understand what I went through for the next 48 hours.

An occasional bloody stool is frequently noted by runners[6] and the incidence of occult bleeding is high.[7] As the amount of bleeding in most cases is small, most athletes are not affected clinically but occasionally iron-deficiency anemia may occur. Reduced iron stores are denoted by a low serum ferritin level (Chapter 37).

The most frequently reported site of exercise-associated gastrointestinal hemorrhage is the fundus

of the stomach. The mechanism underpinning this transitory hemorrhagic gastritis is uncertain. Ischemia may play a role as may direct trauma from the diaphragm. In susceptible individuals, the gastritis may result in part from the general stress of competition along with the associated rise in key stress hormones such as adrenalin (epinephrine) and cortisol. NSAIDs (but not aspirin) contribute to gastrointestinal bleeding in runners.[6, 7] A Mallory–Weiss tear secondary to forceful vomiting may also present with signs of upper gastrointestinal bleeding.

No examples of bleeding from the small intestine have been reported. However, colonic bleeding has been observed, particularly from the proximal colon.

The etiology of gastrointestinal bleeding associated with exercise is uncertain and is likely to be multifactorial. During exercise, blood flow is diverted from the splanchnic bed to the exercising muscles. Blood flow to the gastrointestinal tract may be reduced by as much as 75% during intense exercise.[8] A number of other factors may contribute to a reduction of blood flow. Such factors include exercise in the fasted state as the absence of nutrients within the intestine reduces the blood flow to that area.

It must be remembered that gastrointestinal bleeding in an athlete is not necessarily associated with exercise and the athlete with obvious gastrointestinal bleeding should be fully investigated to determine the source of the bleeding.

Treatment

If no obvious cause of the bleeding is established, adequate hydration must be ensured to prevent aggravation of the relative ischemia. As the mechanical effect of jarring while running is thought by some to be a contributory factor to gastrointestinal bleeding, the amount of jarring should be reduced with the use of appropriate footwear and avoiding running on hard surfaces.

Those athletes with a known tendency for gastrointestinal bleeding or those who may complain of excessive tiredness and fatigue should have the state of their iron stores assessed by measurement of their serum ferritin levels. Serum ferritin levels of less than 30 ng/mL in women and 50 ng/mL in men indicate reduced iron stores (Chapter 37).

Abdominal pain

Many athletes complain of a sharp, colicky pain in the left or right upper quadrant during strenuous exercise.

This is commonly referred to as a 'stitch'. The exact cause of this common phenomenon is unknown but it may be due to muscle spasm of the diaphragm or trapping of gas in the hepatic or splenic flexure of the colon. This condition has often been thought to be associated with exercise undertaken soon after eating a solid meal. There is no proof of this but avoidance of a solid meal prior to exercise may be an appropriate treatment.

Occasionally, athletes get a 'claudication-type' abdominal pain. This occurs in association with intense, endurance exercise and is thought to occur as a consequence of relative ischemia due to shunting of blood away from the gastrointestinal tract to the exercising muscles.[8] This effect is aggravated by dehydration. A rare cause of abdominal pain is 'cecal slap' on the right psoas muscle.

The possibility of abdominal pain being referred from the thoracic spine should always be considered. A thorough examination of the thoracic spine should be performed in any athlete complaining of abdominal pain. Hypomobility detected in one or more intervertebral segments should be corrected by manual therapy techniques and the effect on the athlete's symptoms noted.

Diarrhea

Diarrhea appears to be more frequent with exercise,[9] especially with long-distance running; as a result the terms 'runner's trots' and 'runner's diarrhea' have been coined to describe the condition. Athletes may complain of an urge to defecate while running and approximately half of those who experience this urge to defecate actually complain of episodes of diarrhea during running.

The incidence of runner's diarrhea seems to be related to the intensity of the exercise and occurs more commonly in competition than in training. The anxiety associated with competition may be a contributory factor.

The exact cause of runner's diarrhea is uncertain. Relative intestinal ischemia, described previously, may be a contributory factor. An increase in intestinal motility may also contribute to the development of diarrhea. Studies of the relationship between intestinal transit time and exercise have shown conflicting results but it would appear that intestinal motility is increased with intense exercise. This increase in gut motility and changes in intestinal secretion and absorption may be related to the increased level of endorphins associated with exercise.

When faced with a patient with diarrhea, the clinician should also seek a history of vitamin and mineral supplementation, or ingestion of caffeine or artificial sweeteners prior to exercise. Each of these may contribute to runner's diarrhea.

 Acute diarrhea is usually due to an infective cause and may be viral or bacterial. This is a particular problem for athletes when they are traveling away from home and is further considered in Chapter 59. In the 24 hours prior to major competition, team physicians generally prescribe norfloxacin (800 mg) or ciprofloxacin (1 g) with loperamide (4 mg) to try to provide rapid symptom relief. Athletes with chronic diarrhea should be fully investigated to exclude any other abnormality (e.g. inflammatory bowel disease).

Treatment

The treatment of athletes with exercise-related diarrhea is often difficult. Dietary changes should include reduction of the fiber content of the diet in the 24 hours prior to intense competitive exercise. If the problem persists, prophylactic antidiarrheal medication, such as loperamide, may be used. However, this should not be used on a regular basis. Antispasmodics (e.g. mebeverine) may be useful. A summary of the management of common gastrointestinal symptoms is shown in Table 47.2.

Table 47.2 Treatment of common gastrointestinal problems

Symptoms	Treatment
Heartburn, reflux, epigastric pain	Avoid solid foods prior to exercise Antacid medication Histamine H_2-receptor antagonist (rarely necessary)
Gastrointestinal bleeding	Ensure adequate hydration Reduce jarring (e.g. good shoes, soft surfaces) Investigate if persistent Increase iron content of diet
Abdominal 'stitch'	Reassure Avoid pre-exercise meal
Runner's diarrhea	Reduce fiber content of food 24 hours prior to run Antidiarrheal medication (e.g. loperamide)

Exercise and gastrointestinal diseases

Lactose intolerance

A limited number of people lack the enzyme lactase, which is necessary for the digestion of lactose or milk sugar. Asian and African populations typically display an absence of lactase. Also, adult lactase has only about 5% of the activity of childhood lactase. Lactose intolerance leads to gastrointestinal disorders resulting in cramps, flatulence and diarrhea.

Athletes suffering from lactose intolerance will need to avoid dairy products, with the possible exception of yoghurt. The lactose in yoghurt is largely broken down by the bacterial cultures present. It is important that athletes who avoid lactose ensure an adequate dietary intake of calcium and protein via alternative sources such as soy-based products, including milks, yoghurts, cheeses and ice-creams. An often unrecognized source of lactose is high protein drinks and sports supplements. Also, temporary lactose intolerance may follow acute infective diarrhea (particularly if caused by rotavirus). Therefore, milk-based products should be among the last to be reintroduced to the athlete's diet after such an episode.

Celiac disease

Celiac disease is characterized by abnormal mucosa in the small intestine induced by a component of the gluten protein of wheat. Barley, rye and oats also contain gluten. Anemia is often seen in athletes with celiac disease due to malabsorption of iron and folate. Howell-Jolly bodies may be seen on the blood film due to folate deficiency.

New prevalence data suggest that symptomatic or latent celiac disease affects up to 1 in 200 people in most Western countries. It may not always present with the classic symptoms of diarrhea and bloating; tiredness is a common presentation (Chapter 52).[10] Laboratory testing may show high levels of IgA anti-endomysial and IgA tissue transglutaminase antibodies. However, any of the IgA tests may be falsely negative in up to 3–5% of celiac patients, mainly in those with associated IgA deficiency.[11] Definitive diagnosis is via multiple small bowel biopsy, showing typical mucosal changes of subtotal villous atrophy.

Athletes diagnosed with celiac disease are given comprehensive lists of alternative high-carbohydrate food sources. Athletes with celiac disease should consult a dietitian for assistance in planning a nutritionally adequate diet.

Irritable bowel syndrome

This very common gastrointestinal disorder causes lower abdominal pain and constipation alternating with diarrhea. The cause is not known but there seems to be a strong association between this condition and the intestinal response to emotional stress (e.g. sporting competition). The clinically popular treatment of symptoms includes a balanced fiber diet together with antispasmodic agents (e.g. dicyclomine).

Prevention of gastrointestinal symptoms that occur with exercise

Many of the gut complaints experienced by runners are a direct result of the physical activity of running, which causes jolting of the gastrointestinal tract and reduced blood supply to the cells. However, some relief can be gained by a number of dietary modifications.

Limit dietary fiber intake prior to competition

To ensure that the gut has minimal food content prior to racing, it is necessary to reduce the fiber content of the diet in the days preceding the race. This means, in the two days prior to the competition, changing from wholemeal and wholegrain varieties of rice, breads and cereals to the more refined alternatives, avoiding fresh fruit and vegetables with skin, legumes and heavy seasonings such as garlic, pepper and curry.

Runners who regularly suffer from diarrhea or the urge to use their bowels regularly during a race may benefit from a liquid nutrition supplement during the last days preceding the competition. This will ensure that the gastrointestinal contents are minimized prior to the race. An alternative approach is to consume only fluids prior to competition on the day of the event.

Avoid solid foods during the last 3 hours prior to the race

To ensure that the stomach is empty, it is important that the pre-event meal is consumed at least 3 hours before the race begins. However, in some athletes with a low GER, the pre-event meal may need to be accompanied by a prokinetic agent (e.g. cisapride) and eaten up to 4–6 hours prior to competition. Fluids, however, should still be consumed in the period leading up to the race.

Select the pre-event meal carefully

This meal should contain negligible amounts of fat and protein so that it will be easily digested by the time the event begins. Select from low-fiber, high-carbohydrate foods such as white rice, white bread, plain pastas, plain breakfast cereals (e.g. cornflakes, rice bubbles) and avoid adding any fats such as margarine, butter or creamy sauces. Simple carbohydrates such as honey, jam and syrup may be used to increase the energy value of the meal. Note that high-fructose foods (e.g. dried fruit, fruit juices, jam, soft drinks/pop) are absorbed slowly, so large volumes may not be well tolerated if the sportsperson has a tendency for gastrointestinal upset.

Prevent dehydration

It is important to drink small amounts frequently during the event, aiming for 500–800 mL per hour. During long events (more than 90 minutes) the athlete should choose a drink that contains some carbohydrate (up to 10% solution) and dilute amounts of sodium and potassium. Concentrated drinks are more likely to cause symptoms. Practice drinking during training so that it becomes a habit in competitions.

Avoid fat and protein intake during exercise

During ultra-endurance events where food may be consumed during the event, select items that contain minimum quantities of protein and fat. Fiber intake needs to be kept low and some runners may find liquid meal replacements a useful option. Boiled white rice, pasta, pancakes with syrup, canned fruit, peeled potatoes, plain dry biscuits and plain rolls or bread all make good choices. Practice food intake during training.

Sample pre-event diet

A sample 24-hour pre-race diet that will help minimize gastrointestinal problems during a race is shown in the box. This plan provides approximately 14 700 kJ (3500 kcal) with 76% of the energy from carbohydrate and less than 20 g of dietary fiber.

Consult a sports psychologist

If pre-race nerves are a likely cause of gastrointestinal problems, it may be helpful to discuss race build-up with a sports psychologist. Proper management of anxiety can not only improve stomach and bowel problems but may also help maximize race performance (Chapter 39).

Breakfast

1 large bowl (2 cups) breakfast cereal with skim milk
2 slices white toast spread with honey
1 cup canned peaches
1 glass 100% apple juice

Snack

3 pancakes (made with low-fat milk) topped with golden syrup
300 mL flavored mineral water

Lunch

2 white bread rolls filled with low-fat cheese
1 tub low-fat fruit yoghurt
2 glasses water

Snack

2 toasted crumpets spread with honey
1 glass 100% pineapple juice

Dinner

2 cups boiled white pasta topped with sauce made from tomato paste and fresh mushrooms
1 slice white bread
1 serve rice pudding (white rice)
3 glasses water

Snack

300 mL nutrition supplement
1 glass lemonade

Recommended Reading

Carter MJ, Lobo AJ, Travis SP. Inflammatory bowel disease section, British Society of Gastroenterology. Guidelines for the management of inflammatory bowel disease in adults. *Gut* 2004; 53(suppl. 5): V1–16.

Ng V, Millard WM. Competing with Crohn's disease. Management issues in active patients. *Physician Sportsmed* 2005; 33(11). Available online: <http://www.physsportsmed.com/issues/2005/1105/millard.htm>, accessed 27 Mar 2006.

Pitsis GC, Fallon KE, Fallon SK, Fazakerley R. Response of soluble transferrin receptor and iron-related parameters to iron supplementation in elite, iron-depleted, nonanemic female athletes. *Clin J Sport Med* 2004; 14(5): 300–4.

References

1. Bi L, Triadafilopoulos G. Exercise and gastrointestinal function and disease: an evidence-based review of risks and benefits. *Clin Gastroenterol Hepatol* 2003; 1(5): 345–55.

2. Casey E, Mistry DJ, MacKnight JM. Training room management of medical conditions: sports gastroenterology. *Clin Sports Med* 2005; 24(3): 525–40, viii.

3. Shawdon A. Gastro-oesophageal reflux and exercise. Important pathology to consider in the athletic population. *Sports Med* 1995; 20(2): 109–16.

4. Brouns F, Senden J, Beckers EJ, Saris WH. Osmolarity does not affect the gastric emptying rate of oral rehydration solutions. *J Parenter Enteral Nutr* 1995; 19(5): 403–6.

5. Rogers J, Summers RW, Lambert GP. Gastric emptying and intestinal absorption of a low-carbohydrate sport drink during exercise. *Int J Sport Nutr Exerc Metab* 2005; 15(3): 220–35.

6. Simons SM, Kennedy RG. Gastrointestinal problems in runners. *Curr Sports Med Rep* 2004; 3(2): 112–16.

7. Smetanka RD, Lambert GP, Murray R, Eddy D, Horn M, Gisolfi CV. Intestinal permeability in runners in the 1996 Chicago marathon. *Int J Sport Nutr* 1999; 9(4): 426–33.

8. van Nieuwenhoven MA, Brouns F, Brummer RJ. Gastrointestinal profile of symptomatic athletes at rest and during physical exercise. *Eur J Appl Physiol* 2004; 91(4): 429–34.

9. Rao SS, Beaty J, Chamberlain M, Lambert PG, Gisolfi C. Effects of acute graded exercise on human colonic motility. *Am J Physiol* 1999; 276(5 Pt 1): G1221–6.

10. Feighery C. Fortnightly review: coeliac disease. *BMJ* 1999; 319(7204): 236–9.

11. Gastroenterological Society of Australia. Professional Guidelines. Coeliac Disease. Available online: <http://www.gesa.org.au/members_guidelines/coeliacdisease/index.htm>, accessed 27 Mar 2006.

Diabetes Mellitus

WITH SANDY HOFFMAN AND MATT HISLOP

This chapter proposes to examine two aspects of the relationship between diabetes mellitus and exercise. Firstly, the adjustments the athlete with diabetes might make if he or she wishes to exercise and, secondly, what the risks and benefits are, both in the short term and long term, of exercise to the patient with diabetes.

There are many examples of athletes with diabetes who have been extremely successful. British rower Steven Redgrave developed diabetes at the age of 35 having won gold medals at each of the previous four Olympic games. Following his diagnosis he was able to continue training and competing and won a fifth consecutive gold medal in the Sydney Olympics in 2000.[1]

There are two distinct types of diabetes mellitus: insulin-dependent (type 1) and non-insulin-dependent (type 2).

Type 1 diabetes

Type 1 diabetes (insulin-dependent diabetes mellitus, IDDM), previously known as juvenile-onset diabetes, is thought to be an inherited autoimmune disease in which antibodies are produced against the beta cells of the pancreas. This ultimately results in the absence of endogenous insulin production, which is the characteristic feature of type 1 diabetes. The incidence of type 1 diabetes varies throughout the world but represents approximately 10–15% of diabetic cases in the Western world. The onset commonly occurs in childhood and adolescence but can become symptomatic at any age. Insulin administration is essential to prevent ketosis, coma and death. The aims of treatment are tight control of blood glucose levels and prevention of microvascular and macrovascular complications.

Type 2 diabetes

Type 2 diabetes (non-insulin-dependent diabetes mellitus, NIDDM), previously known as maturity-onset or adult-onset diabetes, is a disease, as the former names suggest, of later onset, linked to both genetic and lifestyle factors. It is characterized by diminished insulin secretion relative to serum glucose levels in conjunction with peripheral insulin resistance, both of which result in chronic hyperglycemia. Approximately 90% of individuals with diabetes have type 2 diabetes and it is thought to affect 3–7% of people in Western countries. The prevalence of type 2 diabetes increases with age. The pathogenesis of type 2 diabetes remains unknown but it is believed to be a heterogeneous disorder with a strong genetic factor. Approximately 80% of individuals with type 2 diabetes are obese.

Type 2 diabetes is characterized by three major metabolic abnormalities:

1. impairment in pancreatic beta cell insulin secretion in response to a glucose stimulus
2. reduced sensitivity to the action of insulin in major organ systems such as muscle, liver and adipose tissue
3. excessive hepatic glucose production in the basal state.

Clinical perspective

Diagnosis

Both type 1 and type 2 diabetes are diagnosed by detection of a fasting (>8 hours) plasma glucose level that exceeds 7 mmol/L (126 mg/dL), or a plasma glucose level greater than 11 mmol/L (200 mg/dL) at

2 hours after an oral glucose challenge (oral glucose tolerance test), or by the appearance of other classic symptoms of diabetes.

Diabetic screening

Prior to commencement or an increase in the intensity of an exercise program in patients with diabetes, a full examination should be performed with particular attention to the sites of diabetic complications—the cardiovascular system, the feet and the eyes.

Ideally patients should have reasonable diabetic control before considering exercise. Long-term diabetic control indicators such as glycosylated hemoglobin (HbA$_{1C}$) and fructosamine allow an objective measure. The HbA$_{1C}$ level allows assessment of the diabetes control in the preceding two to three months, and fructosamine in the preceding three weeks. The actual levels of these markers accepted to indicate reasonable control depends on the laboratory used. The ideal HbA$_{1C}$ level should be less than or equal to 7% for most patients. A blood glucose level diary should be kept, with measurements taken at variable times during the day. Fasting cholesterol and triglyceride levels should also be measured. Assessment of renal function measuring urea, creatinine and electrolyte levels, and urinary protein excretion and creatinine clearance should also be performed.

Examination should focus on the:

1. cardiovascular system—blood pressure including postural drop, heart, presence of carotid bruits, peripheral pulses
2. eyes—retinopathy, glaucoma, cataracts
3. peripheral neuropathy.

Pre-exercise cardiac screening should be thorough. Ischemic heart disease is present in up to 50% of patients with type 2 diabetes at the time of diagnosis and 'chest pain' will not always be present in a diabetic because of the risk of silent ischemia secondary to autonomic neuropathy. Exercise stress testing should be performed if the patient:

- will be undergoing vigorous activity (heart rate >60% of maximum)
- has had type 2 diabetes for more than 10 years
- has had type 1 diabetes for more than 15 years
- is over 35 years of age
- has any coronary artery disease risk factors
- has any micro/macrovascular disease or peripheral vascular disease.

Complications

Both type 1 and type 2 diabetes may result in complications that affect multiple end-organ systems. In particular, diabetes is associated with accelerated atherosclerosis formation, resulting in the risk of acute myocardial infarction increasing by two to three times.[2] Peripheral arterial disease incidence is elevated dramatically and the risk of cerebral stroke doubles. In addition, diabetes can cause retinopathy, nephropathy and autonomic neuropathy (leading to complications such as impaired gastric emptying, altered sweating and potential silent myocardial ischemia), all of which can have serious implications for exercise. The risk of such complications is associated with both the duration of the diabetes and the diabetic control. The life expectancy of someone with diabetes is reduced to two-thirds that of a non-diabetic individual.[3]

Treatment

The treatment of both type 1 and type 2 diabetes depends on the maintenance of near normal blood glucose levels. For those patients with type 1 diabetes, exogenous insulin is essential, in conjunction with management through diet and close monitoring of blood glucose levels. In contrast, only patients with poorly controlled type 2 diabetes require insulin, the majority being managed with a combination of diet, exercise and weight loss. If, however, this is not adequate, a patient with type 2 diabetes may require the use of oral hypoglycemic agents. These agents are used in preference to insulin, the insulin being reserved only for patients in whom adequate control cannot be achieved. For people with either type 1 or type 2 diabetes, a low-fat, carbohydrate-controlled diet with an emphasis on an increased intake of complex carbohydrates and reduced simple carbohydrates is recommended.

Pharmacotherapy in diabetes

Four principle types of insulin are available for patients with type 1 diabetes:

1. Rapid acting: very fast onset (within 5–15 minutes with a peak of action within 1 hour) and short duration (3–5 hours). Examples include insulin lispro and insulin aspart.
2. Short acting: rapid onset of action (within 30 minutes with peak of action between 2–3 hours) and longer duration (5–8 hours). Examples include neutral insulin (e.g. Actrapid, Humulin R).

3. Intermediate acting: slower onset (may take 1–2 hours with peak of action between 4–10 hours) and longer duration (6–18 hours). Examples include lente (Monotard) and Protophane.

4. Long acting: slow onset (2+ hours with peak at 6–20 hours) and long duration (at least 24 hours) allowing a background level of insulin. Examples include ultralente. Insulin glargine is another long-acting insulin that is 'peakless', with onset in about 1.5 hours and a maximum effect at 4–5 hours that is maintained for 11–24 hours.

Exercising diabetics have the options of using a combination of self-administration of the above types of insulin (classically three courses of rapid-acting insulin with meals during the day, and an intermediate- or long-acting insulin at night) or of using a continuous subcutaneous insulin pump allowing for background insulin to be delivered every few minutes in small increments to meet requirements during fasting and sleep, and boluses to be delivered before meals and snacks. The infusion set is replaced every two to three days with a new subcutaneous infusion site. Complications include blockage (and potential unexpected hyperglycemia) and infections, and units are costly to maintain.

In contrast, only patients with poorly controlled type 2 diabetes require insulin. If a trial of a healthy lifestyle for two to three months is unsuccessful in controlling the blood glucose level, oral hypoglycemic agents can be used. If weight continues to be lost while exercising the dose may be reduced or even stopped. Metformin is usually the medication of first choice. It enhances glucose uptake and reduces hepatic glucose output and insulin resistance. Sulfonylureas increase pancreatic insulin production. They can cause hypoglycemia and should be used with caution when undertaking vigorous exercise. If an HbA_{1C} of less than 7% is not achieved after three months of monotherapy, combination therapy should be considered. The most commonly used combination is a sulfonylurea and metformin. These agents are used in preference to insulin, the insulin being reserved only for patients in whom adequate control cannot be achieved.

Dietary management

The importance of a high-carbohydrate, low-fat diet for optimal diabetic control is now well established. Fortunately, this conforms to the guidelines for maximizing athletic performance. Some older patients with type 2 diabetes may have been educated to have a low-carbohydrate diet, which results in depletion of glycogen stores and impairment of performance.

Carbohydrate requirements for exercise vary considerably between individuals and athletes should be encouraged to monitor their blood glucose levels to determine their carbohydrate needs before, during and after exercise (Table 48.1).

Individuals vary considerably in their responses to exercise. Only blood glucose monitoring before, during and after training determines individual needs. Table 48.1 should be used as a starting point or guide only.

Athletes involved in endurance events who are carbohydrate-loading prior to competition may need to increase their insulin dosage to cope with the increased carbohydrate intake. It is then important that carbohydrate is ingested before, during and after the event.

While it is advised that all insulin-dependent diabetic athletes seek individual counseling from a sports dietitian and physician to arrange a specific dietary and training program, there are some important points that all diabetic athletes should be aware of:

- Athletes need to learn the effects of different types of exercise, under different environmental conditions, on their blood glucose levels.
- When exercising away from home, it is important to always carry carbohydrate foods such as fruit, fruit juice, barley sugar or biscuits.
- After vigorous exercise, blood glucose levels may continue to drop for a number of hours. It is important that carbohydrate is ingested when exercise is completed to ensure replenishment of glycogen stores and to prevent hypoglycemia.
- Dehydration may be confused with hypoglycemia. All athletes should be encouraged to consume plenty of fluid before, during and after exercise.
- Alcohol should be discouraged after exercise as it lowers blood glucose levels as well as having a dehydrating effect.
- The best time for training is when blood glucose levels are above fasting level but not high. About 1–2 hours following a meal is ideal.
- If exercise is intermittent, the athlete should take some form of carbohydrate during the breaks to control blood glucose levels and to prevent hunger.
- During long-duration exercise, most diabetic athletes require regular carbohydrate intake in the form of food or liquids.
- Exercise may speed up the absorption of insulin from exercising limbs. This can be counteracted

Table 48.1 Adjustment of food intake with exercise

Activity	Time	Blood glucose level (mmol/L [mg/dL])	Adjustment
Low level	½ hour	<5.5 (<100) >5.5 (>100)	10 g CHO (small serve fruit, bread, biscuits, yoghurt or milk) No extra food
Moderate intensity	1 hour	<5.5 (<100) 5.5–10 (100–180) 10–16.5 (180–300) >16.5 (>300)	20–30 g CHO (1.5–2 serves fruit, bread, biscuits, yoghurt and/or milk) 10 g CHO (small serve fruit, bread, biscuits, yoghurt or milk) No extra food (in most cases) No extra food. Preferably do not exercise as blood glucose level may go up
Strenuous activity	1–2 hours	<5.5 (<100) 5.5–10 (100–180) 10–16.5 (180–300) >16.5 (>300)	45–60 g CHO (1 sandwich and fruit and/or milk or yoghurt) 25–50 g CHO (½ sandwich and fruit and/or milk or yoghurt) 15 g CHO (1 serve fruit, bread, biscuits, yoghurt or milk) Preferably do not exercise as blood glucose level may go up
Varying intensity	Long duration ½–1 day		Insulin may best be decreased (Conservatively estimate the decrease in insulin peaking at time of activity by 10%. A 50% reduction is not common.) Increase carbohydrate before, during and after activity 10–50 g CHO per hour, such as diluted fruit juice

CHO = carbohydrate.

to some extent by injecting into parts of the body away from the exercising muscle (e.g. the abdomen).

Exercise and diabetes

The sports physician should be encouraged to work closely with the endocrinologist when considering exercise prescription for a diabetic patient. The target of an adult should be to achieve *at least* 30 minutes of continuous moderate activity, equivalent to brisk walking five or six days a week, with the flexibility of shorter bouts of more intense activity being considered important. This is provided that cardiovascular and hypertensive problems are taken into account. Heart rate may be an unreliable indicator of exertion because of autonomic neuropathy, and the rating of perceived exertion scales may be more useful.

Although exercise in conjunction with a proper diet and medications is the cornerstone in the treatment of diabetes, special care must be taken in those taking insulin. Both insulin and exercise *independently* facilitate glucose transport across the mitochondrial membrane by promoting GLUT4 transporter proteins from intracellular vesicles. The action of insulin and exercise is also *cumulative*. As such, an exercising type 1 diabetic will have lowered insulin requirements, and may notice up to a 30% reduction in insulin requirements with exercise. Importantly, in the person with

type 1 diabetes, glycemic control may not be improved with regular exercise if changes in the individual's diet and insulin dosage do not appropriately match exercise requirements. In the absence of exercise, even for a few days, the increased insulin sensitivity begins to decline.

It is of extreme importance that those with diabetes monitor their blood glucose levels before and after every work-out. If the work-out is prolonged, or symptoms occur, the blood sugar level should also be taken during the exercise session. If no means exist to identify blood glucose levels before a work-out, then the work-out should be of short duration and low intensity with a glucose supply readily available.

Certain environmental conditions, such as extreme heat or strong winds, should be taken into consideration, as supplemental glucose may be required while exercising under such conditions. In contrast, if exercising when unwell or with a low-grade infection, glucose levels need to be monitored as a relative hyperglycemia may occur.

All patients with diabetes should carry an identification card or bracelet identifying them as having diabetes. They should be educated to be alert to the early signs of hypoglycemia for at least 6–12 hours after exercise. It is essential that they carry glucose tablets or an alternative source of glucose with them at all times. Dehydration during exercise should be prevented by adequate fluid consumption. It is also recommended that the diabetic athlete exercise with somebody else, if possible, in case of adverse reactions.

Benefits of exercise

The benefits of exercise in type 1 diabetics include improved insulin sensitivity, improved blood lipid profiles, decreased heart rate and blood pressure at rest, decreased body weight and possible decreased risk of coronary heart disease.[4] It does not appear that exercise improves glycemic control, however, insulin requirements may be decreased slightly. While exercise may not improve glucose control, the benefits of exercise in those with diabetes occur mainly through reducing the risk factors for cardiovascular disease. People with type 1 diabetes typically live longer if they participate in regular physical activity as a part of their lifestyle.[5]

It is well recognized that exercise reduces the risk of developing type 2 diabetes. There are also considerable benefits for those with type 2 diabetes.[6] A program of regular physical activity can reverse many of the defects in metabolism of both fat and glucose that occur in people with type 2 diabetes.[7]

As noted above, HbA_{1C} is used as an index of long-term blood glucose control. The lower the value, the better. HbA_{1C} is reduced by chronic exercise in people with type 2 diabetes. The evidence for improvement of HbA_{1C} with exercise in type 1 diabetes is not as convincing.

Exercise and type 1 diabetes

Control of blood glucose is achieved in a patient with type 1 diabetes through a balance in the carbohydrate intake, exercise level and insulin dosage. The meal plan and insulin dosage should be adjusted according to the patient's response to exercise. Unfortunately a degree of trial and error is necessary for type 1 diabetics taking up new activities. Frequent self-monitoring should occur, at least until a balance is achieved among diet, exercise and insulin parameters. The ideal pre-exercise blood level is 6.6–10 mmol/L (120–180 mg/dL).[4] Athletes who have blood glucose concentrations exceeding 11 mmol/L (200 mg/dL) and ketones in their urine, or a blood glucose level of more than 16.5 mmol/L (300 mg/dL) regardless of ketone status, should postpone exercise and take supplemental insulin. Those with blood glucose levels less than 5.5 mmol/L (100 mg/dL) require a pre-exercise carbohydrate snack (e.g. sports drink, juice, glucose tablet, fruit).

Exercise of 20–30 minutes at less than 70% Vo_{2max} (e.g. walking, golf, table tennis) requires a rapidly absorbable carbohydrate (15 g fruit exchange or 60 calories) before exercise but needs minimal insulin dosing adjustments.

More vigorous activity of less than 1 hour (e.g. jogging, swimming, cycling, skiing, tennis) often requires a 25% reduction in pre-exercise insulin and 15–30 g of rapidly absorbed carbohydrate exchange before and every 30 minutes after the onset of activity.

Strenuous activity of longer than 1 hour (e.g. marathon running, triathlon, cross-country skiing) will require a 30–80% reduction in pre-exercise insulin and ingestion of two fruit exchanges (30 g or 100–120 calories) every 30 minutes. It is important to remember that excess insulin exacerbates the hypoglycemic effect more during intense rather than moderate exercise.

If early morning activity is to be performed the basal insulin from the evening dose of intermediate-acting insulin may need to be reduced by 20–50%, with checking of the morning blood glucose level. The morning regular-acting insulin dose may also need to be reduced by 30–50% before breakfast, or even omitted if exercise is performed before food. Depending on the intensity and duration of the initial activity and likelihood of further activity, a reduction of 30–50% may be needed with each subsequent meal.

After exercise hyperglycemia will occur, but insulin should still be decreased by 25–50% (because insulin sensitivity is increased for 12–15 hours after activity has ceased). Consuming carbohydrates within 30 minutes after exhaustive, glycogen-depleting exercise allows for more efficient restoration of muscle glycogen. This will also help prevent post-exercise, late-onset hypoglycemia, which can occur up to 24 hours following such exercise.[8]

If exercise is unexpected, then insulin adjustment may be impossible. Instead, supplementation with 20–30 g of carbohydrate, at the onset of exercise and every 30 minutes thereafter, may prevent hypoglycemia. In elite athletes and with intense bouts of exercise, reductions in insulin dosage may be even higher than those listed above. During periods of inactivity (e.g. holidays, recovery from injury), increased insulin requirements are to be expected.

Exercise and type 2 diabetes

Those patients with type 2 diabetes who are managed with diet therapy alone do not usually need to make any adjustments for exercise. Patients taking oral hypoglycemic drugs may need to halve their doses on days of prolonged exercise or withhold them altogether, depending on their blood glucose levels. They are also advised to carry some glucose with them and to be able to recognize the symptoms of hypoglycemia. Hypoglycemia is a particular risk in those people with diabetes taking sulfonylureas due to their long half-lives and increased endogenous insulin production. Biguanides (e.g. metformin) provide less of a problem as they do not increase insulin production.

Diabetes and competition

Diabetic athletes participating in team sports need to have a good knowledge of their normal glucose profile in response to exercise. As competition may require interstate travel and altered eating patterns, the diabetic athlete should practice the match day routine at home and have snacks available as necessary. Good control of blood glucose levels may require regular access to carbohydrate-containing drinks. This not only serves to improve the glucose profile but also aids rehydration during prolonged exercise.

Diabetes and travel

A physician's letter should accompany diabetic travelers stating that they carry insulin, needles and blood glucose testing equipment. Copies of prescriptions should be taken, with medications in their original packaging. Insulin should not be packed into checked luggage, as there is a risk of it being misplaced, and freezing and thawing in the luggage hold. Insulin will generally keep for a month at room temperature. An emergency supply of carbohydrate should be carried by the diabetic.

Travel from north to south generally requires no alteration to insulin doses. East to west travel of more than 5 hours generally requires insulin dose adjustment. East-bound travel results in a shorter day, while west-bound travel a longer one. Travelers should check blood glucose levels at least every 6 hours on the flight. Omitting long-acting insulin for the flight duration and using quick-acting insulin approximately every 6 hours around average meal times is one technique. Once at the destination, quick-acting insulin is used until bedtime, when long-acting insulin is recommenced. Continuous insulin pumps usually require no adjustment, with the pump's clock being adjusted to the destination time on arrival.

High-risk sports

The already high risk in certain sports is increased in diabetics. Hypoglycemic attacks, characterized by inattention or lack of concentration, in sports such as rock and mountain climbing and skydiving have the potential for serious if not fatal injury. The suitability of scuba diving for diabetics has been studied. Military diving is not allowed in Great Britain for those with type 1 diabetes, and in the United States they cannot join the military at all.[9] Scuba diving may be safe with adequate preparation and a skilled partner who can handle trouble with diabetes during the dive.

Exercise and the complications of diabetes

Exercise is often neglected when the secondary complications of diabetes occur. Some unique concerns for the patient with diabetes that warrant close scrutiny include autonomic and peripheral neuropathy, retinopathy and nephropathy. Poor glucose control appears to be associated with an increased occurrence of neuropathy.

Abnormal autonomic function is common among those with diabetes of long duration. The risks of exercise when autonomic neuropathy is present include hypoglycemia, abnormal heart rate and blood pressure responses (e.g. postural drop), impaired sympathetic and parasympathetic nervous system activity and abnormal thermoregulation. Patients with autonomic neuropathy are at high risk of developing complications during exercise. Sudden death and myocardial infarction have been attributed to autonomic neuropathy and diabetes. High-intensity activity should be avoided, as should rapid changes in body position and extremes in temperature. Water activities and stationary cycling are recommended.

Peripheral neuropathy (typically manifested as loss of sensation and of two point discrimination) usually begins symmetrically in the lower and upper extremities and progresses proximally. Podiatric review should occur on a regular basis, and correct footwear can prevent the onset of foot ulcers. Regular close inspection of the feet and use of proper footwear are important and the patient should avoid exercise that may cause trauma to the feet. Feet and toes should be kept dry and clean and dry socks should also be used. Non-weight-bearing activities, such as swimming, cycling and arm exercises, are recommended in those with insensitive feet. Activities that improve balance are appropriate choices.

The incidence of diabetic retinopathy is directly proportional to the severity and duration of the diabetes: 98% of cases of type 1 and 78% of type 2 diabetes will progress to detectable retinopathy in 15 years from the diagnosis. Diabetics with proliferative retinopathy should avoid exercise that increases systolic blood pressures to 170 mmHg and prolonged Valsalva-like activities. Exercise that increases blood pressure may worsen retinopathy. Jarring of the head during exercise in contact sports may cause detachment of the retina. In those with proliferative retinopathy, only submaximal exercise tests should be conducted. Exercise that results in a large increase in systolic pressure (such as weightlifting) can cause retinal hemorrhage. Exercise for these patients could include stationary cycling, walking and swimming. If possible, blood pressure should be monitored during the exercise program. Exercise is contraindicated if the individual has had recent photocoagulation treatment or surgery.

Diabetic nephropathy can be classified according to urinary albumin excretion rates: <20 μg/min (normo-albuminuria); 20–200 μg/min (microalbuminuria); >200 μg/min (overt nephropathy). Patients with microalbuminuria and overt renal disease should undertake light-to-moderate exercise only. Vigorous exercise that results in marked changes in hemo-dynamics should be avoided. These include lifting heavy weights and high-intensity aerobic activities. Activities that are weight-bearing yet low impact are preferable. It is important to wear well-cushioned shoes. Renal patients should be fully evaluated before commencing an exercise program. Fluid replacement is extremely important in these patients. Specific training programs for patients undergoing hemodialysis are advised.

Complications of exercise in the diabetic athlete

The diabetic athlete may suffer hypoglycemia, diabetic ketoacidosis and problems associated with the complications of diabetes. Patients should be encouraged to monitor their blood glucose level before, during and after exercise and to learn their individual patterns of response to exercise of different intensities and durations and to avoid these potentially life-threatening complications.

Hypoglycemia

Hypoglycemia (blood glucose level <3.6 mmol/L [<65 mg/dL]) is the major concern among athletes with type 1 diabetes. The use of too much exogenous insulin will prevent hepatic glucose production, and cause increased glucose uptake into skeletal muscle with a subsequent risk of exercise-induced hypoglycemia. After exercise there is increased insulin sensitivity and reduced glycogen stores, and excess insulin

will increase the risk of post-exercise hypoglycemia. Post-exercise and delayed-onset hypoglycemia can occur up to 4–24 hours after exercise, respectively. The effects are commonly nocturnal with disturbed sleep patterns, altered recovery and impaired performance the following day.

The initial symptoms of hypoglycemia include sweating, headache, nervousness, tremor and hunger. The symptoms of impending hypoglycemia may be difficult to differentiate from symptoms experienced during vigorous exercise. If the hypoglycemia is not corrected, confusion, abnormal behavior, loss of consciousness and convulsions may occur.

At the first indication of hypoglycemia, the athlete should ingest oral carbohydrate in solid or liquid form. Diabetic athletes should carry quickly digestible forms of carbohydrate (e.g. glucose tablets, barley sugar) or have a glucose–electrolyte solution available. The semiconscious or unconscious diabetic patient requires urgent intravenous glucose administration (50 mL of 50% solution).

Nocturnal hypoglycemia may occur following late afternoon or evening training or competition. Symptoms include night sweats, unpleasant dreams and early morning headaches.

Prevention of hypoglycemia depends upon adjustment of the carbohydrate intake and insulin dosage to meet the individual athlete's needs, as discussed above. A continual source of glucose must be available during exercise and, as a rule of thumb, athletes usually require 15–30 g of glucose per half hour of vigorous exercise. Nocturnal hypoglycemia may be prevented by exercising earlier in the day, reducing the evening insulin dose or by consuming a complex carbohydrate prior to going to bed.

Diabetic ketoacidosis in the athlete

Despite increased glucose uptake that occurs in exercise independent of insulin, a relative deficiency of insulin can lead to hyperglycemia, hyperlipidemia and possible diabetic ketoacidosis. Individuals with blood glucose levels of 20–25 mmol/L (364–455 mg/dL) and above are especially at risk of precipitating diabetic ketoacidosis if they exercise vigorously. This occurs because the counter-regulatory hormone response (glucagon, catecholamines, growth hormone and glucocorticoids) to exercise pushes the glucose levels higher and there is insufficient insulin to prevent ketosis. Therefore, an athlete must be aware of his or her diabetic control before exercise. In addition, athletes with so-called brittle diabetes must be very cautious in reducing their insulin dose before exercise.

The presence of ketones in the urine confirms the presence of hypoinsulinemia and thus increases the risk of hyperglycemia and ketosis. Hyperglycemia may manifest as poor concentration, dehydration or even under-performance, and athletes need to be aware of these signs. If the blood glucose level is >17 mmol/L (>309 mg/dL) or 14 mmol/L (255 mg/dL) plus the presence of ketones on urinalysis, then exercise should be avoided until insulin has been administered and metabolic control is re-established. Athletes should not exercise as a way to control high blood glucose levels.

Musculoskeletal manifestations of diabetes

A number of musculoskeletal disorders are found in a higher prevalence in diabetic patients compared to the normal population.[10] The diagnosis of diabetes should always be considered in the patient presenting with the conditions listed below and summarized in Table 48.2.

- *Frozen shoulder (adhesive capsulitis).*[11] This condition appears at a younger age and is usually less painful in patients with diabetes. It is associated with the duration of diabetes and with age. The use of corticosteroid injections may increase blood sugar levels in diabetics over the 24–48 hour period after the injection.
- *Limited joint mobility.*[12] This is also known as diabetic cheiroarthropathy and is characterized by thick, tight, waxy skin mainly on the dorsal aspect of the hands, with flexion deformities of the MCP and IP joints. In the early stages paresthesias and slight pain may develop with symptoms increasing slowly. Treatment consists of optimizing diabetic control and individualized hand therapy.
- *Dupuytren's contracture.*[13] This is palmar or digital thickening, tethering or contracture of

the hands. In diabetics the ring and middle finger are more commonly affected compared with the fifth finger in non-diabetics. Treatment consists of optimizing glycemic control, physiotherapy and surgery if severe.
- *Carpal tunnel syndrome.*[14] This has a prevalence of 11–16% in diabetics; 5–8% of patients with carpal tunnel syndrome have diabetes.
- *Flexor tenosynovitis.*[15] This is fibrous tissue proliferation in the tendon sheath leading to limitation of the normal movement of the tendon. It is associated with the duration of diabetes, but not age, and a corticosteroid injection is often curative.
- *Complex regional pain syndrome type 1.*[16] This is characterized by continuing pain out of proportion to stimuli and vasomotor dysfunction. Other predisposing conditions include hyperthyroidism, hyperparathyroidism and type IV hyperlipidemia.
- *Diffuse idiopathic skeletal hyperostosis (DISH).*[17] This condition is characterized by new bone formation, particularly in the thoracolumbar spine. New bone appears to flow from one vertebra to the next, and is more prominent on the right side of the thoracic vertebra. Ossification of ligaments and tendons can occur elsewhere, including the skull, pelvis, heels or elbows. Twelve to 80% of patients with DISH have diabetes or impaired glucose tolerance. Management consists of education, diabetic control and physiotherapy.
- *Neuropathic (Charcot's) joints.*[18] This results from diabetic peripheral neuropathy and is seen usually in patients over 50 years of age who have had diabetes for many years. The joints affected are weight-bearing joints. Management includes optimizing glycemic control, regular foot care and review, and occasionally surgery.

Table 48.2 Prevalence of musculoskeletal disorders in patients with or without diabetes[10]

Musculoskeletal disorder	With diabetes	Without diabetes
Adhesive capsulitis (frozen shoulder)	11–30%	2–10%
Limited joint mobility	8–50%	0–26%
Dupuytren's contracture	20–63%	13%
Carpal tunnel syndrome	11–16%	0.125%
Flexor tenosynovitis	11%	<1%
Diffuse idiopathic skeletal hyperostosis	13–49%	1.6–13%

- *Diabetic amyotrophy.*[19] This is distinct from other forms of diabetic neuropathy and is characterized by muscle weakness/wasting and by diffuse, proximal lower limb muscle pain, and asymmetrical loss of tendon jerks. The shoulder girdle may be affected but less commonly. It occurs most often in older men with type 2 diabetes and is a diagnosis of exclusion (sinister causes must be sought). Management consists of stabilizing glycemic control and the use of physiotherapy.

Conclusion

The athlete with diabetes needs to have a good understanding of the effects of exercise on blood glucose levels. With regular monitoring and appropriate adjustments to insulin dosage and carbohydrate intake, the athlete with diabetes should be able to participate fully in sporting activities.

Recommended Reading

Bassuk SS, Manson JE. Epidemiological evidence for the role of physical activity in reducing risk of type 2 diabetes and cardiovascular disease. *J Appl Physiol* 2005; 99(3): 1193–204.

Birrer RB, Sedaghat V-D. Exercise and diabetes mellitus. *Physician Sportsmed* 2003; 31(5): 29–41.

La Monte MJ, Blair SN, Church TS. Physical activity and diabetes prevention. *J Appl Physiol* 2005; 99(3): 1205–13.

Smith LL, Burnet SP, McNeil JD. Musculoskeletal manifestations of diabetes mellitus. *Br J Sports Med* 2003; 37: 30–5.

Zinman B, Ruderman N, Campaigne BN, et al; American Diabetes Association. Physical activity/exercise and diabetes. *Diabetes Care* 2004; 27 (suppl. 1): 558–62.

References

1. Gallen IW, Redgrave A, Redgrave S. Olympic diabetes. *Clin Med* 2003; 3(4): 333–7.

2. Garcia MJ, McNamara PM, Gordon T, et al. Morbidity and mortality in diabetes in the Framingham population. A sixteen year follow up study. *Diabetes Care* 1974; 23: 105–11.

3. Campaigne BN, Lampman RM. *Exercise in the Clinical Management of Diabetes.* Champaign, IL: Human Kinetics, 1994.

4. Birrer RB, Sedaghat V. Exercise and diabetes mellitus. *Physician Sportsmed* 2003; 31(5): 29–41.

5. Moy CS, Songer TJ, LaPorte RE, et al. Insulin dependent diabetes mellitus, physical activity and death. *Am J Epidemiol* 1993; 137: 74–81.

6. Boule NG, Haddad E, Kenny GP, et al. Effects of exercise on glycemic control and body mass in type 2 diabetes mellitus. A meta-analysis of controlled clinical trials. *JAMA* 2001; 286: 1218–27.

7. Farrell PA. Diabetes, exercise and competitive sports. *Gatorade Sports Sci Inst Sports Sci Exchange* 2003; 16: 1–6.

8. Colberg SR, Swain DP. Exercise and diabetes control: a winning combination. *Physician Sportsmed* 2000; 28(4): 63–81.

9. Draznin M. Type 1 diabetes and sports participation: strategies for training and competing safely. *Physician Sportsmed* 2000; 28(12): 49–56.

10. Smith LL, Burnet SP, McNeil JD. Musculoskeletal manifestations of diabetes mellitus. *Br J Sports Med* 2003; 37(1): 30–5.

11. Balci N, Balci MK, Tuzuner S. Shoulder adhesive capsulitis and shoulder range of motion in type ii diabetes mellitus: association with diabetic complications. *J Diabetes Complications* 1999; 13: 135–40.

12. Buckingham BA, Uitto J, Sandborg C, et al. Scleroderma-like changes in insulin-dependent diabetes mellitus: clinical and biochemical studies. *Diabetes Care* 1984; 7: 163–9.

13. Gudmundsson KG, Angrimsson R, Sigfusson N, et al. Epidemiology of Dupuytren's disease: clinical, serological, and social assessment. The Reykavik study. *J Clin Epidemiol* 2000; 59: 291–6.

14. Comi G, Lozza L, Galardi G, et al. Presence of carpal tunnel syndrome in diabetics: effect of age, sex, duration and polyneuropathy. *Acta Diabetol Lat* 1985; 22: 259–62.

15. Leden I, Schersten B, Svensson B, et al. Locomotor system disorders in diabetes mellitus. Increased prevalence of palmar flexor tenosynovitis. *Scand J Rheumatol* 1983; 12: 260–2.

16. Marshall AT, Crisp AJ. Reflex sympathetic dystrophy. *Rheumatology (Oxford)* 2000; 39: 401–9.

17. Forgacs SS. Diabetes mellitus and rheumatic disease. *Clin Rheum Dis* 1986; 12: 729–53.

18. Bayne O, Lu EJ. Diabetic Charcot's arthropathy of the wrist. Case report and literature review. *Clin Orthop* 1998; 357: 122–6.

19. Sander HW. Diabetic amyotrophy: current concepts. *Semin Neurol* 1996; 16: 173–8.

The Athlete with Epilepsy

WITH PAUL McCRORY

Epidemiology and nomenclature

Epilepsy affects approximately 2% of the population. In three-quarters of these cases, the diagnosis is made before the age of 21 years. Thus, epilepsy is a relatively common condition that may affect individuals during the years of sport participation.

Epilepsy is a neurological disorder of the brain characterized by recurrent (more than two) seizures. It has been estimated that approximately 10–30% of the population will have a seizure at some time in their lives.[1] However, neither single episodes of seizures during adolescence or adult life, nor febrile convulsions in infancy, constitute a diagnosis of epilepsy.

The terms 'seizure', 'epilepsy', 'convulsion' and 'fit' are often used interchangeably. For the purpose of this chapter, the term 'seizure' will refer to an epileptic seizure and the term 'convulsion' will be used to describe the movements during an episode without implying a specific etiology.

Pathology

A seizure usually occurs suddenly and is the result of an abnormal electrical discharge within the brain. In the vast majority of cases, the cause of the electrical disturbance in the brain is unknown. In a small percentage of cases, either specific genetic inheritance or structural anatomical abnormalities can induce seizures. Cortical scars related to head injuries, stroke and other intracranial injuries may also cause seizures. During the seizure there may be an initial prodromal stage ('aura'), followed rapidly by disturbances in movement and alterations in consciousness.

Epilepsy can be classified by criteria developed by the International League Against Epilepsy (ILAE),[2] which are presently under review.[3] This classification utilizes the electroclinical features of the seizure to make a syndromal or etiological diagnosis, which then has important implications for management. In the broadest sense, the ILAE classification breaks seizures into generalized or focal (depending on the origin of the seizure), and complex or partial (depending upon whether consciousness is preserved during the episode). Outside of neurological practise, the specific epilepsy subtype may be difficult to quantify and subjects are often simply reported to have a generalized seizure. This type of seizure was previously known as 'grand mal' but this term has fallen out of favor and should be avoided.

Generalized tonic–clonic seizure

In the generalized tonic–clonic seizure, the patient usually falls to the ground and goes through a 'tonic' phase of muscle stiffness followed by a 'clonic' phase of muscle twitches prior to resolution of the attack. After the attack, the patient is usually sleepy, confused and may have a headache. The average length of the seizure is usually no more than 30 seconds, although most people who have witnessed someone having a seizure feel that the attack seems to last much longer.

Convulsions that are not due to epilepsy

In addition to the true epilepsy seizures described above, there are other situations where convulsions may occur. These may superficially resemble epilepsy although the etiology of such syndromes is distinctly different. These have the potential to cause confusion for non-neurologists and the eyewitness history usually provides the basis of the diagnosis. The two commonest situations are listed below:

1. Concussive convulsions, where a convulsion may be a manifestation of the concussive impact. Although usually brief and limited to tonic posturing, it may occasionally result in a prolonged convulsion over several minutes. These are benign phenomena and require no specific management beyond that of the underlying concussion (Chapter 13).[4, 5]
2. Convulsive syncope, where convulsive movements (including generalized movements, tongue biting and incontinence) occur in the setting of a syncopal faint.

In both situations the convulsive movements result from reflex phenomena, not epileptic discharge.

Diagnosis of epilepsy

The diagnosis of epilepsy relies primarily upon the clinical history and on the nature of the electroencephalogram (EEG) changes. The most important and useful diagnostic consideration is history from an eyewitness who has seen and can describe the attack, particularly the onset and offset of the seizure. Any patient observed to have a seizure should be referred to a neurologist for assessment.

Investigations

In most cases of a seizure, a neurologist would order an EEG as well as neuroimaging studies (usually MRI). If the EEG is performed within 24 hours of a seizure, its diagnostic sensitivity is increased from 30% to 50% and this may be further improved by performing a 'sleep-deprived' EEG study. MRI is the investigation of choice to adequately image the brain in this circumstance. Specific MRI protocols are necessary to obtain diagnostic information in these cases. Where necessary, these investigations would be supplemented by blood tests to rule out other causes of seizures, such as hypoglycemia, hyper- or hyponatremia (Chapter 53) or hypercalcemia.

Treatment

The role of specific treatment in patients with a single seizure or recurrent seizures (epilepsy) requires an understanding of the nature of the seizure disorder and its natural history as well as individual patient consideration. In some situations, drug treatment should begin after a single seizure. Consideration of lifestyle factors in the overall management is paramount. Specific factors that may lower seizure threshold include sleep deprivation, alcohol and use of recreational drugs. Patients must be specifically counseled about such lifestyle issues when they begin pharmacological therapy.

More than half the individuals taking antiepileptic medication for idiopathic generalized epilepsy can expect to be seizure-free with minimal restriction on their lifestyle. Approximately one-third may have only an occasional seizure, which usually does not greatly limit their lifestyle. The other 20% will have seizures frequently enough to restrict their lifestyle to some extent.

The medications used in the treatment of epilepsy may cause a number of side-effects, including tiredness, poor concentration, impairment of coordination and cognitive impairment. In some cases, medication (e.g. phenytoin) toxicity may result in permanent neurological symptoms.

Exercise prescription

Regular physical activity is advocated for individuals with epilepsy.[6] In general, people with epilepsy report better seizure control when exercising regularly.[7] Occasionally, some individuals will have more seizures with exercise,[8] and hence every case must be treated individually. Persons with epilepsy have no higher injury rate in sport[6] than those without epilepsy and sport participation does not affect serum drug levels.

In a sample of over 200 patients with epilepsy in Norway, exercise patterns were similar to that of the average population.[6] In the majority of the patients, physical exercise had no adverse effects, and over a third of patients claimed that regular exercise contributed to better seizure control. In 10% of patients, exercise appeared to be a seizure precipitant and this applied particularly to those with symptomatic partial epilepsy (i.e. underlying structural brain lesion). The risk of sustaining serious seizure-related injuries while exercising in this population was modest.[6]

There are a number of important considerations when counseling the individual who has epilepsy and wishes to exercise. Patients having frequent seizures must be discouraged from activities such as scuba diving, horseback riding or rock climbing. Sports where any impairment in split-second neuromuscular timing is dangerous (e.g. motor racing or downhill ski racing) should also be avoided. Patients with epilepsy will not be affected adversely by participating in contact sport provided the normal safeguards for participation are followed.

The frequency of seizures is important when considering activities such as swimming, where the potential for serious injury exists if a seizure were to occur. Generally, swimming is allowed under supervision (e.g. with a 'buddy'). Swimming with a companion is a sensible rule for all swimmers, not just those with epilepsy.

The physical and psychological wellbeing of the individual also requires attention. In children, particularly adolescents, participation in activities is important in establishing a good self-image and gaining peer group acceptance. Therefore, it is important to allow the child with epilepsy to pursue many activities. Absolute and relative contraindications to sporting activities are shown in Table 49.1.

Management of a seizure

Observing a seizure can be a frightening experience. For an observer, there is often an overwhelming feeling of helplessness and concern that the patient may die during the seizure. It is important to remember that seizures always terminate spontaneously and that rarely is a seizure life-threatening. Furthermore, the patient experiencing the seizure usually does not feel pain or remember the event.

Any individual observing or supervising an epileptic patient should remember two things when confronted by a seizure. Firstly, the individual must be protected from injury. Secondly, the seizure must be closely observed in order to give an accurate description to the patient's physician. The longstanding convention of trying to put a knotted sheet or spoon in the patient's mouth should be discouraged and the patient should not be physically restrained under most circumstances.

It is important to remember that the shaking will cease spontaneously after a period of time. At the end of this time, the patient breathes normally and appears sleepy. The patient should then be managed as for an unconscious patient (e.g. the ABC of first aid, Chapter 44).

Conclusion

Overall, people with epilepsy are able to participate in sport with few limitations. Occasionally, it is appropriate to restrict certain physical activities. A person with epilepsy must meet certain legal obligations when driving a car. The individual with epilepsy must take his or her medication correctly and ensure a well-balanced eating and sleeping schedule. Family, friends, team mates and coaches must be aware of the epilepsy and understand what to do in the event of a seizure. All these factors will contribute to removing unnecessary barriers to a normal active lifestyle in those with epilepsy.

Recommended Reading

Dubow JS, Kelly JP. Epilepsy in sports and recreation. *Sports Med* 2003; 33(7): 499–516.

Fountain NB, May AC. Epilepsy and athletics. *Clin Sports Med* 2003; 22: 605–16.

Howard GM, Radloff M, Sevier TL. Epilepsy and sports participation. *Curr Sports Med Rep* 2004; 3: 15–19.

Mesad S, Devinsky O. Epilepsy and the athlete. In: Jordan B, Tsaris P, Warren RF, eds. *Sports Neurology*. 2nd edn. Philadelphia: Lippincott-Raven Publishers, 1998: 275–89.

McCrory PR, Berkovic SF. Concussive convulsions. Incidence in sport and treatment recommendations. *Sports Med* 1998; 25: 131–6.

Sahoo SK, Fountain NB. Epilepsy in football players and other land-based contact or collision sport athletes: when can they participate, and is there an increased risk *Curr Sports Med Rep* 2004; 3: 284–8.

Table 49.1 Absolute and relative contraindications to sporting activities in people with epilepsy

Absolute	Relative (with supervision)
Rock climbing	Swimming
Flying	Cross-country skiing
Hang-gliding	Backpacking
Pistol shooting	Cycling
Scuba diving	
Archery	
Sky diving, parachuting	
Motor racing	

References

1. Sander JW, Hart YM, Johnson AL, et al. National General Practice Study of Epilepsy: newly diagnosed epileptic seizures in a general population. *Lancet* 1990; 336: 1267–71.

2. Commission on Classification and Terminology of the International League Against Epilepsy. Proposal for revised classification of epilepsies and epileptic syndromes. *Epilepsia* 1989; 30: 389–99.

3. Engel J, Jr. Classifications of the International League Against Epilepsy: time for reappraisal. *Epilepsia* 1998; 39: 1014–17.

4. McCrory PR, Berkovic SF. Concussive convulsions. Incidence in sport and treatment recommendations. *Sports Med* 1998; 25: 131–6.

5. McCrory PR, Bladin PF, Berkovic SF. Retrospective study of concussive convulsions in elite Australian rules and rugby league footballers: phenomenology, aetiology, and outcome. *Br Med J* 1997; 314: 171–4.

6. Nakken KO. Physical exercise in outpatients with epilepsy. *Epilepsia* 1999; 40: 643–51.

7. Eriksen HR, Ellertsen B, Gronningsaeter H, et al. Physical exercise in women with intractable epilepsy. *Epilepsia* 1994; 35: 1256–64.

8. Schmitt B, Thun-Hohenstein L, Vontobel H, et al. Seizures induced by physical exercise: report of two cases. *Neuropediatrics* 1994; 25: 51–3.

Joint-Related Symptoms without Acute Injury

WITH NICK CARTER

The dictum 'not everything that presents to the sports clinic is sports medicine' should never be forgotten. In daily practise sports clinicians see many patients who have mechanical joint injuries; thus, it can be tempting to attribute a mechanical diagnosis to every patient who presents with a painful or swollen joint. It is, however, wise to maintain an index of suspicion for inflammatory joint disease masquerading as a mechanical condition. For example, a 30-year-old runner may present with recurrent knee swelling but have no convincing history of injury. Swelling is very uncommon in patellofemoral pain (Chapter 28) and a meniscal injury is rare without trauma at that age. Thus, the athlete presents with a single swollen joint but no injury. The clinician should be alert to the possibility that this swollen knee may be caused by an inflammatory condition. In this chapter we discuss the clinical approach to diagnosing patients with the following four common presentations:

1. the single swollen joint
2. low back pain and stiffness
3. multiple joint symptoms
4. joint pain and 'pain all over'.

We also discuss when to use rheumatological investigations and how to interpret them.

The patient with a single swollen joint

In the athlete with a single swollen joint without a history of trauma, a possible inflammatory cause should be considered. Table 50.1 summarizes the differential diagnosis of a single swollen joint.

Table 50.1 Differential diagnosis in the athlete presenting with a single swollen joint without a clear history of trauma

Common conditions	Less common conditions
Reactive arthritis	Pigmented villonodular synovitis
Septic arthritis	Juxta-articular bone tumors
Psoriatic arthritis	Synovial sarcoma
Gout/pseudogout	Monoarticular rheumatoid arthritis
Peripheral ankylosing spondylitis	Acute sarcoidosis
Osteoarthritis	Peripheral enteric arthritis

Clinical perspective

The key to accurate diagnosis of a swollen joint is through taking a careful history and physical examination and having an appropriate index of suspicion. Inflammatory joint problems are characterized by pain, swelling, warmth, redness, night pain and prominent morning stiffness. In all athletes, and especially in children and adolescents, inflammatory, infective or neoplastic conditions should be considered in the light of these symptoms.

History

Many of the inflammatory diseases are associated with extra-articular features that may provide additional clues as to the diagnosis:

- Psoriatic arthritis may be associated with rash, nail dystrophy, tendon insertion pain (enthesopathy) or low back pain.

- A history of inflammatory bowel disease (ulcerative colitis, Crohn's disease or celiac disease) suggests enteropathic arthritis. Urethral discharge or eye inflammation may suggest a reactive arthritis.
- Rheumatoid arthritis is characteristically a small joint (hands, wrists and feet), symmetrical polyarthritis but can present as a single swollen joint in 15% of cases.
- Hypothyroidism, hyperparathyroidism and hemochromatosis may be associated with calcium pyrophosphate dihydrate deposition in articular tissues that may manifest as an acute gout-like presentation ('pseudogout') or may have a subacute or chronic course.
- Previous renal disease or diuretic use may give clues to diagnosing gout.
- Septic arthritis is uncommon in the normal joint but the possibility should be considered in joints recently aspirated or in patients with arthritis, diabetes or impaired immune function.
- A family history of inflammatory arthritis is significant as first-degree relatives of patients with rheumatoid arthritis are four times more likely to develop the condition than the general population.[1]

The clinician must ask about these features as the athlete is unlikely to volunteer them.

Examination

In addition to examining the symptomatic joint, the clinician should perform a general physical examination. This may provide clues to indicate an underlying inflammatory cause. Table 50.2 summarizes important extra-articular signs that may be associated with an acutely swollen joint.

Investigations

Laboratory tests and imaging should be guided by the clinical findings to help confirm or refute a suspected diagnosis. The clinician should avoid blanket screening. Infectious or inflammatory conditions may be associated with elevation of acute-phase reactants (e.g. erythrocyte sedimentation rate [ESR], C-reactive protein [CRP]). Synovial fluid aspiration should be

Table 50.2 Extra-articular signs that may be associated with an acutely swollen joint

System	Sign	Disease
General	Fever	Septic arthritis, acute gout
	Lymphadenopathy	Septic arthritis, malignant bone/soft tissue tumor
Skin/mucous membranes	Psoriasis, nail dystrophy	Psoriatic arthritis
	Erythema nodosum	Acute sarcoidosis
	Tophi	Gout
	Nail fold infarcts, splinter hemorrhages	Rheumatoid arthritis (RA) (vasculitis)
	Circinate balanitis, keratoderma blennorrhagica (Fig. 50.1)	Reactive arthritis (ReA)
	Pyoderma gangrenosum	Enteropathic arthritis (EnA)
	Erythema chronicum migrans	Lyme disease
Eyes	Conjunctivitis	ReA
	Iritis	Ankylosing spondylitis (AS), psoriatic arthritis, EnA
	Dry eyes (and mouth)	Sjogren's syndrome (RA)
Locomotor system	Small hand (MCP, PIP) and foot (MTP) synovitis	RA, psoriatic arthritis, chondrocalcinosis
	Hand (DIP, 1st CMC joints)	Nodal osteoarthritis
	Large (lower limb) joint synovitis	ReA, AS, psoriatic arthritis, EnA
	Restricted lumbar range of motion/ sacroiliac tenderness	AS, ReA, psoriatic arthritis, EnA
	Tender, swollen entheses	AS, ReA, psoriatic arthritis, EnA
	Tenosynovitis	RA, gout
Neurological	Carpal tunnel syndrome	RA

CMC = carpometacarpal; DIP = distal interphalangeal; MCP = metacarpophalangeal; MTP = metatarsophalangeal; PIP = proximal interphalangeal.

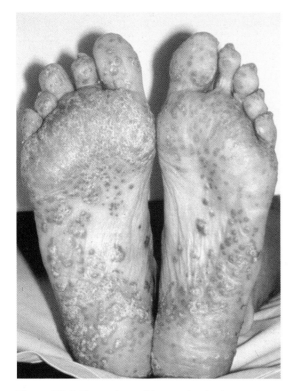

Figure 50.1 Keratoderma blennorrhagica in reactive arthritis

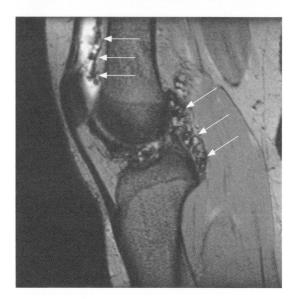

Figure 50.2 MRI scan of pigmented villonodular synovitis of the knee

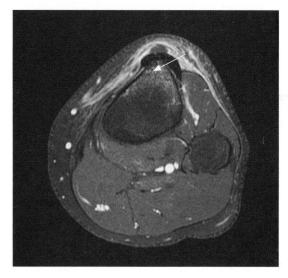

Figure 50.3 MRI scan of osteomyelitis that caused swelling of the knee

considered mandatory in cases of acute monoarthritis. If septic arthritis is suspected, the aspiration must be performed before antibiotics are given. The choice of antibiotic can be adjusted depending on the results of the Gram stain and culture of synovial fluid and blood culture. Uric acid (gout) or calcium pyrophosphate dihydrate (pseudogout) crystals may be detected under polarized light microscopy. It is important to remember that acute crystal arthropathy can be associated with fever and leukocytosis and may mimic septic arthritis. Furthermore, these conditions may coexist. In cases of suspected reactive arthritis, symptoms of urethral discharge should prompt referral to a genitourinary specialist and stool culture may help identify gut infection (e.g. *Shigella*, *Salmonella* or *Campylobacter*).

For non-traumatic acute presentations of a swollen joint, plain radiographs are not indicated as they seldom show more than soft tissue swelling or joint effusion. Plain films may, however, be helpful in identifying bone tumors, erosions or osteoarthritis. MRI remains a powerful tool for patients with traumatic lesions, bone and soft tissue tumors, pigmented villonodular synovitis (Fig. 50.2) and osteomyelitis (Fig. 50.3), and for the early detection of erosions. Chest X-ray may reveal bilateral hilar lymphadenopathy in acute sarcoidosis.

The patient with low back pain and stiffness

A systemic illness is present in up to 10% of patients who present with low back pain. Because patients with low back pain gravitate to sports clinicians for management, it is important that clinicians have an index of suspicion for those patients with a non-mechanical cause for their low back pain.

Clinical perspective

The differential diagnosis of low back pain is broad and is documented in Chapter 21. This differential diagnosis includes inflammatory arthritis of the spine and sacroiliac joints, known as spondyloarthropathy. Spondyloarthropathy is a generic term applied to the clinical, radiological and immunological features shared by the following diseases:

- ankylosing spondylitis
- reactive arthritis following genitourinary or gut infection
- psoriatic arthritis
- enteropathic arthritis (Crohn's disease, ulcerative colitis or celiac disease).

Although patients with these conditions have an increased likelihood of being positive for HLA B27 (see below), a negative result does not eliminate the diagnosis. Spondyloarthropathy has its greatest prevalence in young men and usually achieves near full disease expression by age 35 years; thus, patients commonly present to the sports clinician.

History

Patients with back pain due to spondyloarthropathy complain of pain that is worse at night, with prominent morning stiffness (of 2 hours or more), which is eased with gentle exercise and NSAIDs. This pain pattern is very different from the typical pain pattern of mechanical low back pain (Chapter 21). Buttock or posterior thigh pain may be present, so this symptom does not distinguish the two types of back pain. When the patient describes morning back pain with prominent stiffness, the physician should ask whether there is a past history of psoriasis or nail dystrophy (psoriatic arthritis), inflammatory bowel disease (enteropathic arthritis), or recent genitourinary or gut infection (reactive arthritis). Spondyloarthropathy is characterized by inflammation of the entheses, commonly at the patellar tendon, Achilles tendon and the plantar fascia.

Peripheral joints may be involved with spondyloarthropathy, particularly an asymmetric, lower limb, large joint inflammation. The shoulder or hip is involved in 30% of patients with ankylosing spondylitis. A history of extra-articular involvement such as anterior uveitis (iritis) and the rash of keratoderma

blennorrhagica (Fig. 50.1) or circinate balanitis (reactive arthritis) may provide clues to the specific cause of back pain. It is important that the clinician actively seeks these associations as the athlete may not find them noteworthy to mention. There is often a strong family history of spondyloarthropathy; for example, approximately 6% of siblings of patients with ankylosing spondylitis will develop the condition.[2]

Examination

When examining the patient with back pain and a suspected inflammatory etiology, the clinician should seek tenderness over the sacroiliac joints and pain on sacroiliac springing. Restriction of lumbosacral spine movement becomes evident first in lateral flexion. The clinician should also examine the appendicular skeleton for evidence of enthesopathy or peripheral joint involvement. Thorough inspection of the skin may detect previously unrecognized plaques of psoriasis (Fig. 50.4). The umbilicus, natal cleft and scalp are common sites and these changes may be subtle.[3]

Investigations

The diagnosis of spondyloarthropathy is essentially clinical. Investigations may help confirm or refute a suspected diagnosis and should not be used as a blanket screening tool. There may be a non-specific elevation of acute-phase reactants (ESR, CRP), particularly with peripheral joint involvement, but only one-third to two-thirds of patients with active ankylosing spondylitis mount an acute-phase response. HLA B27 is associated with ankylosing spondylitis in up to 95% of cases and approximately 70% of patients with reactive arthritis and axial involvement. The association is weaker in cases of enteropathic arthritis and psoriatic arthritis, with only about 50% of these

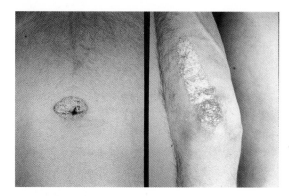

Figure 50.4 Psoriatic plaques of the elbow (right) and umbilicus (left)

patients being HLA B27 positive. As 7% of the general population is positive for HLA B27, there is no place for requesting HLA B27 as a screening tool for back pain (see p. 861).[4]

The diagnosis of ankylosing spondylitis requires sacroiliitis to be evident on plain X-ray. Early changes include sclerosis and erosion of the sacroiliac joints progressing to ankylosis (spontaneous fusion). Concurrently, there may be erosion at the edges of, and squaring of (Fig. 50.5), the vertebral bodies in the thoracolumbar spine progressing to syndesmophyte (bone spurs) formation and bony bridging ('bamboo spine'). As these changes may take up to 10 years to develop,[5] plain radiography is relatively insensitive in identifying inflammatory spine and sacroiliac lesions in athletes with a short history of symptoms. MRI, however, may detect up to 75% of cases of X-ray-negative early sacroiliitis and this may be considered in such cases.[6]

The patient presenting with multiple painful joints

Occasionally patients may attend the sports medicine clinic with multiple joint pain (polyarthralgia) or multiple joint pain with synovitis (polyarthritis). A systematic approach is vital to make an accurate diagnosis. Table 50.3 summarizes the differential diagnosis of the patient presenting with a polyarthritis.

History

The practitioner should begin by distinguishing polyarthritis with joint pain, stiffness and swelling from polyarthralgia alone. Joint inflammation is characterized by night pain, prominent morning stiffness (of at least 60 minutes but often for hours), swelling, warmth and loss of function. In many of these conditions the diagnosis is clinical. A key diagnostic feature is the onset and pattern of joint involvement.

Rheumatoid arthritis symmetrically affects the small joints of the hands (Fig. 50.6), wrists and feet (PIP, MCP, MTP) and in the majority of patients onset occurs over weeks or months.[7] Reactive arthritis (following genitourinary or gastrointestinal infection), on the other hand, is often more rapid in onset and

Table 50.3 Conditions that must be considered when a patient presents with polyarthritis

Common conditions	Less common conditions
Rheumatoid arthritis	Lyme disease

Viral arthritis
  Parvovirus B19
  Epstein-Barr virus
	Viral arthritis
	  Hepatitis B, C
	  Rubella

Polyarticular psoriatic arthritis	Rheumatic fever
Polyarticular reactive arthritis	Enteropathic polyarthritis

Inflammatory
  osteoarthritis
	Overlap syndrome (with
	  inflammatory myositis,
	  scleroderma)

Systemic lupus
  erythematosus
	Polyarticular gout/
	  pseudogout

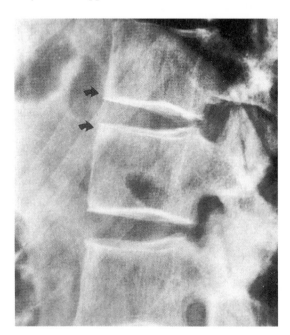

Figure 50.5 Squaring of the vertebral bodies in ankylosing spondylitis

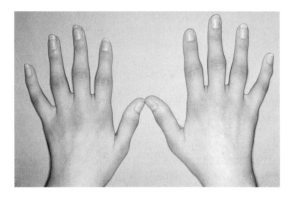

Figure 50.6 Early rheumatoid hands

has a propensity to asymmetric involvement of the large joints of the lower limb together with enthesitis (inflammation at the insertions of tendons, ligaments or capsules) or dactylitis (sausage digits). The duration of symptoms should be recorded.

Parvovirus B19 polyarthritis frequently affects young women who care for small children (mothers or school teachers) who develop parvovirus B19 infection (fifth disease or 'slapped cheek' syndrome). This condition may be indistinguishable from early rheumatoid arthritis. Symptoms and signs usually settle within six weeks, whereas rheumatoid arthritis often follows a chronic and progressive course. The presence or absence of extra-articular manifestations of rheumatological conditions may also aid accurate diagnosis (see Table 50.2). The pattern of joint involvement in polyarticular pseudogout or psoriatic arthritis often resembles rheumatoid arthritis but without nodulosis, vasculitis or other systemic features seen in rheumatoid arthritis.

Examination

Clinical examination requires thorough evaluation of all systems. Many of the extra-articular features are summarized in Table 50.2. The polyarthritis of systemic lupus erythematosus may be associated with alopecia, mouth ulceration, cutaneous vasculitis (local hemorrhages) or a lacy purplish rash referred to as livido reticularis in the young female athlete. The characteristic photosensitive facial rash (Fig. 50.7) in systemic lupus erythematosus is often follicular or sometimes itchy. The overlap connective tissue disorders may be associated with Raynaud's phenomenon, dyspepsia due to esophageal dysmotility, scleroderma of the hands and face, and soft tissue calcification.

Investigations

Investigations should only be requested to help confirm or refute a suspected diagnosis and must be guided by the clinical findings. As with other presentations discussed in this chapter, there is no place for blanket screening tests as these are likely to lead to a high number of false positive results. There may be a non-specific elevation of acute-phase reactants (ESR, CRP). Aggressive rheumatoid arthritis is often associated with a highly elevated ESR in the early stages of disease. The clinical utility of rheumatoid factor and antinuclear antibody tests is discussed below. Rising immunoglobulin (Ig) M antibody titers to *Borrelia burgdorferi* may aid in the diagnosis of Lyme disease when suspected. Likewise, antibody screening may help with the diagnosis of viral arthropathies (parvovirus B19, Epstein-Barr virus and hepatitis).

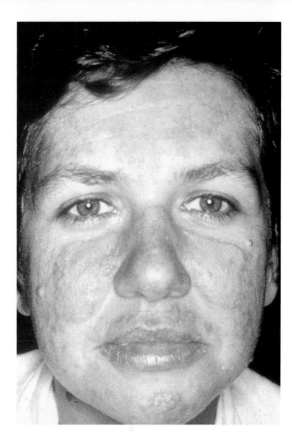

Figure 50.7 Urticarial photosensitive rash in systemic lupus erythematosus

When crystal arthropathy is suspected, the physician should aspirate the joint and arrange for crystal microscopy under polarized light. Radiographs of the hands and feet may detect early erosive change in patients with rheumatoid arthritis (Fig. 50.8) or psoriatic arthritis, a feature rarely seen in systemic lupus erythematosus. A polyarthritis with radiological changes of osteoarthritis and chondrocalcinosis in the menisci or triangular fibrocartilage complex of the wrist may represent calcium pyrophosphate dihydrate deposition disease.

The patient with joint pain who 'hurts all over'

A challenging presentation for any clinician is the evaluation of the athlete with widespread joint or muscle pain who 'hurts all over'. These patients are often frequent attenders and it can be extremely rewarding to provide a diagnosis and the help they need. In many cases, patients with this presentation have little to find

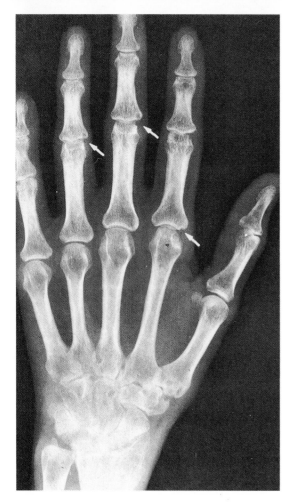

Figure 50.8 Erosive rheumatoid arthritis

Table 50.4 Conditions in patients presenting with polyarthralgia

System	Cause
Drug induced	Quinolones, acyclovir, vitamin A, clofibrate, beta-blockers, statins
Infectious	Viral syndromes, vaccines
Endocrine	Hyper/hypothyroidism, hyperparathyroidism, corticosteroid withdrawal
Autoimmune	Polymyalgia rheumatica, inflammatory myositis
Neoplastic	Leukemia, lymphoma, multiple myeloma, bone metastasis
Psychiatric	Depression, somatization disorder
Other	Fibromyalgia (chronic fatigue syndrome), silicone implant syndrome

on clinical examination. The differential diagnosis of this presentation is broad and includes the conditions listed in Table 50.3. Table 50.4 highlights other possible diagnoses and directs the practitioner towards appropriate clinical evaluation.

Investigations must be directed towards a specific diagnosis but may include blood count with differential white cell count, ESR, plasma immunoglobulin assay and electrophoresis, calcium, phosphate, thyroid function and creatine kinase tests.

Ordering and interpreting rheumatological tests

The indication for and interpretation of the results of commonly requested rheumatological tests cause confusion. In this section we consider five frequently requested investigations: rheumatoid factor (RhF), erythrocyte sedimentation rate (ESR), antinuclear antibodies (ANA), HLA B27 and serum uric acid.

Rheumatoid factor

Rheumatoid factors (RhF) are autoantibodies that react, principally, with a specific Fc antigen of normal IgG. Approximately 80% of patients with rheumatoid arthritis are RhF positive. Vasculitis, nodules and more rapidly progressive erosive disease are all features of patients with high RhF titers. Note that patients with other conditions and up to 5% of healthy young individuals may be RhF positive (15% in the older adult) (Table 50.5). Blanket screening for RhF may therefore yield a high rate of false positives and the request for an RhF test should be reserved for patients with clinical features consistent with rheumatoid arthritis. More recently, additional antibodies such as anti-CCP (anti-cyclic citrullinated peptide) have been identified that

Table 50.5 Conditions with an RhF association

Condition	RhF association (%)
Sjogren's syndrome	90
Rheumatoid arthritis	75–80
Systemic lupus erythematosus	25–50
Pulmonary diseases	10–25
Ankylosing spondylitis/gout	5–10
Normal population	<5

are as sensitive as RhF in rheumatoid arthritis patients though far more specific for the condition. A positive anti-CCP result will yield fewer false positive results[8] and may predict disease severity.[9]

Erythrocyte sedimentation rate

The ESR is simple and cheap to perform. It is a non-specific acute- and chronic-phase reactant, and while very high elevations (>100 mm/h) may indicate malignancy, sepsis or vasculitis (e.g. giant cell arteritis), normal levels do not exclude disease. Confounding factors in the interpretation of the ESR include anemia, polycythemia, abnormal red cell morphology or congestive heart failure. ESR testing is not useful as a screening test in asymptomatic individuals.

Antinuclear antibodies

Autoantibodies that react with various components of the cell nucleus are called antinuclear antibodies (ANA). Almost 100% of patients with systemic lupus erythematosus will be ANA positive but, as with RhF, ANAs are found in individuals with other conditions, such as scleroderma, Sjogren's syndrome, rheumatoid arthritis, inflammatory myositis, Hashimoto's thyroiditis, chronic liver or lung disease, drug-induced lupus and in 15% of healthy older persons. The ANA test should not be used to screen patients with joint pain or presumed systemic illness.

HLA B27

HLA B27 is a normal gene found in up to 8% of normal individuals. HLA B27 is often associated with ankylosing spondylitis, reactive arthritis, psoriatic arthritis and enteropathic arthritis (the spondylo-arthropathies). The prevalence of this allele in different populations is shown in Table 50.6.

Also, 12% of HLA B27 positive siblings of patients with ankylosing spondylitis will develop the condition.[2] In athletes with low back pain, HLA B27 should not be ordered routinely as there is an 8% prevalence of HLA B27 positive alleles in the general population, whereas the prevalence in patients with spondyloarthropathy is approximately 0.5%. Given these pre-test probabilities, the test is more likely to produce a false positive than a true positive result. It is diagnostically valuable when the incomplete syndrome is present or when the pre-test probability that the athlete has the condition lies between 30% and 70%. It has no value for screening (low pre-test probability) or in patients with classic presentations (high pre-test probability).[10]

Table 50.6 Prevalence of the HLA B27 allele

Population	Frequency of HLA B27 (%)
Ankylosing spondylitis	90
Ankylosing spondylitis with iritis	>95
Reactive arthritis (Reiter's syndrome)	75–80

Psoriatic arthritis
  Spondylitis
  Peripheral arthritis
	
	50
	<10

Enteropathic arthritis
  Spondylitis
  Peripheral arthritis
	
	50
	<10

General population	6–8

Serum uric acid

Serum uric acid estimation is primarily used in the diagnosis of gout. Abnormal levels are taken at two standard deviations either side of the mean (range, 150–425 µmol/L [2.5–7 mg/dL]) and therefore 5% of the normal population will have abnormally low or high uric acid levels. Uric acid will reach saturation level in extra-cellular tissues over approximately 380 µmol/L (6 mg/dL) and serum uric acid levels greater than this are associated with an increased risk of gout and kidney stones. During 40% of acute attacks of gout the uric acid level will, however, fall within the reference range. The diagnosis of acute gout cannot be made merely because of the presence of an acutely swollen joint and a high serum uric acid level. The diagnosis depends on the demonstration of uric acid crystals in synovial fluid. Serial uric acid estimations are useful to monitor the effect of hypouricemic drugs.

Recommended Reading

Cush JJ, Kavanaugh AF, Olsen NJ, et al. *Rheumatology: Diagnosis and Therapeutics.* Baltimore, MD: Williams & Wilkins, 1999: 1–559.
A very clear, concise pocket-size guide that clarifies many rheumatological issues for the non-rheumatologist.
Van der Heijde D, Landewe R. Imaging in spondylitis. *Curr Opin Rheumatol* 2005; 17: 413–17.

References

1. Alamanos Y, Drosos AA. Epidemiology of adult rheumatoid arthritis. *Autoimmun Rev* 2005; 4: 130–6.

2. Carter N, Williamson L, Kennedy LG, et al. Susceptibility to ankylosing spondylitis. *Rheumatology (Oxford)* 2000; 39: 445.

3. Gladman DD, Antoni C, Mease P, et al. Psoriatic arthritis: epidemiology, clinical features, course, and outcome. *Ann Rheum Dis* 2005; 64 (suppl. 2): ii, 14–17.

4. Kim TH, Uhm WS, Inman RD. Pathogenesis of ankylosing spondylitis and reactive arthritis. *Curr Opin Rheumatol* 2005; 17: 400–5.

5. Baraliakos X, Landewe R, Hermann KG, et al. Inflammation in ankylosing spondylitis: a systematic description of the extent and frequency of acute spinal changes using magnetic resonance imaging. *Ann Rheum Dis* 2005; 64: 730–4.

6. Oostveen J, Prevo R, den Boer J, et al. Early detection of sacroiliitis on magnetic resonance imaging and subsequent development of sacroiliitis on plain radiography. A prospective, longitudinal study. *J Rheumatol* 1999; 26: 1953–8.

7. Harris E, ed. *Clinical Features of Rheumatoid Arthritis.* Philadelphia: WB Saunders, 2001.

8. Lee DM, Schur PH. Clinical utility of the anti-CCP assay in patients with rheumatic diseases. *Ann Rheum Dis* 2003; 62: 870–4.

9. Riedemann JP, Munoz S, Kavanaugh A. The use of second generation anti-CCP antibody (anti-CCP2) testing in rheumatoid arthritis—a systematic review. *Clin Exp Rheumatol* 2005; 23: S69–S76.

10. Brown M, Wordsworth P. Predisposing factors to spondyloarthropathies. *Curr Opin Rheumatol* 1997; 9: 308–14.

Common Sports-Related Infections

Athletes are subject to the same infections suffered by the rest of the community. Certain circumstances in sport may increase the susceptibility of athletes to infections. Athletes involved in team sports have prolonged close contact with fellow team members, thereby increasing the likelihood of spread of infection. In addition, team members often share food and drink, particularly since the increased use of squeeze bottles during exercise.

In this chapter we describe the infections that are particularly relevant to the sportsperson either because of the serious nature of the infection (e.g. HIV) or because of its prevalence (e.g. upper respiratory tract infection). We then address the question of whether or not athletes have increased susceptibility to infection. Finally, we provide practical advice for the clinician advising an athlete who has an infection whether or not to participate.

Hepatitis

Acute viral hepatitis is a systemic infection predominantly affecting the liver. At least five distinct hepatitis viruses have been identified: hepatitis A (HAV), hepatitis B (HBV), hepatitis C (HCV), hepatitis delta or D (HDV) and hepatitis E (HEV). More than 350 million people worldwide have chronic, lifelong infections of HBV. These carriers are at high risk of serious diseases such as liver cirrhosis and primary liver cancer, which kill more than one million of them a year.[1]

The various types of hepatitis viruses can all produce clinically similar illnesses.[2] While the classic sign is the presence of jaundice (icterus), most cases of acute viral hepatitis are anicteric and result in non-specific symptoms such as fatigue and nausea.

The disease is often misdiagnosed as an influenza-like illness. Those patients who develop icteric disease often experience symptoms such as low-grade fever, anorexia, fatigue, abdominal discomfort and nausea prior to the onset of jaundice.[3]

Most cases of acute viral hepatitis are self-limited and have an excellent prognosis for recovery. The most serious complication is the development of fulminant hepatitis (massive hepatic necrosis). Another potential complication following acute infection with HBV, HCV and HDV (but not HAV or HEV) is the development of chronic hepatitis. With HBV the rate of progression from acute to chronic hepatitis is influenced by the age at which the infection occurs, with a very high rate (90%) for neonatally acquired infections, but only 5% for adult-acquired infections. Acute HCV results in chronic infection in 60–80% of cases.[2]

Athletes are at risk of developing hepatitis mainly as a result of non-sports-related activity (e.g. sexual contact, sharing needles), however, a small theoretical risk of virus contamination during certain types of athletic activity does exist. The mode of transmission of viral hepatitis from an infected individual varies depending upon the specific viral agent, although some overlap does exist (Table 51.1).

Infection with HAV or HEV is likely to occur as a result of exposure to contaminated food or beverages. The risk of infection is particularly high during international travel to areas with poor hygienic conditions where HAV and HEV are endemic.[4] Direct transmission of HAV or HEV during sports participation has not been described,[2] however, outbreaks of hepatitis among groups of athletes have been reported, the most famous of which involved 90 members of an American college's football team after an infected

Table 51.1 Transmission of viral hepatitis[2]

Transmission	HAV	HBV	HCV	HDV	HEV
Fecal–oral	Yes	No	No	No	Yes
Percutaneous	Yes (unusual)	Yes	Yes	Yes	No
Perinatal	No	Yes	Yes	Yes	No
Sexual	Yes (homosexual men)	Yes	Yes	Yes	No

group of children contaminated the drinking water used during practise.[5]

For athletes, exposure to blood-borne pathogens such as HBV and HCV is also much more likely to occur during non-sports-related activities such as unprotected sexual activity, using injectable drugs such as anabolic steroids, sharing personal items such as razors, and tattooing and body piercing. However, there is the potential for horizontal transmission of HBV and HCV while playing sports, especially contact or collision sports.

The blood of an infected athlete may contaminate the skin or mucous membranes of other athletes or staff. Two reports of transmission of HBV among Japanese athletes have been described, one in sumo wrestling[6] and the other in American footballers at the University of Okayama.[7]

There has been only one report of HBV transmission in a non-contact sport.[8] Between 1957 and 1963, 568 cases of HBV were reported among Swedish athletes participating in the sport of orienteering. It was thought that the most likely route of contamination was the use of water contaminated with infected blood to clean the wounds on multiple individuals who were cut by thorns and bushes during the competition.

There have been no documented cases of HCV transmission during sporting activity,[2] but there has been a documented case during bloody fisticuffs which was thought to have occurred when the two participants shared a common handkerchief to wipe their bleeding wounds.[9] There has also been a report of three soccer players from one amateur club contracting HCV as a result of sharing a syringe to inject intravenous vitamin complexes.[10]

It is clear that the risk of transmission of both HBV and HCV during sport is very low, and there is no reason why infected individuals should not be allowed to compete.

Acute viral hepatitis and activity

In those patients with acute viral hepatitis, strict bed rest and avoidance of all physical activity are no longer thought to be necessary. Acute hepatitis infection

should be viewed just as other viral infections and the ability to play should be based upon clinical signs and symptoms such as fever, fatigue or hepatomegaly.[11] Hepatomegaly (80%) and splenomegaly (10–20%) may persist after other symptoms have settled. Contact and collision sports should be avoided until the organomegaly has resolved.[4]

Prevention of viral hepatitis

Safe and effective vaccines against HAV and HBV are available. Athletes working or traveling in countries that have a high or intermediate rate of HAV infection should be vaccinated. Until recently it was only those at increased risk who were advised to have an HBV vaccination course, but recently HBV vaccination has been recommended in all children.[1] Certainly, any athlete involved in a contact or collision sport should be vaccinated.

The hepatitis B vaccine (Engerix-B) is on a zero, one and six month schedule. At this time immunity should be assessed by a blood test. Approximately 90% of people become immune after a course of three injections. If immunity is not present, a further injection should be given. This will increase the chance of developing immunity to approximately 95%.

In those who have not been vaccinated and experience a known or high-risk exposure to HAV or HBV, post-exposure prophylaxis with the respective immune globulin should be administered. Additionally there is now evidence that post-exposure immunization with HBV vaccine can attenuate or prevent acute HBV.

Human immunodeficiency virus (HIV)

HIV is a highly lethal virus transmitted sexually or by contact with blood or blood products. Infection with HIV initially causes a flu-like illness. This is followed by an asymptomatic period characterized by replication of the HIV virus and antibody formation. The length of this period is variable but may last months or years. This is followed by the development of acquired immunodeficiency syndrome (AIDS), which may present as a variety of diseases associated with the suppression of immunity. These include *Pneumocystis carinii* pneumonia, Kaposi's sarcoma, cytomegalovirus infection, cryptosporidiosis or lymphoma.

The presence of HIV antibodies can be detected a short time (usually within three months) after the initial exposure. Practicing safe sex and avoiding direct contact with blood or blood products can reduce the risk of HIV infection. There is an extremely slight risk of acquiring HIV from a contact on the sporting field with an HIV carrier bleeding from an open wound or from bloodstained clothing. This risk has been described as being 'exceedingly low' and is estimated to be between one per million and one per 85 million game contacts.[12]

There are no confirmed reports of HIV transmission during sport, although there has been one possible transmission during a football match[13] and a number of reports of transmission during bloody street fights.[14, 15]

Attention to the guidelines described in the box on page 872 will reduce this risk. Medical personnel attending bleeding players must make every attempt to stop the bleeding and remove all exposed blood. If bleeding cannot be controlled, the player should be removed from the field of play. Medical staff should always wear gloves when treating a bleeding wound.

The optimal level of participation and competition in an HIV-affected athlete remains unknown. Current opinion is that healthy, asymptomatic athletes with HIV may continue in competition and exercise without restriction but should avoid overtraining. Athletes with AIDS may remain physically active and continue training on a symptom-related basis but should avoid strenuous exercise and reduce activity during acute illness.

Infectious mononucleosis

The Epstein-Barr virus causes infectious mononucleosis, also known as glandular fever or 'mono'. The incidence of infectious mononucleosis is highest in adolescence and early adulthood with 1–3% of American college students reported to become infected yearly.[16] Many clinicians believe that the incidence of infectious mononucleosis is higher in athletes who are training intensely but there are no studies to support (or refute) this claim.

The severity of the infection appears to increase with age. Children infected by the Epstein-Barr virus develop a flu-like illness. Adolescents and young adults typically develop symptoms of sore throat, malaise, headache and less commonly myalgia, nausea and vomiting.

Examination of the typical 15–19-year-old patient reveals an exudative pharyngitis and swollen cervical lymph nodes. A fever of 39–40°C (102–104°F) is common. Splenomegaly occurs in about 50% of cases and peaks in the second or third week of the illness. A similar clinical picture may be seen with cytomegalovirus infection, toxoplasmosis and primary infection with HIV. Patients with infectious mononucleosis who are treated with ampicillin or amoxycillin (amoxicillin) often develop a diffuse macular rash. Older patients have an increased tendency to develop complications of infectious mononucleosis such as hepatitis or thrombocytopenia (reduced platelet count).

The virus is spread through close contact, especially saliva (kissing). The incubation period is usually between 30 and 50 days after exposure to the virus and the illness lasts between five and 15 days. However, tiredness may be more prolonged and, in some cases, continue for a number of months.

Investigations usually reveal a moderately raised white cell count ($10-20 \times 10^9$/L [$10-20 \times 10^3$/μL] with an increase in the number of lymphocytes (50% or more of total white blood cell count). Between 10% and 20% of these lymphocytes are usually described as 'atypical'. Mild thrombocytopenia (platelet count $<140 \times 10^9$/L [$<140 \times 10^3$/μL]) occurs in approximately 50% of patients. Liver function test abnormalities occur in approximately 75% of patients. The development of jaundice, however, is uncommon. Enlargement of the spleen may be confirmed on ultrasound.

Confirmation of infectious mononucleosis is usually made serologically. The presence of heterophile antibodies can be seen in 85–90% of acute EBV infections. Most clinical laboratories use some form of latex agglutination method such as the Monospot and Paul Bunnell tests. These tests are usually positive in the second week of illness. False negative results occur but other diagnoses (e.g. cytomegalovirus, HIV, toxoplasmosis) should be considered in the presence of a negative Monospot result.

In the 10–15% who never develop a positive Monospot test result, EBV-specific antibodies are measured. Most laboratories provide immunoglobulin (Ig) M and IgG antibody results. The IgM assay is positive in an acute infection and remains so for one to two months. The IgG antibodies tend to persist for life so are not indicative of current infection, only that a previous infection has occurred.

Treatment of infectious mononucleosis involves symptomatic treatment to reduce fever and sore throat. Infectious mononucleosis is not particularly contagious despite the relatively high incidence in adolescents and young adults. There is no need for isolation of the athlete with infectious mononucleosis. Many people have adequate antibody levels because of childhood exposure.

The athlete with infectious mononucleosis should rest from sporting activity until all acute symptoms have resolved. As there have been a number of case reports of splenic rupture associated with infectious mononucleosis, contact and collision sports should be avoided while the spleen is enlarged. The dilemma for the treating physician is how to determine that the spleen size has returned to normal. If the spleen is palpable, then it is clearly enlarged. However, many enlarged spleens are not palpable.

Ultrasound is used to measure spleen size. Simple linear ultrasonographic measurements are often used, but there is uncertainty as to the normal size. An upper limit of normal of 12 cm (6 in.) length, 7 cm (3.5 in.) width and 4 cm (2 in.) thickness has been proposed, but spleen size varies considerably between individuals, although it correlates reasonably well with body size. Unfortunately, very few individuals have previous ultrasonic measurement of the spleen with which to compare the post-infective size.

The majority of spleen ruptures have occurred within 21 days of the onset of symptoms so there is a case for allowing return to play after that period of time, remembering that there is still a slight possibility of rupture at a later date.

Skin infections

Skin infections occur more commonly in athletes than sedentary individuals.[17] They may be viral (e.g. herpes simplex, molluscum contagiosum, warts), bacterial (e.g. impetigo, folliculitis, otitis externa) or fungal (e.g. tinea, scabies, lice). Sweating, chaffing and occlusive clothing form a perfect environment for skin infections. Any breach in the skin from cuts, abrasions or lacerations increases the risk of infection.

Viral infections

Contact sports such as wrestling or rugby have a higher rate of viral skin infections than non-contact sports.[18] Training environments may promote the transmission of some viral infections via fomites, such as weights, mats, weight benches, pool decks and communal showers.[19]

Herpes simplex virus infections

Herpes simplex virus (HSV-1) skin infections occur in athletes, particularly among wrestlers (herpes gladiatorum) and rugby forwards (herpes rugbeiorum or 'scrum pox'). The virus is transmitted through skin-to-skin contact. Outbreaks have been reported particularly among wrestlers. A review of a recent outbreak suggested that there is a 33% probability of transmission if herpes develops on a sparring partner.[20]

In contact sports, lesions are common on the head and may involve the eyes, leading to conjunctivitis or blepharitis (infection of the eyelids). HSV infections can be extremely painful and may be accompanied by systemic symptoms such as fever and malaise. These symptoms represent the prodrome, but not every episode of HSV has a prodrome. After an incubation period of five to 10 days, asymptomatic shedding of viral particles and the development of clinical lesions may occur. The vesicles rupture quickly and crust over within a few days. Crusted lesions last five to seven days, and may take two to three weeks to heal completely.[18] The diagnosis is made on the typical appearance of the herpes lesions and can be confirmed with viral cultures.

Herpes labialis (cold sores) typically appear at mucocutaneous junctions, especially on the lip. They may affect snow skiers and others who are exposed to cold stress or to increased ultraviolet solar radiation at high altitudes.[21]

Treatment is symptomatic and should begin with oral acyclovir (400 mg three times a day or 200 mg five times a day for seven to 10 days) immediately with the onset of prodromal symptoms. The earlier the antiviral is taken, the more effective it is. Topical acyclovir is not helpful. The athlete with herpes simplex skin infection should not play sport and should avoid contact sport until the lesions have healed.

As HSV is not eliminated, recurrences may occur, particularly at times of undue physical or psychological stress. Recurrent attacks are usually milder, lasting only five days. Treatment is the same but a shorter course (five days).

HSV is highly contagious and no-one should compete in a contact sport until the scabs have dried and there are no further vesicles, ulcers or drainage. In the United States where high school and college wrestling is a popular sport, organizations have imposed strict rules. The National Collegiate Athletic Association's (NCAA) rules include that:[22]

- the athlete must be free of systemic symptoms (fever, malaise)

- the athlete must be free of any new lesions for 72 hours
- no moist lesions and all lesions must have a firm, adherent crust
- the athlete must be using appropriate antiviral medication for 120 hours (five days) before competition
- covering active lesions is not acceptable.

None of these recommendations, however, are evidence-based. On the basis of virus shedding studies in herpes genitalis, the athlete can probably return to competition four to seven days after a recurrent outbreak,[23] whereas others recommend removing the athlete from practise and competition for eight days.[24]

Molluscum contagiosum

Characterized by discrete white to skin-colored, umbilicated papules that are 3–5 mm (~0.25 in.) in diameter, molluscum contagiosum affects mainly children and is caused by a virus from the Poxviridae family.[18] The papules are more common in swimmers, gymnasts and wrestlers, and are commonly seen on the hands, forearms and face. They are generally asymptomatic and spread by skin-to-skin contact.

Treatment is generally recommended, particularly if an athlete participates in a contact sport. The infection is self-limited but may take months or even years to resolve without treatment.[18] The most common method of treatment is application of liquid nitrogen or curettage. Lesions should be covered while playing contact sport.

Warts

Warts or verrucae are caused by infection with various forms of the human papilloma virus (HPV). They are commonly seen on the hands and feet and tend to be hard and have a verrucous surface. Infectivity is low, but warts are transmitted either by direct skin-to-skin contact or through fomites such as swimming pool decks and showers. Warts are frequently spread by autoinoculation from shaving, scratching or other skin trauma. Plantar warts can be painful and should be treated.

Visual inspection is usually sufficient for diagnosis. The main challenge is distinguishing a wart from a callus. Warts do not retain the normal fingerprint lines on the hands and feet that corns and calluses do. A wart on the surface of the foot can also be distinguished from a callus by paring the lesion down with a no.15 blade. Warts will have 10 to 15 pinpoint black spots that are thrombosed capillaries. Once the wart has been pared down it can be treated with liquid nitrogen.

Athletes can return to competition as soon as warts have been treated, but the warts should remain covered until completely resolved.[18]

Bacterial skin infections

Certain bacterial infections can be found in epidemic numbers in athletes.

Impetigo

A *Staphylococcus* or *Streptococcus* skin infection that is easily spread from person to person, impetigo is particularly common in sports with close skin-to-skin contact, such as wrestling and the various football codes. Impetigo has two different presentations: bullous and non-bullous. The bullous form typically begins as multiple fluid-filled vesicles that either coalesce or individually enlarge, forming blister-like lesions that eventually collapse centrally. The center has the classic honey-crusted lesion that, when removed, reveals erythematous plaques draining serous fluid.

Non-bullous impetigo originates as small vesicles or pustules with erythematous bases and honey-colored crusts which also drain fluid. Breaks in the skin provide an avenue for bacterial invasion. Patients are typically afebrile, but enlarged lymph glands may be present.[25]

In most cases the diagnosis is made clinically and confirmed with bacterial cultures when necessary. Impetigo may resolve spontaneously but when the disorder is widespread treatment should be implemented, either with topical or oral (flucloxacillin, cephalexin) antibiotics. Local debridement of the crusts with soap and water is helpful.

All lesions should be covered during contact sport. The NCAA wrestling guidelines state that the athlete must take antibiotics for 72 hours before competition and be free from any new skin lesion for 48 hours.[22]

Folliculitis and furunculosis

Folliculitis is a superficial infection of the upper portion of the hair follicle and surrounding areas characterized by mildly tender papules or pustules surrounded by erythema. Furunculosis is an infection of the deeper hair follicle cavity and the lesions usually contain pus.

Furuncles or boils are large, well-defined, erythematous and fluctuant nodules that commonly occur in areas of increased sweating and friction, such as the buttock, belt line, anterior thigh and axilla.[25] Both folliculitis and furunculosis are caused by *Staphylococcus aureus*. Widespread infection should be treated with anti-staphylococcal antibiotics (e.g. flucloxacillin 500 mg three times a day for 10–14 days). Boils and abscesses require incision and drainage.

Pseudomonas or 'hot tub' folliculitis is usually contracted in spas or hot tubs. Symptoms appear from 6 hours to five days after bathing in contaminated water and include generalized malaise, low-grade fever and headache, accompanied by a pustular rash commonly appearing in the axilla, perineum, or buttocks. The rash is usually self-limiting and disappears after seven to 14 days. These infections are prevented by adequate filtration and chlorination of the baths. Folliculitis may also occur after a vigorous massage (especially when insufficient lubricants are used) or after leg waxing or shaving.

Otitis externa

Otitis externa, an infection of the external auditory canal common in swimmers, is caused by either *Pseudomonas* or *S. aureus*. This is sometimes known as 'swimmer's ear'. Otitis externa presents as a painful itch or discharge from the external ear. Pain is aggravated by traction on the tragus of the ear. The external auditory canal is usually swollen and tender and may be filled with debris.

Treatment is by irrigation to remove purulent debris, protection from exposure to water and mechanical trauma (e.g. avoiding ear plugs) and liberal application of corticosporin drops (polymyxin B, neosporin and hydrocortisone) over a cotton wick. There is a high incidence of recurrent infection. Recurrences may be limited by the use of drying agents such as 5% acetic acid (Aquaear) before and after swimming and the insertion of water-resistant ear plugs. Another simple preventive measure is shaking water out of the ear after swimming and drying the area with a hair dryer.

Fungal skin infections

Fungal skin infections are common among athletes due to the presence of sweat.

Tinea

The two most common fungal skin infections are tinea pedis ('athlete's foot') and tinea cruris ('jock itch'). These infections cause irritation and itching between the toes and in the groin area, respectively.

Topical antifungal cream (e.g. clotrimazole, miconazole, ketoconazole) is effective in most cases of tinea pedis. This should be applied two to three times per day over the affected toes for two to four weeks. Moist infections between the toes resolve more quickly with the addition of drying powders. Preventive measures include regular changes of socks, shorts and underwear, the use of foot powders, and regular cleaning of shower facilities. Resistant cases should be referred to a dermatologist for alternative topical agents or oral medications.

Onychomycosis

Onychomycosis, typically caused by *Tricophyton rubrum* or *Tricophyton mentagrophytes*, is common among athletes, particularly those who swim in pools, use communal showers, or have chronic tinea pedis and wear occlusive footwear.[26] The infection results from migration of the fungus under the distal nail plate leading to a nail bed infection that results in discoloration of the nail plate. Subungual debris then forms and the nail plate becomes distorted, thickened and separated from the nail bed. Over time the nail plate becomes brittle and crumbles.[27] Treatment requires a long-term commitment with either an oral antifungal agent or topical nail lacquer.

Scabies

Scabies mites are easily transmitted through skin-to-skin contact. Once on the skin surface the mite burrows into the epidermis, but symptoms may not arise until three to four weeks after exposure.[27]

Infestation manifests as small linear burrows and/or vesicles characteristically in axillary skin folds, finger and toe web spaces, the flexor surface of the wrists, the extensor surface of the elbows and knees, periumbilicus, genitalia, buttocks and lateral foot. The most prominent symptom is severe itching.

Confirmation of the diagnosis can be made by direct microscopic visualization of mites from an infected papule. Topical therapy is nearly 100% effective.

Pediculosis (lice)

Lice can occur on the body (pediculosis corporis), head (pediculosis capitis) and genitalia (pediculosis pubis) and are spread by close physical contact.[27] Once a person is infested, it can take up to 10 days for the nit (louse egg) to hatch. Patients may describe night-time itching and may develop an inflammatory reaction to scratching. As bites emerge, they appear as 2–4 mm (<0.25 in.) red papules on an erythematous base. Diagnosis can be confirmed by direct visualization. Various medications for head lice are available over the counter. Most involve application to the scalp once and, if required, again seven days later. In addition, a fine comb should be used to remove nits, and all clothing, bed linen and sporting equipment should be washed and dried in a hot dryer or discarded.

Viral respiratory infections

Infections of the upper and lower respiratory tracts are common, especially during winter months. Viruses commonly involved are the adenovirus, influenza virus, echovirus, cytomegalovirus and rhinovirus. They may cause rhinitis, pharyngitis, bronchitis or pneumonia. Treatment is usually aimed at control of the accompanying fever and a reduction of symptoms. Some symptomatic treatments are contained in the list of substances banned by the World Anti-Doping Agency (WADA) (Chapter 61). Antibiotics should not be used unless bacterial infection is suspected.

Influenza

Influenza is a common viral infection occurring in winter months. There are a number of strains of influenza virus and the predominant strain tends to vary from year to year.

Influenza can be a debilitating illness with systemic symptoms such as fever, malaise and myalgia. It is recommended that susceptible individuals, such as the elderly, have an annual influenza vaccination.

Athletes may wish to have an annual influenza vaccination as the illness may result in their missing a considerable period of competition and training. Athletes involved in team sports may wish to be vaccinated because of the possibility of spread among team members. The vaccination should be performed during autumn. Some recently developed anti-influenza drugs are showing promise as a possible treatment for those who are in the early stages of the illness.

Travelers' diarrhea

Diarrhea is commonly associated with travel to foreign countries. Limited attacks of diarrhea occur frequently among athletes in international competition. Agents that may cause travelers' diarrhea include *Escherichia coli*, *Campylobacter*, rotavirus, *Salmonella*, *Shigella* and *Giardia lamblia*.

The high incidence of diarrhea among travelers is thought to be due to changes in the normal bacterial flora of the food and water in foreign countries. The traveler is exposed to different bacteria to which he or she is not already immune.

The attack of diarrhea usually occurs in the first week after arrival and commonly lasts between 24 and 48 hours. It is often associated with mild fever, abdominal pain and malaise. Although the majority of these illnesses settle quickly, athletic performance may be affected during the attack and for some time afterwards.

Because of the potential effect on performance, attention has been paid to possible methods of prevention of travelers' diarrhea. Avoidance of local water and raw foods that may have been washed in water (e.g. salads) is recommended. However, in spite of these precautions infection may still occur.

The use of freeze-dried cultures or yoghurt may reduce the possibility of infection. Antibiotic prophylaxis of traveler's diarrhea remains controversial.[28] When deciding whether or not to use this approach, the athlete and physician must take into account any underlying medical illnesses, the importance of the competition, compliance of the traveler with food precautions and individual preference. Antibiotics may cause mild, or in some cases serious, allergic reactions. Recommended antibiotics include norfloxacin (400 mg/day) and ciprofloxacin (500 mg/day). These should be commenced on arrival in the foreign country and continued until the athlete has returned home for 48 hours. Trimethoprim sulfamethoxazole and doxycycline were popular in the 1990s but resistance is common now. Bismuth subsalicylate is less effective than antibiotic prophylaxis.

Treatment of traveler's diarrhea includes appropriate fluid and electrolyte replacement. Antidiarrheal medications (e.g. loperamide) are recommended for symptomatic relief. Norfloxacin (800 mg to start and then 400 mg twice daily for three days) or ciprofloxacin (1000 mg initially, then 500 mg twice daily for three days) can shorten symptoms and they are indicated if diarrhea is severe, dysenteric or persists for more than 48 hours. If diarrhea persists for more than five to seven days, giardiasis should be considered and this can be treated with a single dose of tinidazole (2 g). More persistent diarrhea should be investigated.

Exercise and infection

There is considerable debate regarding the relationship between exercise and infection. It is important to, firstly, consider the relationship between exercise and the immune system, then examine whether there is an increased incidence of infection associated with intense exercise, and finally to consider when an athlete can train and play with an infection.

Exercise and the immune system

The immune system can be considered as two complementary parts.[29] First is the innate immune system, which is non-specific regarding host defense. Its components include the skin, mucous membranes, phagocytes, natural killer (NK) cells, cytokines and complement factors. The latter two elements control and mediate immune function and help activate T- and B-lymphocytes, key parts of the acquired immune system. In contrast to the innate system, the acquired system protects the body against specific infectious agents during both initial and subsequent attacks.[29]

The body's first line of defense consists of skin and mucous membranes, which can be impaired by temperature, wind, sun, humidity and trauma. Many upper respiratory pathogens are airborne and affected by airflow patterns, mechanical barriers, and ciliary action in the respiratory tract.[29]

During exercise, the athlete switches from nasal to mouth breathing, and this can increase deposition of harmful articles in the lower respiratory tract. It also causes increased cooling and drying of the respiratory mucosa, which slows ciliary movement and increases mucous viscosity.[30]

NK cells express spontaneous cytolytic activity against cells infected with viruses.[29] NK cell counts increase 150–300% immediately after high-intensity exercise lasting less than 1 hour. Within 30 minutes of the end of such high-intensity exercise, however, NK cell counts fall below pre-exercise levels.[31] NK cell activity increases by 40–100% in response to acute exercise of less than 1 hour in duration, and falls to 25–40% below pre-exercise levels 1–2 hours into recovery time. Intense exercise lasting longer than 1 hour causes no rise in NK cell activity. There is, however, a more profound and sustained drop in NK cell activity in recovery, which is likely to be a cortisol-induced effect.[32]

Macrophages phagocytose foreign particles, present antigens to lymphocytes, and produce lymphocyte-stimulating cytokines.[30] Acute strenuous exercise increases the macrophage count and several aspects of macrophage function. Long-term training seems to attenuate the macrophage response to acute exercise, but the resulting macrophage function is still greater than in untrained subjects.[31]

Cytokines are produced by and mediate communication between immune and non-immune cells, and are divided into proinflammatory and anti-inflammatory types. Proinflammatory cytokines such as tumor necrosis factor (TNF)-α, interleukin (IL)-1 and IL-6 are increased with acute exercise. IL-6 levels can increase up to 100-fold after a marathon. Anti-inflammatory cytokines such as IL-10 and IL-1 receptor antagonist (IL-1ra) also increase with exercise.

Neutrophils are capable of phagocytosis both alone and in response to antigen-dependent defenses.[29] Neutrophil counts increase with acute exercise, most likely due to demargination, and several hours after exercise, a cortisol-induced phenomenon. Acute moderate exercise increases neutrophil activity, but acute intense exercise suppresses it.[31] Endurance training reduces several aspects of neutrophil function compared with being sedentary. It seems that long-term moderate training increases neutrophil counts whereas intense training decreases them.[31]

The acquired portion of the immune system has the ability to form a memory and attack specific foreign particles that have invaded the body previously. The main components of this system are T- and B-lymphocytes and plasma-cell-secreted antibodies. Overall, lymphocyte counts increase with acute exercise. Lymphocyte counts and B-cell function are decreased after intense exercise, but not after moderate exercise.

Antibody production, most notably IgA, is impaired by intense, prolonged exercise.[29] Cross-country skiers have low baseline salivary IgA levels, which further decline after racing. Studies of longitudinal changes in salivary IgA levels in swimmers have yielded conflicting results.[29] IgG does not seem to be affected as much by intense training, although some elite athletes show a small decrease during peak training.[30]

Among T-lymphocytes are the CD4+ (T-helper) and CD8+ (T-suppressor) cells. A ratio of CD4+ to CD8+ cells of 1.5:1 is considered necessary for proper cellular immune function. Heavy exercise decreases this ratio by decreasing CD4+ cells and increasing CD8+ cells. A decreased CD4+ count also diminishes cytokine output, which decreases NK cell and macrophage activation, and B-cell proliferation.[30]

Researchers have named the brief immunosuppression after acute, intense physical activity, when ciliary action, mucosal IgA levels, NK cell count and activity, T-lymphocyte count, and CD4+ to CD8+ ratio are decreased, as the immunological 'open window' during which an athlete may be more susceptible to infection.

Exercise and infections

Given the measurable changes in the immune system with exercise, are athletes more susceptible to infections? A number of studies have been performed examining the incidence of upper respiratory tract infection and exercise. The results are conflicting, although there is some evidence that intense training is associated with a higher level of infection.[29]

Nieman[33] has proposed the J curve (Fig. 51.1). According to this theory, regular moderate exercise decreases the risk of upper respiratory tract infection to below that of sedentary individuals, whereas strenuous intense exercise increases the risk above that of sedentary individuals. The exact frequency, duration, type and intensity of exercise required to optimally lower one's risk of infection, or to adversely increase the risk of infection, remains to be determined.[29]

Foster[34] proposed identifiable parameters of training which related to illness. He related the incidence of common illness to indices of training load and noted a correspondence between spikes in the indices of training and subsequent (within 10 days) illness, and computed individual thresholds that allowed for optimal explanation of illnesses. On these calculations, 84% of illnesses could be explained by a preceding spike in training load above the individual training threshold. However, 55% of the excursions above the threshold were accomplished without a related illness. A subsequent study failed to support Foster's theory.[35]

Infection and athletic performance

Infection or subclinical infection is commonly used to explain poor athletic performance. Infection may compromise muscle enzyme activity and muscle strength. Impaired muscle metabolism has also been demonstrated using MRI. Exercise performed during illness also requires greater cardiopulmonary effort. These findings may theoretically lead to a detrimental effect of infection on performance.

A number of studies have been performed at the Australian Institute of Sport in Canberra examining the relationship between mild illness and sporting performance. An initial study in elite swimmers did not show any statistically significant decrease in performance in competition in those who had suffered a minor illness in the month leading up to competition.[36] In a group of elite middle-distance and distance runners, illness-affected runners reported a higher perceived training intensity. However, laboratory-based measures of performance showed little change in physical work capacity.[35] A third study in another group of elite swimmers suggested that mild illness had a trivial effect on the competitive performances of female swimmers, and a substantial though small harmful effect in male swimmers. In this study it was noted that although the mean harmful effects were trivial to small, the chances of harm for individuals were substantial.[37]

Should an athlete train during illness?

One of the most difficult dilemmas facing the clinician and the athlete is to decide whether or not to train and/or compete in the presence of a viral illness.

It is important to differentiate those athletes suffering from viral illness into two groups—those with symptoms restricted to one system, usually the upper respiratory tract, and those with generalized symptoms. An athlete with an upper respiratory tract infection manifesting itself as a sore throat, runny nose or headache, who is afebrile, should be allowed to continue with mild-to-moderate training below 80% of Vo_{2max}. Modification of the training program may involve increased skill training with less anaerobic or endurance training for the period of the illness.

Those athletes with systemic symptoms of general malaise, excessive fatigue, muscle pains and tenderness, temperature in excess of 38°C (100°F) or a resting heart rate greater than 10 beats above normal should avoid any athletic activity until the systemic symptoms and signs return to normal or near normal. Activity should then be gradually resumed.

Engaging in intense exercise during an infection has been associated with an increased risk of heat exhaustion,[38] post-viral fatigue syndrome,[39, 40] and viral myocarditis.[41]

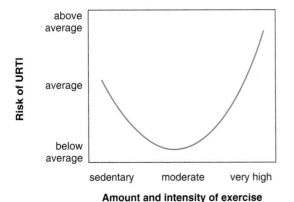

Figure 51.1 The association between exercise and susceptibility to upper respiratory tract infection[33]

This differentiation between the two forms of viral illness is known as the 'neck check'.[38, 42] In other words, if symptoms are above the neck (runny nose, nasal congestion, sore throat) and not associated with symptoms below the neck (fever, malaise, muscle aches, severe cough, gastrointestinal), then the athlete may commence training at half intensity for 10 minutes. If symptoms do not worsen, then the training session can continue as tolerated.

There is no evidence that exercise will affect the severity or duration of an illness.[43]

 If symptoms of viral illness are generalised, athletes should not train intensely or compete. If they are confined to one area (e.g. sore throat), then they can train moderately.

National position statements on infectious diseases

Sports medicine authorities in Australia, the United States and Canada have all produced national position statements on infectious diseases, with particular reference to HIV and hepatitis B. These are summarized below.

A number of blood-borne infectious diseases can be transmitted during body contact and collision sports. The more serious include HIV (AIDS) and hepatitis infections. These diseases may be spread by contact with infected:

- blood
- saliva (not for HIV)
- perspiration (not for HIV)
- semen and vaginal fluids.

The following recommendations will reduce the risk of disease transmission. All open cuts and abrasions must be reported and treated immediately.

Players

1. It is the players' responsibility to maintain strict personal hygiene as this is the best method of controlling the spread of these diseases.
2. It is strongly recommended that all participants involved in contact sport be vaccinated with hepatitis B vaccine.
3. Players with prior evidence of these diseases must obtain advice and clearance from a physician prior to participation.

Team areas

1. It is the clubs' responsibility to ensure that the dressing rooms be clean and tidy. Particular attention should be paid to hand basins, toilets and showers. Adequate soap, paper hand towels, brooms and disinfectants must be available at all times.

2. Communal bathing areas (e.g. spas) should be strongly discouraged.
3. Spitting or urinating in team areas must not be permitted.
4. All clothing, equipment and surfaces contaminated by blood must be considered potentially infectious and treated accordingly. Clothing soiled with blood and other body fluids should be washed in hot, soapy water.
5. Sharing of towels, face washers and drink containers should be avoided.
6. All personnel working in team areas should be vaccinated against hepatitis B.
7. In all training areas, open cuts and abrasions must be reported and treated immediately.

Referees and game officials

1. These officials must report all open cuts and abrasions at the first available opportunity.
2. Those who officiate in body contact and collision sports should be vaccinated against hepatitis B.
3. All contaminated clothing and equipment must be replaced prior to the player being allowed to resume play.
4. If bleeding should recur, the above procedure must be repeated.
5. If bleeding cannot be controlled and the wound securely covered, the player must not continue in the game.

Education

1. There is an obligation upon all relevant sporting organizations to provide suitable information on associated risk factors and prevention strategies for these diseases.

2. The safe handling of contaminated clothing, equipment and surfaces must be brought to the attention of all players and ancillary staff.
3. In the event of a player, official or member of the ancillary staff being found to be suffering from such a blood-borne disease (e.g. hepatitis B, HIV), that person cannot resume training or play, nor be involved in any team or match, until cleared by his or her local medical officer or the team physician.

Recommended Reading

American Academy of Pediatrics. Human immunodeficiency virus and other blood-borne viral pathogens in the athletic setting. *Pediatrics* 1999; 104: 1400–3.

American Medical Society for Sports Medicine and American Orthopaedic Society for Sports Medicine. Position statement on HIV and other blood-borne pathogens in sports. *Clin J Sport Med* 1995; 5: 199–204.

Anish EJ. Viral hepatitis: sports-related risk. *Curr Sports Med Rep* 2004; 3: 1200–6.

Centers for Disease Control and Prevention. National Prevention Information Network. HIV/AIDS and Sports. 1996. Available online: <http://www.cdcnpin.org/scripts/hiv/index.asp>.

Canadian Academy of Sports Medicine. Position statement. HIV as it relates to sport. Revised 1999. Available online: <http://www.casm-acms.org/PositionStatements/HIVEng.pdf>.

Cyr P. Viral skin infections. *Physician Sportsmed* 2004; 32(7): 33–8.

Doolittle R. Pharyngitis and mononucleosis. In: Fields KB, Fricker PA, eds. *Medical Problems in Athletes*. Malden, MA: Blackwell Science, 1995; 11–20.

Harrington DW. Viral hepatitis and exercise. *Med Sci Sports Exerc* 2000; 32(suppl. 7): S422–S430.

Howe WB. Preventing infectious disease in sports. *Physician Sportsmed* 2003; 31(2): 23–9.

International Federation of Sports Medicine (FIMS). FIMS position statement. AIDS and sports. 1997. Available online: <http://www.fims.org/default.asp?PageID=120975716>.

Johnson R. Herpes gladiatorum and other skin diseases. *Clin Sports Med* 2004; 23: 473–84.

Kordi R, Wallace WA. Blood borne infections in sport: risks of transmission, methods of prevention, and recommendations for hepatitis B vaccination. *Br J Sports Med* 2004; 38: 678–84.

Landry GL, Chang C. Herpes and tinea in wrestling. *Physician Sportsmed* 2004; 32(10): 34–41.

Levy JA. Common bacterial dermatoses. *Physician Sportsmed* 2004; 32(6): 33–9.

Mackinnon LT. *Advances in Exercise Immunology*. Champaign, IL: Human Kinetics, 1999.

Metz JP. Upper respiratory tract infections: who plays, who sits? *Curr Sports Med Rep* 2003; 2: 84–90.

Midgley A, McNaughton LR, Sleap M. Infection and the elite athlete: a review. *Res Sports Med* 2003; 11: 235–59.

Nieman DC. Exercise, the immune system and infectious disease. In: Garrett WE, Kirkendall DT, eds. *Exercise and Sports Science*. Philadelphia: Lippincott, Williams & Wilkins, 2000.

Nieman DC. Current perspective on exercise immunology. *Curr Sports Med Rep* 2003; 2: 239–42.

Sports Medicine Australia. Policy on infectious diseases with particular reference to HIV (AIDS) and viral hepatitis (B, C etc.). 1997. Available online: <http://www.sma.org.au/pdfdocuments/InfDisease.pdf>.

Winokur RC, Dexter WW. Fungal infections and parasitic infestations in sports. *Physician Sportsmed* 2004; 32(10): 23–33.

Woods J, Davis J, Smith J, et al. Exercise and cellular innate immune function. *Med Sci Sports Exerc* 1999; 31: 57–66.

World Health Organization. Hepatitis B. 2002. Available online: <http://www.who.int/mediacentre/factsheets/fs204/en/>.

References

1. World Health Organization. Hepatitis B. 2002. Available online: <http://www.who.int/mediacentre/factsheets/fs204/en/>.

2. Anish EJ. Viral hepatitis: sports-related risk. *Curr Sports Med Rep* 2004; 3: 100–6.

3. Mezey E. Diseases of the liver. In: Barker LR, Burton JR, Zieve PD, eds. *Principles of Ambulatory Medicine*. 5th edn. Baltimore: Williams & Wilkins, 1999; 529–40.

4. Harrington DW. Viral hepatitis and exercise. *Med Sci Sports Exerc* 2000; 32: S422–S430.

5. Morse LJ, Bryan JA, Hurley JP, et al. The Holy Cross College football team hepatitis outbreak. *JAMA* 1972; 219: 706–8.

6. Kashiwagi S, Hayashi J, Ikematsu H, et al. An outbreak of hepatitis B in members of a high school sumo wrestling club. *JAMA* 1982; 248: 213–14.

7. Tobe K, Matsuura K, Ogura T, et al. Horizontal transmission of hepatitis B virus among players of an American football team. *Arch Intern Med* 2000; 160: 2541–5.

8. Ringertz O, Zetterberg B. Serum hepatitis among Swedish track finders. *N Engl J Med* 1967; 276: 540–6.

9. Bourliere M, Halfon P, Quenin Y, et al. Covert transmission of hepatitis C virus during fisticuffs. (a). *Gastroenterology* 2000; 119(2): 507–11.

10. Parana R, Lyra L, Trepo C. Intravenous vitamin complexes used in sporting activities and transmission of HCV in Brazil. *Am J Gastroenterol* 1999; 94: 857–8.

11. American Medical Society for Sports Medicine and American Academy of Sports Medicine. Joint position statement: human immunodeficiency virus and other blood-borne pathogens in sports. *Clin J Sport Med* 1995; 5: 199–204.

12. Brown L, Drotman P, Chu A, et al. Bleeding injuries in professional football: estimates of the risk of HIV transmission. *Ann Intern Med* 1995; 122: 271–5.

13. Torre D. Transmission of HIV-1 infection via a sports injury. *Lancet* 1990; 335: 1105.

14. Ippolito G, Del Paggio P, Arici C, et al. Transmission of zidovudine-resistant HIV during a bloody fight. *JAMA* 1994; 272: 433–4.

15. O'Farrell N, Tovey SJ. Transmission of HIV-1 infection after a fight. *Lancet* 1992; 339: 246.

16. Brodski AL, Heath CW. Infectious mononucleosis: epidemiological patterns at United States colleges and universities. *Am J Epidemiol* 1972; 96: 87–93.

17. Beck C. Infectious diseases in sports. *Med Sci Sports Exerc* 2000; 32(7): S431–S438.

18. Cyr PR. Viral skin infections. Preventing outbreaks in sports settings. *Physician Sportsmed* 2004; 32(7): 33–8.

19. Rush S. Sports dermatology. *ACSM Health Fitness J* 2002; 6(4): 24–6.

20. Anderson BJ. The epidemiology and clinical analysis of several outbreaks of herpes gladiatorum. *Med Sci Sports Exerc* 2003; 35(11): 1809–14.

21. Brenner IK, Shek PN, Shephard RJ. Infection in athletes. *Sports Med* 1994; 17(2): 86–107.

22. Bubb RG. *Wrestling Rules and Interpretations*. Indianapolis: The National Collegiate Athletic Association, 2002.

23. Anderson BJ. The effectiveness of valacyclovir in preventing reactivation of herpes gladiatorum in wrestlers. *Clin J Sport Med* 1999; 9(2): 86–90.

24. Johnson R. Herpes gladiatorum and other skin diseases. *Clin Sports Med* 2004; 23: 473–84.

25. Levy JA. Common bacterial dermatoses. *Physician Sportsmed* 2004; 32(6): 33–9.

26. Seraly MF, Fuerst ML. Diagnosing and treating onychomycosis. *Physician Sportsmed* 1998; 26(8): 58–67.

27. Winokur RC, Dexter WM. Fungal infections and parasitic infestations in sports. *Physician Sportsmed* 2004; 32(10): 23–33.

28. Young MA, Fricker PA, Maughan RJ, et al. The traveling athlete: issues relating to the Commonwealth Games, Malaysia, 1998. *Clin J Sport Med* 1998; 8: 130–5.

29. Metz JP. Upper respiratory tract infections: who plays, who sits? *Curr Sports Med Rep* 2003; 2: 84–90.

30. Shepard RJ, Shek PN. Exercise, immunity, and susceptibility to infection. A J-shaped relationship? *Physician Sportsmed* 1999; 27(6): 47–71.

31. Woods J, Davis J, Smith J, et al. Exercise and cellular innate immune function. *Med Sci Sports Exerc* 1999; 31: 57–66.

32. Nieman D. Nutrition, exercise and immune system function. *Clin Sports Med* 1999; 18: 537–48.

33. Nieman D. Is infection risk linked to exercise workload? *Med Sci Sports Exerc* 2000; 32(7): S406–S411.

34. Foster C. Monitoring training in athletes with reference to overtraining syndrome. *Med Sci Sports Exerc* 1998; 30: 1164–8.

35. Fricker PA, Pyne DB, Saunders PU, et al. Influence of training loads on patterns of illness in elite distance runners. *Clin J Sport Med* 2005; 15(4): 246–52.

36. Pyne DB, McDonald W, Gleeson M, et al. Mucosal immunity, respiratory illness, and competitive performance in elite swimmers. *Med Sci Sports Exerc* 2001; 33: 348–53.

37. Pyne DB, Hopkins WG, Batterham AM, et al. Characterising the individual performance responses to mild illness in international swimmers. *Br J Sports Med* 2005; 39(10): 752–6.

38. Primos WA Jr. Sports and exercise during acute illness. Recommending the right course for patients. *Physician Sportsmed* 1996; 24(1): 44–4.

39. Budgett R. Fatigue and underperformance in athletes: the overtraining syndrome. *Br J Sports Med* 1998; 32(2): 107–10.

40. Parker S, Brukner P. Chronic fatigue syndrome and the athlete. *Sports Med Train Rehabil* 1996; 6: 269–78.

41. Friman G, Wesslen L. Infections and exercise in the high-performance athletes. *Immunol Cell Biol* 2000; 78: 510–22.

42. Eichner E. Infection, immunity, and exercise: what to tell your patients. *Physician Sportsmed* 1993; 21: 125.

43. Weidner T, Schurr T. Effect of exercise on upper respiratory tract infection in sedentary subjects. *Br J Sports Med* 2003; 37: 304–6.

The Tired Athlete

WITH KAREN HOLZER

Persistent tiredness, often accompanied by a feeling of lethargy and impaired sporting performance, is a frequent presenting symptom to a sports medicine practitioner. These symptoms may be the primary reason for a visit to the practitioner or may be an additional complaint of a sportsperson presenting with an injury, commonly an overuse injury.

There are many possible causes of persistent tiredness and/or impaired performance in sportspeople. A list of possible causes is shown in Table 52.1. Athletes in heavy training are constantly tired but can usually differentiate between normal, 'healthy' tiredness and abnormal tiredness, particularly when this is accompanied by a deterioration in training and competition performance. 'Healthy' tiredness is usually easily reversed with a day or two of reduced training or rest. This chapter addresses the problem of the athlete with persistent tiredness whose symptoms do not disappear after a brief period of rest.

History

The degree of tiredness should be established from the history.

- Does the patient fall asleep during the day?
- Is there a constant feeling of fatigue or does tiredness occur only during or after training?
- Is the tiredness constant or intermittent? If it is intermittent, does it occur only at a particular venue, which may indicate an allergy, or only in hot weather, which may indicate dehydration?

Table 52.1 Causes of persistent tiredness in sportspeople

Common	Less common	Not to be missed
Overtraining syndrome	Dehydration	Malignancy
Viral illness	Asthma/exercise-induced asthma	Cardiac problems
Upper respiratory tract infection	Deficiency—magnesium, zinc, vitamin B	Bacterial endocarditis
Infectious mononucleosis	Allergic disorders	Cardiac failure
(glandular fever or 'mono')	Jet lag	Diabetes
Inadequate carbohydrate intake	Anemia	Renal failure
Depletion of iron stores	Psychological stress	Neuromuscular disorders
Inadequate protein intake	Anxiety	Malabsorption
Insufficient sleep	Depression	Infections
Chronic fatigue syndrome	Medications	Hepatitis A, B, C
	Beta-blockers	HIV
	Anxiolytics	Malaria
	Antihistamines	Eating disorders
	Spondyloarthropathies	Anorexia
	Hypothyroidism	Bulimia
		Pregnancy
		Post-concussive syndrome

- How long has tiredness been present? Was the onset of tiredness related to any particular event, such as an associated viral illness or an overseas trip?
- Are there associated symptoms such as a sore throat or discomfort with swallowing, which may indicate an upper respiratory tract infection or infectious mononucleosis?
- Are there respiratory symptoms, such as a post-exercise cough or chest tightness, that may indicate exercise-induced asthma or a lower respiratory tract infection?

Training diary

A comprehensive training history is a crucial diagnostic aid. Note, the volume and intensity of training and, in particular, any recent changes in either of these parameters. It is important to take a weekly training history to judge whether or not there is sufficient recovery time between intense training sessions. The athlete should also be asked whether any active recovery is undertaken (Chapter 7). Also, it is essential to examine the overall training cycle over a period of weeks or months. The concept of periodization is discussed in Chapter 6. Discover what stage of the cycle the athlete is at and what the forthcoming program entails.

Other factors to note include:

- the amount of sleep and bed rest—swimmers, who tend to rise early to train, are particularly susceptible to lack of sleep, and many sportspeople, especially those studying or in employment, find it difficult to get adequate rest and sleep
- the athlete's social life, which may regularly intrude on sleep
- other commitments (such as sponsors' functions)—it is difficult for many athletes to combine training with the demands of a job, study and social life.

Psychological factors

Any psychosocial factors that may be contributing to the athlete's tiredness should also be noted. These may be related to either the athlete's sporting performance or to other aspects of his or her life. Typical sport-related problems may be a fear of a major impending competition, concern about poor training performance or a fear of failure. Factors unrelated to sport may include anxiety or depression related to work, study or relationships (Chapter 39).

Nutrition diary

Inadequate fluid intake may contribute to the development of fatigue, especially in hot weather. Fluid intake before, during and after training should be noted.

There are a number of possible dietary causes of persistent tiredness and, thus, a full dietary history should be taken. This involves the athlete completing a seven-day food diary, which is subsequently analyzed to ensure an adequate carbohydrate, protein and iron intake (Chapter 37). The athlete should also be questioned about eating habits to detect eating disorders (e.g. anorexia, bulimia).

Medical causes

In addition to the multitude of sport-related causes of persistent tiredness, there are numerous medical causes of this symptom. A full medical history should include:

- past history, history of allergies and current medications
- attention to any cardiac symptoms such as palpitation, ankle edema or chest pain, which may indicate the presence of bacterial endocarditis or cardiac failure
- cough, shortness of breath or wheeze, which suggest asthma or respiratory infection
- gastrointestinal symptoms such as diarrhea, which raise the possibility of malabsorption
- a neuromuscular problem, which may be inferred by the presence of muscle weakness
- a history of travel within the previous few months, which may indicate a tropical infection such as malaria
- a history of frequent, heavy menstrual bleeding, which suggests iron deficiency and anemia
- a history of absent periods, which may be due to pregnancy and an unrecognized cause of tiredness, or weight loss, which is suggestive of an eating disorder.

Examination

A full physical examination must be performed to exclude any of the possible medical causes of persistent tiredness. Inspection should determine the presence of anemia or jaundice. Examination includes assessment of the upper respiratory tract and cervical lymph nodes; a thorough cardiovascular examination, including resting pulse, blood pressure and examination of the heart; respiratory examination to exclude the presence of a chest infection or asthma; and examination of the abdomen with particular attention to palpation of the liver and spleen. The practitioner should also note any evidence of endocrine disease such as hypothyroidism or diabetes. A neurological examination should be performed if indicated by the history.

Investigations

Although the history and examination are the most important contributors to the diagnosis of the tired athlete, a number of investigations are performed as part of the routine work-up of this athlete. Other investigations may be indicated from the history or examination.

Urine should be routinely tested for the presence of glucose, blood and protein. Necessary tests include a full blood examination, including a blood film, iron studies (iron, ferritin, transferrin and transferrin receptor saturation), and vitamin B_{12} and folate levels.

Zinc, magnesium, urea and electrolyte levels and liver function tests may be added if clinically indicated, as may thyroid function tests.

If a viral illness is suspected, investigations may include a Paul Bunnell test or Monospot test for infectious mononucleosis, serological examination for cytomegalovirus and Epstein-Barr virus and, if indicated, hepatitis and HIV serological examination. A chest X-ray may be performed if there is a clinical suspicion of a cardiac or respiratory tract abnormality.

Lung spirometry may be useful if exercise-induced asthma is suspected from the clinical history and examination. Comparison of lung function tests pre and post exercise or other challenge tests for exercise-induced asthma should be performed. If an allergy is suspected, skin sensitivity tests and RAST blood tests may be useful.

A summary of the history, examination and investigations used in the diagnosis of the tired athlete is shown in the box below.

Summary of history, examination and investigations of the tired athlete

History

Duration of tiredness
Degree of tiredness
Timing of symptoms
Association with viral illness
Associated symptoms
Training diary
Amount of sleep and rest
Time commitments
Psychological problems
Fluid intake
Dietary history
Menstrual history
Work/personal stress
Associated medical problems
Medications
Allergies

Examination

Full medical examination including:
- pallor
- resting pulse
- blood pressure
- upper respiratory tract including sinuses
- heart
- lungs
- liver/spleen/lymph nodes

- thyroid
- others as indicated

Investigations

Urine testing:
- blood
- glucose
- protein

Routine blood tests:
- hemoglobin
- white cell count
- blood film
- erythrocyte sedimentation rate (ESR)/ C-reactive protein (CRP)
- urea, electrolytes
- serum ferritin/transferrin receptor saturation level
- vitamin B_{12} and folate
- thyroid function tests

Selective blood tests:
- infectious mononucleosis (Paul Bunnell, Monospot)
- vitamins and minerals (zinc, magnesium)
- serology (Epstein-Barr virus, cytomegalovirus, hepatitis, HIV)

Chest X-ray/ECG/echocardiography
Lung spirometry/eucapnic voluntary hyperpnea (pre and post exercise)

Overtraining syndrome

The overtraining syndrome is a common cause of persistent tiredness in athletes. It may have disastrous consequences for the serious athlete. It is important to clarify exactly what is meant by certain terms. The terms 'overtraining', 'overreaching', 'overtraining syndrome', 'burnout' and 'staleness' have all been used in association with this condition and need to be clarified.

Overtraining is a process of excessive training in high performance athletes that may lead to persistent fatigue, performance decrements, neuroendocrine changes, alterations in mood states and frequent illness, especially upper respiratory tract infections.

The *overtraining syndrome* is a neuroendocrine disorder that may result from the process of overtraining and reflects accumulated fatigue during periods of excessive training with inadequate recovery.

The term *overreaching* describes similar symptoms (fatigue, performance decrements, mood state changes) but of a more transitory nature. Thus, overreaching is resolved with short periods of rest or recovery training, usually within a two-week period, whereas overtraining may require months or occasionally years. *Burnout* and *staleness* are other terms previously used to describe overtraining.

Development of the overtraining syndrome

Overreaching is often utilized by athletes during a typical training cycle to enhance performance. Intense training, in the short term, can result in a decline in performance; however, when incorporated with appropriate periods of recovery, a 'supercompensation' effect may occur, with the athlete exhibiting an enhanced performance when compared with the baseline level.[1]

The overtraining syndrome develops when there is failed adaptation to overload training (Chapter 6) due to inadequate regeneration. A combination of excessive training load and inadequate recovery time results in short-term overtraining or overreaching. The overreaching is associated with impaired performance. If, at this stage, the athlete rests and has time to regenerate, the symptoms disappear and supercompensation may occur.

Unfortunately, some athletes react to impaired performance by increasing the intensity of their training. This leads to further impairment of performance, which may, in turn, result in the athlete increasing training further. A vicious cycle develops and leads to the overtraining syndrome. This progression is demonstrated in Figure 52.1.

The initial symptom of the overtraining syndrome is usually fatigue but, in time, other symptoms develop. There are a large number of symptoms associated with the overtraining syndrome, although few of these have been clearly documented as reliable and valid indicators of the syndrome.[2] Some of the physiological variables used as indicators of overtraining include:

- performance decrements despite continued training
- decreased economy of effort during exercise or decreased work rate at lactate threshold
- persistent fatigue
- cardiovascular changes such as increased early morning heart rate or resting blood pressure
- hematological changes such as decreased serum ferritin concentration
- hormonal changes such as decreased catecholamine production or alterations in the ratio of serum free testosterone to cortisol
- frequent illness such as upper respiratory tract infection
- persistent muscle soreness
- loss of body mass.

Psychological and behavioral variables often associated with the overtraining syndrome include:

- mood state changes as shown by the Profile of Mood States (POMS)[3]
- apathy, lack of motivation
- loss of appetite
- sleep disturbances
- high self-reported stress levels
- irritability or depression.

The only parameters consistently shown in scientific studies[2] to be associated with overtraining are:

- performance decrements
- persistent high fatigue ratings
- decreased maximal heart rate
- changes in the blood lactate threshold, lactate concentration at a given work rate or maximal blood lactate level
- neuroendocrine changes such as elevated resting plasma noradrenalin (norepinephrine) levels and decreased noradrenalin (norepinephrine) excretion
- high self-reported stress levels and sleep disturbances.

Physiological changes

Performance decrements of 10% as well as an inability to maintain training loads are not unusual. In one large

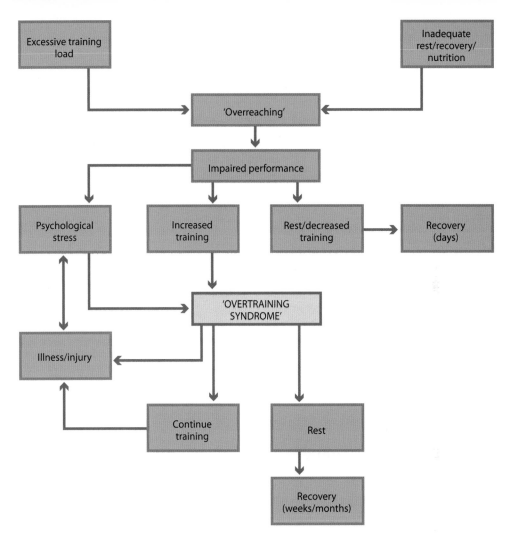

Figure 52.1 The development of the overtraining syndrome

study, training pace decreased 11–15%, competition pace decreased 6–17%, and training distance 43–71% in overtrained distance runners.[4] Deterioration in performance is an essential criterion for the diagnosis of overtraining; it is not sufficient as a single marker of the syndrome because performance also may be adversely affected by short-term fatigue.[2] In general, measurements of time to fatigue will show greater changes in exercise capacity as a result of overreaching and overtraining,[1] however, these tests are not an accurate performance indicator as they do not truly reflect the demands of competition.

Although many athletes and coaches have found the early morning heart rate or resting heart rate useful indicators of overtraining,[5] most scientific studies have

failed to confirm this relationship.[6] However, there is good evidence that maximal heart rate (measured at maximal work rate in a progressive exercise test) decreases by 5–10 beats per minute during overreaching/overtraining in endurance athletes.[7] Heart rate variability (HRV), the term used to describe the oscillation in the interval between consecutive heart beats, has also been suggested as an indicator of overtraining, but limited research has thus far failed to confirm this correlation.[1]

Biochemical changes

Resting blood lactate levels do not appear to change in overtrained athletes, however, decreased blood lactate concentrations at maximal work rate have been consistently noted in overreached/overtrained athletes.[8]

Skeletal muscle glycogen depletion has been associated with overtraining in swimmers,[7] however, a study in cyclists showed no evidence of depletion.[8] Other biochemical markers such as creatine kinase, urea and iron levels have been considered as possible indicators of overtraining, although findings have been inconsistent.[1]

Overreaching and overtraining can also occur in power athletes, such as weightlifters. Decreases in muscle strength and endurance may be seen in association with fatigue.[9]

Hormonal changes

Basal urinary catecholamine excretion has been reported to be significantly reduced in overtrained athletes,[10] and catecholamine excretion was negatively correlated to fatigue ratings. Furthermore, following a period of recovery, catecholamine excretion returned to baseline values.[10] Both Hooper et al.[6] and Lehmann et al.[11] observed increased resting noradrenalin levels in athletes who were thought to be overtrained, or who had undergone a period of increased training that resulted in performance incompetence.

Although resting cortisol levels do not appear to change with overtraining, maximal cortisol responses appear to be reduced. Both Snyder et al.[8] and Urhausen et al.[12] have reported reduced maximal cortisol levels in overreached athletes.

The response of both total and free testosterone levels in overreached athletes is contradictory. Flynn et al.[13] observed decreased total and free testosterone levels in conjunction with a decease in performance following a period of intensive training. However, Vervoorn et al.,[14] although also reporting lower testosterone levels in rowers following an intense period of training, found these changes in the absence of overtraining. A further study found no significant differences in resting testosterone levels during normal training and a state of overreaching, with an associated reduction in performance.[12]

Testosterone and cortisol are thought to have opposing effects on muscle metabolism, protein synthesis and growth.[2] The ratio of free testosterone to cortisol is suggested to indicate the balance between androgenic–anabolic activity (testosterone) and catabolic activity (cortisol), and has been suggested as a diagnostic tool for overtraining. Both cortisol and testosterone are released in response to high-intensity aerobic and anaerobic exercise, and it is believed that the ratio of testosterone to cortisol is an indicator of the positive and negative effects of training due to the opposing effects that the hormones have on growth, protein synthesis and muscle metabolism.[15] A decrease in the testosterone:cortisol ratio of 30% or more has been suggested as an indicator of overtraining. However, studies have failed to support the usefulness of this ratio; the ratio has been shown to be unchanged in overreached athletes,[12] and decreased in athletes who show no performance decrements following intensive training.[14] It has been suggested, however, that if followed over time in individual athletes, the ratio of these hormones may give an indication of the athlete's adaptive response to short-term physiological strain.[16]

Immunological changes

Although there are numerous anecdotal reports of increased susceptibility to illness and infections in athletes who are overtrained, there is little scientific evidence to substantiate this.

A number of studies have been performed measuring peripheral leukocyte counts both during periods of intense training that have resulted in overreaching and in athletes diagnosed as overtrained; in all these studies, except one, a change in leukocyte count has not been demonstrated in overtrained individuals.[1] The single study that demonstrated a change found a significant decline in the leukocyte count when training was increased.[17]

Although resting peripheral blood lymphocyte counts also do not appear to be influenced by overtraining, it has been suggested that the activation of the lymphocytes may be increased.[1] Neutrophil numbers have been reported to be both unchanged and increased during periods of intensified training; however, neutrophil function has not been assessed in overreached athletes, so the role of the neutrophil in immune dysfunction is not known. Natural killer cell numbers appear to be unaltered in athletes showing symptoms of overreaching.[1]

Salivary IgA, an important factor in host defense, has been used to study the mucosal immune system response to overtraining. Salivary IgA levels have been shown to be reduced in athletes with symptoms of overtraining compared with those athletes who were well trained.[18] A further study also reported lower, but not significantly significant, levels of IgA after intensified training.[19]

The production of glutamine, an important substrate for cells of the immune system, especially lymphocytes, macrophages and possibly natural killer cells, is usually increased during periods of immunological challenge.[20] Plasma glutamine levels have been found to be lowered in overtrained athletes,[21, 22] although a lowered glutamine level was not associated with any increase in upper respiratory tract infections in overtrained swimmers.[21] It has been suggested that low glutamine levels after prolonged exercise may result in a reduction in immune function and a subsequent increased risk of infection; however, there is still no evidence to link low glutamine levels with impaired immune function and increased susceptibility to illness or infection.[1]

Psychological changes

Psychological symptoms associated with overtraining include anxiety, depression, apathy, lack of motivation, irritability, inability to relax and lack of self-confidence. In athletes, the Profile of Mood States (POMS)[3] has been used to quantify total mood disturbance. The specific POMS scores of tension and depression have been shown to be higher in overtrained swimmers,[23] but also in swimmers after increased training without any evidence of overtraining.[24, 25] Self-ratings of wellbeing have correlated well with overtraining and may be a predictor of its onset.

Central fatigue and overtraining

Although the exact biochemical and metabolic changes fundamental to the development of the overtraining syndrome have not been clearly established, changes within the central nervous system appear to play an important role in the development of chronic fatigue and many of the other common signs and symptoms that are frequently seen in the overtraining syndrome, such as disrupted sleep, changes in appetite and weight, irritability, impaired concentration, decreased motivation and depressed mood. It has been suggested that alterations in brain neurotransmitters (e.g. serotonin) and the central effects of peripherally released inflammatory mediators (e.g. cytokines) are important in the development of the overtraining syndrome.[26]

Serotonin has been shown to influence central fatigue and depression, and it has been suggested that it may also play a role in the overtraining syndrome. It has been proposed that overtraining can result in chronically diminished concentrations of branched-chain amino acids and increased plasma free tryptophan levels.[26] Tryptophan is a metabolic precursor to serotonin. The central nervous system, in turn, influences the peripheral neuroendocrine milieu through two hormonal axes:

the hypothalamic–pituitary–adrenocortical (HPA) axis and the sympathetic–adrenal medullary (SAM) axis.[27] The end products of these axes—catecholamines and glucocorticoids—have been implicated in the overtraining syndrome.[28] As a consequence of the hypothalamic and pituitary dysfunction, overtrained athletes may experience decreased pituitary release of thyroid-stimulating hormone, reduced pituitary adrenocorticotrophic response to corticotropin-releasing hormone, and alterations in growth hormone. There is also evidence of reduced intrinsic activity of the sympathetic nervous system in the later stages of the overtraining syndrome.[29]

Ultimately it may be changes in noradrenergic, serotonergic or dopaminergic activity in the hypothalamus and pituitary gland that occur with the prolonged stress of overtraining that lead to alterations in the HPA and SAM axes.[30] Circulating cytokines, released in association with a state of chronic systemic inflammation induced by overtraining, may also bind to receptors in the hypothalamus and also impact on the HPA and SAM axes.[28]

Many of the signs and symptoms that characterize the overtraining syndrome are remarkably similar to those of clinical depression, and unfavorable changes in global mood, behavior and cognition are a consistent finding in athletes with the overtraining syndrome. It may be difficult to clinically distinguish between the two conditions.[26] Armstrong and VanHeest[27] have proposed using an antidepressant such as the selective serotonin reuptake inhibitor (SSRI) fluoxetine as a treatment for the overtraining syndrome and describe the dramatic effect the use of such a medication had on the running fortunes of the great American distance runner Alberto Salazar who had suffered from the overtraining syndrome for more than a decade.

Monitoring of overtraining

Unfortunately, no single test can detect overtraining in the athlete. However, there are a number of parameters, both clinical and laboratory, which in combination may enable the athlete to be monitored in order to prevent the development of full-blown overtraining syndrome.

Probably the simplest and most effective means of monitoring overtraining is self-analysis by athletes themselves. Daily documentation should include sources and ratings of stress, fatigue, muscle soreness, quality of sleep, irritability and perceived exertion during training or standardized exercise. An example of the contents of a daily diary is shown in the box on page 882.

Blood parameters such as red and white blood cell counts, hemoglobin level, hematocrit, urea and ammonia levels are not usually abnormal during overtraining. Changes in exercise blood lactate concentration and blood lactate threshold have been shown to be good indicators of overtraining but are influenced by many other factors and are probably only useful if assessed repeatedly. The POMS test as mentioned above may be a useful predictor of overtraining but is not a reliable diagnostic tool.

Prevention of overtraining

The prevention of overtraining is discussed in previous chapters. It requires maintenance of the correct balance between training load (Chapter 6) and recovery/regeneration (Chapter 7). The most important component of prevention is awareness of the problem, particularly among coaches. Education of coaches in the science of training will lead to fewer athletes developing this syndrome. Periodization of training, allowing sufficient regeneration time within the training program and the use of regenerative techniques such as massage, hydrotherapy and relaxation as well as higher fluid and carbohydrate intakes are all being used increasingly by serious athletes to enable them to cope with high training loads.

Certain groups of athletes appear to be at an increased risk of developing the overtraining syndrome. An athlete new to a particular sport may train overzealously, and an athlete who is achieving some initial success may be encouraged to train even harder. An athlete may be led into overtraining by trying to train with better athletes. It may also be dangerous to follow the training program of an established 'champion' whose training log may have been published in a magazine or passed into sporting folklore.

The athlete who does not have a coach or training group to set training programs is far more likely to overtrain. The support of a sensible, experienced coach or training partner is the best means of maximizing performance and avoiding overtraining.

Early recognition that an athlete may be developing the overtraining syndrome may enable the practitioner or coach to take the immediate measures to avoid further progression. Close liaison between coach and the clinician is essential (Chapter 1). The coach can provide feedback on the athlete's condition and details of the past, present and intended training program.

In patients who present with a relatively brief history of overtraining, complete rest is recommended in the short term and the athlete is advised to get as much sleep as possible over the next 48 hours. Often this can be done over a weekend. If the syndrome is not severe, this may be sufficient and the athlete may recover and begin the week with renewed vigor.

If this brief period of rest does not reduce the athlete's fatigue, the overtraining syndrome has developed. This may take weeks or months to resolve. Treatment includes rest, attention to dietary and fluid intake and psychological support.

Viral illness

Viral illness is a common cause of persistent tiredness in the athlete. The immunological changes that occur as a result of prolonged intense training may result in the athlete having an increased susceptibility to viral illness, especially upper respiratory tract infections.

The athlete with a viral illness presents the sports medicine practitioner with a number of dilemmas.

- Should the athlete be allowed to continue intense training?
- Will continued intense training result in aggravation of the symptoms and the development of a more serious illness?
- If the decision is made to avoid intense training, is light training or no training preferable?
- If the athlete is about to compete, will performance be impaired as a result of this viral illness and, in team sports, will this affect the performance of the team and should a replacement be sought?
- If the athlete does have time off from training due to a viral illness, when is it appropriate to resume training and at what level?

In these situations, each case must be considered on its merits. However, when an athlete presents with a viral illness and has an elevated temperature, intense training is contraindicated as there may be the potential for serious illness to develop (e.g. myocarditis) or the athlete may prolong the illness or develop post-viral fatigue syndrome. In an athlete with a mild temperature, light training is permissible and may, in fact, have a positive effect. In this case, the pulse rate should be kept below 70% of the maximum heart rate. When the viral illness is accompanied by systemic symptoms (e.g. muscle pain), training is contraindicated.

The conundrum of whether or not to compete with a viral illness is almost impossible to solve. In most cases, performance will be impaired when an athlete has a viral illness. However, there are anecdotal reports of excellent sporting performances in athletes who apparently competed while ill.

Recurrent viral illnesses may indicate a specific immune deficiency, most commonly an IgG3 subclass deficiency.[31] IgA and IgM deficiencies are less common.[32] Specific viral infections (e.g. infectious mononucleosis, hepatitis, HIV) are considered in Chapter 51.

Nutritional deficiencies

Depletion of iron stores

Depletion of body stores of iron is a common cause of tiredness, particularly in swimmers and endurance athletes. Athletes are susceptible to iron deficiency for a number of reasons, including inadequate iron intake, increased iron loss and inadequate absorption of dietary iron (Chapter 37). Special groups with a greater risk of iron deficiency are menstruating females, any athlete who diets and adolescent athletes.

Runners and endurance athletes are at high risk of iron deficiency due to a combination of increased gastrointestinal and genitourinary blood loss, loss of iron in sweat and an increase in hemolysis in runners, swimmers and rowers. The hemolysis is believed to be due to an increase in the destruction of the older, more fragile red blood cells, and is thought to be contributed to by altered flow dynamics in vigorous sports and an increase in body temperature.

Iron deficiency is further contributed to by an inadequate dietary intake, commonly seen in distance runners and vegetarians.

Athletes rarely develop frank anemia, which will clearly result in tiredness and impaired performance due to a reduced oxygen-carrying capacity in the blood. However, some athletes with hemoglobin levels within the 'normal' range may have relative anemia,

in other words, their hemoglobin level is too low for them and they have mild anemia.

An earlier stage of iron deficiency involves depletion of iron stores, primarily from the bone marrow. This can also result in tiredness and impaired performance, probably because of the important role of iron as a cofactor in muscle metabolism.

Serum ferritin measurement is a good indicator of body iron stores and serum transferrin receptor levels of the transmission of iron-bearing transferrin to cells. Elevated levels of ferritin represent increased iron stores, however, elevated transferrin receptor levels are a reflection of tissue iron needs. The combination of both ferritin and transferrin receptor levels provides the most sensitive measurement of the iron status of an athlete.[33] Both ferritin and transferrin receptor levels should be measured regularly in athletes training intensely. Female endurance athletes who eat little or no red meat are particularly susceptible to this condition. We regard serum ferritin levels of less than 30 µg/L (30 ng/mL) in females and less than 50 µg/L (50 ng/mL) in males, and/or the transferrin receptor level of greater than 2.4 mg/L as evidence of reduced body iron stores and thus a possible cause of tiredness and impaired performance.

Athletes with symptoms of lethargy and poor performance, in combination with low ferritin levels and/or increased transferrin receptor levels, should attempt to increase their iron intake. Referral to a dietitian may be required. Exclusion of a gastrointestinal or genitourinary cause of iron loss is important. Oral supplementation with ferrous gluconate, sulfate or lactate may be required and appears to be effective.[34, 35] Absorption is best between meals and may be improved with the intake of vitamin C (Chapter 37). Often gastrointestinal intolerance or poor absorption of oral iron may necessitate the administration of parental iron.

Glycogen depletion

Chronic glycogen depletion is an important cause of fatigue in the athlete. Glycogen is the storage form of carbohydrate and the major source of energy for the athlete. Glycogen stores are depleted after an intense bout of exercise, such as a heavy training session. If the glycogen stores are not adequately replenished prior to the next training session, they will become further depleted. Over a period of intense training and inadequate glycogen repletion, a state of chronic glycogen depletion will develop. In this state there is inadequate energy available for intense exercise, resulting in fatigue and impaired performance.

Replenishment of glycogen stores is achieved with a diet high in complex carbohydrates, as described in Chapters 7 and 37. It is important to note that the sooner carbohydrate is taken following the bout of exercise, the more effective is the replenishment of glycogen stores. Therefore, athletes should replenish their glycogen stores immediately after exercise with a source of complex carbohydrate such as fruit, cereal or high-carbohydrate drinks.

Inadequate protein intake

Inadequate protein intake is another potential cause of persistent tiredness in the athlete, although the mechanism by which these symptoms are produced is not clear. Protein is an energy source providing 10% of the energy needs through conversion of amino acids to glucose. Adequate protein is essential to replace protein broken down by muscle contraction. Good sources of protein in the diet include lean meat, poultry, fish and eggs. Protein intake is discussed further in Chapters 7 and 37.

Chronic fatigue syndrome

Chronic fatigue syndrome (CFS) is a controversial condition, the existence of which is hotly debated within the medical profession. The term itself was first used in 1988 but the syndrome has existed for much longer. It has previously been known as neurasthenia and myalgic encephalomyelitis (ME). The term CFS has been adopted to define a sufficiently homogeneous group of patients to allow research into etiology, pathogenesis, natural history and management. As the word 'syndrome' suggests, CFS is not recognized as a distinct disease process.

Definition

A number of definitions of CFS have been proposed. All include the concept of fatigue that interferes with activities of daily living and is of at least six months' duration. The Center for Disease Control (CDC) in Atlanta has defined CFS as the presence of:[36]

- clinically evaluated, unexplained, persistent or relapsing fatigue that is of new or definite onset; is not the result of ongoing exertion; is not alleviated by rest; and results in a substantial reduction of previous levels of occupational, educational, social or personal activities and
- four or more of the following symptoms that persist or recur during six or more consecutive

months of illness and that do not predate the fatigue:
— self-reported impairment in short-term memory or concentration
— sore throat
— tender cervical or axillary nodes
— muscle pain
— multijoint pain without redness or swelling
— headaches of a new pattern or severity
— unrefreshing sleep
— post-exertional malaise of at least 24 hours.

Etiology

CFS is more common in females, high achievers and professionals and more common in young adults. CFS is widespread in affluent settings and virtually unreported in developing countries.

Research to date has not identified any clear etiology for CFS. It is unlikely that chronic fatigue has a single etiology in an individual patient. There are likely to be predisposing states, predisposing factors and perpetuating factors all operating to produce abnormal prolonged pathological fatigue. Predisposing states might include a positive family history, trait anxiety, depression, coping styles and family factors. Fatigue symptoms might be perpetuated by secondary gain or learned behavior.

Acute infectious illnesses are clearly important precipitating factors in many cases, more often a viral respiratory tract illness than infectious mononucleosis. Orthostatic hypotension has been associated with CFS, however, this may be a product of the deconditioning associated with the syndrome rather than a causative factor.

Studies have reported immunological abnormalities such as decreased T-cell responses to mitogens in vitro and immunological subclass G abnormalities in cases of CFS; however, as immune abnormalities have been found in psychological disorders, these findings are non-specific.

Symptoms

The most prominent symptom of CFS is usually overwhelming fatigue, especially after exercise. Other common symptoms include headaches, sore throat, enlarged lymph nodes, muscle pain especially after exercise, unrefreshing sleep, chest and abdominal pains.

The diagnosis of CFS is difficult to confirm in the absence of any definitive sign or test. It is often a diagnosis of exclusion. The other problem with the diagnosis of CFS is that there are a number of conditions whose symptoms overlap with those of CFS. The two most significant are fibromyalgia and depression. The major presenting symptom in fibromyalgia is usually widespread muscle and joint pain but fatigue is nearly always present. Fibromyalgia is characterized by the presence of multiple tender points in the muscles. Trigger points are also frequently seen in patients with CFS and form an important part of the treatment. Fatigue is often the primary presenting symptom in patients with depression and many of the symptoms described in CFS are found in depressive patients.

Management

Management of the patient with CFS (or fibromyalgia and depression) is a considerable challenge for the practitioner. The natural history of CFS is of a very gradual improvement over a period of months and sometimes years. Treatment should be oriented towards psychological support and symptom relief. It is essential that the treating practitioner acknowledges that the patient has a real problem and is prepared to give the patient a diagnosis. It is important to give the patient plenty of time and both the patient and those close to her (or him) will have many questions. We recommend seeing the patient at least weekly in the initial treatment phase and later on a less frequent but still regular basis.

Exercise is the cornerstone of treatment of chronic fatigue.[37] This may seem strange when one considers that post-exercise fatigue and muscle pain are two of the most significant features of the disease but a slow, graduated increase in activity is an essential part of management. The exercise program may have to commence at a 'ridiculously' low level considering the history of some athletes. But it should commence at a level that the patient can achieve comfortably with minimal or no adverse effects in the 24–48 hours post-exercise. The increase in activity should be very gradual and if adverse symptoms develop, the patient should return to the previous level of activity and build up even more slowly.

In a six-month randomized blinded prospective trial[38] in 96 individuals with CFS, it was found that a graded exercise program significantly improved both health perceptions and the sense of fatigue whereas the use of an antidepressant (fluoxetine) improved depression only. Another study of 66 patients with CFS also demonstrated a positive effect with graded aerobic exercise.[39]

Many drug treatments have been advocated but with little evidence of their efficacy. Simple analgesics may be helpful and we recommend the use of a tricyclic antidepressant (e.g. amitryptiline 10–25 mg) in a single nocte dose. This drug seems to improve sleep quality and patients will usually wake up more refreshed as a result.

Many nutritional supplements have also been advocated but again there is no evidence of their efficacy. We have found the treatment of muscle trigger points with dry needling to be helpful in reducing muscle pains and headaches in a number of patients with CFS.

CFS and the sportsperson

It has been suggested that the incidence of CFS is higher in athletes than in the normal population.[40] Certainly a number of high-profile athletes have been diagnosed with the condition. One problem in the athlete is the overlap in symptoms between the overtraining syndrome and CFS.[41] It may be that the etiology of the two conditions is similar, with both having a neurotransmitter effect on central fatigue. Athletes who appear to be particularly prone to developing CFS are those who are attempting to combine a high level of commitment to their sport with full-time work, social and family commitments. The other group who appear vulnerable are those athletes who continue to train and/or compete at an intense level when they are suffering from a viral illness. We have seen a number of athletes with debilitating CFS whose onset appears to have coincided with such an episode.

Other causes of tiredness

A number of psychological problems are associated with a feeling of excessive tiredness. The two most common states are anxiety and depression. These problems may be related to the athlete's sporting endeavors or, alternatively, may be quite unrelated. The presence of eating disorders such as anorexia nervosa and bulimia should also be considered.

Hypothyroidism is more common than most realize, occurring in 1% of adults, with subclinical disease in 5%. The condition can affect any organ system. Hypothyroidism is characterized by a general slowing of body processes and can present as chronic fatigue, cold intolerance, weight gain and, in women, menorrhagia.[42] It is often associated with high cholesterol levels. An elevated serum thyroid stimulating hormone level is a sensitive indicator and patients with this condition generally respond well to treatment with levothyroxine.

Diabetes, neuromuscular disorders and cardiac problems are all associated with excessive tiredness. Exercise-induced asthma may occasionally present with tiredness as the major symptom rather than the more typical cough, chest tightness or shortness of breath post exercise.

A number of medications may cause excessive tiredness. These include beta-blockers, antihistamines, diuretics, anticonvulsants, sedatives and muscle relaxants.

Summary

Excessive tiredness is a common problem among athletes in hard training. While overtraining, a viral illness or a nutritional deficiency (especially iron) are the most likely causes, other causes should always be considered. A thorough history, comprehensive examination and appropriate use of investigations will usually lead to the correct diagnosis.

Recommended Reading

Armstrong LE, VanHeest JL. The unknown mechanism of the overtraining syndrome. *Sports Med* 2002; 32(3): 185–209.

Beard J, Tobin B. Iron status and exercise. *Am J Clin Nutr* 2000; 72(suppl.): 594S–597S.

Halson SL, Jeukendrup AE. Does overtraining exist? An analysis of overreaching and overtraining research. *Sports Med* 2004; 34(14): 967–81.

Hawley CJ, Schoene RB. Overtraining syndrome. A guide to diagnosis, treatment and prevention. *Physician Sportsmed* 2003; 31(6): 25–31.

Kreider RB, Fry AC, O'Toole ML, eds. *Overtraining in Sport.* Champaign, IL: Human Kinetics, 1998.

Mackinnon LT, Hooper SL. Overtraining and overreaching: causes, effects, and prevention. In: Garrett WE, Kirkendall DT, eds. *Exercise and Sports Science.* Philadelphia: Lippincott, Williams & Wilkins, 2000.

Moeller JL. The athlete with fatigue. *Curr Sports Med Rep* 2004; 3: 304–9.

Pearce PZ. A practical approach to the overtraining syndrome. *Curr Sports Med Rep* 2002; 1: 179–83.

Shepard RJ. Chronic fatigue syndrome. An update. *Sports Med* 2001; 31(3): 167–94.

References

1. Halson SL, Jeukendrup AE. Does overtraining exist? An analysis of overreaching and overtraining research. *Sports Med* 2004; 34(14): 967–81.

2. Mackinnon LT, Hooper SL. Overtraining and overreaching: causes, effects, and prevention. In: Garrett WEJ, Kirkendall DT, eds. *Exercise and Sports Science.* Philadelphia: Lippincott, Williams & Wilkins, 2000.

3. McNair BM, Lorr M, Doppleman LE. *Profile of Mood States Manual.* San Diego: Educational & Industrial Testing Service, 1971.

4. Barron JL, Noakes TD, Levy W, et al. Hypothalamic dysfunction in overtrained athletes. *J Clin Endocrinol Metab* 1985; 60: 803–6.

5. Dressendorfer RH, Wade CE, Scaff Jr JH. Increased morning heart rate in runners: a valid sign of overtraining? *Physician Sportsmed* 1985; 13(8): 77–92.

6. Hooper SL, Mackinnon LT, Gordon RD, et al. Hormonal responses of elite swimmers to overtraining. *Med Sci Sports Exerc* 1993; 25(6): 741–7.

7. Costill DL, Flynn MG, Kirwan JP, et al. Effects of repeated days of intensified training on muscle glycogen and swimming performance. *Med Sci Sports Exerc* 1988; 20: 249–54.

8. Snyder AC, Kuipers H, Cheng B, et al. Overtraining followed intensified training with normal muscle glycogen. *Med Sci Sports Exerc* 1995; 27: 1063–70.

9. Fry AC, Kraemer WJ, van Borselen F, et al. Performance decrements with high-intensity resistance exercise overtraining. *Med Sci Sports Exerc* 1994; 26: 255–9.

10. Lehmann MJ, Foster C, Dickhuth HH, et al. Autonomic balance hypothesis and overtraining syndrome. *Med Sci Sports Exerc* 1998; 30(7): 1140–5.

11. Lehmann M, Schnee W, Scheu R, et al. Decreased nocturnal catecholamine excretion: parameter for an overtraining syndrome in athletes. *Int J Sports Med* 1992; 13: 236–42.

12. Urhausen A, Gabriel HH, Kindermann W. Impaired pituitary hormonal response to exhaustive exercise in overtrained endurance athletes. *Med Sci Sports Exerc* 1998; 30(3): 407–14.

13. Flynn MG, Pizza FX, Boone JB Jr, et al. Indices of training stress during competitive running and swimming seasons. *Int J Sports Med* 1994; 15: 21–6.

14. Vervoon C, Quist AM, Vermulst LJ, et al. The behaviour of

the plasma free testosterone/cortisol ratio during a season of elite rowing training. *Int J Sports Med* 1991; 12(3): 257–63.

15. Mackinnon LT, Hooper SL, Jones S, et al. Hormonal, immunological and hematological responses to intensified training in swimmers. *Med Sci Sports Exerc* 1997; 29: 1637–45.

16. Urhausen A, Gabriel H, Kindermann W. Blood hormones as markers of training stress and overtraining. *Sports Med* 1995; 20: 251–76.

17. Lehmann MJ, Wieland H, Gastmann U. Influence of an unaccustomed increase in training volume vs intensity on performance, hematological and blood chemical parameters in distance runners. *J Sports Med Phys Fitness* 1997; 37(2): 110–16.

18. Mackinnon LT, Hooper S. Mucosal (secretory) immune system responses to exercise of varying intensity and during overtraining. *Int J Sports Med* 1994; 15: S179–S183.

19. Halson SL, Lancaster GI, Jeukendrup AE, et al. Immunological responses to overreaching in cyclists. *Med Sci Sports Exerc* 2003; 35(5): 854–61.

20. Rowbottom DG, Keast D, Morton AR. The emerging role of glutamine as an indicator of exercise stress and overtraining. *Sports Med* 1996; 21(2): 80–97.

21. Mackinnon LT, Hooper SL. Plasma glutamine and upper respiratory tract infection during intensified training in swimmers. *Med Sci Sports Exerc* 1996; 28(3): 285–90.

22. Parry-Billings M, Budgett R, Koutedakis Y, et al. Plasma amino acid concentrations in the overtraining syndrome: possible effects on the immune system. *Med Sci Sports Exerc* 1992; 24(12): 1353–8.

23. Hooper SL, Mackinnon LT, Hanrahan SJ. Mood states as an indication of staleness and recovery. *Int J Sport Psych* 1997; 28: 1–12.

24. O'Connor PJ, Morgan WP, Raglin JS. Psychobiologic effects of 3d of increased training in female and male swimmers. *Med Sci Sports Exerc* 1991; 23(9): 1055–61.

25. Morgan WP, Costill DL, Flynn MG, et al. Mood disturbance following increased training in swimmers. *Med Sci Sports Exerc* 1988; 20(4): 408–14.

26. Anish EJ. Exercise and its effects on the central nervous system. *Curr Sports Med Rep* 2005; 4: 18–23.

27. Armstrong LE, VanHeest JL. The unknown mechanism of the overtraining syndrome: clues from depression and psychoneuroimmunology. *Sports Med* 2002; 32(3): 185–209.

28. Smith LL. Cytokine hypothesis of overtraining: a physiological adaptation to excessive stress? *Med Sci Sports Exerc* 2000; 32: 317–31.

29. Uusitalo ALT. Overtraining: making a difficult diagnosis and implementing targeted treatment. *Physician Sportsmed* 2001; 29(5): 35–50.

30. Budgett R. Fatigue and underperformance in athletes: the overtraining syndrome. *Br J Sports Med* 1998; 32: 107–10.

31. Reid VL, Gleeson M, Williams N, et al. Clinical investigation of athletes with persistent fatigue and/or recurrent infections. *Br J Sports Med* 2004; 38: 42–5.

32. Fallon KE. Inability to train, recurrent infection, and selective IgM deficiency. *Clin J Sport Med* 2004; 14: 357–9.

33. Feelders RA, Kuiper-Kramer EP, Van Eijk HG. Structure, function and clinical significance of transferrin receptors. *Clin Chem Lab Med* 1999; 37: 1–10.

34. Brutsaert TD, Hernandez-Cordero S, Rivera J, et al. Iron supplementation improves progressive fatigue resistance during dynamic knee extensor exercise in iron-depleted, nonanaemic women. *Am J Clin Nutr* 2003; 77: 441–8.

35. Verdon F, Burnand B, Stubi CL, et al. Iron depletion without anemia and physical performance in young women. *BMJ* 2003; 326: 1124–31.

36. Fukuda K, Straus SE, Hickie I, et al. The chronic fatigue syndrome: A comprehensive approach to its definition and study. International chronic fatigue syndrome study group. *Ann Intern Med* 1994; 121: 953–9.

37. McCully KK, Sisto SA, Natelson BH. Use of exercise for treatment of chronic fatigue syndrome. *Sports Med* 1996; 21(1): 35–48.

38. Wearden AJ, Morriss RK, Mullis R, et al. Randomised, double-blind, placebo-controlled treatment trial of fluoxetine and graded exercise for chronic fatigue syndrome. *Br J Psychiatry* 1998; 172: 485–90.

39. Fulcher KY, White PD. Randomised controlled trial of graded exercise in patients with the chronic fatigue syndrome. *BMJ* 1997; 314: 1647–52.

40. Parker S, Brukner P. Is your sportsperson suffering from chronic fatigue syndrome? *Sport Health* 1994; 12(1): 15–17.

41. Shephard R. Chronic fatigue syndrome: an update. *Sports Med* 2001; 31(3): 167–94.

42. Lathan SR. Chronic fatigue? Consider hypothyroidism. *Physician Sportsmed* 1991; 19(10): 67–70.

Exercise in the Heat

WITH TIMOTHY NOAKES

Because sporting activity may occur in hot conditions, sports medicine clinicians must be well versed in both prevention and management of heat-associated illness. Humans can only survive core temperatures greater than 41°C (106°F) for short periods and protein denatures at a body temperature of 45°C (113°F).

Fortunately, of all mammals, humans have developed an almost unmatched capacity to sweat, providing our species with one of the greatest capacities to lose heat during exercise and thus safely to regulate our body temperatures even during exercise of long duration in environmental conditions that would otherwise be considered extreme. This was brilliantly shown by the performance of the 40 kg Japanese runner, Mizuki Noguchi, who won the 2004 Athens Olympic Marathon for women in a time of 2 h 26 min 20 s despite the extreme environmental conditions—35°C with moderate humidity.

Some have argued that this remarkable sweating capacity of humans must have developed for some evolutionary purpose. Thus, Heinrich has proposed that as humans are savanna-adapted animals, the reason for our highly developed sweating response is because it provides us with an advantage, most likely to perform prolonged exercise in the heat According to Heinrich, 'We don't need a sweating response to outrun predators, because that requires relatively short, fast sprinting, where accumulating a heat load is, like a lactic acid load, acceptable. What we do need sweating for is to *sustain* running in the heat of the day—the time when most predators retire into the shade'.[1] Heinrich also notes that modern hunter-gatherers, like the !Kung Bushmen (San) of Southern Africa, do not carry food or water with them (on 30 km hunts in the heat) because that 'hinders

their ability to travel'.[1] The first documentation of just such a hunt recorded that the !Kung San do not begin these long hunts lasting 4–6 hours unless the desert temperature is in excess of 40°C (104°F) (with low humidity);[2] the preferred hunting temperature is 42–45°C (108–113°F).

Despite this remarkable ability of some humans to exercise in such heat without health risk, on occasion, heat injury, in particular heatstroke, occurs to persons exercising in much less severe environmental conditions when the total heat load cannot explain why heatstroke developed. This suggests that individual susceptibility, rather than the environmental conditions, plays a much more important role in the development of this condition than has previously been acknowledged.

In this chapter we briefly review the physiology of heat gain and heat loss before discussing the diagnosis and management of three common presentations in the heat—heatstroke, exercise-associated collapse and cramps. As these names suggest, only the former is truly related to heat! Finally, we discuss an important differential diagnosis of heatstroke—hyponatremia. This condition results from fluid overload.[3, 4]

Mechanisms of heat gain and loss

Heat is produced by both endogenous sources (muscle activity and metabolism) and exogenous sources (transfer to the body when environmental temperature exceeds body temperature). The rate of heat production and the risk of heatstroke should be greatest in those who run the fastest and have the highest work rate (i.e. in short-distance rather than marathon events). Heat loss occurs by conduction, convection, radiation or evaporation. At rest, when environmental temperature is below body temperature, thermal balance is maintained by convection of heat to the skin surface and radiation of heat to the environment.

As an individual starts to exercise and produce more heat, sweating provides compensatory heat loss through evaporation. When the environmental temperature equals or exceeds body temperature, sweating is the predominant mechanism of heat loss;[5] athletes exercising in these conditions rely almost exclusively on evaporative heat loss to regulate body temperature.

The effectiveness of sweating to cool the body is affected by humidity. In a dry environment, sweat is evaporated. A humid environment, in which there is a high level of water vapor in the air, limits the evaporation of sweat and its cooling effect. Therefore, the combination of high temperature and high humidity is particularly dangerous. Athletes should avoid exercising in these conditions if possible. In extreme environmental conditions, when the humidity is high and the temperature is in excess of about 33°C (91°F), core temperature can increase substantially even in relatively short-distance races (6–15 km). Heavier athletes are particularly at risk because they produce more heat and have greater difficulty losing that heat adequately than do lighter athletes when both exercise at the same velocity in humid conditions.[6] In contrast, because they produce less heat when exercising at the same velocity as heavier athletes, small athletes are especially advantaged when competing in prolonged events in the heat.[6–8] For example, the 52 kg world marathon record holder Paula Radcliffe was unable to finish the Athens 2004 Olympic Marathon, which was won by an athlete who was 12 kg lighter and whose best marathon time in cooler conditions was substantially slower than Radcliffe's best.

The effects of humidity as well as the effects of solar and ground radiation, air temperature and wind speed are included in the wet bulb globe temperature (WBGT) index. This index is used to determine the amount of activity that should be undertaken in hot conditions. It is recommended that endurance events, especially those involving high intensities of exercise (4–21 km), should not be held when the WBGT index exceeds 28°C (82°F).[9] In practical terms, a WBGT index of 28°C (82°F) approximates a dry bulb temperature of 28°C (82°F) with 100% humidity.

Clinical perspective

Appropriate clinical assessment of the athlete who presents after exercising in the heat is the cornerstone of good management. In the past, there has been a tendency to initiate treatment before making a rational diagnosis. This position was taken partly because of the problem of high rates of admission to the medical tent at major events and partly because it was assumed that all athletes who collapsed were dehydrated and needed immediate intravenous hydration. The former problem can be overcome by a system of triage at events (Chapter 60), and the latter assumption is not evidence-based.[10] Thus, the emergency treatment of life-threatening conditions, including heatstroke and hyponatremia, can safely be delayed for 1 or 2 minutes while the rectal temperature is measured and a reasonable working diagnosis is established. The obvious exception is cardiac arrest, which occurs uncommonly, and the diagnosis of which is unambiguous.

The criteria for determining the severity of collapse are shown in Table 53.1. The initial assessment is based on the athlete's level of consciousness and knowledge of where in the race the athlete collapsed.

 Patients who are seriously ill show alterations in their level of consciousness and almost always collapse before completion of the race (Fig. 53.1).

In addition, the cause of illness in persons who collapse during the race is usually quite easily determined

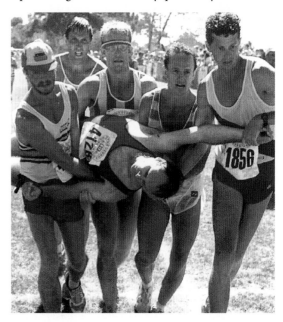

Figure 53.1 Collapse *before* the finish line suggests a serious cause of collapse. Exercise-associated collapse occurs *after* the athlete has completed the race, crosses the finish line, and stops voluntarily.

Table 53.1 Guidelines for determining the severity of the collapsed athlete's condition

Non-severe	Severe
Immediate assessment	Immediate assessment
Conscious	Unconscious or altered mental state
Alert	Confused, disoriented, aggressive
Rectal temperature: <40°C (104°F)	Rectal temperature: >40°C (104°F)
Systolic blood pressure: >100 mmHg	Systolic blood pressure: <100 mmHg
Heart rate: <100 beats/min	Heart rate: >100 beats/min
Specialized assessment	Specialized assessment
Blood glucose level: 4–10 mmol/L (72–180 mg/dL)	Blood glucose level: <4 or >10 mmol/L (<72 or >180 mg/dL)
Serum sodium concentration: 135–148 mmol/L (135–148 mEq/L)	Serum sodium concentration: <135 or >148 mmol/L (<135 or >148 mEq/L)
Body weight loss: 0–5%	Body weight loss: >10%
	Body weight gain: >2%

and forms part of the physician's standard medical training.

Measuring rectal temperature, blood pressure and heart rate provides additional diagnostic information. In longer races (>25 km) when hypoglycemia is more likely, a glycometer should also be used. In mass events of much longer duration (>4 hours), including ultramarathons, equipment for measuring the serum sodium concentration must be available so that potentially lethal exercise-related hyponatremia can be diagnosed expeditiously. Intravenous therapy should only be considered after a serum sodium concentration greater than 135 mmol/L (>135 mEq/L) has been measured. It is no longer defensible *not* to measure the serum sodium concentration in an athlete admitted to a medical tent after a sporting event of 4 or more hours and in whom there is evidence of some alteration in the level of consciousness.[11]

Whether or not the athlete is conscious or unconscious is the most important sign guiding the differential diagnosis. If the athlete is unconscious, the initial differential diagnosis is between a medical condition not necessarily related to exercise, for example, cardiac arrest, grand mal epilepsy, subarachnoid hemorrhage or diabetic coma, and an exercise-related disorder, most especially heatstroke, hyponatremia or severe hypoglycemia. The latter is an uncommon cause of exercise-related coma in non-diabetic subjects. If the athlete is unconscious, the crucial initial measurement is the rectal temperature, followed by heart rate and blood pressure. If the rectal temperature is above 41°C (106°F), the diagnosis is heatstroke and the patient must be cooled immediately (see below) and the cooling continued until the rectal temperature stabilizes at 38°C (100°F) or lower.

If the rectal temperature is below 40°C (104°F) in an unconscious patient, the blood pressure and pulse rate are not grossly abnormal, and there is no other obvious medical condition, the probability is that the athlete has exercise-associated hyponatremia or, rarely, another electrolyte abnormality such as hypochloremia also causing cerebral edema.

 Note that 'dehydration' in the range measured in athletes during marathon and other endurance or ultraendurance events does not cause unconsciousness.

Heatstroke—a temperature above 41°C (106°F)

When running, the metabolic rate is a function of running speed and body mass; thus, the highest rectal temperatures are usually seen in the fastest runners competing in events of 8–21 km. In such runners, the rectal temperatures may increase to 40.5°C (104.9°F) without symptoms or evidence of heat-related illness.[12, 13] Higher rectal temperatures are usually associated with symptoms that include dizziness, weakness, nausea, headache, confusion, disorientation and irrational behavior, including aggressive combativeness or drowsiness progressing to coma. Examination reveals the patient is hypotensive and has tachycardia. The presence or absence of sweating does not influence the diagnosis. The tachycardia and hypotension are initially due to a low peripheral resistance in the face of an elevated cardiac output.[14] Recovery of cardiovascular function occurs with normalization of the cardiac output and with an increase in peripheral vascular resistance.

If, during exercise, a previously healthy athlete shows marked changes in mental functioning, for example, collapse with unconsciousness or a reduced level of consciousness (stupor, coma) or mental stimulation (irritability, convulsions), in association with a rectal temperature above 41°C (106°F), the diagnosis of heatstroke is confirmed and warrants immediate initiation of cooling.

Management of heatstroke

The more rapidly the rectal temperature is reduced to 38°C (100°F) the better the prognosis. The patient should be placed in a bath of ice water for 5–10 minutes. The body temperature should decrease to 38°C (100°F) within this time.[15] Care must be taken to avoid inducing hypothermia as rectal temperature lags behind the core temperature. Shivering indicates that core temperature has decreased to 37°C (99°F) or below. Although there is no evidence that dehydration is the single critical factor causing heatstroke, intravenous fluids may be given to correct the expected dehydration and to assist in stabilizing the hyperkinetic circulation. Thus, 1–1.5 L of a 0.5% or 0.9% saline solution can be given initially, in part to ensure rapid venous access should this be required. However, cardiac function is compromised in hyperthermia and aggressive fluid therapy can induce pulmonary edema. Mortality from heatstroke should be zero in healthy athletes who are cooled promptly. Indeed, it is usual for athletes to be fully recovered and ambulatory within 30–60 minutes of collapse, providing they are correctly and expeditiously treated and they do not have a predisposing medical condition that explains their increased individual susceptibility to heatstroke (exercise-induced malignant hyperpyrexia).

 It is the delay in initiating cooling that makes heatstroke a potentially fatal condition.

Is hospital admission indicated?

The medical team must decide whether or not to admit the athlete to hospital for further observation after his or her temperature has been reduced to below 38°C (100°F). There is a tendency for rectal temperature to increase after cooling; this increase may not be noticed if the patient returns home without appropriate supervision. An increasing rectal temperature after cessation of exercise and appropriate cooling indicates ongoing heat-generating biochemical processes in muscle unrelated to exercise that may be related to conditions such as malignant hyperthermia.

Hospital admission is always required if the patient fails to regain consciousness within 30 minutes of appropriate therapy that returns the rectal temperature to 38°C (100°F). Patients who regain consciousness rapidly, whose cardiovascular system is stable and whose rectal temperature does not increase in the first hour after active cooling ceases usually do not need hospital admission. Thus, the decision as to whether hospital admission is needed can usually be made within an hour of the patient reaching medical treatment.

An absolute indication for hospital admission would be a failure to achieve cardiovascular stability during that time. A persisting tachycardia and hypotension in the supine, head-down position suggests that cardiogenic shock is developing. As heatstroke is such an uncommon complication of exercise, its presence should raise the possibility that other factors may be operative. These include genetic predisposition, unaccustomed drug use or subclinical viral infection. Indeed, in such cases the question must be asked: Is the hyperthermia the cause of the condition or merely a sign of another potentially more serious condition?

Complications of heatstroke

Heatstroke may be associated with damage to one or more body systems, as shown in Table 53.2. Whether the hyperthermia of heatstroke directly causes this damage or whether it is merely an accompanying feature of another disease syndrome that has yet to be properly described needs to be considered.[3] It appears that there is an individual susceptibility to heatstroke. Malignant hyperthermia, which is usually activated by certain general anesthetic agents, may also be triggered by other stimuli, perhaps including exercise. The biochemical abnormality resides in skeletal muscle, where it may activate uncontrolled metabolism and hyperthermia and ultimately an extensive, and potentially fatal, rhabdomyolysis (degeneration of skeletal muscle). The process can only be reversed by a specific drug, dantrolene sodium, or, less often, by rapid whole-body cooling. A number of deaths among high-profile professional athletes in the United States who died within 16–24 hours of the onset of 'heatstroke' despite receiving appropriate medical care raises the strong possibility that:

1. they were not suffering from heatstroke but from some other condition of which the hyperthermia was merely a diagnostic 'red herring'
2. because of a hereditary or acquired predisposition, exercise may be one factor that

Table 53.2 Complications of heatstroke

System	Abnormality
Cardiovascular	Arrhythmias Myocardial infarction Pulmonary edema
Neurological	Coma Convulsion Stroke
Gastrointestinal	Liver damage Gastric bleeding
Hematological	Disseminated intravascular coagulation
Muscular	Rhabdomyolysis
Renal	Renal failure

triggers the development of this fatal condition in these susceptible individuals

3. focusing solely on lowering the body temperature may not be enough to save the lives of these predisposed individuals—rather, attempts must be made to prevent the rhabdomyolysis, which appears to be the immediate cause of the critical complications (acute renal failure and cardiac arrest) that ultimately cause death.

Patients suffering rhabdomyolysis present with brown-colored urine accompanied by muscle weakness, swelling and pain. The skin may become discolored because of hemorrhages and the muscles have a 'doughy' feel. The urine contains high levels of myoglobin, which causes the brown discoloration and granular casts. Serum creatine kinase activity is also high. Laboratory tests may reveal elevated levels of potassium and uric acid and, in severe cases, evidence of disseminated intravascular coagulation. This condition requires urgent intensive care treatment.

Exercise-associated collapse

Exercise-associated collapse describes the common type of collapse that occurs in athletes who successfully complete endurance events without distress but who suddenly develop symptoms and signs of postural hypotension when they stop exercising. This condition has been referred to as 'heat syncope' and 'heat exhaustion' but we avoid these terms as the condition is benign and the rectal temperature is never sufficiently elevated to suggest a diagnosis of heatstroke. If the rectal temperature is elevated and the patient has an altered level of consciousness,

heatstroke is the correct diagnosis. The largest modern study of subjects who required medical attention after long-distance events found that only a tiny proportion of participants had markedly elevated rectal temperatures, indicating heatstroke, and few without heatstroke required hospitalization.[16]

This phenomenon of collapse after completing a sporting event in the heat occurs because the sudden cessation of exercise induces postural hypotension by causing blood to 'pool' in the dilated capacitance veins in the lower limb when the 'second heart' action of the lower limb musculature stops. In addition, there may be abnormal perfusion of the splanchnic circulation, with loss of a large fluid volume into the highly compliant splanchnic veins. The problem is a precipitous fall in the central (rather than circulating) blood volume and, hence, atrial filling pressures.[17–19] Since athletes collapse after exercise, dehydration cannot be a factor as fluid loss sufficient to impair cardiovascular function must produce its effects before the athlete completes the race and not after the race has been completed when the stress on the cardiovascular function is reducing.

The early publications referring to this condition did not find elevated rectal temperatures and used the terms 'heat exhaustion', 'heat prostration' or 'heat syncope' to describe the condition of collapse due to postural hypotension that develops in people who exercise in the heat. Unfortunately, this terminology has been misinterpreted to indicate that the collapse is caused by elevated body temperature and failure of heat regulation, which is not the case. Rather the condition is caused by the persistence into recovery of the low state of peripheral vascular resistance present during exercise. In addition, Noakes has drawn attention to the possible action of the Barcroft-Edholm reflex in this condition.[20] In 1945 Barcroft and Edholm showed that a sudden reduction in the right atrial pressure, in their case induced by venesection but analogous to the sudden reduction in atrial pressure that will result when the muscle pump becomes inactive on the cessation of exercise, induced a sudden and atavistic reduction in peripheral vascular resistance leading to hypotension and syncopy.[21] Restoration of the right atrial filling pressure reversed this vasodilation by increasing the peripheral vascular resistance.

The diagnosis of exercise-associated collapse can be made on the basis of a typical history, findings of a postural hypotension reversed by lying supine with the pelvis and legs elevated (Trendelenberg position), and the exclusion of readily identifiable medical syndromes such as diabetes and heatstroke (Chapter 44).

Management of exercise-associated collapse

As patients with exercise-associated collapse are conscious, they can be encouraged to ingest fluids orally during recovery. Sports drinks containing both glucose (4–8%) and electrolytes (Na: 10–20 mM) are appropriate provided the athlete does not also have evidence of fluid overload. The patients should lie with their pelvis and legs elevated. Nursing patients in this head-down position is always dramatically effective, producing a more stable cardiovascular system within 30–90 seconds and, usually, instant reversal of symptoms as a result of reversal of the Barcroft/Edholm reflex. The symptoms of dizziness, nausea and vomiting associated with this condition may result simply from a sudden reduction in blood pressure, especially as there is a dramatic fall from the elevated blood pressure maintained during exercise. Generally, recovery occurs within 10–20 minutes in persons nursed in the head-down position. Most athletes with exercise-associated collapse will be able to stand and walk unaided within 10–30 minutes of appropriate treatment and can be encouraged to leave the facility at that time.

Few, if any, athletes with exercise-associated collapse are sufficiently dehydrated to show the usual clinical signs of dry mucous membranes, loss of skin turgor, sunken eyeballs and an inability to spit. Some clinicians advocate intravenous therapy when these signs are present but we only use intravenous therapy in athletes who continue to have increased heart rates (>100 beats/min) and hypotension (<110 mmHg) when lying supine with the legs and pelvis elevated above the level of the heart.

Cramps

Heat cramps were first described among coal miners in 1923, eventually becoming known as 'miner's', 'fireman's', 'stoker's', 'cane-cutter's' or simply 'heat' cramps. The popular belief that cramps are caused by severe dehydration and large sodium chloride losses that develop during hot conditions has no scientific basis.[22–24] After a lifetime studying sodium balance in persons exercising in desert heat, Epstein and Sohar concluded that salt-deficiency heat cramps had never been proven to exist and illustrated 'christening by conjecture'.[25] Cramps can occur at rest or during or after exercise undertaken in any environmental conditions; they are specific neither to exercise, nor to exercise in the heat. The more modern hypothesis proposes that cramps probably result from alterations in spinal neural reflex activity activated by fatigue in susceptible individuals (Chapter 2).[22–24] The term 'heat cramps' should be abandoned as it clouds understanding of the possible neural nature of this connection.

Management of cramps

Stretching out the muscle to length is one effective therapy. Application of ice and physiotherapy of the affected muscle may also help. The Boston Marathon medical team treats muscle cramps with intravenous normal saline, and intravenous magnesium therapy has been used in the Hawaiian Ironman Triathlon, but clinical trials of either treatment have yet to be published.

Fluid overload: hyponatremia

Hyponatremia is perhaps the most important differential diagnosis in athletes who seek medical attention at an event undertaken in the heat, particularly at an ultramarathon. Thus, any athlete who becomes unconscious during or after ultradistance running or triathlon races and whose rectal temperature is not elevated should be considered to have symptomatic hyponatremia (hyponatremic encephalopathy) until measurement of the serum sodium concentration refutes the diagnosis. We emphasize that dehydration does not cause unconsciousness until it is associated with renal failure with uremia or hepatic failure.[10] To achieve such a weight loss as a result of dehydration, a 50 kg athlete would require 10 hours of high-intensity exercise at a sweat rate of 1 L per hour without any fluid replacement. Such a performance seems improbable in modern sporting events in which fluid is provided usually every 1–3 km and athletes are typically advised to drink 'as much as tolerable during exercise'. In contrast the !Kung San have been known to exercise for 6 hours in 45°C (113°F) desert heat without fluid replacement and without obvious detrimental effects other than some evidence of fatigue.[2] It is much more likely that athletes encouraged to drink 'as much as tolerable' during exercise in order to prevent 'dehydration' will present with fluid overload.[11, 26]

Athletes with hyponatremic encephalopathy and serum sodium concentrations below 129 mmol/L (129 mEq/L) are overhydrated by between 2 L and 6 L.[27, 28] The physician should be alerted to this diagnosis in a patient with an altered level of consciousness. If the patient is conscious, he or she may complain of feeling bloated or 'swollen'. A helpful clinical sign is that rings, race identification bracelets and watchstraps feel and are noticeably tighter. The race bracelet is a particularly useful indicator, as it is usually loose fitting before a race.

Management of hyponatremia

Under no circumstances should any hypotonic or isotonic fluids be given to unconscious or semiconscious athletes with hyponatremia. Rather, patients with hyponatremia require some or all of the following interventions dependent on the degree to which they have developed encephalopathy secondary to cerebral edema: fluid restriction; diuretics; intravenous hypertonic (3–5%) saline at rates of about 100 mL/h.[11] As the condition is due in part (see below) to abnormal secretion of arginine/vasopressin (antidiuretic hormone [ADH]) in the face of hypotonicity and fluid overload, diuresis may be delayed even in patients with quite mild hyponatremia. The use of a diuretic may be justified to initiate diuresis. Providing hypotonic or isotonic fluids to patients who are unconscious because of cerebral edema delays recovery and may produce a fatal result, as appears to have happened in isolated cases in recent years.[29–31]

In summary, it is essential that physicians caring for athletes with hyponatremia are aware of the correct management of this condition. The current management includes:

- bladder catheterization to monitor the rate of urine production during recovery—spontaneous recovery will occur if adequate amounts of urine (>500 mL/h) are passed. (*Note*: A high urine sodium concentration in the face of hyponatremia is diagnostic of inappropriate secretion of arginine/vasopressin [ADH], one of the three cardinal requirements for the development of this condition, see below).
- no fluids by mouth—salt tablets and sodium-containing foods can be given
- high sodium (3–5%) solutions given intravenously provided they are infused slowly (50–100 mL/h)
- use of diuretics.

Etiology of exercise-associated hyponatremia and hyponatremic encephalopathy

 The seminal paper describing the first cases of exercise-associated hyponatremia in 1985 concluded, on the basis of the history, the clinical findings and the estimated sodium and water balance during exercise in those athletes, that the etiology of the hyponatremia was due to overhydration.[32]

The article also concluded that the intake of hypotonic fluids in excess of that required to balance sweat and urine losses may be hazardous in some individuals.

A second study published in 1991[27] unambiguously resolved the issue of what causes exercise-associated hyponatremic encephalopathy. In this study, each of eight athletes who collapsed with exercise-associated hyponatremia was fluid overloaded by 1.22–5.92 L. The athletes conservatively estimated that their fluid intakes during exercise ranged from 0.8 to 1.3 L/h, compared with maximum values of 0.6 L/h in athletes with normal serum sodium concentrations. It was also found that the athletes' sodium losses (153 ± 35 mmol) were not larger than those of athletes who maintained normonatremia during exercise. Thus, this study concluded that exercise-associated hyponatremia results from fluid retention in athletes who consume abnormally large fluid volumes during prolonged exercise. It was also noted that because the potential dangers of severe dehydration and, thus, the need to drink adequately during prolonged exercise have been so well publicized, some athletes may consume dangerously large volumes of water during prolonged exercise.

Despite this unequivocal evidence presented 20 years earlier,[33] and subsequently confirmed by a large prospective clinical trial,[26] a number of influential sports medicine organizations began to advocate that athletes should drink 'as much as tolerable' during exercise. At the same time the theory evolved that exercise-associated hyponatremia was due to large unreplaced sodium losses in sweat (Fig. 53.2) and that the condition could therefore be prevented by the ingestion of sports drinks during exercise.

However, the first international consensus statement on exercise-associated hyponatremia[11] has concluded that the role of sodium loss in the development of exercise-associated hyponatremia has yet to be established. Rather, the study of Noakes et al.[3] concludes that three factors explain why the range of serum sodium concentrations after exercise is so variable even when the weight change is the same (Fig. 53.3). Thus, to develop exercise-associated hyponatremia subjects must:

1. over-drink, usually by drinking in excess of 750 mL per hour for at least 4 hours during exercise
2. fail adequately to suppress the inappropriate secretion of the water-retaining hormone arginine/vasopressin (ADH) and
3. either inappropriately osmotically inactivate circulating serum ionized sodium or fail

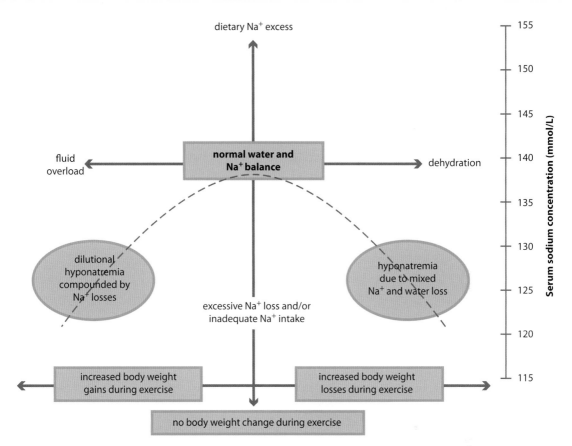

Figure 53.2 A theoretical diagram of how the serum sodium (Na⁺) concentration might alter with changes in sodium and fluid balance. It was proposed that weight loss during exercise would cause hyponatremia as a result of dehydration and large, unreplaced sodium losses (right side of the diagram). In contrast, excessive drinking leading to weight gain would reduce the serum sodium concentration by the dilution of the equally reduced whole-body sodium content in an expanded volume of total body water. A plot of serum sodium concentration versus body weight change during exercise would be an inverted U shape. ADAPTED FROM ARMSTRONG LE, ED. *PERFORMING IN EXTREME ENVIRONMENTS*. CHAMPAIGN, IL: HUMAN KINETICS, 2000: 103–35, FIGURE 6.4.

to mobilize osmotically inactive sodium to maintain a normal serum sodium concentration in an expanded total body water.

The conclusion of these findings is that the avoidance of over-drinking is the sole factor required to prevent exercise-associated hyponatremia.[11] Furthermore, the ingestion of sports drinks plays no role in this prevention because:

1. sports drinks are markedly hypotonic with a low sodium concentration (about one-seventh the serum sodium concentration). Thus, their ingestion adds substantially more water than sodium to the body. Since exercise-associated hyponatremia is due to fluid overload, the inappropriate ingestion of large volumes of sports drinks will compound the hyponatremia

2. exercise-associated hyponatremia is always also due to inappropriate secretion of arginine/vasopressin (ADH). The action of ADH on the kidney is to produce water retention and sodium diuresis.[3] Thus, the ingestion of any fluid regardless of its sodium content will cause further fluid retention, with excretion of all the sodium present in the ingested fluid.

3. the internal osmotically inactive sodium stores exceed, by an order of magnitude, the amount of sodium that might be ingested from a sports drink during prolonged exercise. Thus, appropriate mobilization of these stores will

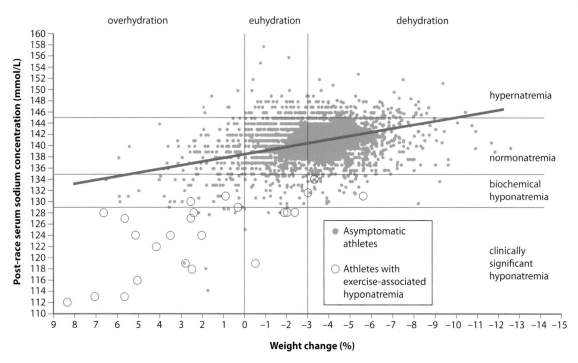

Figure 53.3 In a study of 2135 athletes, Noakes and colleagues[3] found that weight gain during exercise was significantly, and linearly, associated with a lower serum sodium concentration after racing (*P* < 0.0001). The data points formed a line, not an inverted U shape, indicating that hyponatremia was due to excessive fluid consumption.

ADAPTED FROM NOAKES TD, ET AL.[3]

prevent exercise-associated hyponatremia, regardless of how much sodium is ingested by mouth during exercise.

Other causes of exercise-related collapse in hot weather

Heatstroke and exercise-associated collapse are the most likely causes of distress or collapse while exercising in hot weather. It is, however, important to consider other possible causes of distress or collapse that may also occur in these conditions. A list of possible causes of collapse and the likely circumstances surrounding that collapse is shown in Table 53.3. This highlights the importance of determining the rectal temperature as the first step in the assessment of the collapsed athlete in hot weather. A rectal temperature above 40°C (104°F) indicates that heat illness is the most likely cause of collapse. A rectal temperature below 40°C (104°F) should encourage the clinician to consider other causes of collapse.

It is important to remember that athletes suffering from hyperthermia and hypothermia may present in the same event. The faster runners with their increased

heat production may present with hyperthermia, while slower runners, particularly those who have stopped to a walk, may present later in the day with hypothermia. The possibility of hypothermia is increased if a cold wind is present or if the temperature drops over the duration of the event. Cold-related illness is discussed in Chapter 54.

Heat acclimatization

Athletes are able to cope much better with hot or humid conditions if they are acclimatized.[34, 35] The human body adjusts to exposure to hot conditions by increasing blood volume and venous tone and, particularly, by alterations to the sweating mechanism. The main ways in which the sweating mechanism is affected are by:

- earlier onset of sweating
- increased amount of sweating
- increased dilution of the sweat (lower sodium concentration).

These changes result in increased heat loss for a given set of environmental conditions and a smaller rise in body temperature.

Table 53.3 Other causes of collapse

Cause	Associated features
Hypoglycemia	Diabetic using medication Poor carbohydrate loading and intake High alcohol intake prior to event
Hyponatremia	Ultraendurance event Large amounts of plain water
Hypothermia	Slow athlete in endurance event Cold wind (change of weather)
Drug toxicity	Athlete using social or performance-enhancing drugs (e.g. cocaine, amphetamines)
Ischemic heart disease/ arrhythmia	Previous history of cardiac disease Family history High risk factor profile
Stroke	Older athlete Hypertensive athlete
Convulsions/coma	Epilepsy Head injury Hyponatremia
Head injury	Contact sport

There is considerable dispute regarding the ideal length of time required for heat acclimatization, although a minimum of two weeks is probably required when coming from a cool climate to a hot or humid climate. One problem that reduces the effectiveness of heat acclimatization is that in the week or two prior to a major event, the athlete is often tapering (i.e. reducing the amount of training). While there is some effect on heat acclimatization in the rested state, it may be necessary to perform relatively intensive exercise to maximize acclimatization. Therefore, exposure to the warmer environment should occur for a minimum of two weeks.

A number of other factors affect acclimatization. If the athlete wishes to compete in a hot and humid environment, it is necessary to acclimatize for both heat and humidity. Training in a hot, dry environment provides only partial acclimatization for a hot, humid environment. Another factor affecting heat acclimatization is the presence or absence of air conditioning. To maximize acclimatization, the athlete should be exposed to the environmental conditions 24 hours a day. If the only exposure to the hot conditions is during training and the athlete

then returns to an air-conditioned environment, the effectiveness of acclimatization is reduced. Therefore, it is recommended that athletes spend a minimum of two weeks acclimatizing at the site of competition or in an environment very similar to that anticipated for competition. Some intense training should be performed during this period and air conditioning should be restricted to night-time for sleeping and adequate recovery.

Although it is possible to assist the acclimatization process by exercising in a heat chamber for 3 hours per day prior to departure, it is only partially effective and should be used as an adjunct to rather than as a replacement for full acclimatization. Wearing impermeable clothing while exercising may also make a small contribution to acclimatization.

Recommended Reading

Holtzhausen LM, Noakes TD. Collapsed ultraendurance athlete: proposed mechanisms and an approach to management. *Clin J Sport Med* 1997; 7: 292–301.

Noakes TD. Hyperthermia, hypothermia and problems of hydration. In: Shephard RJ, Åstrand PO, eds. *Endurance in Sport*. Oxford: Blackwell Scientific, 2000: 591–613.

Noakes TD. *Lore of Running*. 4th edn. Champaign, IL: Human Kinetics, 2003.

References

1. Heinrich B. *Racing the Antelope*. New York: Harper Collins, 2001.
2. Foster D, Foster D. *Africa. Speaking with Earth and Sky*. Cape Town: David Philip Publishers, 2005.
3. Noakes TD, Sharwood K, Speedy D, et al. Three independent biological mechanisms cause exercise-associated hyponatremia: evidence from 2,135 weighed competitive athletic performances. *Proc Natl Acad Sci U S A* 2005; 102(51): 18550–5.
4. Noakes TD. Mind over matter: deducing heatstroke pathology. *Physician Sportsmed* 2005; 33(10): 44–6.
5. Bracker MD. Environmental and thermal injury. *Clin Sports Med* 1992; 11: 419–36.
6. Dennis SC, Noakes TD. Advantages of a smaller bodymass in humans when distance-running in warm, humid conditions. *Eur J Appl Physiol Occup Physiol* 1999; 79(3): 280–4.
7. Marino FE, Mbambo Z, Kortekaas E, et al. Advantages of smaller body mass during distance running in warm,

Guidelines for the prevention of heat illness

Most cases of heat illness could be prevented if the following guidelines are followed.

1. Perform adequate conditioning. The athlete must have trained appropriately and be conditioned for the planned activity.

2. Undergo acclimatization if competing in unaccustomed heat or humidity.

3. Avoid adverse conditions. Event organizers should ensure that high intensity or endurance events should not take place in adverse conditions of heat or humidity. If events are to occur in hot climates, they should take place in the early morning before conditions deteriorate.

4. Alter training times. Unless trying to acclimatize, the athlete should avoid exercise at the hottest time of the day.

5. Wear appropriate clothing. In hot conditions, athletes should wear a minimal amount of loose-fitting, light-colored clothing. An open weave or mesh top is ideal. Many athletes choose to remove their top during training in hot conditions. This has the advantage of allowing better heat loss from sweating but is counterbalanced by an increased heat gain from the environment.

6. Drink appropriate amounts of fluids before the event. The athlete should ensure that he or she is adequately hydrated in the 24 hours prior to the event. A good method of confirming this is to ensure that urine output is clear and of good volume. Fluids should be drunk right up until the commencement of exercise. It is recommended that 500 mL of fluid be drunk in the half hour prior to exercise in the heat. Remember, however, that humans are unable to 'store' fluid. Thus, a fluid intake in excess of requirements is unnecessary before the race.

7. There is no evidence that fluid ingestion during exercise can prevent heatstroke in those predisposed to develop the condition. Nor is there any published evidence that dehydration is an important factor predisposing to heatstroke or the development of illness in athletes who have some access to such fluids during exercise.[33, 36] It has been shown that fluid ingestion during exercise in the laboratory may reduce the rectal temperature somewhat[37] but that this effect may be a result of the inadequate convective cooling usually present in indoor exercise.[38] When exercise is undertaken in the laboratory in environmental conditions that reproduce the conditions in out-of-door exercise, high rates of fluid ingestion are not required to prevent this additional increase in rectal temperature. Rather, drinking to the dictates of thirst (ad libitum) produces an optimum result.[38]

8. To minimize the uncomfortable sensations of thirst and so to optimize performance during exercise, athletes can be assured that they need drink only according to the dictates of their thirst (ad libitum)[36]. Usually, rates of ad-libitum fluid ingestion during exercise may vary between 200 and 800 mL per hour; much higher amounts are not uncommon in athletes who develop exercise-associated hyponatremia.[27, 39] Interestingly, elite athletes appear to drink sparingly during exercise, suggesting that superior athletic ability may be associated with a reduced dipsogenic drive during exercise. This would clearly be an advantageous evolutionary adaptation in early human hunter-gathers like the !Kung San who, since they have no access to fluid during hunting, will not be disabled by the development of intolerable thirst and hence have to terminate their hunt prematurely. For exercise up to 1 hour in duration, plain water is appropriate. For exercise lasting longer than 1 hour, a dilute glucose and electrolyte solution should be used (Chapter 37).

9. Ensure athletes and officials are well educated. It is important that event organizers, coaches and athletes understand the importance of adequate hydration, the danger of water intoxication, and the need to avoid excessive environmental conditions.

10. Provide proficient medical support. A well-equipped, well-trained medical team should be present at all endurance events occurring in hot or humid conditions. The guidelines for the medical coverage of an endurance event are discussed in Chapter 60.

humid environments. *Pflugers Arch* 2000; 441(2–3): 359–67.

8. Marino FE, Lambert MI, Noakes TD. Superior performance of African runners in warm humid but not in

cool environmental conditions. *J Appl Physiol* 2004; 96(1): 124–30.

9. Armstrong LE, Epstein Y, Greenleaf JE, et al. American College of Sports Medicine position stand. Heat and cold

illnesses during distance running. *Med Sci Sports Exerc* 1996; 28(12): i–x.

10. Noakes TD. Hyperthermia, hypothermia and problems of hydration. In: Shephard RJ, Åstrand PO, eds. *Endurance in Sport*. Oxford: Blackwell Scientific, 2000: 591–613.

11. Hew-Butler T, Almond C, Ayus JC, et al. Consensus statement of the 1st International Exercise-Associated Hyponatremia Consensus Development Conference, Cape Town, South Africa 2005. *Clin J Sport Med* 2005; 15(4): 208–13.

12. Maughan RJ. Thermoregulation in marathon competition at low ambient temperature. *Int J Sports Med* 1985; 6: 15–19.

13. Noakes TD, Myburgh KH, du Pliess J, Lang L, van der Riet C, Schall R. Metabolic rate, not percent dehydration predicts rectal temperature in marathon runners. *Med Sci Sports Exerc* 1991; 23: 443–9.

14. O'Donnell TF Jr, Clowes GH Jr. The circulatory requirements of heat stroke. *Surg Forum* 1971; 22: 12–14.

15. Armstrong LE, Crago AE, Adams R, Roberts WO, Maresh CM. Whole-body cooling of hyperthermic runners: comparison of two field therapies. *Am J Emerg Med* 1996; 14: 355–8.

16. Roberts WO. A 12-year summary of Twin Cities Marathon injury. *Med Sci Sports Exerc* 1996; 28: S123.

17. Holtzhausen LM, Noakes TD, Kroning B, de Klerk M, Roberts M, Emsley R. Clinical and biochemical characteristics of collapsed ultra-marathon runners. *Med Sci Sports Exerc* 1994; 26(9): 1095–101.

18. Holtzhausen LM, Noakes TD. The prevalence and significance of post-exercise (postural) hypotension in ultramarathon runners. *Med Sci Sports Exerc* 1995; 27(12): 1595–601.

19. Holtzhausen LM, Noakes TD. Collapsed ultraendurance athlete: proposed mechanisms and an approach to management. *Clin J Sport Med* 1997; 7(4): 292–301.

20. Noakes TD. The forgotten Barcroft/Edholm reflex: potential role in exercise associated collapse. *Br J Sports Med* 2003; 37(3): 277–8.

21. Barcroft H, Edholm OG. On the vasodilatation in human skeletal muscle during post-haemorrhagic fainting. *J Physiol* 1945; 104: 161–75.

22. Schwellnus MP. Skeletal muscle cramps during exercise. *Physician Sportsmed* 1999; 27(12): 109–15.

23. Schwellnus MP, Nicol J, Laubscher R, Noakes TD. Serum electrolyte concentrations and hydration status are not associated with exercise associated muscle cramping (EAMC) in distance runners. *Br J Sports Med* 2004; 38(4): 488–92.

24. Sulzer NU, Schwellnus MP, Noakes TD. Serum electrolytes in Ironman triathletes with exercise-associated muscle cramping. *Med Sci Sports Exerc* 2005; 37(7): 1081–5.

25. Epstein Y, Sohar E. Fluid balance in hot climates: sweating, water intake, and prevention of dehydration. *Public Health Rev* 1985; 13(1–2): 115–37.

26. Almond CS, Shin AY, Fortescue EB, et al. Hyponatremia among runners in the Boston Marathon. *N Engl J Med* 2005; 352(15): 1550–6.

27. Irving RA, Noakes TD, Buck R, et al. Evaluation of renal function and fluid homeostasis during recovery from exercise-induced hyponatremia. *J Appl Physiol* 1991; 70(1): 342–8.

28. Speedy DB, Noakes TD, Rogers IR, et al. Hyponatremia in ultradistance triathletes. *Med Sci Sports Exerc* 1999; 31(6): 809–15.

29. Garigan TP, Ristedt DE. Death from hyponatremia as a result of acute water intoxication in an Army basic trainee. *Mil Med* 1999; 164(3): 234–8.

30. Noakes TD. Perpetuating ignorance: intravenous fluid therapy in sport. *Br J Sports Med* 1999; 33(5): 296–7.

31. Thompson J, Wolff A. Hyponatremic encephalopathy in a marathon runner. *Chest* 2003; 124(suppl.): 313S.

32. Noakes TD, Goodwin N, Rayner BL, Branken T, Taylor RK. Water intoxication: a possible complication during endurance exercise. *Med Sci Sports Exerc* 1985; 17(3): 370–5.

33. Noakes T, Speedy D. Case proven: exercise-associated hyponatraemia is due to overdrinking. So why did it take 20 years before the original evidence was accepted? *Br J Sports Med* 2006; 40: in press.

34. Sparling PB. Expected environmental conditions for the 1996 Summer Olympic Games in Atlanta. *Clin J Sport Med* 1995; 5(4): 220–2.

35. Sparling PB. Environmental conditions during the 1996 Olympic Games: a brief follow-up report. *Clin J Sport Med* 1997; 7(3): 159–61.

36. Noakes T. Drinking guidelines for exercise: what is the evidence that athletes should either drink 'as much as tolerable' or 'to replace all the weight lost during exercise' or 'ad libitum'. *J Sports Sci* 2006; 24: in press.

37. Montain SJ, Coyle EF. Influence of graded dehydration on hyperthermia and cardiovascular drift during exercise. *J Appl Physiol* 1992; 73(4): 1340–50.

38. Saunders AG, Dugas JP, Tucker R, Lambert MI, Noakes TD. The effects of different air velocities on heat storage and body temperature in humans cycling in a hot, humid environment. *Acta Physiol Scand* 2005; 183(3): 241–55.

39. Hew T. Response to the letter to the editor by Roy J. Shephard, MD, PhD, DPE. *Clin J Sport Med* 2003; 13: 192–3.

Exercise at the Extremes of Cold and Altitude

WITH MICHAEL KOEHLE

Exercise in the cold

Activities in which cold injuries are likely to occur include those involving water immersion (e.g. swimming, scuba diving, boating, triathlons), those commonly performed in alpine environments (e.g. skiing), and those that require prolonged activity (e.g. marathons, ultraendurance events). Hypothermia, a central or core temperature of 35°C (95°F) or lower, occurs when the body loses more heat than it generates.

Generation of body heat

Humans function optimally in a relatively narrow temperature range. At ambient air temperatures above 28°C (82°F), heat produced by basal metabolism maintains the core temperature at 37°C (99°F). In conditions below this temperature, the body must produce additional heat to remain thermoneutral. Such heat production can be achieved by greater physical activity and autonomically mediated shivering, a physiological response of healthy individuals in a moderate environment.

Shivering involves involuntary muscular contractions in response to cold and uses energy stores quickly. The capacity to shiver lessens as local glycogen stores are depleted. The intensity of shivering is generally related to the rate of change of temperature. Shivering results in decreased muscular coordination and, therefore, impairs sporting performance. Non-shivering thermogenesis occurs in young children because of metabolism of brown fat but this mechanism is not available to adults, who have little brown fat.

Heat loss

Heat transfer occurs mainly from the skin and is therefore regulated by the circulation, the amount of insulation and perspiration. Heat loss occurs through conduction, convection, radiation and evaporation.

Conduction

Conduction occurs because of direct contact with a cold object or air. Heat transfer is related to the area of contact and the relative heat conductance of the objects. Conduction is most important in water immersion, as the conductivity of water is approximately 23 times that of air. Conduction may also be important when lying on cold wet ground.

Convection

Convection relates to the movement of air close to the body. This is normally low when wearing clothes but may be important in windy conditions with temperatures up to 20°C (68°F). It is also significant in sports such as cycling and running.

Radiation

Radiation involves the emission of heat energy to nearby objects. This occurs from uncovered skin and is the greatest source of heat loss under normal conditions. In cold conditions, however, the amount of heat loss through radiation is less as the skin temperature approximates the environmental temperature.

Evaporation

Heat lost as sweat on the external skin or clothing is converted from liquid to gas by evaporation.

Evaporation forms part of the body's insensible water losses that occur continually. Evaporation is increased in dry, windy conditions and may go unnoticed. An evaporative heat loss occurs when water is evaporated from the outside of a wetsuit in windy conditions. Heat is also lost through feces, urine and respiration.

Minimizing heat loss

Several factors help minimize heat loss. Peripheral vasoconstriction reduces external heat loss and increases the thickness of the shell of insulation but it is not effective in the head and scalp. Clothing helps reduce heat loss and curling the body into a ball to reduce the exposed surface area may minimize this even further. Keeping still also prevents heat loss. Lean athletes may be at a disadvantage with exposure to cold because fat provides insulation.

Measurement of body temperature

Direct measurement of core temperature is not practical. Thus, indirect measures are made at the tympanic membrane (intermediate zone) or the skin or mouth (peripheral zone). Measuring low temperatures requires a low-reading thermometer (below 32°C [90°F]).

Oral temperature is unreliable as it may be affected by wind, rain, external temperature and recent ingestion of food. It may, however, be a useful screening exercise as the core temperature will never be lower than the oral temperature. If the oral temperature is above 35°C (95°F), hypothermia can be excluded. It is necessary to leave the thermometer in the mouth for at least 3 minutes and the temperature should not be taken within 30 minutes of ingestion of hot or cold food.

Measurement of axillary temperature is also not reliable as it may be affected by skin temperature. Axillary temperature is usually 1–1.5°C (1.8–2.7°F) below core temperature and becomes less reliable in cold conditions.

Measurement of rectal temperature is the most commonly performed procedure to assess hypothermia. It is necessary to leave the thermometer in the rectum for at least 3 minutes at a depth of 10 cm (4 in.). Rectal temperature represents the temperature of the circulation supplying 'intermediate' tissues. Measurement of tympanic membrane temperature is less accurate and may be affected by water or wax in the ear as well as the surrounding skin temperature.[1]

In an outdoor emergency, if a thermometer is not available, the best means of assessing body temperature is to feel an area of the body that is not normally cold. It is important to remember that skin temperature is a poor guide to core temperature. Skin temperatures can drop to as low as 21–23°C (70–73°F) before any decrease in core temperature is detected.

Effects of hypothermia

Cardiovascular effects

Vasoconstriction may lead to fluid shifts by increasing the central blood volume, thus causing a cold diuresis. This diuresis, in conjunction with the increased fluid loss from respiration and sweat during exercise, may reduce total circulating volume. Upon rewarming, peripheral vessels dilate and cause a fluid shift to the periphery with a further reduction in central circulation. When combined with a cold myocardium, this may lead to circulatory collapse.

Decreased cardiac output occurs because of a combination of reduced circulatory volume, myocardial depression and impaired electrical conductance. Impaired conductance results in a decreased heart rate and ECG/EKG changes with prolongation of all intervals. The presence of a J wave in the ST segment is indicative of hypothermia. Atrial fibrillation may occur and usually reverts with rewarming. Ventricular fibrillation may occur and may be refractory to treatment at very low temperatures.

Respiratory effects

Cold exposure results in hyperventilation with a resultant respiratory heat and water loss. This may contribute to dehydration and bronchospasm.

A decrease in core temperature is also associated with a reduction in airway protective mechanisms and subsequent increased risk of aspiration. There is, however, no direct damage to the lung from exposure to cold due to the effective heating and humidifying mechanism of the upper airway.

Other effects

Delayed nerve conduction and neuromuscular transmission causes numbness, impaired coordination and cognition. This may persist for some hours or even days after the core temperature returns to normal.

Muscle stiffness and weakness associated with hypothermia may lead to an increased risk of muscle tears. Adequate warm-up and stretching should be performed prior to muscular activity in cold conditions. Excessive shivering may lead to poor voluntary muscular control and increased fatigue. Hypothermia may inhibit glycolysis and fat metabolism. Renal function can be impaired due to decreased renal blood flow,[2] and coagulopathies can occur.[3]

Clinical features

The clinical features of hypothermia vary depending on the degree of reduction in core temperature. These are listed in Table 54.1.

General principles of managing hypothermia

Management of the hypothermic athlete requires:

- recognition of the problem
- removal from cold, windy or wet conditions
- gentle and minimal handling
- measurement of the core temperature
- insulation to prevent further heat loss
- provision of nutritional and fluid support
- assessment for the presence of other conditions (e.g. frostbite)
- possible passive or active rewarming
- possible transportation to a medical facility.

Methods to achieve rewarming

Passive rewarming

Passive rewarming involves insulating the patient adequately to allow metabolic heat to rewarm slowly from within. If the patient can be removed from the cold environment, then it is advisable to remove all wet clothing and cover the whole body, including the head, with dry blankets.

If removal from the cold environment is not possible, wet clothing should only be removed if it can be done in a gentle fashion without exposing the bare patient to wind or rain. This minimizes the risk of movement inducing ventricular fibrillation. This is usually not possible. If the wet clothing is not removed, the patient should be placed in a plastic bag from the neck downwards to prevent any evaporative loss and to avoid wetting any dry insulation placed over the wet clothes. A second plastic bag placed over the dry insulation will keep it dry from subsequent exposure to rain. If none of the above is possible, a group of fully clothed people closely surrounding the patient is helpful ('penguin effect').[4]

Space blankets are commonly used in the treatment of hypothermia. However, in cold conditions, radiant heat loss is minimal compared with conductive loss, especially with poor insulation and high winds. Space blankets, therefore, provide little added protection, are easily torn by twigs, shred easily and are highly flammable.

In cases of moderate and severe hypothermia, passive rewarming is the safest way to rewarm[5] unless the patient is in a highly monitored intensive care unit with experienced skilled staff. Metabolic heat production initially increases with shivering and then decreases with decreasing temperature to 50% of a normal rate at 24°C (75°F). This heat production can rewarm the patient at 0.5–1°C (1–1.8°F) per hour even in profound hypothermia.

External active rewarming

Active rewarming may be by external or internal methods. External active rewarming is recommended in cases of mild hypothermia but should be avoided in severe hypothermia. There are a number of different means of external active rewarming, including a hot air or water-circulating blanket, hot packs to the axillae, groin and torso or a hot tub. Warming should be ideally directed to the trunk to reduce the risk of core temperature afterdrop, a phenomenon caused by cold blood returning from the extremities to the core.

Table 54.1 Clinical features of hypothermia

Mild (33–35°C [91–95°F])	Moderate (31–32°C [88–90°F])	Severe (<31°C [<88°F])
Cold extremities	Apathy, poor judgment	Inappropriate behavior
Shivering	Reduced shivering	Total loss of shivering
Tachycardia	Weakness and drowsiness	Cardiac arrhythmias
Tachypnea	Slurred speech and amnesia	Pulmonary edema
Urinary urgency	Dehydration	Hypotension and bradycardia
Mild incoordination	Increased incoordination and clumsiness Fatigue	Reduced level of consciousness Muscle rigidity

Internal active rewarming

Internal active rewarming can be performed in a hospital setting. Techniques that may be used include extracorporeal blood warming, cardiopulmonary bypass, airway warming and warm intravenous infusion. In severe hypothermia, active rewarming in a highly monitored intensive care unit with experienced staff can increase survival; however, in circumstances less than that, active rewarming may be both dangerous and counterproductive.

Other rewarming methods

Drugs play little or no role in the treatment of complicated hypothermia. Exercise is not helpful in anything but very mild hypothermia. Exercise depletes glycogen and therefore eventually inhibits shivering. Exercise also increases the rate of heat loss.

Treatment of hypothermia in sport

Although sporting activity generally provides sufficient body heat to keep the athlete warm, hypothermia may occur as a result of the following situations:

- an accident or injury
- exhaustion
- dehydration
- immersion (accidental or deliberate).

Sports with a particularly high risk of cold injury include endurance running, skiing or cycling, mountaineering, hiking, caving, windsurfing, kayaking and scuba diving. Insufficient clothing may provide inadequate protection from the environment, particularly near the end of a long race when running speed and heat production are reduced. Frostbite can occur in low temperatures, especially when combined with high wind speed.

The risk of hypothermia in athletes is increased by a lack of knowledge, lack of communication, pushing oneself to exhaustion, ignoring early warning signs, poor psychological and physical preparation and inadequate protection from the weather. Cold wind increases heat loss in proportion to wind speed, that is, wind chill factor. Note that if the temperature is –1°C (30°F) in still air, wind speeds of 16, 32 and 48 km/h reduce the temperature to –9°C (16°F), –14°C (7°F) and –19°C (–2°F), respectively.[6] Cyclists and skiers can generate these wind chill factors on a still day.

Hypothermia is a medical emergency and therapy should be instituted at once. Athletes presenting with hypothermia must have their temperature measured with a low-reading thermometer and managed according to whether they have mild, moderate or severe hypothermia. We discuss each of these conditions and a specific form of hypothermia—that associated with cold-water immersion.

Treatment of mild hypothermia

A patient with mild hypothermia (33–35°C [91–95°F]) should be removed from the cold, insulated appropriately and given a warm, sweet drink. Alcohol should be avoided. This patient will safely rewarm with or without active rewarming. The application of external heat may make him or her feel more comfortable. Heat should be applied to the torso, axillae and groin only and the patient should be continually monitored. Mild activity may be performed provided the rectal temperature remains close to 35°C.

Treatment of moderate hypothermia

The patient with moderate hypothermia (31–32°C [88–90°F]) should also be removed from the cold and insulated appropriately. In the field setting, the patient should not be rewarmed actively until the rectal temperature is rising and is above 34°C (93°F). The patient should be continually monitored, if possible, for the presence of hypotension and arrhythmias. Active rewarming can be performed in the hospital setting with continuous monitoring, intravenous rehydration and the availability of resuscitation equipment. Moderate hypothermia is not usually life-threatening itself; however, these patients are at risk of progressing to severe hypothermia, which has a significant mortality.

Treatment of severe hypothermia

The patient with severe hypothermia (<31°C [<88°F]) should be handled as little and as gently as possible as the risk of ventricular fibrillation is considerable. The treatment of the severely hypothermic patient depends on the availability of appropriate facilities. If the patient can be transported quickly and safely with minimal handling, he or she should be transferred to a hospital equipped with an intensive care unit. In this setting, active rewarming can begin.

The severely hypothermic patient may often appear dead but on closer observation may have an extremely slow heart rate (as low as 6 beats per minute) and a slow respiration rate. These patients must not be mistaken for being in asystole as cardiopulmonary resuscitation may precipitate ventricular fibrillation.

Patients suffering from severe hypothermia should never be considered to be dead until they are warm and dead.[7, 8]

Treatment of immersion hypothermia

Immersion hypothermia usually results from rapid cooling in a non-exhausted patient. Other major dangers to a victim of immersion are impaired swimming performance and immediate cardiorespiratory responses due to cold. The patient should be gently removed, in the horizontal position if possible, from the water with particular attention paid to signs of cardiovascular collapse when the hydrostatic support of the patient's blood pressure is removed. If the rectal temperature is below 31°C, the patient should be treated in the same way as any patient with severe hypothermia. If the rectal temperature is above 32°C and the patient has been in the water less than 3 hours, rapid rewarming can begin, as significant fluid shifts should not have occurred.[9] It is important to remember when insulating the patient that sweat may reduce the effectiveness of the insulating material and that evaporation from the outer surface of a wetsuit may cause considerable heat loss.

Frostbite

Frostbite involves crystallization of fluids in the skin or subcutaneous tissue after exposure to subfreezing temperatures (<−0.6°C [<31°F]). With low skin temperature and dehydration, cutaneous blood vessels constrict and limit circulation because the viscosity of blood increases. Water is drawn out of the cells and ice crystals cause mechanical destruction of skin and subcutaneous tissues. It most commonly occurs in the periphery, with the fingers and toes being most affected.[10] The tip of the nose and ears and the tissue of the cheek are also affected. Cross-country ski races are postponed if the temperature at the coldest point in the course is less than −20°C (−4°F) because of the severe wind chill generated at race pace.[6]

Frostbite can be classified as:

- superficial or mild, involving the skin and subcutaneous tissue only, or
- deep or severe, involving the full skin thickness and deeper tissues.

Clinical features

Patients with superficial frostbite complain of a burning local pain with numbness. On examination, the skin is initially pale and grey and becomes red after thawing. Superficial serous bullae (blisters) may be present; hemorrhagic blisters represent subdermal damage.

Local thawing by contact with direct body heat can treat superficial frostbite. The injured part should not be directly rubbed as sloughing may occur. No attempt should be made to thaw the injured part unless it is certain that refreezing will be prevented. Refreezing results in a far more serious injury.

Deep frostbite is initially extremely painful and then becomes numb. The body part affected appears as a frozen block of hard, white tissue with areas of gangrene and deep hemoserous blisters if severe. The affected part should be rapidly rewarmed in a hot water bath of temperature 39–41°C (102–106°F). A whirlpool bath with added antiseptic is ideal. The rewarming process is often acutely painful and requires analgesia. Radiant heat from a fire or radiator should not be used as skin burns may occur. The tissue should continue to be warmed until it becomes soft and pliable and normal sensation returns. Appropriate tetanus prophylaxis is indicated.[11] The serous blisters contain thromboxanes and prostaglandins that damage underlying tissue. These serous blisters should be debrided and treated topically with aloe. Hemorrhagic blisters should be left intact. Ibuprofen 400 mg orally twice a day is recommended to prevent further prostaglandin-mediated tissue damage.[11]

Intravenous infusion of low-molecular-weight dextran may help reduce swelling and maintain vasodilatation. Prophylactic parenteral penicillin should be administered for 72 hours.[11] It is important to salvage as much tissue as possible. Debridement should be delayed for days to weeks when obvious demarcation has occurred. Contractures and compartment syndromes may develop and should be treated appropriately.

Prevention of cold injuries

The majority of cold injuries are preventable if general guidelines are followed and the athlete benefits from the specific strategies that have been developed for cold weather activities.

General guidelines

The following guidelines apply to all activities where hypothermia has the potential to occur:

1. Plan adequately.
2. Communicate plans to others.
3. Avoid activity inappropriate for fitness level.
4. Avoid activity to exhaustion.

5. Avoid dehydration.
6. Ensure adequate nutrition.
7. Warm up appropriately.
8. Wear appropriate clothing for weather conditions.
9. Cancel activity or seek shelter if appropriate. Note that the American College of Sports Medicine recommends that if the ambient dry bulb temperature is below −20°C (−4°F), race directors should consider canceling or rescheduling races.[6]

Athletes should wear appropriate clothing for the particular environmental conditions. It is advisable to wear a number of layers of clothing rather than one thick layer. This will enable the athlete to remove layers of clothing when exercising in warmer conditions and therefore reduce sweating. It also enables the athlete to put on additional clothing if the temperature or level of activity drops. Clothing should be made of a good insulating material such as wool, synthetic fleece or polypropylene. Use of cotton garments should be avoided.

In rain or snow, adequate waterproof outer clothing should be worn. The outer jacket should also offer adequate protection against wind. Recommended materials include nylon and Gore-Tex. In cold conditions, extremities such as the head, face and hands should be covered. Synthetic or wool socks should be worn instead of cotton.

Running and cycling

Runners and cyclists are at particular risk of cold injuries because they usually wear a minimum of clothing, are exposed to an increased wind chill factor and often prefer to train alone. Dehydration and exhaustion are also common.

As mentioned in Chapter 53, it is possible to see cold and heat injuries in the same endurance events. Slower participants are susceptible to cold injuries.

Mountaineers, hikers and cavers

These athletes are at particular risk of hypothermia due to increased convective and conductive heat loss.[12] Often, when exercising in a group, the least fit person is at risk of developing cold injuries. This person may have excessive sweating, hyperventilation and peripheral vasodilatation resulting in exhaustion, dehydration and increased heat loss.

It is important for other members of the party to observe for the early signs of cold injury (e.g. shivering, dysarthria, delayed cerebration). The group's plans should constantly be reviewed taking into account the latest environmental conditions and forecasts and the state of the individual members of the party.

Back-country and cross-country skiing

The cross-country skier is at a high risk of cold injury due to exposure to a cold environment and the potential for fatigue and injury. Clothing with effective thermal insulation including leg covers is essential. It is important to keep the inner garments dry. If clothing becomes wet, it should be changed promptly while the individual is still alert. The cross-country skier should never ski alone.

Water sports

In surface water sports (e.g. windsurfing, kayaking), wind and spray may contribute to cold injuries. Exhaustion may occur quickly and the windsurfer may be some distance from shore when this occurs. Cold injuries can be prevented by the use of wetsuits with coverings for extremities (e.g. hood, gloves, boots). Knowledge of weather conditions is important and the sport should not be performed alone.

Divers should also always dive with a partner. The dive should be planned taking into consideration the water temperature and the degree of insulation provided by the wetsuits. It is important to conserve energy in order to reduce heat losses. The diver (or partner) must be vigilant for the early signs of cold injury.[13]

Exercise at altitude

Many active people enjoy traveling to altitude for recreation. Altitude illness can occur at altitudes above 3000 m (10 000 ft) and can cause significant morbidity among travelers to altitude. The life-threatening manifestations of altitude illness—high-altitude cerebral edema and high-altitude pulmonary edema—occur in 0.1–4.0% of visitors to altitude.[14] A larger proportion of travelers experience milder symptoms. While not life-threatening, these can be severe enough to interfere with trip participation and enjoyment. Fortunately, altitude illness is preventable, and proper pre-trip counseling can play a role in reducing morbidity and mortality at altitude.

Itinerary

One of the most important determinants of an individual's risk of altitude illness is the itinerary. Rate of ascent is a strong predictor for acute mountain sickness.[15] Those who ascend slowly, allowing for gradual acclimatization, have a lower likelihood of developing acute mountain sickness (odds ratio 3.0 for faster ascent).[15] Sleeping altitude is monitored when assessing the rate of ascent as large increases in sleeping altitude pose the greatest risk of altitude illness. Various guidelines have been proposed for graded ascent, ranging from 300 m to 600 m (1000–2000 ft) of ascent per night[16, 17] when above 3000 m (10 000 ft). Additionally, at least one night at an intermediate altitude (1500–2500 m [5000–8000 ft]) on the way to very high altitude is recommended for acclimatization.[14] No controlled studies have been conducted that demonstrated an ideal ascent rate. A recommended ascent rate of no more than approximately 400 m (1300 ft) per night should be followed. Approximately every 1000 m (3200 ft), an additional rest day is recommended where the traveler sleeps at the same altitude for two consecutive nights.

Daytime acclimatization hikes to higher altitudes are permitted and encouraged in those travelers who are not exhibiting signs and symptoms of altitude illness. This 'climb high, sleep low' approach has long been used to accelerate acclimatization by intermittently exposing the individual to a higher dose of hypoxia.

Travelers with more rigid itineraries often ascend too quickly or while symptomatic or sick in order to meet external deadlines. Although 40% of trekkers in the Nepal Himalayas are in organized groups, they account for 80% of medical evacuations.[18] Patients should be encouraged to have a flexible itinerary, with room for extra rest days to allow for illness or other setbacks.

Previous altitude history

Patients with a previous history of altitude illness are at increased risk of recurrence.[15, 19] Susceptible individuals should follow a more conservative itinerary (aiming for 300 m [1000 ft] increments in sleeping altitude). These individuals should also strongly consider chemoprophylaxis, especially if they are returning to an altitude at which they were previously ill (discussed later).

The effect of recent previous altitude exposure is a matter of much debate. In laboratory models of deacclimatization,[20] hypoxic ventilatory response seems to recede after only one week. However, observational studies suggest that altitude exposure in the previous two months provides a significant degree of protection from acute mountain sickness.[15] The protection from high-altitude pulmonary edema seems to be much shorter lasting. Re-entry high-altitude pulmonary edema[21, 22] is a phenomenon whereby high-altitude residents develop pulmonary edema after a brief trip to low altitude. These residents would presumably be well acclimatized to their home altitude, but apparently do not retain any protection from high-altitude pulmonary edema when they briefly descend. It therefore appears that previous altitude exposure may provide some protection from acute mountain sickness, but not from high-altitude pulmonary edema.

Patient characteristics and previous medical history

Gender is not believed to be a risk factor for acute mountain sickness.[23, 24] There does appear to be a slight overrepresentation of male patients with high-altitude pulmonary edema.[14] Although early work suggested that older travelers might have some slight protection from acute mountain sickness, there is insufficient data using current definitions of altitude illness to confirm this finding.[25] One hypothesis for the mechanism of this phenomenon involves cerebral atrophy. Brain swelling within a rigid cranium may play a role in the pathophysiology of high-altitude cerebral edema and acute mountain sickness.[26] The cerebral atrophy associated with aging may be therefore mildly protective against acute mountain sickness.

High-altitude pulmonary edema has some unique medical risk factors. The pathophysiology of high-altitude pulmonary edema involves increased pulmonary vascular pressures, possibly related to heterogeneous hypoxic pulmonary vasoconstriction. Therefore, conditions that increase pulmonary vascular pressure, such as unilateral pulmonary artery hypertension[26, 27] and primary pulmonary hypertension[27] increase the risk of an individual developing high-altitude pulmonary edema.

Asthma

Asthma is not a risk factor for altitude illness. Asthmatics tend to have fewer symptoms while at moderate altitude. The improvement in clinical status is believed to be due to thinner air and a relative dearth of pollutants and lung irritants in the air.[28] (At extreme altitude, airway heat loss may aggravate asthma.) Before intense physical efforts, patients should pre-medicate with bronchodilators (and possibly inhaled corticosteroids), especially if they have known exercise-induced bronchospasm.[29] Rapid ascent to an altitude of 3000 m (10 000 ft) or more should be avoided in those with moderate or severe asthma.[29]

Refractive eye surgery

Patients who have had refractive eye surgery may have visual difficulties while traveling at altitude (especially above 5000 m [16 400 ft]). There are several reports of visual disturbances after scalpel radial keratotomy at high altitude.[30, 31] The more recent laser procedures (laser PRK and LASIK) have resulted in fewer complications. A recent study of mountaineers with LASIK demonstrated that some still had symptoms such as blurring and dry eyes while traveling above 5000 m (16 400 ft).[32] Exacerbation of dry eye is the presumed mechanism of these disturbances.[33] Patients should be cautioned about possible visual problems and should bring artificial tears for daily instillation while at moderate altitude and above. If visual blurring does occur, they should not ascend any further.

Hormones and pregnancy

The effectiveness of oral contraceptive pill (OCP) regimens is not believed to be altered at altitude.[24] Mountain travelers often suffer diarrhea or other conditions requiring concurrent medication therapy that may interfere with the efficacy of OCPs. Patients should be cautioned to use a second method of contraception in these situations.

There is also a theoretical risk that combination OCPs might have the potential of increasing the risk of thrombosis at altitude (especially when combined with conditions which can commonly occur such as dehydration, polycythemia and stasis). To date, there have been no reports of deep vein thrombosis in this group.[24] At sea level, third-generation OCPs (containing desorgestrel or gestodene) have a higher risk of thrombosis than second-generation OCPs (relative risk 1.7),[34] which may be preferable for sojourners to altitude.

There are some specific concerns for pregnant women at altitude. With travel at altitude, comprehensive medical care is often unavailable. Furthermore, medication options for acute mountain sickness prevention are more limited in pregnant women. For example, sulfonamides (such as acetazolamide) are contraindicated in the first trimester and after 36 weeks of pregnancy. Pregnancy-specific conditions that may be affected by altitude include spontaneous abortion, pre-eclampsia, gestational hypertension, placental abruption and intrauterine growth restriction (IUGR). The data relevant to these conditions are limited and usually derived from studies of high-altitude residents (as opposed to sojourners), who may have different risk profiles. The Union Internationale des Associations d'Alpinisme (UIAA) consensus paper[24] has the following recommendations regarding pregnant women:

- those at risk of spontaneous abortion, preeclampsia, IUGR and placental abruption should avoid high-altitude exposure
- pregnant women should allow two to three days for acclimatization prior to exercising at altitude, waiting two weeks before performing strenuous exercise
- chronic hypertension, anemia, smoking and cardiopulmonary disease are contraindications for travel to altitude after 20 weeks' gestation.

General preventive measures

Exertion

Exertion is an independent risk factor for acute mountain sickness.[35] Because both exertion and cold can increase pulmonary vascular pressure, they are both believed to worsen high-altitude pulmonary edema.[36] Travelers are therefore encouraged to adopt a regular even pace and avoid overexertion while at altitude. They should also be encouraged to bring appropriate clothing and equipment for the cold weather.

Hydration

Some recent research indicates that dehydration may also potentiate acute mountain sickness.[37] The air at altitude is dry, respiratory rate is higher, and mouth breathing is more common. These factors increase insensible losses at altitude. Travelers should therefore consume at least 3–4 L of water and clear non-caffeinated, non-alcoholic beverages per day while trekking or climbing. On rest days, fluid requirements would be slightly less. A good guideline is to aim for the urine to be clear.

Infections

Upper respiratory tract infections are extremely common at altitude. There is some evidence that these infections may increase the risk of acute mountain sickness,[38] and high-altitude pulmonary edema.[39] At altitude, upper respiratory tract infections may also increase the potential for dehydration (through increased insensible losses). Travelers should be counseled to modify their rate of ascent when they contract an upper respiratory tract infection, allowing more time for rest and acclimatization. They should also be monitoring their fluid intake to avoid dehydration.

Diet

A high-carbohydrate diet is recommended for altitude travelers.[40] Presumably, the etiology of this benefit is related to an elevated respiratory quotient (V_{CO_2}/V_{O_2}) from the metabolism of carbohydrates over fats. Increasing carbon dioxide production leads to increased ventilation, and improved arterial oxygen saturation.

One of the later manifestations of altitude acclimatization is increased red blood cell production. Adequate iron stores are required to allow for the new heme pigment production. Those who may have low iron stores (e.g. vegetarians, menstruating women) should consider iron supplementation to facilitate this process.[41]

Ultraviolet light

With ascent, ultraviolet light exposure increases by approximately 4% per 300 m (1000 ft).[17] By this formula, there would be approximately 70% more ultraviolet radiation at Everest Base Camp than at sea level. This increased radiation is compounded by radiation reflected off any snow that is present. Because of this reflected radiation, individuals can get sunburns in unlikely places such as the underside of the nose or chin. Travelers should be advised of the increased risk of sunburn and snow blindness (ultraviolet keratitis) at altitude. They should bring appropriate sun-protective clothing, hats, sun block and lip balm. Sunglasses with adequate face protection (glacier glasses or wraparound glasses are best) are essential for the prevention of snow blindness. If traveling with guides or porters, the traveler should ensure that they are also adequately equipped for sun and cold protection. As many cases of snow blindness occur after the patient's sunglasses have been broken or lost, it is a good idea to bring an extra pair of sunglasses for the traveling group.

Prophylactic medications

In certain conditions, prophylactic medications may be warranted. Individuals who are at higher risk of altitude illness should consider taking medications for prophylaxis. These individuals are those with a previous history of an altitude illness, with an aggressive itinerary, or with other risk factors mentioned above. Different medication regimens are used for prevention of acute mountain sickness/high-altitude cerebral edema than for high-altitude pulmonary edema.

Acute mountain sickness

Acetazolamide is a medication that is legendary among climbers and trekkers. Over the years, there has been a lot of experience with using acetazolamide in the prevention of acute mountain sickness. There have also been several high-quality studies demonstrating its efficacy.[42–45] In these studies, a dose of 250 mg orally twice a day has been shown to be effective in reducing the incidence of acute mountain sickness. A low-dose regimen (125 mg orally twice a day) reduced the incidence of acute mountain sickness.[44] The relative risk reduction at this dosage level was approximately 50% (one case prevented for every eight people treated). When a dose of 125 mg twice daily was compared to 250 mg twice daily by Carlsten et al.,[45] the lower dose was not significantly different from placebo.

A meta-analysis of several studies concluded that a dose of 750 mg twice daily was the only effective dose, however, it was limited by varying ascent rates and final altitudes among studies as well as excluding studies that did not dichotomize outcomes into presence or absence of altitude illness. The optimal dose of acetazolamide for the prevention of acute mountain sickness that minimizes adverse effects has yet to be clarified. A prospective study, comparing different dosages at the same ascent rate, is required to address this controversy properly.

Acetazolamide is contraindicated in many travelers to altitude, including those with an allergy to sulfonamides and those with glucose-6-phosphate dehydrogenase deficiency. Pregnant and breastfeeding women should also avoid this medication. Furthermore, acetazolamide should not be taken in conjunction with salicylates as there is an increased risk of central nervous system depression and metabolic acidosis.

Dexamethasone is an appropriate alternative for acute mountain sickness prophylaxis in those who cannot tolerate acetazolamide. The recommended prophylactic dose is 8 mg daily (usually divided twice daily).[46] For prophylaxis, these medications need only be taken until the traveler reaches a stable altitude (and is asymptomatic at that altitude). Once descent has begun, these medications are not required.

Other xenobiotics have been proposed for acute mountain sickness prophylaxis. Ginkgo biloba initially showed some promise in smaller initial studies, but two recent high-quality studies have shown no benefit over placebo.[43, 47] Both coca and garlic have been proposed as possible prophylactic therapies. There have been no published studies of either intervention. Coca can also increase the risk of acute coronary syndrome among users,[48] a devastating complication in a remote area. None of these alternative therapies can be recommended for the prevention of acute mountain sickness.

High-altitude pulmonary edema

Several medications have been shown to be efficacious in the prevention of recurrent high-altitude pulmonary edema. Nifedipine (20 mg sustained-release preparation three times a day),[49] tadalafil (10 mg twice a day),[50] dexamethasone (8 mg twice a day)[50] and salmeterol (two puffs twice a day)[51] have all been examined. Unfortunately, no powerful studies have yet been done to compare each of these four therapies. The decision of which medication to prescribe should probably be based on tolerance and mitigation of adverse events.

Sleep at altitude

Visitors to high altitude often have poor sleep marked by frequent arousals and periodic breathing.[52] Sleep quality and periodicity improve with acclimatization at moderate altitudes, but may persist at extreme elevations.[52] Both acetazolamide and benzodiazepines have been used effectively to improve sleep quality at altitude.

Acetazolamide acts to reduce respiratory alkalosis, and hence respiratory periodicity. It has long been used to improve the sleep quality at high altitude.[53] The standard dose of acetazolamide for improving sleep is 125 mg orally every 4 hours.

Temazepam (10 mg orally) improves both subjective[54, 55] and objective measures of sleep quality in travelers to altitude.[56] It is an appropriate alternative in those patients unable to take acetazolamide.

Specific issues for athletes

Although sporting events can often take place at moderate altitude (e.g. the Mexico City Olympics were held at 2240 m [7300 ft]), it is rare that they would occur above 3000 m (10 000 ft) where altitude illness is a risk. However, some ski resorts (e.g. in Colorado) are high enough to cause altitude illness among visitors.

Altitude presents a few unique challenges to competing athletes. The hypoxia can cause decrements in performance, particularly in endurance events. With drier air and more ultraviolet light exposure, athletes can be at an increased risk of dehydration and sunburn. Full acclimatization can take weeks to months, but a short acclimatization period at the altitude of competition prior to the event is beneficial for performance. This should be of at least 48 hours in duration and preferably longer if scheduling permits.[57] During this acclimatization period, rest and hydration status should be prioritized. A high-carbohydrate diet would also be beneficial (as mentioned above).

Intermittent hypoxic exposure (e.g. sleeping in a hypoxic tent) is commonplace among elite endurance athletes. These repeated exposures to simulated altitude have been shown to increase the ventilatory response to hypoxia, and might prove beneficial by 'pre-acclimatizing' athletes to altitude before arrival.

Conclusion

Exposure to altitude can lead to altitude illness and/or exacerbation of pre-existing medical conditions. Many of these situations are preventable through appropriate planning or pharmaceutical intervention. A thorough medical history combined with analysis of the itinerary is a key step in the prevention of medical problems at altitude. Altitude also provides unique challenges to the competing athlete that can be mitigated with appropriate preparation and acclimatization.

Recommended Reading

Auerbach P. *Wilderness Medicine: Management of Wilderness and Environmental Emergencies.* 4th edn. St Louis: Mosby, 2001.

Butcher JD, Gambrell RC. Hypothermia. In: Fields KB, Fricker PA, eds. *Medical Problems in Athletes.* Malden, MA: Blackwell Science, 1997: 285–92.

Krakauer J. *Into Thin Air: a Personal Account of the Mount Everest Disaster.* New York: Anchor Books, 1998.

Laskowski-Jones L. Responding to winter emergencies. *Dimens Crit Care Nurs* 1999; 18: 13–22.

Marsigny B, Lecoq-Jammes F, Cauchy E. Medical mountain rescue in the Mont-Blanc massif. *Wilderness Environ Med* 1999; 10: 152–6.

References

1. Cattaneo CG, Frank SM, Hesel TW, El-Rahmany HK, Kim LJ, Tran KM. The accuracy and precision of body temperature monitoring methods during regional and general anesthesia. *Anesth Analg* 2000; 90(4): 938–45.

2. Yoshitomi Y, Kojima S, Ogi M, Kuramochi M. Acute renal failure in accidental hypothermia of cold water immersion. *Am J Kidney Dis* 1998; 31(5): 856–9.

3. Ulrich AS, Rathlev NK. Hypothermia and localized cold injuries. *Emerg Med Clin North Am* 2004; 22(2): 281–98.

4. Blows WT. Crowd physiology: the 'penguin effect'. *Accid Emerg Nurs* 1998; 6(3): 126–9.

5. Nielsen HK, Toft P, Koch J, Andersen PK. Hypothermic patients admitted to an intensive care unit: a fifteen year survey. *Dan Med Bull* 1992; 39(2): 190–3.

6. Armstrong LE, Epstein Y, Greenleaf JE, et al. American College of Sports Medicine position stand. Heat and cold illnesses during distance running. *Med Sci Sports Exerc* 1996; 28(12): i–x.

7. Bolte RG, Black PG, Bowers RS, Thorne JK, Corneli HM. The use of extracorporeal rewarming in a child submerged for 66 minutes. *JAMA* 1988; 260(3): 377–9.

8. Southwick FS, Dalglish PH Jr. Recovery after prolonged asystolic cardiac arrest in profound hypothermia. A case report and literature review. *JAMA* 1980; 243(12): 1250–3.

9. Golden FS, Tipton MJ, Scott RC. Immersion, near-drowning and drowning. *Br J Anaesth* 1997; 79(2): 214–25.

10. Cattermole TJ. The epidemiology of skiing injuries in Antarctica. *Injury* 1999; 30(7): 491–5.

11. Murphy JV, Banwell PE, Roberts AH, McGrouther DA. Frostbite: pathogenesis and treatment. *J Trauma* 2000; 48(1): 171–8.

12. Christensen ED, Lacsina EQ. Mountaineering fatalities on Mount Rainier, Washington, 1977–1997: autopsy and investigative findings. *Am J Forensic Med Pathol* 1999; 20(2): 173–9.

13. White LJ, Jackson F, McMullen MJ, Lystad J, Jones JS, Hubers RH. Continuous core temperature monitoring of search and rescue divers during extreme conditions. *Prehosp Emerg Care* 1998; 2(4): 280–4.

14. Basnyat B, Murdoch DR. High-altitude illness. *Lancet* 2003; 361(9373): 1967–74.

15. Schneider M, Bernasch D, Weymann J, Holle R, Bartsch P. Acute mountain sickness: influence of susceptibility, preexposure, and ascent rate. *Med Sci Sports Exerc* 2002; 34(12): 1886–91.

16. Murdoch D. How fast is too fast? Attempts to define a recommended ascent rate to prevent acute mountain sickness. *Int Soc Mountain Med Newsletter* 1999; 9(1): 3–6.

17. Hackett P, Roach R. High-altitude medicine. In: Auerbach P, ed. *Wilderness Medicine: Management of Wilderness and Environmental Emergencies.* 4th edn. St Louis: Mosby, 2001: 1–37.

18. Shlim DR, Gallie J. The causes of death among trekkers in Nepal. *Int J Sports Med* 1992; 13(suppl. 1): S74–S76.

19. Bartsch P, Bailey DM, Berger MM, Knauth M, Baumgartner RW. Acute mountain sickness: controversies and advances. *High Alt Med Biol* 2004; 5(2): 110–24.

20. Katayama K, Sato Y, Shima N, et al. Enhanced chemosensitivity after intermittent hypoxic exposure does not affect exercise ventilation at sea level. *Eur J Appl Physiol* 2002; 87(2): 187–91.

21. Hultgren HN, Marticorena EA. High altitude pulmonary edema. Epidemiologic observations in Peru. *Chest* 1978; 74(4): 372–6.

22. Scoggin CH, Hyers TM, Reeves JT, Grover RF. High-altitude pulmonary edema in the children and young adults of Leadville, Colorado. *N Engl J Med* 1977; 297(23): 1269–72.

23. Gaillard S, Dellasanta P, Loutan L, Kayser B. Awareness, prevalence, medication use, and risk factors of acute mountain sickness in tourists trekking around the Annapurnas in Nepal: a 12-year follow-up. *High Alt Med Biol* 2004; 5(4): 410–19.

24. Jean D, Leal C, Kriemler S, Meijer H, Moore LG. Medical recommendations for women going to altitude. *High Alt Med Biol* 2005; 6(1): 22–31.

25. Honigman B, Theis MK, Koziol-McLain J, et al. Acute mountain sickness in a general tourist population at moderate altitudes. *Ann Intern Med* 1993; 118(8): 587–92.

26. Hackett PH, Roach RC. High altitude cerebral edema. *High Alt Med Biol* 2004; 5(2): 136–46.

27. Naeije R, De Backer D, Vachiery JL, De Vuyst P. High-altitude pulmonary edema with primary pulmonary hypertension. *Chest* 1996; 110(1): 286–9.

28. Smith JM. The use of high altitude treatment for childhood asthma. *Practitioner* 1981; 225(1361): 1663–6.

29. Cogo A, Fischer R, Schoene R. Respiratory diseases and high altitude. *High Alt Med Biol* 2004; 5(4): 435–44.

30. Mader TH, White LJ. Refractive changes at extreme altitude after radial keratotomy. *Am J Ophthalmol* 1995; 119(6): 733–7.

31. White LJ, Mader TH. Refractive changes with increasing altitude after radial keratotomy. *Am J Ophthalmol* 1993; 115(6): 821–3.

32. Dimmig JW, Tabin G. The ascent of Mount Everest following laser in situ keratomileusis. *J Refract Surg* 2003; 19(1): 48–51.

33. Mader TH, Tabin G. Going to high altitude with preexisting ocular conditions. *High Alt Med Biol* 2003; 4(4): 419–30.

34. Kemmeren JM, Algra A, Grobbee DE. Third generation oral contraceptives and risk of venous thrombosis: meta-analysis. *BMJ* 2001; 323(7305): 131–4.

35. Roach RC, Maes D, Sandoval D, et al. Exercise exacerbates acute mountain sickness at simulated high altitude. *J Appl Physiol* 2000; 88(2): 581–5.

36. Reeves JT, Wagner J, Zafren K, Honigman B, Schoene RB. Seasonal variation in barometric pressure and temperature in Summit County: effect on altitude illness. In: Sutton JR, Houston CS, Coates G, eds. *Hypoxia and Molecular Medicine.* Burlington VT: Queen City Printers, 1993: 275–81.

37. Cumbo TA, Basnyat B, Graham J, Lescano AG, Gambert S. Acute mountain sickness, dehydration, and bicarbonate clearance: preliminary field data from the Nepal Himalaya. *Aviat Space Environ Med* 2002; 73(9): 898–901.

38. Murdoch DR. Symptoms of infection and altitude illness among hikers in the Mount Everest region of Nepal. *Aviat Space Environ Med* 1995; 66(2): 148–51.

39. Durmowicz AG, Noordeweir E, Nicholas R, Reeves JT. Inflammatory processes may predispose children to high-altitude pulmonary edema. *J Pediatr* 1997; 130(5): 838–40.

40. Hansen JE, Hartley LH, Hogan RP 3rd. Arterial oxygen increase by high-carbohydrate diet at altitude. *J Appl Physiol* 1972; 33(4): 441–5.

41. Hannon JP, Chinn KS, Shields JL. Effects of acute high-altitude exposure on body fluids. *Fed Proc* 1969; 28(3): 1178–84.

42. Dumont L, Mardirosoff C, Tramer MR. Efficacy and harm of pharmacological prevention of acute mountain sickness: quantitative systematic review. *BMJ* 2000; 321(7256): 267–72.

43. Gertsch JH, Basnyat B, Johnson EW, Onopa J, Holck PS. Randomised, double blind, placebo controlled comparison of ginkgo biloba and acetazolamide for prevention of acute mountain sickness among Himalayan trekkers: the prevention of high altitude illness trial (PHAIT). *BMJ* 2004; 328(7443): 797.

44. Basnyat B, Gertsch JH, Johnson EW, Castro-Marin F, Inoue Y, Yeh C. Efficacy of low-dose acetazolamide (125 mg bid) for the prophylaxis of acute mountain sickness: a prospective, double-blind, randomized, placebo-controlled trial. *High Alt Med Biol* 2003; 4(1): 45–52.

45. Carlsten C, Swenson ER, Ruoss S. A dose-response study of acetazolamide for acute mountain sickness prophylaxis in vacationing tourists at 12,000 feet (3630 m). *High Alt Med Biol* 2004; 5(1): 33–9.

46. Rock PB, Johnson TS, Larsen RF, Fulco CS, Trad LA, Cymerman A. Dexamethasone as prophylaxis for acute mountain sickness. Effect of dose level. *Chest* 1989; 95(3): 568–73.

47. Chow T, Browne V, Heileson HL, Wallace D, Anholm J, Green SM. Ginkgo biloba and acetazolamide prophylaxis for acute mountain sickness: a randomized, placebo-controlled trial. *Arch Intern Med* 2005; 165(3): 296–301.

48. Mittleman MA, Mintzer D, Maclure M, Tofler GH, Sherwood JB, Muller JE. Triggering of myocardial infarction by cocaine. *Circulation* 1999; 99(21): 2737–41.

49. Oelz O, Maggiorini M, Ritter M, et al. Prevention and treatment of high altitude pulmonary edema by a calcium channel blocker. *Int J Sports Med* 1992; 13 (suppl. 1): S65–S68.

50. Clarenbach CF, Christ AL, Senn O, et al. Dexamethasone and tadalafil prevent HAPE and subclinical alterations in lung function and nocturnal oxygenation associated with pulmonary interstitial fluid accumulation. *High Alt Med Biol* 2005; 5(4): 478.

51. Sartori C, Allemann Y, Duplain H, et al. Salmeterol for the prevention of high-altitude pulmonary edema. *N Engl J Med* 2002; 346(21): 1631–6.

52. Weil JV. Sleep at high altitude. *High Alt Med Biol* 2004; 5(2): 180–9.

53. Sutton JR, Houston CS, Mansell AL, et al. Effect of acetazolamide on hypoxemia during sleep at high altitude. *N Engl J Med* 1979; 301(24): 1329–31.

54. Dubowitz G. Effect of temazepam on oxygen saturation and sleep quality at high altitude: randomised placebo controlled crossover trial. *BMJ* 1998; 316(7131): 587–9.

55. Leverment J, Nickol A, Richards P, et al. Effect of temazepam on subjective measures (sleep quality and acute mountain sickness score, AMS) at high altitude. *High Alt Med Biol* 2005; 5(4): 492.

56. Nickol A, Richards P, Seal P, et al. Effect of temazepam on objective measures (sleep disordered breathing and next day performance) at high altitude. *High Alt Med Biol* 2005; 5(4): 496.

57. Weston AR, Mackenzie G, Tufts MA, Mars M. Optimal time of arrival for performance at moderate altitude (1700 m). *Med Sci Sports Exerc* 2001; 33(2): 298–302.

Exercise Prescription for Health

WITH PEKKA KANNUS AND TERESA LIU-AMBROSE

Even though the benefits of exercise are widely known, the great majority of the developed world remains sedentary. In the United States, one in four individuals reported doing no leisure time physical activity.[1] In Great Britain, one in six are physically inactive.[2] A great number of chronic conditions are associated with physical inactivity and a review entitled 'Waging war on modern chronic diseases: primary prevention through exercise biology' argues cogently that almost 30% of annual deaths would be preventable with a primary prevention approach through physical activity.[3]

We feel that the sports clinician is ideally placed to wage the war on physical inactivity for several reasons. Firstly, all the members of the sports medicine team (Chapter 1) are aware that physical inactivity is the enemy and most have already adopted a healthy lifestyle. Secondly, sports clinicians, be they primary care physicians, physiotherapists or massage therapists, work with the inactive as well as the active and, thus, are well placed to influence many people to take additional exercise if it is needed.

Thirdly, sports medicine practitioners have an expertise in musculoskeletal medicine and familiarity with exercise that is an advantage when prescribing exercise. For example, a sports physician or physiotherapist may assess a patient with osteoporosis and back pain and realize that the pain is coming from a hypomobile facet joint. There is no contraindication to exercise prescription—merely a need for treatment (Chapters 10, 21). A physician less familiar with musculoskeletal medicine may have thought that the pain was directly related to osteoporosis or its complications and, thus, proscribed exercise.

The aim of this chapter is to refresh those unfamiliar with exercise prescription with the basic concepts

so that they may feel more confident in counseling a patient appropriately. Many medical practitioners are not confident about their ability to prescribe exercise for patients.[4] We outline the approach to pre-exercise assessment and then detail aerobic and resistance exercise prescription. We illustrate standard resistance exercises so that they can be photocopied for patients' benefit. We discuss exercise prescription for the elderly patient as this large segment of our population can benefit enormously from exercise prescription. Finally, we illustrate how to prescribe exercise for four common afflictions: hypertension, cardiac event, osteoarthritis and osteoporosis.

Pre-exercise evaluation

Before prescribing exercise, the practitioner must take a history and perform a physical examination just as he or she would when prescribing medication. To extend the analogy, the clinical assessment may indicate that special tests are needed before therapy (in this case an exercise program) can begin.

Establish lifestyle goals

A good place to start the history is by asking the patient to outline his or her goal(s) related to the exercise program. Be clear as to whether the aim is to prevent risk of a disease, slow progression of complications of a disease or improve quality of life that has been compromised by a chronic disease. The aim will influence the exercise prescription itself and how progress is to be measured.

The history should include a thorough medical review to seek any possible contraindications to exercise. Screening programs such as the Physical Activity

Readiness Questionnaire (PAR-Q)[5] help the exercise specialist who does not feel medically qualified to assess the patient. The healthcare practitioner will seek to identify any abnormalities in the cardiovascular, pulmonary, musculoskeletal, metabolic or endocrine systems that should prevent physical activity. Previous and current physical activity levels are reviewed, as is the use of medications, alcohol and cigarettes. Cholesterol screening should be undertaken where indicated. Patients taking diuretics should have potassium levels checked. As discussed in Chapter 45, whether or not an exercise stress test with ECG/ EKG is indicated remains a controversial issue and the reader is directed to two excellent monographs on this subject.[6, 7]

Discuss activity preferences and interests

To be successful, an exercise program must be tailored to the patient's interests. Thus, the practitioner needs to ask about sporting and activity preferences and profile. A lifestyle questionnaire (Fig. 55.1) can aid in developing a program that is both individually appropriate and interesting.

Lifestyle questionnaire

Name of participant: **Date:**

1. Indicate the physical activities that you participated in over the last month during your leisure time.

	Frequency	Duration (minutes)				Intensity		
	Number of occasions over the last month	1–15	15–30	31–60	60+	Light	Medium	Heavy
		Average number of activity minutes spent on each occasion				*Slight change from normal state*	*Some perspiration, faster than normal breathing*	*Heavy perspiration, heavy breathing*
Walking for exercise	_____	❏	❏	❏	❏	❏	❏	❏
Bicycling	_____	❏	❏	❏	❏	❏	❏	❏
Swimming	_____	❏	❏	❏	❏	❏	❏	❏
Jogging/running	_____	❏	❏	❏	❏	❏	❏	❏
Home exercises	_____	❏	❏	❏	❏	❏	❏	❏
(Ice) skating	_____	❏	❏	❏	❏	❏	❏	❏
Cross-country skiing	_____	❏	❏	❏	❏	❏	❏	❏
Tennis	_____	❏	❏	❏	❏	❏	❏	❏
Golf	_____	❏	❏	❏	❏	❏	❏	❏
Popular dance	_____	❏	❏	❏	❏	❏	❏	❏
Baseball/softball	_____	❏	❏	❏	❏	❏	❏	❏
Alpine skiing	_____	❏	❏	❏	❏	❏	❏	❏
Ice hockey	_____	❏	❏	❏	❏	❏	❏	❏
Bowling	_____	❏	❏	❏	❏	❏	❏	❏
Exercise classes	_____	❏	❏	❏	❏	❏	❏	❏
Racquetball	_____	❏	❏	❏	❏	❏	❏	❏
Curling	_____	❏	❏	❏	❏	❏	❏	❏
Others: please specify								
_____	_____	❏	❏	❏	❏	❏	❏	❏
_____	_____	❏	❏	❏	❏	❏	❏	❏
_____	_____	❏	❏	❏	❏	❏	❏	❏

Figure 55.1 Lifestyle questionnaire

2. How long have you been doing some physical activity in your leisure time at least once a week?
   - ❏ I don't do an activity each week
   - ❏ For less than 3 months
   - ❏ From 3 months to just under 6 months
   - ❏ For more than 6 months

3. If you want to participate more in physical activities than you do now, why aren't you able to? (Check at most three reasons.)
   - ❏ I don't want to participate more
   - ❏ Ill health
   - ❏ Injury or handicap
   - ❏ Lack of energy
   - ❏ Lack of time because of work/school
   - ❏ Lack of time because of other leisure activities
   - ❏ Costs too much
   - ❏ No facilities nearby
   - ❏ Inadequate facilities
   - ❏ No leaders available
   - ❏ Requires too much self-discipline
   - ❏ Lack necessary skills
   - ❏ Other _____

4. If you wanted to participate more in physical activities, which of the following would increase the amount of physical activity you do? (Check at most three.)
   - ❏ Nothing
   - ❏ Better or closer facilities
   - ❏ Different facilities
   - ❏ Less expensive facilities
   - ❏ More information on the benefits
   - ❏ Organized fitness classes available
   - ❏ Employer- or union-sponsored activities available
   - ❏ Organized sports available
   - ❏ Organized fitness classes available
   - ❏ Fitness test with personal activity program available
   - ❏ People with whom to participate
   - ❏ Common interest of family
   - ❏ Having necessary equipment
   - ❏ Common interest of friends
   - ❏ More leisure time
   - ❏ More energy
   - ❏ More self-discipline
   - ❏ Better health

5. Here is a list of reasons why some people do physical activities during their leisure time. How important is each of these to *you*?

	Very important	Of some importance	Of little importance	Of no importance
To feel better mentally and physically	❏	❏	❏	❏
To be with other people	❏	❏	❏	❏
For pleasure, fun or excitement	❏	❏	❏	❏
To control weight or to look better	❏	❏	❏	❏
To move better or to improve flexibility	❏	❏	❏	❏
As a challenge to my abilities	❏	❏	❏	❏
To relax or reduce stress	❏	❏	❏	❏
To learn new things	❏	❏	❏	❏
Because of advice to improve general health	❏	❏	❏	❏
Because of physician's order for therapy or rehabilitation	❏	❏	❏	❏
Other _____	❏	❏	❏	❏

6. How important is each of the following to you in gaining a feeling of wellbeing?

	Very important	Of some importance	Of little importance	Of no importance
Adequate rest and sleep	❏	❏	❏	❏
A good diet	❏	❏	❏	❏
Low calorie snacks between meals	❏	❏	❏	❏
Maintenance of proper weight	❏	❏	❏	❏
Participation in social and cultural activities	❏	❏	❏	❏
Control of stress	❏	❏	❏	❏
Regular exercise, sports or games	❏	❏	❏	❏
Being a non-smoker	❏	❏	❏	❏
Adequate medical and dental care	❏	❏	❏	❏
Positive thinking/meditation	❏	❏	❏	❏

7. Comparing yourself to others of your own age and sex, would you say you are:
   ❑ more fit?　　　　　　　　❑ less fit?　　　　　　　　❑ as fit?

8. In the past year, what physical activities have you stopped doing? (Do not include those stopped due to a change in the season.)
   ❑ None or list activity/ies

   _____

   Why did you stop doing this activity?

   _____

   _____

   Why did you stop doing this activity?

   _____

9. What physical activities would you like to start in order to improve your fitness and health?
   ❑ None or list activity/ies

   _____

   What is the main reason you have not yet started this?

   _____

   _____

   What is the main reason you have not yet started this?

   _____

   _____

   What is the main reason you have not yet started this?

   _____

10. With whom do you/would you *usually* do your physical activities in your leisure time?
    ❑ No-one　　　　　　　　　❑ Friends　　　　　　　　❑ Immediate family or relatives
    ❑ Co-workers　　　　　　　❑ Classmates at school　　❑ Others

11. At what time do you/would you usually do your physical activities? (Indicate more than one if you usually do activities *more* than once a day.)
    ❑ In the morning　　　　　❑ At lunchtime　　　　　　❑ Immediately after work
    ❑ In the evening　　　　　❑ In the afternoon　　　　❑ At no special time

12. (a) How would you describe your state of emotional wellbeing?
    ❑ Very good　　　　　　　❑ Adequate　　　　　　　❑ Poor
    ❑ Good　　　　　　　　　❑ Very poor
    (b) How do you think this might affect your physical activity/fitness goals?
    ❑ Aid　　　　　　　　　❑ Hinder　　　　　　　　❑ No effect
    Please explain: _____

13. What do you *usually* eat for breakfast? (Usually means at least four days a week.) Check all that apply.
    ❑ I don't eat breakfast　　❑ Bread, danish or donut　❑ Fruit or fruit juice　　❑ Yoghurt
    ❑ Eggs　　　　　　　　　❑ Granola　　　　　　　❑ At least 170 mL milk　❑ Tea/coffee
    ❑ Bacon or other meat,　　❑ Other cereals　　　　❑ Cheese
       fish or poultry

14. In the last year, have you been eating:

	More	Less	Same as before
Sweet food and candies?	❑ More	❑ Less	❑ Same as before
Fruit and vegetables?	❑ More	❑ Less	❑ Same as before
Fats and fried foods?	❑ More	❑ Less	❑ Same as before
Salt and salty foods?	❑ More	❑ Less	❑ Same as before
Meals on a regular basis?	❑ More	❑ Less	❑ Same as before
The same amount of food or calories?	❑ No, more	❑ No, less	❑ Yes, same as before

15. (a) About how many hours of sleep do you *usually* get each day?
   - ❏ Six hours or less
   - ❏ Seven
   - ❏ Eight
   - ❏ Nine
   - ❏ Ten
   - ❏ Eleven hours or more

   (b) Do you think you are getting enough sleep?
   - ❏ Always
   - ❏ Usually
   - ❏ Seldom
   - ❏ Never

16. (a) About how often do you *usually* drink alcohol?
   - ❏ More than once a day
   - ❏ 4–7 times a week
   - ❏ 1–3 times a week
   - ❏ 1–3 times a month
   - ❏ Less than once a month
   - ❏ I don't drink alcohol—go to question 17

   (b) About how many drinks do you usually have at a time?
   Where one drink is:
   - one pint of beer (350 mL)
   - one small glass of wine
   - one shot of liquor/spirits (i.e. 30–45 mL with/without mix)
   - ❏ 1
   - ❏ 2–3
   - ❏ 4–5
   - ❏ 6–7
   - ❏ 8+

17. Which of the following best describes your experience with tobacco? Check all that apply.
   - ❏ I haven't smoked
   - ❏ I currently smoke
     - ❏ cigarettes occasionally
     - ❏ less than ½ pack of cigarettes daily
     - ❏ about a pack of cigarettes daily
     - ❏ two or more packs of cigarettes daily
     - ❏ a pipe, cigar or cigarillo occasionally
     - ❏ a pipe, cigars or cigarillos daily
   - ❏ I stopped smoking
     - ❏ cigarettes recently
     - ❏ cigarettes over a year ago
     - ❏ a pipe, cigars or cigarillos recently
     - ❏ a pipe, cigars or cigarillos over a year ago

18. In general, how would you describe your state of health?
   - ❏ Very good
   - ❏ Poor
   - ❏ Good
   - ❏ Very poor
   - ❏ Average

Physical examination

A complete physical examination includes examination of the neuromuscular system, cardiovascular system and respiratory function. In preparation for physical activity the sports medicine practitioner is ideally trained to assess the biomechanical competence of the spine and the musculoskeletal system in order to prevent musculoskeletal injury associated with activity, and to understand the physiological changes of exercise in patients of all ages (Chapter 6).

Management

It is important at this stage to match the participant's goals with their preferences and abilities. Figure 55.2 is an assessment form for this purpose. If the match between these three elements is an uneasy one, the practitioner must refocus participants on each element and inform them of the benefits and limitations of their choices. The practitioner must discover what facilities and programs are available to the individual, both in the home and in the local community (e.g.

a heated pool may be easily accessible). The action plan worksheet (Fig. 55.3) can assist with the program planning stage. It includes reasonable lifestyle changes and achievable short-term goals. These are both keys to the success of any program.

Contingency plans and follow-up

As in any clinical interaction, it is important to identify personal barriers to achieving the goals set up in the action plan and to have a contingency plan if blocks are encountered. For example, if the participant chooses a combined land and water exercise program, ask them if they have a swimsuit and whether a pool is accessible by bus. Have an alternative plan available should the program be offered on days or at times that are inconvenient. In addition, it is important to ask about social and financial barriers that are often not addressed, for example, the older adult who is responsible for grandchildren thus has very little time to participate. Also, factors such as body image and self-efficacy issues are barriers to physical activity that are less often acknowledged.[8, 9]

Inventory of Lifestyle Needs and Activity Preferences

Lifestyle needs

I feel it is important to me to:
- ❏ like the people I'm with
- ❏ be in a group
- ❏ be independent
- ❏ get to know other people
- ❏ have the other people like me
- ❏ be physically active
- ❏ use my imagination
- ❏ create something
- ❏ find the activity challenging
- ❏ feel safe and secure
- ❏ try something new and different
- ❏ be myself
- ❏ use my talents
- ❏ improve myself and my skills
- ❏ accomplish something
- ❏ relax
- ❏ spend time with my family

- ❏ release energy
- ❏ have common interests with other people
- ❏ be able to contribute something to a group
- ❏ meet many new people
- ❏ be a leader
- ❏ feel confident
- ❏ learn something
- ❏ be in pleasant, attractive surroundings
- ❏ be alone
- ❏ have a structured activity
- ❏ be able to do things at the last minute
- ❏ follow rules
- ❏ be praised
- ❏ have fun and enjoy myself
- ❏ release frustration
- ❏ take a risk

Instructions: Once you have checked the lifestyle needs that are important to you, list the three most important and identify which activities would most probably satisfy those needs.

Lifestyle needs	Activity preferences
1. _____	_____
	_____
	_____
	_____
2. _____	_____
	_____
	_____
	_____
3. _____	_____
	_____
	_____
	_____

Figure 55.2 Assessment form for exercise prescription

Patients should be followed up regularly just as they would if they were being treated with medication. Asking patients about progress and documenting the response will provide them with a positive stimulus. The practitioner can have a substantial influence on the patient's behavior and, thus, should praise improvements liberally. Exercise goals should be examined periodically and adjusted according to progress. Nothing adds to boredom more quickly than performing the same program repetitively. Any pain or discomfort should be noted and treated appropriately, as discussed in Chapters 6 and 10.

Other tips

Encourage participants to involve family or friends in their program goals. Even a casual question from friends such as 'How is your activity program coming along?' may provide the impetus needed to maintain compliance.

Suggest to your patients/clients that they use a 'buddy system' if possible. Also, direct them to a program where strong social support can be established, as studies suggest adherence is improved with group participation.

Action Plan Worksheet   Name: _____   Date: _____

Goals and action steps: **Time frame:**

Goal #1 _____   _____

Action steps

1. _____   _____
2. _____   _____
3. _____   _____

Goal #2 _____   _____

Action steps

1. _____   _____
2. _____   _____
3. _____   _____

Goal #3 _____   _____

Action steps

1. _____   _____
2. _____   _____
3. _____   _____

Prescription for physical activity

Frequency	
Intensity	
Time	
Type	

Comments:		

Success indicators

1. _____
2. _____
3. _____
4. _____
5. _____

Date for next appraisal: _____

Figure 55.3 The action plan worksheet

Components of exercise prescription

In this section we review the components of an exercise program and outline prescription for the healthy adult. This provides a menu to help the practitioner prescribe exercise for patients.

Aerobic activities: endurance training

Aerobic activities improve the capacity of individuals to exercise for long periods. They are generally considered of benefit to the cardiorespiratory system, but multiple systems (e.g. brain, joints) can benefit from aerobic training. Dynamic exercises that use large muscle groups for long duration include walking, jogging, running, swimming, bicycling, cross-country skiing and aerobic dance. Exercises that use the arms as well as the legs include some forms of stationary cycles with movable handlebars, cross-country ski simulators and rowing machines. Low-impact activities such as stationary cycling are ideal for individuals with conditions such as arthritis or poor balance, which may put them at an increased risk of musculoskeletal injury. Swimming is suitable for some people but can aggravate shoulder osteoarthritis if the freestyle stroke is used and knee osteoarthritis with vigorous breast-stroke kicking. A program that provides endurance training while performing some resistance exercise is circuit training. Participants undertake short periods of exercise at a number of stations arranged in a circuit. The continuous nature and high number of repetitions characteristic of this form of exercise may improve both endurance and muscular strength.

Aerobic exercise intensity is measured by heart rate or by rating of perceived exertion. The training rate is 70–85% of maximum heart rate, which can be measured in a maximal test or estimated by subtracting the individual's age from 220. Borg's perceived exertion scale is also a useful way of monitoring intensity.[10] There has been a shift from prescribing vigorous exercise several times a week to prescribing moderate activity daily. The US Surgeon-General's report recommends a total of 30 minutes of moderate activity, such as walking, sweeping or doing housework, daily. Swedish exercise physiologist, Per Åstrand, who can still ride to work aged over 80 years, calculated that 60 minutes per day is required in today's sedentary society.[11]

Resistance training

In addition to its role in increasing muscle bulk and strength, resistance training provides multisystem benefits such as to prevent diabetes, reduce the risk of cardiovascular disease and improve brain function. Resistance training is an integral part of any comprehensive health program and it is vigorously promoted by the American College of Sports Medicine, American Heart Association and the US Surgeon-General's office. Some practitioners are uncomfortable in prescribing resistance training because of a personal unfamiliarity with the subject.[4] Exercise guidance, if there is any at all, consists of 'walk for half an hour a day'. However, the guidelines for resistance exercise prescription are easy to follow.

Current research recommends that healthy persons of all ages and many patients with chronic diseases perform single-set resistance exercise programs of up to 15 repetitions on a minimum of two days per week.[12] Each work-out session should consist of eight to 10 different exercises that train the major muscle groups. Examples are illustrated in Figure 55.4. The prescription should include at least one exercise from each of the six columns in Table 55.1. Single set programs are less time-consuming and should therefore aid with program adherence. They also provide virtually all of the health benefits of multiple set programs.[13] The goal of this type of program is to gain a significant amount of muscle mass, endurance and strength to contribute to overall fitness and health. Patients with chronic diseases (e.g. arthritis) may have to limit range of motion for some exercises and use lighter weights with more repetitions. Patients who have osteoarthritis, or limited range of motion due to previous injury, should perform the activity slowly and give equal time to both the up and down phase of a repetition.

Exercise prescription for the older individual

Older people vary widely in their exercise capacity, so we provide advice for the rather inactive and the generally active person.

Inactive

For older adults who are sedentary, the first goal of exercise prescription is simply to reduce the time spent sitting. Thus, the action plan might be to reduce the amount of time spent watching television. Other suggestions include parking further away at malls and shopping centers, taking the stairs instead of the elevator, or taking a brief walk several times a day. Use the information from the health assessment and lifestyle sheets (Figs 55.1, 55.2) to incorporate the

Table 55.1 Resistance exercises classified by body region

Chest and shoulder region	Upper and lower back	Abdominal region	Arm region	Hip and thigh region	Leg region
Bench press (Fig. 55.4a)	Back extension (Fig. 55.4e)	Bent knee curl-up (Fig. 55.4h)	Arm curl (Fig. 55.4j)	Leg curl (Fig. 55.4l)	Toe (heel) raise (Fig. 55.4p)
Shoulder shrugs (Fig. 55.4b)	Latissimus pull-down (Fig. 55.4f)	Reverse sit-up (Fig. 55.4i)	Triceps pull-down (Fig. 55.4k)	Seated leg press (Fig. 55.4m)	
Seated (overhead) press (Fig. 55.4c)	Bent-over row (Fig. 55.4g)			Half-squat (Fig. 55.4n)	
Upright row (Fig. 55.4d)				Side leg raises (Fig. 55.4o)	

individual's favorite activities. Remember that the aphorism 'start low, go slow' applies in this population as it does in exercise prescription in general. The practitioner should set easily attainable short-term goals and increase the time spent performing moderate activities by no more than 5% per week. The eventual goal is to accumulate 30 minutes a day of moderately intense physical activity on most days of the week.

Generally active

For older people who are generally active, begin by increasing the volume of aerobic exercise or resistance training. Aerobic exercises that are particularly attractive to older individuals are cycling on a stationary bicycle, brisk walking, swimming and water aquatics. The person should warm up (e.g. slow walking) for 5 minutes and stretch slowly for 5–10 minutes before

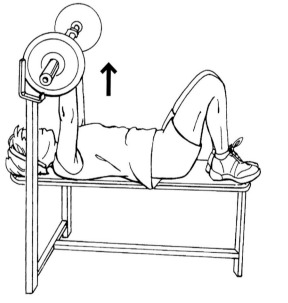
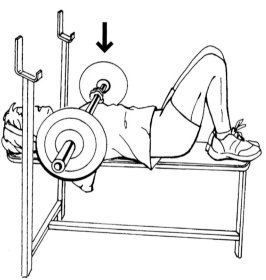

Figure 55.4 Examples of resistance exercises

(a) Bench press

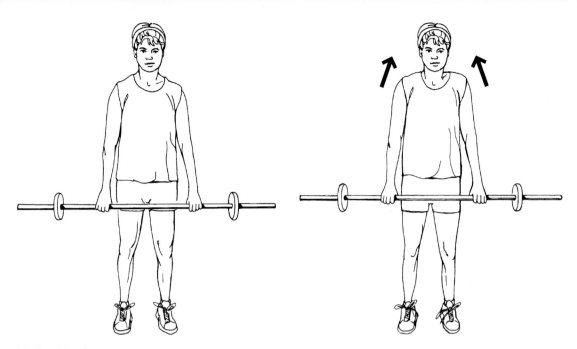

(b) Shoulder shrugs

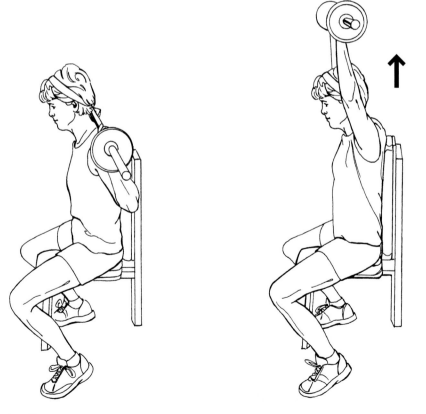

(c) Seated (overhead) press

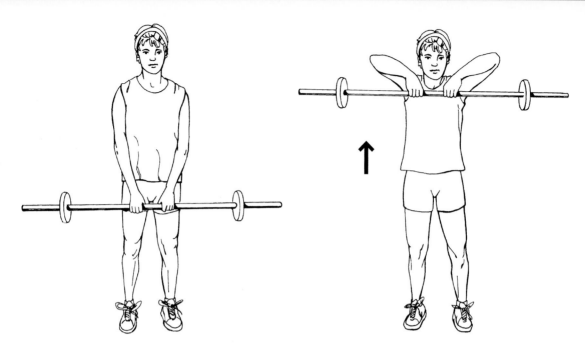

(d) Upright row

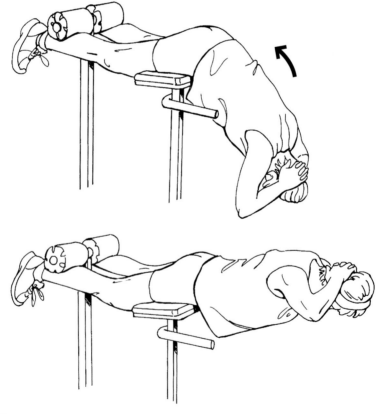

(e) Back extension

exercising at a moderate level—one at which a conversation can be easily maintained. The cool-down after the exercise session should be by walking slowly and stretching for 10–15 minutes.

The person about to undertake resistance training should also perform a warm-up and stretch first. Free weights and commercially available equipment are both suitable for the older person exercising. Proper breathing consists of exhaling during the lift for 2–4 seconds followed by inhaling during the lowering of the weight for 4–6 seconds, working through the entire range of motion (or as tolerated for those with arthritis). The Valsalva maneuver should be avoided, particularly in the elderly who are more prone to postural hypotension and syncope than their younger counterparts. The lifts should be separated by 2 seconds of rest. The goal is to perform one or two sets of eight to 15 repetitions per set with 1–2 minutes of rest between sets. The patient should aim to lift a weight that is 70–80% of a one repetition maximum. One repetition maximum refers to the most he or she can lift through a full range of motion at one time. The resistance should be increased no more frequently than monthly. Strength exercises should be followed by a cool-down and a stretch. The principles

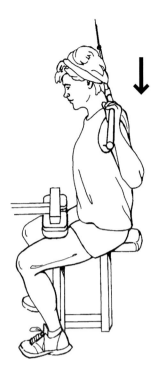

(f) Latissimus pull-down

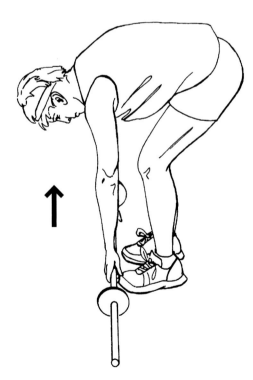
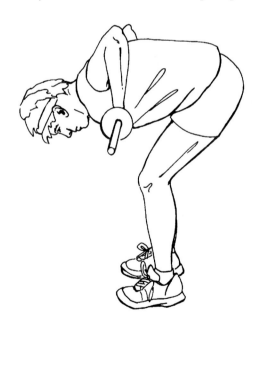

(g) Bent-over row

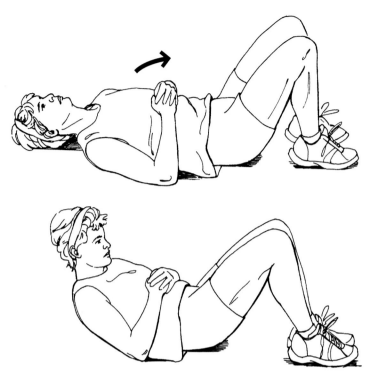

(h) Bent knee curl-up

of follow-up and praise for progress as outlined in the general introduction to exercise prescription apply particularly to seniors, who may feel less confident about their capacity for activity.

Exercise prescription for the patient with hypertension

The general guidelines for exercise prescription, as outlined above, should be followed. Pre-exercise evaluation should be used to identify other risk factors and detect concurrent disease. In many centers, an exercise stress test (Chapter 45) is advised if two risk factors (e.g. male gender, diabetes mellitus, hypercholesterolemia, family history of early coronary artery disease, smoking) are present in an asymptomatic hypertensive individual. This provides an opportunity to measure submaximal and maximal blood pressure responses and exercise capacity. Patients with a systolic blood pressure over 180 mmHg or diastolic pressure above 105 mmHg should have drug therapy initiated before an exercise program proceeds.

Training intensity does not need to be high in the patient with hypertension—it should be maintained within 65–70% of maximum heart rate as measured by the exercise test or from the calculated formula (220 – age). The initial conditioning period should last for 12–16 weeks and then, if blood pressure is adequately controlled, antihypertensive medication can be gradually reduced while the patient is closely observed for rebound hypertension and evidence of myocardial ischemia. This would require biweekly follow-ups.

Resistance training for the cardiac patient

Endurance exercise is promoted as part of cardiac rehabilitation programs and an Australian expert working group, extending the 1996 US Surgeon-General's report on physical activity and health, recommended that:[14]

- people with established clinically stable cardiovascular disease should aim, over time, to achieve 30 minutes or more of moderate intensity physical activity on most, if not all, days of the week
- less intense and even shorter bouts of activity with more rest periods may suffice for those with advanced cardiovascular disease

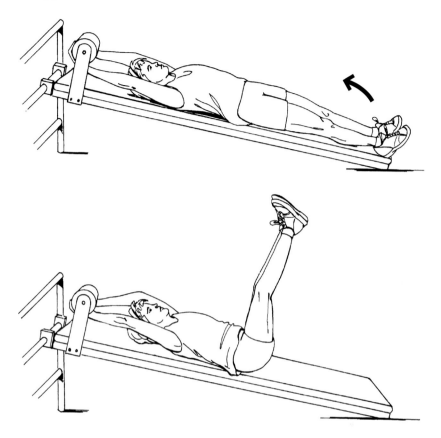

(i) Reverse sit-up

- regular low-to-moderate level resistance activity, initially under the supervision of an exercise professional, is encouraged.

The benefits from regular moderate physical activity for people with cardiovascular disease include augmented physiological functioning, lessening of cardiovascular symptoms, enhanced quality of life, improved coronary risk profile, superior muscle fitness and, for survivors of acute myocardial infarction, lower mortality. The greatest potential for benefit is in those people who were least active before beginning regular physical activity, and this benefit may be achieved even at relatively low levels of physical activity. Medical practitioners should routinely provide brief, appropriate advice on physical activity to people with well-compensated, clinically stable cardiovascular disease.[14]

We alert the reader to the trend towards including resistance training together with endurance activities in this population. Pre-existing guidelines for resistance exercise in cardiac rehabilitation were considered vague and/or overly restrictive, limiting the ability of cardiac rehabilitation programs to help patients achieve their desired levels of daily activity in a timely manner after cardiac events.[15] Like healthy adults, patients who have suffered myocardial infarction need a minimum level of muscular strength to perform activities of daily living but they often lack the confidence or physical strength necessary. The importance of resistance training is increasingly being recognized and the sports medicine practitioner may be asked to provide expertise in prescribing a resistance exercise program for the cardiac patient.

Updated resistance training guidelines for cardiac patients[16] are similar to those for healthy adults. The primary differences are the reduced intensity and slower progression of the training volume for the cardiac patients together with the increased patient monitoring and program supervision.[12] Lighter weights should be used for 10–15 repetitions. Low-risk patients (>7 metabolic equivalent capacity measured by cardiac stress test) can be cleared for heavy resistance training that involves 12–15 repetitions

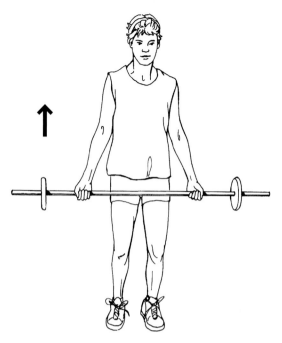
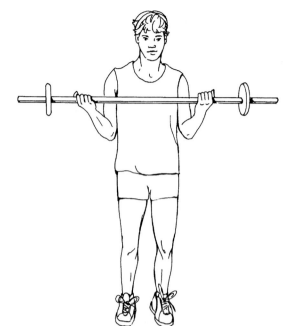

(j) Arm curl

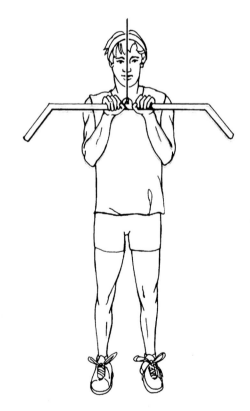
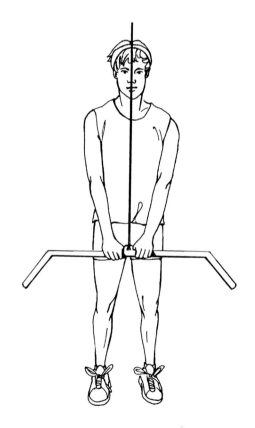

(k) Triceps pull-down

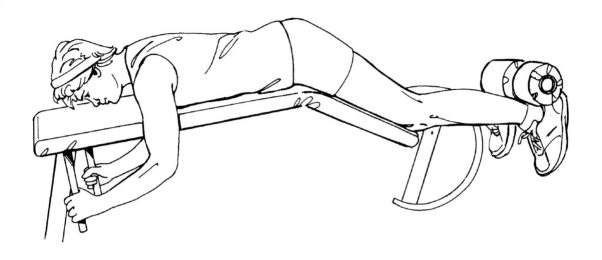

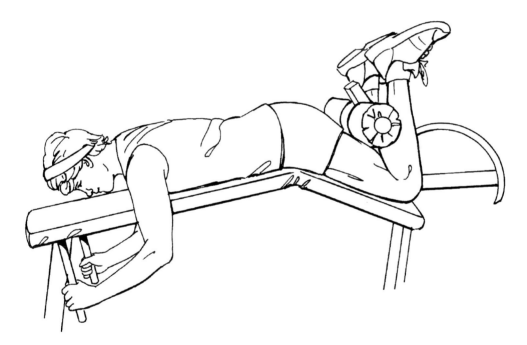

(l) Leg curl

to fatigue. More high-risk patients should keep their fatigue to a moderate level. Given that beta-blockers can alter the normal hemodynamic response to exercise, patients should monitor their level of exertion, and there is increasing use of Borg's rating of perceived exertion (RPE) scale[17] to monitor the patient's level of exertion when training.[16] An RPE range of 11–15 is frequently used in cardiac rehabilitation settings to prescribe dynamic exercise (such as walking on a treadmill) intensity.

Exercise prescription in patients with osteoarthritis

Osteoarthritis of both the knee and the hip are important non-fatal conditions that cause pain and

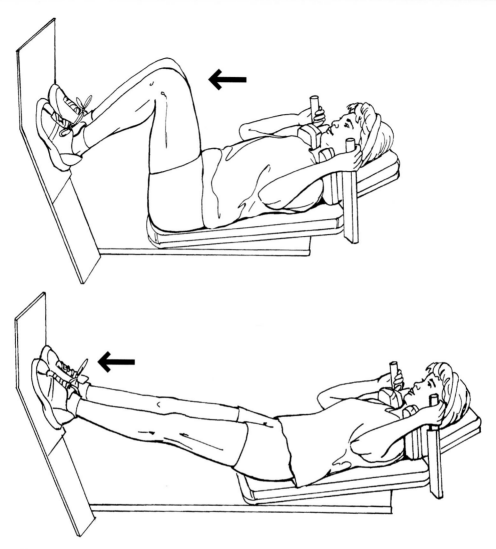

(m) Seated leg press

limit activity in older people. There are no cures or disease-modifying agents for osteoarthritis and, thus, the goal of treatment is to reduce pain and disability and improve quality of life.[18] The American College of Rheumatology has published guidelines for the treatment of knee osteoarthritis that suggest that exercise is an important part of therapy. Exercise programs provided modest improvements in measures of disability, physical performance and pain in the knee[18–20] and the hip.[19] Unfortunately, there are insufficient data to outline the optimal protocol. Both resistance and exercise programs have proven helpful, as was a mixture of several types of therapy.[20]

One successful exercise protocol consisted of a three-month facility-based walking program and then a 15-month home-based walking program. The facility-based program consisted of 12–15 participants meeting with an exercise instructor three times per week and walking on an indoor track. For the home program, which was also prescribed thrice weekly, most participants walked on pavement along streets or in nearby parks. The exercise leader contacted subjects regularly. Each aerobic session consisted of 10 minutes for each of warm-up and warm-down that bracketed a 40-minute walk at between 50% and 70% of their heart rate reserve as determined by a screening exercise test.

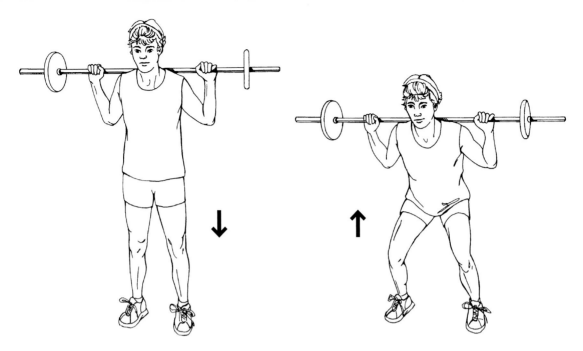

(n) Half squat

The resistance training was arranged along parallel lines to the aerobic exercise training with respect to the distribution of time spent at the facility and time spent on a home program and attention given to warm-up and warm-down. The 40-minute resistance training program consisted of two sets of 12 repetitions of nine exercises: leg extension, leg curl (Fig. 55.4l), step-up, heel raise (Fig. 55.4p), chest fly, upright row (Fig. 55.4d), seated press (Fig. 55.4c), arm curl (Fig. 55.4j) and a pelvic tilt exercise. Weight was begun at the lowest possible level (about 1 kg [2.2 lb]) and increased in a stepwise fashion as long as the participant could complete two sets of 10 repetitions. Once a plateau was reached, weight was increased after patients successfully completed two sets of 12 repetitions for three consecutive days. Although much more research is needed to test the various modalities of exercise for osteoarthritis of these joints,[21] this protocol provides a basis from which practitioners can prescribe exercise.

Exercise prescription in patients with osteoporosis

Most types of activity programs are preferable to a sedentary lifestyle for patients with osteoporosis and should be encouraged. Exercise sessions should begin with a 20-minute warm-up, comprising 10 minutes of gentle stretching and range of motion activity followed by 10 minutes of aerobic exercises. For cardiovascular exercises, targeted heart rate should be 60% of maximum heart rate (220 – age) for a beginner or a deconditioned woman and 70–75% for those in more intermediate health. Weight training with light free weights and rubber tubing can then be incorporated. As per standard resistance training, the exercises should target the major muscle groups. Effective upper arm exercises include pushing against a wall or pulling and twisting against a partner.[22] Quadriceps strength can be improved with a wall slide (squat) exercise or by practicing standing from a seated position. Trunk stabilization (i.e. core stability) exercises are often introduced in the crook lying position and progressed to sitting and standing. Trunk stabilization exercises target the recruitment of transversus abdominis and the internal and external obliques rather than rectus abdominis. Due to the propensity to develop a kyphotic posture with osteoporosis, back posture correction exercises should also be emphasized and can be done standing, in a chair or prone.

Balance exercises can be introduced initially by having individuals hold a tandem stance for 10 seconds with their eyes open while holding onto the kitchen counter for support. Other balance exercises include single leg stance with eyes open (then eyes

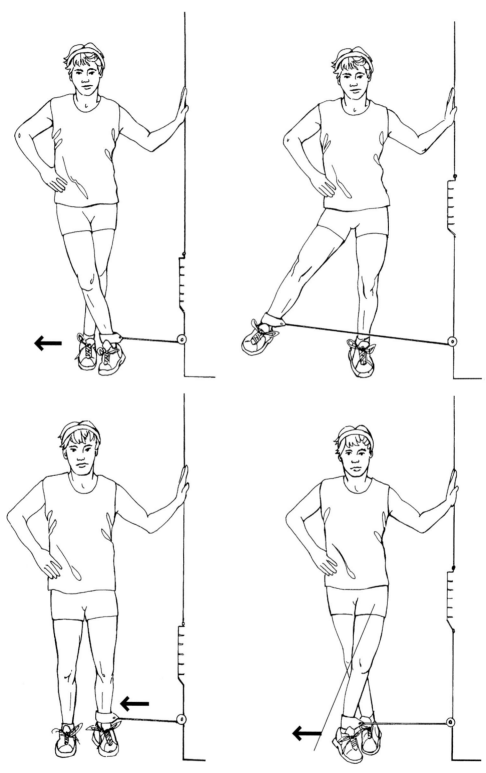

(o) Side leg raises

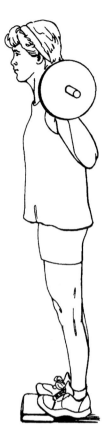 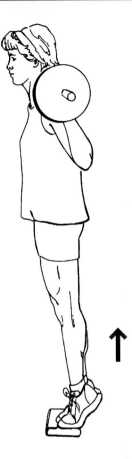

(p) Toe (heel) raise

closed), tandem forward walking, walking backwards, and tandem backwards walking.

The exercise program should conclude with a 15-minute cool-down period and warm-down stretches can be done sitting on the floor.

Remember also that the assessment for exercise prescription should allow the practitioner to discover what activities the client values. Many popular activities require some degree of strength, flexibility, endurance, balance and coordination. For example, a good line dancing class emphasizes posture and the attributes listed, is fun, and does not require a partner.

Community-based exercise program for osteoporosis

'Osteofit' is an exercise-based program devised by staff of the British Columbia Women's Health Center Osteoporosis Program in Vancouver, Canada. This community-based program for women and men aims to reduce participants' risk of falling and improve their functional ability and thereby enhance their quality of life. It differs from typical seniors' exercise classes by specifically targeting posture, balance, gait, coordination, and trunk and pelvic stabilization rather than general aerobic fitness.

A typical class consists of a warm-up, the work-out and a relaxation component, which are outlined below. 'Osteofit' classes also include 'Osteofit tips', a 5-minute health education topic that the instructor shares with participants.

The work-out itself consists of strengthening and stretching exercises intended to improve posture by combating medially rotated shoulders, chin protrusion (excessive cervical extension), thoracic kyphosis and loss of lumbar lordosis. Exercises to improve balance and coordination may progress from heel raises and toe pulls to the mildly challenging two-legged heel–toe rock and the more challenging tandem walks and obstacle courses. Pelvic stabilization is trained using leg exercises (e.g. hip abduction and extension) or balance exercises. After appropriate training and progression through less challenging positions, trunk stabilization is addressed when the participant is cued and positioned to do all standing exercises with resistance for the arms (e.g. biceps curls) and shoulders (e.g. lateral arm raises). The abdominal muscles are strengthened in their function as stabilizers rather than as prime movers. Exercises to improve functional ability include chair squats and getting up and down off the floor.

Upper and lower body activities are alternated to reduce the risk of tendinopathy. If the class includes more than one set of an exercise, the sets are separated by a short rest period. Repetitions are kept to between eight and 16 and weights are relatively light so that participants do not work to fatigue with each set. The exercises are arranged so that the less strenuous exercises, such as hamstring stretching, are at the end of the work-out. The last few minutes of the class are devoted to relaxation techniques such as deep breathing, progressive muscle tensing and relaxing, and visualizations to a background of soft music and/or nature sounds. 'Osteofit' is one form of safe and effective exercise for a population that is at high risk of osteoporotic fracture.[23, 24]

Exercise prescription in practise: a case study

We provide a case report of a 75-year-old woman with osteoporosis who participated in a six-month program of high-intensity, twice-weekly resistance training.[24, 25]

Case report

Mrs S was a 75-year-old woman who lived with her husband. She had a history of falls and low trauma fractures to her wrists. According to Mrs S, her nickname among her family and close friends was 'Betty Broken Bones'. Due to her fear of sustaining further fall-induced fractures, Mrs S was reluctant to partake in regular exercise. As a result, Mrs S was quite deconditioned and her physical state was negatively affecting her quality of life. For example, for the past two years, Mrs S was no longer able to take bubble baths, something she immensely enjoyed, due to her inability to get in and out of the bathtub safely.

In 2002, Mrs S decided she was going to participate in a six-month program of high-intensity, twice-weekly resistance training.[24] The protocol for the resistance training program was progressive and of high intensity; it aimed to increase muscle strength in the extremities and trunk. Both a Keiser Pressurized Air system and free weights were used to provide the training stimulus. Mrs S underwent a two-week familiarization period with the equipment and the exercises. The exercises included: biceps curls (Fig. 55.4j), triceps extension (Fig. 55.4k), seated row, latissimus dorsi pull-downs (Fig. 55.4f), mini-squats, mini-lunges, hamstring curls (Fig. 55.4l), calf raises (Fig. 55.4p) and gluteus maximus extensions on a mat. The intensity of the training stimulus was initially set at 50–60% of one repetition maximum as determined at week two, with a work range of two sets of 10–15 repetitions, and progressed to 75–85% of one repetition maximum at a work range of six to eight repetitions (two sets) by week four. The training stimulus was increased using the seven repetition maximum method,[26] when two sets of six to eight repetitions were completed with proper form and without pain or discomfort. Squats, lunges and gluteus maximus extensions, however, did not follow the above guideline. These three exercises were performed initially with body weight and loading was increased only when proper form was maintained for two sets of 10 repetitions.

Over the course of the six-month period, Mrs S found that she had the strength and confidence to once again enjoy her bubble baths. Mrs S also found she was more confident in her own abilities. After completing the six-month resistance training program and research study, Mrs S decided to continue with resistance training at her local community center with a friend she met through training. When Mrs S was interviewed again at the end of 2005, a full three years after taking on resistance training as a research participant, she stated she had not fallen since 2002 and was still enjoying her bubble baths daily!

Recommended Reading

Booth FW, Chakravarthy MV, Gordon SE, Spangenburg EE. Waging war on physical inactivity: using modern molecular ammunition against an ancient enemy. *J Appl Physiol* 2002; 93(1): 3–30.

Booth FW, Gordon SE, Carlson CJ, Hamilton MT. Waging war on modern chronic diseases: primary prevention through exercise biology. *J Appl Physiol* 2000; 88(2): 774–87.

Briffa TG, Maiorana A, Sheerin NJ, Stubbs AG, Oldenburg BF, Sammel NL, Allan RM. Physical activity for people with cardiovascular disease: recommendations of the National Heart Foundation of Australia. *Med J Aust* 2006; 184(2): 71–5.

Christmas C, Andersen RA. Exercise and older patients: guidelines for the clinician. *J Am Geriatr Soc* 2000; 48: 318–24.

Kujala UM. Evidence for exercise therapy in the treatment of chronic disease based on at least three randomized controlled trials—summary of published systematic reviews. *Scand J Med Sci Sports* 2004; 14(6): 339–45.

Kujala UM. Benefits of exercise therapy for chronic diseases. *Br J Sports Med* 2006; 40(1): 3–4.

McKay HA, Macdonald H, Reed KE, Khan KM. Exercise interventions for health: time to focus on dimensions, delivery, and dollars. *Br J Sports Med* 2003; 37(2): 98–9.

Pedersen BK, Saltin B. Evidence for prescribing exercise as therapy in chronic disease. *Scand J Med Sci Sports* 2006; 16(suppl. 1): 3–63.

Pollock ML, Franklin BA, Balady GJ, et al. AHA Science Advisory. Resistance exercise in individuals with and without cardiovascular disease: benefits, rationale, safety, and prescription. An advisory from the Committee on Exercise, Rehabilitation, and Prevention, Council on Clinical Cardiology, American Heart Association; position paper endorsed by the American College of Sports Medicine. *Circulation* 2000; 101: 828–33.

References

1. Cooper DL. Year 2000 fitness objectives for the nation: the physician's role. *Clin Sports Med* 1991; 10(1): 223–6.

2. Fentem PH. Exercise in the prevention of disease. *Br Med Bull* 1992; 48(3): 630–50.

3. Booth FW, Gordon SE, Carlson CJ, Hamilton MT. Waging war on modern chronic diseases: primary prevention through exercise biology. *J Appl Physiol* 2000; 88(2): 774–87.

4. Petrella RJ, Wight D. An office-based instrument for exercise counseling and prescription in primary care. The Step Test Exercise Prescription (STEP). *Arch Fam Med* 2000; 9(4): 339–44.

5. Thomas S, Reading J, Shephard RJ. Revision of the Physical Activity Readiness Questionnaire (PAR-Q). *Can J Sport Sci* 1992; 17(4): 338–45.

6. Fardy PS, Yanowitz FG. *Cardiac Rehabilitation, Adult Fitness, and Exercise Testing*. Baltimore, MD: Williams & Wilkins, 1995.

7. Durstine L. *ACSM's Exercise Management For Persons With Chronic Diseases and Disabilities*. Champaign, IL: Human Kinetics, 1997.

8. Teixeira PJ, Going SB, Houtkooper LB, et al. Exercise motivation, eating, and body image variables as predictors of weight control. *Med Sci Sports Exerc* 2006; 38(1): 179–88.

9. Vertinsky P. 'Run, Jane, run': central tensions in the current debate about enhancing women's health through exercise. *Women Health* 1998; 27(4): 81–111.

10. Borg E, Kaijser L. A comparison between three rating scales for perceived exertion and two different work tests. *Scand J Med Sci Sports* 2006; 16(1): 57–69.

11. Astrand PO. 1992 J. B. Wolffe Memorial Lecture. 'Why exercise?' *Med Sci Sports Exerc* 1992; 24(2): 153–62.

12. Feigenbaum MS, Pollock ML. Prescription of resistance training for health and disease. *Med Sci Sports Exerc* 1999; 31: 38–45.

13. Starkey DB, Pollock ML, Ishida Y, et al. Effects of resistance training volume on strength and muscle thickness. *Med Sci Sports Exerc* 1996; 28: 1311–20.

14. Briffa TG, Maiorana A, Sheerin NJ, et al. Physical activity for people with cardiovascular disease: recommendations of the National Heart Foundation of Australia. *Med J Aust* 2006; 184(2): 71–5.

15. Adams J, Cline MJ, Hubbard M, McCullough T, Hartman J. A new paradigm for post-cardiac event resistance exercise guidelines. *Am J Cardiol* 2006; 97(2): 281–6.

16. Pollock ML, Franklin BA, Balady GJ, et al. AHA Science Advisory. Resistance exercise in individuals with and without cardiovascular disease: benefits, rationale, safety, and prescription. An advisory from the Committee on Exercise, Rehabilitation, and Prevention, Council on Clinical Cardiology, American Heart Association; position paper endorsed by the American College of Sports Medicine. *Circulation* 2000; 101(7): 828–33.

17. Borg GAV. Psychophysical bases of perceived exertion. *Med Sci Sports Exerc* 1982; 14: 377–81.

18. Ettinger WH Jr, Burns R, Messier SP, et al. A randomized trial comparing aerobic exercise and resistance exercise with a health education program in older adults with knee osteoarthritis. The Fitness Arthritis and Seniors Trial (FAST). *JAMA* 1997; 277(1): 25–31.

19. Van Baar ME, Dekker J, Oostendorp RAB, et al. The effectiveness of exercise therapy in patients with osteoarthritis of the hip or the knee: a randomized clinical trial. *J Rheumatol* 1998; 25: 2432–9.

20. Messier SP, Loeser RF, Miller GD, et al. Exercise and dietary weight loss in overweight and obese older adults with knee osteoarthritis: the Arthritis, Diet, and Activity Promotion Trial. *Arthritis Rheum* 2004; 50(5): 1501–10.

21. Van Baar ME, Assendelft WJJ, Dekker J, Oostendorp RAB, Bijlsma JWJ. Effectiveness of exercise therapy in patients with osteoarthritis of the hip or knee. A systematic review of randomized clinical trials. *Arthritis Rheum* 1999; 42: 1361–9.

22. Simkin A, Ayalon J, Leichter I. Increased trabecular bone density due to bone loading exercises in postmenopausal osteoporotic women. *Calcif Tissue Int* 1987; 40: 59–63.

23. Carter ND, Khan KM, McKay HA, et al. Community-based exercise program reduces risk factors for falls in 65- to 75-year-old women with osteoporosis: randomized controlled trial. *Can Med Assoc J* 2002; 167(9): 997–1004.

24. Liu-Ambrose T, Khan KM, Eng JJ, Janssen PA, Lord SR, McKay HA. Resistance and agility training reduce fall risk in women aged 75 to 85 with low bone mass: a 6-month randomized, controlled trial. *J Am Geriatr Soc* 2004; 52(5): 657–65.

25. Liu-Ambrose TY, Khan KM, Eng JJ, Gillies GL, Lord SR, McKay HA. The beneficial effects of group-based exercises on fall risk profile and physical activity persist 1 year postintervention in older women with low bone mass: follow-up after withdrawal of exercise. *J Am Geriatr Soc* 2005; 53(10): 1767–73.

26. Braith RW, Graves JE, Leggett SH, Pollock ML. Effect of training on the relationship between maximal and submaximal strength. *Med Sci Sports Exerc* 1993; 25(1): 132–8.

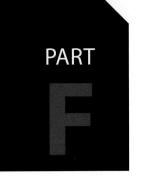

PART

F

Practical Sports Medicine

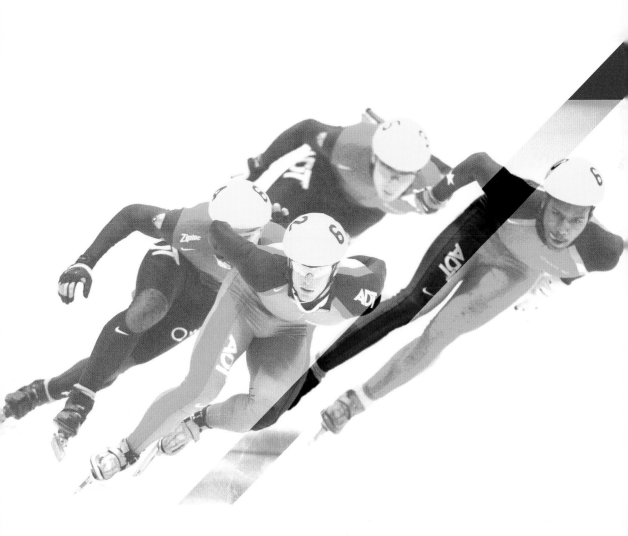

The Preparticipation Physical Evaluation

WITH SANDY HOFFMAN

A preparticipation physical evaluation (PPE) should take place for competitive athletes of all ages, genders and levels of organized sports competition. The primary objectives of a PPE are to provide a structured environment in which to identify and maintain the health and safety of an athlete and to identify illnesses, injuries or chronic medical conditions that may endanger an individual athlete's health and safety, or the health and safety of those with whom they practice and compete.[1] The PPE can also be used as a guide to help competitive athletes with chronic medical conditions participate to their fullest extent and provide an access point for general healthcare.

A PPE is often a mandatory administrative requirement of an athletic association for organized sports participation. There is a wide variation throughout the world in how these examinations are performed, including questions asked, physical examination components performed, and the level of training of practitioners conducting these examinations.

This chapter will discuss the objectives of the PPE as well as presenting a format for conducting a thorough evaluation. Participation clearance will also be discussed. The reader is referred to Chapters 40–43 for details regarding special populations such as the older and younger athlete, the female athlete and the disabled athlete.

Objectives

Detection of life-threatening or disabling conditions is a daily challenge for healthcare practitioners, and a primary objective of the PPE. Many medical conditions that are life-threatening are difficult to detect and are dependent on the level of experience of the practitioner performing the examination, as well as the conditions under which the examination is performed. Developing worldwide uniformity in the approach to a comprehensive PPE may help define and improve the ability to achieve this goal in a typically younger and 'healthier' population.[1–7]

Another primary objective of the PPE is to screen for conditions that may predispose a competitive athlete to injury or illness. There is no literature to support the concept that performance of a PPE predicts who will develop an orthopedic injury, or prevents or reduces the severity of an orthopedic injury in an athlete.[8] Furthermore, in a case series of 158 athletes with sudden death, the cardiovascular abnormality responsible for death was prospectively identified in only one athlete.[9] Despite the lack of evidence that the PPE as currently conducted is able to prevent injury or illness, early recognition and treatment of such may minimize time lost from training and competition, an important goal of a competitive athlete.

The PPE can also serve as a vehicle to meet administrative requirements of an athletic association or governing body for eligibility to participate in competitive athletics. In the United States, a PPE is a required condition to participate in organized sports at the high school and collegiate levels. Italy requires compulsory annual medical clearance to compete in organized sports at many levels,[5] and the PPE requirements are different in Australia.[2] In addition, there are numerous country-specific legal statutes that govern the rights of athletes to participate, as well as the confidentiality of medical records obtained during performance of a PPE.

For many athletes the PPE serves as an entry point into a healthcare system, especially for adolescents, allowing an opportunity to provide quality and cost-effective healthcare, determine general health, and initiate discussion on health-related topics. At higher levels of competition it may also provide an opportunity to assess psychological, social and nutritional factors that may affect performance, gather baseline data related to performance such as muscle strength and flexibility, and develop a rehabilitation plan for any pre-existing injury to maximize performance. The PPE also affords the opportunity for the sports medicine team and athletes to meet and develop a working relationship and to initiate counseling and education regarding injury and illness prevention, high-risk behaviors, nutrition and hydration, environmental issues, as well as other aspects of training and performance. Lastly, the PPE can provide a forum for clinicians to advise participants on appropriate sports in which to participate, especially for those athletes with disabilities.[10]

Who should undergo the PPE

The PPE was developed for competitive athletes at the high school, college and elite amateur and professional levels. Recently Maron et al.[11] have proposed recommendations for preparticipation screening and assessment of cardiovascular disease at the masters athlete level. In the broader context, however, all persons who begin a new activity program should have a 'PPE' tailored to their age, ability and anticipated 'athletic' endeavor. This chapter, however, will focus on the competitive athlete and the reader is referred to Chapter 55 on how to develop an exercise prescription for all 'athletes'.

Who should perform the PPE

The Team Physician Consensus Statement from the American College of Sports Medicine makes recommendations at the collegiate level for which practitioners should perform the PPE.[12] Skills in both musculoskeletal evaluation, as well as cardiac auscultation, may require that more than one clinician perform components of the examination. In the United States, laws vary from state to state as to the educational and experiential skills that a practitioner needs to perform a PPE. International and professional athletes are governed by their athletic organizations as to who is considered qualified to perform a PPE.

When to perform the PPE

Timing of the PPE ideally should occur at least six to eight weeks prior to the beginning of the practise season to allow time for appropriate rehabilitation of injuries or to evaluate and treat medical conditions.

The required frequency of the PPE varies according to the governing bodies of various athletic organizations and the age of the athlete.[2, 4, 6] Generally it is recommended that a comprehensive PPE be performed at entry to middle school, high school and college, any time an athlete transfers to a new school, and at least every two years in younger athletes.[1] An interim comprehensive history that includes the integral components of the American Heart Association screening guidelines,[13] height, weight, blood pressure, and a problem-focused examination is also recommended. The optimal frequency for elite amateur, professional and masters athletes has yet to be determined.

Where to conduct the PPE

Office-based examinations are more costly but provide privacy and the opportunity for continuity of care, especially if there is a previously established provider–patient relationship. If the provider, however, has not had adequate training in components of the PPE, particularly in musculoskeletal and cardiac examination, the visit may end up focusing more on health maintenance and developmental concerns than on the particular athletic endeavor.

A station-based examination is inexpensive and designed to have a sports focus, but lacks continuity of care and often does not allow an athlete an opportunity to explore developmental issues or risk-taking behaviors. The PPE working group has developed tips to improve the coordinated medical team approach to a PPE, including having the team physician coordinate the process, as well as having clinicians with various expertise available.[1]

What to include in the PPE

History

A thorough medical history is crucial to the preparticipation evaluation of competitive athletes. Various questionnaires have been developed for athletes of all ages and levels of competition. Controversy exists as to whether the PPE should cover a broad range of topics, including health promotion and risk behaviors, or be limited to orthopedic and cardiac conditions. The Preparticipation Evaluation Working Group has developed an evaluation form that includes most conditions that could affect the health and safety of athletes.[1] This form also includes follow-up questions on substance use, mental health, and general safety issues that they recommend be discussed face-to-face with the clinician performing the examination.

Younger athletes are encouraged to complete the history form prior to the evaluation with an adult to help ensure accuracy. A web-based PPE has been used on a small scale with collegiate and high school athletes in the United States,[14, 15] and has the potential to facilitate research on the effectiveness of the PPE as currently performed.

The essential components of the history include a thorough system review for acute or chronic medical and orthopedic conditions, and a sports participation history, including the use of protective equipment, use of medications and supplements, allergies, and a menstrual history for female athletes. Questions regarding immunization status, dietary status and health-risk behaviors are often included (Table 56.1).

Physical examination

The physical examination component of the PPE should be performed by skilled clinicians with a particular focus on cardiovascular, neurological and orthopedic abnormalities that would identify athletes at high risk of disability or death. Baseline data should also be obtained on blood pressure, weight, height and organ function in case of injury or illness (Table 56.2).

Table 56.1 Important components of the history

Past history	**Neurological**
• Ever been denied participation	• Head, facial or dental injury
• Chronic medical conditions	• Confusion or memory loss after a head injury
• Hospitalizations, surgeries	• Numbness, tingling or inability to move arms or legs after being hit
• Unpaired organ (eye, testicle, kidney)	• Headaches with or immediately after exercise
• Medications, supplements	
Allergies	**Eyes**
• Medications	• Glasses or contact lenses
• Foods	• Use of protective eyewear
• Bees, wasps, other	**General**
Cardiovascular	• History of heat illness
• Syncope, near syncope (during or after activity)	• History of sickle-cell trait or disease
• Chest pain	**Dietary**
• Palpitations	• Weight loss/gain
• Heart murmur	• Satisfaction with current weight
• High blood pressure	• Dietary habits, limit or control certain foods
• Fatigue	**Females**
• Shortness of breath with exertion	• When menstruation commenced
• Family history of sudden cardiac death (or unexpected drowning)	• How many menses in last 12 months
• Family history of premature coronary disease	• Last menstrual period, prior menstrual period
Orthopedic	**Immunizations**
• Injury (sprain, strain)	• Tetanus
• Broken bones, dislocated joints or stress fracture	• Hepatitis A, B
• Brace	• Meningococcal
Respiratory	• Influenza
• Exercise-related wheezing, cough, difficulty breathing	• Others (dependent on travel history)
Infectious diseases	**Health-risk behaviors**
• Recent infectious mononucleosis	• Tobacco, alcohol, drugs
• Herpes skin infection	• Sexual history

Table 56.2 Important components of the physical examination

General

- Height
- Weight

Eyes, ears, nose, throat

- Visual acuity
- Pupil symmetry
- Ear canals and tympanic membranes
- Nasal septum, polyps
- Teeth
- Throat lesions

Lungs

- Breath sounds
- Chest expansion
- Contour of thoracic cage

Cardiovascular system

- Blood pressure in both arms
- Radial and femoral pulses
- Heart rate, rhythm
- Murmurs (systolic/diastolic and grade)
- Stigmata of Marfan's syndrome

Abdomen

- Tenderness
- Organomegaly
- Masses

Skin

- Rashes
- Lesions

Genitalia (males only)

- Testicles, masses
- Hernia

Musculoskeletal (symmetry, range of motion, strength, flexibility, balance)

- Neck, back
- Shoulder
- Elbow, wrist, hand
- Hip
- Knee
- Ankle, foot
- Gait

Diagnostic tests

Cardiovascular testing

The prevalence of cardiovascular diseases capable of causing sudden death in young athletes is estimated to be very low, although it differs in various parts of the world.[15, 16] A thorough history and physical examination based on the American Heart Association screening recommendations remains the cornerstone of the cardiac preparticipation screening.[13, 17] Reviews of high school[4] and collegiate[6] PPE forms used in the United States, however, demonstrate a significant lack of essential components in most questionnaires.

Much interest has been generated in the use of diagnostic testing to assist in screening for cardiovascular conditions that may predispose an athlete to sudden cardiac death. Routine diagnostic testing with an ECG/EKG has been performed as part of the PPE in Italy for many years and has been found useful in identifying athletes with hypertrophic cardiomyopathy.[3, 5] The ECG is a relatively easy and inexpensive test to perform, but the sensitivity and specificity are too low to be used as a screening test in a young population.[18] Atherosclerotic coronary disease is the most common form of heart disease in masters athletes and a routine screening ECG is recommended for this population as part of their PPE.[11]

Echocardiography and exercise stress testing are not suggested for routine screening, however, these diagnostic tests may be indicated in certain populations such as masters athletes, particularly if they are undertaking sudden vigorous training,[11] and for athletes with abnormalities on a resting ECG.

It is important to recognize that further testing and referral should be considered for any athlete who has a personal or family history of sudden cardiac death or premature coronary disease. Symptoms of syncope, unexplained exertional dyspnea or chest pain should be thoroughly evaluated[19] as they may be an early sign of one of the genetic cardiovascular diseases (Table 56.3). Additional testing should also be undertaken if the athlete has a heart murmur, hypertension, or abnormalities suggestive of Marfan's syndrome or coarctation of the aorta.

Neurological testing

No evidence-based guidelines exist as to the requirements for assessment of a previous head injury during

Table 56.3 Genetic cardiovascular diseases

Hypertrophic cardiomyopathy (HCM)
Arrhythmogenic right ventricular cardiomyopathy (ARVC)
Marfan's syndrome
Ion channel diseases
Long-QT syndrome (LQTS)
Brugada syndrome
Catecholaminergic polymorphic ventricular tachycardia (CPVT)

the PPE.[20] Consensus expert recommendations exist, however, for the use of a baseline cognitive assessment such as the Prague sport concussion assessment tool (SCAT) as well as baseline neuropsychological testing, particularly for those athletes in high-risk sports such as Rugby, soccer, ice hockey, and American football.[21]

Other diagnostic tests

Other diagnostic tests may be appropriate for selected athletes (Table 56.4).

Table 56.4 Miscellaneous diagnostic tests

Urinalysis
Hemoglobin and ferritin levels
Hepatitis B, C and HIV antibodies
Bone mineral density
Peak flow and pulmonary function
Body fat composition
Isokinetic muscle testing
Biomechanical analysis and gait assessment
Video analysis of technique

Why do the PPE for competitive athletes? What is 'clearance'?

The objective of the PPE is to allow athletes to participate in their sport of choice safely, without harm to themselves or others. If an athlete cannot safely participate in his or her chosen sport with treatment of a medical or orthopedic condition, even on a limited basis, determination should be made as to what activities he or she can compete in. Classification of activities based on dynamic (volume load) or static (pressure load) demands on the left ventricle[22] and degree of physical contact[23] can help the clinician guide athletes into appropriate activities based on their general health and cardiovascular status. Tables 56.5 and 56.6 provide examples of sports based on strenuousness and degree of contact. Detailed recommendations that contain expert consensus regarding 'clearance' for a particular competitive sport have been developed by several groups.[1, 11, 19, 23–25] As in all aspects of medicine, reliance on current consensus guidelines, good medical practice, and the athlete's overall health should be considered when making individual decisions about participation.[26]

Conclusions

An ideal screening test is one that screens for a condition that is prevalent and causes morbidity and mortality, is accurate, practical, cost-effective, safe, and identifies conditions that are treatable.

The PPE as currently performed may not be an ideal evidence-based screening tool for prevention of illness and injury in athletes. Some authors suggest a move towards a history and examination that contains an overview of an athlete's entire health status, including age-appropriate preventive health services such as tobacco cessation. The PPE, however, should not replace comprehensive health maintenance visits

Table 56.5 Examples of sports classified by strenuousness

High/moderate dynamic and static	High/moderate dynamic and low static	High/moderate static and low dynamic	Low static and low dynamic
Rugby	Soccer	Gymnastics	Curling
Downhill skiing	Swimming	Sailing	Golf
Wrestling	Table tennis	Archery	Bowling
Ice hockey	Volleyball	Diving	Cricket
Water polo	Squash	Auto racing	

Table 56.6 Examples of sports classified by contact

Contact/collision	Limited contact	Non-contact
Rugby	Gymnastics	Curling
Ice hockey	Snowboarding	Golf
Soccer	Skiing	Swimming
Water polo	Volleyball	Bowling
Wrestling	Handball	Table tennis

for athletes unless it incorporates components of such into its format.[27]

Considerations for improving the way a PPE is performed include developing a common format, determining optimal frequency, and measuring the effectiveness of the delivery of healthcare services performed during a PPE.[1,2,5,7] Electronic implementation of a PPE questionnaire has been attempted at the high school and collegiate levels in the United States,[14,15] providing the beginning of a database from which we may gather information, measure effectiveness of our current process, and develop a PPE that focuses on how sports participation influences an individual athlete's short- and long-term health. A more focused, systematic, standardized PPE, tailored to specific populations, that is age and developmentally specific, is a goal of sports medicine practitioners throughout the world.

Recommended Reading

Preparticipation Physical Evaluation Working Group. *Preparticipation Physical Evaluation Monograph.* 3rd edn. Minneapolis: McGraw-Hill Healthcare Information, 2004.

References

1. Preparticipation Physical Evaluation Working Group. *Preparticipation Physical Evaluation Monograph.* 3rd edn. Minneapolis: McGraw-Hill Healthcare Information, 2004.
2. Brukner P, White S, Shawdon A, et al. Screening of athletes: Australian experience. *Clin J Sports Med* 2004; 14: 169–77.
3. Corrado D, Basso C, Schiavon M, Thiene G. Screening for hypertrophic cardiomyopathy in young athletes. *N Engl J Med* 1998; 339: 364–9.
4. Glover DW, Maron BJ. Profile of preparticipation cardiovascular screening for high school athletes. *JAMA* 1998; 279: 1817–19.
5. Pelliccia A, Maron BJ. Preparticipation cardiovascular examination of the competitive athlete perspectives from the 30-year Italian experience. *Am J Cardiol* 1995; 75: 827–9.
6. Pfister GC, Puffer JC, Maron BJ. Preparticipation cardiovascular screening for US collegiate student-athletes. *JAMA* 2000; 283: 1597–9.
7. Wingfield K, Matheson GO, Meeuwisse WH. Preparticipation evaluation: an evidence-based review. *Clin J Sport Med* 2004; 14: 109–14.
8. Hulkower S, Fagan B, Watts J, Ketterman E. Do preparticipation clinical exams reduce morbidity and mortality for athletes? *J Fam Pract* 2005; 54: 28–32.
9. Maron BJ, Shirani J, Poliac LC, et al. Sudden death in young competitive athletes. Clinical, demographic, and pathological profiles. *JAMA* 1996; 276: 199–204.
10. Patel DR, Greydanus DE. The pediatric athlete with disabilities. *Pediatr Clin North Am* 2002; 49: 803–27.
11. Maron BJ, Araujo CG, Thompson PD, et al. Recommendations for preparticipation screening and the measurement of cardiovascular disease in masters athletes: an advisory for healthcare professionals from the Working Groups of the World Heart Federation, the International Federation of Sports Medicine, and the American Heart Association on Exercise, Cardiac Rehabilitation, and Prevention. *Circulation* 2001; 103: 327.
12. Herring SA, Bergfeld JA, Boyd J, et al. Team Physician Consensus Statement. Available online: <www.acsm.org>.
13. Maron B, Thompson P, Puffer J, et al. Cardiovascular preparticipation screening of competitive athletes: a statement for health professionals from the Sudden Death Committee (clinical cardiology) and Congenital Cardiac Defects Committee (cardiovascular disease in the young), American Heart Association. *Circulation* 1996; 94: 850–6.
14. Meeuwisse WH, Matheson GO. Prevalence of positive responses on sports participation screening in Ohio students. *Clin J Sports Med* 2003; 13: 381.
15. Peltz JE, Haskell W, Matheson GO. A comprehensive and cost-effective preparticipation exam implemented on the World Wide Web. *Med Sci Sport Exerc* 1999; 31: 1727–40.
16. Maron BJ. Sudden death in young athletes. *N Engl J Med* 2003; 349: 1064–75.
17. Maron BJ, Douglas PS, Graham TP, et al. 36th Bethesda Conference. Task Force 1: Preparticipation screening and diagnosis of cardiovascular disease in athletes. *J Am Coll Cardiol* 2005; 45: 1322–6.
18. Beckerman J, Wang P, Hlatky M. Cardiovascular screening of athletes. *Clin J Sport Med* 2004; 14: 127–33.
19. Maron BJ, Chaitman BR, Ackerman MJ, et al. Recommendations for physical activity and recreational sports participation for young patients with genetic cardiovascular diseases. *Circulation* 2004; 109: 2807–16.
20. McCrory P. Preparticipation assessment for head injury. *Clin J Sport Med* 2004; 14: 139–44.
21. McCrory P, Johnston K, Meeuwisse W, et al. Summary and agreement statement of the 2nd International Conference on Concussion in Sport, Prague 2004. *Br J Sports Med* 2005; 39: 196–204.
22. Mitchell JH, Haskell WL, Raven PB. Classification of sports. *Med Sci Sports Exerc* 1994; 26(suppl.): S242–S245.
23. American Academy of Pediatrics Committee on Sports Medicine and Fitness. Medical conditions affecting sports participation. *Pediatrics* 2001; 107: 1205–9.

24. Pellicia A, Fagard R, Bjornstad HH, et al. Recommendations for competitive sports participation in athletes with cardiovascular disease. A consensus document from the Study Group of Sports Cardiology of the Working Group of cardiac rehabilitation and Exercise Physiology and the Working Group of Myocardial and Pericardial Diseases of the European Society of Cardiology. *Eur Heart J* 2005; 26: 1422–45.

25. Maron BJ, Zipes DP. 36th Bethesda Conference. Introduction: eligibility recommendations for competitive athletes with cardiovascular abnormalities—general considerations. *J Am Coll Cardiol* 2005; 45: 1318–21.

26. Mitten MJ, Maron BJ, Zipes DP. 36th Bethesda Conference Task Force 12: legal aspects of the 36th Bethesda Conference recommendations. *J Am Coll Cardiol* 2005; 45: 1373–5.

27. US Department of Health and Human Services, Centers for Disease Control and Prevention: Assessing Health Risk Behaviors Among Young People: Youth Risk Behavior Surveillance System, 2004. Available online: <http://www.cdc.gov/yrbss>.

Screening the Elite Athlete

Screening the competitive athlete is an important component of the sports medicine team's job. It involves taking a comprehensive history and examination with additional tests if appropriate. Screening differs from a preparticipation examination (Chapter 56) in that it is oriented both towards health and performance.

Aims of medical screening

The medical screening of high performance athletes has a number of aims:

1. Ensure optimal medical health
   (a) Recognize previously undiagnosed medical problems, such as cardiac murmurs, exercise-induced asthma, anorexia nervosa, Marfan's syndrome, depression
   (b) Assess the status of known medical problems, such as asthma, diabetes, epilepsy
2. Ensure optimal musculoskeletal health
   (a) Assess any current injury
   (b) Assess the deficit(s) resulting from any previous injury
   (c) Identify unrecognized injury
3. Optimize performance (nutrition, psychology, biomechanics)
4. Injury prevention
   (a) Assess the presence of any predisposing factors to musculoskeletal injury, such as lack of flexibility, muscle weakness/imbalance, impaired proprioception, abnormal biomechanics
5. Review medications and vaccinations
6. Baseline data collection
   (a) Obtain baseline data, such as muscle strength, joint range of motion, blood tests, neuropsychological testing, to compare pre- and post-concussion results, or bone density measurement
7. Develop professional relationship with athlete
8. Education

Benefits of screening

There are a number of advantages to be gained from screening the athlete in addition to the above-mentioned factors. Screening provides an opportunity for the athlete to be examined by a physician, sometimes for the first time in many years. Young athletes are usually healthy and rarely seek assistance from a medical practitioner. The athletic screening may be the first time that a physician has listened to the athlete's heart since birth. It may be the first time the athlete's blood pressure or urine have ever been tested.

The screening process gives the clinical team an opportunity to develop a relationship with the athlete that may stand them in good stead in the future. A knowledge of the athlete's personal details, including family, job and other personal habits, may provide useful information in the future management of the athlete. Screening also gives the opportunity for the clinical team to offer advice regarding the prevention of injuries (e.g. the need for warm-up and stretching), to emphasize the importance of early reporting of injuries and appropriate initial management, to discuss possible symptoms of overtraining and the various methods of preventing overtraining, and to give advice regarding diet and psychological techniques.

When should athletes be screened?

Athletes should be screened at the earliest opportunity. This may be prior to or immediately after they join a high-level squad or team. A full screening should be performed initially. Subsequent modified screening, usually concentrating on musculoskeletal problems and focusing on areas that may have proved a problem in the preceding season, should be performed each year between the end of one season and the commencement of training for the following season. This allows adequate time for any specific treatment, such as surgery or rehabilitation, to be performed before the resumption of intense training.

The screening protocol

The proposed protocol is shown in Figure 57.1 (pp. 949–53; this is also available as a downloadable PDF file at <www.clinicalsportsmedicine.com>). The first page contains the athlete's personal details and consent form, along with the outcome summary to be filled in by the examining physician. Page two is completed by the physician with recommendations and suggested follow-up. Pages one and two can then be used as a summary to be distributed to the appropriate personnel following the screening. Pages three and four are to be filled in by the athlete, preferably prior to coming in for screening, or else in the waiting room. We recommend that younger athletes, in particular, fill in the form with the help of a parent or guardian if possible. The final page is a summary of the examination findings and is filled in by the examining physician.

Cardiovascular screening

Statistics regarding the incidence of sudden death in sport in Australia are not available, but episodes of sudden unexplained death during exercise occur and are often reported in the media. We assume that the rate of sudden death is similar to that in other countries (approximately 1 in 200 000). Anecdotal evidence indicates that, similar to the experience in other countries, cardiac causes comprise the vast majority of sudden deaths in athletes. The most common cardiac abnormalities associated with sudden death in young (<35 years old) athletes are hypertrophic cardiomyopathy (HCM), coronary artery abnormalities, myocarditis, arrhythmias, valve abnormalities and aortic rupture.

Basic screening to detect those at risk of sudden cardiac death include a careful history and physical examination. A family history of sudden death under the age of 60 or a history of episodes of unexplained syncope or palpitations warrant further investigation.

Seto[1] claims that personal and family history can reveal 64–78% of conditions that would prohibit or alter sports participation. However, the American Heart Association found that the combination of history and physical examination was unable to detect serious cardiovascular diseases.[2] According to Maron et al.,[3] detection of HCM by standard screening is unreliable because most patients have the non-obstructive form of this disease, characteristically expressed by only a soft heart murmur or none at all. Furthermore, most athletes with HCM do not experience syncope or have a family history of premature sudden death due to the disease.

The addition of a 12-lead ECG to the screening process enhances the detection of certain cardiovascular abnormalities. The ECG is abnormal in about 95% of patients with HCM. The major drawback of the use of ECGs in screening, aside from the expense, is the high frequency of abnormal findings associated with normal physiological adaptations of an athlete's heart to training.[3]

A two-dimensional echocardiogram is the principal diagnostic tool for the detection of HCM and will also detect most, but not all, important cardiac lesions. However, the considerable expense of the echocardiogram means that it would cost hundreds of thousands of dollars to detect one previously undiagnosed case.

In Italy approximately five million sports participants undergo a preparticipation screening including an ECG each year. Its efficacy for detecting cardiac abnormalities that may result in sudden cardiac death has not been investigated. A recent review of the program by Pigozzi et al.[4] stated that the usefulness of 12-lead ECG for identifying cardiovascular disease in highly trained athletes is limited. Based on the large proportion of false positive abnormal ECGs found in the athletic population (40%) in Italy, the diagnostic power of the ECG was low (sensitivity 50%, positive predictive value 7%).

We do not perform routine ECGs as part of our medical screening but if there is any symptom or sign suggestive of cardiovascular disease, then an ECG and frequently an echocardiogram will be ordered. In sports such as basketball and volleyball, we look closely for the presence of clinical features of Marfan's syndrome.

The questions relating to cardiovascular problems in our questionnaire are adapted from those recommended by the American Heart Association:[3]

- Have you ever passed out, become dizzy or had chest pain during or after exercise?
- Has anyone in the family died suddenly and unexpectedly before the age of 50?

- Have you ever had a heart abnormality or murmur diagnosed by a doctor?
- Have you ever had an abnormal heart rate, palpitations or irregular heart beats?
- Have you had high blood pressure or high cholesterol?
- Has a physician ever denied or restricted your participation in sport for heart problems?
- Have any of your relatives ever had cardiomyopathy, Marfan's syndrome, long QT syndrome or significant heart arrhythmia?

Medical health

Generally, fit, young athletes have very little occasion to visit a physician. Some of the athletes will not have been to see a physician for many years and may not have a regular general practitioner, especially if their sporting prowess has resulted in them moving from their home town. The examining physician should not assume that basic medical procedures such as auscultation of the heart and blood pressure measurement have ever been performed on the athlete. The screening questionnaire necessarily focuses on the more common conditions affecting young athletes.

Asthma and exercise-induced asthma have a significant prevalence of under- and over-diagnosis, as well as under- and over-treatment. As a result and especially recently with the International Olympic Committee (IOC) and World Anti-Doping Agency (WADA) restrictions on the use of beta-2 agonists, the detection of asthma is a high priority. The efficacy of different methods of screening for the presence of asthma and exercise-induced asthma are described in Chapter 46. The standard questions in our protocol are:

- Do you have asthma, chest tightness, wheezing or coughing spells during or after exercise?
- Have you been tested in an accredited laboratory?

Obviously, there is almost an unlimited amount of questions that could be included in a health questionnaire in an attempt to detect some abnormality. Apart from the cardiovascular and respiratory questions mentioned above, we include the following questions in our questionnaire:

- Do you have a history of concussion or loss of consciousness?
- Have you ever suffered a heat-related illness (e.g. dizziness, cramps, blurred vision, disorientation, collapse)?

- Do you have any problems with your skin (e.g. rashes, moles, acne)?
- Do you have a chronic illness or see a physician regularly for any particular problem (e.g. diabetes, epilepsy, thyroid problems, bowel disorder)?
  Please list:
- Have you ever had surgery or required hospitalization?
  Please list, including approximate dates:

In addition, urinalysis is a simple screening tool for the presence of diabetes.

Menstrual abnormalities are commonly associated with intense athletic activity in females and may lead to significant bone loss resulting in stress fractures and osteoporosis. Therefore, it is important to include questions designed to detect abnormal menstruation in the questionnaire:

- Have you started your periods? _____
  If so, what age _____?
- Date of your last gynecological examination/ PAP smear _____ / _____ / _____
- Have you ever missed your period for more than 6 months?
- Does your menstruation affect your performance?

In our clinical experience, the incidence of mild depression among high level athletes is quite significant. The medical screening presents an opportunity for the athlete to discuss their depression. If the athlete complains of excessive fatigue, depression should be considered among other possible causes of fatigue.

- Have you, or a close relative, ever suffered from depression?
- Have you ever suffered from excessive fatigue or overtraining?

Musculoskeletal screening

Time constraints do not allow a comprehensive assessment of all joints and muscles. The aim of musculoskeletal screening, therefore, is to assess recovery from any previous injury and to assess the presence of proven (very few) or suspected risk factors for future injury. Athletes involved in sports associated with a high risk of specific joint or muscle injuries (e.g. swimmers' shoulders, pitchers' elbows) should have specific assessments performed on these areas.

A full injury history should be taken and any deficits remaining post-injury should be fully assessed with a view to designing a rehabilitation program to restore full function. Frequently, athletes will have resumed full athletic participation following a significant injury and yet still have considerable limitations in strength, range of movement, proprioception and so on.

The questionnaire asks the athlete to describe the nature and date of any previous injury and list any residual problems. They are asked to describe the nature, date and symptoms of any current injury.

Optimize performance

The medical screening process is an opportunity to assess areas that may not necessarily impact on health but may affect performance. Examples of these are nutrition, psychology and biomechanics. A brief assessment of these areas may suggest a problem which can then be followed up by the appropriate expert.

Athletes in sports in which competitors have to be under a specified weight (e.g. wrestling, boxing) or sports where being thin is thought to have some aesthetic (gymnastics) or performance (distance running) advantage may be at an increased risk of unhealthy eating or the development of an eating disorder.

- Do you have problems making weight for your sport?
- Do you follow any special diet (e.g. vegetarian, weight loss, Pritikin)?
- Have you ever had a nutritional deficiency diagnosed (e.g. iron, vitamin B_{12})?

Injury prevention

There is very little research evidence showing associations between the presence of certain risk factors and particular injuries. An example would be the presence of menstrual abnormalities or an eating disorder leading to the development of stress fractures.[5] Clinical experience suggests additional possible relationships. The medical screening process is an opportunity to identify potentially correctable risk factors and implement measures designed to reduce that risk. It is also an opportunity to ensure that appropriate equipment, such as helmets, mouthguards and shin pads, is used in relevant sports.

- Do you wear orthoses?
- Do you wear any protective equipment when playing your sport?

Medications and vaccinations

The medical screening is an opportunity to review the use of medications—both prescription and over-

the-counter drugs—as well as supplements. The list of banned substances produced by WADA and the IOC is regularly changed and athletes need to be aware of the most recent changes.

- Do you take any prescribed medicine? _____ Please list type and dose:
- Do you have any 'over-the-counter' supplements/medication/herbal remedies? ____ Please list:
- Have you notified your national sporting organization (NSO)?
- Do you have any allergies to any medication, insects or other agents?

The screening also presents an opportunity to check the vaccination status of the athlete.

- Vaccinations (please put dates if you have had any of the following):

Tetanus:_____ Rubella
Influenza: _____ (German
Typhoid: _____ measles):_____
Hepatitis A:_____ Hepatitis B:_____
Yellow fever: _____ Chickenpox:_____
Meningitis C: _____ Polio: _____
(Hepatitis A and B may be in a combination vaccine, usually a series of three injections over 6 months.)
(Measles, mumps and rubella is a combination vaccine, part of usual childhood series.)

Baseline data collection

In certain sports, particularly at elite level, regular monitoring of hematological and biochemical parameters is performed to detect early evidence of deficiencies. An example would be the monitoring of serum ferritin levels in female endurance athletes.

In contact sports such as football, team physicians are increasingly using neuropsychological testing to monitor recovery from concussion. A team physician might wish to perform baseline testing before the season to use as a comparison in the recovery process.

Develop professional relationship with the athlete

The medical screening process on entry into a professional team or institute program gives an opportunity for the team physician to commence his or her professional relationship with the athlete. It enables the physician to become fully aware of the athlete's past history and gives an insight into the athlete. The athlete is given the opportunity to list on the form any issues that he or she would like to discuss with the physician.

Education

The medical screening presents an opportunity for the physician to educate the athlete on such issues as injury prevention (stretching, warm-up), immediate injury management (RICE), nutrition, appropriate equipment, the use of medications and supplements, vaccinations and so on.

Problems

There are a number of problems inherent in the medical screening program. As mentioned previously there is no uniformity of protocols. Some are very long (up to 40 pages of questionnaire, with full muscle and joint examinations) and are therefore time consuming for both athlete and physician, resulting in compliance issues.

In some cases multiple screenings are performed by different organizations on the same athlete. For example, an elite 18-year-old basketballer in Australia may have screenings as part of his professional team, his state or national institute of sport, the national basketball team and the Australian Olympic team. All will probably be slightly different and represent a waste of time and resources.

Another issue is that of follow-up. Often an extensive screening is performed with various recommendations emanating from it. Unfortunately there is frequently no mechanism for follow-up. We recommend that the examining physician or Chief Medical Officer (CMO) follow up with the athlete either by telephone or in person approximately six weeks after the screening to ensure that the recommended actions have taken place.

Who has access to the data from the screening? The athlete? The team or organization? The examining physician? The information obtained from medical screening is bound by the same confidentiality restrictions as any medical information.

Certainly, the athlete has the right to the information. How that is presented to the athlete is another area of controversy. Athletes who are traveling constantly (e.g. tennis player or golfer on international circuit) should have the screening information in

their possession at all times so that the treating practitioner can be made aware of any problems. It has been suggested that the traveling athlete should have a 'medical passport' (hard copy and CD-ROM) containing all relevant information.

The confidential medical information obtained at the screening should not be distributed to the team or institute administration. It should be held by the CMO of the organization and passed on at the CMO's discretion to relevant medical and paramedical practitioners as required for the optimal management of the athlete.

Recommended Reading

Brukner PD, White S, Shawdon A, Holzer K. Screening of athletes—the Australian experience. *Clin J Sport Med* 2004; 14(3): 169–77.

Fallon KE. Utility of hematological and iron-related screening in elite athletes. *Clin J Sport Med* 2004; 14(3): 145–52.

Gabbe BJ, Bennell KL, Wajswelner H, et al. Reliability of common lower extremity musculoskeletal screening tests. *Phys Ther Sport* 2004; 5: 90–7.

Holzer K, Brukner PD. Screening of athletes for exercise-induced asthma. *Clin J Sport Med* 2004; 14(3): 134–8.

References

1. Seto CK. Pre-participation cardiovascular screening *Clin Sports Med* 2003; 22: 23–35.

2. Maron BJ. The young competitive athlete with cardiovascular abnormalities: causes of sudden death, detection by preparticipation screening, and standards for disqualification. *Cardiac Electrophysiol Rev* 2002; 6: 100–3.

3. Maron BJ, Thompson PD, Puffer JC, et al. Cardiovascular preparticipation screening of competitive adults. *Circulation* 1996; 94: 850–6.

4. Pigozzi F, Spataro A, Faganani F, et al. Preparticipation screening for the detection of cardiovascular abnormalities that may cause sudden death in competitive athletes. *Br J Sports Med* 2003; 37: 4–5.

5. Bennell KL, Malcolm SA, Thomas SA, et al. Risk factors for stress fractures in track and field athletes: a 12 month prospective study. *Am J Sports Med* 1996; 24: 810–18.

ATHLETE MEDICAL INFORMATION
(ATHLETE TO COMPLETE)

NAME: _____ D.O.B: _____

ADDRESS: _____

HOME PHONE: _____ MOBILE: _____

EMAIL: _____

SPORT: _____ EVENT/POSITION: _____

Next of kin: _____ Relationship to you: _____

Phone no: _____

Local physician's name & contact details: _____

Physiotherapist's name & contact details: _____

Consent:

- I agree to undertake this procedure in order to enable medical staff to ensure I am fit to train and compete.
- I am aware that some information may require clarification or follow-up with my treating physician and physiotherapists, and agree to the release of relevant information to these people.
- I am aware that medical fitness issues may be discussed with my coach.
- I understand that the information contained in this form is otherwise confidential and can only be released with my consent.

Name: _____ Signature: _____ Date: _____

Parent/guardian signature if athlete under 18 years of age: _____ Date: _____

PHYSICIAN USE ONLY

Outcome of screening

Physician:

Yes No

❑ ❑ Is the athlete medically fit to compete and train in a high performance program?

❑ ❑ Are there any medical issues that warrant further assessment?

❑ ❑ Are any further vaccinations required?

Copy sent to:

❑ GP ❑ Physiotherapist ❑ Coach ❑ Strength Coach ❑ NSO or ASDA

❑ Other _____

Physician's name _____ Signature _____ Date _____

RECOMMENDATIONS (PHYSICIAN TO COMPLETE):

Physician: _____

Relevant medical issues: _____

Figure 57.1 Medical screening protocol

Referrals made: _____

_____

Athlete: (e.g. to get blood tests, make optometry appointment) _____

_____

Physiotherapist/Physical therapist: _____

_____

_____

Strength and conditioning coach: _____

_____

_____

Coach: _____

_____

_____

Any other issues: _____

_____

_____

Date of follow-up: _____ / _____ / _____   ❑ Visit   ❑ Phone   ❑ Letter

| **ATHLETE MEDICAL INFORMATION** |
| (ATHLETE TO COMPLETE PRIOR TO SCREENING APPOINTMENT) |

Yes	No	Unsure	
❑	❑	❑	Have you ever passed out, become dizzy or had chest pain during or after exercise?
❑	❑	❑	Has anyone in the family died suddenly and unexpectedly before the age of 50?
❑	❑	❑	Have you ever had a heart abnormality or murmur diagnosed by a doctor?
❑	❑	❑	Have you ever had an abnormal heart rate, palpitations or irregular heart beats?
❑	❑	❑	Have you had high blood pressure or high cholesterol?
❑	❑	❑	Has a physician ever denied or restricted your participation in sport for heart problems?
❑	❑	❑	Have any of your relatives ever had cardiomyopathy, Marfan's syndrome, long QT syndrome or significant heart arrhythmia?
❑	❑	❑	Do you have asthma, chest tightness, wheezing, or coughing spells during or after exercise?
❑	❑	❑	Have you been tested in an accredited laboratory?
❑	❑	❑	Do you have a history of concussion or loss of consciousness?
❑	❑	❑	Have you ever suffered a heat-related illness (e.g. dizziness, cramps, blurred vision, disorientation, collapse)?
❑	❑	❑	Do you have any problems with your skin (e.g. rashes, moles, acne)?
❑	❑	❑	Do you have a chronic illness or see a physician regularly for any particular problem (e.g. diabetes, epilepsy, thyroid problems, bowel disorder)? Please list: _____
❑	❑	❑	Have you ever had surgery or required hospitalization? Please list, including approximate dates: _____
❑	❑	❑	Do you take any prescribed medicine? Please list type and dose: _____

❏ ❏ ❏ Do you use 'over-the-counter' supplements/medication/herbal remedies?
Please list: _____

❏ ❏ ❏ Have you notified your national sporting organization?
❏ ❏ ❏ Do you have any allergies to any medication, insects or other agents?
❏ ❏ ❏ Do you wear corrective lenses or glasses?
❏ ❏ ❏ Do you smoke?
❏ ❏ ❏ Do you drink alcohol?
❏ ❏ ❏ Have you, or a close relative, ever suffered from depression?
❏ ❏ ❏ Have you ever suffered from excessive fatigue or overtraining?
❏ ❏ ❏ Do you wear orthoses?
❏ ❏ ❏ Do you wear any protective equipment when playing your sport?

Nutrition:
❏ ❏ ❏ Do you have problems making weight for your sport?
❏ ❏ ❏ Do you follow any special diet (e.g. vegetarian, weight loss, Pritikin)?
❏ ❏ ❏ Have you ever had a nutritional deficiency diagnosed (e.g. iron, vitamin B_{12})?

Female:
❏ ❏ ❏ Have you started your periods?   If so, what age _____ ?
Date of your last gynecological examination/PAP smear _____ / _____ / _____
❏ ❏ ❏ Have you ever missed your period for more than 6 months?
❏ ❏ ❏ Does your menstruation affect your performance?

VACCINATIONS

Please put dates if you have had any of the following:
Tetanus: _____ Rubella (German measles): _____ influenza: _____
Typhoid: _____ Hepatitis A: _____ Hepatitis B: _____ Yellow fever: _____
Chickenpox: _____ Meningitis C: _____ Polio: _____
(Hepatitis A and B may be in a combination vaccine, usually a series of three injections over 6 months.)
(Measles, mumps and rubella is a combination vaccine, part of usual childhood series.)

Family Medical History
Is there a family history of (*please circle*):
Yes No Unsure
❏ ❏ ❏ Heart disease
❏ ❏ ❏ Cancer
❏ ❏ ❏ Arthritis
❏ ❏ ❏ Diabetes
❏ ❏ ❏ Stroke, high blood pressure
❏ ❏ ❏ Marfan's syndrome
❏ ❏ ❏ Glaucoma or other eye disease

Specify details: _____

Injuries

Yes No Unsure
❏ ❏ ❏ Have you had any injuries/medical conditions that have interfered with your sporting career?

For each injury/condition, state:

Nature of injury _____ Date of injury _____ Any residual problems? _____

_____

_____

_____

_____

_____

_____

Yes   No   Unsure

❏   ❏   ❏   Do you have any current injuries?

Nature of injury _____ Date of injury _____

_____

_____

_____

_____

_____

Do you wish to discuss any health or sports medicine issues with the physician? If yes, please detail below.

_____

_____

_____

_____

_____

EXAMINATION
(TO BE COMPLETED BY PHYSICIAN)

Mandatory

CVS   Blood pressure (sitting)

             Pulse rate and rhythm

             Heart size

             Heart sounds, including murmurs (supine and standing)

             Femoral artery pulses

RESPIRATORY   Auscultation   ❏ Normal   ❏ Abnormal (clarify below)

MUSCULOSKELETAL ASSESSMENT OF ANY INJURED REGION

_____

_____

_____

_____

Optional (as indicated by questionnaire responses)

ANTHROPOMETRY Height ———————— cm   Weight ———————— kg   BMI ————————

ENT	NORMAL	ABNORMAL (clarify below)
ABDOMINAL	NORMAL	ABNORMAL (clarify below)
NEUROLOGICAL	NORMAL	ABNORMAL (clarify below)
SKIN (sun damage, suspicious nevi, acne)	NORMAL	ABNORMAL (clarify below)
MARFAN'S ASSESSMENT	NORMAL	ABNORMAL (clarify below)
BIOMECHANICS (pronation/supination or asymmetry)	NORMAL	ABNORMAL (clarify below)
OPTOMETRY (acuity, color blindness, fundoscopy)	NORMAL	ABNORMAL (clarify below)
BLOODS (indicated by history)	NORMAL	ABNORMAL (clarify below)
URINALYSIS	NORMAL	ABNORMAL (clarify below)
SPIROMETRY	NORMAL	ABNORMAL (clarify below)

ADDITIONAL NOTES FROM EXAMINATION:

_____
_____
_____
_____
_____
_____
_____
_____
_____
_____
_____
_____
_____
_____
_____
_____
_____
_____

Name of Examiner ———————————— Signature ———————————— Date ————————

Providing Team Care

WITH JILL COOK, PETER HARCOURT AND CHRIS MILNE

One of the most challenging yet enjoyable aspects of sports medicine is involvement in team care. Working with a team provides opportunities to:

- belong to a team and share in its successes and failures
- work closely with athletes on a regular basis
- implement preventive strategies
- manage acute injuries from the time of injury
- closely monitor the progress of injuries
- learn and develop decision-making skills in a competitive environment
- work closely with other clinicians and disciplines and thereby develop your own skills (e.g. massage, nutrition advice)
- liaise closely with the coaching and fitness staff and understand the demands placed on them
- better understand the demands of the particular sport
- understand the psychological pressures on the players
- fully appreciate the importance of team dynamics.

Many of the skills gained in the team environment can be incorporated into one's own office practise.

The off-field team

The size and make-up of the medical support team will depend on a number of factors, including the size of the sporting team, the standard of competition and financial considerations. Frequently, the support team will consist of one individual who may be either a physician, physiotherapist, massage therapist or trainer. Specialists from various branches of medicine can contribute to the sports medicine team[1, 2] as, of course, does the family medicine practitioner, who represents the largest category of medical team care provision. Specialized sports medicine training is now available in many countries.[3-6] A sole practitioner should develop a network of supporting practitioners who can assist where additional professional management is indicated.

Professional sporting teams often employ a medical support team that consists of representatives of different sports medicine disciplines. Whoever is responsible for assembling such a team must ensure not only that all the individuals have high professional standards but also that they work well as a team, as some practitioners are more suited to this than others. The ethical issues facing professional teams' clinicians are different from a clinician working as a volunteer for a local sporting team (see also Chapter 62).[7-13]

If possible, the professional sporting team should have access to the services of a sports physician, physiotherapist, massage therapist, podiatrist, dietitian, psychologist, orthopedic surgeon and sports trainer as well as the coaching and fitness staff. If specific areas of responsibility are clearly defined, this will help avoid conflict. Ideally, one member of this team should be the leader and take ultimate responsibility for difficult management decisions and the smooth running of the group.

Coaching and fitness staff

Clinicians caring for a team have multiple responsibilities. Although their unarguable primary responsibility is to the athlete, they also have responsibilities to the coach, team management and fellow support staff. Thus, the medical team should liaise closely with the coaching and fitness staff for the athletes' benefit.

Fitness staff should be included in the regular meetings of the sports medicine team so that a coordinated approach is maintained and the team clinicians should have input into training programs as part of an injury prevention strategy (see Chapter 6). It is particularly important that medical and fitness staff collaborate closely in injury rehabilitation so that a player's post-injury rehabilitation transfers seamlessly from the physiotherapist/athletic trainer's care to that of the conditioning coach when appropriate. Unfortunately, cases have arisen where the player receives conflicting instructions from 'competing' members of the rehabilitation team!

Pre-season assessment

As team sports have a distinct playing season, all players should be reviewed at the end of a season to plan appropriate individual treatment and rehabilitation for the off-season and to arrange how this will be monitored by the sports clinician. Similarly, there should be full assessment of all team members at the beginning of pre-season training. New recruits should be evaluated as soon as possible. The pre-season assessment consists of a comprehensive history and examination, looking for evidence of medical illness, a full musculoskeletal assessment and further tests, if necessary. The assessment is described further in Chapters 56 and 57 and will often be carried out in conjunction with a fitness assessment.

Educate team members

Working with a team provides an ideal opportunity to educate athletes and also coaches. Pre-season assessment provides one opportunity. Other teaching moments arise during follow-up consultations or treatments and in regular brief talks given to the team by the sports medicine practitioners. Experienced team clinicians have found that relevant topics of education include:

- injury prevention strategies (e.g. appropriate warm-up, stretching, strength programs, protective equipment)
- the importance of players reporting injuries early
- the importance of the first 24 hours in acute injury management
- a request that the players report any other treatment being received for their injuries
- nutritional advice (Chapter 37).

 In many cases the most important education for athletes in sports that are subject to drug testing is:

- advice regarding permitted and banned medications—team members should be told that it is essential that they do not take any medication without checking first with the medical staff.

Other essentials

Issues such as the quality of the medical facilities, thorough record-keeping, respect for athletes' confidentiality, availability of equipment and having an active presence around the team all contribute to being a successful team practitioner.

Facilities

Adequate facilities are essential. If possible, there should be a separate, well-equipped room at training and competition venues to enable proper assessment and treatment of injuries to take place. This room should have a door that can separate it from the rest of the training venue when privacy and confidentiality are required. The room should contain a good light source, a couch and appropriate equipment and medications.

It is the responsibility of the sports medicine team to ensure that adequate first-aid equipment is present at both training and competition venues (Chapter 44). This includes:

- stretchers (including an appropriate stretcher for the transport of spinal injuries)
- resuscitation equipment, such as an automatic external defibrillator
- an Air-Viva for oxygen, as well as splints, bandages and crutches
- an adequate supply of ice.

There should also be easy access for an ambulance if required, and a telephone with emergency numbers (ambulance, nearest hospital) must be readily available.

Record-keeping

As in all medical practice, records are important for patient care and medico-legal purposes. It becomes particularly important when more than one member of the medical team is involved in the treatment of a patient. Excellent software programs allow the practitioner to maintain records on a laptop computer.

This is particularly useful when there are various training venues or when traveling with the team (Chapter 59).

Confidentiality

It is essential that members of the sports medicine team do not discuss a player's medical problems with other team members, officials or the media without the player's express permission. The British Olympic Association has published a position statement on athlete confidentiality[8] that clearly tells coaches, managers, administrators and other team officials that the athlete comes first![8, 9] A key platform of the code of conduct states: 'Coaches wish to be informed of athletes' problems. This can only occur with the consent of the individual athlete.' The British Olympic Association has produced a consent form (see box) that other sporting bodies may consider using. The code emphasizes that even if the athlete has signed a consent form, he or she may still withhold consent for any specific consultation, test or treatment.

Athlete consent form as proposed by the British Olympic Association[9]

Athlete consent form

I agree/do not agree to relevant details from consultations, test or treatments undertaken by .... in (year/season) .... being released to (e.g. coach/performance director/member of support staff) ....

I realize that refusal to give consent for the release of details will not affect my access to medical care, treatment or testing. It cannot be guaranteed that others will not use this refusal of consent in relation to selection.

Consent can be withdrawn at any time, and only notice of its withdrawal will be released to those specified above.

I have read the notes on informed consent and fully understand them.

Signed...

Date...
(to be signed also by parent or guardian for those under 18 years)

The 'team clinician's bag'

The contents of the 'team clinician's bag' will vary depending on the type of sport, the access to other facilities and the clinician's own preferences. Some suggested contents for the 'team clinician's bag' for a sports clinician responsible for a contact sport team without immediate access to more sophisticated facilities are listed in the box (p. 957).

Being part of the 'team chemistry'

To be effective, the members of the sports medicine team must attend training sessions and competition. In this way, the medical team members gain an understanding of the physical and psychological demands placed on athletes. It also enables them to observe specific training routines and techniques, which in turn may lead to an increased understanding of the mechanism of injury. This assists the clinician in devising a sport-specific rehabilitation program. Regular attendance also means that the clinician is likely to be present when an acute injury occurs and is therefore able to institute appropriate therapy. The final advantage of being in constant attendance is an increased acceptance by the team members and other officials of the clinician as a valuable part of the team.

Recommended Reading

Apple D. Team physician—bad ethics, bad business, or both? *Orthopedics* 2002; 25(1): 16, 26.

Attarian DE. The team physician: ethics and enterprise. *J Bone Joint Surg Am* 2001; 83A(2): 293.

Bennell K, Webb G. Educating Australian physiotherapists: striving for excellence in sport and exercise medicine. *Br J Sports Med* 2000; 34: 241–3.

Mass participation event management for the team physician: a consensus statement. *Med Sci Sports Exerc* 2004; 36(11): 2004–8.

No pain, no gain. The dilemma of a team physician. *Br J Sports Med* 2001; 35(3): 141–2.

Sideline preparedness for the team physician: consensus statement. *Med Sci Sports Exerc* 2001; 33(5): 846–9.

Team physician consensus statement. *Am J Sports Med* 2000; 28(3): 440–1.

The team physician and conditioning of athletes for sports: a consensus statement. *Med Sci Sports Exerc* 2001; 33(10): 1789–93.

Tucker AM. Ethics and the professional team physician. *Clin Sports Med* 2004; 23(2): 227–41, vi.

The 'team clinician's bag'

Diagnostic instruments

Oral/rectal thermometer
Stethoscope
Blood pressure cuff
Ophthalmoscope
Otoscope
Pencil torch

Sutures/dressings

Needle holders
Forceps
Scissors—nail clippers, small
    sharp scissors and tape
    scissors
Scalpel
Scalpel blades
Syringes (2 mL, 5 mL, 10 mL)
Needles (23, 21, 16 gauge)
Sutures—nylon 3/0, 4/0, 5/0,
    6/0; dexon 3/0
Suture cutters
Local anesthetics—1%
    lignocaine (lidocaine)
—1% lignocaine (lidocaine)
    with adrenalin
    (epinephrine)
—marcaine
Steri-strips (3 mm [0.12 in.],
    6 mm [0.25 in.])
Alcohol swabs
Gauze swabs
Dressing packs
Antiseptic solution
    (povidone iodine)
Tincture of benzoin
Melolin dressing pads
Dressing strips
Bandaid plastic strips
Crepe bandages
Tube gauze

Medications

Oral analgesics (e.g.
    paracetamol
    [acetaminophen], aspirin)
Injectable analgesics (e.g.
    pethidine [meperidine],
    morphine)
NSAIDs
Antibiotics (e.g. amoxycillin
    [amoxicillin], erythromycin,
    flucloxacillin, doxycycline,
    metronidazole)
Antacid tablets
Antinausea (e.g.
    prochlorperazine [oral/IM])
Antidiarrheal (e.g.
    loperamide)
Fecal softeners
Antihistamines
Bronchodilators (e.g.
    salbutamol inhaler,
    beclomethasone inhaler)
50% glucose solution
Sedatives
Throat lozenges
Cough mixture (e.g. senega
    and ammonia)
Creams/ointments: antifungal,
    antibiotic, corticosteroid,
    anti-inflammatory
Eye/otic antibiotic drops
Tetanus toxoid

Equipment

Oral airway
Bolt cutters/screwdriver
Air splints
Triangular bandage (sling)
Tongue depressors
Cotton-tipped applicators
Rigid sports tape (2.5 cm
    [1 in.], 3.8 cm [1.5 in.], 5 cm
    [2 in.])

Hypoallergenic tape
Dressing retention tape
Elastic adhesive bandage
    (2.5 cm [1 in.], 5 cm
    [2 in.])
Compression bandage (5 cm
    [2 in.], 7.5 cm [3 in.], 10 cm
    [4 in.])
Adhesive felt
Adhesive foam
Blister pads
Adhesive spray
Coolant spray
Finger splints
Cervical collar, soft and hard
Sterile gloves, goggles, mask
Eye kit including irrigation
    solution, fluorescein, eye
    patches, local anesthetic
    and antibiotic eye drops,
    contact lens container
    (Chapter 15)
Sunscreen
Massage oil/heat rubs
Intravenous fluid and giving
    sets

Other

Urine reagent strips
Safety pins
Tampons
Contaminated needle
    container
Spare shoelaces
Batteries
Safety razor
Plastic bags (for ice)
Heel raises
Heel wedges
Arch supports
List of banned substances

References

1. Abernethy L, MacAuley D, McNally O, McCann S. How important is sport and exercise medicine to the accident and emergency specialist? A study in the UK and Ireland. *Emerg Med J* 2003; 20(6): 540–2.

2. Dubey SG, Roberts C, Adebajo AO, Snaith ML. Rheumatology training in the United Kingdom: the trainees' perspective. *Rheumatology (Oxford)* 2004; 43(7): 896–900.

3. Thompson B, MacAuley D, McNally O, O'Neill S. Defining the sports medicine specialist in the United Kingdom: a Delphi study. *Br J Sports Med* 2004; 38(2): 214–17.

4. Kannus P, Parkkari J. Sports and exercise medicine in Finland. *Br J Sports Med* 2000; 34(4): 239–40.

5. Brukner P. Sports medicine in Australia [editorial]. *Med J Aust* 1993; 158(8): 511–12.

6. Fricker P. Sports medicine education in Australia. *Br J Sports Med* 2000; 34(4): 240–1.

7. DiCello N. No pain, no gain, no compensation: exploiting professional athletes through substandard medical care administered by team physicians. *Cleve State Law Rev* 2001; 49(3): 507–38.

8. British Olympic Association. The British Olympic Association's position statement on athlete confidentiality. *Br J Sports Med* 2000; 34: 71–2.

9. MacAuley D, Bartlett R. The British Olympic Association's position statement on athlete confidentiality. *Br J Sports Med* 2000; 34: 1–2.

10. Orchard JW, Fricker PA, Brukner P. Sports medicine for professional teams. *Clin J Sport Med* 1995; 5(1): 1–3.

11. Tucker AM. Ethics and the professional team physician. *Clin Sports Med* 2004; 23(2): 227–41, vi.

12. Warren RF. The professional team physician, 1984–present. *Pediatr Ann* 2002; 31(1): 71–2.

13. Apple D. Team physician—bad ethics, bad business, or both? *Orthopedics* 2002; 25(1): 16, 26.

Traveling with a Team

WITH JILL COOK, PETER HARCOURT AND CHRIS MILNE

Traveling with a team presents the sports medicine practitioner with a considerable challenge. While friends and colleagues may consider that you are heading off on a glamorous trip, the reality is that providing quality medical support for a traveling team is stressful and exhausting.[1, 2] Being a successful member of a touring team (Fig. 59.1) requires far more than good professional skills.

The traveling sports clinician often has to fill a number of roles. These may include physician, physiotherapist, massage therapist, podiatrist, trainer, fitness adviser, dietitian, psychologist, assistant team manager, assistant coach, statistician, travel coordinator and baggage supervisor. Traveling with a team often involves working long hours in less than ideal conditions with athletes and coaches who are under great stress due to the demands of competition and travel. It also involves extended periods of time away from family and work.

The success, or otherwise, of the sports clinician traveling with a team depends on preparing carefully, working long hours, developing multiple treatment skills and having well-developed interpersonal skills and personal coping mechanisms.

Preparation

Adequate planning is the key to a successful trip. Preparation includes researching the destination, providing advice for team members and obtaining supplies. It also requires thorough self-preparation.

Things to do before travel

- Be well-versed about the travel destination. Climate, altitude, level of pollution, accommodation, food, water, vaccination requirements, security and the level of medical support at the destination must all be anticipated.[3-5] If the competition is at altitude or in the heat, acclimatization will be necessary (Chapter 53). This may entail arriving well before the competition begins.
- Obtain details about the team's accommodation. In hot climates, air-conditioning may be an advantage for comfort although it may delay heat acclimatization. Sleeping arrangements must be adequate. Particularly tall athletes require extra-long beds. Try to guarantee a dedicated medical room when traveling with a large team. If this is not possible, the clinician

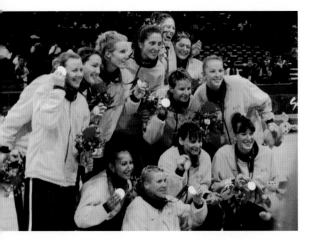

Figure 59.1 Success on the road! Although traveling with a team requires great personal sacrifice, the sports medicine practitioner can contribute to athletes' achieving their dreams

should have a hotel room to himself or herself which doubles as a treatment room and permits players to be treated with privacy and confidentiality as needed.

- Research the type of food available at the venue. If there is not sufficient high-carbohydrate food available or if the food is likely to be unfamiliar and unappetizing, it may be possible to have appropriate meals prepared. It may also be necessary to bring food, both in solid and liquid form, from home.
- Discover whether the water supply is of good quality and if there is a risk of gastrointestinal infections, especially 'traveler's diarrhea'. This will affect planning and determination of whether precautionary measures are needed.
- Vaccination requirements vary considerably between countries. Cholera and typhoid vaccinations are required in certain countries, particularly in Asia, South America and Africa.[6, 7] Travel to tropical areas may require malaria prophylaxis. Immunizations for the athlete are listed in Table 59.1. The vaccination and malaria prophylaxis requirements are constantly changing and up-to-date information should be obtained from local or national travel advisory services and from databases such as the websites of the World Health Organization and the Centers for Disease Control and Prevention in Atlanta (see Recommended Websites, p. 967). This is particularly important for illnesses where the disease pattern is rapidly evolving (e.g. the severe acute respiratory syndrome [SARS] outbreak in 2003, the avian flu which began in 2005).
- Assess medical support services, such as ambulance and hospitals, at the destination. Travel insurance, including medical cover, should be arranged for all team members.

Assessing team members' fitness

- Contact all team members, including coaches and officials, prior to departure to ask about present and past injuries and illnesses. Often officials provide a traveling clinician with much anxiety because of medical conditions such as coronary artery disease. Attempts must be made to treat injuries prior to departure. This not only benefits the athlete but reduces the subsequent load on the medical team. It may be necessary to liaise with the player's own treating clinician.
- In many cases the team will assemble at a predeparture camp. The medical support team should attend the camp to meet athletes and officials, perform comprehensive assessments and initiate treatment for any medical or musculoskeletal problem.
- Prior to departure, the clinician should ask whether the coach and officials expect non-medical tasks to be performed during the forthcoming trip. This may include responsibility for warm-ups, nutrition advice and attention to strength and conditioning. Videotaping has been needed at times! These possibly unfamiliar roles may need some brushing up.

Advice for team members

A vital part of the preparation is to provide advice for the team members about air travel (see p. 964), minimization of the effects of jet lag, precautions required with food and drink during the tour, heat acclimatization, drugs and sexual activity. This advice may be given prior to departure by hand-outs, email or team websites. This provides background information but it should be supplemented by team or individual discussions either at the predeparture

Table 59.1 Immunizations for the athlete

Basic (essential)	Recommended	Regional (depends on travel destination)
Tetanus	Hepatitis A (frequent international travel)	Malaria
Diphtheria	Hepatitis B (contact sports especially)	Typhoid fever
Measles	Influenza (annual vaccination)	Japanese encephalitis
Mumps		Cholera
Rubella		Rabies
Poliomyelitis		*Meningococcus* Yellow fever

camp or at a team meeting soon after arrival at the destination.

Diet

It is not easy for athletes to maintain good dietary practises when traveling. In some situations, it may be difficult to obtain sufficient amounts of appropriate foods. Fast food outlets are convenient but often supply high-fat foods inadequate in carbohydrate. Athletes should be advised as to wise food choices and which snacks may be appropriate. In addition, athletes often eat in village dining rooms or restaurants where buffet-style food is offered. There is a tendency for athletes to overeat in this situation if it is unfamiliar. Since the athlete may also be tapering and so burning up fewer calories, weight gain can occur. Swimmers seem to be particularly susceptible to this problem. Some suggestions regarding suitable meals while traveling are shown in the box below.

Athletes should be advised about the importance of maintaining an adequate fluid intake in hot climates.[5] If there is uncertainty about the quality of the water,

tap water and ice should be avoided and fluid intake restricted to bottled water.

To minimize the risk of traveler's diarrhea, athletes should be advised to wash their hands carefully before meals (using bottled water where necessary), eat only food that has been cooked and avoid shellfish, salads, unpasteurized milk products and unpeeled fruits.

Gender verification

Gender verification is no longer required at most World Championships or the Olympic Games. Staff should check with the relevant International Federation.

Drug testing

If drug testing is to be performed, team members must be reminded that certain medications, including many over-the-counter medications used in the treatment of coughs and colds, are banned (Chapter 61). It is vital that no athlete takes any medication without checking with the medical support team. It is also important to explain the drug testing procedure as this may be

---

Breakfast

- Avoid overeating at buffet-style breakfasts
- Wholegrain cereal with low-fat milk
- Fresh, tinned or dried fruit
- Pancakes, raisin bread, toast, muffins or crumpets topped with jam, honey, golden syrup
- Low-fat yoghurt or Fromage Frais
- Grilled tomatoes or baked beans on toast
- Fresh fruit juice, tea, coffee (in moderation)

Lunch

- Avoid high-fat choices such as French fries, pies, pastries, fried fish or chicken
- Sandwiches, rolls, bagels or pita bread with low-fat fillings (e.g. tuna, skinless chicken, egg, turkey, salad)
- Thick crust pizza with low-fat toppings—avoid salami, ham, sausage, pepperoni
- Steamed rice with stir-fried vegetables
- Plain hamburger with salad—no egg, bacon, onion or cheese
- Chicken souvlaki or doner kebab with salad
- Fruit juices, low-fat milk, mineral water

Dinner

- Avoid dishes described as fried, crispy, breaded, creamed, buttery or au gratin. Look for dishes

described as steamed, boiled, grilled, poached, chargrilled or 'in its own juice'
- Ask for sauces and butter on the side. Request extra bread, potato, rice and pasta
- Find restaurants that offer Italian foods such as pasta, salad and thick pizza. Select pasta dishes with low-fat sauces such as marinara, napolitana or vegetarian. Avoid butter on bread and excessive dressing
- From Asian restaurants, select rice or noodles with vegetables and lean chicken or beef
- Barbecued chicken (skin removed) with corn, baked potato and salad
- Thick vegetable or minestrone soup with bread, crackers or muffins
- Grilled fish with baked potato, rice, pasta and vegetables
- Fresh fruit, sorbet or gelati for desserts
- Limit alcohol and always ask for a jug of iced water or bottled water (commercial sports drinks may provide a readily available source of electrolyte as well as fluid)
- Check that the seal of drinks has not been broken, especially if buying drinks from potentially dubious sources (e.g. some roadside stalls)
- Visit the kitchen and talk to the chef. Look for fresh and recently cooked food

---

stressful, particularly for younger or inexperienced athletes. If possible, a member of the medical team should accompany the athlete to the drug test, both to provide emotional support and to ensure that the correct testing procedure is followed. Up-to-date information about drug testing and banned substances can be obtained from National Sporting Organizations and Olympic Federations. Telephone inquiry hotlines have been established in many countries and some are listed in Table 59.2. Remember to discuss illicit drug use such as marijuana or ecstasy and how this may be detected in drug testing.

Sexual activity

Team members should be warned of the dangers of acquiring sexually transmitted infections such as gonorrhea, chlamydia, hepatitis B or HIV. Abstinence guarantees prevention but condoms should be made available.

The medical bag

The next step in the preparation for travel is to assemble the medical kit of equipment and supplies. The contents of the medical kit will vary depending on the make-up of the medical support team, the size of the overall team, the destination and the local facilities available. It is advisable to be as self-sufficient as possible when traveling with a team. Obtaining equipment and medications in a foreign country may be difficult, time-consuming and expensive. The suggested contents for a medical kit for a sports clinician accompanying a team to overseas competition are shown in the box opposite. Athletes should be advised that it is their responsibility to provide any

Table 59.2 Contact details for obtaining drug information in various countries

Country	Drug information hotline telephone number/website address
Australia	(02) 6206 0200/<www.asda.org.au>
Canada	1 800 672 7775/<www.cces.ca> (613) 748 5755
Great Britain	0171 380 8029 (UK Sports Council) 0181 864 0609 or 0181 992 1963 (British Olympic Association Medical Centre)
New Zealand	0800 DRUGFREE = 0800 378 437
South Africa	(12) 841 2686/2639 (SA Institute for Drug-Free Sport)
United States	(800) 233 0393

supplements (e.g. vitamin, mineral or carbohydrate supplements) they may wish to take but the clinician should ensure that banned substances are not inadvertently included by an athlete.

 When traveling internationally, take a written inventory of the contents of each bag for customs purposes. A non-confrontational response to customs checks usually works best! Do not carry narcotic analgesics; tramadol is effective for severe pain and is subject to fewer restrictions in most countries.

Clinician's hip bag

A small hip bag[8] is a useful way to carry small quantities of basic medical supplies when traveling by airplane; this contains the essentials to provide team members symptom relief until hold baggage can be accessed. Note that even small nail scissors are not permitted in cabin baggage.

The precise contents will vary according to individual team needs, but consider including:

- simple analgesics (e.g. paracetamol [acetaminophen], soluble aspirin)
- adhesive plasters (e.g. bandaids)
- nose spray (e.g. oxymetazoline)
- throat lozenges
- antiemetic (e.g. metoclopramide, prochlorperazine buccal tablets)
- antidiarrheal (e.g. loperamide)
- sedatives (e.g. triazolam) on long night flights.

Self-preparation

Finally, it is important for the clinician to prepare himself or herself for travel. Because trips are always extremely busy, it is important to be well rested and in good health prior to departure. It is also important to spend time with loved ones prior to departure, especially for lengthy trips. A summary of the guidelines for preparation for travel with a team is shown below.

1. Information
   (a) Venue
      (i) climate
      (ii) altitude
      (iii) pollution
      (iv) accommodation
      (v) food
      (vi) security
      (vii) water
      (viii) vaccination requirements

Contents of the medical bag for interstate and international travel

Diagnostic instruments

Oral/rectal thermometer
Stethoscope
Blood pressure cuff
Ophthalmoscope
Otoscope
Pencil torch

Sutures/dressings

Needle holders
Forceps
Scissors: nail clippers, small sharp
    scissors and tape scissors
Scalpel
Scalpel blades
Syringes (2 mL, 5 mL, 10 mL)
Needles (23, 21, 16 gauge)
Sutures: nylon 3/0, 4/0, 5/0, 6/0;
    dexon 3/0
Suture cutters
Local anesthetics:
    1% lignocaine (lidocaine)
    1% lignocaine (lidocaine) with
        adrenalin (epinephrine)
    marcaine
Steri-strips (3 mm [0.12 in.], 6 mm
    [0.25 in.])
Alcohol swabs
Gauze swabs
Dressing packs
Antiseptic solution (povidone
    iodine)
Tincture of benzoin
Melolin dressing pads
Dressing strip
Bandaid plastic strips
Crepe bandages
Tube gauze

Medications

Oral analgesics (e.g. paracetamol
    [acetaminophen], aspirin)

Injectable analgesics (e.g.
    pethidine [meperidine],
    morphine)
Adrenalin (epinephrine) for
    anaphylaxis
NSAIDs
Antibiotics (e.g. amoxycillin
    [amoxicillin], erythromycin,
    flucloxacillin, doxycycline,
    metronidazole)
Antacid tablets
Antinausea (e.g.
    prochlorperazine [oral/IM])
Antidiarrheal (e.g. loperamide)
Oral contraceptive pill
Fecal softeners
Antihistamines
Bronchodilators (e.g. salbutamol
    inhaler, beclomethasone
    inhaler)
50% glucose solution
Sedatives and hypnotics
Throat lozenges
Cough mixture (e.g. senega and
    ammonia)
Creams/ointments: antifungal,
    antibiotic, corticosteroid,
    anti-inflammatory
Eye/otic antibiotic drops
Tetanus toxoid

Equipment

Oral airway
Bolt cutters/screwdriver
Air splints
Triangular bandage (sling)
Tongue depressors
Cotton-tipped applicators
Rigid sports tape (2.5 cm
    [1 in.], 3.8 cm [1.5 in.],
    5 cm [2 in.])
Hypoallergenic tape
Dressing retention tape

Elastic adhesive bandage
    (2.5 cm [1 in.], 5 cm [2 in.])
Compression bandage (5 cm
    [2 in.], 7.5 cm [3 in.], 10 cm
    [4 in.])
Adhesive felt
Adhesive foam
Blister pads
Adhesive spray
Coolant spray
Finger splints
Cervical collar, soft and hard
Sterile gloves, goggles, mask
Eye kit including irrigation
    solution, fluorescein, eye
    patches, local anesthetic and
    antibiotic eye drops, contact
    lens container (Chapter 15)
Sunscreen
Massage oil/heat rubs
Electrotherapy (e.g. TENS,
    portable laser)
Portable couch
Alarm clock
Intravenous fluid and giving sets

Other

Urine reagent strips
Safety pins
Tampons
Contaminated needle
    container
Spare shoelaces
Flexible orthoses
Batteries
Safety razor
Plastic bags (for ice)
Heel raises
Heel wedges
Arch supports
List of banned substances
Transformer and dual voltage
    connector (if appropriate)

(ix) malaria prophylaxis
(x) available medical support
(b) Team members
    (i) past and present illnesses and
        injuries

2. Advice
    (a) air travel
    (b) jet lag
    (c) food
    (d) drink

(e) drugs
(f) gender verification
(g) infectious diseases
3. Medical kit
(a) medication
(b) tape, bandages, etc.
(c) other (e.g. nutritional supplements)

Air travel and jet lag

Air travel is an important part of professional and international sport. Short-distance air travel (up to 3 hours) does not appear to present any problems to the athlete.[9] On the other hand, extended air travel, as may be required for major events such as Olympic Games or World Championships, can provide significant problems.

Jet lag, when the body is unable to adapt rapidly to a time zone shift and normal body rhythms lose synchrony with the environment, is aggravated by a number of factors in addition to the amount of time zone change.[10–12] Factors that appear to increase the severity of jet lag include traveling east rather than west, age, impaired health, lack of previous travel experience, sleep deprivation, dehydration, stress, alcohol and excessive food intake.[13–17]

The trip can be made significantly more comfortable if the team management plans ahead to obtain seats on less busy flights that minimize stopovers and time spent waiting for connections. Advanced planning also permits players' preferred food options, such as low salt, low fat, vegetarian, seafood or 'sports meals', to be available for them on the flight. Especially on international flights with connections that have more than a 1 hour break, the team may try to negotiate entry into the airport club lounges for all the athletes.

Whether or not pharmacological agents such as short-acting hypnotics (e.g. triazolam 0.25–0.5 mg) or melatonin (5 mg taken at night) reduce the impact of jet lag remains unclear.[18, 19] Most team doctors traveling with Super 14 Rugby teams advocate the use of triazolam 0.25–0.5 mg for travel on a long night-time sector. Some team members may require additional doses for a few days after arriving at the destination if travel has occurred over more than about six time zones.

The Cochrane Collaboration concluded that 'Melatonin is remarkably effective in preventing or reducing jet-lag, and occasional short-term use appears to be safe. It should be recommended to adult travelers flying across five or more time zones, particularly in an easterly direction, and especially if they have experienced jet-lag on previous journeys'.[18]

 PRACTISE PEARL Consistent with these data, we recommend that, if possible, upon arrival at the destination, athletes spend some time outdoors, rather than indoors, during the sunlight hours so that natural light can have a physiological effect on resetting circadian rhythm.

Experienced practitioners and many successful sportspeople suggest that low-intensity physical activity early after arrival helps promote adjustment to the new time zone.

Experienced air travelers have developed a series of guidelines to minimize the adverse effects of long-distance travel. These have been phrased in the second person in the box opposite so that they may be photocopied and given to athletes.

The medical room

A medical room should be established soon after arrival. Ideally, this should be a large room separated from any bedrooms. Hours of treatment should be specified so that the practitioner has adequate time for meal and exercise breaks. This must be strictly enforced as athletes have a tendency to extend these hours. An appointment sheet enables athletes to plan their treatment and it also provides a record of treatment. The clinician should ensure that athletes know the room number of the medical staff in case of emergencies at night. It is important that the team manager knows how to contact the medical staff if the room is unattended. It also helps to obtain an athlete room list from the team manager.

For trips involving a single venue, a portable examination couch (treatment table) is valuable for the comfort of both the athlete and treating clinician. A low soft bed may not be an appropriate site for massage or spinal mobilization. On trips involving multiple venues, the advantages of having a treatment couch must be weighed up against the inconvenience of transporting the couch. When traveling with two clinicians, the compromise is often to take one portable table and use the hotel bed as a second treatment site for electrotherapy, massage and so on.

Illness

Traveler's diarrhea

Traveler's diarrhea, the most common infectious illness encountered when on the road with a team, is generally due to non-viral pathogens such as enterotoxigenic *Escherichia coli*, *Salmonella*, *Shigella*, *Campylobacter* or *Giardia lamblia*. Strategies for

Guidelines to make long-distance travel as straightforward as possible

1. If you have control of flight times, consider arriving at your final destination late afternoon.[12]
2. In the days prior to departure, adjust your eating, sleeping and training times towards those of the destination. Once the trip begins, set your watch to the time at the destination and be guided by that as to when you eat and sleep, and try to remain active.
3. The timing of sleep on long flights can help a lot to minimize jet lag once you arrive at the destination. For a morning arrival, try to sleep in the hours before arrival. For an evening arrival, try to sleep earlier in the flight depending on its duration. When it is time to sleep, recline the seat fully, ensure you are warm and use the pillows provided or an inflatable pillow. Eyeshades and earplugs may be useful.
4. When organizing seating on the plane, try to get your preferred seat either at check-in or by swapping with a team mate or official. Tall players will often be provided the exit row; this has additional leg room. Some players prefer the aisle seat because of ease of access to the bathroom and opportunities to walk. Some athletes find it easier to sleep in window seats.
5. Plan ways to avoid boredom during long flights and have any material you need (e.g. your favorite books, iPod, DVDs, CDs, card sets) in your cabin luggage. Hopefully the movies will be good ones!
6. It is important to be active when possible. Regular walking in the aisle reduces risk of deep venous thrombosis, permits a chance to get extra water from the water fountain and can also provide you an opportunity to stretch (e.g. near some exits). Take advantage of stopovers to stretch and walk. Jogging or more aerobic exercises are not recommended as your muscles will be tight and your joints stiff.
7. If you think the airline food may not be to your liking (e.g. taste, fat content of many 'snacks'), bring some of your own food. Consume some fruit if possible.
8. The dry atmosphere of the aircraft cabin tends to lead to dehydration, which may be aggravated by drinking coffee or alcohol, both of which have a diuretic effect. Ask for additional rehydrating drinks as needed. Most appropriate drinks are water, mineral water, fruit juice or lemonade. Caffeine-containing drinks, such as coffee, tea or cola, and alcohol should be avoided. Excessive sparkling fluids (e.g. soft drinks [pop] or sparkling mineral water) can lead to abdominal discomfort in the low-pressure cabin environment.
9. Remember to stay calm when traveling. Long-distance travel is inevitably associated with delays at airline check-ins, customs or due to inclement weather and mechanical problems. Adopt a relaxed attitude to these delays—they are beyond your control.
10. Upon arrival at the destination, adopt local time and eating habits. Make every effort to stay awake during the day even if you feel very tired. Some exercise can help if you feel likely to doze off. Where possible, we advocate you avoid using sleeping tablets as they delay acclimatization of normal circadian patterns. On arrival, weather permitting, try to spend some time in the natural sunlight to help your body adjust to the new time zone.

decreasing risk of exposure to infection were discussed in the dietary advice above (p. 961). Although all antibiotics have the potential to cause occasional adverse side-effects, it may be advisable to use them prophylactically when traveling to high-risk areas for major competitions. Examples of short-term prophylaxis used by some teams include either 500 mg ciprofloxacin daily, 100 mg doxycycline daily or the combination of 800 mg sulfamethoxazole with 160 mg trimethoprim daily.[5] Note that the first two of these choices can produce photosensitivity.

Traveler's diarrhea is usually mild and self-limiting but may occasionally be severe and distressing. Any illness near the time of competition is particularly disturbing for the athlete. The condition should be treated aggressively with loperamide, two tablets initially and then one tablet with each loose bowel action until symptoms abate. At the same time, the player should drink dilute fluid to prevent dehydration. The most suitable fluid intake is a glucose–electrolyte solution made up with bottled water. If symptoms persist or are accompanied by systemic symptoms such as fever or sweating, treatment is commenced with antibiotics such as doxycycline (200 mg stat then 100 mg 12 hourly) or norfloxacin (400 mg twice daily for three days).

Upper respiratory tract infections

Upper respiratory tract infections are also common among traveling athletes. Moving from one environment to another exposes the athlete to different strains of respiratory viruses. Air travel and accommodation in air-conditioned hotels also increase the risk of upper respiratory tract infections. At events where drug testing is taking place, therapeutic options for the treatment of these infections are limited. Antihistamines may be helpful. Throat lozenges and corticosteroid nasal sprays can provide symptomatic relief. Early intervention with antibiotics should be considered.

There is some concern in a team situation of the possibility of cross-infection between team mates. Any team member with a significant viral or bacterial infection should be isolated to minimize the risk of spread throughout the team. This may involve the infected team member having to sleep in a room away from other athletes and careful handling of water bottles and towels.

Injury

A good time to implement injury prevention strategies, such as warm-up, stretching, strength maintenance and massage, is when a team is on the road. Traveling with a team also permits early intensive treatment of injuries, which, in conjunction with the high motivation of athletes, often results in some dramatic responses.

While on tour, the sports clinician may need to provide the services of other health professionals (multiskilling). For instance, if the sole clinician is a physician, he or she needs to be able to use electrotherapeutic modalities, and provide soft tissue therapy and spinal mobilization in the treatment of soft tissue injury. Similarly, a physiotherapist traveling with a team needs to have a broader understanding of medical issues than one who works exclusively in an office. Every opportunity should be taken to acquire the necessary skills before going on tour. However, the clinician who travels with a team cannot be an expert in all areas of medicine. If faced with a problem beyond one's knowledge and experience, it is advisable to seek assistance, either locally from another clinician or by telephone or email from a colleague at home.

Drug testing

The sports clinician must be familiar with the drug-testing rules for the particular competition, including the list of banned drugs and the testing procedure (Chapter 61). The clinician should attempt to meet the chief medical officer in charge of drug testing prior to the event. The medical support team needs to remind athletes constantly that they must not take any medication without approval.

Sometimes a conflict will arise when the clinician needs to decide whether to stay with an athlete who is to be drug tested (which may involve a wait of some hours) or to return to the team's accommodation to treat other athletes. This should be discussed with players and the coaching staff prior to the situation arising but may need to be decided according to the needs of each situation.

Local contacts

It is best to contact local medical officials before arrival if possible and modern communication has made this increasingly easier. National consulates and embassies may provide useful sources of information about the quality of local medical personnel and facilities. Upon arrival and before competition begins, the traveling practitioner should meet local medical support staff. As well as facilitating immediate care of the athletes, this provides an opportunity to exchange ideas with clinicians from different backgrounds.

Psychological skills

One of the main roles of the medical team while on tour is to provide psychological support to the rest of the team.[20] Travel can be extremely stressful to team members and this may be compounded by the stress of high-level competition. There is a tendency for team members, coaches and officials alike to unburden their problems onto the medical staff. These problems may be related to poor performance or, alternatively, to personal problems, sometimes involving other members of the team. Personal conflicts within a team are common, particularly when the team is unsuccessful. It is important that the members of the medical support team retain a positive and professional attitude at all times.

The medical support team is expected to adopt a leadership role in team situations. The most difficult situation for medical team members is in situations of conflict, particularly between the coach and one or more team members. It is essential that the medical team gives the coach their full support, while at the same time using their psychological and interpersonal skills to resolve conflict if possible.

Personal coping skills

The medical support team should adopt certain personal skills to enable them to cope with the stresses of traveling with a team.[20] Adequate preparation is an essential component of success on tour. It is also important to control the hours of work to ensure adequate time for meals, exercise and sleep. It may also, on occasion, be necessary to give priority to certain team members who may play more important roles in a team sport. This needs to be explained to all team members. It is important at all times to adopt a positive mental attitude in spite of any excessive physical or emotional demands of the job. On return from traveling with a team, it is time to rest and spend quality time with family and friends. This is the ideal time to review the tour and submit a tour report. It is also important to consider ways in which performance could be improved if further travel opportunities arise.

Why some clinicians 'fail' on tour

There are a number of problems for the medical support team associated with a traveling team. These include the long hours, the demanding nature of the work, complex group dynamics, the stress of competition, the need to perform multiple roles and the lack of back-up professional support. These problems all contribute to the relatively high failure rate of medical support team members, as perceived by coaches, officials and other team members.

Recommended Websites

Communicable Diseases Australia: <http://www.cda.gov.au/about.htm>

US Centers for Disease Prevention and Control: <http://www.cdc.gov>

World Health Organization (WHO): <http://www.who.int/topics/en/>

WHO site on avian influenza: <http://www.who.int/csr/disease/avian_influenza/en/>

WHO site on SARS: <http://www.who.int/csr/sars/en/>

Recommended Reading

Brown DW. Medical issues associated with international competition. Guidelines for the traveling physician. *Clin Sports Med* 1998; 17: 739–54.

A practical summary of the issues by a very experienced soccer physician. Particularly enlightening on the psychological aspects of team dynamics.

Manfredini R, Manfredini F, Fersini C, et al. Circadian rhythms, athletic performance, and jet lag. *Br J Sports Med* 1998; 32: 101–6.

Milne C. Medical problems on tour. *Phys Ther Sport* 2002; 3: 97–109.

An article for physiotherapists who provide team coverage.

Walker E, Williams G, Raeside F, Calvert L. *ABC of Healthy Travel*. 5th edn. London: BMJ Books, 1997.

Easily accessible information, consistent with other titles in this series.

World Health Organization. *International Travel and Health: Situation as on 1 January 2005*. Geneva: WHO, 2005.

Internationally respected publication, updated annually.

Postolache T, ed. *Sports Chronobiology. An Issue of Clinics in Sports Medicine 24-2*. New York: Saunders, 2005.

Young M, Fricker P, Maughan R, et al. The traveling athlete: issues relating to the Commonwealth Games, Malaysia, 1998. *Clin J Sport Med* 1998; 8: 130–5.

An excellent summary, particularly for athletes traveling to hot and humid countries.

References

1. Milne C. New Zealand Olympic experience—Sydney 2000. *Br J Sports Med* 2001; 35: 281.
2. Milne C, Shaw M, Steinweg J. Medical issues relating to the Sydney Olympic Games. *Sports Med* 1999; 28: 287–98.
3. Gioulekas D, Damialis A, Papakosta D, et al. 15-year aeroallergen records. Their usefulness in Athens Olympics, 2004. *Allergy* 2003; 58: 933–8.
4. Sparling PB. Environmental conditions during the 1996 Olympic Games: a brief follow-up report. *Clin J Sport Med* 1997; 7: 159–61.
5. Young M, Fricker P, Maughan R, et al. The travelling athlete: issues relating to the Commonwealth Games, Malaysia, 1998. *Br J Sports Med* 1998; 32: 77–81.
6. Pollack RJ, Marcus LC. A travel medicine guide to arthropods of medical importance. *Infect Dis Clin North Am* 2005; 19: 169–83.
7. Siedenburg J, Perry I, Stuben U. Tropical medicine and travel medicine: medical advice for aviation medical examiners concerning flight operations in tropical areas. *Aviat Space Environ Med* 2005; 76: A1–30.
8. Milne C. The doctor's hip bag: advice sheet. *NZ J Sports Med* 2003; 31: 39.
9. Steenland K, Deddens JA. Effect of travel and rest on performance of professional basketball players. *Sleep* 1997; 20: 366–9.

10. Recht LD, Lew RA, Schwartz WJ. Baseball teams beaten by jet lag. *Nature* 1995; 377: 583.

11. Lemmer B, Kern RI, Nold G, et al. Jet lag in athletes after eastward and westward time-zone transition. *Chronobiol Int* 2002; 19: 743–64.

12. Waterhouse J, Edwards B, Nevill A, et al. Identifying some determinants of 'jet lag' and its symptoms: a study of athletes and other travellers. *Br J Sports Med* 2002; 36: 54–60.

13. Atkinson G, Drust B, Reilly T, et al. The relevance of melatonin to sports medicine and science. *Sports Med* 2003; 33: 809–31.

14. Cardinali DP, Bortman GP, Liotta G, et al. A multifactorial approach employing melatonin to accelerate resynchronization of sleep-wake cycle after a 12 time-zone westerly transmeridian flight in elite soccer athletes. *J Pineal Res* 2002; 32: 41–6.

15. Manfredini R, Manfredini F, Conconi F. Standard melatonin intake and circadian rhythms of elite athletes after a transmeridian flight. *J Int Med Res* 2000; 28: 182–6.

16. Sando B. Olympic medicine. *Lancet* 2003; 362 (suppl): s50–1.

17. Youngstedt SD, O'Connor PJ. The influence of air travel on athletic performance. *Sports Med* 1999; 28: 197–207.

18. Herxheimer A, Petrie KJ. Melatonin for the prevention and treatment of jet lag. *Cochrane Database Syst Rev* 2005; issue 4. Available online: <http://cochrane.org/reviews/end/ab001520.html>.

19. Petrie KJ, Powell D, Broadbent E. Fatigue self-management strategies and reported fatigue in international pilots. *Ergonomics* 2004; 47: 461–8.

20. Brown DW. Medical issues associated with international competition. Guidelines for the traveling physician. *Clin Sports Med* 1998; 17: 739–54, vi.

Medical Coverage of Endurance Events

WITH TIMOTHY NOAKES

The organizers of endurance events are obliged to provide medical coverage both to enable competitors to have immediate access to optimal management of medical problems and to relieve the burden on local medical services. These endurance events may include marathons, ultramarathons, triathlons and 'ironman' triathlon events, as well as long-distance events such as walking, swimming, cycling and cross-country skiing. Many of these events will have large numbers of competitors with varying degrees of fitness.

Blisters, bruises, lacerations and muscle cramps are the cause of a large number of presentations to the medical tent at these events. Overuse injuries may develop or may be aggravated in athletes by competing in an endurance event, whereas traumatic injuries may occur as a result of a fall in a crowded running field or from a bike, for example. Thermal injuries (heatstroke or hypothermia) are common in endurance events (Chapters 53 and 54). As there is the possibility of cardiovascular collapse during such events, appropriate facilities must be available.

The precise details of the medical services required will depend on the particular sport, the duration and intensity of the activity and the prevailing environmental conditions. Medical teams that have worked at endurance events for years are able to predict the expected numbers of casualties. It is vital to keep medical records for all athletes treated at a particular event and to analyze these data for historical trends (Table 60.1). We will consider a marathon foot race with 1000 competitors as the basis for our recommendations. The figures should be adjusted according to the type of events and the number of competitors.

Table 60.1 The expected percentage of race starters likely to be admitted to the central medical care facility at a sporting event with 1000 competitors[1]

Activity	Percentage of race starters
Running	
42 km	2–20
21 km	1–5
Ultratriathlon >200 km	15–30
Cycling	5
Cross-country skiing	5

Race organization

Specific pre-race strategies to enhance the safety of the competitors include the following:

1. Schedule the race at a time of year and day when environmental conditions will not adversely affect performance or health. The medical director of the race should have the authority to cancel the race should adverse weather conditions prevail. The American College of Sports Medicine position statement recommends that if the wet bulb globe temperature index is above 28°C (82°F) or if the ambient dry bulb temperature is below –20°C (–4°F), organizers should consider canceling or rescheduling the event.[2]
2. Ensure adequate provision of carbohydrate-containing fluids en route, as this is essential.
3. Plan the race course so that the start and finish are in an area large enough to accommodate all spectators and race finishers, medical facilities

and quick get-away routes for emergency vehicles. Place first-aid stations along the route at points allowing for rapid access by emergency vehicles and ideally about 3–5 km apart.

4. Set preparticipation screening and qualification standards to ensure that unfit and inexperienced athletes do not place themselves at undue medical risk during the event.

5. Provide pre-race seminars for participants by medical personnel, as this can reduce the number of casualties. Advice may include:
   (a) correct training
   (b) consumption of sufficient carbohydrate before the race
   (c) eating a pre-race breakfast and drinking approximately 500–800 mL of a 4–7% carbohydrate solution every hour during the race
   (d) warning of the dangers of competing during or shortly after a febrile illness or while taking medications.

6. Ensure registration forms include questions regarding past and present medical history. This enables identification of, for example, athletes with diabetes, asthma and coronary artery disease. Such athletes could be sent specific information advising them on safety precautions such as wearing a medical bracelet.

7. Implement an 'impaired competitor' strategy. Strategically positioned first-aid helpers should be permitted to stop athletes who appear ill and unable to finish the course. There should be vehicles to transport these competitors to the finish line.

8. Advise the local hospital emergency department of the forthcoming race and the likely number and nature of casualties.

9. Hold meetings between the various members of the medical team (see below).

10. Ensure an emergency transport service is available to bring problem cases to the central medical facility or to the nearest hospital emergency facility. Helicopter evacuation has proven invaluable for prompt treatment of athletes suffering cardiac arrest and other life-threatening conditions.

The medical team

A medical director of appropriate expertise should be appointed a number of months prior to the staging of an endurance event to work closely with the event director. Early appointment of a medical director permits him or her to implement the pre-race strategies outlined above.

The medical director is responsible for the preparation of medical services and the supervision of the medical team on the day of the event. As endurance events are commonly held over a large area, communication between the different members of the medical team is the highest priority. The medical director should ensure adequate means of communication are available through the use of a two-way radio system or cellular network system.

The medical team should consist of appropriately trained doctors (sporting injuries and medical emergencies), physiotherapists, sports/athletic trainers, nurses, podiatrists and masseurs. For an endurance event with 1000 competitors, the medical team should number approximately 20, of which at least one-third should be doctors. Approximately 60% of the medical team should be situated in the medical areas near the finishing line, 10% of the medical team should be at the finish line itself, 20% of the medical team should be distributed at the first-aid stations along the route and 10% of the medical team should be patrolling the route in road cars, bicycles or ambulances. In shorter events, a greater proportion of the medical team should be situated near the finish line.

The medical team should practice performing emergency procedures, athlete evacuation and rapid assessment of the collapsed athlete prior to the event. At peak periods in a large race of 10 000–20 000 competitors, it is common to have four to six athletes requiring attention every minute—a much faster rate of admission than even the busiest inner-city trauma centers. Thus, the medical team must have procedures well rehearsed. This preparation period also provides the medical director the opportunity to ensure that all caregivers are using the most recent, evidence-based guidelines for the management of casualties.[3, 4] In large events(>3000 competitors) or in adverse environmental conditions, at least one fully equipped mobile intensive care ambulance should be in attendance near the finish line. In small events, the ambulance service should be notified that the event is taking place.

First-aid stations

First-aid stations should be placed en route at strategic positions, providing a stretch and massage facility for cramping muscles, first aid (plasters, bandaids) for chafing skin and blistered feet, and identification of the at-risk runner who is confused or delirious.

These stations provide a center from which athletes can be transported to the central medical facility or to a nearby hospital emergency department. Thus, stations should be positioned in areas that have good access to exit routes as needed.

In running events, first-aid stations should be about 3–5 km apart. Practitioners skilled in treating common musculoskeletal problems and administering emergency first aid should staff these. A doctor should staff each of a number of first-aid stations. All first-aid stations should be in communication with the medical director. In larger events, a road car or ambulance should patrol the course with a doctor in attendance.

Drink stations are usually situated next to first-aid stations. It is important that the two be separated by at least 50 m so that the large crowds passing through the drink stations do not interfere with first-aid management. Additional drink stations should be situated at approximately 2–2.5 km intervals in events such as a marathon.[5, 6] For events lasting less than 1 hour, water is the fluid of choice for rehydration. For longer events, a glucose–electrolyte drink is preferred in order to improve endurance and to prevent hypoglycemia.

Medical facility at the race finish

The layout of the central medical station will depend on the facilities available to the race organizers. Figure 60.1 shows the floor plan of the medical facility at the end of the 56-km Two Oceans ultramarathon foot race held annually in Cape Town, South Africa.[1] The green and red zones are for non-severe and severe cases, respectively. Other areas are allocated for the diagnostic laboratory, physiotherapy, medical supplies and toilets.

Note that the red zone for emergencies such as cardiovascular collapse, hypothermia and heatstroke is best located immediately adjacent to the triage station. The red zone can be constructed to afford a degree of privacy for distressed or seriously ill patients and permit discrete measurement of rectal temperatures. This area should be staffed by emergency

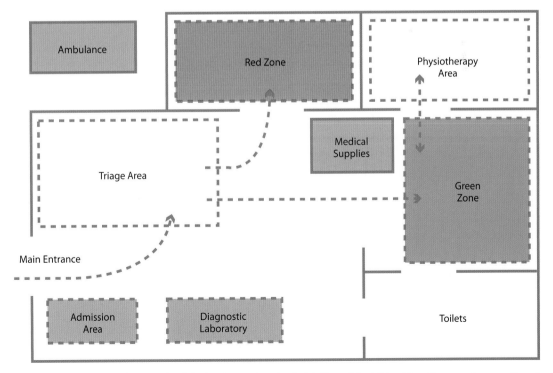

Figure 60.1 Floor plan of the medical facility located at the finish line of the 56-km Two Oceans ultramarathon foot race held in Cape Town, South Africa

trained doctors and nurses. An ambulance should be located next to the red zone to allow rapid transport of emergency cases.

The benefit of this type of system over the undifferentiated medical tent that was prevalent in the past is that potentially lethal emergencies are much less likely to be overlooked in the general hustle and bustle of athletes with numerous important but not life-threatening musculoskeletal problems. Figure 60.2 provides guidelines for the activities that need to be completed in each of the areas.

The equipment needs for a race medical center include the following:

1. Chairs and tables for the computer operator at the admission area, for the laboratory technologist and the diagnostic equipment, and for the other medical equipment and drugs.
2. Stretchers for transporting collapsed athletes from the race finish to the medical facilities. These are also used for athletes to lie on in the green and red zones. Stretchers must be

rigid so the foot can be elevated and collapsed athletes can be nursed, at least initially, in the head-down position (Chapter 53). Some A-frame stands are needed to elevate the foot of the stretcher. These are removed once the athlete's cardiovascular status has normalized.
3. Blankets for each stretcher. These allow for discrete measurement of rectal temperature (Chapter 53) and treatment of hypothermia (Chapter 54).
4. Plastic baths large enough to accommodate the torso of 40–90 kg (6.3–14.5 stone) athletes. These are filled with ice water and are used to treat heatstroke (Chapter 53).
5. Refrigerator facility—a mobile refrigerator truck is ideal for large races.
6. Computer terminal linked to the race finish.
7. Blood electrolyte and sodium analyzers. Ideally, serum sodium and potassium concentrations should be measured in all patients. However, this is essential in all subjects who are diagnosed as 'dehydrated'

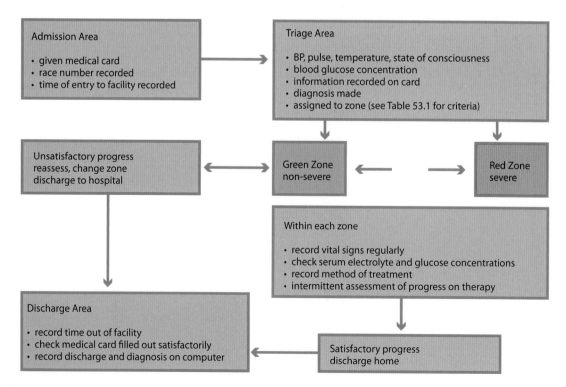

Figure 60.2 Suggested flow chart for the management of athletes once they enter the central medical facility (see Fig. 60.1)

and in need of intravenous fluids. A serum sodium concentration below 130 mmol/L (130 mEq/L) indicates that the athlete is more likely over- rather than under-hydrated.

8. Bins for rubbish and 'sharps'.

9. Toilet facilities.

10. Medications and equipment. Table 60.2 lists the resuscitation and medical equipment and Table 60.3 the medications required to cope with the expected emergency conditions. A pharmacist should be present to control the distribution of medications.

11. Given that over 60% of runners requiring attention after a marathon require physiotherapy services, it is ideal if a separate physiotherapy area can be set aside from the central medical facility. Many endurance events also provide a massage tent for athletes. As there are often a large number of minor foot injuries associated with endurance running events, the presence of a podiatrist is of great assistance also.

Additional supplies required for the medical tents and first-aid stations are shown in the boxes on page 974.

Table 60.2 Essential resuscitation and diagnostic tools for an endurance sporting event with 1000 competitors

Resuscitation tools	Diagnostic tools
Oral airways (sizes 6–8)	Stethoscopes (5)
Resuscitation masks (disposable)	Sphygmomanometers for blood pressure measurement (5)
Defribrillator	Rectal thermometers (5 with disinfectant)
Oxygen cylinder/mask (2)	Torches
	Ophthalmoscope and otoscope
	Glucometers for blood monitoring (2)
	Reflex hammer
	Blood electrolyte analyzer
	Urine sticks
	Peak flow meter (1)

Table 60.3 Basic medications required in the medical facility at endurance sporting events with 1000 competitors

Mode of administration	Medication
Injectable	Atropine (0.4 mg/mL)
	Dexamethasone (4 mg/mL)
	Morphine sulfate 15 mg/cc
	Dextrose 50%
	Adrenalin (epinephrine) (1:1000) (1 mg/mL)
	Salbutamol for nebulizer
	Metoclopramide
	Cardiac resuscitation drugs: atropine, lignocaine (lidocaine), frusemide
	Xylocaine (local anesthetic)
	Tetanus toxoid
Inhalation	Salbutamol inhaler
Oral	Paracetamol (acetaminophen) (500 mg)
	Sublingual glyceryl trinitrate (nitroglycerin) (0.4 mg)
	Isordil spray
	Chlorzoxazone tablets (500 mg)
	Loperamide capsules (2 mg)
Topical	Propacaine (0.5%) eye anesthetic
	Water-soluble lubricant
	Povidone iodine
	Tincture of benzoin

Supplies required for medical stations at the finish line of a marathon with 1000 competitors

Surgical instruments and disposables
Scissors
Latex gloves
Syringes (3 mL, 5 mL, 10 mL)
Needles (18, 21, 25 gauge)
Steri-strips, bandaids
Skin disinfectant
Adhesive bandages
Gauze pads
Suture equipment (disposable)
Space blanket
Fluid administration sets; cannulas, poles, giving
    sets (10)
Normal saline for intravenous use (10 × 1 L)
5% dextrose for intravenous use (2 × 1 L)
Haemacel for intravenous use (2 × 1 L)

Other equipment

Ice and plastic bags (100 kg of ice)
Water (500 L)
Glucose–electrolyte drink (to make 250 L)
Cups (2000)
Towels
Blankets (10) and space blankets
Rigid-frame stretchers (10)
Nebulizer (2)
Inflatable arm and leg splints (2 each)
Slings (5)
Rigid strapping tape (various sizes)
Elastic bandages (various sizes)
Tape scissors
Dressing packs (10)
Eye pads
Petroleum jelly
Pens and paper for record collection
Laptop computer for data entry
Athletic trainer's kit
Podiatrist's kit (scalpel, sharp scissors,
    disinfectant, skin care pad, adhesive felt)

Supplies required at a first-aid station along a marathon course with 1000 competitors

Stretchers (5)
Blankets (5)
10 cm (4 in.) and 15 cm (7.5 in.) elastic bandages
    (6 each)
Gauze pads
Rigid strapping tape
Dressing packs (5)
Skin disinfectant
Inflatable arm and leg splints (1 each)
Athletic trainer's kit
Petroleum jelly
Pen and paper for record collection

Conclusion

The risks associated with endurance events can be reduced with adequate preparation, good medical coverage on the day of the event and, most importantly, education of the competitors. Educating the competitors regarding some of the pitfalls of competing in an endurance event will not only improve their performance but will also reduce the risk of any major problem developing.

Medical input into the planning of the event is essential. The risk of thermal injury is reduced if the event is held at a time that is likely to avoid extremes of heat or cold. Events held in warmer climates should be commenced early in the morning or in the evening. Adequate facilities and equipment should be provided with well-stocked, regular drink stations along the route.

The presence of experienced, trained medical and paramedical staff to deal with any emergency will dramatically reduce the risk of serious problems. A functional layout of the medical facility can permit rapid, appropriate care of all race participants.

Recommended Reading

Hew-Butler T, Almond C, Ayus JC, et al. Exercise-Associated Hyponatremia (EAH) Consensus Panel. Consensus statement of the 1st International Exercise-Associated Hyponatremia Consensus Development Conference, Cape Town, South Africa 2005. *Clin J Sport Med* 2005; 15(4): 208–13.

Noakes, TD. *The Lore of Running*. 4th edn. Champaign: Human Kinetics, 2003.

Speedy DB, Noakes TD, Kimber NE, et al. Fluid balance during and after an ironman triathlon. *Clin J Sport Med* 2001; 11(1): 44–50.

Speedy DB, Noakes TD, Boswell T, Thompson JM, Rehrer N, Boswell DR. Response to a fluid load in athletes with a history of exercise induced hyponatremia. *Med Sci Sports Exerc* 2001; 33(9): 1434–42.

References

1. Holtzhausen LM, Noakes TD. Collapsed ultraendurance athlete: proposed mechanisms and an approach to management. *Clin J Sport Med* 1997; 7(4): 292–301.

2. Armstrong LE, Epstein Y, Greenleaf JE, et al. American College of Sports Medicine position stand. Heat and cold illnesses during distance running. *Med Sci Sports Exerc* 1996; 28(12): i–x.

3. Noakes TD, Sharwood K, Speedy D, et al. Three independent biological mechanisms cause exercise-associated hyponatremia: evidence from 2,135 weighed competitive athletic performances. *Proc Natl Acad Sci U S A* 2005; 102(51): 18550–5.

4. Hew-Butler T, Almond C, Ayus JC, et al. Exercise-Associated Hyponatremia (EAH) Consensus Panel. Consensus statement of the 1st International Exercise-Associated Hyponatremia Consensus Development Conference, Cape Town, South Africa 2005. *Clin J Sport Med* 2005; 15(4): 208–13.

5. Speedy DB, Rogers IR, Noakes TD, et al. Diagnosis and prevention of hyponatremia at an ultradistance triathlon. *Clin J Sport Med* 2000; 10(1): 52–8.

6. Reid SA, Speedy DB, Thompson JM, et al. Study of hematological and biochemical parameters in runners completing a standard marathon. *Clin J Sport Med* 2004; 14(6): 344–53.

Drugs and the Athlete

The use of performance-enhancing drugs is probably the major problem facing sport today. Despite intense efforts by sporting bodies and the medical profession to eliminate the problem, drug taking to assist sports performance remains widespread.

The International Olympic Committee's (IOC) definition of doping is:

> ...the use of an expedient (substance or method) which is potentially harmful to athlete's health and/or capable of enhancing their performance, or the presence in the athlete's body of a prohibited substance or evidence of the use thereof or evidence of the use of a prohibited method.

A look at the history of drug use in sport shows that drug use is not a recent phenomenon.

Historical perspective

Drugs were used to enhance performance in ancient civilizations. The ancient Greeks used mushrooms, while the Roman wrestlers used special mixtures of herbs to improve performance. A favorite mixture among ancient Egyptian athletes is said to have been the rear hooves of an Abyssinian ass, ground up, boiled in oil and flavored with rose petals and rosehip.

The use of performance-enhancing substances has even resulted in the introduction of two commonly used words in our language. The Norwegian warriors, the Berserkers, fortified themselves with psychoactive mushrooms that so wildly affected their behavior that the word 'berserk' is now part of our language. Indigenous South African tribes used a local liquor called 'dop' as a stimulant, leading to the use of the word 'doping', which has come to be used as a general term to describe the use of chemical means to enhance performance.

Reports of doping were common in the 19th century. Substances used included caffeine, alcohol, glyceryl trinitrate (nitroglycerine), opium and strychnine. The first reported drug-related death occurred in 1896 when an English cyclist died of an overdose of 'trimethyl'. Thomas Hicks ran to victory in the Olympic marathon of 1904 in St Louis with the help of raw egg, injections of strychnine, and doses of brandy administered to him during the race.

The origins of the current epidemic of drug use among sportspeople can be traced back to the introduction of various substances during World War II. Amphetamines were introduced to US troops to help keep them awake at the battlefront. Following the war, some sportspeople began to use amphetamines. This problem came to public attention when Danish cyclist, Kurt Jensen, died from a heat-related illness at the 1960 Rome Olympics. The misuse of amphetamines and nicotinic acid contributed significantly to his death. A further indication of the amphetamine problem was shown by the death, in front of a huge television audience, of British cyclist Tommy Simpson in the 1967 Tour de France. These deaths and the widespread allegations of drug taking at the 1964 Tokyo Olympics led the IOC to establish a Medical Commission in 1967 and to ban the use of pharmaceutical agents to enhance performance.

Around the same time, sensitive gas chromatography drug-testing techniques were introduced by Arnold Beckett in London. The IOC commenced drug testing at the 1968 Olympics in Mexico but it was not until the 1972 Olympics in Munich that full-scale testing was commenced. Seven athletes, including four medalists, had positive test results to stimulants or narcotics.

The use of anabolic steroids can be traced back to 1927 when Fred Koch, an organic chemist at the University of Chicago, developed a form of testosterone by extracting the hormone from bull's testicles and treating it with benzene and acetone. The substance produced aggressive behavior and masculine characteristics in animals. The first reported use of testosterone in humans came during World War II when German storm-troopers used it to enhance their aggressiveness.

It was alleged that Soviet athletes used anabolic steroids in the 1952 Olympics in Helsinki and these allegations were substantiated by one of the Russian team physicians two years later at the World Weightlifting Championships in Vienna. Western athletes began to use anabolic steroids after the release of dianabol in 1958. The use of anabolic steroids, especially by power athletes, became widespread in the late 1960s and 1970s.

A reliable test method was finally developed in 1974 and the IOC added anabolic steroids to its list of prohibited substances in 1975. This resulted in a marked increase in the number of drug-related disqualifications in the late 1970s, notably in strength-related sports such as throwing events and weightlifting. Since the fall of the Communist regime in the former German Democratic Republic, it has become evident that athletes from that nation were subjected to a systematic doping program.

In 1983, caffeine and testosterone were added to the prohibited list. In that year, improved testing techniques instituted at the Pan American Games at Caracas resulted in a number of weightlifters being disqualified for steroid use. Many athletes, on hearing of the increased sensitivity of the tests, elected to return home rather than compete. In 1985, beta-blockers, diuretics and glucocorticosteroids were added to the prohibited list of substances.

At the 1988 Seoul Olympics, the positive test result for anabolic steroids on 100 m winner Ben Johnson focused world attention on the continuing problem of drug abuse in sports and resulted in renewed international attempts to stamp out the use of performance-enhancing drugs in sport. In Australia, the Australian Sports Drug Agency (ASDA) was established. The emphasis by this doping control agency is on random and out-of-competition drug testing of athletes.

The first allegations regarding blood doping were made about Finnish distance runners in the 1970s. At the 1984 Olympics, members of the US cycling team admitted to blood doping, and Finnish distance runner Marti Vaino tested positive for anabolic steroids, apparently as a result of reinfusing blood that had been extracted some time earlier. The IOC banned blood doping as a method in 1986, but had no reliable method for its detection until recently.

With blood doping banned, athletes sought other ways of increasing their levels of hemoglobin. One method was by injecting erythropoietin (EPO) and this was included in the IOC's list of prohibited substances in 1990, even though an EPO detection test, based on a combination of blood and urine analysis, was only developed in time for the Sydney Olympics in 2000.

In 1998, a large number of prohibited medical substances was found in a raid during the Tour de France. The scandal led to a major reappraisal of the role of public authorities in anti-doping affairs. At that time, a number of organizations, many with conflicts of interest, were involved in developing policies and sanctions. The IOC convened the World Conference of Doping in Sport in Lausanne, Switzerland in February 1999 and the delegates produced the Lausanne Declaration on Doping in Sport.

As a result of this Declaration, the World Anti-Doping Agency (WADA) was established in November 1999 to promote and coordinate the fight against doping in sport internationally. WADA was set up under the initiative of the IOC with the support and participation of intergovernmental organizations, governments, public authorities, and other private and public bodies fighting against doping in sport. WADA consists of equal representatives from the Olympic Movement and public authorities.

In the past decade there have been reports that traditional 'sports' drugs (particularly body-building agents) have been used in other settings. For example, drugs banned in sports have been used in gymnasiums as well as in security and military services. In addition, these agents appear to have found a niche in the entertainment industry, where physique and public image are important.

Why athletes take drugs

Unfortunately, there has been little research into this question but there are a number of possible reasons why athletes take performance-enhancing drugs:

- knowledge or a belief that their competitors are taking drugs
- a determination to do anything possible to attain success
- direct or indirect pressure from coaches, parents and peers

- pressure from government and/or authorities themselves (e.g. Eastern block countries during the 1960s to 1990s)
- lack of access to legal and natural methods to enhance performance (e.g. nutrition, psychology, recovery)
- community attitudes and expectations regarding success and performance
- financial rewards
- influence from the media in facilitating these expectations and rewards.

It is likely that a combination of the above factors is present in most athletes who take drugs.

Prohibited substances

WADA is responsible for producing and maintaining the World Anti-Doping Code containing the Prohibited List of Substances, which contains those substances and methods that are banned either at all times or in competition only. Substances will be added to the list if they satisfy any two of the following three criteria:

1. the potential for enhanced performance
2. the potential for being detrimental to health
3. they violate the spirit of sport.

The list is reviewed annually and an updated list commences on 1 January each year. The list that took effect on 1 January 2006 contains five classes of *substances* that are prohibited both in and out of competition, another four classes of substances prohibited in competition only, three *methods* prohibited in and out of competition, and two substances prohibited in particular sports (see box).

In addition, WADA monitors certain other substances (in 2006, stimulants and narcotics) to detect patterns of misuse; this may lead to these substances being added to the Prohibited List in the future.

Athletes may have illnesses or conditions which require them to take banned medications. In these cases the athlete may apply for a Therapeutic Use Exemption (TUE) from their National Anti-Doping Organization of their International Federation to obtain authority to use the substance. WADA does not grant TUEs but may consider appeals related to the granting or denying of a TUE.

A summary of the prohibited classes of drugs, their medical usage, effect on performance and side-effects is shown in Table 61.1.

WADA's list of prohibited substances and methods (as at 1 January 2006)

Prohibited classes of substances (in and out of competition)

S1. Anabolic agents
S2. Hormones and related substances, mimetics and analogs
S3. Beta-2 agonists
S4. Agents with anti-estrogenic activity
S5. Diuretics and other masking agents

Prohibited classes of substances (in competition only)

S6. Stimulants
S7. Narcotics
S8. Cannabinoids
S9. Glucocorticosteroids

Prohibited methods (in and out of competition)

M1. Enhancement of oxygen transfer
M2. Chemical and physical manipulation
M3. Gene doping

Substances prohibited in particular sports

P1. Alcohol
P2. Beta-blockers

Prohibited classes of substances

Anabolic agents

S1: Anabolic agents

Anabolic agents are prohibited.
1. Anabolic androgenic steroids (AAS)
   (a) exogenous AAS: e.g. danazol, fluoxymesterone, gestrinone, 4-hydroxytestosterone, mesterolone, metenolone, methandienone, methyl-1-testosterone, methylnortestosterone, methyltestosterone, nandrolone, 19-norandrostenedione, norethandrolone, oxymesterone, stanozolol, tetrahydrogestrinone, and other substances with a similar chemical structure or similar biological effect

continues

(b) endogenous AAS: e.g. androstenediol, androstenedione, dihydrotestosterone, prasterone, testosterone and their metabolites and isomers

For endogenous substances, a sample will be deemed to contain a prohibited substance if the concentration so deviates from the range of values normally found in humans that it is unlikely to be consistent with normal endogenous production.

If the sample is in the normal range but there are serious indications of a possible use of a prohibited substance, such as comparison to reference steroid profiles, further investigation will be carried out.

When a testosterone/epitestosterone (T/E) ratio is greater than 4:1, further investigation may be conducted

Other anabolic agents: clenbuterol, tibolone, zeranol, zilpaterol.

Source: WADA. The 2006 Prohibited List. International Standard. Available online: <http://www.wada-ama.org/rtecontent/document/2006_LIST.pdf>.

Anabolic androgenic steroids

Androgens are steroid hormones that are secreted primarily by the testes but also by the adrenal glands and ovaries. Testosterone is the principal androgen responsible for the development of the primary sexual characteristics in utero and during the neonatal period. It is also responsible for the development of the pubertal secondary sexual characteristics and it contributes to the increase in height and amount of skeletal muscle at that time. Testosterone promotes aggressive behavior, which is possibly due to direct stimulation of brain receptors. It also plays a role in sexual orientation.

Anabolic androgenic steroid (AAS) hormones are derivatives of testosterone. The structure of the testosterone molecule can be adjusted to maximize either the androgenic or anabolic effect. Athletes generally abuse those agents that have maximum anabolic effect while minimizing the androgenic side-effects. A large number of different AAS hormones have been synthesized.

Examples of prohibited AASs are shown in the box above. The exogenous ones are synthetic analogs of testosterone and the endogenous ones are naturally occurring and are involved in the metabolic pathways of testosterone.

The clinical uses of anabolic steroids are limited. They may be used as hormone replacement for primary and secondary hypogonadism, Klinefelter's syndrome and occasionally delayed puberty. They have also been used to treat disturbances of nitrogen balance and muscular development, and several other non-endocrine diseases, including several forms of anemia, hereditary angioneurotic edema and breast carcinoma. Steroids increase lean body mass in patients with chronic obstructive pulmonary disease and HIV, and they may have a role in the treatment of muscular dystrophy and several dermatological diseases.[1]

The use of AASs in certain sports, particularly power sports such as weightlifting, power lifting,[2] sprinting and throwing, is widespread, as is their use by body builders.[3] The use of AASs in footballers varies in the different codes of football. There would appear to be a high incidence of use in players of American football with a lower incidence in players of other football codes.

While the incidence of AAS use is highest in elite athletes, there is a disturbingly high incidence among recreational and high school athletes.[4-7] This may be related to a desire to increase sporting performance or to improve body image. In 1987, the first US national study of AAS use at a high school level found that 6.6% of male seniors had used the drugs; 38% of those users had commenced before turning 16 years of age.[4] Subsequent studies have confirmed that 4–6% (range 3–12%) of US high school boys have used AASs at some time, as have 1–2% of US high school girls.

AASs are taken orally or by intramuscular injection. More recently, transdermal patches, buccal tablets, nasal sprays, gels and creams are being used as the delivery mechanisms.[8]

AASs are usually used in a cyclical manner with periods of heavy use, generally lasting six to 12 weeks, alternating with drug-free periods lasting from one to 12 months. The aim of the drug-free periods is to reduce the side-effects of the drugs; whether this is the case remains unknown.

AAS users follow a 'pyramid' regimen, which commences with a low daily dose and gradually increases to a high dose then back down to a lower dose, and/or a 'stacking' regimen, in which several different types of anabolic steroids, oral and/or injectable, are taken simultaneously. The purpose behind the 'stacking' regimen is to achieve receptor saturation with a lower total androgen dose than would be required if only one compound were used. Users hope that this regimen may reduce the incidence of side-effects. Commonly, a combination known as 'pyramid stacking' is used. The dosages taken by AAS users varies but those wishing

Table 61.1 Prohibited drugs and their effects

Type of drug (examples)	Medical usage	Effect on performance	Side-effects
Anabolic steroids			
Methandrostenolone, stanozolol, nandrolone	Hypogonadism, severe osteoporosis, breast carcinoma	Increased muscle bulk, increased muscle strength, possibly improving anticatabolic effect, recovery	Acne, baldness, gynecomastia, decreased sperm production, testes size and sex drive, increased aggression, liver abnormalities, hypertension, hypercholesterolemia
Hormones and related substances			
Erythropoietin (EPO)	Anemia secondary to chronic renal disease	Increased endurance	Increased blood viscosity, myocardial infarction
Human growth hormone (hGH)	Dwarfism, short stature	Anecdotal evidence only	Allergic reactions, diabetogenic effect, acromegaly
Insulin-like growth factor (IGF-1)	Dwarfism, diabetes mellitus type 2	Anecdotal evidence only	Acromegaly, organomegaly, hypoglycemia
Insulin	Diabetes	Anecdotal evidence only	Hypoglycemia
Human chorionic gonadotrophin (hCG)	Hypogonadism	May increase endogenous production of steroids	Gynecomastia
Adrenocorticotropic hormone (ACTH)	Steroid-responsive conditions	Euphoria	As in corticosteroids
Beta-2 agonists			
Salbutamol, terbutaline	Asthma, exercise-induced bronchospasm	Possible anabolic effects	Tachycardia, tremor, palpitations
Agents with anti-estrogenic activity			
Aromatase inhibitors (anastrozole, aminoglutethamide)	Breast cancer	Used to counter gynecomastia	Joint aches, stiffness
Selective estrogen receptor modulators (SERMS) (tamoxifen)	Breast cancer, osteoporosis	Males: used with AAS to prevent gynecomastia Females: muscle bulk (anecdotal evidence)	Females: masculinization Deep venous thrombosis
Clomiphene, cyclofenil	Anovulatory infertility	Increases gonadotrophin-releasing hormone (GnRH) and endogenous testosterone (anecdotal evidence)	Bloating, stomach pains, blurred vision, headaches, nausea and dizziness

Table 61.1 Prohibited drugs and their effects *continued*

Type of drug (examples)	Medical usage	Effect on performance	Side-effects
Diuretics			
Frusemide, hydrochlorothiazide, chlorothiazide	Hypertension, edema, congestive cardiac failure	Rapid weight loss, decreases concentration of drugs in urine	Electrolyte imbalance, dehydration, muscle cramps
Stimulants			
Amphetamines (dexamphetamine, dimethylamphetamine)	Narcolepsy, ADHD	May delay fatigue, increased alertness	Anxiety, insomnia, dizziness, euphoria, headache, nausea, vomiting, confusion, psychosis, hypertension, addiction
Ephedra	Dietary supplements for weight loss	Large doses improve cycling performance Additive effect with caffeine	Hypertension, arrythmias, seizure, cerebrovascular accident
Cocaine	Nasal anesthetic	Increased alertness	Impaired hand–eye coordination, aggression, cardiac and cerebral abnormalities
Narcotics			
Pethidine, morphine	Moderate-to-severe pain	No evidence of improved performance, may be able to compete with injury	Nausea, vomiting, dizziness, respiratory depression, addiction
Cannabinoids			
Marijuana, hashish	Palliative care, chronic pain	Negative effect	Impaired psychomotor skills, altered perception of time, impaired concentration
Glucocorticosteroids			
Prednisolone	Widely used anti-inflammatory Severe asthma	Euphoria Effect on performance unknown	Cushingoid symptoms
Enhancement of oxygen transfer			
Blood doping	Nil	Improves endurance	Transfusion reaction, increased blood viscosity
Artificial oxygen carriers (hemoglobin oxygen carriers, perfluorocarbon emissions)	Rapid blood volume expansion Following acute blood loss	Improved endurance (no evidence)	

AAS = anabolic androgenic steroids; ADHD = attention deficit hyperactivity disorder.

to bulk up frequently use dosages 10–100 times the physiological dose.

Different AASs are used at different times of the training program depending on the phase of activity being performed. Certain AASs are regarded by their users (e.g. body builders) as more appropriate for specific aims, such as increased muscle definition. AAS users may use other drugs (e.g. diuretics, anti-estrogens, human chorionic gonadotrophin [hCG] and anti-acne medications) to counteract the common side-effects of AAS.

Most AASs are obtained through a black market that exists through gymnasiums, health centers and increasingly on the Internet (e.g. <http://www.pharmaeurope.com>, viewed 22 December 2005). Information (and misinformation!) is readily available in pamphlets, niche-market magazines and, of course, the Internet.

Testosterone precursors (e.g. dehydroepiandrosterone [DHEA]) and designer steroids (e.g. tetrahydrogestrinone [THG]) have recently received considerable publicity (see p. 985).

Effect on performance

Anabolic steroids have a threefold effect.

1. *Anabolic effect.* This is due to the induction of protein synthesis in skeletal muscle cells. AASs attach to specific cytoplasmic receptors in muscle cells and this complex then activates the nucleus to synthesize ribosomal and messenger RNA and initiate the process of protein synthesis. This anabolic effect continues during steroid treatment. An additional anabolic effect may occur indirectly through increased levels of endogenous growth hormone associated with AAS administration.

2. *Anticatabolic effect.* This is mediated in two ways. AASs may reverse the catabolic effects of glucocorticosteroids released at times of training stress and they may improve the utilization of ingested protein, thereby increasing nitrogen retention. This effect depends on adequate protein intake. Athletes in heavy training, especially weight training, are in a catabolic state. This is associated with the release of glucocorticosteroids and increased nitrogen utilization. When intense training is combined with insufficient recovery time or inadequate protein intake, a chronic catabolic state may develop. This can be associated with impaired training and competition performance and the development of overuse injuries. Anabolic

steroids may reverse this catabolic state, and permit an increased training load.

AAS use appears to increase muscle size and muscle strength but only when certain conditions are met. For anabolic steroids to be effective in increasing muscle size and strength, the athlete taking the steroids must perform intense weight training and have an adequate protein intake. If these conditions are met, an increase in muscle size and strength will result.

3. *Enhancement of aggressive behavior.* Increased aggression may encourage a greater training intensity and may also be advantageous during competition in sports such as weightlifting and contact sports. However, there may also be negative psychological effects, as discussed below.

There is considerable evidence that testosterone administration combined with weight training leads to an increase in lean body mass and a decrease in body fat.[9–11] This effect appears to be dose-related. The change in muscle mass with testosterone use is due to muscle fiber hypertrophy and increases in myonuclear number.[12]

Studies have demonstrated a 5–20% increase in baseline strength, depending on the drugs and dose used as well as the administration period.[1]

While the majority of anabolic steroid use has been by athletes in power events, there is anecdotal evidence of a positive effect of anabolic steroids on endurance exercise. Firstly, the anticatabolic effect may improve recovery from heavy training, thus reducing the likelihood of injury and allowing the athlete to undertake greater volume and intensity of training. Secondly, anabolic steroids have a stimulatory effect on bone marrow, which may result in an increased production of red blood cells, thus improving the oxygen-carrying capacity of the blood.

Long-term treatment of certain anemias with AASs has shown an increase in hemoglobin concentrations, but the majority of studies have failed to show any improvement in endurance performance with AAS.[1]

The above effects of anabolic steroids occur in both males and females.

Side-effects

Side-effects of anabolic steroid usage are extremely common and can be particularly significant in women.

The majority of side-effects are reversible on cessation of the drug(s). However, a number of serious side-effects have been reported with anabolic steroid use, in some cases leading to death. The mortality rate among elite power lifters suspected of steroid abuse was significantly higher (12.9%) than that of a control population (3.1%).[13] Another study investigating the deaths of 34 known users of the drugs concluded that AAS use was associated with an increased risk of violent death from impulsive, aggressive behavior or depressive symptoms.[14]

An additional health risk associated with the use of AASs is that of infection associated with needle sharing.[1] HIV, hepatitis B and C, and abscesses have been documented among anabolic steroid injectors who share needles[15] and one study found that 25% of adolescent AAS users shared needles.[15]

As yet, the long-term effects of prolonged anabolic steroid usage are unknown. However, as athletes who abuse these compounds often administer doses as high as 100 times the usual therapeutic dose, there must be serious concerns for side-effects and toxicity. As well as this, a number of violent crimes, including domestic violence, which have resulted in death, have been attributed to 'roid rage'. A list of the common and less common side-effects of anabolic steroid usage is shown in Table 61.2.

Toxicity in both sexes

1. *Liver.* As many as 80% of individuals using those androgens that have a 17-methyl substitution on the steroid molecule have developed liver disorders, including hyperbilirubinemia and elevated liver enzyme levels.[16] These changes can be reversed with cessation of the drug. However, continued administration can lead to biliary obstruction and jaundice. This may take up to three months to reverse when steroid use is ceased. The responsible steroid compounds are mainly oral and include stanozolol and oxymethalone. Intermittent administration of these compounds has been shown to lower the incidence of these symptoms. The carbon-17 esters such as testosterone and nandrolone are not associated with these liver problems as these substances are administered by injection and bypass the liver. The use of anabolic steroids to treat various medical illnesses has been occasionally associated with the development of other liver abnormalities, such as peliosis hepatis (blood-filled cysts in the liver),[17, 18] as well as benign and malignant hepatic tumors.[19, 20]

2. *Tumors.* There have been occasional cases of tumors reported in athletes using anabolic

Table 61.2 Side-effects of anabolic steroids

Common	Less common
Both sexes	
Acne	Peliosis hepatis
Alopecia	Hepatoma/
Abnormal liver enzymes	hepatocarcinoma
Lowered HDL level	Wilms' tumor
Raised LDL level	Coronary artery disease
Elevated triglyceride level	Tendon ruptures
Hypertension	Psychosis
Reduced humoral	Acute schizophrenia
immunity	? Addiction
Irritability	? Leukemia
Aggression	
Mood swings	
Changes in libido	
? Addiction	
Males	
Decreased sperm	? Cancer of the prostrate
production	
Decreased testicle size	
Decreased FSH, LH	
Gynecomastia	
Females	
Menstrual irregularities	Deepening of voice
	Male pattern baldness
	Hirsuitism
	Clitoromegaly
	Breast shrinkage
Adolescents	
Increased facial/body hair	Phallic enlargement
Acne	Male pattern baldness
Premature closure of	Deepening of voice
epiphyses	Abnormal psychosocial
	maturation

FSH = follicle stimulating hormone; HDL = high-density lipoprotein; LDL = low-density lipoprotein; LH = luteinizing hormone.

steroids. These include Wilms' tumor, carcinoma of the prostate and leukemia. It is not possible to prove a direct relationship between the development of these tumors and anabolic steroid usage.

3. *Lipids.* Changes in lipid profiles are commonly seen with anabolic steroid usage.[21–23] Lowered levels of high-density lipoprotein (HDL) cholesterol and raised levels of low-density lipoprotein (LDL) cholesterol are seen. A lowered HDL:LDL ratio is a risk factor for the development of coronary heart disease but as yet

there is no convincing evidence of an increased incidence of coronary heart disease in anabolic steroid users.[24] These lipid changes appear to be reversed on cessation of the drug(s).[25]

4. *Hypertension.* Raised blood pressure is commonly seen in association with anabolic steroid usage,[23, 26] although the changes are not consistent. The increase in blood pressure also usually reverts to normal on cessation of use. The elevation in blood pressure may be secondary to sodium and water retention. Isolated cases of myocardial infarction[27, 28] and cerebrovascular accident[27–29] have been reported in association with anabolic steroid use. There is serious concern about the possible long-term sequelae of anabolic steroid use, in particular, the possibility of an increased incidence of coronary artery disease in the light of the persistent findings of elevated blood pressure, decreased HDL levels and increased LDL levels. Whether or not these transient effects are negated by the return to normal values in times of steroid abstinence remains to be seen.

5. *Immunity.* There is evidence that humoral immunity is reduced with steroid use. Lowered levels of IgG, IgM and IgA have been noted. The clinical significance of these changes is uncertain.

6. *Skin.* Skin changes are common with anabolic steroid usage and are related to excessive sebum production.[30, 31] These changes include acne, rosacea, sebaceous cysts, furunculosis, folliculitis and increased body and facial hair. Care should be taken with the treatment of severe acne with either tetracyclines or isotretinoin as these drugs may aggravate pre-existent liver damage.

7. *Psychological.* Mild psychological effects, such as irritability, mood swings, changes in libido and increased aggression, are common with anabolic steroid usage.[32, 33] AAS use directly causes significant disturbances in personality profile.[34] Another study showed that AAS users reported being significantly less in control of their aggression than did controls.[35]

Violent behavior may occur in susceptible individuals and psychiatric abnormalities such as acute schizophrenia and transient psychoses are not uncommon.[36] It would appear that anabolic steroids may also become both psychologically and physically addictive.[37] Withdrawal may lead to depression, fatigue, decreased sex drive, insomnia and anorexia.

Toxicity in males

A reduction in testicular size and sperm volume appears to be common with anabolic steroid use due to a negative feedback effect resulting in decreased pituitary production of follicle stimulating hormone (FSH) and luteinizing hormone (LH).[38] Testicular volume is reduced on average by 20%, and sperm production is severely reduced and commonly ceases altogether. The popular usage of human chorionic gonadotrophin (hCG) in conjunction with anabolic steroids to avoid testicular atrophy does not appear to be effective, although it has been suggested that clomiphene may successfully restore AAS-induced pituitary–gonadal dysfunction.[39]

These side-effects appear to be reversible on cessation of anabolic steroids. However, decreased sperm production may take three months to return to normal.

Ironically, one of the side-effects of anabolic steroid usage is feminization. This occurs as a result of peripheral conversion of AAS to estrogens. Plasma estradiol levels rise considerably with anabolic steroid usage. This feminization manifests itself as gynecomastia (development of breast tissue in males). Body builders use tamoxifen to counteract this estrogen effect and, as a result, increase the androgenic side-effects, but there is no evidence for its effectiveness.[40]

Toxicity in females

In female athletes, menstrual irregularities frequently occur with anabolic steroid use. Other symptoms can include deepening of the voice, male pattern baldness, hirsutism, altered libido, uterine atrophy and an enlarged clitoris. These changes may be irreversible. Anabolic steroids taken in pregnancy can cause fetal abnormalities or miscarriage.

Toxicity in adolescents

Anabolic steroid usage during adolescence in both sexes is commonly associated with acne, increased facial and body hair and premature closing of the epiphyseal plates.[41, 42] Other changes that may be seen during adolescence include phallic enlargement, male pattern baldness, deepening of the voice and abnormal psychosocial maturation.

Testosterone precursors

It has been suggested that testosterone precursors or prohormones such as androstenedione ('andro') and dehydroepiandrosterone (DHEA) may have an ergogenic effect by increasing testosterone levels.

Androstenedione

Androstenedione is a relatively weak steroid available in many over–the-counter nutritional supplements. It is an immediate precursor to testosterone as well as estradiol and estrone. Its anabolic activity is one-fifth to one-tenth of testosterone. Although some studies have shown that androstenedione use will lead to increased testosterone levels, there is no evidence that it will significantly increase strength or lean body mass.[8] Adverse effects include gynecomastia and increased risk of cardiovascular disease secondary to increased levels of estrogen, and a significant reduction of HDL cholesterol.

Dehydroepiandrosterone (DHEA)

DHEA is also a testosterone precursor and secreted by the adrenal gland.[43] It has been promoted to increase muscle mass and weight loss. Its use was publicized by the US baseballer, Mark McGwire, who admitted to using DHEA during the season in which he set the home run scoring record. DHEA does not enhance serum testosterone concentration or increase strength.[44] Although there is some evidence of a weight loss effect in rats, the only human study into the effectiveness of DHEA in weight loss failed to show any benefit.[45] Due to the potential for androgenic effects, DHEA is not recommended for young children and women.[8]

Tetrahydrogestrinone (THG)

It has been suspected for many years that laboratories were working on developing a designer steroid that would prove undetectable. THG, a newly developed designer steroid, was discovered in 2003 when a track and field coach gave the contents of a used syringe to drug testing authorities. The drug was subsequently analyzed and its chemical structure determined. A test to detect the presence of THG was developed and past urine samples of a number of elite track athletes analyzed and found to be positive.[46]

THG was created with the dual purpose of imparting anabolic steroid effects to athletes, and allowing those athletes to avoid detection by standard doping control drug testing. The primary reason THG went undetected in urine samples was that it tends to break down when prepared for analysis by the standard anabolic steroid screen.[47] Once it was suspected that the steroid was disintegrating during standard testing, a more sensitive assay process was used.

THG has been shown to be chemically and pharmacologically related to the specifically listed anabolic steroids gestrinone and trenbolone on the WADA Prohibited List. In vitro studies have suggested that THG may be a potent anabolic agent, although the in vivo potency will depend upon the steroid's circulating half-life and its binding to sex hormone-binding globulin.[48]

The discovery of a previously unknown designer steroid raises the concern that other undetectable substances are being used. Another designer steroid, desoxy-methyl testosterone, has subsequently been discovered.

Clenbuterol

Clenbuterol, which is considered both an anabolic agent and a beta-2 agonist, has been used as an ergogenic aid but there is no scientific evidence in humans to support the animal studies that showed increased lean mass.[49] Side-effects include tremor and tachycardia. There are anecdotal reports of sudden death in two body builders.[49]

Hormones and related substances

S2: Hormones and related substances

The following substances, including other substances with a similar chemical structure or similar biological effect, and their releasing factors are prohibited:

1. Erythropoietin (EPO)
2. Growth hormone (hGH), insulin-like growth factors (e.g. IGF-1), mechano growth factors (MGFs)
3. Gonadotrophins (LH, hCG), prohibited in males only
4. Insulin
5. Corticotrophins

Unless an athlete can demonstrate that the abnormal concentration was due to a physiological or pathological condition, a sample will be deemed to contain a prohibited substance where the concentration of the prohibited substance or its metabolites and/or relevant ratios or markers in the athlete's sample so exceeds the range of values normally found in humans that it is unlikely to be consistent with normal endogenous production.

If a laboratory reports, using a reliable analytical method, that the prohibited substance is of exogenous origin, the sample will be deemed to contain a prohibited substance and shall be reported as an adverse analytical finding.

> The presence of other substances with a similar chemical structure or similar biological effect, diagnostic marker or releasing factors of a hormone listed above or of any other finding which indicates that the substance detected is of exogenous origin, will be deemed to reflect the use of a prohibited substance and shall be reported as an adverse analytical finding.
>
> Source: WADA. The 2006 Prohibited List. International Standard. Available online: <http://www.wada-ama.org/rtecontent/document/2006_LIST.pdf>.

Erythropoietin

EPO is a naturally occurring hormone secreted by the kidney. It stimulates the bone marrow and increases red blood cell production. This leads to an increase in red blood cell mass, hemoglobin and hematocrit. Its main therapeutic use has been in patients with anemia due to conditions such as chronic renal failure, cancer chemotherapy or HIV (patients on zidovudine), and also for surgical patients to minimize the need for blood transfusions.[50]

Recombinant EPO (rhEPO) became available in the late 1980s and was used by some athletes competing in endurance sports. There have been incidents in the past two decades in which athletes have either admitted taking or tested positive to EPO, particularly in cycling and cross-country skiing, the most publicized being the 1998 Tour de France where the Festina team was caught with huge amounts of EPO.

As EPO causes an increased red cell mass, an extra oxygen-carrying capacity is created, which permits an increase in energy production by aerobic oxidation of glucose and free fatty acids.[51, 52] This is the most efficient means of energy production and limits anaerobic production, which is inefficient and leads to fatigue. Aerobic oxidation is the most important energy source for endurance athletes. EPO provides the benefits of blood doping without the risk of blood transfusion.

EPO has been shown to increase hemoglobin levels by 11%[53] and improve $V_{O_{2max}}$ (7%)[54] and exercise tolerance (17% increased time for run to exhaustion).[55]

The main side-effect of EPO is hyperviscosity of the blood due to a raised hematocrit. This raises the risk of myocardial infarction and cerebrovascular accident, the risk being increased with dehydrating endurance exercise. The unexplained death of 18 otherwise healthy cyclists between 1997 and 2000 has

been linked to EPO, but there is no concrete evidence to support this theory.[50]

Less serious side-effects of EPO use include fever, nausea, headache, anxiety and lethargy. Seizures have been reported in 2–3% of patients in the first 90 days of therapy.[50]

Some sports have introduced safety cut-offs for hematocrit levels (e.g. 50%) as an indirect means of restricting the use of EPO.[56] This is unsatisfactory due to the wide variations in 'normal' hematocrit levels and the number of factors that can affect the value.[57] Athletes may then manipulate their drug intake to ensure that they are just below the allowed limit.

Recently it has become possible to detect the use of EPO by athletes. Testing for EPO was introduced at the 2000 Sydney Olympics and involved a combination of blood and urine tests.[58]

Two cross-country skiers were stripped of their medals at the 2002 Winter Olympic Games in Salt Lake City after testing positive for darbepoetin, a new recombinant version of EPO.

Human growth hormone

Human growth hormone (hGH) is a polypeptide hormone produced by the anterior pituitary. It is also called somatotrophic hormone and somatotrophin. It is essential for normal growth and development.

Growth hormone exerts its effect on all cells in the body. It is anabolic in nature and causes an increased rate of protein synthesis and concurrent reduction in protein catabolism. It produces mobilization and increased use of fatty acids for energy and thus increases lean tissue mass and decreases fat mass. It causes a decreased rate of glucose utilization. Growth hormone also produces accelerated growth. In the skeletally immature, stature is increased and prolonged treatment results in gigantism. When the epiphyses are closed, linear growth ceases and hGH produces acromegaly.

Another important action of hGH is the stimulation of the insulin-like growth factor-1 (IGF-1) in the liver, which synergizes with hGH to produce many of its effects. Exercise stimulates the production of hGH five- to tenfold, whereas starvation decreases its production.[59]

hGH is species specific and bovine and porcine hormones have no effect in humans. Since 1985 recombinant hGH has been produced. Prior to this hGH was derived from cadavers and this led to several cases of Creutzfeldt–Jakob disease in the recipients.

The medical use of hGH is limited to the treatment of 'dwarfism' and replacement therapy in growth-deficient children. It may have a role for children with Turner's syndrome and for people with chronic renal insufficiency. It is only available in the injectable form.

Athletes use hGH because of its alleged anabolic effects, that is, increased muscle mass and decreased fat mass.[60] A number of scientific studies have not shown a link between hGH use and increased muscle strength or improved exercise performance[61, 62] and therefore some scientists are adamant that there is absolutely no anabolic effect from hGH.[63] However, these studies include very small sample sizes and use doses of hGH which are probably considerably less than those used by athletes; no studies have evaluated the use of a combination of hGH and AAS, a common practise among athletes. Further studies must be done before we can finally determine whether hGH has an anabolic effect.

Adverse reactions are well documented and include gigantism in the younger athlete, acromegaly in the adult athlete, hypothyroidism, hypercholesterolemia, ischemic heart disease, congestive cardiac failure, cardiomyopathy, myopathies, arthritis, diabetes mellitus, impotence, osteoporosis, menstrual irregularities and Creutzfeldt–Jakob disease. Although recombinant hGH has no risk of Creutzfeldt–Jakob disease, 'black market' sources of hGH are often derived from cadavers.

In 1996 the IOC launched a program called Human Growth Hormone 2000 (HGH 2000) with the aim of developing a reliable screening test to detect exogenous hGH by the time of the Sydney Olympic Games in 2000. Despite considerable funding, the difficulties proved insurmountable and the test was not ready by the Sydney Games. There were a number of reasons for the difficulty. Firstly, hGH is a naturally occurring hormone, with varying levels between individuals of different ages, sexes and activity levels. Secondly, hGH release is stimulated by exercise and varies in concentration throughout the day in each individual, and thirdly, no reliable marker for hGH level is excreted in the urine, therefore a blood test must be used.[59] Since 2000 further progress has been made and it is now possible to perform a blood test to detect the presence of hGH.

Insulin-like growth factors

Growth hormone effects on the growth of bones and cartilage and on protein metabolism are brought about indirectly by stimulation of the liver and other tissue to release somatomedins (growth factors). The principal somatomedin is insulin-like growth factor (IGF-1/somatomedin C). IGF-1 results in an increase in glucose and amino acid uptake and inhibits apoptosis (programmed cell death). It enhances lipolysis indirectly by insulin suppression and it may be linked to carcinogenesis (increased IGF-1 receptors have been found in tumors of the lung, breast and Wilms' tumor of the kidney).

Clinical applications are limited but include some types of dwarfism and growth problems in children, and in people with diabetes mellitus type 2, and it may have a role in kidney disease, catabolic states, osteoporosis, atherosclerosis and osteoarthritis.

IGF-1 is used by athletes with the aim of increasing muscle mass, but studies have failed to show any increase. In addition, supplementation of IGF-1 appears to be associated with moderate-to-severe hypoglycemia, decreased growth hormone secretion, a shift from lipid to carbohydrate oxidation for energy, and a general disruption of the insulin/glucagon system.[64] There is some evidence that it is the IGF binding protein-3 that is more closely related to overall growth than IGF-1 itself.[65] There is also some disturbing evidence to suggest that IGF-1 is mitogenic. Elevated IGF-1 levels have been linked to prostate, colorectal and lung cancers.[66]

Human chorionic gonadotrophin

hCG is produced by the placenta and is a glycoprotein hormone produced in large amounts during pregnancy and also by certain types of tumors. It has a very similar structure to LH and has the same biological activity except that it has a much longer half-life. hCG mainly stimulates sex steroid hormone biosynthesis in the gonads. Thus, in the female, hCG can substitute for the ovulatory surge of LH and ovulation and also maintain the corpus luteum for the production of progesterone, mainly in pregnancy. In the male, hCG can replace LH in stimulation of the interstitial cells within the testes to produce testosterone.

The therapeutic uses of hCG are limited. It can be used to stimulate ovulation in females and has been used to induce puberty in adolescent males who have delayed sexual development. It is mainly abused by male athletes as it increases the endogenous production of both testosterone and epitestosterone without increasing the urinary testosterone-to-epitestosterone ratio above the normal levels. Its other main use is to attempt to maintain testicular volume in the male athlete using anabolic steroids, which leads to inhibition of pituitary LH and FSH secretion and consequently loss of testicular volume. However, as it is FSH that maintains testicular volume, using hCG is unlikely to be effective. In the female athlete it is unlikely to give any benefit.

The main side-effect of hCG is gynecomastia, probably from raised estrogen secretion from the testes. The drug combination of hCG and anabolic steroids causes headaches, depression and edema.

hCG and LH were prohibited in all athletes but following problems with elevated hCG levels in females who were either currently pregnant or had recently miscarried, since 2006 they are prohibited in male athletes only. An elevated level of hCG in the male is a doping offence unless it can be shown to be due to a physiological or (very rarely) a pathological condition such as a tumor.

Insulin

Insulin is a small hormone produced in the pancreas whose main role is in carbohydrate metabolism. Insulin is anabolic in nature causing cell growth, increasing both glucose and amino acid uptake by cells and increased protein synthesis. It also decreases protein catabolism. Insulin also increases lipogenesis by promoting fatty acid synthesis and storage in adipose tissue. The main clinical use for insulin is for treating people with diabetes mellitus type 1.

Athletic use of insulin is mainly found in the power sports—weightlifting and body building. In one report, as many as 25% of AAS users concurrently use insulin.[67] The method of insulin abuse appears to be relatively simple and spread by word of mouth. Most users inject 10 IU of regular insulin after exercise and then consume sugar-containing foods and drinks. As insulin has a half-life of 4 minutes in the human body, it vanishes rapidly and would be very difficult to detect. Even when detected it is impossible to distinguish from the athlete's own insulin.

The anabolic properties of insulin used in the hypoinsulinemic state (diabetic) are well recognized, however, the concept of a hyperinsulinemia-induced anabolic state is much less well supported.[68] Physiological hyperinsulinemia reportedly stimulates amino acid transport in human skeletal muscle. Although insulin inhibits protein breakdown, stimulation of bulk protein synthesis during hyperinsulinemia is observed only when concomitant hyperaminoacidemia occurs.[69]

The use of insulin in this situation is potentially very dangerous. Unrecognized hypoglycemic attacks can cause permanent neurological deficit and even death.[68]

Corticotrophins

Adrenocorticotropic hormone (ACTH) is also known as corticotrophin or adrenocorticotrophin and is secreted by the anterior pituitary gland. Its main effect is on the adrenal cortex. Three major steroid hormones are produced in the adrenal cortex. These are:

1. aldosterone (mineral corticoid)
2. cortisol (glucocorticoid effect)
3. DHEA (androgenic effect) (see p. 985).

ACTH stimulates secretory activity in those cells that produce cortisol and androgens. It is abused in order to increase the secretion of the adrenal androgens, which are moderately active male sex hormones. These are converted to testosterone in extra-adrenal tissues, which accounts for much of their androgenic activity. ACTH abuse also increases cortisol levels and this in turn stimulates gluconeogenesis, which raises blood glucose levels. This is achieved by mobilization of amino acids, mainly from muscle for conversion to glucose in the liver and also by decreasing glucose utilization by the cells. Thus, the ergogenic effect of ACTH is negligible as its catabolic effects cancel out its anabolic effects. In fact, ACTH has no ergogenic benefit and is detrimental to performance. It is because of a belief in increased performance within the athletic community that it is placed on the Prohibited List.

Beta-2 agonists

S3: Beta-2 agonists

All beta-2 agonists including their D- and L-isomers are prohibited.

As an exception, formoterol, salbutamol, terbutaline and salmeterol when administered by inhalation require an abbreviated TUE (ATUE). Despite the granting of any form of TUE a concentration of salbutamol greater than 1000 ng/mL will be considered an adverse analytical finding unless the athlete proves that the abnormal result was the consequence of the therapeutic use of inhaled salbutamol.

Source: WADA. The 2006 Prohibited List. International Standard. Available online: <http://www.wada-ama.org/rtecontent/document/2006_LIST.pdf>.

Beta-2 agonists are used widely, mainly in their aerosol forms, in the treatment of asthma. When given systemically by tablet or injection, beta-2 agonists may have anabolic effects and their use is therefore prohibited. They are not permitted to be given by the oral or intravenous route.

Side-effects include:

- nervousness
- tremor

- tachycardia
- palpitation
- headache
- nausea
- vomiting
- sweating.

The side-effects are minimized when the drugs are given by inhalation. An abbreviated Therapeutic Use Exemption (ATUE) is required for the use of the four permitted inhaled beta-2 agonists (formoterol, salbutamol, terbutaline and salmeterol). Confirmation of the diagnosis of asthma or exercise-induced asthma may be required (Chapter 46).

Agents with anti-estrogenic activity

> **S4: Agents with anti-estrogenic activity**
>
> The following classes of anti-estrogenic substances are prohibited.
> 1. Aromatase inhibitors including, but not limited to, anostrozole, letrozole, aminoglutethimide, exemestane, formestane, testolactone.
> 2. Selective estrogen receptor modulators (SERMS) including, but not limited to, raloxifene, tamoxifen, toremifene.
> 3. Other anti-estrogenic substances, including, but not limited to, clomifenil, cyclofenil, fulvestrant.
>
> Source: WADA. The 2006 Prohibited List. International Standard. Available online: <http://www.wada-ama.org/rtecontent/document/2006_LIST.pdf>.

Aromatase inhibitors lower the amount of estrogen in the body, whereas drugs such as the selective estrogen receptor modulators (SERMs) block the estrogen receptors.

The anti-estrogen drugs such as tamoxifen and clomiphene are used by both male and female athletes for different reasons. Male athletes primarily use tamoxifen in conjunction with AASs to prevent the development of gynecomastia. Tamoxifen also increases testosterone levels in males and is advertised as a body fat reducer.

In females, there is evidence that tamoxifen is used as an ergogenic agent, particularly by body builders.[70] By blocking the estrogen receptors in a woman's body, tamoxifen leaves testosterone unopposed. This could lead to masculinization.

Tamoxifen has a number of harmful effects in females. It has been shown to increase the risk of venous thromboembolic events. As it is related to diethylstilbestrol (DES), women who became pregnant while taking the drug may be at increased risk of giving birth to a child with congenital defects.

Diuretics and other masking agents

> **S5: Diuretics and other masking agents**
>
> Masking agents include but are not limited to:
> - diuretics
> - epitestosterone
> - probenecid
> - alpha-reductase inhibitors (e.g. finasteride, dutasteride)
> - plasma expanders (e.g. albumin, dextran, hydroxyethyl starch)
>
> Diuretics include: acetazolamide, amiloride, bumetanide, canrenone, chlorthalidone, ethacrynic acid, frusemide, indapamide, metolazone, spironolactone, thiazides (e.g. bendroflumethiazide, chlorothiazide, hydrochlorothiazide), triamterene and related substances.
>
> Source: WADA. The 2006 Prohibited List. International Standard. Available online: <http://www.wada-ama.org/rtecontent/document/2006_LIST.pdf>.

Clinically, diuretics are used in the treatment of hypertension, fluid retention and congestive cardiac failure. Side-effects from their use include dehydration, hypotension, muscle cramps and electrolyte disturbances. Athletes use diuretics in order to lose weight rapidly prior to competition in sports where weight limits are set. These sports include boxing, wrestling, weightlifting, judo, light-weight rowing; they are also used by jockeys.

The use of diuretics may be combined with other dehydration techniques such as use of a sauna, exercise in hot conditions and food and water restrictions. These practises may result in rapid dehydration and electrolyte imbalances, which may be harmful to the athlete, particularly if practiced on a regular basis. Diuretics are also used to aid the excretion or dilute the presence of illegal substances in the urine.

Epitestosterone is taken by athletes who are also taking testosterone or AASs in an attempt to normalize their testosterone/epitestosterone (T/E) ratio, where an abnormally high ratio is used as an indication of illegal drug use (see above). Probenecid is a drug used clinically to increase the uptake of penicillin administered intramuscularly. It is used by athletes to accelerate the excretion of prohibited substances.

Finasteride is used clinically in the treatment of symptomatic benign prostatic hypertrophy and male pattern baldness. As male pattern baldness is one of the side-effects of the use of testosterone and its related substances, finasteride may be used to reduce that side-effect.

Plasma volume expanders such as hydroxyethyl starch (HES) dilute the concentration of hemoglobin and erythrocytes. A number of Finnish cross-country skiers were found to be using HES at the 2001 World Championships and subsequently disqualified.

Stimulants

S6: Stimulants

The following stimulants are prohibited in competition: adrafinil, adrenalin (epinephrine),[a] amfepramone, amiphenazole, amphetamine, amphetaminil, benzphetamine, bromantan, carphedon, cathine,[b] clobenzorex, cocaine, cropopamide, crotetamide, cyclazodone, dimethylamphetamine, ephedrine,[c] etamivan, etilamphetamine, etilefrine, famprofazone, fenbutrazate, fencamfamine, fencamine, fenetylline, fenfluramine, fenproporex, furfenorex, heptaminol, isometheptene, levmethamfetamine, meclofenoxate, mephentermine, mesocarb, methamphetamine(D-), methylenedioxyamphetamine, methylenedioxymethamphetamine, p-methylamphetamine, methylephedrine, methylphenidate, modafinil, nikethamide, norfenafrine, norflenfluramine, octopamine, ortetamine, oxilofrine, parahydroxyamphetamine, pemoline, pentetrazol, phendimetrazine, phenmetrazine, phenpromethamine, phentermine, prolintane, propylhexedrine, selegiline, sibutramine, strychnine and other substances with a similar chemical structure or similar biological effects.

(a) Adrenalin (epinephrine) associated with local anesthetic agents or by local administration (e.g. nasal, ophthalmological) is not prohibited.
(b) Cathine is prohibited when its concentration in urine is greater than 5 µg/mL.
(c) Each of ephedrine and methylephedrine is prohibited when its concentration in urine is greater than 10 µg/mL.
Source: WADA. The 2006 Prohibited List. International Standard. Available online: <http://www.wada-ama.org/rtecontent/document/2006_LIST.pdf>.

The stimulants are a broad group of substances and include central nervous system stimulants, sympathomimetic agents and cocaine. Until 2004 all stimulants were on the Prohibited List. In 2004 bupropion, caffeine, phenylephrine, phenylpropanolamine, pipadrol, pseudoephedrine and synephrine were removed from the Prohibited List and placed on the Monitoring Program. The major stimulants remaining on the banned list are the amphetamines, cocaine, ephedrine and modafinil.

Amphetamines

Amphetamines were first used clinically in the 1930s for their stimulatory effects in the treatment of narcolepsy. Their clinical use nowadays is restricted to the treatment of narcolepsy and childhood hyperactive syndromes such as attention deficit hyperactivity disorder (ADHD).[71] They have been widely used in sport to delay fatigue and increase alertness, although their use appears to have diminished in recent years, possibly due to adverse publicity regarding side-effects. There is some evidence that the use of amphetamines may enhance speed, power, endurance and concentration.

The 'benefits' of amphetamine use must be weighed against the adverse effects. Acute behavioral side-effects are common with the use of amphetamines. These include central nervous system excitation as demonstrated by irritability, insomnia, restlessness, dizziness or a tremor. Occasionally, more severe effects such as confusion, paranoia, delirium and uncontrolled aggression may occur. Systemic side-effects include hypertension, angina, vomiting, abdominal pain and occasional cerebral hemorrhage. Some deaths of sportspeople have resulted, even when 'normal' doses of amphetamines have been used, when undertaking maximal physical activity. Chronic use of amphetamines is associated with central nervous system related symptoms such as uncontrolled involuntary movements. Amphetamines are addictive and withdrawal is associated with fatigue, lethargy and depression.

There has been considerable controversy over the granting of TUEs for amphetamines on the basis of required treatment for ADHD. The granting of TUEs in ADHD is mostly confined to children. The previous requirements involved requiring children to cease their ADHD treatment on weekends or other occasions to allow them to compete but this was considered unreasonable after expert advice deemed it to have negative effects on symptom control. Currently, the granting of TUEs for children with ADHD is well documented and accepted.

The use of stimulants in the treatment of adult-onset ADHD remains controversial primarily because recognition of the clinical entity itself is relatively recent. It appears that with the release of a new non-stimulating medication (e.g. atoxematine) for adult ADHD the problem of no alternative treatment may be solved.

Ephedra

Ephedra is a shrub that grows mainly in desert or arid regions and is native to Northern China and Inner Mongolia. Different species vary in the amount of ephedrine alkaloids, the content of which produces the pharmacological effects of ephedra. The most common alkaloid is ephedrine, which generally constitutes 40–90% of the alkaloid content. This is the major ephedra alkaloid found in over-the-counter supplements. Pseudoephedrine is the next most common alkaloid and is less potent. It is produced synthetically and is used in many over-the-counter and prescription medications as a nasal decongestant. Norephedrine and norpseudoephedrine are minor alkaloid components.

The main use of ephedra, especially in the United States, is in dietary supplements. A review of case reports showed that 60% of users of ephedra-containing supplements were women and that the major reasons for its use were weight loss (59%), improved athletic performance (16%), and increased energy (6%).[72] There is some physiological basis for the use of ephedra as a weight loss medication and some data showing a modest increase in weight loss, although only over a six month period.[73]

The performance-enhancing effects of ephedrine and pseudoephedrine have been extensively studied. Normal dosages of both substances do not appear to enhance performance.[74] Large doses of pseudoephedrine enhance cycling performance, and the combination of ephedrine and caffeine has been shown to enhance performance[75] and carry the most risk.

Following an increasing number of reports of adverse events, including hypertension, arrhythmias, myocardial infarction, seizure, cerebrovascular accidents and death, the US Food and Drug Administration made it illegal for manufacturers to sell dietary supplements containing ephedrine.

Similarly, phenylpropanolamine, another commonly used dietary supplement, was voluntarily withdrawn from the market after its use was found to be an independent risk factor for hemorrhagic stroke in females.

Cocaine

Cocaine is more a community drug problem rather than a drug for performance enhancement. It emerged in the 1960s to become a major health problem. Recently, the introduction of 'crack', a purer form of cocaine, has increased the risks associated with its use.

Cocaine has a minimal performance-enhancing effect because of the brief duration of its action. Decreased fatigue has been noticed and cocaine use causes increased activity and talkativeness. The main feeling produced by cocaine is one of euphoria and a sense of wellbeing. The mood elevation appears similar to that produced by amphetamines but is far more transient. The feeling of euphoria is usually followed soon after by a feeling of dysphoria and craving. This may be overcome by another dose of cocaine. Tachyphylaxis occurs following repeated use.

The positive effects on athletic performance are minimal and may be associated with heightened arousal and increased alertness with low doses. Detrimental effects on performance are reported more frequently and include impaired hand–eye coordination, distorted sense of time and inappropriate aggression.

The side-effects of cocaine are numerous and include:

- serious cardiovascular problems, such as myocardial infarction, cardiac arrhythmia
- cerebral hemorrhage
- convulsions
- similar behavioral changes to amphetamine users.

The normal clinical use of cocaine is restricted to its use as a topical anesthetic agent in eye and nose surgery but it cannot be used in sport as a topical anesthetic. Its use is illegal in most countries and possession of cocaine can carry heavy penalties.

Modafinil

In the 2003 World Track and Field Championships Kelli White was disqualified after her victories in the 100 m and 200 m sprints when she tested positive for the presence of modafinil, which she claimed she was taking for the treatment of narcolepsy. At the time modafinil was not specifically listed on the Prohibited List, but the International Association of Athletics Federations (IAAF) considered that modafinil fell under the category 'and related substances' for stimulants and recommended that she be stripped of her medals. Modafinil is not a classic psychostimulant and it is not clear if it is a performance-enhancing agent.[76] Those who are prescribed modafinil in the treatment of narcolepsy should apply for a TUE, which requires the diagnosis of narcolepsy to be confirmed by one of the accepted methods (e.g. sleep studies in an accredited institution).

Narcotics

> ### S7: Narcotics
>
> The following narcotics are prohibited in competition: buprenorphine, dextromoramide, diamorphine (heroin), fentanyl and its derivatives, hydromorphone, methadone, morphine, oxycodone, oxymorphone, pentazocine, pethidine and related substances.
>
> Source: WADA. The 2006 Prohibited List. International Standard. Available online: <http://www.wada-ama.org/rtecontent/document/2006_LIST.pdf>.

Narcotics are derivatives of the opium poppy and include morphine, pethidine and diamorphine (heroin). They are commonly used in the management of moderate-to-severe pain.

As well as their analgesic effect, narcotics may cause:

- mood disturbances
- drowsiness
- mental clouding
- constipation
- nausea
- vomiting.

In high doses they may cause:

- respiratory depression
- hypotension
- muscle rigidity
- addiction
- significant withdrawal effects.

Narcotics have no ergogenic effect but have the potential to mask pain and permit athletes to compete with musculoskeletal injuries. For this reason, they are included on the list of prohibited substances.

Codeine, dextromethorphan, dextropropoxyphene, dihydrocodeine, diphenoxylate, ethylmorphine, pholcodine, propoxyphene and tramadol are permitted.

Cannabinoids

> ### S8: Cannabinoids
>
> Cannabinoids (e.g. marijuana, hashish) are prohibited in competition.
>
> Source: WADA. The 2006 Prohibited List. International Standard. Available online: <http://www.wada-ama.org/rtecontent/document/2006_LIST.pdf>.

The products of the cannabis plant such as marijuana, hashish, hash oil, sensemilla and others are considered to be the most popular illicit drug in the world. The most important compound contained in the plant is the cannabinoids, in which the substance delta-9-tetrahydrocannabinol (THC) is the most significant compound due to its psychoactive properties. The rate of absorption of THC by the lungs is very high. Maximal blood concentrations are obtained after 3–8 minutes, the onset of action on the central nervous system is observed in approximately 20 minutes and the peak effect in 2–4 hours. Duration of action for psychoactive effects is 4–6 hours.

For occasional users cannabinoid metabolites can be detected in urine up to five to seven days after the exposure. In chronic users it may be detected as long as 30 days after the last exposure.

From 1989 cannabis has been included on the list of drugs subject to certain restrictions. A concentration in the urine of carboxy-THC greater than 15 ng/mL has been used to allow for the possible effect of passive smoking. In the 1998 Nagano Winter Olympics, snowboarder Ross Rebagliati tested positive for cannabinoids, was suspended and subsequently reinstated.

Cannabinoids have a negative effect on sports performance through impairment of psychomotor skills, altered perception of time and impaired concentration. They may also have a negative effect on exercise performance.[77] The well-recognized 'amotivational' syndrome associated with long-term marijuana use may be particularly damaging to a sporting career.

Glucocorticosteroids

> ### S9: Glucocorticosteroids
>
> All glucocorticosteroids are prohibited in competition when administered orally, rectally or by intravenous or intramuscular injection. Their use requires a TUE.
>
> *continues*

Topical preparations when used for dermatological, aural/otic, nasal, buccal cavity and ophthalmological disorders are not prohibited and do not require any form of TUE.

Other routes of administration (e.g. inhalation) require an abbreviated TUE (ATUE).

Source: WADA. The 2006 Prohibited List. International Standard. Available online: <http://www.wada-ama.org/rtecontent/document/2006_LIST.pdf>.

Glucocorticosteroids are used widely in medicine for their anti-inflammatory effect. Oral glucocorticosteroids are prohibited because of their potential ergogenic effect. Some studies have shown that large doses of intravenous glucocorticosteroids increase cardiac output. There has been some speculation that large doses of oral glucocorticosteroids may also increase cardiac output but the evidence is inconclusive. However, it is known that large doses of oral glucocorticosteroids can cause mood elevation, euphoria, restlessness and increased motor activity. Some athletes have been suspected of taking large doses of glucocorticoids in an effort to enhance performance. This is concerning, not only because of the potential ergogenic effect but also because of the serious side-effects related to corticosteroid use.

Prohibited methods

Enhancement of oxygen transfer

M1: Enhancement of oxygen transfer

The following are prohibited:
1. Blood doping, including the use of autologous, homologous or heterologous blood or red blood cell products of any origin.
2. Artificially enhancing the uptake, transport or delivery of oxygen, including but not limited to perfluorochemicals, efaproxiral (RSR13) and modified hemoglobin products (e.g. hemoglobin-based blood substitutes, microencaspsulated hemoglobin products).

Source: WADA. The 2006 Prohibited List. International Standard. Available online: <http://www.wada-ama.org/rtecontent/document/2006_LIST.pdf>.

Blood doping

Blood doping is the administration of blood or red blood cells to an athlete to increase the red blood cell mass. This may be autologous (infusion with the athlete's own blood) or homologous (infusion with appropriately cross-matched donated blood).

The usual method of blood doping is to withdraw two units of an athlete's own blood four to six weeks prior to competition. This allows time for the red blood cell count to return to normal prior to reinfusing the blood a day or two before competition. The aim of this procedure is to increase the red blood cell mass and therefore increase the oxygen-carrying capacity of the blood. Improved endurance may occur as a result of blood doping.[78, 79]

Blood doping has been prohibited since 1984 but its use dropped dramatically when recombinant EPO became available in 1987.[80] Recently with the advent of testing for EPO blood doping has again become popular. Only recently has a reliable method been developed for its detection. The American cyclist Tyler Hamilton was one of the first athletes to be found guilty of blood doping in 2004.

Side-effects do occur with blood doping as they do with any transfusion, especially if donated blood is used. Allergic reactions may occur and there is an increased risk of blood-borne diseases such as hepatitis B and C and HIV. In addition, blood doping has been reported to increase the blood viscosity significantly and this may lead to some serious health risks due to sludging of blood, particularly in the cerebral circulation.

The production of recombinant EPO led to the practise of blood doping being abandoned by athletes, however, since the advent of a reliable blood test for the detection of EPO, blood doping has again become popular.

Artificial oxygen carriers

Artificial oxygen carriers or 'blood substitutes' are being developed to serve as a temporary replacement for transfused red blood cells in the prevention of ischemic tissue damage and hypovolemic shock. Two main types are available: hemoglobin oxygen carriers (HBOCs) and perfluorocarbons (PFCs).

Hemoglobin oxygen carriers

HBOCs have been developed as hemoglobin substitutes in recent years for use when a rapid expansion of blood volume is needed in acute blood loss following severe injury, surgery, or severe hemolytic anemia when human blood is unavailable, time necessary to undertake a proper cross-match is short, or the risk of blood infection is high.[81]

As the free hemoglobin molecule is inherently unstable, biochemical modifications have been made to the molecule. Three principle approaches have been used to stabilize and modify tetramic hemoglobin: polymerization using polyaldehydes, conjugation of polymers to the surface of the hemoglobin, or cross-linking the alpha- and beta-dimers of the protein.[82]

Hemoglobin is available from three different sources: bovine blood, human blood and genetic engineering. Bovine blood is cross-linked by glutaraldehyde, thus preventing the breakdown of hemoglobin. It can readily release oxygen into the tissues and is relatively inexpensive. One study of its effect on exercise performance, although significantly flawed, showed increased oxygen uptake and lowered lactate levels compared to autologous transfusion.[83]

HBOCs have several advantages. They can be pasteurized and ultrafiltered and so are safe from infection, they are readily available and easy to store with a long shelf life of up to 2 years, all blood types are compatible, and they have only one-third the viscosity of blood.[81] The main disadvantage is that they only last 12–48 hours in the body, compared with 120 days for blood cells. There is some evidence of high pulmonary and peripheral blood pressure associated with their use.[82]

There have been rumors of their use in sport but no definitive evidence.

Perfluorocarbon emulsions

PFCs, a group of synthetic compounds similar to teflon, are hydrocarbons to which fluorine atoms have been added. They are extremely inert, inexpensive to produce, and are made up in a sponge-like emulsion containing very small particles, 0.2 μm in diameter, which can deliver oxygen to the tissues through very small blood vessels. They are capable of physically dissolving large amounts of oxygen in plasma.[81]

Unlike hemoglobin, PFCs do not bind oxygen. The amount of oxygen that can be carried in solution is directly proportional to the gas partial pressure. A high partial pressure gradient is required to dissolve a large quantity of oxygen in the PFCs, and such gradients are also necessary between PFC and tissue in order to achieve a biologically useful degree of oxygen unloading. This precludes their use where supplemental oxygen is not available.[82]

The first generation PFCs (e.g. Fluosol-DA) proved unsatisfactory, but the second generation products (Oxygent, Oxyfluor) using improved technology and containing higher concentrations of the active agent in the emulsion show promise.

As yet, no study had investigated the performance-enhancing effects of PFCs, however, they have been found to improve oxygen delivery to the tissue under many conditions.

Detection

It would be futile to analyze urine samples in search of PFCs and most HBOCs since they are not processed by the kidney and/or the urinary excretion is too low and variable. The presence of an artificial oxygen carrier in the blood will be easily detected as long as the sample is taken soon after competition.[82]

Chemical and physical manipulation

> **M2: Chemical and physical manipulation**
>
> 1. Tampering, or attempting to tamper, in order to alter the integrity and validity of samples collected during doping controls is prohibited. These include but are not limited to catheterization, urine substitution and/or alteration.
> 2. Intravenous infusions are prohibited, except as legitimate acute medical treatment.
>
> Source: WADA. The 2006 Prohibited List. International Standard. Available online: <http://www.wada-ama.org/rtecontent/document/2006_LIST.pdf>.

Chemical and physical manipulation is the use of substances and/or methods that alter, attempt to alter or may reasonably be expected to alter the integrity and validity of urine samples used in doping controls. These include, without limitation:

- catheterization
- sample substitution and/or tampering.

The success or failure of the use of a prohibited substance or method is not material. It is sufficient that the said substance or procedure was used or attempted for the infraction to be considered as consummated.

WADA has prohibited procedures that interfere with the content or collection of urine samples used for drug testing such as the use of catheters to substitute urine. There have been a number of cases of athletes who have been disqualified from competition when they have been caught substituting urine from a coach, relative or fellow athlete in order to avoid having their own urine tested. This use of surrogate urine is prohibited and there have been examples where the athlete has subsequently been caught out because the surrogate urine has contained a prohibited substance that was being used by a friend or relative at the time of the test!

Current testing procedures are structured in such a way that the risk of substituting surrogate urine is minimal. The athlete is accompanied by a chaperone (of the same gender) so that the urine sample is provided under direct observation and the chance of substituting alternative urine is virtually impossible. However, athletes still use ingenious methods to avoid detection.

Intravenous infusions are no longer allowed by WADA except as a legitimate acute medical treatment. However, there is not, as yet, an accepted definition of 'acute medical treatment'.

Gene doping

> **M3: Gene doping**
>
> The non-therapeutic use of cells, genes, genetic elements, or of the modulation of gene expression, having the capacity to enhance performance, is prohibited.
>
> Source: WADA. The 2006 Prohibited List. International Standard. Available online: <http://www.wada-ama.org/rtecontent/document/2006_LIST.pdf>.

Gene doping or gene transfer technology to improve athletic performance is a serious threat to the integrity of elite sport. The principle of gene therapy is based on the delivery to a cell of a therapeutic gene that may compensate for an absent or abnormal gene. In general, DNA is used as the genetic material. This genetic material encodes for a therapeutic protein and needs to be delivered to the cell nucleus to be active. In order to deliver the genetic material, this material can be encapsulated into a virus such as an adenovirus or retrovirus, or into a lipid such as a liposome. The viruses are crippled so that they are no longer pathogenic. The encapsulated genetic material is mostly referred to as a vector and is introduced into the body by direct injection into the target organ or administered by aerosol for lung delivery.

Depending on the nature of the promoter and the vector used for delivery, the protein expression may be of short (days/weeks) or long (weeks/years) duration. The expressed protein may be confined to the cell that was treated (e.g. muscle) or may be released into the circulation.

Examples of potential areas for gene doping to improve athletic performance are EPO for endurance performance and IGF-1 for muscle strength. An adenovirus was used to deliver the EPO gene in mice and monkeys and this boosted the hematocrit from 49% to 81% in the mice and from 40% to 70% in the monkeys. The effects lasted over a year in the mice and for 12 weeks in the monkeys.[84] Mice injected with the IGF-1 gene showed a 15% increase in muscle bulk.[85]

Detecting gene doping will be very difficult. Engineered genes are likely to look identical with endogenous gene products. Detection of associated viral particles may be possible but that would involve muscle biopsies. Labeling of gene transfer products with genetic 'bar codes' may be another option but would require the cooperation of scientists, the pharmaceutical and biotech industries and public authorities.[86]

WADA, in collaboration with the Karolinska Institute and the Swedish Sports Confederation, held a workshop meeting in Stockholm on the subject of gene doping in sport in December 2005. The meeting was the second such meeting sponsored by WADA, the first being the workshop held at the Banbury Center, Long Island, New York, in March 2002. The Stockholm meeting included more than 50 participants from 15 countries and included geneticists and other biomedical scientists, ethicists, public policy experts, representatives of the IOC, and the broad international sports community.

The following principles and conclusions were agreed upon:

- Clinical results indicate that gene transfer for the purpose of therapy (gene therapy) now represents a proven, although very immature and still experimental field of human medicine and is an important area of biomedical research with great promise for the uniquely effective correction of many other serious and intractable human diseases.
- Clinical research in human gene therapy is filled with many recognized and unrecognized pitfalls and dangers. All gene transfer procedures in human subjects and patients should be required to abide by established principles and codes

governing gene transfer in human subjects, with special emphasis on full disclosure of the nature and dangers of a procedure and fully informed consent by participants. Such manipulations should also be carried out strictly in accordance with existing local and national rules and regulations for gene transfer in human subjects.

- The participation of physicians and other licensed professionals in gene transfer procedures that are not fully compliant with such standards of human clinical research and human experimentation should be considered medical malpractice and/or professional misconduct.

- Greater interactions should be encouraged among the sports community, professional scientific organizations, licensing agencies and clinical research oversight bodies to stimulate awareness of the potential illicit use of gene transfer techniques for athletic and other enhancement purposes and to develop appropriate sanction mechanisms for illegal or unethical application of gene transfer in sport. Public discussion on the prospect of gene-based enhancement should be promoted.

- The vigorous research program that has been instituted by WADA has led to significant progress towards a better understanding of the genetic and physiological effects of doping and of scientifically rigorous methods for more effective detection of pharmacological and gene-based doping. Scientific progress made through the WADA-supported research studies that were summarized at the conference suggests that new detection methods are likely to emerge and will help to prevent tainting of sport by gene doping. Research programs instituted by WADA and other anti-doping organizations should be supported. Academic, private and government research organizations should be encouraged to dedicate resources to further progress to deter gene doping.

- The use of genetic information to select for or to discriminate against athletes should be strongly discouraged. This principle does not apply to legitimate medical screening or research.

- Sports organizations at all levels, from student and amateur levels to international elite levels, should promote knowledge about the potential dangers associated with the misuse of genetic manipulations for athletic enhancement.

Classes of drugs banned in certain sports

Alcohol

P1: Alcohol

Alcohol (ethanol) is prohibited in competition only in the following sports. Detection will be conducted by analysis of breath and/or blood. The doping violation threshold for each Federation is reported.

- Aeronautic (FAI)   0.20 g/L
- Archery (FGITA, IPC)   0.10 g/L
- Automobile (FIA)   0.10 g/L
- Billiards (WCBS)   0.20 g/L
- Boules (CMSB, IPC bowls)   0.10 g/L
- Karate (WKF)   0.10 g/L
- Modern pentathlon (UIPM)
  (for disciplines involving shooting)   0.10 g/L
- Motorcycling (FIM)   0.10 g/L
- Powerboating (UIM)   0.30 g/L

Source: WADA. The 2006 Prohibited List. International Standard. Available online: <http://www.wada-ama.org/rtecontent/document/2006_LIST.pdf>.

Alcohol generally has a negative effect on athlete performance, impairing reaction time, hand–eye coordination, accuracy, balance, gross motor skills and strength.[87]

Beta-blockers

P2: Beta-blockers

Unless otherwise specified, beta-blockers are prohibited in competition only, in the following sports:
- Aeronautic (FAI)
- Archery (FGITA, IPC) (also prohibited out of competition)
- Automobile (FIA)
- Billiards (WCBS)
- Boules (CMSB, IPC bowls)
- Bridge (FMB)
- Chess (FIDE)
- Curling (WCF)
- Gymnastics (FIG)
- Modern pentathlon (UIPM) (for disciplines involving shooting)

continues

- Motorcycling (FIM)
- Nine-pin bowling (FIQ)
- Sailing (ISAF) (for match race helms only)
- Shooting (ISSF, IPC)
- Skiing/snowboarding (FIS) in ski jumping, freestyle aerials/halfpipe and snowboard halfpipe/big air
- Wrestling (FILA)

Beta-blockers include, but are not limited to, the following: acebutolol, alprenolol, atenolol, betaxolol, bisoprolol, bunolol, carteolol, carvedilol, celiprolol, esmolol, labetalol, levobunolol, metipranolol, metoprolol, nadolol, oxyprenolol, pindolol, propranolol, sotalol, timolol.

Source: WADA. The 2006 Prohibited List. International Standard. Available online: <http://www.wada-ama.org/rtecontent/document/2006_LIST.pdf>.

Beta-blockers are drugs commonly used in the treatment of hypertension, angina, arrhythmia, migraine, anxiety, tremor and following myocardial infarction. Their anxiolytic and anti-tremor effects resulted in their use in the sports of shooting and archery where steadiness of hand and arm is important.

Beta-blockers do not show any other positive effect on performance, in fact, they may have negative effects on both anaerobic and aerobic endurance. Side-effects may include fatigue, depression, nightmares, bronchospasm and sexual dysfunction. Alternative treatments to beta-blockers are available for most of the clinical conditions mentioned.

Specified substances

The Prohibited List identifies specified substances that are particularly susceptible to unintentional anti-doping rule violations because of their general availability in medicinal products or are less likely to be successfully abused as doping agents (see box).

Therapeutic use of a prohibited substance

Athletes may have illnesses or conditions that require them to take particular medications. If the medication an athlete is required to take to treat an illness or condition happens to fall under the Prohibited List, a TUE may give that athlete the authorization to take the needed medicine.

The criteria necessary to be fulfilled to grant 'therapeutic use' are:

Specified substances

A doping violation involving such substances may result in a reduced sanction provided that the ... athlete can establish that the use of such a specified substance was not intended to enhance sports performance ...

Specific substances include:
- all inhaled beta-2 agonists except clenbuterol
- probenecid
- cathine, cropropamide, crotetamide, ephedrine, etamivan, famprofazone, heptaminol, isometheptene, levmethamfetamine, meclofenoxate, p-methylamphetamine, methylephedrine, niketamide, norfenefrine, octopamine, ortetamine, oxilofrine, phenpromethamine, propylhexedrine, selegiline, sibutramine
- cannabinoids
- all glucocorticosteroids
- alcohol
- all beta-blockers.

Source: WADA. The 2006 Prohibited List. International Standard. Available online: <http://www.wada-ama.org/rtecontent/document/2006_LIST.pdf>.

- the athlete would experience significant health problems without taking the prohibited substance or method
- the therapeutic use of the substance would not produce significant enhancement of performance and
- there is no reasonable therapeutic alternative to the use of the otherwise prohibited substance or method.

WADA has issued an International Standard for the granting of TUEs. The Standard states that all International Federations and National Anti-Doping Organizations must have a process in place whereby athletes with documented medical conditions can request a TUE, and have such a request appropriately dealt with by a panel of independent physicians called a Therapeutic Use Exemption Committee (TUEC).

Those athletes wishing to take a prohibited substance can begin treatment only after receiving the authorization notice from the relevant organization. TUEs are granted for a specific medication with a defined dosage and specific length of time.

The process is considerably simpler for two groups of drugs:

1. glucocorticosteroids by non-systemic routes (e.g. intramuscular, intra-articular injection)
2. beta-2 agonists by inhalation (formoterol, salbutamol, salmeterol, terbutaline).

For these drugs, an abbreviated TUE (ATUE) form is submitted to the relevant organization and the athletes can begin treatment as soon as the form has been received by the relevant organization.

Permitted substances

Drug groups permitted by WADA
Antibiotics
Antidepressants
Antidiarrheals
Antihistamines
Antihypertensives (excluding beta-blockers)
Antinauseants
Aspirin (ASA), paracetamol (acetaminophen), codeine, dextropropoxyphene
Eye medications
NSAIDs
Oral contraceptives
Skin creams and ointments
Sleeping tablets

Recently deleted drugs

As mentioned above a number of drugs have been removed from the Prohibited List over the past few years and are now being monitored by WADA to detect possible patterns of misuse. The two most controversial omissions have been caffeine and pseudoephedrine.

Caffeine

Caffeine is the most commonly used drug in the world. It occurs naturally in more than 60 plants and is contained in coffee, tea, chocolate, cola and various beverages. Until 2004, caffeine was on the Prohibited List with urine levels above 12 µg/mL deemed illegal. This was thought to be the equivalent of six to eight cups of coffee. A typical cup of brewed coffee contains about 100 mg of caffeine, the same amount as an Australian No Doz tablet. Interestingly, an American No Doz tablet contains 200 mg of caffeine. For many years athletes in various sports have been using caffeine in doses below the banned level.

A list of the amounts of caffeine contained in various foods and drinks is shown in Table 61.3.

The effect of caffeine on sporting performance has been widely studied. The vast majority of research demonstrates that caffeine improves muscle contractility, work output, time to exhaustion, and performance during prolonged, moderate- to high-intensity activities lasting 30–120 minutes.[88] There is less convincing evidence for a beneficial effect of caffeine in short-term exercise, although there are clearly some ergogenic benefits during intense exercise lasting at least 1 minute, but to a lesser degree than for prolonged exercise.[88]

Caffeine is widely used in high-intensity intermittent scenarios such as a football match, but the effect on performance is unclear. One study from Boston looked at intermittent high-intensity activity in the laboratory setting and found a positive effect for caffeine,[89] but the laboratory conditions failed to mimic those of a football match.

There are various theories as to how caffeine works to help performance. The majority of available research suggests that adenosine receptor antagonism is the primary mode of action for caffeine's ergogenic effects rather than the long-held belief that it was due to glycogen sparing.[88] Because caffeine can improve concentration, reduce fatigue and enhance alertness, it has been suggested that some of its benefits on performance may be derived from its psychological effects. There is also the possibility of a placebo effect, in other words, if an athlete believes a caffeine tablet will help, then it may do so.

Table 61.3 Caffeine contained in various foods and drinks

Food or drink	Serve	Caffeine content (mg)
Instant coffee	250 mL	60
Brewed coffee	250 mL	80–100 (variable)
Tea	250 mL	30
Hot chocolate	250 mL	5–10
Chocolate	60 g bar	5–15
Coca-Cola	375 mL can	50
Red Bull energy drink	250 mL can	80
V energy drink	250 mL can	50
Lift Plus	250 mL can	36
Black Stallion	250 mL can	80

Coffee contains many substances in addition to caffeine and it is possible that some of these may counter the performance enhancing effect of caffeine. There is some evidence that caffeine taken alone in the form of a tablet is a more effective performance enhancer than caffeine taken in coffee.

There are some areas of activity in which caffeine may have a negative effect. Large doses of caffeine impair fine motor control and technique, which may impair performance. Over-arousal may lead to interference with recovery and sleep patterns, which may interfere with the ability to recover between training competitions.

Other side-effects include palpitations, increased stomach acidity, restlessness, anxiety, tremors and increased muscle tension. Ingestion of caffeine has long been thought to lead to dehydration but studies have failed to support this theory.[88]

There are concerns that since caffeine has been removed from the Prohibited List its use in sport has increased dramatically. If WADA decides that this increased use is of sufficient concern to take action, it is faced with a dilemma. Banning caffeine totally would be impossible. It would mean that no athlete could have a coffee or cola 24–48 hours prior to a game. Another alternative would be to reintroduce the 12 µg/mL urine level beyond which it becomes a doping offence. The problem with this level is that the performance-enhancing effect of caffeine occurs at dosages below that which would exceed the urine level. Most research has shown that the positive effect of caffeine occurs at a dosage of 3–6 mg/kg of body weight, in other words, between 200 and 400 mg in the average athlete.

Non-intentional doping in sports

When athletes test positive for a banned substance, they frequently deny the claim and allege circumstances other than intentional doping. Typical defenses include that their drink had been spiked, passive inhalation of drug smoke or inadvertently taking a nutritional supplement or food that contained a prohibited substance.

Studies have shown that it is possible that an individual could produce detectable levels of cannabinoids in urine samples only after extremely severe conditions of passive exposure to marijuana smoke. The IOC has in the past required a urine concentration of carboxy-THC of greater than 15 µg/L. It is most unlikely that such a level could be obtained through passive exposure.[90] Similarly, only individuals exposed to passive cocaine smoke under extremely harsh conditions would show cocaine metabolites in a urine sample.

Research has indicated that both poppy seed-containing food[91] and herbal cocoa tea[92, 93] can produce levels of morphine and cocaine metabolites above the allowed limit. Studies have also shown that it is possible to yield illegal positive results for anabolic agents after consumption of meat originating from animals treated with anabolic agents.[94]

A number of studies have shown that there is a significant number of 'nutritional supplements' which contain substances other than those described on the label and that a number of these are prohibited substances such as prohormones or anabolic steroids.[90] The IOC has reported that 14.8% of some 650 products sampled contained levels of banned substances sufficient to result in a positive urine sample. None of the substances carried warnings or product information on the contents.[95] Athletes should be wary of ingesting these supplements.

Biotransformation products of permitted substances can also cause an athlete to test positive. One example is the permitted analgesic codeine, which is metabolized to morphine at levels above the threshold.

Drug testing

Drug testing has become commonplace in both amateur and professional sport. The clinician providing services to the team or individual must be familiar with the list of prohibited substances and the drug testing procedure itself. The athlete is entitled to have a representative present to confirm that the correct testing procedures have taken place. Often the representative is the team clinician.

Testing procedure

Selection

An athlete can be selected for a drug test at any time (including while injured and/or post-operatively).

Notification

An athlete can be notified of their selection for a drug test by a drug control official either:

- in person (at any time, in or out of competition)
- by telephone (out of competition)
- by written notice (out of competition).

The criteria for deciding which athlete is tested vary from event to event. At some competitions, placegetters will be tested, at others, competitors are selected randomly, while at other times, certain events may be targeted for testing.

Presenting for a drug test

The drug control official records the athlete's details on a notification form, which is then signed by the athlete. A copy is kept by the athlete for his/her records.

In the presence of the chaperone the athlete may:

- receive necessary medical attention
- attend a victory ceremony
- fulfil media commitments
- compete in further events
- warm-down
- eat or drink (at his/her own risk)—during competition events sealed drinks are provided and it is recommended that athletes only consume these fluids until after the testing is completed.

Sample collection

The athlete is required to provide a urine sample in the direct view of a drug control official who is the same gender as the athlete. The athlete's representative is not permitted to observe the actual collection of the sample, only the testing procedures and paperwork.

A minimum of 80 mL of urine is required for a competition test and 60 mL for an out-of-competition test. (If there is insufficient sample, the initial sample will be sealed with a temporary seal and additional urine sample(s) will be collected and mixed with the original sample until there is sufficient.) Following the collection of the sample, the athlete will return to the doping control area, where a second doping control official will be present, as well as the athlete's representative if there is one accompanying them, to complete the sealing of the sample and paperwork.

The athlete will be asked to select a sample collection kit, which consists of two bottles (labeled 'A' and 'B' with identifying numbers) housed in a sealed polystyrene outer case. It is important that the athlete, and his/her representative, checks that the kits are sealed correctly, that the bottles are clean and that the lids are suitable.

Splitting, sealing and labeling of the sample

The athlete will be asked to pour a measured amount of urine into both the A and B bottles, leaving a small amount behind for the drug control official to test the pH and/or specific gravity. The athlete will seal the bottles with the self-sealing, one-use only, lids

provided. The sample code number of the kit will be identified and recorded on the drug testing form.

Checking pH and concentration of sample

The drug control official will check the pH and/or specific gravity of the sample. If the urine pH is less than 5 or greater than 9, or the urine has a specific gravity of less than 1.010, a second specimen is required. If the second specimen is also outside this range, then the test will still proceed.

Final paperwork

At this stage, the competitor provides the medical declaration. The medical declaration is extremely important. The competitor is asked to list all medications taken in the previous week, including over-the-counter medications, prescription drugs and other substances taken by mouth, injection, inhalation or suppository.

This list should include all vitamins, amino acids and other supplements. It is vitally important that this list be completed accurately as all substances taken in that period are likely to show up in the laboratory test.

The competitor, his or her representative and the drug control officer then check all the written information and, if satisfied, sign the drug testing form. The competitor is given a copy of the form.

The sealed samples and the section of paperwork that does not disclose the athlete's name are then sent in a sealed bag to an accredited laboratory where the sample is analyzed using gas chromatography and mass spectrometry.

Initially only the A sample is analyzed. If the laboratory finds a possible positive test result in the sample in the A bottle, it informs the drug testing agency, which then informs the competitor that a possible positive test result has been recorded. The competitor, or a representative, is then entitled to be present at the unsealing and testing of the B sample. If the B sample also proves positive, the relevant sporting organizations are informed. It is the responsibility of the relevant sporting organization to determine what penalty/sanctions are to be applied following a report of a positive test result. The testing agency does not determine the penalty to apply.

WADA has designated penalties to which most sporting bodies now adhere.

Ethical dilemmas

Most drug taking among athletes does not involve contact with the medical profession. A flourishing black market both of medical and veterinary products gives athletes relatively easy access to these drugs. However, many athletes concerned about the reported effects of these drugs will seek a medical opinion before commencing these drugs. This gives the clinician an excellent opportunity to counsel the athlete.

It also may provide an ethical dilemma for the clinician. While it is clear that no clinician should prescribe prohibited drugs or facilitate their use, the dilemma arises when an athlete, accepting that the clinician will not actually prescribe the drugs, asks that their drug usage be monitored for possible side-effects.

There are conflicting arguments as to whether clinicians should become involved in the monitoring of drug use by athletes. On the one hand, many feel that to do so would be to encourage the use of prohibited substances. On the other hand, others feel that clinicians have a duty to monitor patients and that if this is ignored, athletes may be at increased risk of developing serious problems. The medical profession continues to monitor other forms of drug abuse, such as tobacco and alcohol, both of which have significant morbidity and mortality. This is an ethical dilemma for each individual clinician to resolve.

However, there is opportunity to:

- determine *why* athletes wish to take the drug—for example, do they want to be bigger or do they believe that other athletes they are competing against are using performance-enhancing substances
- discuss all other aspects of their sporting performance and any external pressures that are being applied by parents, coaches, other competitors, officials or media
- give an honest appraisal of substances they are taking or may wish to take
- explore other permitted options, including nutrition, massage, sports psychology and training methods
- discuss the ethical issues of drug usage in athletes—the use of drugs is a form of cheating.

Clinicians are reminded that there are medical board rulings on the prescription of anabolic steroids for non-medical reasons. These vary from state to state and country to country. Clinicians need to be aware that the use of many substances has documented physical and psychological adverse effects. Ultimately, the decision remains one for the individual clinician with due reference to the guidelines and regulations of the medical board of the state in which he/she practices.

The battle against drugs

The sporting community is waging a constant battle against the use of drugs in sport. In the 1970s and 1980s, drug use became widespread, particularly in elite and professional sport. The turning point of the battle against drug use may have been the sensational disqualification of 100 m sprinter Ben Johnson at the 1988 Seoul Olympic Games. This single event focused attention on the problem of drug use and encouraged governments and sporting bodies to address the problem. As a result of this event and subsequent government inquiries, random internationally verified, out-of-competition drug testing is available and used in many countries. This is an extremely costly exercise but essential if drug taking is to be reduced. Countries such as Australia and Canada have taken the lead in the fight against doping. Unfortunately, not all countries are as enthusiastic and vigilant, and many international countries do not have random out-of-competition testing as part of their normal testing procedures. This creates an inequitable situation for international sports competition.

The athletes and their chemists will always find new drugs to take. For instance, the development of masking agents and new short-acting, rapidly eliminated anabolic agents creates a challenge for the testing authorities. The introduction of both blood and urine sample collection will help towards the detection of a wider range of performance-enhancing substances, including the use of some recombinant hormonal substances such as hGH and EPO. While random testing has been a significant step in the battle against drugs, the battle is far from over.

The sporting community must remain vigilant to stamp out all drug use in sport. The athletes themselves are desperate to eliminate all cheating from among their fellow competitors but they will require the unqualified support of their sporting organizations and the testing authorities internationally in order to achieve a level playing field in international sport.

There are four important principles to be followed if drug use is to be prevented.

1. We must be honest with athletes about the advantages and side-effects of drugs.
2. We must educate our athletes, particularly school-age athletes, about the problems associated with drug taking (including alcohol and tobacco).
3. Random, internationally verified, out-of-competition drug testing must be carried out regularly.

4. Society's attitude that winning is the only thing that matters must be gradually changed.

The last point will be the hardest battle to win.

The role of the team clinician

The team clinician has an extremely important role to play in the prevention and management of doping problems. The primary role of the team clinician should be education of team members. This should involve regular briefings, especially prior to the season. Topics covered should include:

- the Prohibited List (available at <http://www.wada-ama.org/rtecontent/document/2006_LIST.pdf>)
- prescription drugs:
  — athletes must inform clinicians that they are subject to drug testing and ensure that the clinician confirms that the medication being prescribed does not contain any banned substance
  — if the clinician is uncertain, suggest contacting the national anti-doping agency for confirmation
- inadvertent doping:
  — checking the contents of all medications, especially over-the-counter substances and supplements
  — if uncertain, contact the national anti-doping agency for confirmation
- drug testing protocols:
  — especially the importance of listing all medications including supplements
- travel:
  — be aware while traveling in foreign countries that drugs with the same or similar brand names in one country may have a different composition in another country
  — always ensure that you take your own regular medications with you.

Recommended Reading

American Academy of Pediatrics. Adolescents and anabolic steroids: a subject review. *Pediatrics* 1997; 99(6): 904–8.

American College of Sports Medicine. Stand on the use of anabolic androgenic steroids in sport. Indianapolis: *American College of Sports Medicine*, 1984.

Bahrke MS, Yesalis CE. *Performance-Enhancing Substances in Sport and Exercise*. Champaign, IL: Human Kinetics, 2002.

Bahrke MS, Yesalis CE, Kopstein AN, et al. Risk factors associated with anabolic-androgenic steroid use among adolescents. *Sports Med* 2000; 229(6): 397–405.

Bohn AM, Khodaee M, Schwenk TL. Ephedrine and other stimulants as ergogenic aids. *Curr Sports Med Rep* 2003; 2: 220–3.

Bouchard R, Weber AR, Geiger JD. Informed decision-making on sympathomimetic use in sport and health. *Clin J Sport Med* 2002; 12: 209–24.

Corrigan B. DHEA and sport. *Clin J Sport Med* 2002; 12: 236–41.

Corrigan B. Beyond EPO. *Clin J Sport Med* 2002; 12: 242–4.

Dean H. Does exogenous growth hormone improve athletic performance? *Clin J Sport Med* 2002; 12: 250–3.

Earnest CP. Dietary androgen 'supplements'. Separating substance from hype. *Physician Sportsmed* 2001; 29(5): 63–79.

Evans NA. Current concepts in anabolic-androgenic steroids. *Am J Sports Med* 2004; 32(2): 534–42.

Foster ZJ, Housner JA. Anabolic-androgenic steroids and testosterone precursors: ergogenic aids and sport. *Curr Sports Med Rep* 2004; 3: 234–41.

Goldman B. *Death in the Locker Room*. South Bend, IN: Icarus Press, 1984.

Graham TE. Caffeine and exercise. Metabolism, endurance and performance. *Sports Med* 2001; 31(11): 785–807.

Houlihan B. *Dying to Win. Doping in Sport and the Development of Anti-Doping Policy*. Strasbourg: Council of Europe Publishing, 1999.

Keisler BD, Hosey RG. Ergogenic aids: an update on ephedra. *Curr Sports Med Rep* 2005; 4: 231–5.

Kutscher EC, Lund BC, Perry PJ. Anabolic steroids. A review for the clinician. *Sports Med* 2002; 32(5): 285–96.

Landry GL. Ephedrine use is risky business. *Curr Sports Med Rep* 2003; 2: 1–2.

Leigh-Smith S. Blood boosting. *Br J Sports Med* 2004; 38: 99–101.

Malvey TC, Armsey TD. Tetrahydrogestrinone: the discovery of a designer steroid. *Curr Sports Med Rep* 2005; 4: 227–30.

Mendoza J. The war on drugs in sport: a perspective from the front line. *Clin J Sport Med* 2002; 12: 254–8.

Paluska SA. Caffeine and exercise. *Curr Sports Med Rep* 2003; 2: 213–19.

Parssinene M, Seppala T. Steroid use and long-term health risks in former athletes. *Sports Med* 2002; 32(2): 83–94.

Schumacher YO, Ashenden M. Doping with artificial oxygen carriers. An update. *Sports Med* 2004; 34(3): 141–50.

Stacy JJ, Terrell TR, Armsey TD. Ergogenic aids: human growth hormone. *Curr Sports Med Rep* 2004; 3: 229–33.

Voy R. *Drugs, Sports and Politics*. Champaign, IL: Leisure Press, 1991.

Yesalis C. *Anabolic Steroids in Sport and Exercise*. 2nd edn. Champaign, IL: Human Kinetics, 2000.

Yesalis CE, Bahrke MS. Anabolic-androgenic steroids and related substances. *Curr Sports Med Rep* 2002; 1: 246–52.

Yesalis CE, Cowart VS. *The Steroids Game*. Champaign, IL: Human Kinetics, 1998.

Yonamine M, Garcia PR, Moreau RL. Non-intentional doping in sports. *Sports Med* 2004; 34(11): 697–704.

Recommended Websites

Australian Sports Drug Agency website: www.asda.org.au.

WADA. Athlete Guide. 3rd edn. <http://www.wada-ama.org/rtecontent/document/WADA_Athlete-Guide_ENG.pdf>.

WADA. Athletes and medications. Q&As. <http://www.wada-ama.org/rtecontent/document/meds_qas_en.pdf>.

World Anti-Doping Agency (WADA): <http://www.wada-ama.org>.

References

1. Hartgens F, Kuipers H. Effects of androgenic-anabolic steroids in athletes. *Sports Med* 2004; 34(8): 513–54.

2. Yesalis CE III, Herrick RT, Buckley WE, et al. Self-reported use of anabolic-androgenic steroids by elite power lifters. *Physician Sportsmed* 1988; 16(12): 91–8.

3. Lindstrom M, Nilsson AL, Katzman PL, et al. Use of anabolic-androgenic steroids among body builders—frequency and attitudes. *J Intern Med* 1990; 227: 407–11.

4. Buckley WE, Yesalis CE, Friedl KE, et al. Estimated prevalence of anabolic-androgenic steroid use among male high school seniors. *JAMA* 1988; 260: 3441–5.

5. Corbin CB, Feyrer-Melk SA, Phelps C, et al. Anabolic steroids: a study of high school athletes. *Pediatr Exerc Sci* 1994; 6: 149–58.

6. Melia P, Pipe A, Greenberg L. The use of anabolic-androgenic steroids by Canadian students. *Clin J Sport Med* 1996; 6: 9–14.

7. Terney R, McLain LG. The use of anabolic steroids in high school students. *Am J Dis Child* 1990; 144: 99–103.

8. Yesalis CE, Bahrke MS. Anabolic-androgenic steroids and related substances. *Curr Sports Med Rep* 2002; 4: 246–52.

9. Bhasin S, Storer TW, Berman N, et al. The effects of supraphysiological doses of testosterone on muscle size and strength in normal men. *N Engl J Med* 1996; 335: 1–7.

10. Forbes GB, Porta CR, Herr BE, et al. Sequence of changes in body composition induced by testosterone and reversal of changes after drug is stopped. *JAMA* 1992; 267: 397–9.

11. Giorgi A, Weatherby RP, Murphy PW. Muscular strength, body composition, and health responses to the use of testosterone enanthate: a double blind study. *J Sci Med Sport* 1999; 2: 341–55.

12. Sinha-Hikim I, Artaza J, Woodhouse L, et al. Testosterone-induced increase in muscle size in healthy young men is associated with muscle fiber hypertrophy. *Am J Physiol Endocrinol Metab* 2002; 283: E154–E164.

13. Parsinnen M, Seppala T. Steroid use and long-term health risks in former athletes. *Sports Med* 2002; 32(2): 83–94.

14. Thiblin I, Lindquist O, Rais J. Cause and manner of death among users of anabolic androgenic steroids. *J Forensic Sci* 2000; 45: 16–23.

15. Rich JD, Dickinson BP, Feller A, et al. The infectious complications of anabolic-androgenic steroid injection. *Int J Sports Med* 1999; 20: 563–6.

16. Ishak KG, Zimmerman HJ. Hepatotoxic effects of the anabolic/androgenic steroids. *Semin Liver Dis* 1987; 7(3): 230–6.

17. Bagheri SA, Boyer JL. Peliosis hepatis associated with androgenic-anabolic steroid therapy. A severe form of hepatic injury. *Ann Intern Med* 1971; 81: 610–18.

18. Cabasso A. Peliosis hepatis in a young adult bodybuilder. *Med Sci Sports Exerc* 1994; 26(1): 2–4.

19. Creagh TM, Rubin A, Evans DJ. Hepatic tumours induced by anabolic steroids in an athlete. *J Clin Pathol* 1988; 41: 441–3.

20. Klava A, Super P, Aldridge M, et al. Body builder's liver. *J R Soc Med* 1994; 87: 43–4.

21. Cohen LI, Hartford CG, Rogers GG. Lipoprotein (a) and cholesterol in body builders using anabolic androgenic steroids. *Med Sci Sports Exerc* 1996; 28(2): 176–9.

22. Ebenbichler CF, Sturm W, Ganzer H, et al. Flow-mediated endothelium-dependent vasodilatation is impaired in male body builders taking anabolic-androgenic steroids. *Atherosclerosis* 2001; 158: 483–90.

23. Kuipers H, Wijnen JA, Hartgens F, et al. Influence of anabolic steroids on body composition, blood pressure, lipid profile, and liver functions in body builders. *Int J Sports Med* 1991; 12: 413–18.

24. Melchert RB, Welder AA. Cardiovascular effects of androgenic-anabolic steroids. *Med Sci Sports Exerc* 1995; 27(9): 1252–62.

25. Hartgens F, Kuipers H. Body composition, cardiovascular risk factors and liver function in long-term androgenic-anabolic steroids using body builders three months after drug withdrawal. *Int J Sports Med* 1996; 17: 429–33.

26. Riebe D, Fernhall B, Thompson PD. The blood pressure response to exercise in anabolic steroid users. *Med Sci Sports Exerc* 1992; 24(6): 633–7.

27. Ferenchick GS, Adelman S. Myocardial infarction associated with anabolic steroid use in a previously healthy 37-year-old weight lifter. *Am Heart J* 1992; 124(2): 507–8.

28. Sullivan ML, Martinez CM, Gennis P, et al. The cardiac toxicity of anabolic steroids. *Prog Cardiovasc Dis* 1998; 41: 1–15.

29. Mochizuki RM, Richter KJ. Cardiomyopathy and cerebrovascular accident associated with anabolic-androgenic steroid use. *Physician Sportsmed* 1988; 18(11): 109–14.

30. Scott MJ. Cutaneous side-effects of anabolic androgenic steroid use. *Clin Sports Med* 1989; 1: 5–16.

31. Kiraly CL. Androgenic-anabolic steroid effects on serum and skin surface lipids, on red cells, and on liver enzymes. *Int J Sports Med* 1988; 9: 249–52.

32. Bahrke MS, Yesalis CE III, Wright JE. Psychological and behavioural effects of endogenous testosterone levels and anabolic-androgenic steroids among males. *Sports Med* 1990; 10(5): 303–37.

33. Choi PYL, Parrott AC, Cowan D. Adverse behavioural effects of anabolic steroids in athletes: a brief review. *Clin Sports Med* 1989; 1: 183–7.

34. Cooper CJ, Noakes T, Dunne T, et al. A high prevalence of personality traits in chronic users of anabolic-androgenic steroid users. *Br J Sports Med* 1996; 30: 246–50.

35. Midgley SJ, Heather N, Davies JB. Levels of aggression among a group of anabolic-androgenic steroid users. *Med Sci Law* 2001; 41: 309–14.

36. Lubell A. Does steroid abuse cause—or excuse—violence? *Physician Sportsmed* 1989; 17(2): 176–85.

37. Kashkin KB, Kleber HD. Hooked on hormones? An anabolic steroid addiction hypothesis. *JAMA* 1989; 262(22): 3166–70.

38. Jarow JP, Lipshultz LI. Anabolic steroid-induced hypogonadotropic hypogonadism. *Am J Sports Med* 1990; 18(4): 429–31.

39. Tan RS, Vasudevan D. Use of clomiphene citrate to reverse premature andropause secondary to steroid abuse. *Fertil Steril* 2003; 79: 203–5.

40. Friedl KE, Yesalis CE. Self-treatment of gynecomastia in bodybuilders who use anabolic steroids. *Physician Sportsmed* 1989; 17(3): 67–79.

41. Wilson JD. Androgen abuse by athletes. *Endocr Rev* 1988; 9(2): 181–99.

42. Rogol AD, Yesalis CE III. Anabolic-androgenic steroids and athletes: what are the issues? *J Clin Endocrinol Metab* 1992; 74(3): 465–9.

43. Corrigan B. DHEA and sport. *Clin J Sport Med* 2002; 12: 236–41.

44. Brown GA, Vukovich MD, Reifenrath TA, et al. Effects of anabolic precursors on serum testosterone concentrations and adaptations to resistance training in young men. *Int J Sport Nutr Exerc Metab* 2001; 10: 340–59.

45. Welle S, Jozefowicz R, Statt M. Failure of dehydroepiandrosterone to influence energy and protein metabolism in humans. *J Clin Endocrinol Metab* 1990; 71: 1259–64.

46. Caitlin DH, Sekera MH, Ahrens BH, et al. Tetrahydrogestrinone discovery, synthesis, and detection in urine. *Rapid Commun Mass Spectrom* 2004; 18: 1245–9.

47. Malvey TC, Armsey TD. Tetrahydrogestrinone: the discovery of a designer steroid. *Curr Sports Med Rep* 2005; 4: 227–30.

48. Death AK, McGrath KCY, Kazlauskas R, et al. Tetrahydrogestrinone is a potent androgen and progestin. *J Clin Endocrinol Metab* 2004; 89: 2498–500.

49. Prather ID, Brown DE, North P, et al. Clenbuterol: a substitute for anabolic steroids? *Med Sci Sports Exerc* 1995; 27(8): 1118–21.

50. Scott J, Phillips GC. Erythropoietin in sports: a new look at an old problem. *Curr Sports Med Rep* 2005; 4: 224–6.

51. Audran M, Gareau R, Matecki S, et al. Effects of erythropoietin administration in training athletes and possible indirect detection in doping control. *Med Sci Sports Exerc* 1999; 31(5): 639–45.

52. Ekblom B. Blood doping and erythropoietin. The effects of variation in hemoglobin concentration and other related factors on physical performance. *Am J Sports Med* 1996; 24(6): S40–S42.

53. Berglund B, Ekblom B. Effect of recombinant erythropoietin treatment on blood pressure and some hematological parameters in healthy men. *J Intern Med* 1991; 229: 125–30.

54. Birkeland KI, Stray-Gundersen J, Hemmersbach P, et al. Effect of rhEPO administration on serum levels of STFR and cycling performance. *Med Sci Sports Exerc* 2000; 32: 1238–43.

55. Ekblom B, Berglund B. Effect of erythropoietin administration on maximal aerobic power. *Scand J Med Sci Sports* 1991; 1: 88–93.

56. O'Toole ML, Douglas PS, Douglas W, et al. Hematocrits of triathletes: is monitoring useful? *Med Sci Sports Exerc* 1999; 31(3): 372–7.

57. Scumacher YO, Schmid A, Lenz T, et al. Blood testing in sports: hematological profile of a convicted athlete. *Clin J Sport Med* 2001; 11: 115–17.

58. Kazlauskas R, Howe C, Trout G. Strategies for rhEPO detection in sport. *Clin J Sport Med* 2002; 12: 229–35.

59. Dean H. Does exogenous growth hormone improve athletic performance? *Clin J Sport Med* 2002; 12: 250–3.

60. Crist DM, Peake GT, Egan PA, et al. Body composition response to exogenous GH during training in highly conditioned adults. *J Appl Physiol* 1988; 65(2): 579–84.

61. Stacy JJ, Terrell TR, Armsey TD. Ergogenic aids: human growth hormone. *Curr Sports Med Rep* 2004; 3: 229–33.

62. Yarasheki KE, Zachwieja JJ, Angleopoulos TJ, et al. Short-term growth hormone does not increase muscle protein

synthesis in experienced weightlifters. *J Appl Physiol* 1993; 74: 3073–6.

63. Rennie MJ. Claims for the anabolic effects of growth hormone: a case of the emperor's new clothes? *Br J Sports Med* 2003; 37: 100–5.

64. Adams G. Insulin-like growth factor in muscle growth and its potential abuse by athletes. *Br J Sports Med* 2000; 34: 412–13.

65. Baxter RC. Insulin-like growth factor (IGF)-binding proteins: interactions with IGFS and intrinsic bioactivities. *Am J Physiol* 2000; 278: E967–E976.

66. Grimberg A, Cohen P. Role of insulin-like growth factors and their binding proteins in growth control and carcinogenesis. *J Cell Physiol* 2000; 183: 1–9.

67. Rich JD, Dickinson BP, Merriman MA, et al. Insulin use by bodybuilders. *JAMA* 1998; 279: 161–3.

68. Evans PJ, Lynch RM. Insulin as a drug of abuse in body building. *Br J Sports Med* 2003; 37: 356–7.

69. Banadonna RC, Saccomani MP, Cobelli C, et al. Effect of insulin on system A amino acid transport in human skeletal muscle. *J Clin Invest* 1993; 91: 514–21.

70. Seeheusen DA, Glorioso JE. Tamoxifen as an ergogenic agent in women body builders. A case report. *Clin J Sport Med* 2002; 12: 313–14.

71. Hickey G, Fricker P. Attention deficit hyperactivity disorder, CNS stimulants and sport. *Sports Med* 1999; 27(1): 11–21.

72. Geiger JD. Adverse effects associated with supplements containing ephedra alkaloids. *Clin J Sport Med* 2002; 12: 263.

73. Shekelle P, Hardy MA, Morton S, et al. Efficacy and safety of ephedra and ephedrine for weight loss and athletic performance: a meta-analysis. *JAMA* 2003; 289: 1537–45.

74. Bohn AM, Khodaee M, Schwenk TL. Ephedrine and other stimulants as ergogenic aids. *Curr Sports Med Rep* 2003; 2: 220–5.

75. Bell DG, Jacobs I, Zamecnik J. Effects of caffeine, ephedrine, and their combination on time to exhaustion during high intensity exercise. *Eur J Appl Physiol* 1996; 81: 428–33.

76. Kaufman KR, Gerner R. Modafinil in sports: ethical considerations. *Br J Sports Med* 2005; 39(4): 241–4.

77. Renaud AM, Cormier Y. Acute effects of marihuana smoking on maximal exercise performance. *Med Sci Sports Exerc* 1986; 18(6): 685–9.

78. Jones M, Pedoe DST. Blood doping—a literature review. *Br J Sports Med* 1989; 23(2): 84–8.

79. Sawka MN, Joyner MJ, Miles DS, et al. American College of Sports Medicine position stand. The use of blood doping

as an ergogenic aid. *Med Sci Sports Exerc* 1996; 28(6): i–viii.

80. Leigh-Smith S. Blood boosting. *Br J Sports Med* 2004; 38: 99–101.

81. Corrigan B. Beyond EPO. *Clin J Sport Med* 2002; 12: 242–4.

82. Schumacher YO, Ashenden M. Doping with artificial oxygen carriers. *Sports Med* 2004; 34(3): 141–50.

83. Hughes GS, Yancey EP, Albrecht R, et al. Hemoglobin-based oxygen carrier preserves submaximal exercise capacity in humans. *Clin Pharmacol Ther* 1995; 58: 434–43.

84. Svensson E, Black H, Dugger D, et al. Long term erythropoietin expression in rodents and non-human primates following intramuscular ingestion of a replication-defective adenoviral vector. *Hum Gene Ther* 1997; 8: 1797–806.

85. Barton-Davis E, Shoturma D, Musaro A, et al. Viral mediated expression of insulin like growth factor 1 blocks the ageing-related loss of skeletal muscle function. *Proc Natl Acad Sci U S A* 1998; 95: 15603–7.

86. McCrory P. Super athletes or gene cheats? *Br J Sports Med* 2003; 37: 192–3.

87. O'Brien CP. Alcohol and sport. Impact of social drinking on recreational and competitive sports performance. *Sports Med* 1993; 15(2): 71–7.

88. Paluska SA. Caffeine and exercise. *Curr Sports Med Rep* 2003; 2: 213–19.

89. Trice I, Haymes EM. Effects of caffeine ingestion on exercise-induced changes during high-intensity, intermittent exercise. *Int J Sport Nutr* 1995; 5(1): 37–44.

90. Yonamine M, Garcia PR, Moreau RLM. Non-intentional doping in sports. *Sports Med* 2004; 34(11): 697–704.

91. elSohly HN, elSohly MA, Stanford DF. Poppy seed ingestion and opiates urinalysis: a closer look. *J Anal Toxicol* 1990; 14: 308–10.

92. Jackson GF, Saady JJ, Poklis A. Urinary excretion of benzoylecgonine following ingestion of health Inca tea. *Forensic Sci Int* 1991; 49(1): 57–64.

93. Jenkins AJ, llosa T, Montoya I, et al. Identification and quantitation of alkaloids in cocoa tea. *Forensic Sci Int* 1996; 77: 179–86.

94. Kicman AT, Cowan DA, Myhre L, et al. Effect on sports drug tests of ingesting meat from steroid (methenolone)-treated livestock. *Clin Chem* 1994; 40(11): 2084–7.

95. International Olympic Committee. *IOC Nutritional Supplements Study Points to Need for Greater Quality Control.* Lausanne: IOC, 2002. Available online: <http://www.olympic.org>.

Ethics and Sports Medicine

The broad goal of medical ethics is to improve the quality of patient care by identifying, analyzing and attempting to resolve the ethical problems that arise in the practise of clinical medicine.[1] In addition, the increased professionalism of sport has raised numerous significant ethical issues in sports medicine. Influences such as the practitioner's employer (sports team or organization), the athlete's desire to play with pain and injury, and the economic consequences of playing or not playing all complicate medical decisions.[2, 3]

Five of those contentious areas are discussed below:

1. conflict of interest
2. confidentiality
3. performance-enhancing drugs
4. infectious diseases
5. ethics in sport.

It is to be hoped that we have come a long way over the last few decades. For example, in the 1970s, an Australian football star said:

> I know that a football club doctor would never have the audacity to tell you the truth ... Front up in the medical room with severe internal bleeding and they will say something like 'it's just a scratch—you'll be right'. I guess that's why they have football club doctors and why players should never go to anyone else.
>
> *The Age* (Melbourne), 6 July 1979

In 1981, however, the World Medical Association (WMA) adopted a declaration to act as a guideline to clinicians treating athletes. The declaration was subsequently amended at WMA Assemblies in 1987 and 1993. The Federation International de Sports Medicine (FIMS) simplified the code into three principles:[4]

1. Always make the athlete a priority.
2. Never do harm.
3. Never impose your authority in a way that impinges on the individual right of the athlete to make his or her own decision.

Conflict of interest

The goal of most patients is usually to reduce suffering and prolong healthy life. Athletes, especially professional athletes, have as their priority a desire to perform. A major objective for a sports clinician is to support athletic achievement.[2] As a result of the dynamics of professional sports, medical decision making can be affected by a host of factors not normally encountered in standard practise.

Decision making can potentially be affected by pressures exerted from a variety of sources that may influence both clinicians and the patient/players. A professional team clinician should recognize these potential influences and their effect on ethical medical decision making. These pressures may come from players, management and coaches, and the clinicians themselves.[5]

The team clinician may come under pressure to allow the athlete to play from a number of different sources. The players themselves are usually the greatest potential source of pressure on the clinician. Athletes are highly motivated. An athlete may prefer to risk his or her health for the sake of participation and success in the game, motivated by machismo, peer pressure, pride, institutional pressures, and also economic considerations.[6] However, it has been shown that athletes, as a group, significantly underestimate the disruptive effects of injury.[7]

Pressure may also come also from the coach, team mates, parents or team administration. This pressure can take several forms, including pressuring the athletes who will in turn attempt to influence the clinician's decision making. Other forms of pressure may come about from direct or indirect questioning of the clinician's decisions, or scrutinizing the medical care of the team with comments to the media.[3] Management could directly attempt to affect decisions by threatening replacement of the team clinician.[5] Team clinicians treating athletes must keep those powerful motivators in mind when determining the extent of an injury and the time needed for recovery.

A danger that may befall the unwary team physician is the 'fan syndrome'. Its principal symptom is the distortion of proper clinical judgment when the clinician may be influenced by his or her desire to see the team succeed. This can be manifested in many ways. The clinician's desire to see the team succeed may propel a decision to declare a leading athlete fit for a crucial competition when further recuperation from injury is in order. Such may be the clinician's desire to remain on good terms with the team's management that he or her is influenced to provide advice which accords with what will please rather than what may be dispassionately appropriate. The insidious nature of the 'fan syndrome' is that very rarely will a clinician be aware that his or her behavior is affected by it.[8]

Team clinicians inevitably benefit from team success. There may be financial benefits as the staff earn bonuses for success and may have their contracts increased for the following season; they may get the opportunity for travel to play-off games and end-of-season trips based on success; they may get increased media exposure if the team progresses to a high-profile game and their professional reputation may be enhanced (rightly or wrongly) if the team is successful.

The sum of these pressures may affect a clinician's judgment and lead to a vulnerability to litigation. There have been instances in a number of countries of team clinicians being sued.

The clinician's duty: the team or the athlete?

The clinician employed by the professional team, either on a salary or, more commonly, on a contract, has an inherent conflict of interest. Is the primary duty of the clinician to the athlete or the team?

In most situations the interests of the team and the athlete coincide. What is best for the athlete is usually best for the team. However, situations may arise where there may be short-term benefit to the team to the detriment of the athlete's health. This conflict is considered further below under the heading confidentiality.

The overriding duty of the team clinician is always to the athlete. This is true regardless of how much pressure the team clinician feels under from the coaches, other members of the team and parents. The team clinician is required to give full disclosure to the athlete (and the parents if appropriate) regarding the extent of the injury, the nature of the injury, proper rehabilitation, and the consequences of injuries.[9]

If the wellbeing of the athlete is in conflict with an interest of a third party, the wellbeing of the athlete is always paramount.[10] Instituting a policy that the team clinician has the final say regarding any player's participation[9] minimizes potential conflicts between the medical team and coaches and other members of the team administration.

The coaches and other members of the administration associated with the team should all be aware that the team clinician makes the ultimate determination regarding the decision of whether an injured athlete can return to play.

If, after full disclosure, the legally competent athlete, or the parents in the case of a minor athlete, insist on contravening the clinician's recommendation, the team clinician should ask the player (or parent) to sign an exculpatory waiver.

Local anesthetic injection and administration of analgesics

In professional sport, local anesthetic administration is commonplace, but there has been a reluctance to disclose the extent of the prevalence of these injections (Scenario 1).[11] The most common way of administering these drugs such as lignocaine (lidocaine) is by injection into or around the painful area. The most common site and conditions for which local anesthetics are used are AC joint injury, iliac crest contusion (hip pointer), a rib contusion or fracture, or an undisplaced finger fracture. Other conditions for which local anesthetic injections have been used include the plantar fascia (Scenario 1), stress fractures, ankle ligament sprains, tennis elbow and adductor muscle tears.

Analgesics ('pain killers') are also thought to be commonly used in professional sport. These range from simple oral analgesics such as paracetamol

Scenario 1

A professional footballer suffering from plantar fasciitis prior to an important match requests a pain-killing injection from the team clinician. The footballer plays after receiving the pain-killing injection and ruptures the plantar fascia.

(acetaminophen) to more powerful oral medications including substances such as codeine, to injectable analgesics such as ketorolac. A survey of National Football League team clinicians documented that 28 of the 30 responding teams used ketorolac during the season. Medical staff that used the drug treated an average of 15 different players over the course of the season, with the range from 2 to 35.[12]

There are two issues at stake in these situations. The clinician must firstly consider whether playing with the injury may make the injury worse. In most cases the answer is 'yes'. Also, the clinician must consider whether playing with an injury would place the player at an increased risk of other injuries. And whether a player 'carrying' an injury would place other players at increased risk of injury.

Does the situation change if the team clinician has an employment agreement with the team or not; the player is professional or amateur; it is an important/less important game; the player is a key player/lesser player; the request comes from the athlete or the coach or the team administration; or if the athlete is under age?

What if the athlete is under age? What is the role of the parents in the decision making? Can we assume that they are acting in the best interests of the child? What if the player wants to rest and the parents insist he or she plays?

Without the pain from the injured area acting as a warning symptom, players will not be aware that they may be aggravating the injury until the effect of the injection wears off. The clinician and the athlete must weigh up the potential advantages and disadvantages of playing. In professional sport this may be affected by the importance of the occasion, and on whether it is a one-off game such as the final game of the season, after which the player may have an extended time to recover, or whether the injury will require weekly anesthetic injections for a number of weeks to enable the player to continue playing. It may be that continuing to play after an injection may prevent the injury from healing.

The other concern is the long-term effects of continuing to play after an anesthetic or analgesic. Pain may be considered the body's mechanism to alert patients to the potential for damage.

Short-term gain, long-term pain

Frequently there is a conflict between short-term advantage and the potential for long-term problems. Scenarios 2 and 3 are typical examples.

Scenario 2

A star footballer sustains a torn meniscus three weeks before the start of finals/play-offs. The tear is clearly amenable to repair, but this would mean an extended period off sport and no finals/play-offs. A partial menisectomy would almost certainly allow the player to return for the finals/play-offs, but is associated with a much higher risk of subsequent osteoarthritis.

Scenario 3

A professional footballer injures his knee, tearing the anterior cruciate ligament (ACL). In addition, he has significant damage to the articular osteochondral surface. The footballer has an ACL reconstruction (Chapter 27) and is keen to resume playing. He asks for advice.

Scenario 3 is a common one which provides a significant ethical dilemma for team clinicians and orthopedic surgeons. There is a general acceptance in the sporting and medical communities that a torn ACL is no longer a career-ending injury and that athletes should be able to return to high-level competition somewhere between four and 12 months after ACL reconstruction. Recently, however, we[13] and others[14] have expressed concern about the long-term consequences of facilitating return to sport after these injuries.

As described previously, the incidence of long-term osteoarthritis following injuries such as a torn meniscus and torn ACL is significant. It is likely that returning to high-level, high-intensity sport following these injuries would accelerate this process. Clinicians need to discuss these possible adverse effects with their athletes prior to them returning to sport. This emphasizes the importance of informed consent.

Informed consent

Informed consent is of vital importance throughout medicine, particularly in the light of ethical and legal concerns. Informed consent is 'the voluntary agreement by a patient to a proposed health care management approach after proper and adequate information is conveyed to the patient about the proposed management, including potential risks and benefits and alternative management options'.[15]

The potential risks and benefits of a particular course of action need to be explained in a relaxed atmosphere away from distractions. When practical, the clinician should always give players an opportunity to go away and think about it, preferably with some relevant written material, and offer the opportunity of another discussion to answer any queries they may have.

Informed consent in the context of a professional athlete has its particular challenges. It is complicated by some of the issues already mentioned, pressure from coaches, management, agent, family and others who stand to benefit from the athlete's continued participation in their sport. The injured athlete is under pressure to 'do what is best for the team'. An athlete who acts contrary to this, seeks outside advice, chooses non-traditional therapies, refuses to play while still hurting or otherwise attempts to act autonomously is considered petulant, uncommitted and indifferent to the goals of the team. Within professional sports, the number of injured players who have been so labeled is legion.[16]

The athlete will invariably receive information about the possible courses of action from a variety of sources. The internet is now a major source of medical information for patients. Unfortunately, there is no means of separating unscientific information from that which is based on good scientific evidence. Personal testimonials carry a lot of weight with athletes, who will often be more influenced by the experience of a colleague, or a well-publicized experience of a high-profile player, than the advice given by their practitioner. The athlete usually does not appreciate that every case is different.

Another potential difficulty is decisions being made in the middle of a game such as whether or not to have an injection. Fully informed consent is not practical in this circumstance, but this does not excuse the clinician from making a good faith attempt at educating the player on the risks and benefits, and documenting the discussion in the medical record.

Documentation is essential. Ideally, documentation should be provided to the athletes explaining the risks and benefits of a particular course of action. The athlete and the clinician should both sign a document stating that the athlete has been given certain information and advice.

Occasionally the athlete will decide not to heed the advice of the clinician and go ahead with a course of action contrary to what has been advised. Of course, this is the right of the athlete as it is the right of any patient. However, it is essential that it be documented that the athlete is acting against the advice of the practitioner.

Guidelines for resolution of conflict of interest

The guidelines for a clinician to follow for the resolution of conflict of interest include:

- player's health is paramount
- informed consent
- full disclosure
- exculpatory waiver
- team clinician contract
- player contract
- care with the media.

Confidentiality

Patient confidentiality is fundamental to the practise of medicine. The professional codes of conduct of medical and paramedical practitioners limits their freedom to report injuries, illnesses and other problems to anyone else other than the individual directly concerned. How does this affect the team clinician? Scenarios 4 and 5 provide examples.

> **Scenario 4**
>
> During the last training session before a major game, a player sustains a mild hamstring strain, which is not noticed by the coaching staff. The player presents for treatment, tells the clinician 'in confidence', and begs the clinician not to inform the coach.

> **Scenario 5**
>
> A professional player has a career-threatening injury. You are asked by team management to help conceal the injury as it wishes to trade the player.

The athlete and the team clinician have a confidential clinician–patient relationship. But when management pays a team clinician, this may change the relationship between clinician and athlete. The team clinician has two masters to serve: the athlete–patient and the team management.

The American Medical Association admonishes clinicians 'not to reveal confidences entrusted to them unless required to do so by law or, if necessary, to protect the welfare of the individual or community'.[17]

In the case of professional or collegiate team clinicians, because of the salaries or scholarships received by the athletes, management may have access to their records. This access is deemed by some to be appropriate. Therefore, discussing the condition of the athlete with management would also probably be viewed as appropriate.[18]

Before examination the team clinician should remind the athlete that he or she is acting on behalf of the team. Permission must be sought from the athlete to disclose relevant information regarding the athlete's medical or physical condition to appropriate team officials.[19] What if the athlete asks to speak to the clinician 'in confidence', or after telling the clinician some information asks that it be kept confidential?

While it is clear that team clinicians have the right to inform team management of relevant injuries, there is a gray area about what is appropriate. Issues such as drug or alcohol use, personal issues, and psychiatric or psychological problems may all impact on the player's performance and yet the consequences of revealing these problems to the team management may impact negatively on the careers of the players/patients.

It is strongly advised that all players and medical staff sign written agreements prior to the season which make it absolutely clear that the team clinician has the player's permission to divulge information to the team coach/management if appropriate. This has the unfortunate consequence that the player is more likely to seek advice and/or treatment away from the team medical staff.

The British Olympic Association (BOA) has a different view on this question. Just prior to the Sydney Olympic Games, the BOA published a position statement on athlete confidentiality.[20] This argues that coaches can only be informed of an athlete's problems with the consent of the individual athlete. In relation to contracts, the BOA statement said that medical support staff who sign a contract with the governing body may be in breach of their professional code of conduct if they breach their duties of confidentiality. It suggested that athletes who had signed a general consent form could still withhold consent for any specific consultation, test or treatment.

The media

Relationships with the media are another potential problem for the team clinician as sports medicine information can be personally and/or financially damaging to the athlete. The team clinician should always have the permission of the player and, if appropriate, team management before divulging details of injuries to the media.

It is much safer for the clinicians not to talk to the media at all and leave all communication regarding injuries to the team media spokesperson.

Performance-enhancing drugs

It is clear that since the 1980s a significant minority of sports clinicians have played a role in administering performance-enhancing drugs to athletes. The most extreme example occurred in the systemized doping practises of the East German regime of the 1970s and 1980s.[21] Other prominent examples of clinicians mediating doping were the Ben Johnson steroid case at the 1988 Olympics, and the 1998 Tour de France erythropoietin (EPO) scandal (Chapter 61). There has always been a small number of clinicians who encouraged the use of drugs, particularly anabolic steroids.

There were a number of different rationales for this support. Some used the patient autonomy notion that the non-medical use of drugs is simply a matter of personal liberty and individual experimentation and that if athletes are aware of possible adverse reactions and are willing to accept the risks in the hope of other rewards there should be no reason not to prescribe the drugs. Some argued that as other performance-enhancing techniques were allowed drugs were no different, others argued that given that steroid use was widespread there was no point trying to prevent it, and others argued the harm minimization line that clinicians have an obligation to monitor the effects of steroids in the same way as they monitor the potential harmful effects of alcohol and smoking. One suspects that others were influenced by their desire to become associated with elite sportspeople.

It is interesting to note the comments of Californian clinician Robert Kerr, who was a well-known supplier of anabolic steroids in the 1980s. Kerr ceased prescribing steroids, stating that while his intention was to steer athletes clear of black market steroids of dubious quality and to minimize the medical risks of taking steroids by prescribing so-called safe types and dosages, he was duped by his patients because they went to the black market for additional steroids and used far more than the dosages he prescribed.[22]

While it is now illegal to prescribe anabolic steroids in a number of countries such as Australia, it is not illegal to give advice about how to alleviate some of the harmful effects of steroid use, just as clinicians and other healthcare providers give information to intravenous drug users about how to avoid becoming infected with the human immunodeficiency virus (HIV).

By monitoring are you giving de facto approval? Are you facilitating this player's drug use? Scenario 6 provides an example. Monitoring steroid use may allow a clinician to develop a relationship with an athlete that will give the opportunity to help the athlete stop using anabolic steroids. Clinicians are much more effective in changing attitudes about steroid use if they give balanced information about the potential benefits as well as the risks of using anabolic steroids.[23]

Scenario 6

An athlete asks you to monitor his or her anabolic steroid use with regular examinations and blood tests.

A team clinician should be careful not to give the athlete the impression that he or she condones the use of steroids or other performance-enhancing drugs and should make it clear that the opposite is true. This information should be documented in the athlete's record.

We concur with Kennedy's advice[24] that the proper medical response to a request to prescribe or monitor drug use is to provide accurate information and advice in a non-judgmental manner.

Athletes will not seek help or advice about drugs from a team clinician whom they cannot trust to keep their confidence. However, the confidentiality of the clinician–patient relationship allows the clinician to assure athletes that disclosures, discussions and treatments will remain confidential. Clinicians, however, have a duty to warn third parties of impending harm related to an athlete's drug use, and a team clinician's public duty to warn may override the private duty of confidentiality.

Scenario 7

You become aware that a player in your team is taking anabolic steroids. The team is regularly drug tested.

Scenario 7 provides another example. The situation in this scenario places the team clinician in a difficult position. Let us assume, firstly, that the player himself/herself has told you he/she is taking steroids. Does your duty to the team to prevent the adverse effects of a positive drug test result override patient confidentiality? Is the situation different if a third party has informed you? If so, do you approach the player and say that you have heard a rumor and offer advice regarding the personal dangers and the implications for the team?

According to the BOA's position statement, 'a refusal to consent to disclosure must be respected even in the event of an athlete taking a prohibited substance'.[20]

Or, if you confront the player and he/she refuses to stop taking the steroids, what should you do? There are two components to this question. Firstly, it is the clinician's duty to counsel the athlete regarding the dangers of taking anabolic steroids. The second, more difficult, ethical question is whether the clinician should inform team management of the player's anabolic drug use on the basis that a positive drug test may have disastrous implications for the player, the team and team management (possibly including the team clinician if it is known that the clinician was aware of the drug taking).

We believe that patient confidentiality is paramount but attempts should be made to encourage the player to admit his or her drug taking.

Scenario 8

You become aware that one of your athletes is taking a banned substance which cannot currently be detected by drug testing.

What about the situation in Scenario 8 where a new 'undetectable' drug becomes available. How does this situation change Scenario 7 now that there is no risk of testing positive for a drug? There is no longer the risk of embarrassment/shame/penalty that would result from a positive drug test result but you are still aware that one of the players in your care is acting against the laws of the game. Again, patient confidentiality is paramount unless the physical health of another person is endangered.

Infectious diseases

Several questions arise in this contentious area. Can an bbhathlete with HIV, hepatitis B or hepatitis C compete? Is this a medical, ethical or legal problem? This is probably a decision for the sporting body with input from medical, legal and advocacy groups.[25]

In the 1990s in Melbourne an amateur Australian Rules footballer who admitted to being HIV positive was refused permission to play. The player's appeal on the grounds of discrimination was heard at the State Civil and Administrative Tribunal. The *Equal Opportunity Act 1995* provides that a person must not discriminate against another person by excluding such other person from participating in a sporting activity. However, another section of the Act provides that discrimination on the basis of impairment may be permitted if such discrimination is reasonably necessary to protect the health or safety of any person.

The Tribunal found that although there was a statistical risk of transmission of HIV from the player to another player or official, the prospects of such transmission were so low that the Tribunal granted the player permission to play with the proviso that appropriate precautions be taken to protect players from such transmission as far as possible.[26]

Scenario 9 raises similar confidentiality issues to those discussed previously. The clinician must determine whether the public interest outweighs patient confidentiality. The infected player may be a risk to both team mates and opponents.

Scenario 9

An athlete tells you in strict confidence that he or she is HIV, hepatitis B or hepatitis C positive.

The type of sport being played influences the risk of bleeding and may, thus, affect the decision. Sports are divided into combat (e.g. boxing), contact (e.g. football), collision (e.g. basketball), and non-contact (e.g. tennis, golf). Combat, contact and collision sports have higher risks of transmission than non-contact sports.

Ethics in sport

The sports clinician has an important role to play in sport in providing quality medical care. The clinician can also play an important role in sport in general. Currently, many condemnable practises are associated with sport. These include: violence; hazardous training practices; drug use; emotional, physical and sexual abuse; cheating and antisocial behavior.

In the battle to eradicate drug use in sport, the team clinician plays an important role,[27] although until society's attitude towards success changes markedly it is doubtful whether the use of education and widespread drug testing will ever eradicate the problem.[28]

As sports medicine clinicians, we have unique ethical responsibilities for the athletes in our care, the sports organizations we work for, and the ideals of fair play and fair competition.[29] It is easy at times, when caught up in the pressure of competition, to lose sight of the full range of responsibilities. Sports clinicians are in a unique position to intervene with patients, speak out with respect to rules, drugs and violence, and develop and adhere to a sports medicine code of ethics.

Recommended Reading

Bunch WH, Dvonch VM. Informed consent in sports medicine. *Clin Sports Med* 2004; 23: 183–93.

Gallup EM. *Law and the Team Physician*. Champaign, IL: Human Kinetics,1995.

Grayson E. *Ethics, Injuries and the Law in Sports Medicine*. Oxford: Butterworth Heinemann, 1999.

Matheson G. Can team physicians buy credibility? *Physician Sportsmed* 2001; 29(12): 3.

Mitten M. Emerging legal issues in sports medicine: a synthesis, summary and analysis. *St Johns Law Rev* 2002; 76(1): 5–86.

Opie H. Medico-legal issues in sport: the view from the grandstand. *Sydney Law Rev* 2001; 375: 375–6.

Pipe A, Best T. Drugs, sport, and medical practice. *Clin J Sport Med* 2002; 12: 201–2.

Rubin A. Team physician or athlete's doctor. *Physician Sportsmed* 1998; 26(7): 27–9.

Salomon B. Ethics in the locker room: the challenges for team physicians. *Occupat Med* 2002; 17: 693.

Tucker AM. Ethics and the professional team physician. *Clin Sports Med* 2004; 23: 227–41.

References

1. Singer PA. Recent advances. Medical ethics. *BMJ* 2000; 321: 282–5.

2. Bernstein J, Perlis C, Bartolozzi AR. Normative ethics in sports medicine. (a). *Clin Orthop* 2004; 420: 309–18.

3. Polsky SD. Winning medicine: professional sports team doctors' conflicts of interest. *J Contemp Health Law Policy* 1998; 14(2): 503–29.

4. Federation International de Sports Medicine. FIMS code of ethics in sports medicine 1997. Available online: <http://www.fims.org/about/positions/ethics.cfm>.

5. Tucker AM. Ethics and the professional team physician. *Clin Sports Med* 2004; 23: 227–41.

6. King JHJ. The duty and standards of care for team physicians. *Houston Law Rev* 1981; 18(4): 657–704.

7. Crossman J, Jamieson J, Hume K. Perceptions of athletic injuries by athletes, coaches, and medical professionals. *Percept Mot Skills* 1990; 71: 848–50.

8. Opie H. The team doctor/athlete legal relationship. *Sports Med Train Rehabil* 1991; 2: 287–99.

9. Gallup EM. *Law and the Team Physician*. Champaign, IL: Human Kinetics, 1995.

10. King JHJ. The duty and standards of care for team physicians. *Houston Law Rev* 1981; 18(4): 657–704.

11. Orchard J. The use of local anaesthetic injections in professional football. *Br J Sports Med* 2001; 35: 212–13.

12. Tokisk JM, Powell ET, Schlegel TF, et al. Ketorolac use in the National Football League. *Physician Sportsmed* 2002; 30(9): 19–25.

13. Brukner P. Return to play. A personal perspective. *Clin J Sport Med* 2005; 15: 459.

14. Myklebust G, Bahr R. Return to play guidelines after anterior cruciate ligament surgery. *Br J Sports Med* 2005; 39(3): 127–31.

15. Medical Defence Association of Victoria. *Medicine and the Law. A Practical Guide for Doctors*. Melbourne: MDAV, 2005.

16. Bunch WH, Dvonch VM. Informed consent in sports medicine. *Clin Sports Med* 2004; 23: 183–93.

17. American Medical Association. Year end review, medicine by the book. *AMA News* 1989; 6 Jan: 1–28.

18. Berry R, Wong G. Application of legal principles to persons involved in sports. In: *Law and the Business of the Sports Industries: Common Issues in Amateur and Professional Sports*. 2nd edn. Westport, CT: Greenwood Press, 1986.

19. Mitten MJ. Emerging legal issues in sports medicine: a synthesis, summary and analysis. *St Johns Law Rev* 2002; 76(1): 5–86.

20. British Olympic Association. The British Olympic Association's position statement on athlete confidentiality. *Br J Sports Med* 2000; 34: 71–2.

21. Franke WW, Berendonk B. Hormonal doping and androgenization of athletes: a secret program of the German Democratic Republic government. *Clin Chem* 1997; 43(7): 1262–79.

22. Duda M. Do anabolic steroids pose an ethical dilemma for us physicians. *Physicians Sportsmed* 1986; 14(11): 173–5.

23. Salva P, Bacon G. Anabolic steroids: interest among parents and nonathletes. *Southern Med J* 1991; 84(5): 552–6.

24. Kennedy MC, Kennedy JR. Ethics of prescribing drugs to enhance sporting performance. *Med J Aust* 1999; 171: 204–5.

25. Magnusson R, Opie H. HIV and hepatitis in sport: a legal framework for resolving hard cases. *Monash Univ Law Rev* 1994; 214: 243–4.

26. Opie H. Medico-legal issues in sport: the view from the grandstand. *Sydney Law Rev* 2001; 375: 375–6.

27. Pipe A. Drugs, sport and the new millennium. *Clin J Sport Med* 2000; 10: 7–8.

28. Yesalis CE, Bahrke MS, Wright JE. Societal alternatives to anabolic steroid use. *Clin J Sport Med* 2000; 10: 1–6.

29. Pipe A. Reviving ethics in sport. Time for physicians to act. *Physician Sportsmed* 1998; 26(6): 39–40.

Index